Emotion and Decision-Making Explained

Edmund T. Rolls
Oxford Centre for Computational Neuroscience
Oxford, England

OXFORD
UNIVERSITY PRESS

OXFORD
UNIVERSITY PRESS

Great Clarendon Street, Oxford, OX2 6DP,
United Kingdom

Oxford University Press is a department of the University of Oxford.
It furthers the University's objective of excellence in research, scholarship,
and education by publishing worldwide. Oxford is a registered trade mark of
Oxford University Press in the UK and in certain other countries

First Edition published in 2014
Impression: 1

Published in the United States of America by Oxford University Press
198 Madison Avenue, New York, NY 10016, United States of America

British Library Cataloguing in Publication Data
Data available

Library of Congress Control Number: 2013947967

ISBN 978–0–19–965989–0

As printed and bound by
CPI Group (UK) Ltd, Croydon, CR0 4YY

Preface

What produces emotions? Why do we have emotions? How do we have emotions? Why do emotional states feel like something? How do we take decisions? This book seeks explanations of emotion and decision-making by considering these questions.

One of the distinctive properties of this book is that it develops a conceptual and evolutionary approach to emotion (see for example Chapters 2 and 3). This approach shows how cognitive states can produce and modulate emotion, and in turn how emotional states can influence cognition. Another distinctive property is that this book links these approaches to studies on the brain, at the level of neuronal neurophysiology, which provides much of the primary data about how the brain operates; but also to neuropsychological studies of patients with brain damage; to functional magnetic resonance imaging (fMRI) (and other neuroimaging) approaches; and to computational neuroscience approaches. The author's research is in all these areas, and this may help the approach to emotion and decision-making described here to span many levels of investigation. Another distinctive property of this book is that it extends the search beyond emotional value, to economic value, to how decisions are then taken, between for example stimuli that have different value. The empirical evidence that is brought to bear is largely from non-human primates and from humans, because of the considerable similarity of their visual and emotional systems associated with the great development of the prefrontal cortex and temporal lobes in primates, and because the overall aim is to understand how emotion and decision-making are implemented in the human brain, and the neuropsychiatric disorders that can arise.

To understand how the brain works, including how it functions in emotion and decision-making, it is necessary to combine different approaches, including neural computation. Neurophysiology at the single neuron level is needed because this is the level at which information is exchanged between the computing elements of the brain. Evidence from the effects of brain damage, including that available from neuropsychology, is needed to help understand what different parts of the system do, and indeed what each part is necessary for. Neuroimaging is useful to indicate where in the human brain different processes take place, and to show which functions can be dissociated from each other. Knowledge of the biophysical and synaptic properties of neurons is essential to understand how the computing elements of the brain work, and therefore what the building blocks of biologically realistic computational models should be. Knowledge of the anatomical and functional architecture of the cortex is needed to show what types of neuronal network actually perform the computation. And finally the approach of neural computation is needed, as this is required to link together all the empirical evidence to produce an understanding of how the system actually works. This book utilizes evidence from all these disciplines to develop an understanding of how emotion and decision-making are implemented by processing in the brain.

The overall plan of the book is as follows. Chapter 1 outlines the ways in which this book approaches different types of explanation of emotion, and introduces some of the concepts. Chapter 2 then considers the nature of emotion, producing a theory of emotion, and comparing it to some other theories. Chapter 3 considers the functions of emotion, and leads to a Darwinian theory of the adaptive value of emotion, which helps to illuminate many aspects of brain design and behaviour. Chapter 4 takes the explanation of emotion to the level of how emotion is implemented in the brain. Chapter 5 extends and complements this by extending the approach to motivated behaviour, in which affective responses to sensory stimuli are fundamental in for example appetite and the control of food intake. Chapter 6 extends the approach to the pharmacology of emotion and addiction. Chapter 7 extends the approach further, to sexual behaviour. Chapter 8 then considers how one proceeds beyond assessing affective value, by describing brain mechanisms involved in taking decisions between stimuli of for example different affective value, or between different sensory stimuli. It turns out that the mechanisms of decision-making are used in many different brain areas for different purposes, including perceptual categorization, decisions about actions, memory recall, and short-term memory, and the mechanisms described encompass all of these in a unifying conceptual approach. Chapter 8 also considers confidence in decisions, and how we may be able to correct a decision even before the outcome of the choice has been provided. Chapter 9 describes factors that influence decision-making between stimuli or 'goods' of different value, by describing findings in the field of neuroeconomics. Chapter 10 then considers the issue of emotional feelings, which is part of the much larger issue of consciousness. Chapter 11 then synthesizes some of the points made, including how decisions are made and are influenced by emotions.

Appendix A describes some of the computational framework for understanding how systems in the brain in the form of neural networks perform emotion-related learning. Appendix B provides an overview of many different approaches to decision-making, comparing phenomenological with mechanistic approaches. The treatment in Appendix B includes quantitative descriptions of many of these approaches, including the biologically plausible integrate-and-fire attractor model of decision-making (Section B.5) and its mean-field equivalent (Section B.6). Appendix C provides a Glossary of some of the terms used in the book. The book thus seeks to explain emotions in terms of the following: What produces emotions? Why do we have emotions? How do we have emotions? Why do emotional states feel like something? How do we take decisions?

This book evolved from my earlier books *The Brain and Emotion* (Rolls 1999a) and *Emotion Explained* (Rolls 2005b) in some of the following ways:

Emotion and Decision-Making Explained (2014) updates *Emotion Explained* (2005) with much recent research on emotion and reward value, and then goes beyond this by a treatment in Chapter 9 of economic value from the field of neuroeconomics, and then goes further to provide a substantial treatment of decision-making (Chapter 8 and Appendix B), which includes decision-making between stimuli or goods of different value, but also applies to many types of decision-making. This is a natural extension of my treatment of emotion, for after value has been assessed, choices must be made, both between reinforcing stimuli, and about actions to take given the benefits and the costs.

Emotion and Decision-Making Explained goes beyond the brain mechanisms of emotion, in that it seeks to explain emotions in terms of the following: What produces emotions? (The general answer I propose is rewards and punishers, but with other factors too.) Why do we have emotions? (The overall answer I propose is that emotions are evolutionarily adaptive as they provide an efficient way for genes to influence our behaviour to increase their success.) How do we have emotions? (I answer this by describing what is known about the brain mechanisms of emotion.) Why do emotional states feel like something? This is part of the large problem of consciousness, which I address in Chapter 10.

Emotion and Decision-Making Explained also goes beyond the brain mechanisms of emotion by developing my approach and theory of the nature of emotion, and comparing my approach to a range of different approaches to the nature of emotion, including the approaches of Antonio Damasio, Joseph LeDoux, Jaak Panksepp, and appraisal theorists such as Klaus Scherer.

Another way in which this book goes beyond brain mechanisms of emotion is to propose in Chapter 3 a Darwinian account of why animals (including humans) have emotions. The theory will I believe stand the test of time, in the same way as Darwin's theory of evolution by natural selection, and argues that emotions have the important evolutionary role of enabling genes to specify the goals (i.e. the rewards etc. that produce emotions) for actions, rather than the actions themselves. The advantage of this Darwinian design is that although the genes specify the goals, the actual actions are not prespecified by the genes, so that there is great flexibility of the actions themselves. This provides a new approach to the nature vs nurture debate in animal behaviour, for it shows how genes can influence behaviour without specifying a fixed, instinctive, behavioural response. I hope that this will make the book of interest to a wide audience, including many interested in evolution and evolutionary biology.

Although in evolution Darwinian processes lead to gene-defined goals, it is also the case that in humans, goals may be influenced by other processes, including cultural processes. Indeed, some goals are defined within a culture, for example writing a novel like one by Tolstoy vs one by Virginia Woolf. But it is argued that it is primary reinforcers specified by genes of the general type shown in Table 2.1 on page 20 that make us want to be recognized in society because of the advantages this can bring, to solve difficult problems, etc., and therefore to perform actions such as writing novels (see further Ridley (2003) Chapter 8, Ridley (1993b) pp. 310 ff, Laland & Brown (2002) pp. 271 ff, and Dawkins (1982)). Indeed, culture is influenced by human genetic propensities, and it follows that human cognitive, affective, and moral capacities are the product of a unique dynamic known as *gene-culture coevolution* (Gintis 2011, Gintis 2007).

We may also note that the theory that genes set many goals for action does not mean that our behaviour is determined by genes. Modern evolutionary theory has led to the understanding that many traits, particularly behavioural ones, may have some genetic basis but that does not mean that they will inevitably appear, because much depends on the environment (Dawkins 1995, Ridley 2003). Further, part of the power of the theory of emotion described here is that in evolution genes specify rewards and punishers that are goals for action, but do not specify the actions themselves, which are flexible and can be learned. Further, it is shown in Chapter 10 that in humans (and other animals) with a reasoning capability, the reasoning can over-ride the gene-specified rewards to produce behaviour that is in the interests of the individual, the phenotype, and not the genes, and such behaviour is therefore even much less influenced (not 'determined') by genes.

Emotion and Decision-Making Explained further goes beyond the brain mechanisms of emotion with a treatment (in Chapter 4) of the many different learning processes that become engaged in relation to emotion. The book also includes a formal treatment (in Appendix 1) of reinforcement learning and temporal difference (TD) learning, which are increasingly being used to understand emotion-related learning, as well as its brain mechanisms.

Emotion and Decision-Making Explained goes beyond the brain mechanisms of emotion with a treatment of the functions of affective states in motivated behaviour (including hunger, and sexual behaviour), and indeed proposes a fundamental and simple relation between emotion and motivation. The role of sexual selection in the evolution of affective behaviour is included in Chapter 7.

The book includes findings from the rapidly developing field of neuroeconomics in Chapter 9.

Indeed, in this book, I show how it is now possible to follow processing in the brain from the sensory representation and perception of objects including visual and taste objects that are independent of reward value; to brain regions where reward value (both outcome value and expected value) are represented, which are crucial components of decision-making; to brain mechanisms that actually implement the choice part of the decision-making, with a mechanism that is common to categorization and decision-making in other brain systems and cortical areas. I believe that this represents a major advance in neuroscience that we are able to understand at the level of mechanisms all of these processes, and to see how they are linked together in the brain to implement much of our behaviour. Moreover, all of this neural understanding is linked to an understanding of the adaptive value of this organization of behaviour, how emotion is a key component, and even how the subjective feeling of pleasure may arise and be related to these processes.

At the same time, *Emotion and Decision-Making Explained* does consider research on how emotion is implemented in the brain, including much new research in the areas of neurophysiology, and functional neuroimaging, neuropsychiatry, and clinical neuropsychology in humans. This treatment of the brain mechanisms of emotion is important not only for providing a basis for understanding disorders of emotion, but also turns out to be important in unravelling the many different ways in which emotions can influence our behaviour, because the different brain mechanisms themselves are being unravelled. The book includes a theory of how the orbitofrontal cortex supports rapid reversals of emotional behaviour, by using a short-term memory network for the current rule which acts in a biased competition mode to influence neurons known to be present in the orbitofrontal cortex. This helps to provide a contrast between the functions of the orbitofrontal cortex and amygdala in emotion. A description of the theory is given in Chapter 4.

Appendix 1 includes a treatment of autoassociation attractor networks that can maintain stable activity in a brain region, and provide a basis for understanding decision-making mechanisms in the brain. Appendix 1 also shows how interacting attractor networks help to provide a foundation for understanding the interactions between mood, and cognition and memory.

The book links to research in psychiatry, with for example discussions of the impulsive behaviour that is a feature of borderline personality disorder, to research in neurology, with for example assessment of the effects on emotion of damage produced by discrete lesions of the human brain, and to research in neuropsychiatry, by introducing recent approaches based on stochastic neurodynamics to the understanding and treatment of schizophrenia and obsessive-compulsive disorder.

Emotion and Decision-Making Explained also goes beyond the brain mechanisms involved in emotion, by addressing (in Chapter 10) emotional feelings, part of the much larger problem of consciousness. One issue developed here is the concept that there is a credit assignment problem if a multiple step plan does not succeed, and that higher-order thoughts provide a solution to this problem. The book also describes many recent functional neuroimaging investigations in which it has been possible to show that the activations of some brain regions are directly correlated with subjective feelings of affective states such as *pleasure*.

Our understanding of emotion, decision-making, and the mechanisms of brain function, described in this book have wider implications, to for example aesthetics, ethics, and the philosophy of mind, and these wider implications are developed in *Neuroculture: On the Implications of Brain Science* (Rolls 2012d). My book *Memory, Attention, and Decision-Making* (Rolls 2008b) shows how some of the neural mechanisms described in this book, and a number of others, provide a unifying computational neuroscience approach to understanding many aspects of brain function, including short-term memory, long-term memory, top-down attention, visual object recognition, and information representation in the brain, as well as decision-making. *Memory, Attention, and Decision-Making* (Rolls 2008b) includes Appendices that may be useful for those wishing an introduction to the computational neuroscience mechanisms involved in many aspects of brain function. *The Noisy Brain: Stochastic Dynamics as a Principle of Brain Function* (Rolls & Deco 2010) describes in detail stochastic dynamics in the brain, how it can be understood with the techniques of theoretical physics, how it contributes to many aspects of brain function and behaviour, and how it provides new approaches to the cognitive changes that occur with aging, and to psychiatric disorders such as schizophrenia and obsessive-compulsive disorder. The present book replaces *Emotion Explained* (Rolls 2005b) except for *Emotion Explained* Chapter 6 on Thirst, and Chapter 7 on Brain-Stimulation Reward, and both of these Chapters are available at `http://www.oxcns.org`.

It is hoped that this book will be of interest to all those interested in what emotions are, why we have them, how we have them, their disorders, and how we take decisions based on emotions, as well as on rational thinking, and even how we choose between these types of decision-making.

 Part of the material described in the book reflects research performed over many years in collaboration with many colleagues, whose tremendous contributions are warmly appreciated. The contributions of many will be evident from the references cited in the text. In addition, I have benefited enormously from the discussions I have had with a large number of colleagues and friends, many of whom I hope will see areas of the text that they have been able to illuminate. Much of the work described would not have been possible without financial support from a number of sources, particularly the Medical Research Council of the UK, the Human Frontier Science Program, the Wellcome Trust, the McDonnell-Pew Foundation, and the Commission of the European Communities.

The book was typeset by the author in LaTeX using the WinEdt editor.

The cover shows the painting 'Adam and Eve' painted in c. 1528 by Lucas Cranach the Elder (Uffizi Gallery, Florence), which provides an early interpretation of early human emotions, and emotion-related decision-making. This book provides a more recent, scientific, approach to emotions, and to decision-making.

Updates to the publications cited in this book and .pdf files of many papers are available at `http://www.oxcns.org`.

Edmund T. Rolls dedicates this work to the overlapping group: his family, friends, and colleagues: *in salutem praesentium, in memoriam absentium.*

Contents

1 Introduction: the issues

1.1 Introduction

What are emotions? Why do we have emotions? What is their adaptive value? What are the brain mechanisms of emotion, and how can disorders of emotion be understood? Why does it feel like something to have an emotion? Why do emotions sometimes feel so intense? This book aims to provide answers to all these questions. When we know what emotions are, why we have them, how they are produced by our brains, and why it feels like something to have an emotion, we will have a broad-ranging explanation of emotion. This is part of what is referred to in the title of this book *Emotion and Decision-Making Explained.*

We can similarly ask what motivates us: What is motivation? How is motivation controlled? How is motivation produced and regulated by the brain? What goes wrong in motivational disorders, for example in appetite disorders which produce overeating and obesity? How do these motivational control systems operate to ensure that we eat approximately the correct amount of food to maintain our body weight, or drink just enough to replenish our thirst? What are some of the underlying reasons for the different patterns of sexual behaviour found in different animals and humans? Why (and how) do we like some types of touch (e.g. a caress), and what is the relation of this to motivation? What brain processes underlie addiction? What is the relation between emotion, and motivational states such as hunger, appetite, and sexual behaviour? It turns out that the explanations for motivational behaviour are in many ways similar to those for emotional behaviour, and therefore I also treat motivation in this book.

Some of the aims of the book are to explain emotions in terms of the following: What produces emotions? (The general answer I propose is reinforcing stimuli, that is rewards and punishers.) Why do we have emotions? (The overall answer I propose is that emotions are evolutionarily adaptive as they provide an efficient way for genes to influence our behaviour to increase their fitness.) How do we have emotions? (I answer this by describing what is known about the brain mechanisms of emotion.) Why do emotional states feel like something? This is part of the large problem of consciousness, which I address in Chapter 10.

Emotion and motivation are linked by the property that both involve rewards and punishers. Emotions can be thought of as states elicited by rewards or punishers. A full definition of emotion, and theory of emotion, with a starting point as the relation to rewards and punishers is described in Chapter 2. Motivation can be thought of as a state in which a reward is being sought, or a punisher is being avoided or escaped from. This is made clear in Chapters 2, 3, 5, and 7. Because of the importance of reward and punishment for emotion and motivation, I define in Section 1.2 reward and punishment, and describe some of the types of learning that involve rewards and punishers. This is useful groundwork for what follows in the rest of this book. However, for those who wish in a first reading to skip the definitions in Section 1.2 (which are provided to ensure that there is a firm foundation for understanding emotion and motivation), it may be useful simply to think of a reward as something for which an animal (which includes humans) will work, and a punisher as something that an animal will work to escape from or avoid.

Some stimuli are innately rewarding or punishing and are called primary reinforcers (for example no learning is necessary to respond to pain as aversive), while other stimuli are learned or secondary reinforcers (for example the sight of a chocolate cake is not innately rewarding, but may become a learned reinforcer, for which we may work, by the process of association learning between the sight of the cake and its taste, where the taste is a primary reward or reinforcer). This type of learning, which is important in emotion and motivation, is called stimulus–reinforcement association learning. (A better term is stimulus–reinforcer association learning, where reinforcer is being used to mean a stimulus that might be a reward or a punisher.)

1.2 Rewards and punishers, and learning about rewards and punishers: instrumental learning and stimulus–reinforcer association learning

A reward is something for which an animal (including of course a human) will work. A punisher is something that an animal will work to escape or avoid (or that will decrease the probability of actions on which it is contingent). In order to exclude simple reflex-like behaviour, the concept invoked here by the term 'work' is to perform an arbitrary behaviour (called an operant response) in order to obtain the reward or avoid the punisher. An example of an operant response might be putting money in a vending machine to obtain food, or for a rat pressing a lever to obtain food. In these cases, the food is the reward. Another example of an operant response might be moving from one place to another in order to escape from or avoid an aversive (punishing) stimulus such as a cold draught. If the aversive stimulus starts and then the response is made, this is referred to as *escape* from the punisher. If a warning stimulus (such as a flashing light) indicates that the punisher will be delivered unless the operant response is made, then the animal may learn to perform the operant response when the warning stimulus is given in order to *avoid* the punisher.

Because the definitions of reward and punisher make it a requirement that it must be at least possible to demonstrate learning of an arbitrary operant response (made to obtain the reward or to escape from or avoid the punisher), we see that learning is implicit in the definition of reward and punisher. (Merely swimming up a chemical gradient towards a source of food as occurs in single cell organisms is called a taxis as described in Chapter 3; it does not require learning, and does not make the food qualify as a reward under the definition.) In that rewards and punishers do imply the ability to learn what to do to obtain the reward or escape from or avoid the punisher, we call rewards and punishers 'reinforcers'.

This introduction leads to the definition of instrumental **reinforcers** as stimuli that if their occurrence, termination, or omission is made contingent upon the making of an action, alter the probability of the future emission of that action (as a result of the contingency (i.e. dependency) on the response). The alteration of the probability of an action (or behavioural response) is the measure that instrumental learning has taken place to obtain a goal. A positive reinforcer (such as food) increases the probability of emission of an action on which it is contingent; the process is termed **positive reinforcement**, and the outcome is a reward (such as food). A negative reinforcer (such as a painful stimulus) increases the probability of emission of an action which causes the negative reinforcer to be omitted (as in active avoidance) or terminated (as in escape), and the procedure is termed **negative reinforcement**. In contrast, **punishment** refers to procedures in which the probability of an action is decreased. Punishment thus describes procedures in which an action decreases in probability if it is followed by a painful stimulus, as in passive avoidance. Punishment can also be used to refer to a procedure involving the omission or termination of a reward ('extinction' and 'time out' respectively), both of which decrease the probability of actions (Gray 1975, Mackintosh

1983, Dickinson 1980, Lieberman 2000, Mazur 2012). My argument is that an affectively positive or 'appetitive' stimulus (which produces a state of pleasure) acts operationally as a **reward**, which when delivered acts instrumentally as a positive reinforcer, or when not delivered (omitted or terminated) acts to decrease the probability of actions on which it is contingent. Conversely I argue that an affectively negative or aversive stimulus (which produces an unpleasant state) acts operationally as a **punisher**, which when delivered acts instrumentally to decrease the probability of actions on which it is contingent, or when not delivered (escaped from or avoided) acts as a negative reinforcer in that it then increases the probability of the action on which its non-delivery is contingent[1].

Reinforcers, that is rewards or punishers, may be unlearned or **primary reinforcers**, or learned or secondary reinforcers. An example of a primary reinforcer is pain, which is innately a punisher. The first time a painful stimulus is ever delivered, it will be escaped from, and no learning that it is aversive is needed. Similarly, the first time a sweet taste is delivered, it can act as a positive reinforcer, so it is a primary positive reinforcer or reward. Other stimuli become reinforcing by learning, because of their association with primary reinforcers, thereby becoming '**secondary reinforcers**'. For example, a (previously neutral) sound that regularly precedes an electric shock can become a secondary reinforcer. Animals will learn operant responses (actions) reinforced by the secondary reinforcer, for example jumping to a place where the secondary reinforcer is not present or terminates. Secondary reinforcers are thus important in enabling animals to avoid primary punishers such as pain.

There is a close relation of all these processes to emotion, for as we will see in Chapter 2, fear is an emotional state that might be produced by a sound that has previously been associated with an electric shock. Shock in this example is the primary punisher, and fear is the emotional state that occurs to the tone stimulus as a result of the learning of the stimulus (i.e. tone)–reinforcer (i.e. shock) association. Another example of a secondary reinforcer is a visual stimulus associated with the taste of a food. For example, the first time we see a new type of food we do not treat the sight of the new visual stimulus as reinforcing, but if the stimulus has a good taste, the sight of the object becomes a positive secondary reinforcer, and we may choose the food when we see it in future by virtue of its association with a primary reinforcer. This type of learning is thus called stimulus–reinforcer association learning. (The operation is often referred to as stimulus–reinforcement association learning.) This type of learning is very important in many emotions, because it is as a result of this type of learning that many previously neutral stimuli come to elicit emotional responses, as in the example of fear above.

Unconditioned reinforcing stimuli often elicit autonomic responses. (Autonomic responses are those mediated through the autonomic nervous system, via the vagus and sympathetic nerves, which affect smooth muscle.) Examples include alterations of heart rate and of blood pressure which might be produced by a painful stimulus; and salivation which might be produced by the taste of food. Many endocrine (hormonal) responses are also mediated through the autonomic nervous system and so are autonomic responses, for example the release of adrenaline (epinephrine) from the adrenal gland during emotional excitement. Previously neutral stimuli, such as the sound in our previous example, can by pairing with unconditioned stimuli, such as shock in the previous example, come by learning the association, to produce learned autonomic responses. In the example the tone might by pairing with shock come to elicit a change in heart rate, and sweating. This type of learning is called **classical**

[1]Note that my definition of a punisher, which is similar to that of an aversive stimulus, is of a stimulus or event that can either decrease the probability of actions on which it is contingent, or increase the probability of actions on which its non-delivery is contingent. The term punishment is restricted to situations where the probability of an action is being decreased.

conditioning, and also **Pavlovian conditioning** after Ivan Pavlov who performed many of the original studies of this type of learning, including learned salivation to the sound of a bell that predicted the taste of food. It is a type of learning that is very similar to stimulus–reinforcer association learning, except that in the case of classical conditioning the responses involved are autonomic and endocrine responses.

In the case of stimulus–reinforcer association learning, the effects of the learning are mediated through the skeletal motor system, in that actions are performed that are instrumental in enabling animals to obtain rewards or avoid punishers, and are described as voluntary in humans. A key difference between **instrumental learning** and classical conditioning apart from the response systems involved lies in the contingencies that operate. In classical conditioning the animal has no control over whether the unconditioned stimulus is delivered (as in the experiments of Pavlov just described). In contrast, the whole notion of instrumental learning is that what the animal does is instrumental in determining whether the reinforcer (the goal) is obtained, or escaped from or avoided. Both types of learning are important in emotions because (as we will see in Chapter 2) instrumental reinforcers produce emotional responses, but also typically produce autonomic responses that therefore typically occur during emotional states, and indeed mediate important effects of emotions such as preparing the body for action by increasing heart rate etc.

A more detailed description of the nature of classical (Pavlovian) conditioning and instrumental learning, and how both are related to emotion, is provided in Section 4.6.1.

Motivation refers to the state an animal is in when it is willing to work for a reward or to escape from or avoid a punisher. So for example we say that an animal is motivated to work for the taste of food, and in this case the motivational state is called hunger. The definition of motivation thus implies the capacity to perform any, arbitrary, operant response in order to obtain the reward or escape from or avoid the punisher. By implying an operant response, we exclude simple behaviours such as reflexes and taxes (such as swimming up a chemical gradient), as described above and in Chapter 2. By implying learning of any response to obtain a reward (or avoid a punisher), motivation thus focuses on behaviours in which a goal is defined. Motivation is one of the states that are involved in the large area of brain design related to the fundamental issue of how goals for behaviour are defined, and an appropriate behaviour is selected, as described in this book and brought together into a theory in Chapter 2.

1.3 The approaches taken to emotion and motivation: their causes, functions, adaptive value, and brain mechanisms

To explain emotion, and motivation, a number of different approaches are taken, and some of these need some introduction. To examine the causes of emotion, the environmental stimuli and situations that elicit emotions are identified. This is part of the subject of Chapter 2. It is shown how the different environmental stimulus conditions that produce emotions provide the basis for a classification of different emotions. Understanding the functions of emotion also provides part of the explanation of why we have emotions, and many of the functions of emotion are described in Chapter 3. These functions of emotion explain in part the adaptive value of emotion, and give part of an explanation about why emotion has evolved. However, it turns out that emotions provide a fundamental solution to the issue of how genes design brains to produce behaviour that is advantageous to the genes, and this deep understanding of the adaptive value of emotion, and in a sense the cause of emotion, is elaborated in Chapter 3. When considering the adaptive value of emotion in the context of evolution, we must remember that animals are generally social, and that evolution may have led to the development of special reward and punishment systems to help to produce emotional behaviour that is adaptive in social situations. This area, of understanding and explaining aspects of social behaviour in terms of its evolutionary adaptive value, is the field of sociobiology and evolutionary psychology (Buss 2012), and this approach is introduced especially in the context of sexual behaviour in Chapter 7.

Another major approach taken to explain emotion and motivation, and their underlying reward and punishment systems, is in terms of the brain mechanisms that implement them. Understanding the brain processing and mechanisms of behaviour is one way to ensure that we have the correct explanation for how the behaviour is produced. Another important reason for investigating the actual brain mechanisms that underlie emotion and motivation, and reward and punishment, is not only to understand how our own brains work, but also to have the basis for understanding and treating medical disorders of these systems.

It is because of the intended relevance to understanding human emotion and its disorders that emphasis is placed in this book on findings from research in non-human primates, including monkeys, as well as in humans. This is important, for many of the brain systems that are involved in emotion and motivation have undergone considerable development in primates (e.g. monkeys and humans) compared to non-primates (for example rats and mice).

For example, the temporal lobe has undergone great development in primates, and several systems in the temporal lobe are either involved in emotion (e.g. the amygdala), or provide some of the main sensory inputs to brain systems involved in emotion and motivation. In particular, the amygdala and the orbitofrontal cortex, key brain structures in emotion, both receive inputs from the highly developed temporal lobe cortical areas, including those involved in invariant visual object recognition and face identity and expression processing.

Another example is that the prefrontal cortex has also undergone great development in primates, and one part of it, the orbitofrontal cortex, is very little developed in rodents, yet is one of the major brain areas involved in emotion and motivation in primates including humans. Indeed, it has been argued that the granular prefrontal cortex is a primate innovation, and the implication of the argument is that any areas that might be termed orbitofrontal cortex in rats (Schoenbaum, Roesch, Stalnaker & Takahashi 2009) are homologous only to the agranular parts of the primate orbitofrontal cortex (shaded mid grey in Fig. 1.1), that is to areas 13a, 14c, and the agranular insular areas labelled Ia in Fig. 1.1 (Wise 2008, Passingham & Wise 2012). It follows from that argument that for most areas of the orbitofrontal and medial prefrontal cortex in humans and macaques (those shaded light grey in Fig. 1.1), special consideration must be given to research in macaques and humans. As shown in Fig. 1.1, there may be no cortical area in rodents that is homologous to most of the primate including human orbitofrontal cortex (Preuss 1995, Wise 2008, Passingham & Wise 2012).

The development of some of these cortical areas has been so great in primates that even evolutionarily old systems such as the taste system appear to have been rewired, compared with that of rodents, to place much more emphasis on cortical processing, taking place in areas such as the orbitofrontal cortex (Rolls & Scott 2003, Scott & Small 2009, Small & Scott 2009) (Fig. 4.2). In primates, the reward value of the taste is represented in the orbitofrontal cortex in that the responses of orbitofrontal taste neurons are modulated by hunger in just the same way as is the reward value or palatability of a taste. In particular, it has been shown that orbitofrontal cortex taste neurons stop responding to the taste of a food with which a monkey is fed to satiety, and that this parallels the decline in the acceptability of the food (see Fig. 4.22) (Rolls, Sienkiewicz & Yaxley 1989b). In contrast, the representation of taste in the primary taste cortex of primates (Scott, Yaxley, Sienkiewicz & Rolls 1986b, Yaxley, Rolls & Sienkiewicz 1990) is not modulated by hunger (Rolls, Scott,

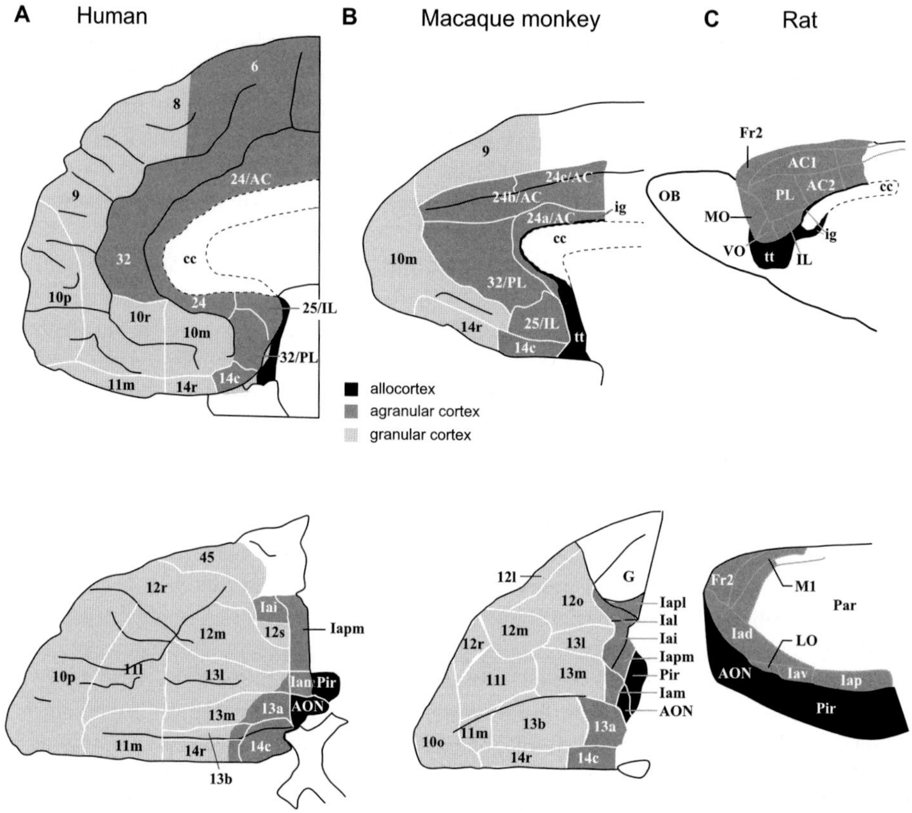

Fig. 1.1 Comparison of the orbitofrontal (below) and medial prefrontal (above) cortical areas in humans, macaque monkeys, and rats. (A) Medial (top) and orbital (bottom) areas of the human frontal codex (Ongur et al. 2003). (B) Medial (top) and orbital (bottom) areas of the macaque frontal cortex (Carmichael and Price 1994). (C) Medial (top) and lateral (bottom) areas of rat frontal cortex (Palomero-Gallagher and Zilles 2004). Rostral is to the left in all drawings. Top row: dorsal is up in all drawings. Bottom row: in (A) and (B), lateral is up; in (C), dorsal is up. Not to scale. Abbreviations: AC, anterior cingulate cortex; AON, anterior olfactory 'nucleus'; cc, corpus callosum; Fr2 second frontal area; Ia, agranular insular cortex; ig, induseum griseum; IL, infralimbic cortex; LO, lateral orbital cortex; MO, medial orbital cortex: OB, olfactory bulb; Pr, piriform (olfactory) cortex; PL, prelimbic cortex; tt, tenia tecta; VO, ventral orbital cortex; Subdivisions of areas are labelled caudal (c); inferior (i), lateral (l), medial (m); orbital (o), posterior or polar (p), rostral(r), or by arbitrary designation (a, b). (After Passingham and Wise (2012). (a) Adapted from Dost Ongur, Amon T. Ferry, and Joseph L. Price, Architectonic subdivision of the human orbital and medial prefrontal cortex, *Journal of Comparative Neurology*, 460 (3), pp. 425–49 Copyright ©2003 Wiley-Liss, Inc. (b) Adapted from S. T. Carmichael and J. L. Price, Architectonic subdivision of the orbital and medial prefrontal cortex in the macaque monkey, *Journal of Comparative Neurology*, 346 (3), pp. 366-402 Copyright ©1994 Wiley-Liss, Inc. (c) Adapted from Palomero-Gallagher N. and Zilles K., Isocortex, in *The Rat Nervous System* 3e, ed. G. Paxinos, p.729–57 ©2004, Elsevier Academic Press.)

Sienkiewicz & Yaxley 1988, Yaxley, Rolls & Sienkiewicz 1988). Thus in the primary taste cortex of primates (and at earlier stages of taste processing including the nucleus of the solitary tract), the reward value of taste is not represented, and instead the identity of the taste is represented (see Section 5.4.2). The importance of cortical processing of taste in primates, first for identity and intensity in the primary taste cortex, and then for reward value in the orbitofrontal cortex, is that both types of representation need to be interfaced to visual and other processing that requires cortical computation. For example, it may have adaptive value to be able to represent exactly what taste is present, and to link it by learning to the sight and location of the source of the taste, even when hunger and reward is not being produced, so that the source of that taste can be found in future, when it may have reward value. In line with cortical processing to dominate the processing of taste in primates, there is no modulation of taste responsiveness at or before the primary taste cortex, and the pathways for taste are directly from the nucleus of the solitary tract in the brainstem to the taste thalamus and then to the taste cortex (Fig. 4.2). In contrast, in rodents such as the rat, the nucleus of the solitary tract connects to a pontine taste area, the parabrachial nucleus, that is not present in primates (Rolls & Scott 2003, Scott & Small 2009, Small & Scott 2009). The rodent pontine taste area then not only has connections to the thalamus and thus to the cortex, but also has direct connections to many subcortical areas important in appetite control, including the amygdala and hypothalamus (Section 5.4.2.4). Moreover, in rodents, satiety reduces the responsiveness of neurons in the nucleus of the solitary tract to the taste of food by approximately 30%, so that taste processing in rodents is from the first synapse in the brain confounded by reward value, by hedonics. That makes the taste system of rodents very difficult to understand functionally for different functions are not separated (taste identity and intensity vs hedonics), and makes the taste system of rodents a poor one with which to understand primate including human taste reward processing. This evidence emphasizes the importance of understanding the evidence from primates including humans, even in a system such as the taste system that one might think is evolutionarily so old (Section 5.4.2.4).

Another reason for focusing interest on the primate brain is that there has been great development of the visual system in primates, and this itself has had important implications for the types of sensory stimuli that are processed by brain systems involved in emotion and motivation. One example is the importance of face identity and face expression decoding, which are both important in primate emotional behaviour, and indeed provide an important part of the foundation for much primate social behaviour. These are among the reasons why emphasis is placed on brain systems in primates, including humans, in the approach taken here. The overall medically relevant aim of the research described in this book is to provide a foundation for understanding in humans the brain mechanisms of emotion, motivation, and decision-making, and thus their disorders, including depression, anxiety, addiction, sociopathy, borderline personality disorder, schizophrenia, eating disorders, and decision-making disorders including pathological gambling.

When considering brain mechanisms involved in emotion and decision-making, findings with human brain imaging are described. These approaches include functional magnetic resonance imaging (fMRI) to measure changes in brain oxygenation level locally (using a signal from deoxyhaemoglobin) to provide an index of local brain activity, as well as positron emission tomography (PET) studies to estimate local regional cerebral blood flow, again to provide an index of local brain activity. It is, however, important to note that these functional neuroimaging approaches provide rather coarse approaches to brain function, in that the spatial resolution is seldom better than 3 mm, so that the picture given is one of 'blobs on the brain', which give some indication of what is happening where in the brain, and what types of dissociation of functions are possible.

However, because there are millions of neurons in each of the areas that can be resolved with functional neuroimaging, such imaging techniques give rather little evidence on how the brain works. For this, one needs to know what information is represented in each brain area at the level at which information is exchanged between the computing elements of the brain, the neurons (brain cells). One also needs to know how the representation of information (for example about stimuli or events in the world) changes from stage to stage of the processing in the brain, to understand how the brain works as a system. It turns out that one can 'read' this information from the brain by recording the activity of single neurons, or groups of single neurons (Rolls & Treves 2011). The reason that this is an effective procedure for understanding what is represented is that each neuron has one information output channel, the firing of its action potentials, so that one can measure the full richness of the information being represented in a region by measuring the firing of its neurons. This can reveal fundamental evidence crucial for understanding how the brain operates (Rolls 2008b). For example, neuronal recording can reveal all the information represented in an area even if parts of it are encoded by relatively small numbers, perhaps a few percent, of its neurons. (This is impossible with brain-imaging techniques, which also are susceptible to the interpretation problem that whatever causes the largest activation is interpreted as 'what' is being encoded in a region).

Neuronal recording also provides evidence for the level at which it is appropriate to build computational models of brain function, the neuronal network level. Such neuronal network computational models consider how populations of neurons with the connections found in a given brain area, and with biologically plausible properties such as learning rules for altering the strengths of synaptic connections between neurons, actually could perform useful computation to implement the functions being performed by that brain area (Rolls 2008b). This approach should not really be considered as a metaphor for brain operation, but as a theory of how each part of the brain operates. The neuronal network computational theory, and any model or simulation based on it, may of course be simplified to some extent to make it tractable, but nevertheless the point is that the neuron-level approach, coupled with neuronal network models that analyse the functions of populations of neurons, together provide some of the fundamental elements for understanding how the brain actually works. For this reason, emphasis is also placed in this book on what is known about what is being processed in each brain area as shown by recordings from neurons. Such evidence, in terms of building theories and models of how the brain functions, can never be replaced by brain imaging evidence, although these approaches do complement each other very effectively. The approach to brain function in terms of computations performed by neuronal networks in different brain areas is the subject of the books *Neural Networks and Brain Function* by Rolls & Treves (1998), *Computational Neuroscience of Vision* by Rolls & Deco (2002), *Memory, Attention, and Decision-Making: A Unifying Computational Neuroscience Approach* by Rolls (2008b), and *The Noisy Brain: Stochastic Dynamics as a Principle of Brain Function* by Rolls & Deco (2010). The reader is referred to these books for more comprehensive accounts of this biologically plausible approach to brain function. It can be described as a mechanistic approach to understanding brain function, in that the underlying computational processes that underlie behaviour and thought must be explicitly understood (and are the 'proximate' causes of behaviour), and must be placed in the context of the evolutionary adaptive value of those mechanisms, the 'ultimate' causes of the behaviour. In this book, some of the neurophysiological evidence and its computational implications for understanding how our brains work to produce emotion and motivation, and the nature of their adaptive value, are described.

This allows me to state what is implied by the title of this book, *'Emotion and Decision-Making Explained'*. In terms of emotion, this is explained in this book at the 'proximate' level of causation (Mayr 1961, Tinbergen 1963) in terms of the neuronal mechanisms in the orbitofrontal cortex, anterior cingulate cortex, amygdala, and connected brain regions. At the 'ultimate' level of causation, the level of adaptive value in evolution (Mayr 1961, Tinbergen 1963), emotion is explained as an efficient and simple way for genes to influence behaviour for their own 'selfish' reproductive success, by specifying the rewarding and punishing goals for instrumental action with the resulting states being emotional states (Chapters 2 and 3). This is simpler and more efficient in terms of evolutionary adaptive value than for genes to specify the actions, the behavioural responses, to be produced by stimuli (Chapter 3).

In terms of decision-making, this is explained at the 'proximate' level of causation in terms of the attractor cortical neuronal network mechanisms described in Chapter 8 and Appendix B that implement decision-making. An attractive feature of this explanation is that it is essentially the same type of cortical mechanism that is used in other cortical areas for long-term memory (e.g. the hippocampus episodic memory and temporal lobe semantic memory systems (Rolls 2008b, Rolls 2010b, Treves & Rolls 1994)) and for short-term memory (Rolls 2008b, Rolls, Dempere-Marco & Deco 2013). Moreover, the mechanism described for decision-making is a neuronal mechanism that specifies how the decision is taken in terms of the neuronal and neuronal network mechanisms (Wang 2002, Rolls & Deco 2010, Deco, Rolls, Albantakis & Romo 2013) (see Chapter 8 and Appendix B), and is different in this respect from a mathematical model such as a drift diffusion model that does not specify the neuronal mechanisms and so sets up artificial constructs for the source of the noise, the threshold at which a decision may be said to have been reached, etc. (Ratcliff & Rouder 1998, Ratcliff, Zandt & McKoon 1999, Gold & Shadlen 2007). Another advantage of an explanation at the proximate level of the biological mechanism rather than a mathematical model is that an explanation at the biological level facilitates insight into biological factors that may influence the mechanisms, such as drug treatments for neuropsychiatric states such as schizophrenia and obsessive-compulsive disorder (Rolls & Deco 2010, Rolls, Loh, Deco & Winterer 2008d, Rolls, Loh & Deco 2008c, Rolls 2012b). Decision-making is explained at the 'ultimate' level of explanation by the evolutionary adaptive value of having accurate continuously graded representations of the decision variables such as value so that they can be represented precisely, and then following this by a non-linear choice mechanism that falls into one of two or more possible and stable decision states, so that behaviour and even the agonist and antagonist muscles are not being pulled in different directions simultaneously. Part of the evolutionary adaptive value of the attractor network decision-making mechanism described in Chapter 8 is that it implements a short-term memory mechanism that enables the decision to be maintained for some time so that behaviour can be directed for some time towards implementing the decision. Another part of the evolutionary adaptive value of the attractor network decision-making mechanism described in Chapter 8 is that although it makes a choice that is stable and is maintained for some time, the actual choice made can be influenced by noise in the brain, which as shown in Chapter 8 and by Rolls & Deco (2010) can be advantageous, including avoidance of predators, and creative thought. Decisions can be made by other brain systems with different neuronal mechanisms, for example by the direct mutual inhibition between neurons that is implemented in the basal ganglia as described in Chapter 6. However, the mechanism using direct mutual inhibition by neurons does not have the evolutionary adaptive value of maintaining the decision on-line using a short-term memory implemented by the recurrent excitatory connections in cortical networks, and indeed that is part of the 'ultimate' explanation for the value of cortical attractor decision-making networks as described in Chapter 8.

Thus both emotion and decision-making are provided with explanations at the 'proximate' and 'ultimate' levels in this book, and this is a point being made by the title of this book. Of course our understanding is not perfect, and there is much exciting research to be performed, but the point is that we can at least address both emotion and decision-making at the proximate and ultimate levels of causation, and that is the aim of this book. Moreover, considering emotion and decision-making together is also useful, for after a value (which is relevant to emotion) has been computed by the brain, a decision is usually needed based on the values of the choices that are currently available for what to do next.

One of the main points made in this section is that rapid progress is being made now in understanding emotion and motivation, and part of this advance is related to the fact that we are just starting to be able to understand how the brain actually works, in terms of how its neuronal networks transform inputs into behaviour. Given that this basis for understanding how our own brains work does depend very much on understanding in detail how the brains of relatively close relatives, non-human primates such as monkeys, work, research on non-human primate brain information processing is quite crucial. We are beginning to understand how this works, and one aim of this book is to show how that research together with research in humans is leading towards a fundamental understanding of emotion and motivation, which are seen to be at the heart of brain design. That understanding is important for understanding the rich variety of human emotional behaviour, its relation to our rational (reasoning) brain systems, and also for understanding and treating disorders in emotion and motivation.

1.4 Reward, punishment, emotion, and motivation: the plan of the book

It may be useful to make it clear why the brain mechanisms of both emotion and motivation (with the examples of motivated behaviour considered being hunger, thirst, addiction, and sexual behaviour), and of decision-making, are being considered together in this book. The reason is that for both emotion and motivation, rewards and punishers are assessed in order to provide the goals for behaviour. Operation of the brain to evaluate rewards and punishers is the fundamental solution of the brain to interfacing sensory systems to action selection and execution systems. Computing the reward and punisher value of sensory stimuli, and then using selection between different rewards and avoidance of punishers represented in a common scale of value that takes into account costs appears to be the fundamental design that brains use in order to produce appropriate behaviour (see Chapter 2). The behaviour selected can be thought of as appropriate in the sense that it is based on the sensory systems and reward decoding that our genes specify (through the process of natural selection) in order to maximize their fitness (reproductive potential). Having reward and punishment systems is the solution that evolution has developed to produce appropriate behaviour. It happens that motivational and emotional behaviour are the types of behaviour in which rewards and punishers operate. However, once reward value, and the costs associated with each potential goal, have been evaluated, choices between these rewards, the potential goals for behaviour, must be made. Major advances in our understanding of the brain mechanisms involved in decision-making have been made in the last few years (Rolls 2008b, Wang 2008, Rolls & Deco 2010, Deco, Rolls, Albantakis & Romo 2013), and it is now possible in this book to link from reward valuation (the realm of emotion) into how decisions are then made between different rewards, and this is an important advance possible since my book *Emotion Explained* (Rolls 2005b).

Considering both emotional and motivational behaviour in this book means that we can describe many of the principles that underlie the decoding of many types of rewarding and punishing stimuli, which have in common that they produce affective states. We can also see how the common currency of the value of each specific type of reward works to enable different rewards to be compared in a decision-making process. We can also see how the reward value of all the different potential rewards that our genes specify is kept within a comparable range, so that we select different behaviours as appropriate. That is, we can examine many of the different ways in which the reward value of different sensory stimuli is modulated, both by internal signals as physiological needs are satisfied, and in addition to some extent by sensory-specific satiety (the mechanism by which repeating one reward causes it gradually to decrease its reward value somewhat, assisting the selection of other rewards in the environment).

However, perhaps the most important reason for treating reward and punishment systems, and the brain systems dealing with rewards and punishers, together is that we can develop an overall theory of how this set of issues, which might sometimes appear mysterious, is actually at the heart of brain design. Much of sensory processing, at least through the brain systems that are concerned with object identification (whether by sight, sound, smell, taste, or touch), can be seen to have the goal of enabling the correct reward value to be decoded and represented after the object has been identified. This means for example that in vision, representations of objects that can be accessed regardless of the view of the object shown, the size of the object on the retina, etc., must be formed. Moreover, these invariant representations of objects must be encoded in an appropriate way for the brain to associate in simple neuronal networks the object with primary (unlearned) reinforcers, such as the taste associated with the object, or the pain produced by the object. The actual motivational and emotional parts of the processing, the parts where the reward or punisher value is made explicit in the representation, should indeed no longer be seen as mysterious or perhaps superfluous aspects of brain processing. Instead, they are at the heart of which behavioural actions are selected, and how they are selected. Moreover, a large part of the brain's action and motor systems can be seen as having the goal in systems-level design of producing behaviour that will obtain the rewards decoded from sensory (and memory) inputs by the motivational and emotional systems of the brain. In particular, the implication is that the action systems for implicit (unconscious) behaviour have as part of their design principle the property that they will perform actions to optimize the output of the reward and punishment systems involved in motivation and emotion. Put another way, the brain systems involved in motivation and emotion must pass reward or punisher signals to decision-making systems, and then to the action systems, which must be built to attempt to obtain and maximize the reward signals being received; to switch behaviour from one reward to another as the reward values being received alter; and to switch behaviour also if signals indicating possible punishers are received (see Chapter 4). Two types of decision-making are fundamental to this process. The first is the ability to take decisions between different rewards or potential goals for action, and this must take into account the positive as well as the negative aspects of a rewarding stimulus. Decisions of this type, value-based decision-making, appears to utilize value information from the orbitofrontal cortex, and to take place in the next cortical tier, the medial prefrontal cortex area 10 which is just anterior to the orbitofrontal cortex (Rolls & Grabenhorst 2008, Grabenhorst & Rolls 2011). The second type of decision is about which action to take given the costs of different actions to obtain each reward. An important area in this type of reward-action decision-making appears to be the anterior cingulate cortex (Rushworth, Noonan, Boorman, Walton & Behrens 2011, Grabenhorst & Rolls 2011) (see Section 4.7).

This book is thus intended to uncover some of the most important and fundamental aspects and principles of brain function and design. The book is also intended to show that the way in which the brain works in motivation and emotion can be seen to be the result of natural selection operating to select genes that optimize our behaviour by building into us the appropriate reward and punisher systems, and the appropriate rules for the operation of these systems.

The plan of the book is that we consider in Chapters 2 and 3 the major issue of emotion, and its functions. These chapters address the explanation of emotion by defining emotion, and elucidating its functions. Another part of the explanation of emotion is how it actually works, that is how it is implemented in the brain, which is described in Chapter 4. By understanding its mechanisms, we not only understand better the different processes that contribute to emotion, but also we provide a fundamental basis for starting to understand many disorders of emotion, including for example depression, and how they can be treated. Affective (emotional) states, and rewards, are involved in motivated behaviour such as eating, addiction, and sexual behaviour, and we consider these in Chapters 5, 6, and 7. These topics provide many clear examples of how the pleasantness or reward value of stimuli reflect a fundamental aspect of the design of both the brain and behaviour, and help to show the rewards, and punishers, that actually influence many aspects of our behaviour. In Chapter 8 and Appendix B I consider how the brain takes decisions, and how confidence in our decisions is reflected by the machinery of the brain. Appendix B provides a quantitative account of decision-making systems in the brain, and their relation to more phenomenological models. These chapters address decision-making between rewards of different value, but also address much more generally decision-making as a process in the brain, which utilizes the same type of computational process for 'decisions' or categorization in sensory systems, and in memory systems during the recall of a memory (Rolls 2008b). Chapter 9 extends the treatment of decision-making beyond decisions between stimuli of affective value, to decisions between stimuli of different economic value and utility, as investigated using approaches in neuroeconomics. In Chapter 10 the issue of emotional feelings, which is part of the large issue of consciousness, is considered, together with the brain processing involved in conscious feelings.

The aims of this book are thus to explain emotion, motivation, and decision-making in terms of:

1. What produces emotions? The answer developed in Chapter 2 is that emotions are produced by rewards and punishers.

2. Why do we have emotions? The most fundamental, and thoroughly Darwinian, explanation, developed in Chapter 3, is that the evolutionary adaptive value of emotions is that they provide an efficient way for genes to influence our behaviour to increase their (the genes') success.

3. How do we have emotions, that is, what are the brain and body processes that implement emotions, and motivational states such as hunger? These processes are described in Chapters 4–7.

4. How do we take decisions, whether between rewards with different values, or between actions with different benefits and costs, or more generally, when we need to perform a non-linear categorization of inputs, including sensory inputs, and memory recall? These processes are described in Chapters 8 and 9, and in Appendix B.

5. Why do emotional states feel like something, which is part of the very large problem of consciousness. This is considered in Chapter 10.

2 The nature of emotion

2.1 Introduction

What are emotions? This is a question in which almost everyone is interested. There have been many answers, many of them surprisingly unclear and ill-defined. William James (1884) was at least clear about what he thought. He believed that emotional experiences were produced by sensing bodily changes, such as changes in heart rate or in skeletal muscles (the muscles involved in voluntary movements). His view was that "We feel frightened because we are running away". But he left unanswered the crucial question even for his theory, which is: Why do some events make us run away (and according to him then feel emotional), whereas others do not?

A more modern theory is that of Frijda (1986), who argues that a change in action readiness is the central core of an emotion. Oatley & Jenkins (1996) (page 96) make this part of their definition too, stating that "the core of an emotion is readiness to act and the prompting of plans" (see also Keltner, Oatley & Jenkins (2013)). But surely subjects in reaction time experiments in psychology who are continually for thousands of trials altering their action readiness are very far indeed from having normal or strong emotional experiences? Similarly, we can perform an action in response to a verbal request (e.g. open a door), yet may not experience great emotion when performing this action. Another example might be the actions that are performed in driving a car on a routine trip – we get ready, and many actions are performed, often quite automatically, yet little emotion occurs. So it appears that there is no necessary link between performing actions and emotion. This may not be a clear way to define emotion. Even more action-related is the approach of Panksepp (1998, 2011a), who treats emotions as fixed action patterns elicited as motor responses to stimuli. This is in complete contrast to the present approach, which is that emotions are states elicited by instrumental reinforcers, which have the evolutionary utility of specifying the goals for actions, and are states in their own right, which specify what actions may hope to achieve, but in which the action is arbitrary, that is, not specified by the emotional state. The difference is a key one: Panksepp would have stimuli eliciting actions, as in a type of reflex. I in contrast hold that stimuli decoded as reinforcers elicit intervening states, emotional states, and that these states, representing values attained or not yet attained, maintain the goals for actions. My theory provides a role for these intervening states, the emotional states, whereas Panksepp's approach (1998) does not need emotional states, just fixed actions to releasing stimuli, akin to earlier ethological approaches (Tinbergen 1951, Tinbergen 1963).

Because it is important to be able to specify what emotions are, in this chapter we consider a systematic approach to this question. Part of the approach is to ask what causes emotions. Can clear conditions be specified for the circumstances in which emotions occur? This is considered in Section 2.2. Continuing with this theme, when we have come to understand the conditions under which emotions occur, does this help us to classify and describe different emotions systematically, in terms of differences between the different conditions that cause emotions to occur? A way in which a systematic account of different emotions can be provided is described in Section 2.3. A major help in understanding emotions would be provided by understanding what the functions of emotion are. It turns out that emotions have quite a number of different functions, each of which helps us to understand emotions a little more clearly. These different functions of emotion are described in Chapter 3. Understanding the different functions of emotion helps us to understand also the brain mechanisms of emotion, for it helps us to see that emotion (or more precisely, stimuli that elicit emotions) can operate to influence several different output systems of the brain.

These analyses leave open though a major related question, which is why emotional states feel like something to us. This it transpires is part of the much larger, though more complex, issue of consciousness, and why anything should feel like something to us. This aspect of emotional feelings, because it is part of the much larger issue of consciousness, is deferred until Chapter 10.

In Chapter 2, in considering the functions of emotions, the idea is presented that emotions are part of a system that helps to enable certain classes of stimuli, broadly identified as rewarding and punishing stimuli (i.e. aversive stimuli or 'punishers'), to be treated as goals for action systems. Part of the idea is that this enables a simple interface between such stimuli and actions, in which any action can be performed to achieve the goal. This is an important area in its own right, which goes to the heart of why animals are built to respond to rewards and punishers, and to have emotions.

The suggestion made in this book is that we now have a way of systematically approaching the nature of emotions, their functions, and their brain mechanisms. Doubtless in time there will be changes and additions to the overall picture. But the suggestion is that the ideas and theory presented here do provide a firm and systematic foundation for understanding emotions, their functions, and their brain mechanisms in a well-founded evolutionary context.

2.2 The outline of a theory of emotion

I will first introduce the essence of the definition of emotion that I propose. *The definition of emotions is that emotions are states elicited by rewards and punishers, that is, by instrumental reinforcers.* As described in Section 1.2, a reward is anything for which an animal will work. A punisher is anything that an animal will work to escape or avoid, or that will suppress actions on which it is contingent[2]. I note that any change in the regular delivery of a reward or a punisher acts as an instrumental reinforcer. The force of 'instrumental' in this definition is that the emotional states are seen as defining the goals for arbitrary behavioural actions, made to obtain the instrumental reinforcer. This is very different from classical conditioning, in which a response, typically autonomic, may be elicited to a stimulus, without any need for an intervening state (see further Section 4.6.1). The relevant states elicited by the instrumental reinforcers are those with the particular functions described in Chapter 3.

An example of an emotion might thus be happiness produced by being given a reward, such as a hug, a pleasant touch, praise, winning a large sum of money, or being with someone whom one loves. All these things are rewards, in that we will work to obtain them. Another example of an emotion might be fear produced by the sound of a rapidly approaching bus when we are cycling, or the sight of an angry expression on someone's face. We will work to avoid such stimuli, which are punishers. Another example might be frustration, anger, or sadness produced by the omission of an expected reward such as a prize, or the termination of a reward such as the death of a loved one. Another example might be relief, produced by the omission or termination of a punishing stimulus, for example the removal of a painful stimulus, or sailing out of danger. These examples indicate how emotions can be produced by the delivery, omission, or termination of rewarding or punishing stimuli, and go some way to

[2] A full definition in terms of instrumental reinforcement contingencies is given below.

indicate how different emotions could be produced and classified in terms of the rewards and punishers received, omitted, or terminated.

Before accepting this proposal, we should consider whether there are any exceptions to the proposed rule. Indeed, at first this may appear to be a rather reductionist hypothesis about what produces emotions. However, one way to test the suggested definition of the events that cause emotions is to ask whether there are any rewards or punishers that do not produce emotions. Conversely, we should ask whether there are any emotions that are produced by stimuli, events, or remembered events that are not rewarding or punishing. If we cannot find exceptions, then we should accept the suggestion as a useful identification, summary, and working definition of the conditions that produce emotions. Therefore in the next few pages we consider the questions: 'Are any emotions caused by stimuli, events, or remembered events that are not rewarding or punishing? Do any rewarding or punishing stimuli not cause emotions?' But first it is worth pointing out that in fact many approaches to or theories of emotion have in common that part of the process involves 'appraisal' (e.g. Frijda (1986), Oatley & Johnson-Laird (1987), Lazarus (1991), Izard (1993), Stein, Trabasso & Liwag (1994), Scherer, Schorr & Johnstone (2001), Scherer (2009), and Moors, Ellsworth, Scherer & Frijda (2013)). This is part, for example, of the suggestion made by Oatley & Jenkins (1996), who on page 96 write that "an emotion is usually caused by a person consciously or unconsciously evaluating an event as relevant to a concern (a goal) that is important; the emotion is felt as positive when a concern is advanced and negative when a concern is impeded" (see also Keltner et al. (2013)). The concept of appraisal presumably involves in all these theories assessment of whether something is rewarding or punishing, that is whether it will be worked for or avoided. The description in terms of reward or punisher, that is in terms of states elicited by instrumental reinforcers, adopted here simply seems much more precisely and operationally specified.

The idea that rewards and punishers, that is instrumental reinforcers, are the stimuli that produce emotions has a considerable history, with origins that can be traced back to Watson (1929, 1930), Harlow & Stagner (1933), and Amsel (1958, 1962). More recently, the approach was developed by Millenson (1967), Larry Weiskrantz (1968), and Jeffrey Gray (1975, 1981). We can introduce some of the emotions that result from different reinforcement contingencies as follows. Consider the emotional effects of delivery of a 'reward' : a state such as pleasure or happiness will be produced. An example might be receiving a prize for excellent work. Now consider the emotional effects of delivery of a 'punisher' : pain or fear may be produced. For example, fear is an emotional state that might be produced by a sound that has previously been associated with a painful electrical shock. Shock in this example is the primary reinforcer, and fear is the emotional state that occurs to the tone stimulus as a result of the learning of the stimulus (i.e. tone)–reinforcer (i.e. shock) association. The tone in this example is a conditioned stimulus because of stimulus–reinforcer association learning, and has secondary reinforcing properties in that actions will be made to escape from it that are instrumental in avoiding the primary reinforcer, shock.

The converse reinforcement contingencies produce the opposite effects on behaviour, and produce different emotions. The omission or termination of a reward ('extinction' and 'time out' respectively) reduce the probability of responses, and may produce the emotions of frustration, disappointment, or rage. (Imagine not receiving a prize that you deserved.) Behavioural responses followed by the omission or termination of a punisher increase in probability (this pair of reinforcement operations being termed 'active avoidance' and 'escape', respectively), and are associated with emotions such as relief.

The classification of emotions in terms of reinforcement contingencies is developed further in Section 2.3, and more formal definitions of rewards and punishers, and how they are related to learning theory concepts such as reinforcement, instrumental learning, and punishment are provided next, and are elaborated further in Sections 1.2 and 4.6.1.

Instrumental reinforcers are stimuli that, if their occurrence, termination, or omission is made contingent upon the making of an action, alter the probability of the future emission of that action (Gray 1975, Mackintosh 1983, Dickinson 1980, Lieberman 2000, Mazur 2012). Rewards and punishers are instrumental reinforcing stimuli. The notion of an action here is that an arbitrary action, e.g. turning right vs turning left, will be performed in order to obtain the reward or avoid the punisher, so that there is no pre-wired connection between the response and the reinforcing stimulus. Some stimuli are primary (unlearned) reinforcers (e.g., the taste of food if the animal is hungry, or pain); while others may become reinforcing by learning, because of their association with such primary reinforcers, thereby becoming 'secondary reinforcers'. This type of learning may thus be called 'stimulus–reinforcer association', and occurs via an associative learning process. A positive reinforcer (such as food) increases the probability of emission of a response on which it is contingent, the process is termed **positive reinforcement**, and the *outcome* is a reward (such as food). A negative reinforcer (such as a painful stimulus) increases the probability of emission of a response that causes the negative reinforcer to be omitted (as in active avoidance) or terminated (as in escape), and the procedure is termed **negative reinforcement**. In contrast, **punishment** refers to procedures in which the probability of an action is decreased. Punishment thus describes procedures in which an action decreases in probability if it is followed by a painful stimulus, as in passive avoidance. Punishment can also be used to refer to a procedure involving the omission or termination of a reward ('extinction' and 'time out' respectively), both of which decrease the probability of responses (Gray 1975, Mackintosh 1983, Dickinson 1980, Lieberman 2000, Mazur 2012). The learning of which action to perform to achieve the goal is 'action–outcome' learning. My argument is that an affectively positive or 'appetitive' stimulus (which produces a state of pleasure) acts operationally as a **reward**, which when delivered acts instrumentally as a positive reinforcer, or when not delivered (omitted or terminated) acts to decrease the probability of actions on which it is contingent. Conversely I argue that an affectively negative or aversive stimulus (which produces an unpleasant state) acts operationally as a **punisher**, which when delivered acts instrumentally to decrease the probability of responses on which it is contingent, or when not delivered (escaped from or avoided) acts as a negative reinforcer in that it then increases the probability of the action on which its non-delivery is contingent[3].

The link between emotion and instrumental reinforcers being made is partly an operational link. Most people find that it is not easy to think of exceptions to the statements that emotions occur after rewards or punishers are given (sometimes continuing for long after the eliciting stimulus has ended, as in a mood state); or that rewards and punishers, but not other stimuli, produce emotional states. But the link is deeper than this, as we will see, in that the theory has been developed that genes specify primary reinforcers in order to encourage the animal to perform arbitrary actions to seek particular goals, thus increasing the probability of their own (the genes') survival into the next generation (Rolls 1999a, Rolls 2005b). The emotional states elicited by the reinforcers have a number of functions, described below, related to these processes. The presence of an intervening state produced by the stimulus associated with a primary reinforcer (e.g. the sight of food, or a tone associated with shock) in instrumental learning that provides a goal for an action is a key concept in my theory, for the intervening state is an affective or emotional state (Rolls 2013d). Further, motivation can now be understood as a state in which the goal (i.e. the instrumental reinforcer) is being sought. Motivational states thus have affective value. Philip Teitelbaum understood this, and reserved the term

[3]Note that my definition of a punisher, which is similar to that of an aversive stimulus, is of a stimulus or event that can either decrease the probability of actions on which it is contingent, or increase the probability of actions on which its non-delivery is contingent. The term punishment is restricted to situations where the probability of an action is being decreased.

'motivation' for states in which an instrumental reinforcer or goal was being sought. If in contrast the behaviour is a reflex such as protruding a proboscis when short of food, then we would not call this motivated behaviour.

Before considering how different emotions are related to different reinforcement contingencies in Section 2.3, I clarify a matter of terminology about moods vs emotions. A useful convention to distinguish between emotion and a mood state is as follows. An emotion consists of cognitive processing that results in a decoded signal that an environmental event (or remembered event) is reinforcing, together with the mood or affective state produced as a result. If the mood state is produced in the absence of the external sensory input and the cognitive decoding (for example by direct electrical stimulation of the brain (Rolls 2005b)), then this is described only as a mood state, and is different from an emotion in that there is no object in the environment towards which the mood state is directed. (In that emotions are produced by stimuli or objects, and thus emotions 'take or have an object', emotional states are examples of what philosophers call intentional states.) It is useful to emphasize that there is great opportunity for cognitive processing (whether conscious or not) in emotions, for cognitive processes will very often be required to determine whether an environmental stimulus or event is an instrumental reinforcer (see further Section 2.4).

2.3 Different emotions

As introduced in Section 2.2, the different emotions can in part be described and classified according to whether the instrumental reinforcer is positive or negative, and by the reinforcement contingency. An outline of such a classification scheme, elaborated by Rolls (1990b, 1999a, 2000a, 2005b) is shown in Fig. 2.1. Movement away from the centre of the diagram represents increasing intensity of emotion, on a continuous scale. The diagram shows that emotions associated with the delivery of a reward (S+) include pleasure, elation and ecstasy. Of course, other emotional labels can be included along the same axis. Emotions associated with the delivery of a punisher (S–) include apprehension, fear, and terror (see Fig. 2.1). Emotions associated with the omission of a reward ($\underline{S+}$) or the termination of a reward (S+!) include frustration, anger and rage. Emotions associated with the omission of a punisher ($\underline{S-}$) or the termination of a punisher (S–!) include relief. Although the classification of emotions presented here (and by Rolls (1986a, 1986b, 1990b, 1999a, 2005b)) differs from earlier theories, the approach adopted here of defining and classifying emotions by instrumentally reinforcing effects is one that has been developed in a number of earlier analyses (e.g. Millenson (1967), and Gray(1975, 1981); see Strongman (2003)).

I should make it clear that the scheme shown in Fig. 2.1 is not intended to be a dimensional scheme. [A dimensional scheme is one in which independent factors or dimensions have been identified that account for the major and independent sources of variation in a data set. Some investigators work to show that these dimensions can be interpreted both biologically (for example as differing in autonomic, endocrine, or arousal-related ways) and psychologically (e.g. as representing anger vs fear), as described in Section 2.6.3.] However, the import of what is shown in Fig. 2.1 is to set out a set of logical possibilities of ways in which reinforcement contingencies can vary, and to show how they may be related to some different types of emotion. I emphasize that there are many different types of instrumental reinforcer, as will be shown with Table 2.1, and that each reinforcer is capable of acting by many of the types of contingency summarized in Fig. 2.1, with each reinforcer producing its own specific and different type of emotion.

It is actually a possibility that the four directions shown in Fig. 2.1 are at least partly independent from each other, and that a four-dimensional space is spanned by what is shown

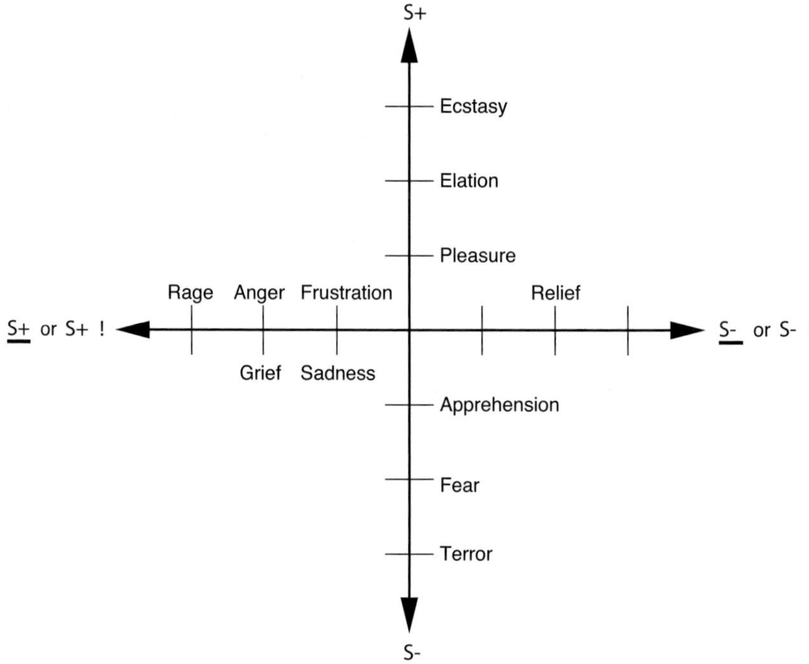

Fig. 2.1 Some of the emotions associated with different reinforcement contingencies are indicated. Intensity increases away from the centre of the diagram, on a continuous scale. The classification scheme created by the different reinforcement contingencies consists with respect to the action of (1) the delivery of a reward (S+), (2) the delivery of a punisher (S–), (3) the omission of a reward (S+) (extinction) or the termination of a reward (S+!) (time out), and (4) the omission of a punisher (S–) (avoidance) or the termination of a punisher (S–!) (escape). Note that the vertical axis describes emotions associated with the delivery of a reward (up) or punisher (down). The horizontal axis describes emotions associated with the non-delivery of an expected reward (left) or the non-delivery of an expected punisher (right). The diagram summarizes emotions that might result for one reinforcer as a result of different contingencies. Every separate reinforcer has the potential to operate according to contingencies such as these. This diagram does not imply a dimensional theory of emotion, but shows the types of emotional state that might be produced by a specific reinforcer. Each different reinforcer will produce different emotional states, but the contingencies will operate as shown to produce different specific emotional states for each different reinforcer.

in Fig. 2.1. For example, sensitivity to (that is the ability to respond to) reward (S+) could be at least partly independent from sensitivity to punishers (S–), sensitivity to non-reward (S+ and S+!), and sensitivity to non-delivery of a punisher (S– and S–!). The dimensions or independent ways in which emotions may differ from each other could thus span 4 dimensions even with what is shown in Fig. 2.1, and these ways are expanded greatly as shown by the following further effects that make different emotions different to each other.

One important point about Fig. 2.1 is that there are a large number of different primary reinforcers, and that for example the reward label S+ shows states that might be elicited by just one type of reward, such as a pleasant touch. There will be a different reward axis (S+) and non-reward axis (S+ and S+!) for each type of reward (e.g. pleasant touch vs sweet taste); and, correspondingly, a different punisher axis (S–) and non-punisher axis (S– and S–!) for each type of punisher (e.g. pain vs bitter taste).

Different reinforcement contingencies can thus be used to classify a wide range of emotions. However, some of my tutorial pupils at Oxford sometimes expressed the view that reinforcement contingencies alone might not be able to account for the full range of human emotions. I therefore set out for them ways in which a system based on reinforcement contingencies could be developed in a number of different ways to give an account of most emotions. This extended set of ways of accounting for different emotions was published in 1986 (Rolls 1986a, Rolls 1986b), and developed a little in later publications (e.g. Rolls (1995a, 1999a, 2005b)). It is described, and elaborated further next. If the reader can think of any emotions that cannot be accounted for by a combination of the ways described next, then it would be interesting to consider what further extensions might be needed.

1. **Reinforcement contingency**
The first way in which different classes of emotion could arise is because of different reinforcement contingencies, as described above and indicated in Fig. 2.1.

2. **Intensity**
Second, different intensities within these classes can produce different degrees of emotion (see above and Millenson (1967)). For example, as the strength of a positive reinforcer being presented increases, emotions might be labelled as pleasure, elation, and ecstasy. Similarly, as the strength of a negative reinforcer being presented increases, emotions might be labelled as apprehension, fear, and terror (see Fig. 2.1). It may be noted here that anxiety can refer to the state produced by stimuli associated with the non-delivery of a reward; or with the delivery of a punisher (Gray 1987).

3. **Multiple reinforcement associations**
Third, any environmental stimulus might have a number of different reinforcement associations. For example, a stimulus might be associated with both reward and punishment, allowing states such as conflict and guilt to arise. The different possible combinations greatly increase the number of possible emotions.

4. **Different primary reinforcers**
Fourth, emotions elicited by stimuli associated with different primary reinforcers will be different even within a reinforcement category (i.e. with the same reinforcement contingency), because the original reinforcers are different. Thus, for example, the state elicited by a stimulus associated with a reward such as the taste of food will be different from that elicited by a reward such as being groomed. Indeed, it is an important feature of the association memory mechanisms described here that when a stimulus is applied, it acts as a key which ‘looks up’ or recalls the original primary reinforcer with which it was associated (Rolls 2008b). Thus emotional stimuli will differ from each other in terms of the original primary reinforcers with which they were associated.

A summary of many different primary reinforcers is provided in Table 2.1, and inspection of this will help to show how some different emotions are produced by different primary reinforcers. For example, from Table 2.1 it might be surmised that one of the biological origins of the emotion of jealousy might be the state elicited in a male when his partner is courted by another male, because this threatens his parental investment in the offspring he raises with his partner, as described in Chapter 7. Jealousy in females would arise in a corresponding way, especially if her resources were threatened. Examples of how further emotions including guilt, shame, anger, forgiveness, envy and love may arise in relation to particular primary reinforcers are provided later in this section, throughout this chapter, in Chapters 3 and 7, and in many other places in this book.

Table 2.1 Some primary reinforcers, and the dimensions of the environment to which they are tuned

Taste	
Salt taste	reward in salt deficiency
Sweet	reward in energy deficiency
Bitter	punisher, indicator of possible poison
Sour	punisher
Umami	reward, indicator of protein; produced by monosodium glutamate and inosine monophosphate
Tannic acid	punisher; it prevents absorption of protein; found in old leaves; probably somatosensory not gustatory (Critchley and Rolls 1996)
Odour	
Putrefying odour	punisher; hazard to health
Pheromones	reward (depending on hormonal state)
Somatosensory	
Pain	punisher
Touch	reward
Grooming	reward; to give grooming may also be a primary reinforcer.
Washing	reward
Temperature	reward if tends to help maintain normal body temperature; otherwise punisher
Visual	
Snakes, etc.	punisher for, e.g., primates
Youthfulness	reward, associated with mate choice
Beauty, e.g. symmetry	reward
Secondary sexual characteristics	rewards
Face expression	reward (e.g. smile) or punisher (e.g. threat)
Blue sky, cover, open space	reward, indicator of safety
Flowers	reward (indicator of fruit later in the season?)
Auditory	
Warning call	punisher
Aggressive vocalization	punisher
Soothing vocalization	reward (part of the evolutionary history of music, which at least in its origins taps into the channels used for the communication of emotions)

Table 2.1 continued **Some primary reinforcers, and the dimensions of the environment to which they are tuned**

Reproduction	
Courtship	reward
Sexual behaviour	reward (different reinforcers, including a low waist-to-hip ratio, and attractiveness influenced by symmetry and being found attractive by members of the other sex, are discussed in Chapter 7).
Mate guarding	reward for a male to protect his parental investment. Jealousy results if his mate is courted by another male, because this may ruin his parental investment
Nest building	reward (when expecting young)
Parental attachment (love)	reward (good for the parent's genes both when the attachment is to the other parent or an infant)
Infant attachment to parents (love)	reward (good for the infant's genes)
Crying of infant	punisher to parents; produced to promote successful development
Power, status, wealth, resources	Attractive to females, who may benefit from resources for their offspring. Attractive to males as they make males attractive to females.
Body size	Large in males may be attractive to females as a signal for the provision of protection and of the ability of her male offspring to compete for a mate. Small in females may be attractive to males as a neotenous sign of youth, and therefore fertility
Other	
Novel stimuli	rewards (encourage animals to investigate the full possibilities of the multidimensional space in which their genes are operating)
Sleep	reward; minimizes nutritional requirements and protects from danger
Altruism to genetic kin	reward (kin altruism)
Altruism to other individuals	reward while the altruism is reciprocated in a 'tit-for-tat' reciprocation (reciprocal altruism). Forgiveness, honesty, and altruistic punishment are some associated heuristics. May provide underpinning for some aspects of what is felt to be moral.
Altruism to other individuals	punisher when the altruism is not reciprocated
Group acceptance, reputation	reward (social greeting might indicate this). These goals can account for why some cultural goals are pursued
Control over actions	reward
Play	reward
Danger, stimulation, excitement	reward if not too extreme (adaptive because of practice?)
Exercise	reward (keeps the body fit for action)
Mind reading	reward; practice in reading others' minds, which might be adaptive
Solving an intellectual problem	reward (practice in which might be adaptive)
Storing, collecting	reward (e.g. food)
Habitat preference, home, territory	reward
Some responses	reward (e.g. pecking in chickens, pigeons; adaptive because it is a simple way in which eating grain can be programmed for a relatively fixed type of environmental stimulus)
Breathing	reward

5. **Different secondary reinforcers**

A fifth way in which emotions can be different from each other is in terms of the particular (conditioned) stimulus that elicits the emotion, and the situation in which it occurs. Thus, even though the reinforcement contingency and even the unconditioned reinforcer may be identical, emotions will still be different cognitively, if the conditioned stimuli that give rise to the emotions are different (that is, if the objects of the emotion are different). For example, the emotional state elicited by the sight of one person may be different from that elicited by the sight of another person because the people, and thus the cognitive evaluations associated with the perception of the stimuli, are different. In another example, not obtaining a monetary reward in a gambling task might lead to frustration, but being blocked by another person from obtaining a reward might lead to anger directed at the person.

Thus evolution may have shaped different reinforcers to contribute in different ways and depending on the environmental circumstances to the exact emotion produced. For example, some emotions may be related to social reinforcers (e.g. love, anger, envy, and breaking rules of society so that shame is produced, see further Section 11.3 and Rolls (2012d)), others to non-social reinforcers (such as fear of a painful stimulus), and others to solving difficult problems. By taking into account the nature of the primary reinforcer, the nature of the secondary reinforcer, and the environmental circumstances in which these apply, many different emotions can thus be accounted for, and cognitive factors taken into account. The common underlying basis of emotion remains however that it is related to goals/instrumental reinforcers, and the reinforcement contingencies that operate. The variety of different goals, and the contingencies and environmental situations in which they occur, combine to contribute to the richness in the variety of emotional states.

The gene-specified reinforcer approach to emotion advocated in this book is somewhat different to the domain-specific (vs domain general) approach of some evolutionary biologists (see Nesse (2000a)). In the domain-specific approach, a modular approach to different emotions may be taken, and the temptation is to end with a large number of specialized emotional systems, each promoting particular types of action. In contrast, in the approach described here, different genes build different reinforcement systems that define the goals for actions, and arbitrary actions appropriate for reaching the goal (i.e. instrumental actions) are then performed, with action–outcome learning guiding the actions produced. This can result in a rich variety of actions being selected in different emotion-provoking situations, without a tendency to suggest that particular perhaps instinctive actions are coupled to particular emotions. (Indeed, fixed action patterns, where responses such as pecking by the herring gull of its parent's red spot on the beak to obtain regurgitated food from the parent (Tinbergen 1951), or pecking responses in birds that lead to the ingestion of grain, or even unconditioned approach towards a releasing stimulus, do not count in the present analysis as involving emotional states, for no states are needed to intervene between the stimulus and the response. In contrast, with the goal for an action being specified by gene-specified instrumental reinforcers, there is a need for a state to intervene between the decoding of the reinforcer and the completion of the action made possibly over many minutes to obtain the reinforcer (Rolls 2013d).) Instead, 'instinct' is, I argue, involved in the process whereby the *goals* for actions, which are reinforcing stimuli, are specified by genes as a result of natural selection, and the behavioural response itself, the particular action, is not specified or 'determined' (see further Section 3.5).

Further, in the approach described here, modular neural systems useful for face identification, face expression recognition, and head gesture and movement may evolve because of the different specialized computational requirements for each and the importance of minimizing wiring length in the brain (see Section 4.4 and Rolls (2008b)), and because the presence of these systems helps to provide representations that are useful in defining which stimulus or object-related events in the environment are associated with primary reinforcers.

6. **The behavioural responses that are available**

A sixth possible way in which emotions can vary arises when the environment constrains the types of behavioural response that can be made. For example, if an active behavioural response can occur to the omission of an expected reward, then anger might be produced and directed at the person who prevented the reward being obtained, but if only passive behaviour is possible, then sadness, depression or grief might occur (see Fig. 2.1).

By realizing that these six possibilities can occur in different combinations, it can be seen that it is possible to account for a very wide range of emotions, and this is believed to be one of the strengths of the approach described here. It is also the case that the extent to which a stimulus is reinforcing on a particular occasion (and thus an emotion is produced) depends on the prior history of reinforcements (both recently through processes that include sensory-specific satiety, and in the longer term), and that the current mood state can affect the degree to which a stimulus (a term that includes cognitively decoded events and remembered events) is reinforcing (see Section 4.12).

If we wish to consider the number of independent ways in which emotions may differ from each other (for comparison with the 'dimensional' theories described in Section 2.6.3) we see immediately that a vast subtlety of emotions can be systematically described using the approach described here. For example, based on the four different reinforcement contingencies shown in Fig. 2.1 we have four at least potentially independent 'dimensions', which are combined with perhaps another 100–500 independently varying (in that they are gene-specified) primary reinforcers, some of which are included in Table 2.1. These are combined with constraints to the actions that may be possible when a reinforcer is received (the 'coping potential' of appraisal theorists), which potentially at least doubles the number of emotions that can be described. We add further combinatorial possibilities by noting (point 3 above) that a given stimulus in the world may have many different reinforcement associations producing states such as conflict. The possible number of different emotions can be further multiplied by the fact that each primary reinforcer may have associated with it almost any neutral stimulus to produce a secondary reinforcer.

The resulting number of emotional states that can be described and categorized is clearly enormous, even if we do not assume that each of the above factors operates strictly independently. For example, it is likely that if a gene were to specify a particular reward as being particularly intense in an individual, for example the pleasantness of touch, then omitting (S+) or terminating (S+!) this reward might also be expected to be particularly intense, so the contributions of reinforcement contingency and identity of the primary reinforcer might combine additively rather than multiplicatively. Even if there is only partial independence of the different processes 1–6 above, and of variation within each process, then nevertheless many different emotions can be systematically classified and described. It does of course remain an interesting issue of how the processes described above do combine, and of the extent to which a few factors actually do account for a great deal in the variation between different emotions. For example, if in an individual's sensitivity to non-reward is generally much more intense than the individual's sensitivity to reward, then this will shape the emotions in that individual, and account for quite a deal of the variance between that individual's emotional states. Such a factor might also account for quite an amount of the variation in emotions and personality between individuals (see Section 2.7).

Some examples of how different emotions might be classified using the above criteria now follow. **Fear** is a state that might be produced by a stimulus that has become a secondary reinforcer by virtue of its learned association with a primary negative reinforcer such as pain (see Fig. 2.1). **Anger** is a state that might be produced by the omission of an expected reward, frustrative non-reward, when an active behavioural response is possible (see Fig. 2.1). (In particular, anger may occur if another individual prevents an expected reward from being obtained.) **Guilt** may arise when there is a conflict between an available reward and a rule or law of society. **Jealousy** is an emotion that might be aroused in a male if the faithfulness of his partner seems to be threatened by her liaison (e.g. flirting) with another male. In this case the reinforcement contingency that is operating is produced by a punisher, and it may be that males are specified genetically to find this punishing because it indicates a potential threat to their paternity and paternal investment, as described in Chapters 7 and 3. Similarly, a female may become jealous if her partner has a liaison with another female, because the resources available to the 'wife' useful to bring up her children are threatened. Again, the punisher here may be gene-specified, as described in Chapter 3. **Envy** or **disappointment** might be produced if a prize is obtained by a competitor. In this case, part of the way in which the frustrative non-reward is produced is by the cognitive understanding that this is a competition in which there will be a winner, and that the person has set himself or herself the goal of obtaining it.

The partial list of primary reinforcers provided in Table 2.1 should provide readers with a foundation for starting to understand the rich classification scheme for different types of emotion that can be classified in this way.

Many other similar examples can be surmised from the area of evolutionary psychology (see e.g. Ridley (1993a), Buss (2012, 2003), and Barrett, Dunbar & Lycett (2002)). For example, there may be a set of reinforcers that are genetically specified to help promote social cooperation and even reciprocal altruism. Such genes might specify that emotion should be elicited, and behavioural changes should occur, if a cooperating partner defects or 'cheats' (Cosmides & Tooby 1999). Moreover, the genes may build brains with genetically specified rules that are useful heuristics for social cooperation, such as acting with a strategy of 'generous tit-for tat', which can be more adaptive than strict 'tit-for-tat', in that being generous occasionally is a good strategy to help promote further cooperation that has failed when both partners defect in a strict 'tit-for-tat' scenario (Ridley 1996). Genes that specify good heuristics to promote social cooperation may thus underlie such complex emotional states as feeling forgiving.

It is suggested that many apparently complex emotional states have their origins in designing animals to perform well in such sociobiological and socioeconomic situations (Ridley 1996, Glimcher 2003, Glimcher 2004, Glimcher, Camerer, Fehr & Poldrack 2009, Glimcher 2011a) (Chapter 9). Indeed, many principles that humans accept as ethical may be closely related to strategies that are useful heuristics for promoting social cooperation, and emotional feelings associated with ethical behaviour may be at least partly related to the adaptive value of such gene-specified strategies. These ideas are developed in Section 11.3 and by Rolls (2012d).

These examples indicate that an emotional state can be systematically specified and classified using the six principles described above in this Section. The similarity between particular emotions will depend on how close they are in the space defined by the above principles.

2.4 Refinements of the theory of emotion

The definition of emotions given above, that they are states produced by instrumental reinforcing stimuli, and have particular functions, is refined now.

First, when positively reinforcing (rewarding) stimuli (such as the taste of food or water) are relevant to a drive state produced by a change in the *internal milieu* (such as hunger and thirst), then we do not normally classify these stimuli as emotional, though they do produce pleasure, and indeed we describe the state they produce as affective (see Chapter 5). In contrast, emotional states are normally initiated by reinforcing stimuli that have their origin in the external environment, such as an (external) noise associated with pain (delivered by an external stimulus). We may then have identified a class of reinforcers (in our example, food) that we do not want to say cause emotions. This then is a refinement of the definition of emotions given above. Fortunately, we can encapsulate the set of reinforcing stimuli that we wish to exclude from our definition of stimuli that produce emotion. They are the set of external reinforcers (such as the sight of food) that are relevant to motivational states such as hunger and thirst, which are controlled by internal need-related (i.e. homeostatic) signals such as the concentration of glucose in the plasma (see Chapter 5). However, there is room for plenty of further discussion and refinement here. Perhaps some people (especially French people?) might say that they do experience emotion when they savour a wonderful food. There may well be cultural differences here in the semantics of whether such reinforcing stimuli should be included within the category that produce emotions.

Another area for discussion is how we wish to categorize the reinforcers associated with sexual behaviour. Such stimuli may be made to be rewarding, and to feel pleasurable, partly because of the internal hormonal state. Does this mean that we wish to exclude such stimuli from the class that we call emotion-provoking, in the same way that we might exclude food reward from the class of stimuli that are said to cause emotion, because the reward value of food depends on an internal controlling signal? I am not sure that there is a perfectly clear answer to this. But this may not matter, as long as we understand that there are some rewarding stimuli that some may wish to exclude from those that cause emotional states.

Second, emotional states can be produced by *remembered reinforcing stimuli*. (Indeed, when we remember stimuli or events, many of the cortical areas activated by the original sensory stimulus are also activated by the remembered stimuli or events. This is the case for most of the cortical areas in each sensory system, apart perhaps from the first (Rolls 1989b, Rolls & Treves 1998, Rolls 2008b). Thus if we recall a particular event, and this leads to reinstatement of activity in the higher parts of the visual system, this activity will provide inputs to the later parts of the brain involved in emotion, so that emotional states may then be produced.

Third, the stimulus that produces the emotional state does not have to be shown to be a reinforcer when producing the emotional state – it simply has to be *capable of being shown to have instrumental reinforcing properties*. An emotion-provoking stimulus can act as a reward or punisher, and is a goal for possible action.

Fourth, the definition given provides great opportunity for *cognitive processing* (whether conscious or not) in emotions, for cognitive processes will very often be required to determine whether an environmental stimulus or event is a reward or punisher. Normally an emotion consists of this cognitive processing that results in a decoded signal that the environmental event is reinforcing, together with the mood state produced as a result. If the mood state is produced in the absence of the external sensory input and the cognitive decoding (for example by direct electrical stimulation of the amygdala (Rolls 1975, Rolls 1999a, Rolls 2005b), then this is described only as a mood state, and is different from an emotion in that there is no object in the environment towards which the mood state is directed. The external reinforcing stimulus may alter the mood state very rapidly, and then the firing of the neurons that represent the mood state may gradually return back to their baseline firing rate, depending on the time course of the emotional state that is produced by the external reinforcing stimulus.

While discussing *mood*, it is worth pointing out that mood may be a particularly difficult state for the brain to maintain at a relatively constant level. In sensory systems the situation is different, for most sensory systems work by contrast, rather than absolute level. For example, early in the visual system it is the difference in brightness levels present at an edge, rather than the absolute brightness, that is signaled. This is achieved by a process of lateral inhibition, which means that neighbouring neurons effectively inhibit each other. The result is that it is only at a dark–light boundary, where there is contrast, that neurons are firing. (In fact the firing will be fast on the bright side of the edge, and low, below a spontaneous level of firing, on the dark side of the edge. In the middle of a large bright area few neurons will be active, because the nearby neurons will be inhibiting each other.) However, for mood, the situation may be different. Here, the absolute firing rates of the neurons that represent mood state must be set to fire at the appropriate rate for long periods. Any drift in firing rates would represent a change of mood level. The situation for a brain system that represents mood may thus be different from that involved in most sensory and motor processing in the brain, both because in sensory systems it is the local contrast of firing rate that is important, not the absolute level, and because in sensory systems the inputs keep changing, so that it is not necessary to maintain an absolute value for long. The difficulty of maintaining a constant absolute level of firing in neurons may contribute to 'spontaneous' mood swings, depression that occurs without a clear external cause, and the multiplicity of hormonal and transmitter systems that seem to be involved in the control of mood (see Chapters 4 and 6).

Having said this, it also seems to be the case that there is some '*regression to a constant value*' for emotional states. What I mean by this is that we are sensitive to some extent not just to the absolute level of reinforcers being received, but also to the change in the rate, probability, or magnitude of reinforcers being received. This is well shown by the phenomenon of *positive and negative contrast* effects with rewards. Imagine that an animal is working at a moderate rate for a moderate reward. If the reward is suddenly increased, the animal will work very much harder for a period (perhaps lasting for minutes or longer), but will then gradually revert back to work at a rate close to that at which the animal was working for the moderate reinforcement. This is called positive contrast (see Fig. 2.2). A comparable contrast effect is seen when the reward magnitude (or rate at which rewards are obtained, or the probability of obtaining rewards) is reduced – there is a negative overshoot in the rate of working for a time, but then the rate reverts back to a value close to that at which the animal worked for the moderate reward. This phenomenon is adaptive. It is evidence that animals are in part sensitive to a change in reinforcement, and this helps them to 'climb reward gradients' to obtain better rewards. In effect, regardless of the absolute level of reinforcement being received, it is adaptive to be sensitive to a change in reinforcement. If this were not true, an animal receiving very little reinforcement but then obtaining a small increase in positive reinforcement might still be working very little for the reward. But it is much more adaptive to work hard in this situation, as the extra little bit of reward might make the difference between survival or not, and might lead the animal in the direction of even better rewards if what has just been done leads to an improvement in rewards. A similar phenomenon may be evident in humans. People who have very little in the way of rewards, who may be poor, have a poor diet, and may suffer from disease, may nevertheless not have a baseline level of happiness that is necessarily very different from that of a person in an affluent society who in absolute terms apparently has many more rewards. This may be due in part to resetting of the baseline of expected rewards to a constant value, so that we are especially sensitive to *changes* in rewards (or punishers), to optimize climbing of the gradient. Similar phenomena are treated in neuroeconomics under the heading of *relative value* (Section 9.5.3).

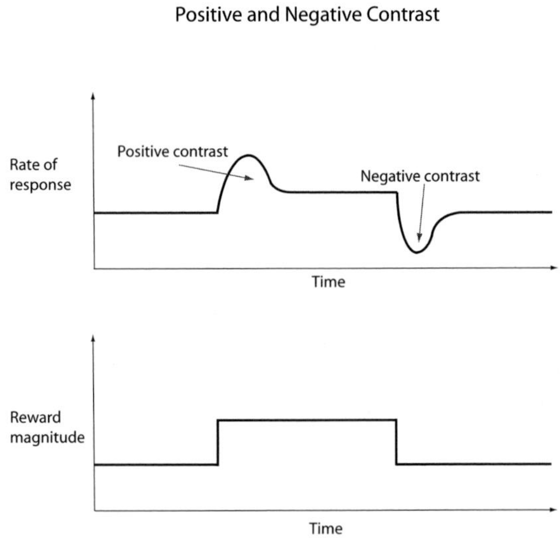

Fig. 2.2 Positive and negative contrast. If the magnitude of a moderate reward (positive reinforcer) is increased, then the rate of working increases markedly, but then drops back to a rate just greater than that to the moderate reinforcer. The positive overshoot is positive contrast. The converse happens if the magnitude of the reward is decreased.

Fifth, in a case where the sight of a stimulus associated with pain produces fear, some philosophers categorize fear as an emotion, but not pain. The distinction they make may be that primary (unlearned) reinforcers do not produce emotions, whereas secondary reinforcers (stimuli associated by stimulus–reinforcement learning with primary reinforcers) do. They describe the pain as a sensation. But neutral stimuli (such as a table) can produce sensations when touched. It accordingly seems to be much more useful to categorize stimuli according to whether they are instrumentally reinforcing (in which case they produce emotions), or are not reinforcing (in which case they do not produce emotions). Clearly there is a difference between primary reinforcers and learned reinforcers; but this is most precisely caught by noting that this is the difference, and that it is whether a stimulus is reinforcing that determines whether it is related to emotion. Primary and secondary reinforcers have in common that they produce affective states, whereas neutral, non-reinforcing, stimuli do not produce affective states. The major division thus seems to be between stimuli that produce affective states and those that do not; and it is instrumental reinforcing stimuli that produce affective states.

Sixth, as we are about to see, emotional states (i.e. those elicited by instrumental reinforcers) have many functions, and the implementations of only some of these functions by the brain are associated with emotional feelings (see Chapters 10 and 4, and Rolls (2005b) and Rolls (2012d)). Indeed there is evidence for interesting dissociations in some patients with brain damage between actions performed to reinforcing stimuli and what is subjectively reported. In this sense it is biologically and psychologically useful to consider emotional states to include more than those states associated with feelings of emotion.

Seventh, the role of learning in many emotions should be emphasized. The approach described above shows that the learning of stimulus–reinforcer (i.e. stimulus–reward and stimulus–punisher) associations is the learning involved when emotional states are learned. In so far as the majority of stimuli that produce our emotional states do so as a result of learning, this type of learning, and the brain mechanisms that underlie it, are crucial to the majority of our emotions. This is stimulus-stimulus association learning, where one of the stimuli is the to-be-associated stimulus, and the other stimulus is the primary reinforcer for instrumental learning, such as the taste of food. This, then, provides a theoretical basis for understanding the functions of some brain systems such as the orbitofrontal cortex in emotion, as it is involved in stimulus-reinforcer association learning, as described in Chapter 4. This helps to provide a foundation for understanding the importance of regions of the brain such as the orbitofrontal cortex in emotion. In addition to associations of stimuli with rewards and punishers that act as the goal for instrumental learning, during emotional learning stimuli may also become classically conditioned with unconditioned responses such as autonomic and endocrine responses, and even with skeletal responses such as freezing (see Section 4.6.1.1). Such classically conditioned responses may be adaptive, but are just associations between stimuli and responses, and do not need intervening states in which a goal must be held in mind as the target for an instrumental action to direct behaviour, and so such classically conditioned responses are not considered as requiring emotional states, though they may of course occur during emotional states.

It also follows from this approach towards a theory of emotion that brain systems involved in disconnecting stimulus–reinforcer associations when they are no longer appropriate will also be very important in emotion. Failure of this function would be expected to lead, for example, in frustrating situations to inappropriate perseveration of behaviour to stimuli no longer associated with rewards. The inability to correct behaviour when reinforcement contingencies change would be evident in a number of emotion-provoking situations, such as frustration (i.e. non-reward), and the punishment of previously rewarded behaviour. It will be shown in Chapter 4 that this approach, which emphasizes the necessity, in for example social situations, to update and correct the decoded reinforcement value of stimuli continually and rapidly, also helps to provide a basis for understanding the functions of some brain regions such as the orbitofrontal cortex in emotion.

Eighth, understanding the functions of emotion is also important for understanding the nature of emotions, and for understanding the brain systems involved in the different types of response that are produced by emotional states. Emotion appears to have many functions, which are not necessarily mutually exclusive. Some of these functions are described in Chapter 3.

However, a fundamentally important function of emotion that I will propose in Chapter 3 draws out a close link with the definition given here of emotions as states elicited by instrumental reinforcing stimuli, which are the goals for action. I show in Chapter 3 that genes define the goals for (instrumental) actions, and that this is an important Darwinian, adaptive, aspect of brain design. These goals for action are instrumental reinforcers, and this thus helps us to see that by understanding emotions as states elicited by instrumental reinforcers, we gain important insight into the nature of emotions. The treatment of the nature of emotion given in this chapter is thus seen to be directly relevant to understanding this fundamentally important role of emotion in brain design which is related to the role that reinforcers have in guiding actions.

2.5 Summary of the classification of emotion

The theory of emotion outlined above provides systematic and principled ways to categorize different emotions.

One useful way to categorize emotions is to note that the main dimensions of the space of possible emotional responses can well be specified by the different primary reinforcers, examples of which are given in Table 2.1. Within each of these gene-specified dimensions, different reinforcement contingencies would lead to different emotional states, for example pleasure produced by a given taste, and disappointment (frustrative non-reward) if that taste is not available. Also within each of these reinforcer-defined dimensions the exact nature of the primary reinforcing stimulus, including its intensity and variations in its quality (for example in the nature of its texture if it is a somatosensory stimulus), would lead to differences in the emotion elicited. Also within each gene-specified dimension, many states could be cognitively different depending on which different stimulus (e.g. person) had become associated by learning with the primary reinforcer to become a secondary reinforcer. If we then remember that each secondary reinforcer may have many different reinforcement associations, then we see that very large numbers of possible emotions can be described and categorized in this way. Although the description leads to an enormously large numbers of different categories, nevertheless it is systematic, principled, and fairly complete.

Another possible way to categorize emotions might be by reinforcement contingency. For example we might group together into one category all emotions elicited by frustrative non-reward ($\underline{S+}$ and S+! in Fig. 2.1). Gray (1987) went even further than this, grouping into one category not only the emotions elicited by frustrative non-reward (the non-delivery of rewards), but also those elicited by the delivery of punishers (S– in Fig. 2.1). Part of his reason for combining these two was that both can lead to decreases in behaviour, which led him to believe that there was a "behavioural inhibition system" (which he identified with the hippocampus) common to both. Clearly at some level the processing is inherently different, in that frustrative non-reward implies a neural system that predicts reward and produces an output if that outcome is not realized, whereas punishment may often involve activation of different sensory systems involved in for example pain. The whole operation and pharmacology of the different circuitry involved in frustrative non-reward and in the effects of punishers must at some level be different, and this is likely to be exploitable in treating emotional states that arise in these two different ways, so it may be very helpful not to combine them into a single category.

In general, categorizing emotions by reinforcement contingency alone produces few emotional categories, which is a disadvantage given the many different emotions that can be distinguished, but does have an advantage in producing a rough grouping together of emotional states that do have something in common. However, it should be noted that the reinforcement contingency alone is not a good predictor of the appropriate emotion and emotional behaviour, as shown for example in Fig. 2.1 by the anger that might result from frustrative non-reward if action is possible, and the sadness that might arise if no action is possible to retrieve the lost reward. Further, I note that the axes in Fig. 2.1 refer to only one particular reinforcer (such as a food reward), and are effectively replicated for each different primary reinforcer.

2.6 Other theories of emotion

In the following subsections, I outline some other theories of emotion, and compare them with the above (Rolls') theory of emotion. Surveys of some of the approaches to emotion that have been taken in the past are provided by Strongman (2003) and Keltner, Oatley & Jenkins (2013).

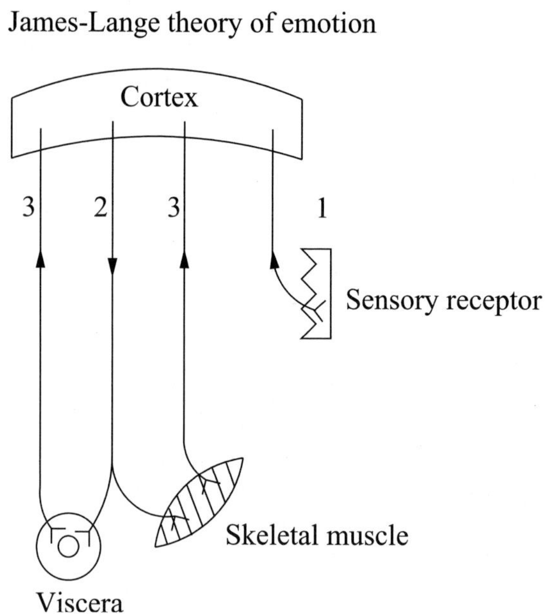

Fig. 2.3 The James–Lange theory of emotion proposes that there are three steps in producing emotional feelings. The first step is elicitation by the emotion-provoking stimulus (received by the cortex via pathway 1 in the Figure) of peripheral changes, such as skeleto-muscular activity to run away, and autonomic changes, such as alteration of heart rate (via pathways labelled 2 in the Figure). The second step is the sensing of the peripheral responses (e.g. altered heart rate, and somatosensory effects produced by running away) (via pathways labelled 3 in the Figure). The third step is elicitation of the emotional feeling in response to the sensed feedback from the periphery.

2.6.1 The James–Lange and other bodily theories of emotion including Damasio's theory

James (1884) believed that emotional experiences were produced by sensing bodily changes, such as changes in heart rate or in skeletal muscles. Lange (1885) had a similar view, although he emphasized the role of autonomic feedback (for example from the heart) in producing the experience of emotion. The theory, which became known as the James–Lange theory, suggested that there are three steps in producing emotional feelings (see Fig. 2.3). The first step is elicitation by the emotion-provoking stimulus of peripheral changes, such as skeleto-muscular activity to produce running away, and autonomic changes, such as alteration of heart rate. But, as pointed out above, the theory leaves unanswered perhaps the most important issue in any theory of emotion: Why do some events make us run away (and then feel emotional), whereas others do not? This is a major weakness of this type of theory. The second step is the sensing of the peripheral responses (e.g. running away, and altered heart rate). The third step is elicitation of the emotional feeling in response to the sensed feedback from the periphery.

The history of research into peripheral theories of emotion starts with the fatal flaw that step one (the question of which stimuli elicit emotion-related responses in the first place) leaves unanswered this most important question. The history continues with the accumulation of empirical evidence that has gradually weakened more and more the hypothesis that peripheral responses made during emotional behaviour have anything to do with producing the emotional behaviour (which has largely already been produced anyway according to the James–Lange theory), or the emotional feeling. Some of the landmarks in this history are as follows.

First, the peripheral changes produced during emotion are not sufficiently distinct to be able to carry the information that would enable one to have subtly different emotional feelings to the vast range of different stimuli that can produce different emotions. The evidence suggests that by measuring many peripheral changes in emotion, such as heart rate, skin conductance, breathing rate, and hormones such as adrenaline and noradrenaline (known in the United States by their Greek names epinephrine and norepinephrine), it may be possible to make coarse distinctions between, for example, anger and fear, but not much finer distinctions (Wagner 1989, Cacioppo, Klein, Berntson & Hatfield 1993, Keltner et al. 2013). However, some recent research has been showing that somewhat different types of emotion (core and body boundary-violation disgust) are associated with somewhat different autonomic activity (Harrison, Gray, Gianaros & Critchley 2010), though whether the feedback from the periphery is causally involved in influencing the emotional state is not clear. Brain processing must of course produce the somewhat different autonomic responses in the first place, and there is evidence that the orbitofrontal and anterior cingulate cortices, perhaps acting via an insular visceral cortex region, are involved in producing autonomic responses (Critchley 2005). Of course there are pathways from the viscera to the brain, and visceral changes can influence the brain (Critchley & Harrison 2013, Gray, Beacher, Minati, Nagai, Kemp, Harrison & Critchley 2012) (Fig. 4.68), but whether those visceral changes are in the normal causal chain for the elicitation of emotional states is much more difficult to prove.

Second, when emotions are evoked by imagery, then the peripheral responses are much less marked and distinctive than during emotions produced by external stimuli (Ekman, Levenson & Friesen 1983, Stemmler 1989, Levenson, Ekman & Friesen 1990). This makes sense in that although an emotion evoked by imagery may be strong, there is no need to produce strong peripheral responses, because no behavioural responses are required.

Third, disruption of peripheral responses and feedback from them either surgically (for example in dogs (Cannon 1927, Cannon 1929, Cannon 1931), or as a result of spinal cord injury in humans (Hohmann 1966, Bermond, Fasotti, Niewenhuyse & Schuerman 1991)), does not abolish emotional responses. What was found was that in some patients there was apparently some reduction in emotions in some situations (Hohmann 1966), but this could be related to the fact that some of the patients were severely disabled (which could have produced its own consequences for emotionality), and that in many cases the patients were considerably older than before the spinal cord damage, and this could have been a factor. What was common to both studies was that emotions could be felt by all the patients; and that in some cases, emotions resulting from mental events were even reported as being stronger (Hohmann 1966, Bermond, Fasotti, Niewenhuyse & Schuerman 1991).

Fourth, when autonomic changes are elicited by injections of, for example, adrenaline or noradrenaline, particular emotions are not produced. Instead, the emotion that is produced depends on the cognitive decoding of the reinforcers present in the situation, for example an actor who insults your parents to make you angry, or an actor who plays a game of hula hoop to make you feel happy (Schachter & Singer 1962). In this situation, the hormone adrenaline or noradrenaline can alter the magnitude of the emotion, but not which emotion is felt. This is further evidence that it is the decoded reinforcement value of the input stimulus or events that determines which emotion is felt. The fact that the hormone injections produced some change in the magnitude of an emotion is not very surprising. If you felt your heart pounding for no explicable reason, you might wonder what was happening, and therefore react more or abnormally.

Fifth, if the peripheral changes associated with emotion are blocked with drugs, then this does not block the perception of emotion (Reisenzein 1983).

Sixth, it is found that in normal life, behavioural expressions of emotion (for example smiling when at a bowling alley) do not usually occur when one might be expected to feel happy because of a success, but instead occur when one is looking at one's friends (Kraut &

Johnson 1979). These body responses, which can be very brief, thus often serve the needs of communication, or of action, not of producing emotional feelings.

Despite this rather overwhelming evidence against an important role for body responses in producing emotions or emotional feelings, Damasio (1994) has effectively tried to resurrect a weakened version of the James–Lange theory of emotion from the 19th century, by arguing with his *somatic marker hypothesis* that after reinforcers have been evaluated, a bodily response ('somatic marker') normally occurs, then this leads to a bodily feeling, which in turn is appreciated by the organism to then make a contribution to the decision-making process[4]. The James–Lange theory has a number of major weaknesses just outlined that apply also to the somatic marker hypothesis.

The somatic marker hypothesis postulates that emotional decision-making is facilitated by peripheral feedback from for example the autonomic nervous system. In a direct test of this, Heims, Critchley, Dolan, Mathias & Cipolotti (2004) measured emotional decision-making using the Iowa Gambling Task (Bechara, Damasio, Damasio & Anderson 1994, Bechara, Tranel, Damasio & Damasio 1996, Bechara, Damasio, Tranel & Damasio 1997, Damasio 1994) (described in Section 4.5.6) in patients with pure autonomic failure. In this condition, there is degeneration of the peripheral autonomic system, and thus autonomic responses are severely impaired, and there can be no resulting feedback to the brain. It was found that performance in the Iowa Gambling Task was not impaired, and nor were many other tests of emotion and emotional performance, including face expression identification, theory of mind tasks of social situations, and social cognition tasks. Thus emotional decision-making does not depend on the ongoing feedback from somatic markers related to autonomic function. Damasio might argue that feedback from the autonomic system is not actually important, and that it is feedback from skeletomotor responses such as arm movements or muscle tension that is important. He might also argue that the autonomic feedback is not usually necessary for emotional decision-making, because it can be 'simulated' by the rest of the brain. However, the study by Heims et al. (2004) does show that ongoing autonomic feedback is not necessary for normal emotional decision-making, and this leaves the somatic marker hypothesis more precarious.

Part of the evidence for the somatic marker hypothesis was that normal participants in the Iowa Gambling Task were described as deciding advantageously before knowing the advantageous strategy (Bechara, Damasio, Tranel & Damasio 1997). The interpretation was that they had implicit (unconscious) knowledge implemented via a somatic marker process that was used in the task, which was not being solved by explicit (conscious) knowledge. Maia & McClelland (2004) (see also Maia & McClelland (2005)) however showed that with more sensitive questioning, normal participants at least had available to them explicit knowledge about the outcomes of the different decks that was as good as or better than the choices made, weakening the arguments of Bechara, Damasio, Tranel & Damasio (1997) and Bechara, Damasio, Tranel & Damasio (2005) that the task was being solved implicitly and using somatic markers. Further evidence on factors that contribute to the effects found in the Iowa Gambling Task are described in Section 4.5.6.

Another argument against the somatic marker hypothesis is that there can be dissociations

[4] In the James–Lange theory, it was emotional feelings that depend on peripheral feedback; for Damasio, it is the decision of which behavioural response to make that is normally influenced by the peripheral feedback. A quotation from Damasio (1994, p190) follows: "The squirrel did not really think about his various options and calculate the costs and benefits of each. He saw the cat, was jolted by the body state, and ran." Here it is clear that the pathway to action uses the body state as part of the route. Damasio would also like decisions to be implemented using the peripheral changes elicited by emotional stimuli. Given all the different reinforcers that may influence behaviour, Damasio (1994) even suggests that the net result of them all is reflected in the net peripheral outcome, and then the brain can sense this net peripheral result, and thus know what decision to take.

between autonomic and other indices of emotion, thus providing evidence that behaviour may not follow from autonomic and other effects. For example, lesions of different parts of the amygdala influence autonomic responses and instrumental behaviour differently, as shown in Section 4.6.3 and Fig. 4.56.

Another major weakness, which applies to both the James–Lange and to Damasio's somatic marker hypothesis, is that they do not take account of the fact that once an information processor has determined that a response should be made or inhibited based on reinforcement association, a function attributed in the theory proposed in this chapter and by Rolls (1986a, 1986b, 1990b, 1999a, 2005b) to the orbitofrontal cortex, it would be very inefficient and noisy to place in the execution route a peripheral response, and transducers to attempt to measure that peripheral response, itself a notoriously difficult procedure. Even for the cases when Damasio (1994) might argue that the peripheral somatic marker and its feedback can be by-passed using conditioning of a representation in, e.g., the somatosensory cortex to a command signal (which might originate in the orbitofrontal cortex), he apparently would still wish to argue that the activity in the somatosensory cortex is important for the emotion to be appreciated or to influence behaviour. (Without this, the somatic marker hypothesis would vanish.) The prediction would apparently be that if an emotional response were produced to a visual stimulus, then this would necessarily involve activity in the somatosensory cortex or other brain region in which the 'somatic marker' would be represented. This prediction could be tested (for example in patients with somatosensory cortex damage), but it seems most unlikely that an emotion produced by a visual reinforcer would require activity in the somatosensory cortex to feel emotional or to elicit emotional decisions. However, Adolphs, Tranel & Denburg (2000b) have pursued this general line of enquiry, and report that the more damage there is to somatosensory cortex, the greater the impairment in the emotional state reported by patients. However, the parts of the somatosensory system that appear to be damaged most frequently in the patients with emotional change are often in the anterior and ventral extensions of the somatosensory cortex in insular and nearby areas, and it would be useful to know whether this damage interrupted some of the connections or functions of the orbitofrontal cortex areas just anterior.

More recently, Damasio has stated the somatic marker hypothesis in a weak form, suggesting that somatic markers do not even reflect the valence of the reinforcer, but just provide a signal that depends on the intensity of the emotion, independently of the type of emotion. On this view, the role of somatic markers in decision-making would be very general, providing, as Damasio says, just a jolt to spur the system on (A.R. Damasio, paper delivered at the 6th Annual Wisconsin Symposium on Emotion, April 2000).

The alternative view proposed here (and elsewhere, Rolls (1986a, 1986b, 1990b, 1999a, 2000a, 2005b)) is that where the reinforcement value of the visual stimulus is decoded, namely in the orbitofrontal cortex and the amygdala, is the appropriate part of the brain for outputs to influence behaviour (via, e.g., the orbitofrontal to cingulate cortex and orbitofrontal-to-striatal connections), and that the orbitofrontal cortex and amygdala, and brain structures that receive connections from them, are the likely places where neuronal activity is directly related to emotional states and to felt emotions (see further Chapter 10 and Rolls (2005b)).

2.6.2 Appraisal theory

Appraisal theory, developed and described by Frijda (1986), Oatley & Johnson-Laird (1987), Lazarus (1991), Izard (1993), Stein, Trabasso & Liwag (1994), Oatley & Jenkins (1996), Scherer (1999), Keltner, Oatley & Jenkins (2013), Scherer (2009) and Moors, Ellsworth, Scherer & Frijda (2013) (see also Scherer (2001), Scherer, Schorr & Johnstone (2001)) generally holds that two types of appraisal are involved in emotion. Primary appraisal holds that "an emotion is usually caused by a person consciously or unconsciously evaluating an event as relevant to a concern (a goal) that is important; the emotion is felt as positive when a concern is advanced and negative when a concern is impeded" (from Oatley & Jenkins (1996), p. 96). As noted above, the concept of appraisal presumably involves assessment of whether something is a reward or punisher, that is whether it will be worked for or avoided. The description in terms of rewards and punishers adopted here simply seems much more precisely and operationally specified. If primary appraisal is defined with respect to goals, it might be helpful to note that goals may just be the reinforcers specified in Rolls' theory of emotion (Rolls 1999a, Rolls 2005b, Rolls 2014d), and if so the reinforcer/punisher approach provides clear definitions of goals (as reinforcers, see Appendix C), which is helpful, precise, and makes a link to what may be specified by genes.

Secondary appraisal is concerned with coping potential, that is with whether for example a plan can be constructed, and how successful it is likely to be.

Scherer (2009) summarizes his approach as follows. He suggests that there are four major appraisal objectives to adaptively react to a salient event:
(a) Relevance: How relevant is this event for me? Does it directly affect me or my social reference group?
(b) Implications: What are the implications or consequences of this event and how do they affect my well-being and my immediate or long-term goals?
(c) Coping Potential: How well can I cope with or adjust to these consequences?
(d) Normative Significance: What is the significance of this event for my self-concept and for social norms and values?
To attain these objectives, the organism evaluates the event and its consequences on a number of criteria or stimulus evaluation checks, with the results reflecting the organism's subjective assessment (which may well be unrealistic or biased) of consequences and implications on a background of personal needs, goals, and values. He states that an important feature of the model is that it does not include overt instrumental behaviour. Instead he sees emotion as a reaction to significant events that prepares action readiness and different types of alternative, possibly conflicting, action tendencies but not as a sufficient cause for their execution. This is a clear difference from my theory, in that my theory is that emotions are states that have a key role in brain design by providing a way for stimuli to produce states that are the goals for instrumental actions (Chapter 3). Of course stimuli that are instrumental reinforcers, goals for action, can also produce adaptive autonomic and skeletomotor reflexes (such as freezing), but these are responses, and can be classically conditioned, but do not require intervening goal-related representations or states, which are emotional and motivational states.

I note that appraisal theory is in many ways quite close to the theory that I outline here and elsewhere (Rolls 1999a, Rolls 2005b), and I do not see them as rivals. Instead, I hope that those who have an appraisal theory of emotion will consider whether much of what is encompassed by primary appraisal is not actually rather close to assessing whether stimuli or events are instrumental reinforcers; and whether much of what is encompassed by secondary appraisal is rather close to taking into account the actions that are possible in particular circumstances, as described above in Section 2.2.

An aspect of some flavours of appraisal theory with which I do not agree is that emotions have as one of their functions releasing particular actions, which seems to make a link with species-specific action tendencies or responses, or 'fixed action patterns' (Tomkins 1995, Panksepp 1998) or more 'open motor programs' (Ekman 2003). I argue in Chapter 3 that rarely are behavioural responses programmed by genes (see Table 2.1), but instead genes optimize their effects on behaviour if they specify the goals for (flexible) actions, that is if they specify rewards and punishers. The difference is quite considerable, in that specifying goals is much more economical in terms of the information that must be encoded in the genome; and in that specifying goals for actions allows much more flexibility in the actual actions that are produced. Of course I acknowledge that there is some preparedness to learn associations between particular types of secondary and primary reinforcers (Seligman 1970), and see this just as an economy of sensory–sensory convergence in the brain, whereby for example it does not convey much advantage to be able to learn that flashing lights (as contrasted with the taste of a food just eaten) are followed by sickness.

2.6.3 Dimensional and categorical theories of emotion

Dimensional and categorical theories of emotion suggest that there are a number of fundamental or basic emotions. Charles Darwin for example in his book *The Expression of the Emotions in Man and Animals* (1872) showed that some basic expressions of emotion are similar in animals and humans. Some of the examples he gave are shown in Table 2.1. His focus was on the continuity between animals and humans of how emotion is expressed.

In a development of this approach, Ekman and colleagues (Ekman 1982, Ekman 1992, Ekman 1993, Ekman, Friesen & Ellsworth 1972, Ekman, Levenson & Friesen 1983) have suggested that humans categorize face expressions into a number of basic categories that are similar across cultures. These face expression categories include happy, fear, anger, surprise, grief and sadness.

A related approach is to identify a few clusters of variables or factors that result from multidimensional analysis of questionnaires, and to identify these factors as basic emotions. (Multidimensional analyses such as factor analysis seek to identify a few underlying sources of variance to which a large number of data values such as answers to questions are related.) The categories of emotions identified in these ways may be supported by correlating them with autonomic measures (e.g. Ekman et al. (1983)).

One potential problem with some of these approaches is that they risk finding seven plus or minus two categories, which is the normal maximal number of categories with which humans normally operate, as described in a famous paper by George Miller (1956). A second problem is that there is no special reason why the first few factors (which account for most of the variance) in a factor analysis should provide a complete or principled classification of different emotions, or of their functions. In contrast, the theory described here does produce a principled classification of different emotions based on reinforcement contingencies, the nature of the primary and secondary reinforcers, etc., as set out in Sections 2.2 and 2.3. Moreover, the present theory links the functions of emotions to the classification produced, by showing how the functions of emotion can be understood in terms of the gene-specified reinforcers that produce different emotions (see Chapter 3).

An opposite approach to the dimensional or categorical approach is to attempt to describe the richness of every emotion (e.g. Ben-Ze'ev (2000)). Although it is important to understand the richness of every emotion, I believe that this is better performed with a set of underlying principles of the type set out above (in Section 2.2), rather than without any obvious principles to approach the subtlety of emotions.

2.6.4 Other approaches to emotion

LeDoux (1992, 1995, 1996, 2011) has described a theory of the neural basis of emotion that is probably conceptually similar to that of Rolls (1975, 1986a, 1986b, 1990b, 1995a, 1999a, 2000a, 2005b) (and this book), except that he focuses mostly on the role of the amygdala in emotion (and not on other brain regions such as the orbitofrontal cortex, which are poorly developed in the rat); except that he focuses mainly on fear (based on his studies of the role of the amygdala and related structures in fear conditioning in the rat); and except that he suggests from his neurophysiological findings that an important route for conditioned emotional stimuli to influence behaviour is via the subcortical inputs (especially auditory from the medial part of the medial geniculate nucleus of the thalamus) to the amygdala, whereas I suggest that cortical processing to the object representation level before the representation is then sent to areas such as the amygdala and orbitofrontal cortex is normally involved in emotion, as emotions normally occur to objects, faces, etc. and not to spots of light or pure tones, which is what are represented precortically (as described on pages 179–180). Further, LeDoux (2011) has emphasized especially reflexes and conditioned reflexes such as autonomic responses and freezing, which I argue have adaptive value or in LeDoux's words survival value, but do not involve intervening states such as representations of goals for actions (i.e. instrumental reinforcers), and which my theory suggests are emotional states.

Panksepp's approach to emotion has its origins in neuroethological investigations of brainstem systems that when activated lead to behaviours like fixed action patterns, including escape, flight and fear behaviour (Panksepp 1998, Panksepp 2011b, Panksepp 2011a). Using evidence from brain stimulation that elicits behaviours, he has postulated that there are a set of basic emotions, including for example Seeking, Rage, Fear, Lust, Care, Panic/Grief and Play. He argued that these are 'natural kinds', things that exist in nature as opposed to being inventions (constructions) of the human mind. My view is that there are not a few basic emotions, that emotions do not involve fixed action patterns as these do not require intervening emotional states to support goal-directed instrumental actions, and that emotions can be classified based on the specific reinforcer, the specific reinforcement contingency, the actions that are available, etc. as described earlier in this chapter in Rolls' theory of emotion. Panksepp's views about consciousness include the postulate that "feelings may emerge when endogenous sensory and emotional systems within the brain that receive direct inputs from the outside world as well as the neurodynamics of the SELF (a Simple Ego-type Life Form) begin to reverberate with each other's changing neuronal firing rhythms" (Panksepp 1998) (p. 309).

Other approaches to emotion are summarized by Strongman (2003) and Keltner et al. (2013).

2.7 Individual differences in emotion, personality, and emotional intelligence

Hans J. Eysenck developed the theory that personality might be related to different aspects of conditioning. He analysed the factors that accounted for the variance in the differences between the personality of different humans (using, for example, questionnaires), and suggested that the first two factors in personality (those which accounted for most of the variance) were introversion vs extraversion, and neuroticism (related to a tendency to be anxious). He performed studies of classical conditioning on groups of subjects, and also obtained measures of what he termed arousal. Based on the correlations of these measures with the dimensions identified in the factor analysis, he suggested that introverts showed greater conditionability (to weak stimuli) and are more readily aroused by external stimulation than extraverts; and that neuroticism raises the general intensity of emotional reactions (see Eysenck & Eysenck (1968) and Eysenck & Eysenck (1985)).

Jeffrey A. Gray (1970) reinterpreted the findings, suggesting that introverts are more sensitive to punishment and frustrative non-reward than are extraverts; and that neuroticism reflects the extent of sensitivity to both reward and punishment (see Matthews & Gilliland (1999)). A related hypothesis is that extraverts may show enhanced learning in reward conditions, and may show enhanced processing of positively valent stimuli (Rusting & Larsen 1998).

Matthews & Gilliland (1999), reviewing the evidence, show that there is some support for both hypotheses about introversion vs extraversion, namely that introverts may in general condition readily, and that extraverts may be relatively more responsive to reward stimuli (and correspondingly, introverts to punishers). However, Matthews & Gilliland (1999) go on to show that extraverts may perform less well at vigilance tasks (in which the subject must detect stimuli that occur with low probability); may tend to be more impulsive; and perform better when arousal is high (e.g. later in the day), and when rapid responses rather than reflective thought is needed (see also Matthews, Zeidner & Roberts (2002)). With respect to neuroticism and trait anxiety, anxious individuals tend to focus attention on potentially threatening information (punishers) at the cost of neglecting neutral or positive information sources; and may make more negative judgements, especially in evaluating self-worth and personal competence (Matthews, Zeidner & Roberts 2002).

More recent evidence comes from functional neuroimaging studies. For example, Canli, Sivers, Whitfield, Gotlib & Gabrieli (2002) have found that happy face expressions are more likely to activate the human amygdala in extraverts than in introverts. In addition, positively affective pictures interact with extraversion, and negatively affective pictures with neuroticism to produce activation of the amygdala (Canli, Zhao, Desmond, Kang, Gross & Gabrieli 2001, Hamann & Canli 2004). This supports the conceptually important point made above that part of the basis of personality may be differential sensitivity to different rewards and punishers, and omission and termination of different rewards and punishers.

The observations just described are consistent with the hypothesis that part of the basis of extraversion is increased reactivity to positively affective (as compared to negatively affective) face expressions and other positively affective stimuli including pictures. The exact mechanisms involved may be revealed in the future by genetic studies, and these might potentially address for example whether genes control responses to positively affective stimuli, or whether some more general personality trait by altering perhaps mood produces differential top-down biasing of face expression decoding systems in the way outlined in Section 4.12.

In one update of this approach, links have been made to behavioural economics by relating loss aversion to greater negative valuation sensitivity compared to positive valuation sensitivity; by suggesting that tendencies to approach or avoid have distinct sensitivities to those of the valuation systems; that approach-avoidance conflict is distinct process from the basic approach and avoidance systems; and linking these to a reinforcer sensitivity theory of personality (Corr & McNaughton 2012).

Another example is the impulsive behaviour that is a part of Borderline Personality Disorder (BPD), which could reflect factors such as less sensitivity to the punishers associated with waiting for rational processing to lead to a satisfactory solution, or changes in internal timing processes that lead to a faster perception of time (Berlin, Rolls & Kischka 2004, Berlin & Rolls 2004) (see Section 4.5.6). It was of considerable interest that the BPD group (mainly self-harming patients), as well as a group of patients with damage to the orbitofrontal cortex, scored highly on a Frontal Behaviour Questionnaire that assessed inappropriate behaviours typical of orbitofrontal cortex patients including disinhibition, social inappropriateness, perseveration, and uncooperativeness. In terms of measures of personality, using the Big Five personality measure, both groups were also less open to experience (i.e. less open-minded). In terms of other personality measures and characteristics, the orbitofrontal and BPD patients performed differently: BPD patients were less extraverted and conscientious and more neurotic and emotional than the orbitofrontal group (Berlin, Rolls & Kischka 2004, Berlin & Rolls 2004, Berlin, Rolls & Iversen 2005). Thus some aspects of personality, such as impulsiveness and being less open to experience, but not other aspects, such as extraversion, neuroticism and conscientiousness, were differentially related to orbitofrontal cortex function.

Daniel Goleman (1995) has popularized the concept of *emotional intelligence*. The rather sweeping definition given was "Emotional intelligence [includes] abilities such as being able to motivate oneself and persist in the face of frustrations, to control impulse and delay gratification; to regulate one's moods and keep distress from swamping the ability to think; to empathize and to hope" (Goleman (1995), p. 34).

One potential problem with this definition of emotional intelligence as an ability is that different aspects within this definition (such as impulse control and hope) may be unrelated, so a unitary ability described in this way seems unlikely. An excellent critical evaluation of the concept has been produced by Matthews, Zeidner & Roberts (2002). They note (p. 368) that in a rough and ready way, one might identify personality traits of emotional stability (low neuroticism), extraversion, agreeableness, and conscientiousness/self-control as dispositions that tend to facilitate everyday social interaction and to promote more positive emotion. (Indeed, one measure of emotional intelligence, the EQ-i (Bar-On 1997), has high correlations with some of the Big Five personality traits, especially, negatively, with neuroticism, and the EQ-i may reflect three constructs, self-esteem, empathy, and impulse control (Matthews et al. 2002).) But these personality traits are supposed to be independent, so linking them to a single ability of emotional intelligence is inconsistent. Moreover, this combination of personality traits might well not be adaptive in many circumstances, so the concept of this combination as an 'ability' is inappropriate (pp. 368–370).

However, the concept of emotional intelligence (Mayer, Roberts & Barsade 2008) does appear to be related in a general way to the usage of the (mainly clinical) term 'alexithymia', in a sense the opposite, which includes the following components: (a) difficulty in identifying and describing emotions and distinguishing between feelings and the bodily sensations of arousal, (b) difficulty in describing feelings to other people, (c) constricted imaginal processes, as evidenced by a paucity of fantasies, and (d) a stimulus-bound externally oriented cognitive style, as evidenced by preoccupation with the details of external events rather than inner emotional experiences (Matthews et al. 2002). In terms of personality, alexithymia converges with the first three dimensions of the Five Factor Model of personality (FFM, the Big Five model), with high N (vulnerability to emotional distress), low E (low positive emotionality), and a limited range of imagination (low O) (Matthews et al. 2002). Indeed, alexithymia is strongly inversely correlated with measures of emotional intelligence, suggesting that emotional intelligence may be a new term that encompasses much of the opposite of what has been the important concept of alexithymia in the clinical literature for more than 20 years (Matthews et al. 2002). Alexithymics have difficulties in identifying face expressions (Lane, Sechrest, Reidel, Weldon, Kaszniak & Schwartz 1996), suggesting some impairments in the fundamental processing of emotion-related information, in particular capacities known to require the orbitofrontal and anterior cingulate cortices (Hornak, Bramham, Rolls, Morris, O'Doherty, Bullock & Polkey 2003). Consistently, it has been found that anterior cingulate cortex activation is correlated across individuals with their ability to recognize and describe emotions induced either by films or by the recall of personal experiences (Lane, Reiman, Axelrod, Yun, Holmes & Schwartz 1998). More generally, alexithymia is associated with reduced activation to emotion-provoking stimuli in the amygdala, anterior/posterior cingulate cortex, and insula, and with increased neural activity in somatosensory and sensorimotor regions (Moriguchi & Komaki 2013). In summary, emotional intelligence, and what is largely its opposite, alexithymia, is probably not a particular ability, is not independent of existing personality measures, but does encompass a number of probably different ways in which individuals may differ in their emotion-related processing (Rolls 2007d).

I do not consider this research area in much more detail. However, I do point out that insofar as sensitivity to rewards and punishers, and the ability to learn and be influenced by rewards and punishers, may be important in personality, and are closely involved in emotion according to the theory developed here, there may be close links between the neural bases of emotion, to be described in Chapter 4, and personality. An extreme example might be that if humans were insensitive to social punishers following orbitofrontal cortex damage, we might expect social problems and impulsive behaviour, and indeed Tranel, Bechara & Denburg (2002) have used the term 'acquired sociopathy' to describe some of these patients.

More generally, we might expect sensitivity to different types of reinforcer (including social reinforcers) to vary between individuals both as a result of gene variation and as a result of learning, and this, operating over a large number of different social reinforcers, might produce many different variations of personality based on the sensitivity to a large number of different reinforcers. Further, insofar as the functions of particular brain regions may be related to particular processes involved in emotion [with evidence for example that the human orbitofrontal cortex is involved in face expression decoding, and in impulsiveness, but not in some other aspects of personality (see Section 4.5.6)], then it may be possible in future to understand different particular modules for inter-relations between reward/punishment and personality systems.

The concept of the relation between differential sensitivity to different types of reward and punisher might produce individuals showing many types of conditional evolutionarily stable strategies (see footnote 13 on page 323), where the conditionality of the strategy might be influenced in different individuals by differential sensitivity to different rewards and punishers. Examples of behaviours that might be produced in this way are included in Chapter 7.

2.8 Cognition and emotion

It may be noted that while the definition of emotions as states elicited by instrumental reinforcers (with particular functions) is operational, it should not be criticized (Katz 2000) as behaviourist. For example, the definition has nothing to do with stimulus–response (habit) associations, but instead with a two-stage type of learning, in which a first stage is learning which environmental stimuli or events are associated with instrumental reinforcers (goals) to represent value, which potentially is a very rapid and flexible process; and a second stage produces appropriate instrumental and arbitrary actions performed in order to achieve the goal (which might be to obtain a reward or avoid a punisher). In the instrumental stage, animals learn about the outcomes of their actions (Section 4.6.1.2 (Dickinson 1994, Pearce 2008, Cardinal, Parkinson, Hall & Everitt 2002, Mazur 2012)).

To determine what is a goal for an action, every type of cognitive operation may be involved. The proposal is that whatever cognitive operations are involved, then if the outcome is that a certain event, stimulus, thought (or any one of these remembered) leads to the evaluation that the event is a reward or punisher, then an emotion will be produced. So cognition is very much included.

Indeed, cognitive operations may produce emotions when operating at three levels of the architecture, as described more fully in Chapter 3. The first is the implicit level (see Fig. 10.4), where a primary reinforcer, or a stimulus or event associated with a primary reinforcer, may lead to emotions. The second level is where a (first-order) syntactic symbol processing system performing "what ... if" computations to implement planning results in identification of a rewarding or punishing outcome. The third level is the higher-order linguistic thought level described in Chapter 10, where thinking about and evaluating the operations of a first-order linguistic processor may result in a reinforcing outcome such as "I should not spend further time thinking about that set of plans, as it would be better now to devote my linguistic resources (which are limited and serial) to this other set of plans".

Another way in which cognition influences emotion is that cognitive states, even at the level of language, can modulate subjective and brain responses to the reward value of affective stimuli, as analysed in Section 4.5.5.7. There an experiment is described in which a word label ('cheese' vs 'body odour') influences the subjective pleasantness ratings, and the activations in olfactory stages at least as early as the secondary olfactory cortex in the orbitofrontal cortex, to a standard test odour (De Araujo, Rolls, Velazco, Margot & Cayeux 2005). An implication of these findings is that language-based cognitive states can influence even relatively early cortical representations of rewards and punishers, and thus potentially modulate how much emotion is felt subjectively to an emotion-provoking stimulus.

I suggest that this top-down modulation of affective representations by cognition occurs in a way that is analogous to top-down attentional effects, which are believed to be implemented by a top-down biased competition mechanism (Rolls & Deco 2002, Deco & Rolls 2003, Deco & Rolls 2005c, Rolls & Stringer 2001b, Rolls 2008b, Rolls 2013a). In this case, the semantic, language-based, representation is the source of the biased competition, and the effect could be not only to bias the early cortical representation of a reward or punisher in one direction or another, but also by providing much or little top-down modulation, to influence how much emotion is felt (see Chapter 10), by modulating the processing of emotion-related stimuli (including remembered stimuli or events) at relatively early processing stages. This could be a mechanism by which cognition can influence how much emotion is felt under conditions in which emotions such as empathy and pity may occur, and when for example reading a novel, attending a play, listening to music, etc. (see Section 11.4). Analysis of the mechanisms by which the top-down biased competition operates are becoming detailed (Desimone & Duncan 1995, Rolls & Deco 2002, Deco & Rolls 2003, Deco & Rolls 2004, Deco & Rolls 2005c, Rolls 2008b, Rolls 2013a), and are included in a model in which a rule module exerts a top-down influence on neurons that represent stimulus–reward and stimulus–punisher combinations to influence which stimulus should currently be interpreted as reward-related (Deco & Rolls 2005a).

Another way in which cognitive factors are related to emotion is that mood can affect cognitive processing, and one of the effects of this is to promote continuity of behaviour (see Chapter 3). One of the mechanisms described (in Section 4.12) utilizes backprojections to cortical areas from the amygdala and orbitofrontal cortex, so that reciprocal interactions between cognition and emotion are made possible.

2.9 Emotion, motivation, reward, and mood

It is useful to be clear about the difference between motivation, emotion, reward, and mood (Rolls 2000a, Rolls 2005b). **Motivation** makes one work to obtain a reward, or work to escape from or avoid a punisher. One example of motivation is hunger, and another thirst, which in these cases are states set largely by internal homeostatically-related variables such as plasma glucose concentration and plasma osmolality (Chapter 5, Rolls (2005b)). A reward is a stimulus or event that one works to obtain, such as food, and a punisher is what one works to escape from or avoid (or which suppresses an action on which its delivery is contingent), such as a painful stimulus or the sight of an object associated with a painful stimulus. Obtaining the reward or avoiding the punisher is the goal for the (instrumental) action. A motivational state is one in which a goal is *desired*. An **emotion** is a state elicited when a goal is obtained, that is by an instrumental reinforcer (i.e. a reward or punisher, or omission or termination of a reward or punisher), for example fear produced by the sight of the object associated with pain. This makes it clear that emotions are states elicited by rewards or punishers that have particular functions.

Of course, one of the functions of emotions is that they are motivating, as exemplified by the case of the fear produced by the sight of the object that can produce pain, which motivates one to avoid receiving the painful stimulus, which is the goal for the action. In that emotion-provoking stimuli or events produce motivation, then arousal is likely to occur, especially for reinforcers that lead to the active initiation of actions. However, arousal alone is not sufficient to define motivation or emotion, in that the motivational state must specify the particular type of goal that is the object of the motivational state, such as water if we are thirsty, food if we are hungry, and avoidance of the painful unconditioned stimulus signalled by a fear-inducing conditioned stimulus.

A **mood** is a continuing state normally elicited by a reinforcer, and is thus part of what is an emotion. The other part of an emotion is the decoding of the stimulus in terms of whether it is a reward or punisher, that is, of what causes the emotion, or in philosophical terminology of what the emotion is about or the object of the emotion. Mood states help to implement some of the persistence-related functions of emotion, can continue when the originating stimulus may be forgotten (by the explicit system described in Chapter 10), and may occur spontaneously not because such spontaneous mood swings may have been selected for, but because of the difficulty of maintaining stability of the neuronal firing that implements mood (or affective) state (see *The Brain and Emotion*, Rolls (1999a), pp. 62, 66; and Rolls (2008b)). Mood states are thus not necessarily about an object.

Thus, motivation may be seen as a state in which one is working for a goal, and emotion as a state that occurs when the goal, a reinforcer, is obtained, and that may persist afterwards. The concept of gene-defined reinforcers providing the goals for action helps to understand the relation between motivational states (or desires) and emotion, as the organism must be built to be motivated to obtain the goals, and to be placed in a different state (emotion) when the goal is or is not achieved by the action. Emotional states may be motivating, as in frustrative non-reward. The close but clear relation between motivation and emotion is that both involve what humans describe as affective states (e.g. feeling hungry, liking the taste of a food, feeling happy because of a social reinforcer), and both are about goals. The Darwinian theory of the functions of emotion developed in Chapter 3 which shows how emotion is adaptive because it reflects the operation of a process by which genes define goals for action applies just as much to motivation (see further Section 3.6), in that emotion can be thought of as states elicited by goals (rewards and punishers), and motivation can be thought of as states elicited when goals are being sought. *By specifying goals the genes must specify both that we must be motivated to obtain those goals, and that when the goals are obtained, further states, emotional states with further functions, are produced.* In this sense, my Darwinian approach to the functions of gene-specified instrumental reinforcers provides a fundamental and unifying approach to emotion and motivation.

2.10 Is the concept of emotion still useful when we understand its mechanisms?

Kralik & Hauser (2000) ask whether it is helpful to maintain the concept of an emotional state when one starts to understand the mechanisms of reward and punisher decoding, the selection of actions, etc. My view is that emotion is a helpful concept, for a number of reasons.

First, the state is produced by clearly defined stimuli (see above).

Second, the state has many different functions, summarized in Chapter 3, so that a model in which a stimulus is connected to a single output is inappropriate. In these circumstances, an intervening state that implements many functions is useful.

Third, one of the functions of emotion is to support the selection of any appropriate action to a reward or punisher, or its omission or termination, as in two-process learning. In the first stage, an emotional state is produced, and in the second stage, any action is selected that is appropriate given the emotional state. For example, if fear is the emotional state produced by a pain-associated stimulus, an action will be selected to escape from or avoid the emotion-provoking stimulus. In that emotion is a state that guides the elicitation of an action to a stimulus, the emotional state is not itself a behavioural response.

Fourth, other functions of emotional states include the biasing of cognitive function to influence the interpretation of future events, which is clearly not a response.

Fifth, emotional states have the important properties that they persist for times in the order of minutes or hours, thus maintaining persistence of behaviour and consistency of action even after the emotion-provoking stimulus has disappeared.

Sixth, the concept of emotional states just described maps neatly onto folk-psychological concepts of emotions, and provides a convenient conceptual level that bridges to the low-level description of exactly how the stimuli are decoded to elicit the state, how the state is maintained, and how it performs its many functions. This point is related to the account I provide for the relation between the mind and the brain in terms of levels of explanation, as described in Section 10.7.

The concept of an emotional state is thus clearly defined in terms of how stimuli elicit the state, and of the many functions of the state including the selection of action. Emotional states are not the stimuli themselves, nor the stimulus decoding, nor the responses finally selected, but consist of on-going states elicited by stimuli in the way described, and performing the functions described. We are indeed starting to understand how the different types of processing involved are implemented in the brain, and these are some of the types of advance described here and elsewhere (Rolls 1999a, Rolls 2005b). But understanding the implementation of the processes involved in emotion does not mean that emotion itself as a useful concept at its own level will disappear.

In addition, understanding 'how' emotion works (a proximate question) will not address a number of important questions about emotion, including the 'why' ('ultimate') questions about for example the evolutionary adaptive value of emotions (see Section 3.1).

2.11 Advantages of the approach to emotion described here (Rolls' theory of emotion)

I now evaluate the advantages of and justifications for starting with the concept that emotions are states elicited by instrumental reinforcers, even though one proposes that a full definition requires the principles summarized in Section 2.2, and incorporating a statement of the functions elicited by those states (Chapter 3).

One advantage is that this definition in terms of rewards and punishers may provide a concise operational definition of the environmental stimuli or events that actually lead to emotions. If we can agree that the environmental conditions that lead to emotions are those that can be described as rewarding or punishing, and that those that are not rewards or punishers do not lead to states that are described as emotional, then we are a long way forward in producing a conceptualization of what emotions may be. No commentators on the *Précis of The Brain and Emotion* (Rolls 2000a) actually produced clear exceptions to this correspondence. If we accept this operational definition, it provides us with a powerful way forward to start to examine emotions (because we accept that they are states elicited by rewards or punishers, and have a useful delimitation of what events produce emotion). This leads directly to an analysis of the brain mechanisms that implement emotions as those brain mechanisms that decode environmental stimuli as primary reinforcers, those brain mechanisms that implement stimulus–reinforcer association learning, and the brain mechanisms that link the resulting emotional states to actions.

A second advantage of this definition is that it enables us to see emotions in the context of what I propose is their most important function, namely as a way to provide a mechanism for the genes to influence behaviour in a brain that evolves by gene selection. It is argued in Chapter 3 that the genes do this by specifying the stimuli or events that the animal is built to find rewarding or punishing, i.e. to find reinforcing, so that the genes specify the goals for action, not the actions themselves. The definition of emotions as states elicited by reinforcers thus links directly to the Darwinian theory I propose for why we have emotions, which is that some genes specify reinforcers, that is goals for action, that will increase the fitness of these genes. It is these particular genes that specify reinforcers that provide the foundation I propose for emotional states. The definition of emotion in terms of states elicited by reinforcers should not be seen thus as behaviourist, but instead as part of a much broader theory that takes an adaptive, Darwinian, approach to the functions of emotion, and how they are important in brain design (see Section 3.5).

A third advantage is that the definition offers a principled way to approach emotion. Different emotions can be classified and understood in terms of different reinforcement contingencies and different reinforcers, and hence directly in terms of their functions. This is recommended as being more advantageous than categorizing emotions based on clusters of variables or factors that result from multidimensional analysis of questionnaires etc., or by correlation with autonomic or face expression measures, which do not lead directly to an understanding of the different functions of different emotions (and run the risk of producing seven plus or minus two categories, cf. Miller (1956)), as described in Section 2.6.3. This definition of emotion also leads to an operational, and thus clearly specified, approach to emotions, whereas approaches such as appraisal theory may suffer from the disadvantage that they quickly become somewhat under-specified and intractable, as described in section 2.6.2. Moreover, this principled way of understanding emotions provides a systematic and fundamental way to approach the brain mechanisms involved in emotion, in that brain regions involved in decoding primary reinforcers, and brain regions involved in learning associations of events to primary reinforcers, can be seen to have a clear information-processing role in emotion. Analysing the information processing performed by each connected stage in the brain provides a fruitful approach to understanding neural computation (Rolls & Treves 1998, Rolls & Deco 2002, Rolls 2008b).

In the context of emotion, this approach is also more principled and systematic than identifying categories of (sometimes ethologically described) behaviour such as playfulness and aggression, and looking for brain centres specialized for each category of behaviour (Panksepp 1998, Panksepp 2011b). The specification of actions such as fixed action patterns (in contrast to goals) by genes is not only genetically expensive, but having brain regions specialized for actions (such as playfulness and rage (Panksepp 1998, Panksepp 2011b)) would lead to a multitude of specialized brain action/emotion systems, with potentially one for every possible type of emotional response. In contrast, specifying emotions as states elicited by reinforcers leaves open and flexible the particular action that may be taken in particular circumstances, and has the great advantage of economy of genetic specification (the genes need only specify what is rewarding and punishing). (Of course, as described above, the type of coping by actions that is possible may influence the emotional state, as in the case of sadness vs anger.)

Specifying emotions in terms of the types of rewards and punishers that elicit the emotion may of course also lead to spatially separated brain systems especially involved in different types of emotion, for the primary reinforcers (such as taste, touch, pain, the failure to receive an expected reward, or a face expression, and learning about these reinforcers) may be decoded and represented in different brain regions. This is because of their different input pathways to the brain, and the utility of forming representations to the object level within each sensory modality before reward value is made explicit in the representation, leading to some specialization of different brain regions and systems in different types of emotion (see Chapter 4).

A fourth advantage of conceptualizing emotions as states elicited by instrumental reinforcers is that this provides an immediate way into understanding the relation between emotion and personality (see Section 2.7).

A complex issue related to one's definition of emotion is where the boundaries for emotional states should be set. Should our definition result in emotions being states that occur in invertebrates such as Aplysia, as suggested by Kupferman (2000)? My own answer to this is to set off from emotions those behaviours that are performed with fixed responses, that is without the possibility for selecting arbitrary types of behaviour as the goals for actions (see Chapter 3). Such fixed-response behaviours include taxes, such as might be performed by a single cell organism swimming up a chemical gradient towards a source of nutrient. Other examples include fixed action patterns, and autonomic and even skeletomotor responses such as freezing, even when conditioned. One reason why these types of behaviour with fixed responses are excluded from emotion (though they may be forerunners to it) is that the behaviour does not occur by elicitation of a persistent or continuing state to a reinforcing stimulus that provides the motivation for (arbitrary) instrumental responses to obtain the goal. (That an instrumental (or operant) response is being made is demonstrated most precisely by the bidirectional criterion that either a response, or its opposite, may be performed as an action to obtain a goal.) It is the intervening persistent state elicited by reinforcing stimuli and the ability to allow stimuli to be interfaced to arbitrary instrumental actions that is one of the prime functions of emotion described here (see Chapter 3), and is therefore incorporated into the definition of emotion. The definition thus provides a clear way of dividing states into emotional or not, as it includes only those states that allow instrumental learning, that is arbitrary actions to be performed to obtain reinforcing outcomes (such as obtaining rewards and avoiding punishers). Although animals that do not perform instrumental learning may not qualify according to this criterion as having emotions, they may of course have states that are precursors to emotions. This discussion thus leads to one possible way to separate animals that have emotions from those that do not, a way that is related to one of the fundamental functions of emotion, but it is realized that the separation made at this point should be seen as a useful separating point with a clear principle underlying it, but not a separating point that need be thought of as more than a useful convention in this context.

3 The functions of emotion: reward, punishment, and emotion in brain design

3.1 Introduction

We now confront the fundamental issue of why we, and other animals, are built to have emotions, as well as motivational states. Biologists would describe this as an 'ultimate' explanation for emotion and motivation. I will propose that we are built to have emotions, and motivational states, because we (and many other animals) use rewards and punishers to guide or determine our behaviour, and that this is a good design for a system that is built by genes where some of the genes are increasing their survival (reproductive success) by specifying the goals for behaviour. The emotions arise and are an inherent part of such a system because they are the states, typically persisting, that are elicited by rewards and punishers and stimuli associated with them, and that are the goals for instrumental actions. I will show that this is a very adaptive way for evolution to design complex animals without having to specify the details of the behavioural responses, the actions, as it is much more flexible in an uncertain environment for responses and actions to be learned.

What results from this analysis is thus a thoroughly Darwinian theory (though not anticipated by Darwin, and operating at the level of individual genes) that places emotion at the heart of brain design because it reflects the way in which genes build our brains in such a way that our genes can specify the goals of our actions, and thus what we do. There is thus a close conceptual link between instrumental learning and emotion, for primary reinforcers (primary rewards and punishers) are the gene-specified goals for our actions, and we use instrumental learning to learn any actions during our life-times that will lead to the gene-specified goals.

In Section 3.2, I outline several types of brain design, with differing degrees of complexity, and suggest that evolution can operate much better with only some of these types of design.

Understanding the functions of emotion is important not only for understanding the nature of emotions, but also for understanding the different brain systems involved in the different types of response that are produced by emotional states. Indeed, answers to 'why' questions in nature (for example, 'Why do we have emotions? What are the functions of emotion?') are important and are 'ultimate' answers. So also are answers to 'how' questions (for example, 'How is emotion implemented in the brain? How do disorders of emotion arise, and how can they be understood and treated?'), which are 'proximate' or mechanistic answers. In fact, answers to proximate questions often suggest answers to ultimate questions, and this was the case in my exploration of the mechanisms for emotion and its functions.

In this book, the question of why we have emotions is a fundamental issue that I answer in terms of a Darwinian, functional, approach, producing the answer that emotions are states elicited by goals (rewards and punishers), and that this is part of an adaptive process by which genes can specify the behaviour of the animal by specifying goals for behaviour rather than fixed responses. I believe that this is approach leads to a fundamental understanding of why we have emotions which is likely to stand the test of time, in the same way that

Darwinian thinking itself provides a fundamental way of understanding biology and many 'why' questions about life (Rolls 2012d).

While considering 'why' (or 'ultimate') questions (which are important in their own right), it may be helpful to place into perspective the approaches taken to understanding the adaptive value of behaviour (Tinbergen 1963) that have led to sociobiology (Wilson 1975) and evolutionary psychology (see Buss (2012)). These approaches are relevant to understanding why we have emotions, including many of the issues discussed in Chapter 7 on sexual behaviour. 'Adaptation' refers to characteristics of living organisms – such as their colour, shape, physiology, and behaviour – that enable them to survive and reproduce successfully in the environments in which they live (Dawkins 1995).

Sociobiology and evolutionary psychology have sometimes been criticized as producing 'just-so' stories in which the purported adaptive explanation for a behaviour seems too facile and untestable (Gould & Lewontin 1979), but we should note that there are rigorous approaches to testing evolutionary hypotheses for the adaptive value of a behaviour or other characteristic (see M. S. Dawkins (1995), Chapter 1) and Buss (2012). The tests include the following:

1. *Making use of existing genetic variation.* A famous example is that of the peppered moth, *Biston betularia*. In its dark form it is found to survive better than the light form when both are released into industrial areas in which the genetically specified black form is better camouflaged (Kettlewell 1955).
2. *Using artificially produced variation.* The variation could be genetically produced, or variation produced in the testing conditions in an experiment. Using the latter approach, Tinbergen, Broekhuysen, Feekes, Houghton, Kruuk & Szule (1967) showed that black-headed gulls' newly born chicks survive better if the parents remove broken egg shells to a good distance from the nest. This supports the hypothesis that the behaviour is adaptive because removing the shells, which are white inside, makes the nest less conspicuous to predators.
3. *The comparative method.* Comparing species in which a trait has evolved genetically and independently can provide good evidence at the correlative level. For example, kittiwakes do not remove hatched egg shells from their nest, and in contrast with black-headed gulls, this is related to the fact that kittiwakes nest in places on cliffs that are inaccessible even to other birds (Cullen 1957).
4. *Adaptation through design features.* If it can be shown that design features such as the bat sonar echolocation system are very well suited to detecting small animals of prey such as moths, then that provides some evidence that the features are genetically selected because of their adaptive value. Even more telling are examples where the behaviour is not as adaptive as it might be – for example, in some schooling fish, the spacing during swimming is not hydrodynamically optimal, and this implies that the details of the behaviour are under selective pressure other than only swimming efficiency (Dawkins 1995).

Thus adaptive accounts of behaviour can be tested, and need not be 'just-so' stories.

We should also note that by no means all behaviour reflects optimal adaptation (see Dawkins (1982) Chapter 3, 'Constraints on Perfection'), for six reasons:
1. There is a *time lag*, and present animals may have evolved under somewhat different selection pressures.
2. *Historical constraints*, which can be important in that natural selection always operates in an 'adaptive landscape' with local optima, not global optima (i.e. natural selection can improve an existing animal, but cannot start from nothing and build towards a particular overall design).

3. *Available genetic variation*, an example of which is that it has not proved possible to breed cattle with more female (cows) than male (bulls) offspring.
4. *Constraints of costs and materials.*
5. Imperfections at one level due to *selection at another level*. An important point here is that evolution through natural selection can be best understood not at the level of what is adaptive for the group or species, but at the level of what increases the fitness of the genes.
6. Mistakes due to *environmental unpredictability* or 'malevolence'. Genes must specify behaviour that is on average good for them, and there are limited numbers of genes that influence behaviour. These constraints mean that genes cannot take into account all possible combinations of environmental contingencies that may arise.

3.2 Brain design and the functions of emotion

3.2.1 Taxes, rewards, and punishers: gene-specified goals for actions, and the flexibility of actions

3.2.1.1 Taxes

A simple design principle is to incorporate mechanisms for taxes into the design of organisms. Taxes consist at their simplest of orientation towards stimuli in the environment, for example the bending of a plant towards light that results in maximum light collection by its photosynthetic surfaces. (When just turning rather than locomotion is possible, such responses are called tropisms.) With locomotion possible, as in animals, taxes include movements towards sources of nutrient, and movements away from hazards such as very high temperatures. The design principle here is that animals have, through a process of natural selection, built receptors for certain dimensions of the wide range of stimuli in the environment, and have linked these receptors to response mechanisms in such a way that the stimuli are approached or escaped from.

3.2.1.2 Rewards and punishers

As soon as we have approach to stimuli at one end of a dimension (e.g. a source of nutrient) and away from stimuli at the other end of the dimension (in this case lack of nutrient), we can start to wonder when it is appropriate to introduce the terms 'rewards' and 'punishers' for the stimuli at the different ends of the dimension. By convention, if the response consists of a fixed response to obtain the stimulus (e.g. locomotion up a chemical gradient), we shall call this a taxis not a reward. If a fixed behavioural response or action pattern such as skeletomotor freezing and autonomic responses are elicited by a stimulus, they may be adaptive, but are essentially stimulus-response reflexes, with no need for an intervening state such as a goal to be reached. On the other hand, if an arbitrary operant response can be performed by the animal in order to approach the stimulus, then we will call this rewarded behaviour, and the stimulus that the animal works to obtain a reward, the goal for the action. (The arbitrary operant response can be thought of as any arbitrary response the animal will perform to obtain the stimulus. It can be thought of as an action.) This criterion, of an arbitrary operant response, is often tested by bidirectionality. For example, if a rat can be trained to either raise its tail, or lower its tail, in order to obtain a piece of food, then we can be sure that there is no fixed relationship between the stimulus (e.g. the sight of food) and the response, as there is in a taxis. Some authors reserve the term 'motivated behaviour' for that in which an arbitrary operant response will be performed to obtain a reward or to escape from or avoid a punisher. If this criterion is not met, and only a fixed response can be performed, then the term 'drive' can be used to describe the state of the animal when it will work to obtain or escape from the stimulus.

We can thus distinguish a first level of approach/avoidance mechanism complexity in a taxis, with a fixed response available for the stimulus, from a second level of complexity in which any arbitrary response (or action) can be performed, in which case we use the term reward when a stimulus is being approached, and punisher when the action is to escape from or avoid the stimulus.

The role of natural selection in this process is to guide animals to build sensory systems that will respond to dimensions of stimuli in the natural environment along which actions of the animals can lead to better survival to enable genes to be passed on to the next generation, which is what we mean by fitness[5]. The animals must be built by such natural selection to perform actions that will enable them to obtain more rewards, that is to work to obtain stimuli that will increase their fitness. Correspondingly, animals must be built to perform actions that will enable them to escape from, or avoid when learning mechanisms are introduced, stimuli that will reduce their fitness. There are likely to be many dimensions of environmental stimuli along which actions of the animal can alter fitness. Each of these dimensions may be a separate reward–punisher dimension. An example of one of these dimensions might be food reward. It increases fitness to be able to sense nutrient need, to have sensors that respond to the taste of food, and to perform behavioural responses to obtain such reward stimuli when in that need or motivational state. Similarly, another dimension is water reward, in which the taste of water becomes rewarding when there is body-fluid depletion (Rolls & Rolls 1982a, Rolls 1999a, Rolls 2005b).

One aspect of the operation of these reward–punisher systems that these examples illustrate is that with very many reward–punisher dimensions for which actions may be performed, there is a need for a selection mechanism for actions performed to these different dimensions. In this sense, rewards and punishers provide a common currency that provides one set of inputs to action selection mechanisms. Evolution must set the magnitudes of each of the different reward systems so that each will be chosen for action in such a way as to maximize overall fitness. Food reward must be chosen as the aim for action if some nutrient depletion is present, but water reward as a target for action must be selected if current water depletion poses a greater threat to fitness than does the current degree of food depletion. This indicates that for a competitive selection process for rewards, each reward must be carefully calibrated in evolution to have the right value on a common scale for the selection process (but not converted into a common currency, see Section 9.5.2). Other types of behaviour, such as sexual behaviour, must be performed sometimes, but probably less frequently, in order to maximize fitness (as measured by gene transmission into the next generation).

There are many processes that contribute to increasing the chances that a wide set of different environmental rewards will be chosen over a period of time, including not only need-related satiety mechanisms that reduce the rewards within a dimension, but also sensory-specific satiety mechanisms, which facilitate switching to another reward stimulus (sometimes within and sometimes outside the same main dimension), and attraction to novel stimuli. (As noted in Sections 3.4.6 and 4.6.5, attraction to novel stimuli, i.e. finding them rewarding, is one way that organisms are encouraged to explore the multidimensional space within which their genes are operating. The suggestion is that animals should be built to find somewhat novel stimuli rewarding, for this encourages them to explore new parts of the environment in which their genes might do better than others' genes. Unless animals are built to find novelty somewhat rewarding, the multidimensional genetic space being explored by genes in

[5]Fitness refers to the fitness of genes, but this must be measured by the effects that the genes have on the organism.

the course of evolution might not find the appropriate environment in which they might do better than others' genes.)

3.2.1.3 Stimulus–response (habit) learning reinforced by rewards and punishers

In this second level of complexity, involving reward or punishment, learning may occur. If an organism performs trial-and-error responses, and as the result of performing one particular response is more likely to obtain a reward, then the response may become linked by a learning process to that stimulus as a result of the reward received. The reward is said to reinforce the response to that stimulus, and we have what is described as stimulus–response or habit learning. The reward acts as a positive reinforcer in that it increases the probability of a response on which it is made contingent. A punisher reduces the probability of a response on which it is made contingent. (It should be noted that this is an operational definition, and that there is no implication that the punisher feels like anything – the punisher just has in the learning mechanism to reduce the probability of responses followed by the punisher.) Stimulus–response or habit learning is typically evident after over-training, and once habits are being executed, the behaviour becomes somewhat independent of the reward value of the goal, as shown in experiments in which the reward is devalued. This is described in more detail in Section 4.6.1 on page 159.

3.2.1.4 Stimulus–reinforcer association learning, and two-factor learning theory for instrumental actions

Two-process learning introduces a third level of complexity and capability into the ways in which behaviour can be guided. Rewards and punishers still provide the basis for guiding behaviour within a dimension, and for selecting the dimension towards which action should be directed.

The first stage of the learning is stimulus–reinforcer association learning, in which the reinforcing value of a previously neutral, e.g. visual or auditory, stimulus is learned because of its association with a primary reinforcer, such as a sweet taste or a painful touch. This learning is of an association between one stimulus, the conditioned or secondary reinforcer, and the primary reinforcer, and is thus stimulus–stimulus association learning. This stimulus–reinforcer learning can be very fast, in as little as one trial. For example, if a new visual stimulus is placed in the mouth and a sweet taste is obtained, a simple approach response such as reaching for the object will be made on the next trial. Moreover, this stimulus–reinforcer association learning can be reversed very rapidly. For example, if subsequently the object is made to taste of salt, then approach no longer occurs to the stimulus, and the stimulus is even likely to be actively pushed away. This process leads to representations of expected value in the orbitofrontal cortex (Chapter 9).

The second process or stage in this type of learning is instrumental learning of an action (or 'operant response') made in order to obtain the stimulus now associated with reward (or avoid a stimulus associated by learning with the punisher). This is action–outcome learning (implemented in brain regions such as the cingulate cortex). The outcome could be a primary reinforcer, but often involves a secondary reinforcer learned by stimulus–reinforcer association learning. The action–outcome learning may be much slower, for it may involve trial-and-error learning of which action is successful in enabling the animal to obtain the stimulus now associated with reward or avoid the stimulus now associated with a punisher. However, this second stage may be greatly speeded if an operant response or strategy that has been learned previously to obtain a different type of reward (or avoid a different punisher) can be used to obtain (or avoid) the new stimulus now known to be associated with reinforcement. It is in this flexibility of the response that two-factor learning has a great advantage over stimulus–

response learning. The advantage is that any response (even, at its simplest, approach or withdrawal) can be performed once an association has been learned between a stimulus and a primary reinforcer. This flexibility in the response is much more adaptive (and could provide the difference between survival or not) than no learning, as in taxes, or stimulus–response learning. The different processes that are involved in instrumental learning are described in more detail in Section 4.6.1.

Another key advantage of this type of two-stage learning is that after the first stage the different rewards and punishers available in an environment can be compared in a selection mechanism, using the common scale of different rewards and punishers for the comparison and selection process (Section 9.5.2). In this type of system, the many dimensions of rewards and punishers are again the basis on which the selection of a behaviour to perform is made.

Part of the process of evolution can be seen as identifying the factors or dimensions that affect the fitness of an animal, and providing the animal with sensors that lead to rewards and punishers that are tuned to the environmental dimensions that influence fitness. The example of sweet taste receptors being set up by evolution to provide reward when physiological nutrient need is present has been given above.

We can ask whether there would need to be a separate sensing mechanism tuned to provide primary (unlearned) reinforcers for every dimension of the environment to which it may be important to direct behaviour. (The behaviour has to be directed to climb up the reward gradient to obtain the best reward, or to climb a gradient up and away from punishers.) It appears that there may not be. For example, in the case of the so-called specific appetites, for perhaps a particular vitamin lacking in the diet, it appears that a type of stimulus–reinforcer association learning may actually be involved, rather than having every possible flavour set up to be a primary reward or punisher. The way that this happens is by a form of association learning. If an animal deficient in one nutrient is fed a food with that nutrient, it turns out that the animal ‘feels better’ some time after ingesting the new food, and associates this ‘feeling better’ with the taste of that particular food. Later, that food will be chosen. The point here is that the first time the animal is in the deficient state and tastes the new food, that food may not be chosen instead of other foods. It is only after the post-ingestive conditioning that, later, that particular food will be selected (Rozin & Kalat 1971). Thus in addition to a number of specific primary (unlearned) reward systems (e.g. sweet taste for nutrient need, salt taste for salt deficiency, pain for potentially damaging somatosensory stimulation), there may be great opportunity for other arbitrary sensory stimuli to become conditioned rewards or punishers by association with some quite general change in physiological state. Another example to clarify this might be the way in which a build-up of carbon dioxide is aversive. If we are swimming deep, we may need to come to the surface in order to expel carbon dioxide (and obtain oxygen), and we may indeed find it very rewarding to obtain the fresh air. Does this mean that we have a specific reward/punisher system for carbon dioxide that can directly guide our actions towards a goal? It may be that too much carbon dioxide has been conditioned to be a negative reinforcer or punisher, because we feel so much better after we have breathed out the carbon dioxide. The implication here is that a number of bodily signals can influence a general bodily state, and we learn to improve the general state, rather than to treat the signal as a specific reinforcer that directs us to a particular goal. Another example might be social reinforcers. It would be difficult to build-in a primary reinforcer system for every possible type of social reinforcer. Instead, there may be a number of rather general primary social reinforcers, such as acceptance within a group, approbation, greeting, face expression, and pleasant touch which are among the primary rewards by association with which other stimuli become secondary social reinforcers.

To help specify the way in which stimulus–reinforcer association learning operates, a list of what may be in at least some species primary reinforcers is provided in Table 2.1 on page 20. The reader will doubtless be able to add to this list, and it may be that some of the reinforcers in the list are actually secondary reinforcers. The reinforcers are categorized where possible by modality, to help the list to be systematic. Possible dimensions to which each reinforcer is tuned are suggested.

3.2.2 Explicit systems, language, and reinforcement

A fourth level of complexity to the way in which behaviour is guided is by processing that includes syntactic operations on semantically grounded symbols (see Section 10.2). This allows multistep one-off plans to be formulated. Such a plan might be: if I do this, then B is likely to do this, C will probably do this, and then X will be the outcome. Such a process cannot be performed by an animal that only performs instrumental actions to obtain a gene-specified reward, or secondary reinforcers. The process may enable an available reward to be deferred for another reward that a particular multistep strategy could lead to. What are the roles of rewards and punishers in such a system?

The language system can still be considered to operate to obtain rewards and avoid punishers. This is not merely a matter of definition, for many of the rewards and punishers will be the same as those described above, those that have been tuned by evolution to the dimensions of the environment that can enable an animal to increase fitness. The processing afforded by language can be seen as providing a new type of strategy to obtain such gene-specified rewards or avoid such punishers. If this were not generally the case, then the use of the language system would not be adaptive: it would not increase fitness.

However, once a language system has evolved, a consequence may be that certain new types of reward become possible. These may be related to primary reinforcers already present, but may develop beyond them. For example, music may have evolved from the system of non-verbal communication that enables emotional states to be communicated to others. An example might be that lullabies could be related to emotional messages that can be sent from parents to offspring to soothe them. Music with a more military character might be related to the sounds given as social signals to each other in situations in which fighting (or co-operation in fighting) might occur. The prosodic quality of voice expression may be part of the same emotion communication system, and brain systems that are activated by prosody may be strongly engaged in women even in tasks that do not require prosody to be analysed (Schirmer, Zysset, Kotz & von Cramon 2004). Then on top of this, the intellectualization afforded by linguistic (syntactic) processing would contribute further aspects to music. Another example here is that solving problems by intellectual means should itself be a primary reinforcer as a result of evolution, for this would encourage the use of intellectual abilities that have potential advantage if used. A further set of examples of how, when a language system is present, there is the possibility for further types of reinforcer, comes from the possibility that the evolution of some mental abilities may have been influenced by sexual selection (see Section 7.7.2).

An additional principle enabled by language is that the rewards and punishers need not be defined only in the interests of the genes, but can be instead in the interests of the individual, the phenotype, as shown in Section 10.3.2.

3.2.3 Special-purpose design by an external agent vs evolution by natural selection

The above mechanisms, which operate in an evolutionary context to enable animals' behaviour to be tuned to increase fitness by evolving reward–punisher systems tuned to dimensions in the environment that increase fitness, may be contrasted with typical engineering design. In the latter, we may want to design a robot to work on an assembly line. Here there is an external designer, the engineer, who defines the function to be performed by the robot (e.g. picking a nut from a box, and attaching it to a particular bolt in the object being assembled). The engineer then produces special-purpose design features that enable the robot to perform this task, by for example providing it with sensors and an arm to enable it to select a nut, and to place the nut in the correct position in the 3D space of the object to enable the nut to be placed on the bolt and tightened. The design engineer also writes the control software that specifies the details of the movements to be made by the robot. This contrast with a real animal allows us to see important differences between these types of control for the behaviour of the system (see also *Neuroculture: On the Implications of Brain Science* Section 2.15 for an analysis of the computational differences between brains and digital computers).

In the case of the animal, there is a multidimensional space within which many optimizations to increase fitness must be performed. The solution to this is to evolve multiple reward–punisher systems tuned to each dimension in the environment that can lead to an increased fitness if the animal performs the appropriate actions. Natural selection guides evolution to find these dimensions. In contrast, in the robot arm, there is an externally defined movement to be performed, of placing the nut on the bolt, and the robot does not need to tune itself to find the goal to be performed. The contrast is between design by evolution that is 'blind' to the purpose of the animal, and design by a designer who specifies the job to be performed (cf. Dawkins (1986b)).

Another contrast is that for the animal the space will be high-dimensional, so that selection of the most appropriate reward for current behaviour (taking into account the costs of obtaining each reward) is needed, whereas for the robot arm, the function to perform at any one time is specified by the designer. Another contrast is that the behaviour, that is the instrumental action, that is most appropriate to obtain the reward must be selected by the animal, whereas the movement to be made by the robot arm is specified by the design engineer.

The implication of this comparison is that operation by animals using reward and punisher systems tuned to dimensions of the environment that increase fitness provides a mode of operation that can work in organisms that evolve by natural selection. It is clearly a natural outcome of Darwinian evolution to operate using reward and punisher systems tuned to fitness-related dimensions of the environment, if arbitrary actions are to be made by the animals rather than just preprogrammed movements such as are involved in tropisms and taxes. This may be the reason why we are built to work for rewards, avoid punishers, have emotions, and feel needs (motivational states). These concepts do not appear to have been developed within selfish gene theory (Dawkins 1976, Dawkins 1982, Dawkins 1986b), and bear on developments in the field of artificial life (see, e.g. Boden (1996)).

The sort of question that some philosophers might ponder is whether if life evolved on Mars it would have emotions. My answer to this is 'Yes', if the organisms have evolved genetically by natural selection, and the genes have elaborated behavioural mechanisms to maximize their fitness in a flexible way, which as I have just argued would imply that they have evolved reward and punisher systems that guide behaviour. They would have emotions in the sense introduced in Chapter 2, in that they would have states that would be produced by rewards or punishers, or by stimuli associated with rewards and punishers (Rolls 2002, Rolls 2005a). It is of course a rather larger question to ask whether our extraterrestrial organisms would have emotional feelings. My answer to this arises out of the theory of consciousness introduced in Chapter 10, and would be 'Only if the organisms have a linguistic system that can think about and correct their first order linguistic thoughts'. However, even if such higher-order thought processes are present, it is worth considering whether emotional feelings might despite these higher-order thoughts not be present. After all, we know that much behaviour can be guided unconsciously, implicitly, by rewards and punishers. My answer to this issue is that the organisms would have emotional feelings; for as suggested above, the explicit system has to work in general for rewards of the type that are rewarding to the implicit system, and for the explicit system to be guided towards solutions that increase fitness, it should feel good when the explicit system works to a correct solution. Otherwise, it is difficult to explain how the explicit system is guided towards solutions that are not only solutions to problems, but that are also solutions that tend to have adaptive value. If the system has evolved so that it feels like something when it is performing higher-order thought processing, then it seems likely that it would feel like something when it obtained a reward or punisher, for this is the way that the explicit, conscious, thoughts would be guided (see Chapter 10 for further explanation).

3.3 Selection of behaviour: cost–benefit 'analysis' of net value

One advantage of a design based on rewards and punishers is that the decoding of stimuli to a reward or punisher value can provide a common scale of value as inputs to the mechanism that selects which behavioural action should be performed. Thus, for example, a moderately sweet taste when little hunger is present would have a smaller reward value than the taste of water when thirst is present. A reward-selection mechanism could thus include in its specification competition between the different rewards, all represented on a common scale of value, with the most active specific reward or value representation indicating the stimulus most likely to be selected for action. As described above, to make sure that different types of reward are selected when appropriate, natural selection would need to ensure that different types of reward would operate on similar scales (from minimum to maximum), so that each type of reward would be selected if it reaches a high value on the common scale (see Section 9.5.2). Mechanisms such as sensory-specific satiety can be seen as contributing usefully to this mechanism which ensures that different types of reward will be selected for action.

However, the action selection mechanisms must take into account not only the relative value of each type of reward, but also the cost of obtaining each type of reward. If there is a very high cost of obtaining a particular reward, it may be better, at least temporarily, until the situation changes, to select an action that leads to a smaller reward, but is less costly. It appears that animals do operate according to such a cost–benefit analysis, in that if there is a high cost for an action, that action is less likely to be performed. One example of this comes from the fighting of deer. A male deer is less likely to fight another if he is clearly inferior in size or signalled prowess (Dawkins 1995). Thus the value of a stimulus or course of action, that is its intrinsic value minus the cost of the actions needed to obtain it and any resulting consequences of obtaining it, needs to be produced in a system that represents net value. Decisions can then be taken between these net value representations, and then actions can be selected as a separate process to obtain the winning stimulus or goal for action.

There may also be a cost to switching behaviour. If the sources of food and water are very distant, it would be costly to switch behaviour (and perhaps walk a mile) every time a mouthful of food or a mouthful of water was swallowed. This may be part of the adaptive value of incentive motivation or the 'salted nut' phenomenon – that after one reward is given early on in working for that reward the incentive value of that reward may increase. This may be expressed in the gradually increasing rate of working for food early on in a meal. By increasing the reward value of a stimulus for the first minute or two of working for it, hysteresis may be built into the behaviour selection mechanism, to make behaviour 'stick' to one reward for at least a short time once it is started.

When one refers to a 'cost–benefit analysis', one does not necessarily mean at all that the animal thinks about it and plans with 'if ... then' multistep linguistic processing the benefits and costs of each possible course of action. Instead, in many cases 'cost–benefit analysis' is likely to be built into animals to be performed with simple implicit processing using heuristics, simple rules that have been selected by evolutionary processes, and which may appear to be short cuts. By this I mean a solution or heuristic that might be found by a genetic algorithm, which may solve the task set, even if in a way that might not have been the way that an engineer or computational neuroscientist would have thought of (Rolls & Stringer 2000). One example would be the incentive motivation just described, which provides a mechanism for an animal to persist for at least a short time in one behaviour without having to explicitly plan to do this by performing as an individual a cost–benefit analysis of the relative advantages and costs of continuing or switching. Another example might be the way in which the decision to fight is made by male deer: the decision may be based on simple processes such as reducing the probability of fighting if the other individual is larger, rather than thinking through the consequences of fighting or not on this occasion. Thus, many of the costs and benefits or rewards that are taken into account in the behaviour selection process may in many animals operate according to simply evaluated rewards and costs built in by natural selection during evolution (Krebs & Kacelnik 1991, Dawkins 1995). Animals may take into account, for example, quite complex information, such as the mean and variance of the rewards available from different sources, in making their selection of behaviour, yet the actual selection may then be based on quite simple heuristics (rules of thumb), such as, 'if resources are very low, choose a reliable source of reward'. It may only be in some animals, for example humans, that explicit, linguistically based multistep cost–benefit analysis can be performed. It is important when interpreting animal behaviour to bear these arguments in mind, and to be aware that quite complex behaviour can result from very simple mechanisms. It is important not to over-interpret the factors that underlie any particular example of behaviour.

Reward and punisher signals provide a common scale of value for different sensory inputs, and can be seen as important in the selection of which actions are performed. Evolution ensures that the different reward and punisher signals are made potent to the extent that each will be chosen when appropriate. For example, food will be rewarding when hungry, but as hunger falls, the current level of thirst may soon become sufficient to make the reward produced by the taste of water greater than that produced by food, so that water is ingested. If however a painful input occurs or is signalled at any time during the feeding or drinking, this may be a stronger signal in the common scale of value, so that behaviour switches to that appropriate to reduce or avoid the pain. After the painful stimulus or threat is removed, the next most rewarding stimulus in the common value scale might be the taste of water, and drinking would therefore be selected.

An implication is that a decision process must be implemented in the brain between options each represented by their net value. (An option is a behaviour that might be chosen – see Chapter 9.) The option of avoiding a painful stimulus would on this net value scale have a high value, and would compete on the option decision process with other options, such as obtaining food, which might have a lower net value that avoiding a painful stimulus. An important point is that these decisions would be taken in a system (such as the orbitofrontal cortex) that represents the *net value of options*, where an option can be thought of as a behaviour that might be selected. It is an important part of brain design that this selection between options in terms of the net reward value of each is a process that happens separately, and before, the system (such as the cingulate cortex) that implements the details of each action by action–outcome learning, where the outcome is the net reward value of the action being learned (see Chapters 4 and 9).

Many of the rewards for behaviour consist of stimuli, or remembered stimuli. Examples of some primary reinforcers are included in Table 2.1. However, for some animals, evolution has built-in a reward value for certain types of response. For example, it may be reinforcing to a pigeon or chicken to peck. The adaptive value of this is that for these animals, simply pecking at their environment may lead to the discovery of food such as grain. Another example might be exercise, which may have been selected to be rewarding in evolution because it keeps the body physically fit (and attractive – see Chapter 7), which could be adaptive. While for some animals making certain responses may thus act as primary reinforcers (see Glickman & Schiff (1967)), this is likely to be adaptive only if animals operate in limited environmental niches. If one is built to find pecking very rewarding, this may imply that other types of response are less able to be made, and this tends to restrict the animal to an environmental niche. In general, animals with a wide range of behavioural responses and strategies available, such as primates, are able to operate in a wider range of environments, are in this sense more general-purpose, are less likely to find that particular responses are rewarding per se, and are more likely to be able to select actions based on which of a wide range of stimuli is most rewarding, rather than based on which response type they are pre-adapted to select.

The overall aim of the cost–benefit analysis in animals is to maximize *fitness*. By fitness we mean the probability that an animal's genes will be passed on into the next generation. To maximize this, there may be many ways in which different stimuli have been selected during evolution to be rewards and punishers (and among punishers we could include costs). All these rewards and punishers should operate together to ensure that over the lifetime of the animal there is a high probability of passing on genes to the next generation; but in doing this, and maximizing fitness in a complex and changing environment, all these rewards and punishers may be expected to lead to a wide variety of behaviour.

Once language enables rewards and punishers to be intellectualized, so that, for example, solving complex problems in language, mathematics, or music becomes rewarding, behaviour might be less obviously seen as adapted for fitness. However, it was suggested above that the ability to solve complex problems may be one way in which fitness, especially in a changing environment, can be maximized. Thus we should not be surprised that working at the level of ideas, to increase understanding, should in itself be rewarding. These circumstances, that humans have developed language and other complex intellectual abilities, and that natural selection in evolution has led problem-solving to be rewarding, may lead to the very rapid evolution of ideas (see also Section 7.7.2).

3.4 Further functions of emotion

The fundamental function of emotion, to enable an efficient way for the goals for actions to be defined by genes during evolution and to be implemented in the brain, has been described in Sections 3.2 and 3.3. The simple brain implementation provided as a result of evolution allows the different goals to be selected and compared by using reward and punisher evaluation or appraisal of stimuli, and of the stimuli that may be obtained by different courses of action. This function allows flexibility of the behavioural responses that will be performed to obtain gene-specified goals. Next we consider some further functions and properties of emotion, and also highlight some particularly interesting examples of the types of emotional behaviour that result from the fundamental operation of emotional systems described above.

3.4.1 Autonomic and endocrine responses

An additional function of emotion is the elicitation of autonomic responses (e.g. a change in heart rate) and endocrine responses (e.g. the release of adrenaline). It is of clear survival value to prepare the body, for example by increasing the heart rate, so that actions such as running which may be performed as a consequence of the reinforcing stimulus can be performed more efficiently. The neural connections from the amygdala and orbitofrontal cortex via the hypothalamus as well as directly towards the brainstem autonomic motor nuclei may be particularly involved in this function (see Chapter 4). The James–Lange theory (see Chapter 2), and theories that are closely related to it in supposing that feedback from parts of the periphery, such as the face (Adelmann & Zajonc 1989) or body (Damasio 1994), leads to emotional feelings, have the major weakness that they do not give an adequate account of how the peripheral change is produced only by stimuli that happen to be emotion-provoking. Perhaps the most important issue in emotion is why only some stimuli give rise to emotions. The way for answering this has been prepared in Chapter 2 by identifying the stimuli that produce emotions as instrumental reinforcers. This prepares the way for answering the question of how emotions are produced, by investigating which parts of the brain decode whether stimuli are reinforcing, and produce responses that include autonomic responses (see Chapter 4).

Mechanisms that lead animals to perform taxes such as swimming up chemical gradients are clearly required extremely early in animal evolution, and indeed are present in single cell animals such as *Amoeba*. At some later time in evolution, when specialized systems are present in the body, the autonomic and endocrine responses just described can be adaptive in enabling the animal to cope effectively with changes in the environment, and it is frequently appropriate for these states of autonomic and or endocrine activation to persist for considerable periods. At this stage in evolution there are thus likely to be brain systems that ensure that autonomic, and probably endocrine, states can be maintained for considerable periods. By this stage in evolution we have two key aspects of processing in place that later become important in emotion, namely guidance of behaviour towards stimuli that are useful (as determined by gene-specification), and guidance of responses away from noxious stimuli; and the persistence of such states after the evoking stimulus has disappeared. Later in evolution, when arbitrary (or operant) instrumental behaviour becomes possible in order to obtain what can now be called instrumental reinforcers, is one convenient stage at which to say that emotions are present. In this sense, the autonomic and endocrine aspects of emotional states may be precursors in evolution to the full emotional states that it is convenient to define as present when arbitrary instrumental actions can be performed to obtain goals.

3.4.2 Flexibility of behavioural responses, because emotions are related to the rewards and punishers that specify the goals for action

A function of emotion inherent in the gene-based theory described above is providing flexibility of behavioural responses, and this function of emotion is elaborated now. The thesis here is that when a rewarding or punishing stimulus in the environment elicits an emotional state, we can perform any appropriate and arbitrary action to obtain the reward, or avoid the punisher. That is, the reward or punisher defines the goal for the action, but does not specify the action itself. The action itself can be selected by the animal as appropriate in the current circumstances as that most appropriate for obtaining the reward or avoiding or escaping from the punisher. This is more flexible than simply learning a fixed behavioural response to a stimulus, which is what was implied by the stimulus–response (S–R) or habit learning theories of the 1930s.

This flexibility of behavioural responses is made very clear when we consider the learning processes that typically occur when emotion-provoking stimuli occur. Let us consider as an example avoidance learning. An example of this might be learning an action to perform when a tone sounds in order to avoid an electrical shock. The learning would take place in two stages, with different processes involved in each stage. In the first stage, stimulus–reinforcer association learning would produce an emotional state such as fear to a tone associated with the shock. This learning stage may be very rapid, and may occur in one trial. (We will see in Chapter 4 that the orbitofrontal cortex and amygdala are especially involved in this type of learning.) The second stage of the avoidance learning would be instrumental learning of an operant response (i.e. an action), motivated by and performed in order to terminate the fear-inducing stimulus. Finding an appropriate action to remove the fear-inducing stimulus may occur by trial-and-error, and may take many trials. This two-stage learning process was suggested as being important for avoidance learning by N. E. Miller and O. H. Mowrer (see Gray (1975) and Section 4.6.1.2).

The suggestion made here is that this general type of two-stage learning process is closely related to the design of animals for many types of behaviour, including emotional behaviour. It simplifies the interface of sensory systems to motor systems. Instead of having to learn a particular response or habit to a particular stimulus by slow, trial-and-error, learning, two-stage learning allows very fast (often one trial) learning of an emotional state to a rewarding or punishing stimulus. Then the action system can operate in a quite general way, sometimes using new trial-and-error learning, but often using many previously learned strategies, to approach the reward or avoid the punisher, which act as goals. This not only gives great flexibility to the interface between the sensory stimulus and an action, but also makes it relatively simple. It means that the reward value of a number of different stimuli can be decoded at approximately the same time. A decision system can then compare the values of the different rewards available, using a common scale of value. (The value of each type of reward on this 'common scale' will be affected by many different factors, such as need state, e.g. hunger; how recently that reward has been obtained; the necessity in evolution to set each type of reward so that it sometimes is chosen if it is important for survival; etc.) The decision system can then choose between the rewards, based on their value, but also on the cost of obtaining each reward (i.e. the net value, see earlier in this chapter). After the choice has been made, the action or motor system can then activate any behavioural responses possible, whether learned or not, in order to maximize the reward signal being obtained. The magnitude of the reward signal being obtained would be indicated just by the firing of the neurons that reflect the value of the reward being obtained (e.g. the taste of a food if hungry, the pleasantness of touch, etc.), as described in Chapters 4–7. The actual way in which the appropriate response or action is learned may depend on response-reinforcer (i.e. action–outcome) association learning, or on some more general type of purposive behaviour that can be learned to obtain goals.

It may be emphasized that emotions are thus an important part of brain design by enabling actions to be selected on the basis of goals, in allowing flexibility of the action performed, but also, and extremely importantly, by enabling a very simple type of one-trial learning, stimulus–reinforcer association learning, which is also very fast, to enable animals to respond to new attractive or dangerous stimuli with learning that may take as little as one trial.

3.4.3 Emotional states are motivating

Another function of emotion is that it is motivating. For example, fear learned by stimulus–reinforcer association formation provides the motivation for actions performed to avoid noxious stimuli. Similarly, positive reinforcers elicit motivation, so that we will work to obtain the rewards. Another example where emotion affects motivation is when a reward becomes no longer available, that is frustrative non-reward (see Fig. 2.1). If an action is possible, then increased motivation facilitates behaviour to produce harder working to obtain that reinforcer again or another reinforcer. If no action is possible to obtain again that reward (e.g. after a death in the family), then as described in Chapter 2, grief or sadness may result. This may be adaptive, by preventing continuing motivated attempts to regain the positive reinforcer that is no longer available, and helping the animal in due course to therefore be sensitive to other potential reinforcers to which it might be adaptive to switch. As described in Chapter 2, if such frustrative non-reward occurs in humans when no action is possible, depression may occur.

A depressed state that lasts for a short time may be seen as being adaptive for the reason just given. However, the depression may last for a very long time perhaps because long-term explicit (conscious) knowledge in humans enables the long-term consequences of loss of the positive reinforcer to be evaluated and repeatedly brought to mind as described in Chapter 10, and this may make long-term (psychological) depression maladaptive. Thus a discrepancy between the evolutionary and current environment caused by the rapid development of an explicit system may contribute to some emotional states that are no longer adaptive.

In an interesting evolutionary approach to depression, Nesse (2000b) has argued that humans may set long-term goals for themselves that are difficult to attain, and may spend years trying to attain these goals. An example of such a goal might be obtaining a particular position in one's career, or professional qualification, which may take years of a person's life. If the goal is not attained, then the lack of the reinforcer may lead to prolonged depression. Humans may find it difficult to reorganize their long-term aims to identify other, replacement and more attainable, goals, and without facility at this reorganization of long-term goals, the depression may be prolonged. The evolutionary aspect of this is that with our long-term explicit planning system (described in Chapter 10) and the value that society places on long-term goals and the status that attaining these may confer, humans find themselves in an environmental situation in which their explicit long-term planning system did not evolve, so that it is not well adapted to identifying goals that are realistic. The explicit system then provides a long-lasting non-reward signal to the emotion system (which in addition did not evolve to deal with such long-lasting non-reward inputs), and this contributes to long-lasting depression. A therapeutic solution would be to help depressed people identify possible precipitating factors such as unachieved long-term goals, and readjust their life aims so that positive reinforcers start to be obtained again, helping to lift the person out of the depression.

In addition to these motivating effects of emotion-provoking stimuli, I also emphasize that my Darwinian view that some genes specify the goals for actions leads not only to an account of emotion, but also to an account of motivation. As described in Chapter 2, motivation does not require an inherently different mechanism to emotion, in that if genes are specifying the reward value of some stimuli ('primary reinforcers'), then the behavioural system must be built to seek to obtain these stimuli (i.e. be motivated to treat them as goals), for otherwise the stimuli would not be operationally describable as rewards. A simple way to think about this is that *motivation is a state in which we are performing instrumental actions to obtain gene-defined goals; and emotions are states that are elicited when those goals are obtained, or are not obtained.*

3.4.4 Communication

Because of its survival value, the ability to decode signals from other animals as being rewarding or punishing is important. The reward or punisher value may in some cases be innate, and in other cases learned. It may also be adaptive to send such signals, and in some cases the sending of such signals may be 'honest' and in other cases 'deceptive'. These communicated signals may indicate for example the extent to which animals are willing to compete for resources, and they may influence the behaviour of other animals (Hauser 1996). Communicating emotional states may have survival value, for example by reducing fighting.

Darwin (1872), in his book entitled *The Expression of the Emotions in Man and Animals* had as a goal emphasizing the similarity, and therefore the possible phylogenetic closeness, of the expressions of man and his closest living relatives, but nevertheless noted the communicative value of such expressions.

The observation that expressions can evoke a response in the receiver underlies the idea that expressions can also be communicative rather than simply outward signs of affect (Chevalier-Skolnikoff 1973). Expression can be seen as a way of inviting/inducing certain responses in the receiver, much as a smile can appease, a laugh can invite participation, and fear could enlist assistance. In non-human primates, expression is used as a tool with which to regulate and maintain social relations. For example, in the macaque if a subordinate grimaces in an aggressive encounter with a dominant, this signals submission. However, the use of expression is not necessarily so straightforward, for if the same expression were to be given by a dominant individual approaching a subordinate, it no longer signals submission but the positive intention of the dominant. In this way, the communicative effect of expression can be said to be context-dependent, and it depends on the age, sex, dominance and kinship of the senders and receivers (Chevalier-Skolnikoff 1973).

Zeller (1987) also describes what may be said to be the manipulation of social relations through facial expression in non-human primates, that is threat faces are given to coerce another into a desired activity, and friendly expressions are given to enlist co-operation from another.

To argue that the expression of emotion is utilized in social communication, then the ability to decode these signals must be demonstrated. That is, are others able to perceive the content of an individual's expression? Humans have been shown to be remarkable in this ability, even cross-culturally (Ekman 1998), and many would say the happiness in a smile and the anger in furrowed brows are intuitively easy signals to understand.

If the facial expression cannot be transmitted, then this might also on this hypothesis be expected to influence the social and emotional behaviour of others. Izard (1971) showed that a rhesus macaque with impaired facial motor nerve (VIII) function received an increased number of aggressive assaults, and that its position in the social dominance hierarchy fell. Further, humans who have difficulties in producing facial expressions (e.g. patients with Bell's palsy or Parkinson's disease) say that their social interactions are made difficult (Sutherland 1997).

A powerful method of looking at adaptation is to compare different groups of related species in order to uncover the evolutionary history (phylogeny) of particular adaptations, and to uncover what particular selection pressures were at work on such adaptations. Such evidence, described in the following, can be used to underscore the communicative value of the expression of emotion. Expression cannot be produced without the relevant facial muscles contracting or relaxing, and therefore expression is dependent on the musculature of the face. The primate order has undergone some dramatic shifts in the evolution of the facial musculature that can be witnessed in the detectable difference in the use of facial expression between the strepsirhines (prosimians) and haplorhines (simians), and the hominoids (apes) and hominids, as follows.

The facial musculature of the strepsirhines is not very differentiated and relatively primitive. Facial innervation is also significantly less (Zeller 1987). Accordingly, the strepsirhines have a meagre set of expressions and a mask-like face (Chevalier-Skolnikoff 1973). In the haplorhines, the muscles of the mid-facial region become more differentiated and afford the face greater expressiveness when compared to the strepsirhines. This can be related to the reduction in the reliance on auditory and olfactory communication, corresponding to the shift from nocturnal to diurnal living. With the great apes, there is a still greater differentiation of the mid-facial muscles, and also the development of new muscles around the mouth. The new muscles offer a mobility that can produce a facial expression which a macaque, for instance, could not perform (Chevalier-Skolnikoff 1973). This trend continues in humans, and the even greater differentiation and the complex interlacing of muscles provide the potential for new movements. For example, the *zygomaticus major* muscle can pull the mouth corners into the human smile (Chevalier-Skolnikoff 1973). Thus, we can see how there have been successive shifts in the muscular differentiation of the face, which has had a concomitant effect on the use of facial expression.

Interestingly, the evolution of the facial anatomy and the expressions that depend on it also correspond to the evolution of sociality through the primate order (Andrew 1963). While the first proliferation of facial expression occurred after the switch to a diurnal way of life, the continuation of this trend accords with the gregariousness of the species. Communication by expression would be more or less pointless in solitary and/or nocturnal species such as the Galago, but would become much more useful in group living, diurnal and terrestrial, species. Consistent with this, highly gregarious and 'socially complex' species of Old World monkeys and apes (e.g. baboons, chimpanzees) have the most exaggerated facial expression repertoire, culminating with that of man. This evidence corroborates the idea that one of the functions of emotion lies in the communicative value of its expression.

Chapter 4 describes the brain systems in the temporal lobe visual cortex, the amygdala, and the orbitofrontal cortex that are specialized for the decoding of face-related information such as expression and identity. Here I note some interesting comparative evidence. Barton & Aggleton (2000) measured the relative volume of the amygdala (by plotting the volume of the amygdala nuclei against medulla volume) across the primate order. They revealed a successive relative enlargement of the cortico-basolateral (CBL) nuclei of the amygdala between the insectivores and the strepsirhines, and strepsirhines and haplorhines. The insectivores were used as a representative of the ancestor of the primate lineage. Further, the size of the CBL group of amygdala nuclei correlated with social group size. Part of the relevance of this is that we know that neurons selectively responsive to faces are found in the basolateral/basal accessory group of amygdala nuclei (Leonard, Rolls, Wilson & Baylis 1985). Thus a part of the amygdala especially concerned with processing face stimuli shows particular evolutionary development through the primates, and correlates with the size of the social group. This evidence is thus also consistent with the importance of communication in social behaviour and emotion, in this case involving probably both face identity and expression.

As social groups are at once both competitive and cooperative, one of the adaptive functions of emotion, and its display, could be to signal, whether honestly or dishonestly, the shifting intentions and dispositions of an individual to another in the social group. Overall, it would be expected that the emphasis on the communicative value of emotion would be greater in species with a socially complex organization, and the evidence above seems to bear this out.

3.4.5 Social attachment

Another area in which emotion is important is in social bonding. Examples of this are the emotions associated with the attachment of the parents to their young, with the attachment of the young to their parents, and with the attachment of the parents to each other (see Section 7.3). In the theory of the ways in which the genes affect behaviour ('selfish gene' theory, see Dawkins (1989), Ridley (2003)), it is held that (because, e.g., of the advantages of parental care) all these forms of emotional attachment have the effect that genes for such attachment are more likely to survive into the next generation. Kin-altruism can also be considered in these terms (see e.g. Dawkins (1989) and Section 7.7.2). In these examples, social bonding is related to primary (gene-specified) reinforcers. In other cases, the emotions involved in social interactions may arise from reinforcers involved in reciprocal altruism, utilizing for example 'tit-for-tat' strategies. In these cases it is crucial to remember which reinforcers are exchanged with particular individuals, so that cheating does not lead to disadvantages for some of those involved. This type of social bonding can be stable when there is a net advantage to both parties in cooperating (see Section 11.3).

Some investigators have argued that the main functions of emotion are in social situations (see Strongman (2003)). While it is certainly the case that many emotions are related to social situations (as can be inferred from Table 2.1), many are not, including for example the fear of snakes by primates, or the fear that is produced by the sight of an object that has produced pain previously.

3.4.6 Separate functions for each different primary reinforcer

It is useful to highlight that each primary (gene-specified) reinforcer (of which a large number are suggested in Table 2.1) not only leads to a different set of emotions, but also implements a different function. A few examples of these functions are elaborated here. This should make it possible for the reader to complete the elaboration for the other primary reinforcers in Table 2.1. Before considering these examples, let us remember that each function is related to the survival value or sexually selected value being provided by the specifying gene by increasing reproductive success for the gene; and that in so far as emotional states are associated with feelings (see Chapter 10), anything that feels pleasant or unpleasant to the organism, and is instrumentally reinforcing, is likely to have survival value, and to implement another function of emotion. (The argument given in Chapter 10 is that stimuli that act as implicit or unconscious rewards may also act to produce pleasant feelings in the explicit or conscious processing system, so that both the implicit and explicit routes to action operate largely consistently.)

One example of a primary reinforcer taken from Table 2.1 is slight novelty, which may feel good and be positively reinforcing because it may lead to the discovery of better opportunities for survival in the environment (e.g. a new food). It is crucial that animals that succeed in the genetic competition that drives evolution have genes that encourage them to explore new environments, for then it is possible for the genes that happen to be present in an individual to explore the large multidimensional space (or more colloquially, range of ways to vary) of the environment in which they might succeed.

Another example from Table 2.1 is gregariousness, which may assist the identification of new social partners, which could provide advantage.

Probably related to the effects of novelty is sensory-specific satiety, the phenomenon whereby pleasant tastes during a meal gradually become less pleasant as satiety approaches (see Chapter 5). This may be an aspect of a more general adaptation to ensure that behaviour does eventually switch from one reinforcer to another.

Although these examples are of positive reinforcers, it is comparably the case that natural selection acting via the reproductive success of genes will lead to the elaboration of other stimuli as punishers when avoiding these stimuli has survival value.

Of course the genes may be misled sometimes and lead to behaviour that does not have survival value, as when for example the non-nutritive sweetener saccharin is eaten by animals. This does not disprove the theory, but only points out that the genes cannot specify correctly for every possible stimulus or event in the environment, but must only on average lead to behaviour feeling pleasant that increases reproductive fitness, i.e. is appropriate for gene survival.

3.4.7 The mood state can influence the cognitive evaluation of moods or memories

Another property of emotion is that the current mood state can affect the cognitive evaluation of events or memories (Blaney 1986, Robinson, Watkins & Harmon-Jones 2013), and this may have the function of facilitating continuity in the interpretation of the reinforcing value of events in the environment. A theory of how this occurs is presented in Section 4.12 'Effects of emotion on cognitive processing and memory'.

3.4.8 Facilitation of memory storage

An eighth function of emotion is that it may facilitate the storage of memories. One way in which this occurs is that episodic memory (i.e. one's memory of particular episodes) is facilitated by emotional states. This may be advantageous in that storage of as many details as possible of the prevailing situation when a strong reinforcer is delivered may be useful in generating appropriate behaviour in situations with some similarities in the future. This function may be implemented in the brain by the relatively non-specific projecting systems to the cerebral cortex and hippocampus, including the cholinergic pathways in the basal forebrain and medial septum (see Section 4.11.5) (Rolls 2008b, Rolls & Treves 1998, Rolls 1999a, Wilson & Rolls 1990a, Wilson & Rolls 1990b, Wilson & Rolls 1990c), and the ascending noradrenergic pathways (see Section 4.11.6).

A second way in which emotion may affect the storage of memories is that the current emotional state may be stored with episodic memories, providing a mechanism for the current emotional state to affect which memories are recalled. In this sense, emotion acts as a contextual retrieval cue, that as with other contextual effects influences the retrieval of episodic memories (Rolls 2008b, Rolls & Treves 1998).

A third way in which emotion may affect the storage of memories is by guiding the cerebral cortex in the representations of the world that are set up. For example, in the visual system, it may be useful to build perceptual representations or analysers that are different from each other if they are associated with different reinforcers, and to be less likely to build them if they have no association with reinforcers. Ways in which backprojections from parts of the brain important in emotion (such as the amygdala) to parts of the cerebral cortex could perform this function are discussed in Section 4.12 'Effects of emotion on cognitive processing and memory'; and by Rolls (2008b).

3.4.9 Emotional and mood states are persistent, and help to produce persistent motivation

A ninth function of emotion is that by enduring for minutes or longer after a reinforcing stimulus has occurred, it may help to produce persistent motivation and direction of behaviour. For example, if an expected reward is not obtained, the persisting state of frustrative non-reward may usefully keep behaviour directed for some time at trying to obtain the reward again.

3.4.10 Emotions may trigger memory recall and influence cognitive processing

A tenth function of emotion is that it may trigger recall of memories stored in neocortical representations. Amygdala and orbitofrontal cortex backprojections to cortical areas could perform this for emotion in a way analogous to that in which the hippocampus could implement the retrieval in the neocortex of recent memories of particular events or episodes (see Rolls

(2008b) and Rolls & Kesner (2006)). This is thought to operate as follows. When a memory is stored in a neocortical area or hippocampus, any mood state that is present and reflected in the firing of neurons in the orbitofrontal cortex or amygdala will become associated with that memory by virtue of the associatively modifiable synaptic connections from the backprojecting neurons onto the neocortical or hippocampal system neurons. Then later, a particular mood state represented by the firing of neurons in the amygdala or orbitofrontal cortex will by the associatively modified backprojection connections enhance or produce the recall of memories stored when that mood state was present. These effects have been formally modelled by Rolls & Stringer (2001b), and are described further in Section 4.12.

One consequence of these effects is that once in a particular mood state, memories associated with that mood state will tend to be recalled and incoming stimuli will be interpreted in the light of the current mood state. The result may be some continuity of emotional state and thus of behaviour. This continuity may sometimes be advantageous, by keeping behaviour directed towards a goal, and making behaviour interpretable by others, but it may become useful in human psychiatric conditions to break this self-perpetuating tendency.

It is useful to have these functions of emotion in mind when considering the neural basis of emotion, for each function is likely to activate particular output pathways from emotional systems associated with it.

3.5 The functions of emotion in an evolutionary, Darwinian, context

In this book (see for example Section 3.2), the question of why we have emotions is a fundamental issue that I answer in terms of a Darwinian, functional, approach, producing the answer that emotions are states elicited by the goals (rewards and punishers) for instrumental actions, and that this is part of an adaptive process by which genes can specify the behaviour of the animal by specifying goals for behaviour rather than fixed responses. The emotional states elicited with respect to the goals depend on the reinforcement contingencies, as illustrated in Fig. 2.1. The states themselves may be the goals for action, such as reducing fear, and additionally maintain behaviour by being persistent, and act in other ways as described in Section 3.4.

This theory of emotion provides I believe a powerful approach to understanding how genes influence behaviour. In much thinking in zoology, an approach has been to understand how genes may determine particular behaviours. For example, Niko Tinbergen (1963, 1951) considered that innate releasing stimuli might elicit fixed action patterns. An example is the herring gull chick's pecking response elicited as a fixed action pattern by the innate releasing stimulus of a red spot on its parent's bill. A successor in this approach in the context of emotion is Panksepp (1998), who specifies fixed action patterns. The instinctive pecking response may be improved by learning (Hailman 1967), but is not an arbitrary, flexible, response as in instrumental, action–outcome, learning (see Section 4.6.1.2). The details of the stimulus, or the context in which it occurs, may be taken into account, to influence the instinctive response (Dawkins 1995), but there is still no arbitrary relation between the stimulus and the action, as in instrumental learning.

In contrast, the most important function of emotion that I propose is for genes to specify the stimuli that are the goals for actions. This means that the genetic specification can be kept relatively simple, in that it is stimuli that are specified by the genes, such as a taste or touch, and this is generally simpler than specifying the details of a response (such as climbing a tree, running along a branch, picking an apple, and placing it into the mouth). It also means that relatively few genetic specifications are needed, for instead of having to encode many relations between particular stimuli and particular behavioural responses, the genes need to span the dimensionality of the stimulus space of primary reinforcers. Examples of some of these primary, gene-encoded, reinforcers are shown in Table 2.1.

Another way in which the genetic specification required can be kept low is that stimulus–reinforcer association learning can then be used to enable quite arbitrary stimuli occurring in the lifetime of an animal to become associated with primary reinforcers by stimulus–reinforcer association learning, and thus to lead to actions.

But the most important advantage conferred by emotion is that the behaviour required need not be genetically specified, for arbitrary actions can be learned in the lifetime of the animal by instrumental, action–outcome, learning to obtain or avoid the goals specified by the genes. The actions are arbitrary operants, in that any action may be made to obtain the goal (see Section 4.6.1.2). Thus the genetic specification of the behaviour that emotion allows is one in which the behaviour is not pre-programmed with respect to the stimulus (as in instinctive behaviour such as fixed action patterns), but instead the action is not specified by the genes, and the goals to which actions are directed are specified by the genes. Of course this does not deny that some behavioural responses are genetically specified as responses, and examples might include pecking to particular stimuli in birds, orientation to and suckling of the nipple in mammals, and some examples of preparedness to learn (see Section 4.6.1.2).

Darwinian natural selection of genes that encode the goals for action (i.e. encode reinforcers) rather than the actions themselves, and thus allows great flexibility of the resulting behaviour, can be thought of as liberating 'The Selfish Gene' (Dawkins 1976, Dawkins 1989). When Richard Dawkins wrote *The Selfish Gene* (Dawkins 1976), he was careful to make it clear that the concept that selection and competition operate at the level of genes (Hamilton 1964, Hamilton 1996) does not lead inevitably to genetic determinism of behaviour. Nevertheless the concept was criticized on these grounds, and Dawkins devoted a whole chapter of *The Extended Phenotype* to addressing this further (Dawkins 1982). The concepts developed in *Emotion and Decision-Making Explained* help to resolve this further, for I argue that an important way in which genes influence behaviour (and in doing so produce emotion), is by specifying the reinforcers, the goals for actions, rather than particular behaviours (Rolls 1999a, Rolls 2005b). This helps to avoid the charge that selfish genes 'determine' the behaviour. Instead, many of the genes that influence behaviour operate by competing with each other in a world of reinforcing stimuli or goals for actions, and thus there is great flexibility in the behaviour that results. We are led to think not of behaviours being inherited or 'determined by selfish genes', but instead of genes exploring by natural selection reinforcers that may guide behaviour successfully so that the fitness of the genes is increased. In this sense, the selfish gene (in particular, those involved in specifying reinforcers) is liberated from directly 'determining' behaviour, to providing goals for (instrumental) actions that can involve completely flexible behaviour made to obtain the goal. In these cases, the heritability of behaviour is best understood as the heritability of reinforcers in a stimulus space not in a behavioural or response space.

An interesting consequence of this fundamental adaptive value of emotion that I propose is that the genetic specification does need to include specification for several synapses through the nervous system from the sensory input to the brain region where the reward or punishment value of the goal stimulus is made explicit in the representation (see footnote 6 on page 71). It is thus a prediction that genes specify the connectivity to the stage of processing in the brain where goals and rewards are specified, so that appropriate actions can be learned to the goals. Evidence is described in Chapters 4 and 5 that the goals may not be made explicit, that is related to neuronal firing, until stages of information processing such as the orbitofrontal cortex and amygdala. An example of this specification is that sweet taste receptors on the tongue must be connected to neurons that specify food reward, and whose responses are modulated by hunger signals (see Chapter 5).

The definition I provide of emotions, that they are states (with particular functions) elicited by instrumental reinforcers (see Chapter 2), thus is consistent with what I see as the most important function of emotion, that of being part of a design by which genes can specify (some) goals or reinforcers of our actions. This means that the theory of emotion that I propose should not be seen as behaviourist, but instead as part of a much broader theory that takes an adaptive, Darwinian, approach to the functions of emotion, and how they are important in brain design. Further, the theory shows how cognitive states can produce and modulate emotion (see Sections 2.8 and 4.5.5.7), and in turn how emotional states can influence cognition (see Section 4.12).

I believe that this approach leads to a fundamental understanding of why we have emotions that is likely to stand the test of time, in the same way that Darwinian thinking itself provides a fundamental way of understanding biology and many 'why' questions about life. This is thus intended to be a thoroughly Darwinian theory of the adaptive value of emotion in the design of organisms.

3.6 The functions of motivation in an evolutionary, Darwinian, context

Motivation may be seen as a state in which one is working for a goal, and emotion as a state that occurs when the goal, a reinforcer, is obtained, and that may persist afterwards. The concept of gene-specified reinforcers providing the goals for action helps the understanding of the relation between motivational states and emotion, as the organism must be built to be motivated to obtain the goals, and to be placed in a different state (emotion) when the goal is or is not achieved by the action. The close but clear relation between motivation and emotion is that both involve what humans describe as affective states (e.g. feeling hungry, liking the taste of a food, feeling happy because of a social reinforcer), and both are about goals. The Darwinian theory of the functions of emotion developed in this chapter, which shows how emotion is adaptive because it reflects the operation of a process by which genes define goals for action, applies just as much to motivation. By specifying goals, the genes must specify both that we must be motivated to obtain those goals, and that when the goals are obtained, further states, emotional states with further functions, are produced. In motivated behaviour, many factors influence how rewarding or punishing the goal is. In terms of motivated states relevant to internal homeostatic needs, the reward or goal value of a sensory stimulus such as the taste of food or water is set up genetically to be influenced by the relevant internal signals, such as plasma glucose concentration or plasma osmolality in the cases of hunger and thirst, as described in Chapter 5 and for thirst in Rolls (2005b). If a gene-specified goal such as the taste of expected food is not obtained, then we are left in a state of frustrative non-reward in which the original goal remains rewarding, which will leave us motivated to still obtain it if it may still be available, or will lead to a learned change in its reward value, and to extinction of that behaviour, if we learn that no action will obtain the goal (see Section 3.4.3).

3.7 Are all goals for action gene-specified?

Finally in this chapter, we can ask whether all goals are gene-specified. An important concept of this chapter has been that part of the adaptive value of emotion is that it is part of the process that results from the way in which genes specify reinforcers, that is the goals for action. Emotions may thus be elicited by primary reinforcers, or by stimuli that become associated by learning with primary reinforcers, i.e. secondary reinforcers. But are there goals related to emotional and motivational states that are not related to goals defined in this way by gene-specified reinforcers?

I think it is likely that most reinforcers can be traced back to a gene-specified goal, even if they are in some cases rather general goals. Some examples of these types of reinforcer (and there are likely to be many others) are included in Table 2.1, such as goals for social cooperation and group acceptance, mind reading, and solving an intellectual problem. However, when an explicit, rational, reasoning system capable of syntactic operations on symbols (as described in Chapter 10) evolves, it is possible that goals that are not very directly related to gene specifications become accepted. This may be seen in some of the effects of culture. Indeed, some goals are defined within a culture, for example writing a novel. But it is argued that it is primary reinforcers specified by genes of the general type shown in Table 2.1 that make us want to be recognized in society because of the advantages this can bring, to solve difficult problems, etc., and therefore to perform actions such as writing novels (see further Chapters 7 and 10, Ridley (2003) Chapter 8, Ridley (1993b) pp. 310 ff, Laland & Brown (2002) pp. 271 ff, Dawkins (1982), and *Neuroculture* Rolls (2012d)). Indeed, culture is influenced by human genetic propensities, and it follows that human cognitive, affective, and moral capacities are the product of a unique dynamic known as *gene-culture coevolution* (Gintis 2007, Bowles & Gintis 2005, Gintis 2003, Boyd, Gintis, Bowles & Richerson 2003).

Nevertheless, there may be cases where the explicit, reasoning, system might specify a goal, and thus lead to emotions, that could not be related to any genetic adaptive value, whether current or specified in evolutionary history. In these cases I would argue that although emotion has evolved and is generally adaptive in relation to gene-specified reinforcers, when the explicit, reasoning, system evolves, this can set up alternative goals that tap into and utilize the existing emotional system for facilitating actions, but with respect to which the goals might be genetically unspecified and even non-adaptive. Indeed, it is argued in Chapters 10 and 11 that much implicit emotion acts in the interests of the genes, whereas reasoning in the explicit system can allow gene-specified rewards to be rejected, in the long-term interests of the individual person, for example to stay alive for a long time (which may not be in the interests of the genes). Thus there can be some goals for action that are not in the interests of the genes.

4 The brain mechanisms underlying emotion

4.1 Introduction

Part of the explanation provided in this book of emotions is the way in which emotions are implemented in our brains. What happens in our brains during emotions? What processes taking place in our brains make us have emotions, and behave the way we do? We start with diagrams to show some of the brain regions we will be discussing. Then there is a short summary of the general principles involved in the brain mechanisms underlying emotion.

Given that emotions can be considered as states elicited by reinforcers (Chapter 2), a principled approach to the brain processes involved in emotion is to consider where primary reinforcers are represented (Section 4.3), where and how potential secondary (learned) reinforcers are represented (Section 4.4), and then the brain regions that implement stimulus–reinforcer, i.e. emotional, learning, considering in turn the orbitofrontal cortex (Section 4.5), amygdala (Section 4.6), and cingulate cortex (Section 4.7). Then we consider output systems for emotion (Section 4.11).

Some of the main brain regions implicated in emotion will now be considered in the light of the introduction given in Chapters 2 and 3 on the nature and functions of emotion. These brain regions include the amygdala, orbitofrontal cortex, cingulate cortex, and basal forebrain areas including the hypothalamus, which are shown in Figs. 4.1 and 4.2. Particular emphasis is placed on investigations of the functions of these regions in primates (usually monkeys and humans), for in primates many areas of the neocortex undergo great development and provide major inputs to these regions, in some cases to parts of these structures thought not to be present in non-primates. One example is the great development of the granular areas of the orbitofrontal cortex, thought not to have a direct homologue in rodents (Wise 2008, Passingham & Wise 2012) (see Fig. 1.1). Another example is the corticalization of taste processing in primates, without the direct connections from brainstem taste relays to subcortical structures found in rodents (see Section 1.3). Another example is the projection from the primate neocortex in the anterior part of the temporal lobe to the basal accessory nucleus of the amygdala (see below). Studies in primates are thus particularly relevant to understanding the neural basis of emotion in humans.

4.2 Overview

The way in which recent studies in primates including humans indicate that the neural processing of emotion is organized is as follows (see Figs. 4.2 and 4.3).

1. In Tier 1 (Fig. 4.2), information is processed to a level at which the neurons represent 'what' the stimulus is, independently of the reward or punishment value of the stimulus. Thus neurons in the primary taste cortex represent what the taste is, and its intensity, but not its reward value. In the inferior temporal visual cortex, the representation is of objects, invariantly with respect to the exact position on the retina, size, and even view. Forming

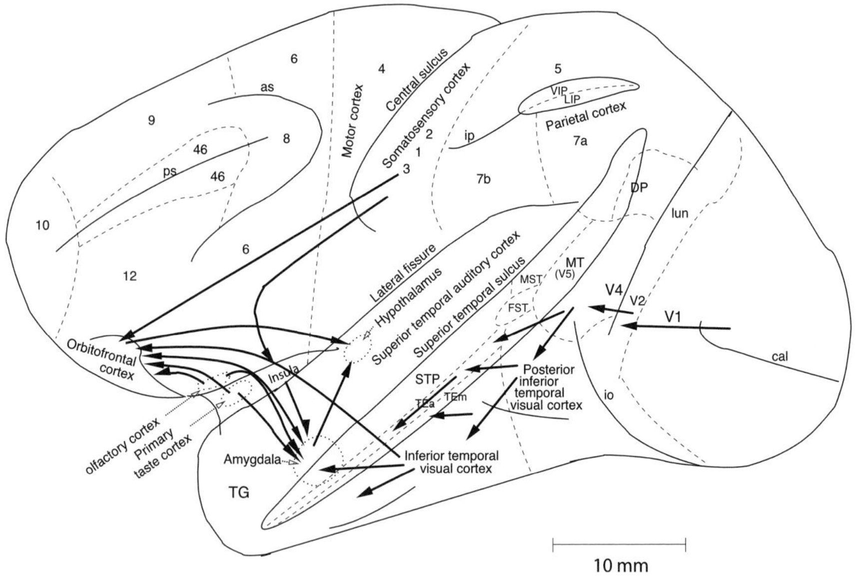

Fig. 4.1 Some of the pathways involved in emotion described in the text are shown on this lateral view of the brain of the macaque monkey. Connections from the primary taste and olfactory cortices to the orbitofrontal cortex and amygdala are shown. Connections are also shown in the 'ventral visual system' from V1 to V2, V4, the inferior temporal visual cortex, etc., with some connections reaching the amygdala and orbitofrontal cortex. In addition, connections from the somatosensory cortical areas 1, 2, and 3 that reach the orbitofrontal cortex directly and via the insular cortex, and that reach the amygdala via the insular cortex, are shown. as, arcuate sulcus; cal, calcarine sulcus; cs, central sulcus; lf, lateral (or Sylvian) fissure; lun, lunate sulcus; ps, principal sulcus; io, inferior occipital sulcus; ip, intraparietal sulcus (which has been opened to reveal some of the areas it contains); sts, superior temporal sulcus (which has been opened to reveal some of the areas it contains). AIT, anterior inferior temporal cortex; FST, visual motion processing area; LIP, lateral intraparietal area; MST, visual motion processing area; MT, visual motion processing area (also called V5); PIT, posterior inferior temporal cortex; STP, superior temporal plane; TA, architectonic area including auditory association cortex; TE, architectonic area including high order visual association cortex, and some of its subareas TEa and TEm; TG, architectonic area in the temporal pole; V1–V4, visual areas V1–V4; VIP, ventral intraparietal area; TEO, architectonic area including posterior visual association cortex. The numerals refer to architectonic areas, and have the following approximate functional equivalence: 1,2,3, somatosensory cortex (posterior to the central sulcus); 4, motor cortex; 5, superior parietal lobule; 7a, inferior parietal lobule, visual part; 7b, inferior parietal lobule, somatosensory part; 6, lateral premotor cortex; 8, frontal eye field; 12, part of orbitofrontal cortex; 46, dorsolateral prefrontal cortex.

invariant representations involves a great deal of cortical computation in the hierarchy of visual cortical areas from the primary visual cortex V1 to the inferior temporal visual cortex (Rolls 2008b, Rolls 2012e). The fundamental advantage of this separation of 'what' processing in Tier 1 from reward value processing in Tier 2 is that any learning in Tier 2 of the value of an object or face seen in one location on the retina, size, and view will generalize to other views etc. Evidence that there is no such clear separation of 'what' from 'value' representations in rodents, for example in the taste system, is described in Sections 1.3 and 5.4.2.4, and this property makes the processing in rodents not only different from that in primates including humans, but also much more difficult to analyse.

2. There are brain mechanisms in Tier 2 that are involved in computing the reward value of primary (unlearned) reinforcers. The primary reinforcers include taste, touch (both pleasant

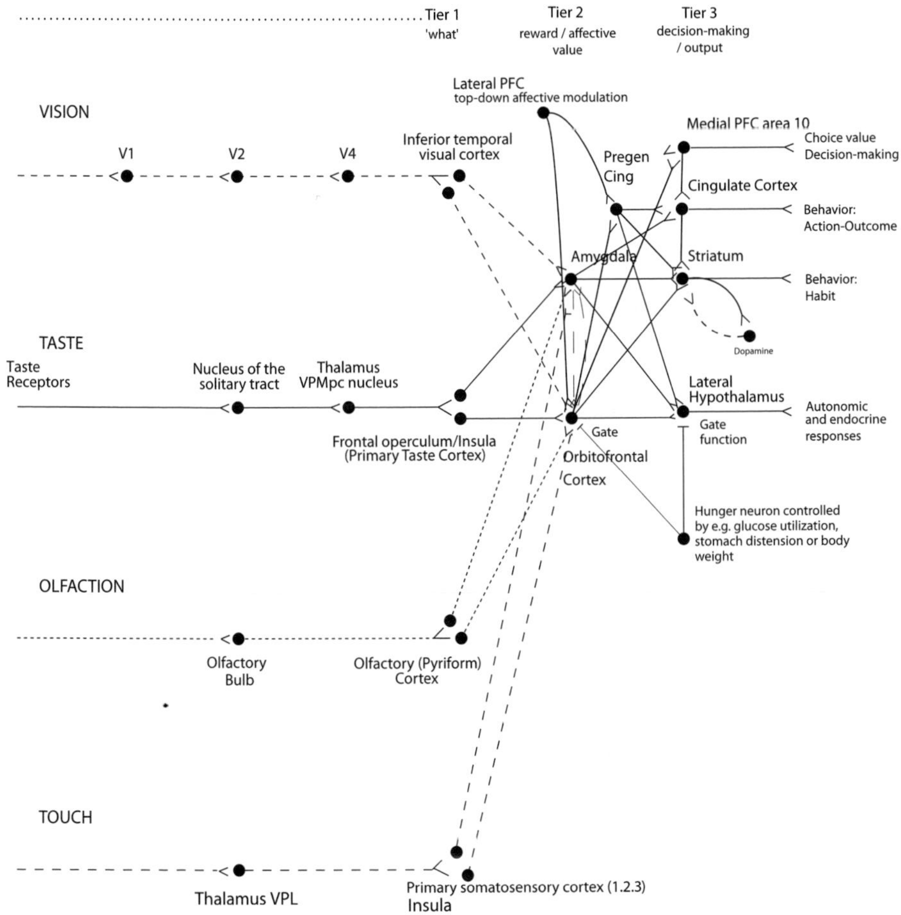

Fig. 4.2 Schematic diagram showing some of the connections of the taste, olfactory, somatosensory, and visual pathways in the brain. V1, primary visual (striate) cortex; V2 and V4, further cortical visual areas. PFC, prefrontal cortex. VPL, ventro-postero-lateral nucleus of the thalamus, which conveys somatosensory information to the primary somatosensory cortex (areas 1, 2 and 3). VPMpc, ventro-postero-medial nucleus pars parvocellularis of the thalamus, which conveys taste information to the primary taste cortex. Pregen Cing, pregenual cingulate cortex. For purposes of description, the stages can be described as Tier 1, representing what object is present independently of reward value; Tier 2 in which reward value is represented; and Tier 3 in which decisions between stimuli of different value are taken, and in which value is interfaced to behavioural output systems.

touch and pain), and to some extent smell, and perhaps certain visual stimuli, such as face expression. There is evidence that there is a representation of the (reward/punishment) value of many primary reinforcers in the orbitofrontal cortex, including taste, positive touch and pain, face expression, face beauty, and auditory consonance/dissonance.

3. Brain regions in Tier 2 are also concerned with learning associations between previously neutral stimuli, such as the sight of objects or of individuals' faces, with primary reinforcers. These brain regions include the amygdala and orbitofrontal cortex. Once the Tier 2 brain regions have determined whether the input is reinforcing, whether primary or secondary, the signal is passed directly to output regions of the brain, with no need to produce and then feed back peripheral body or autonomic responses to the brain.

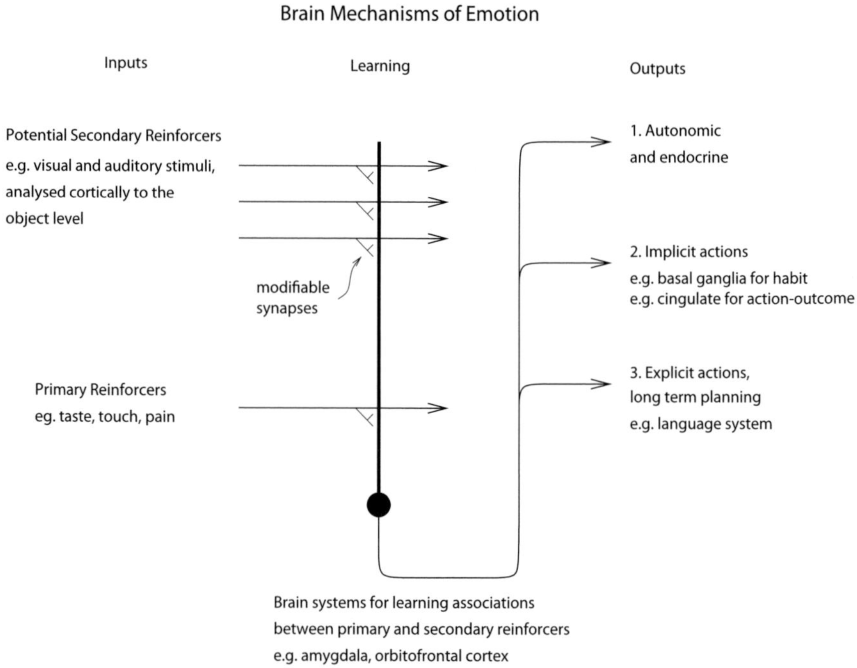

Fig. 4.3 Schematic diagram showing the organization of some of the brain mechanisms underlying emotion, including those involved in learning the reinforcement associations of visual stimuli.

4. In the orbitofrontal cortex in Tier 2, the representation is of the value of stimuli, and actions are not represented. The value of very many different types of stimuli, events or goals are represented separately at the neuronal level, providing the basis for choice between stimuli, and the selection at later stages of processing of appropriate action to obtain the chosen goal.

5. Whereas the orbitofrontal cortex in Tier 2 represents the value of stimuli (potential goals for action) on a continuous scale, an area anterior to this, medial prefrontal cortex area 10 (in Tier 3), is implicated in decision-making between stimuli, in which a selection must be made, moving beyond representation of value on a continuous scale towards a decision between goods based on their value.

6. The brain regions in which the reinforcing, and hence emotional, value of stimuli are represented interface to three main types of output system:

The first is the autonomic and endocrine system, for producing such changes as increased heart rate and release of adrenaline, which prepare the body for action.

The second type of output is to brain systems concerned with performing actions unconsciously or implicitly, in order to obtain rewards or avoid punishers. These brain systems include the basal ganglia for habit ('stimulus-response') behaviour, and the cingulate cortex for action–outcome learning. (The 'outcome' is the reward or punisher that is or is not obtained when the action is performed.)

The third type of output is to a system capable of planning many steps ahead, and for example deferring short-term rewards in order to execute a long-term plan. This system may use syntactic processing to perform the planning, and is therefore part of a linguistic system which performs explicit (conscious) processing, as described more fully in Chapter 10.

4.3 Representations of primary reinforcers, i.e. of unlearned value

Emotions can be produced by primary reinforcers. (Primary reinforcers are unlearned reinforcers, that is they are innately reinforcing.) Other, previously neutral, stimuli, such as the sight of an object, can by association learning with a primary reinforcer come to be a secondary (or learned) reinforcer, which can also produce an emotional response. For these reasons, in order to understand the neural basis of emotion it is necessary to know where in the processing systems in the brain a sensory input comes to be decoded[6] and treated by the rest of the brain (which may try to maximize or minimize its activity) as a primary reinforcer.

4.3.1 Taste

In primates, the evidence that the representation of taste is independent of its rewarding properties as far as and including the primary taste cortex is described in Chapter 5. In the secondary taste cortex, which is part of the orbitofrontal cortex, the representation is of the food reward value of the taste, in that the taste responses of neurons are modulated by hunger in devaluation experiments, and decrease to zero when the animal is satiated, and the taste is no longer rewarding (see Section 4.5.5.1 and Chapter 5). There may be some though a less complete modulation by hunger of neuronal taste responses in the amygdala (see Section 4.6), and in this sense taste reward may be less well represented in the amygdala than the orbitofrontal cortex. Water also has reward value when thirsty, and this value representation reflects neural activity in the primate including human orbitofrontal cortex (Rolls 2005b, De Araujo, Kringelbach, Rolls & McGlone 2003b, Rolls, Sienkiewicz & Yaxley 1989b, Rolls, Yaxley & Sienkiewicz 1990).

4.3.2 Smell

For olfaction, it is known that some orbitofrontal cortex olfactory neurons respond to the smell of food only when a monkey has an appetite for that food (Critchley & Rolls 1996c), and consistent results have been found in humans with functional neuroimaging (O'Doherty, Rolls, Francis, Bowtell, McGlone, Kobal, Renner & Ahne 2000, Gottfried, O'Doherty & Dolan 2003). The responses of these neurons thus reflect the reward value of these food-related olfactory stimuli.

It is not yet known in primates whether this modulation of olfactory neuronal responses occurs at earlier processing stages. However, there is evidence in humans that the primary olfactory cortical areas (including the pyriform cortex and cortico-medial amygdala region) represent the identity and intensity of olfactory stimuli, in that in a functional magnetic resonance imaging (fMRI) investigation, activation of these regions was correlated with the subjective intensity ratings but not the subjective pleasantness ratings of six odours (Rolls, Kringelbach & De Araujo 2003c). In contrast, the reward value of odours is represented in the

[6] By decoding, I mean what is made explicit in the representation. If the firing of neurons (in for example the inferior temporal visual cortex) reflects which object has been seen invariantly with respect to size, position, reward association, etc., then it can be said that representations of objects have been decoded from the sensory information reaching the retina. Although information about which object has been seen is of course present in the retinal neuronal firing, it is not made explicit at this stage of processing. Instead, local contrast over small regions of the retina is made explicit at the retinal level, in that retinal neurons have small concentric receptive fields responsive to small spots of light. If the firing of neurons in, for example, the orbitofrontal cortex reflects whether an object is currently associated with reward, then we can say that the reward value of objects has been decoded by this stage of processing. The most common way for information to be made explicit in the firing is by altering the firing rate of neurons, and any additional information that is available in the relative time of firing of different neurons is minor (Rolls & Treves 2011).

human medial orbitofrontal cortex, in that activation here was correlated with the pleasantness but not intensity ratings of six odours (Rolls, Kringelbach & De Araujo 2003c) (cf. Anderson, Christoff, Stappen, Panitz, Ghahremani, Glover, Gabrieli & Sobel (2003)), and are increased by paying attention to pleasantness but not intensity (Rolls, Grabenhorst, Margot, da Silva & Velazco 2008a). (In rats, there is some evidence that signals about hunger can influence olfactory processing as far peripherally as the olfactory bulb (Pager, Giachetti, Holley & LeMagnen 1972, Pager 1974).)

Some of these primate orbitofrontal cortex olfactory neurons may respond because odours are secondary reinforcers as a result of olfactory-to-taste association learning (Rolls, Critchley, Mason & Wakeman 1996a). Some other olfactory neurons in the orbitofrontal cortex do not alter their responses during olfactory-to-taste association learning (Critchley & Rolls 1996b), and the responses of those olfactory neurons could thus reflect information about whether the odour is a primary reinforcer. However, those neurons could also simply be representing the identity of the odour.

In humans there is some evidence that pheromone-like odours can influence behaviour, though probably not through the vomero-nasal olfactory system, which appears to be vestigial in humans (see Section 7.9). In rodents and many mammals (but not humans and Old World monkeys), signals in an accessory olfactory system which includes the vomeronasal organ and the accessory olfactory bulb could act as primary reinforcers which affect attractiveness and aggression, and act as primary reinforcers (see Section 7.9 and Wyatt (2014)).

4.3.3 Pleasant and painful touch

Experiments have been performed to investigate where in the human touch-processing system (see Figs. 4.1 and 4.2) tactile stimuli are decoded and represented in terms of their rewarding value or the pleasure they produce. In order to investigate this, Rolls, O'Doherty, Kringelbach, Francis, Bowtell & McGlone (2003d) performed functional magnetic resonance imaging (fMRI) of humans who were receiving pleasant, neutral, and painful tactile stimuli. They found that a weak but very pleasant touch of the hand with velvet produced much stronger activation of the orbitofrontal cortex than a more intense but affectively neutral touch of the hand with wood. In contrast, the pleasant stimuli produced much less activation of the primary somatosensory cortex S1 than the neutral stimuli (see Fig. 4.4). It was concluded that part of the orbitofrontal cortex is concerned with representing the positively affective aspects of somatosensory stimuli. Nearby, but separate, parts of the human orbitofrontal cortex were shown in the same series of experiments to be activated by taste and olfactory stimuli. Thus the pleasantness of tactile stimuli, which can be powerful primary reinforcers (Taira & Rolls 1996), is correlated with the activity of a part of the orbitofrontal cortex. This part of the orbitofrontal cortex probably receives its somatosensory inputs via the somatosensory cortex both via direct projections and via the insula (Mesulam & Mufson 1982a, Mesulam & Mufson 1982b). In contrast, the pleasantness of a tactile stimulus does not appear to be represented explicitly in the somatosensory cortex. The indication thus is that only certain parts of the somatosensory input, which reflect its pleasantness, are passed on (perhaps after appropriate processing) to the orbitofrontal cortex by the somatosensory cortical areas. It was also notable that the pleasant touch activated the most anterior (pregenual) part of the anterior cingulate cortex (see Fig. 4.4). In another study, it was found that pleasant, light, slow, rubbing touch to the forearm, which activates C tactile afferent fibres, produces activation in the human orbitofrontal cortex (McCabe, Rolls, Bilderbeck & McGlone 2008, Rolls 2010c, Rolls 2013e).

Warm touch can be pleasant, and cold touch can be unpleasant. In an fMRI investigation we showed that the mid-orbitofrontal and pregenual cingulate cortex have activations that are correlated with the subjective pleasantness ratings made to warm (41°C) and cold (12°C)

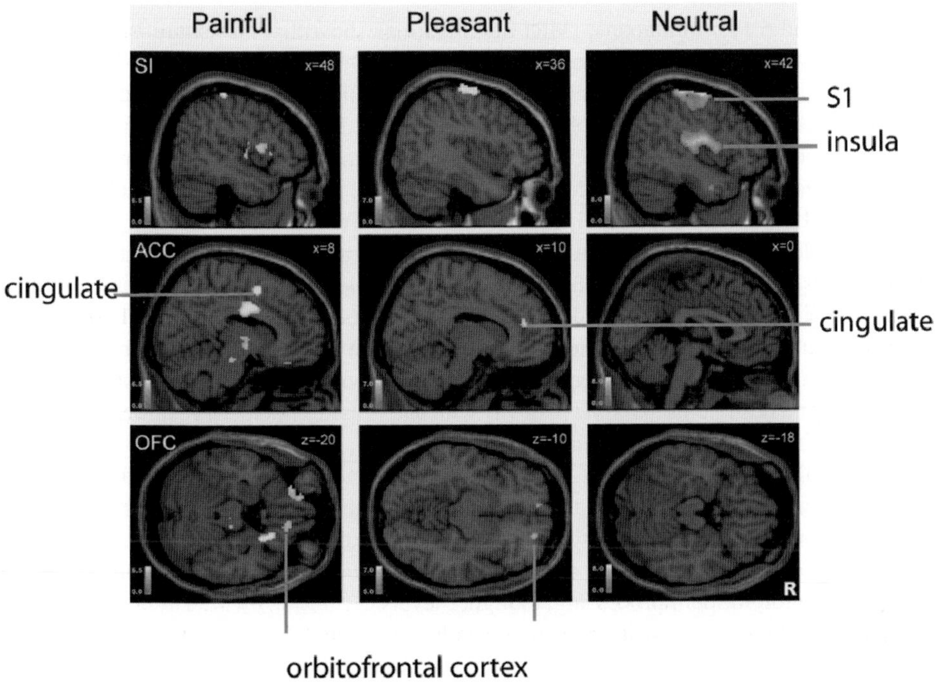

Fig. 4.4 Brain activation to painful, pleasant and neutral touch of the human brain. The top row shows strongest activation of the somatosensory cortex S1/insula by the neutral touch, on sagittal sections (parallel to the midline). The middle row shows activation of the most anterior part of the anterior cingulate cortex by the pleasant touch, and of a more posterior part by the painful touch, on sagittal sections. The bottom row shows activation of the orbitofrontal cortex by the pleasant and by the painful touch, on axial sections (in the horizontal plane). The activations were thresholded at $p<0.0001$ to show the extent of the activations. (See colour plates section.) (This material was originally published in *Cerebral Cortex* 13 (3) Representations of Pleasant and Painful Touch in the Human Orbitofrontal and Cingulate Cortices, pp. 308–17 by E.T. Rolls, J. O'Doherty, M.L. Kringelbach, S. Francis, R. Bowtell and F. McGlone, and has been reproduced by permission of Oxford University Press http://cercor.oxfordjournals.org/content/13/3/308.full.)

stimuli, and combinations of warm and cold stimuli, applied to the hand (Rolls, Grabenhorst & Parris 2008b) (Fig. 4.69 on page 205). Activations in the lateral and some more anterior parts of the orbitofrontal cortex were correlated with the unpleasantness of the stimuli. In contrast, activations in the somatosensory cortex and ventral posterior insula were correlated with the intensity but not the pleasantness of the thermal stimuli. A principle thus appears to be that processing related to the affective value and associated subjective emotional experience of thermal somatosensory stimuli that are important for survival is performed in different brain areas to those where activations are related to sensory properties of the stimuli such as their intensity (Rolls et al. 2008b), consistent with findings in other sensory modalities in primates including humans.

Oral texture can also be pleasant and rewarding. For example, the pleasantness of the fat texture of ice cream, and of cream with strawberries, can be pleasant, with the evolutionary foundation that fat is a source of high energy. Neurons in the primate orbitofrontal cortex respond selectively to the slick oily texture of fat, and represent its reward value in that feeding to satiety with cream selectively reduces to zero the neuronal response to fat (Rolls, Critchley, Browning, Hernadi & Lenard 1999a, Verhagen, Rolls & Kadohisa 2003, Rolls 2011e) (see

Figs. 5.16 and 5.17). In humans, fMRI investigations show that fat texture is represented in areas such as the taste insula and orbitofrontal cortex (De Araujo & Rolls 2004), and that the subjective pleasantness of oral fat texture reflects activations in the orbitofrontal and anterior cingulate cortex (Grabenhorst, Rolls, Parris & D'Souza 2010b).

The issue of where the reinforcing properties of activation of the pain pathways is decoded is complex (Melzack & Wall 1996, Perl & Kruger 1996, Kobayashi 2012, Brodersen, Wiech, Lomakina, Lin, Buhmann, Bingel, Ploner, Stephan & Tracey 2012, Wiech & Tracey 2013). There are clearly specialized peripheral nerves (including C fibres, with some activated via VR1 or capsaicin receptors) that convey painful stimulation to the central nervous system, and perhaps two main brain systems (Julius & Basbaum 2001, Basbaum & Jessell 2013). One is a spino-parabrachial pathway which originates from the superficial dorsal horn in the spinal cord and may have preferential access to brain areas involved in affect such as the amygdala, and the second is the spinothalamic pathway which distributes nociceptive information to parts of the brain involved in both discrimination and affect (Basbaum & Jessell 2013). At the spinal cord level, there are reflexes that enable a limb to be withdrawn from painful stimulation. But the essence of a reinforcer is that it should enable the probability of an arbitrary (that is any) instrumental response or action to be altered. For this learning to occur, it is probably necessary that the activity should proceed past the central gray in the brainstem, which is an important region for pain processing, to higher levels.

There appears to be a focus for pain inputs in part of area 3 of the primary somatosensory cortex, as shown by loss of pain sensation after a lesion to this region (Marshall 1951), and by activation measured in PET studies of regions in the primary and the secondary somatosensory cortex (Coghill, Talbot, Evans, Meyer, Gjedde, Bushnell & Duncan 1994). However, there is evidence that structures as recently developed as the orbitofrontal cortex of primates are important in the subjective aspects of pain, for patients with lesions or disconnection of the orbitofrontal cortex may say that they can identify the input as painful, but that it does not produce the same affective feeling as previously (Freeman & Watts 1950, Melzack & Wall 1996). In the fMRI study of Rolls, O'Doherty, Kringelbach, Francis, Bowtell & McGlone (2003d) painful inputs (produced by a stylus) were also applied to the hand, and we found that the orbitofrontal cortex was more strongly activated by the painful touch than by the neutral touch, whereas the somatosensory cortex was relatively more activated by the physically heavier neutral touch (see Fig. 4.4). This provides evidence that negative (see also Petrovich, Petersson, Ghatan, Ston-Elander & Ingvar (2000)) as well as positive aspects of affective touch are especially represented in the orbitofrontal cortex. In our study, as in many studies (Vogt & Sikes 2000), a part of the anterior cingulate cortex in or near to the cingulate motor area was also activated by pain (see example in Fig. 4.4 and Section 4.7). In another study, multivariate analyses were performed to investigate which voxels of fMRI activations produced by pain-related laser stimuli could predict by decoding whether a stimulus had been perceived as painful. It was found that activations in the primary and secondary somatosensory cortex, anterior insula, dorsolateral and ventrolateral prefrontal cortex, and orbitofrontal cortex were most discriminative (Brodersen et al. 2012).

4.3.4 Visual stimuli

Although most visual stimuli are not primary reinforcers, but may become secondary reinforcers as a result of stimulus–reinforcer association learning, it is possible that some visual stimuli, such as the sight of a beautiful face, of a smiling face or of an angry face, could be primary reinforcers. It has been shown that there is a population of neurons in the cortex in the anterior part of the macaque superior temporal sulcus that categorize face stimuli based on the expression on the face, not based on the identity of the face (Hasselmo, Rolls & Baylis 1989a) (see Section 4.4.5). Thus it is possible that the reinforcing value of face expression could be being decoded by this stage of cortical processing (which is at the same stage approximately as the inferior temporal visual cortex; see Rolls (2008b), Rolls (2011c) and Baylis, Rolls & Leonard (1987)). This cortical region projects into the amygdala, in which face-selective neurons are also found (Leonard, Rolls, Wilson & Baylis 1985). Although it is not yet known whether amygdala face-selective neurons can code for expression or reward as well as identity (Leonard, Rolls, Wilson & Baylis 1985), this does seem likely given that these amygdala neurons receive some of their inputs from the neurons in the cortex in the superior temporal sulcus.

Another population of face-selective neurons is also found in the orbitofrontal cortex (Rolls, Critchley, Browning & Inoue 2006a) (see Section 4.5.5.6), and some of these neurons by being tuned to face expression could represent the primary reinforcing value of a face. Consistent with this, orbitofrontal and cingulate cortex lesions can impair humans' ability to identify the emotional expression in a face (Hornak, Rolls & Wade 1996, Rolls 1999c, Hornak, Bramham, Rolls, Morris, O'Doherty, Bullock & Polkey 2003) (see Section 4.5.6), and the sight of a face expression which is not rewarding and signals that behaviour should be changed activates the lateral orbitofrontal cortex (Kringelbach & Rolls 2003). However, it seems likely that, in addition, at least some of the face-selective neurons in the amygdala and orbitofrontal cortex reflect the secondary reinforcing value of a face, given the role these brain regions play in stimulus–reinforcer association learning (see Sections 4.5 and 4.6).

In humans, it has been found that activation of the orbitofrontal cortex is correlated with the attractiveness of the face being viewed (O'Doherty, Winston, Critchley, Perrett, Burt & Dolan 2003b). This may be an example of a visual primary reinforcer being represented in the orbitofrontal cortex. Systems such as this may contribute to aesthetic appreciation (Rolls 2011d, Rolls 2012d, Ishizu & Zeki 2011, Ishizu & Zeki 2013, Rolls 2014b).

It is possible that some auditory stimuli can be primary reinforcers. Where the reinforcement value may be decoded is not yet known, though auditory neurons that respond to vocalization have been found in the orbitofrontal cortex (Rolls, Critchley, Browning & Inoue 2006a) and amygdala (personal observations), and may also be present in the cingulate cortex (Jurgens 2002, West & Larson 1995); and orbitofrontal and cingulate cortex lesions can impair humans' ability to identify the emotional expression in a voice (Hornak, Rolls & Wade 1996, Hornak, Bramham, Rolls, Morris, O'Doherty, Bullock & Polkey 2003) (see Section 4.5.6). Activations in the human orbitofrontal cortex have been related to consonant (pleasant) vs dissonant musical sounds (Blood, Zatorre, Bermudez & Evans 1999, Blood & Zatorre 2001), and to the resolution of harmony towards pleasant stability (Fujisawa & Cook 2011). A possible evolutionary foundation for dissonance being a primary reinforcer is that dissonant sounds may be produced by the non-linear distortion produced by overloaded vocal cords making shouting angry or warning sounds, in contrast to a soft soothing mother's lullaby.

As discussed in Chapter 3 and Section 4.6.5, novel stimuli are somewhat rewarding and in this sense act as primary reinforcers. The value of this type of reinforcer is that it encourages animals to explore new environments in which their genes might produce a fitness advantage. Neurons that respond to visual stimuli that are associated with rewards, and also to novel stimuli, have been discovered in the primate amygdala, and this evidence suggests that these neurons are involved in the primary reinforcing properties of novel stimuli (Wilson & Rolls 1993, Wilson & Rolls 2005). These neurons may provide inputs to the basal forebrain, probably cholinergic, neurons that project this information to the cerebral cortex, and probably influence arousal and synaptic modification to enhance learning when such stimuli are present (Section 4.11.5). We have also discovered that there is a population of neurons in the primate orbitofrontal cortex that responds to novel visual stimuli (Rolls,

Browning, Inoue & Hernadi 2005a), and these may perform similar functions. (To provide a strong concept about these neurons, we discovered them when a highly familiar visual image loaded into the video framestore incorrectly with a very thin gray line across the image where 2 rows had failed to load correctly, and this was sufficient to make one of these neurons fire on the first such trial only.) Consistent evidence has been found for humans (Petrides 2007).

Further examples of visual primary reinforcers are given in Section 3.2.1.4 and Table 2.1.

Given that primary reinforcers are represented in the orbitofrontal cortex, and that the rewards and punishers provide the goals for action, we should expect that gene specifications of primary reinforcers such as sweet and bitter taste, pleasant and painful touch, etc. should have a genetically specified set of connections all the way to the orbitofrontal cortex. This needs to arrange that for example sweet taste receptors have a molecular recognition mechanism that ensures that sweet taste receptors end up making connections, after many synapses through the taste system, to the correct neurons in the orbitofrontal cortex that will represent the goals for actions that action systems will try to activate by learning the correct actions to activate the reward-specific orbitofrontal cortex neurons. A start has been made on such tracing that specifies which classes of neurons (Rolls & Stringer 2000) should connect to which other classes of neurons in the olfactory system (Mombaerts 2006).

4.4 Representing potential secondary reinforcers

Many stimuli, such as the sight of an object, have no intrinsic emotional effect. They are not primary reinforcers. Yet they can come as a result of learning to have emotional significance. This type of learning is called stimulus–reinforcer association, and the association is between the sight of the neutral visual stimulus (the potential secondary reinforcer) and the primary reward or punisher (for example the taste of food, or a painful stimulus). In that both the potential secondary reinforcer and the primary reinforcer are stimuli, stimulus–reinforcer association learning is a type of stimulus–stimulus association learning.

How are the representations of objects built in the brain, and what is the form of the representation appropriate for it to provide the input stimulus in stimulus–reinforcer association learning? These issues are addressed in detail by Rolls (2008b) and Rolls (2012e), but some of the relevant issues in the present context of how stimuli should be represented if they are to be appropriate for subsequent evaluation by stimulus–reinforcer association learning brain mechanisms are described in this Section (4.4). The description of the functions of brain mechanisms that play a fundamental role in utilizing these representations for emotional learning and processing starts in Section 4.5.

4.4.1 The requirements of the representation

From an abstract, formal point of view we would want the representation of the to-be-associated stimulus, neutral before stimulus–reinforcer association learning, to have some of the following properties:

4.4.1.1 Invariance

The representation of the object should be invariant with respect to physical transforms of the object such as size (which varies with distance), position on the retina (translation invariance), and view. The reason that invariance is such an important property is that if we learned, for example, an association between one view of an object and a reward or punisher, it would be extremely unadaptive if when we saw the object again from a different view we did not have the same emotional response to it, or recognize it as a food with a good taste. We need to learn about the reward and punisher associations of objects, not of particular images with a fixed size and position on the retina. This is the fundamental reason why perceptual processing in sensory systems should proceed to the level at which objects are represented invariantly before the representation is used for emotional and motivation-related learning by stimulus–reinforcer association.

There are only exceptional circumstances in which we wish to learn, or it would be adaptive to learn, associations to stimuli represented early on in sensory processing streams, before invariant representations are computed. There are exceptional cases though, such as it being appropriate to learn an emotional response to a loud sound represented only as tones, as has been studied by LeDoux (1994, 2011) in his model system. We should realize that such cases are exceptions, and that the fundamental design principle is very different, with representations normally being at the object level before there is an interface to emotion learning systems, as described in the work considered below and elsewhere (e.g. Rolls (1986a, 1986b, 1990b, 1999a, 2005b)).

While the example taken has been from vision, the same is true for other modalities. For example, in audition, we would want to make the same emotional decoding to the word 'Fire' independently of whether we hear it spoken (with extremely different pitches) by a child, by a woman, or by a man. This could not be decoded without high-level cortical processing, emphasizing the point that normally we need to have emotional responses to stimuli decoded correctly to the level where an object has been made explicit in the representation.

The capacity for view-invariant representation of objects may be especially well developed in primates, as implied for example by the great development in primates of the parts of the temporal lobe concerned with vision (inferior temporal visual cortex, cortex in the superior temporal sulcus, etc., see Sections 4.4.2 and 4.4.4).

The issue then arises of the organization of vision in non-primates, and whether view-invariant representations are formed when there is a much less well-developed temporal lobe. It may be that for many objects, a sufficiently good representation of objects which is effectively view-invariant can be formed without explicitly computing a view-invariant representation. Take for example the representation of a small fruit such as a raspberry. The nature of this object is that it can be recognized from almost any viewing angle based on the presence of three simple features, (two-dimensional) shape, surface texture, and colour. [Moreover, once one has been identified by, for example, taste, there are likely to be others present locally, and serial feeding (concentrating on one type of food, then switching to another) may take advantage of this.] Thus much behaviour towards objects may take place based on the presence of a simple list of identifying features, rather than by computing true view-invariant representations of objects that look different from different angles (see also Rolls & Deco (2002) Section 8.2.1 and Rolls (2008b)). The sophisticated mechanism present in the primate temporal lobe for computing invariant representations of objects may be associated with the evolution of hands, tool use, and stereoscopic vision, and the necessity to recognize and manipulate objects from different angles to make artefacts. At a slightly simpler level, primates often eat more than 100 different types of food in a day, and the ability to perform view-invariant representations of large numbers of small objects is clearly adaptive in this situation too.

It is certainly of interest that apparently quite complex behaviour, including food selection in birds and insects, may be based on quite simple computational processes, such as in this case object identification based on a list of simple features. We should always be cautious about inferring more complex substrates for behaviour than is really necessary given the capacities. Part of the value of neurophysiological investigation of the primate temporal cortex is that it shows that view-invariant representations are actually computed, even for objects that look very different from different viewing angles (see Section 4.4.2 and Rolls (2008b, 2012e)).

4.4.1.2 Generalization

If we learn an emotional response to an object, we usually want to generalize the emotional response to other similar objects. An example might be the sight of a pin, which, after stimulus–reinforcer association learning, would generalize to the shape of other similar sharp-pointed objects such as a pencil, a pen, etc. Generalization occurs most easily if each object is represented by a population of neurons firing, each perhaps reflecting partly different properties of the object. Then if the object alters a little, in that some of its features change, there will still be sufficient similarity of the representation for it to be reasonably correlated with the original representation.

The way in which generalization occurs in the types of neuronal network found in the brain, and the nature of the representation needed, have been described by Rolls & Treves (1998) and Rolls (2008b). A synopsis of some of the key ideas as they apply most directly to pattern associators, which are types of network involved in learning about which environmental stimuli are associated with reward or with punishment, is provided in Appendix A. The approach is introduced in Fig. 4.5. The unconditioned or primary reinforcer activates the neuron shown (one of many) by unmodifiable synaptic connections (only one of which is drawn in Fig. 4.5). The to-be-conditioned stimulus activates the neuron through a population of modifiable synapses. The association is learned by strengthening those synapses from active conditioned stimulus input axons when the postsynaptic neuron is activated by the primary reinforcer. This is known as the Hebb learning rule (after D. O. Hebb, who in 1949 envisaged a synaptic learning rule of this general form). Later, when only the conditioned stimulus is presented, it activates the postsynaptic neuron through the modified synapses, producing the same firing as that originally produced by the unconditioned stimulus. If the conditioned stimulus is represented by the firing of a set of axons, then we can think of this as a vector. In the same way, we can think of the synaptic weights as another vector. If the input vector matches the weight vector, then the maximal activation of the neuron is produced. If the input vector uses distributed encoding (with perhaps each axon reflecting the presence of one or several features of the object), then a similar vector of firing will represent a similar object. Because many of the strengthened synapses activated by the original stimulus will also be activated by the similar stimulus, the similar stimulus will produce activation of the neuron that is similar to that produced by the original conditioned stimulus. The neuron can thus be thought of as computing the similarity of input patterns of firing, and it is this which results in good generalization (see Appendix A).

This consideration leads to the suggestion that in order to enable good generalization to occur, the to-be-conditioned stimulus, i.e. the potential secondary reinforcer, should be represented with a distributed representation (see further Rolls & Treves (2011)). If, in contrast to a distributed representation, there was a local representation (in which a single neuron would be so specifically tuned that it carried all the information about which stimulus was present), then generalization would be much more difficult. If one learned an association to a single neuron firing that represented the object, then any small alteration of the stimulus would lead to another neuron firing (so that small perceptual differences between stimuli could be represented), and there would be no generalization.

4.4.1.3 Graceful degradation

If there is minor damage to the nervous system, for example if some neurons die or some synapses are lost, there is no catastrophic change in performance. Instead, as the damage becomes more and more major, there is generally a gradual decline in the performance of the function affected. This is known as graceful degradation (and is a form of fault tolerance). Graceful degradation is a simple property of neural networks that use distributed

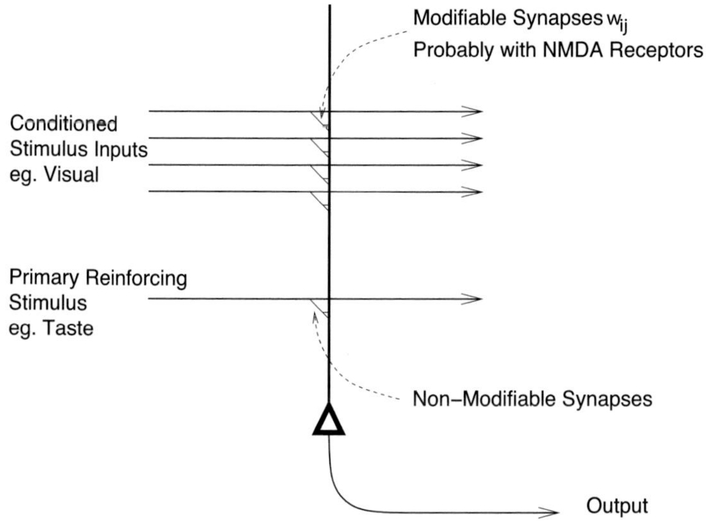

Fig. 4.5 Pattern association between a primary reinforcer, such as the taste of food, which activates neurons through non-modifiable synapses, and a potential secondary reinforcer, such as the sight of food, which has modifiable synapses on to the same neurons. Such a mechanism appears to be implemented in the amygdala and orbitofrontal cortex. (Homosynaptic) long-term depression (see Appendix 1) in a pattern associator in the amygdala could account for the habituating responses to novel visual stimuli which are not associated with primary reinforcers.

representations. It arises in a very similar way to generalization. Because each object is represented by an ensemble (or vector) of neuronal activity, if a few of the input axons or the synapses are damaged, then the remainder of the input axons and synapses can still produce activation of the neuron that approximates the correct activation. [As explained in Appendix A and by Rolls & Treves (1998) and Rolls (2008b), the operation performed by a neuron may be thought of as computing the inner or dot product of the input firing rate vector of neuronal activity and the synaptic weight vector. The result is a scalar value, the activation of the neuron. The dot product effectively measures the similarity of the input firing-rate vector and the stored synaptic-weight vector. Provided that the two vectors use distributed representations, then graceful degradation will occur.] Given that the output of the network is produced in practice not by a single neuron but by a population of neurons, loss of a few output neurons (which of course provide the input to the next stage) does not produce catastrophic degradation either (see further Rolls & Treves (1998), Rolls (2008b), and Appendix A).

4.4.1.4 High capacity

We would like the object representation to convey much information, that is to be capable of representing separately (discriminating between) many different objects. At the same time, we would like this high capacity representation to be readable by a pattern associator of the type just described, which reads out the information from the representation using a dot product operation. It turns out that this can be achieved by a distributed representation of the type found in the brain (Rolls 2008b, Franco, Rolls, Aggelopoulos & Treves 2004, Franco, Rolls, Aggelopoulos & Jerez 2007, Rolls & Treves 2011).

One property of the representation is that each neuron should convey essentially independent information. The implication of this is that the number of stimuli that can be represented increases exponentially with the number of neurons in the population (because information is a log measure). Another property of the representation is that it should be readable by a simple operation such as a dot product, with each input neuron conveying an approximately similar amount of information. (This is described further in Appendix 1. The point is that a binary code would be too compact for the properties required.) It turns out that exactly the type of representation required is built for objects in the visual system, and is found elsewhere in the brain too (see Rolls & Treves (2011), Rolls & Treves (1998), Rolls (2008b), Franco, Rolls, Aggelopoulos & Treves (2004), and Aggelopoulos, Franco & Rolls (2005), and Appendix A). Another advantage of this type of representation is that a great deal of information about which object was shown can be read by taking the activity of any reasonably large subset of the population. This means that neurons in the brain do not need to have an input connection from every neuron in the sending population; and this makes the whole issue of brain wiring during development tractable (Rolls & Treves 1998, Rolls 2008b, Rolls & Stringer 2000, Rolls 2012d, Rolls 2012f).

4.4.1.5 Independence from reward value

It turns out that not only does the inferior temporal visual cortex have a representation of both faces and non-face objects with the properties described above, but also it transpires that the inferior temporal visual cortex does not contaminate its representation of objects (which must be used for many different functions in the brain) by having reward representations associated on to the neurons there (see Section 4.4.2). Instead, because its outputs are used for many functions, the reward value of objects is not what determines the response of inferior temporal cortex neurons. (If it did, then we might go blind to objects if they changed from being rewarding to being neutral. Exactly this change of reward value does occur if we eat a food to satiety, yet we can still see the food, learn about its location even when we are not hungry, etc.) This issue, that the inferior temporal visual cortex is the stage in the object processing stream at which objects become represented, and from which there are major inputs to other parts of the brain which do learn reward and punishment associations of objects, the orbitofrontal cortex and amygdala, is considered next. The reasons for this architectural design are also considered.

4.4.2 Objects, and not their reward and punishment associations or value, are represented in the inferior temporal visual cortex

We now consider whether associations between visual stimuli and reinforcement are learned, and stored, in the visual cortical areas that proceed from the primary visual cortex, V1, through V2, V4, and the inferior temporal visual cortex (see Figs. 4.1 and 4.2). Is the emotional or motivational valence of visual stimuli represented in these regions? A schematic diagram summarizing some of the conclusions that will be reached is shown in Fig. 4.3.

One way to answer the issue just raised is to test monkeys in a learning paradigm in which one visual stimulus is associated with reward (for example glucose taste, or fruit juice taste), and another visual stimulus is associated with an aversive taste, such as strong saline. Rolls, Judge & Sanghera (1977) performed just such an experiment and found that single neurons in the inferior temporal visual cortex did not respond differently to objects based on their reward association. To test whether a neuron might be influenced by the reward association, the monkey performed a visual discrimination task in which the reinforcement contingency could be reversed during the experiment. (That is, the visual stimulus, for example a triangle, to which the monkey had to lick to obtain a taste of fruit juice, was after the reversal associated with saline – if the monkey licked to the triangle after the reversal, he obtained mildly aversive salt solution.) An example of such an experiment is shown in Fig. 4.6. The neuron responded more to the triangle, both before reversal when it was associated with fruit juice, and after reversal, when the triangle was associated with saline. Thus the reinforcement association

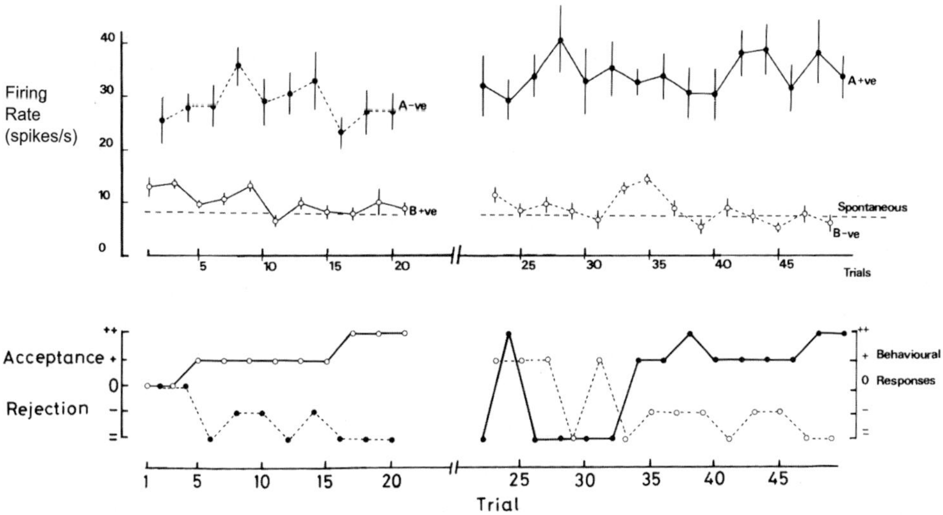

Fig. 4.6 Examples of the responses of a neuron in the inferior temporal visual cortex, showing that its responses (firing rate in spikes/s, upper panel) do not reverse when the reward association of the visual stimuli reverses. For the first 21 trials of the visual discrimination task, visual stimulus A was aversive (–ve, because if the monkey licked he obtained saline), and visual stimulus B was associated with reward (+ve, because if the monkey licked when he saw this stimulus, he obtained fruit juice). The neuron responded more to stimulus A than to stimulus B. After trial 21, the contingencies reversed (so that A was now +ve, and B –ve). The monkey learned the reversal correctly by about trial 35 (lower panel). However, the inferior temporal cortex neuron did not reverse when the reinforcement contingency reversed – it continued to respond to stimulus A after the reversal, even though the stimulus was now +ve. Thus this, and other inferior temporal cortex neurons, respond to the physical aspects of visual stimuli, and not to the stimuli based on their reinforcement association or the reinforcement contingency. (Reprinted from *Brain Research*, 130 (2), E. T. Rolls, S. J. Judge, and Manjit K. Sanghera, Activity of neurones in the inferotemporal cortex of the alert monkey, pp. 229–38, Copyright, 1997, with permission from Elsevier.)

of the visual stimuli did not alter the response to the visual stimuli, which was based on the physical properties of the stimuli (for example their shape, colour, or texture). The same was true for the other neurons recorded in this study.

This conclusion, that the responses of inferior temporal neurons during visual discriminations do not code for whether a visual stimulus is associated with reward or punishment, is also consistent with further findings (Ridley, Hester & Ettlinger 1977, Jarvis & Mishkin 1977, Gross, Bender & Gerstein 1979, Sato, Kawamura & Iwai 1980), including an investigation in which macaques search for food-related stimuli in complex visual scenes (Rolls, Aggelopoulos & Zheng 2003a). In the visual food reward search task the monkeys searched a complex natural visual scene to find and touch one of two objects in order to obtain fruit juice reward. If the wrong object was touched, the monkeys obtained mildly aversive hypertonic saline. The neurons responded to one of the selected stimuli in this experiment, and when the reward/punisher was reversed between the stimuli, the neuron continued to respond independently of whether the stimulus was associated with reward or with the punisher (Rolls, Aggelopoulos & Zheng 2003a). This independence from reward association seems to be characteristic of neurons right through the temporal visual cortical areas, and must be true in earlier cortical areas too, in that they provide the inputs to the inferior temporal visual cortex (Rolls & Deco 2002, Rolls 2008b, Rolls 2012e).

4.4.3 Why reward and punishment associations of objects are not represented early in information processing in the primate brain

The processing stream that has just been considered is that concerned with objects and faces, that is with what is being looked at. Two fundamental points about pattern association networks for stimulus–reinforcer association learning can be made from what we have considered. The first point is that sensory processing in the primate brain proceeds as far as the invariant representation of objects (invariant with respect to, for example, size, position on the retina, and even view), independently of reward vs punisher association. Why should this be, in terms of systems-level brain organization? The suggestion that is made is that the visual properties of the world about which reward associations must be learned are generally objects (for example the sight of a banana, or of an orange), and are not just raw pixels or edges, with no invariant properties, which is what is represented in the retina and the primary visual cortex (V1). The implication is that usually the sensory processing must proceed to the stage of the invariant representation of objects before it is appropriate to learn reinforcer associations. The invariance aspect is important too, for if we had different representations for an object at different places in our visual field, then if we learned when an object was at one point on the retina that it was rewarding, we would not generalize correctly to it when presented at another position on the retina. If it had previously been punishing at that retinal position, we might find the same object rewarding when at one point on the retina, and punishing when at another. This is inappropriate given the world in which we live, and in which our brain evolved, in that the most appropriate assumption is that objects have the same reinforcer association wherever they are on the retina.

The same systems-level principle of brain organization is also likely to be true in other sensory systems, such as those for touch and hearing. For example, we do not generally want to learn that a particular pure tone is associated with a reward or punisher. Instead, it might be a particular complex pattern of sounds such as a vocalization that carries a reinforcement signal, and this may be independent of the exact pitch at which it is uttered. Thus, cases in which some modulation of neuronal responses to pure tones in parts of the brain such as the medial geniculate (the thalamic relay for hearing) (LeDoux 1994, LeDoux 2011) where tonotopic tuning is found, may be rather special model systems (that is simplified systems on which to perform experiments), and may not reflect the way in which auditory-to-reinforcer pattern associations are normally learned. Similar arguments against the normal relevance of subcortical to amygdala processing for emotional stimuli, the so-called 'low-road', apply to emotional blindsight, the ability of blindsight patients with striate cortex damage to respond above chance to emotional expressions even when having no subjective experience of seeing the face (Tamietto, Pullens, de Gelder, Weiskrantz & Goebel 2012). The same may be true for touch in so far as one considers associations between objects identified by somatosensory input, and primary reinforcers. An example might be selecting a food object from a whole collection of objects in the dark.

The second point, which complements the first, is that the visual system is not provided with the appropriate primary reinforcers for such pattern-association learning, in that visual processing in the primate brain is mainly unimodal to and through the inferior temporal visual cortex (see Fig. 4.2). It is only after the inferior temporal visual cortex, when it projects to structures such as the amygdala and orbitofrontal cortex, that the appropriate convergence between visual processing pathways and pathways conveying information about primary reinforcers such as taste and touch/pain occurs (Fig. 4.2). We will later, therefore, turn our attention to the amygdala and orbitofrontal cortex, to consider whether they might be the brain regions that contain the neuronal networks for pattern associations involving primary reinforcers. We note at this stage that in order to make the results as relevant as possible to brain function and its disorders in humans, the system being described is that present in primates such as monkeys. In rats, although the organization of the amygdala may be similar, the areas that may correspond to the primate inferior temporal visual cortex and orbitofrontal cortex are less developed (Section 1.3).

4.4.4 Invariant representations of faces and objects in the inferior temporal visual cortex

4.4.4.1 Processing to the inferior temporal cortex in the primate visual system

A schematic diagram to indicate some aspects of the processing involved in object and face identification from the primary visual cortex, V1, through V2 and V4 to the posterior inferior temporal cortex (TEO) and the anterior inferior temporal cortex (TE) is shown in Fig. 4.7 (Rolls & Deco 2002, Rolls 2008b, Blumberg & Kreiman 2010, Orban 2011, Rolls 2011c, Rolls 2012e). Their approximate location on the brain of a macaque monkey is shown in Fig. 4.8, which also shows that TE has a number of different subdivisions. The different TE areas all contain visually responsive neurons, as do many of the areas within the cortex in the superior temporal sulcus (Baylis, Rolls & Leonard 1987). For the purposes of this summary, these areas will be grouped together as the anterior inferior temporal cortex (IT), except where otherwise stated. There is a host of visual areas in the inferior temporal visual cortex, with those especially relevant in providing inputs to the orbitofrontal cortex which we have studied found approximately 11 to 15 mm anterior to the interaural plane (Baylis, Rolls & Leonard 1987, Rolls 2007a, Rolls 2007f, Rolls 2008b, Rolls 2012e). For comparison, the 'middle face patch' of Tsao, Freiwald, Tootell & Livingstone (2006) was at A6, which is probably part of the posterior inferior temporal cortex (Tsao & Livingstone 2008, Rolls 2011c). Similarly, in humans there are a number of separate visual representations of faces, other body parts, and objects (Spiridon, Fischl & Kanwisher 2006, Weiner & Grill-Spector 2013), with the clustering together of neurons with similar responses influenced by the self-organizing map processes that are a result of cortical design (Rolls 2008b). Many of the studies on neurons in the inferior temporal cortex and cortex in the superior temporal sulcus have been performed with neurons that respond particularly to faces, because such neurons can be found regularly in recordings in this region, and therefore provide a good population for systematic studies (Rolls 2000c, Rolls & Deco 2002, Rolls 2004b, Rolls 2007a, Rolls 2008b, Rolls 2011c, Rolls 2012e).

4.4.4.2 Receptive field size and translation invariance

There is convergence from each small part of a region to the succeeding region (or layer in the hierarchy) in such a way that the receptive field sizes of neurons (for example 1 degree near the fovea in V1) become larger by a factor of approximately 2.5 with each succeeding stage. [The typical parafoveal receptive field sizes found would not be inconsistent with the calculated approximations of, for example, 8 deg in V4, 20 deg in TEO, and 50 deg in inferior temporal cortex (Boussaoud, Desimone & Ungerleider 1991) (see Fig. 4.7)]. Such zones of convergence would overlap continuously with each other (see Fig. 4.7). This connectivity provides part of the basis for the fact that many neurons in the temporal cortical visual areas respond to a stimulus relatively independently of where it is in their receptive field, and moreover maintain their stimulus selectivity when the stimulus appears in different parts of the visual field (Gross, Desimone, Albright & Schwartz 1985, Tovee, Rolls & Azzopardi 1994, Rolls, Aggelopoulos & Zheng 2003a). This is called translation or shift invariance. In addition to having topologically appropriate connections, it is necessary for the connections to have the appropriate synaptic weights to perform the mapping of each set of features, or object, to the same set of neurons

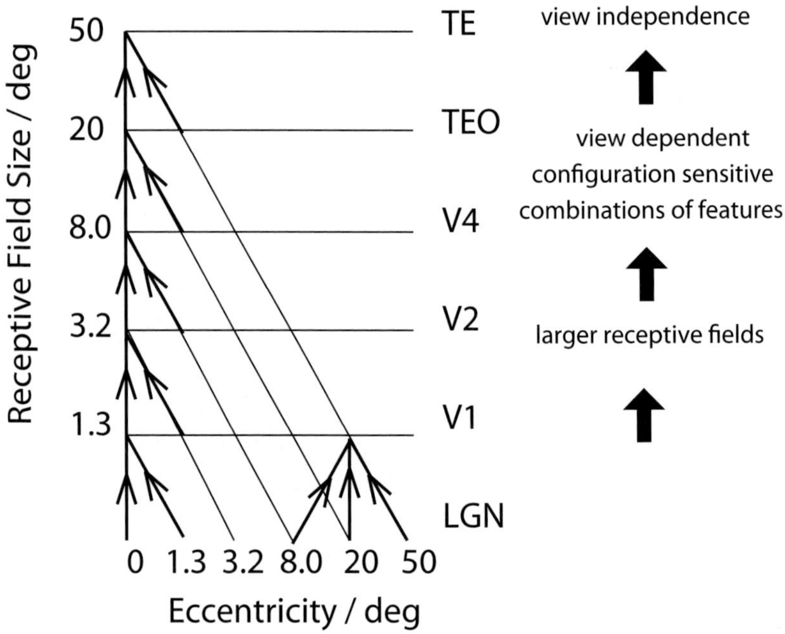

Fig. 4.7 Schematic diagram showing convergence achieved by the forward projections in the visual system, and the types of representation that may be built by competitive networks operating at each stage of the system from the primary visual cortex (V1) to the inferior temporal visual cortex (area TE) (see text). LGN, lateral geniculate nucleus. Area TEO forms the posterior inferior temporal cortex. The receptive fields in the inferior temporal visual cortex (for example in the TE areas) cross the vertical midline (not shown).

in IT. How this could be achieved is addressed in the computational neuroscience models described by Wallis & Rolls (1997), Rolls & Deco (2002), Rolls (2008b) and Rolls (2012e) which learn by making use of the spatio-temporal continuity that characterizes objects when they are viewed.

4.4.4.3 Reduced translation invariance in natural scenes, and the selection of a rewarded object

Until relatively recently, research on translation invariance considered the case in which there is only one object in the visual field. What happens in a cluttered, natural, environment? Do all objects that can activate an inferior temporal neuron do so whenever they are anywhere within the large receptive fields of inferior temporal neurons? If so, the output of the visual system might be confusing for structures that receive inputs from the temporal cortical visual areas (see Fig. 4.9). If one of the objects in the visual field was associated with reward, and another with punishment, would the output of the inferior temporal visual cortex to emotion-related brain systems be an amalgam of both stimuli? If so, how would we be able to choose between the stimuli, and have an emotional response to one but not perhaps the other, and select one for action and not the other?

To investigate how information is passed from the inferior temporal cortex (IT) to other brain regions to enable stimuli to be selected from natural scenes for action, Rolls, Aggelopoulos & Zheng (2003a) analysed the responses of single and simultaneously recorded IT neurons to stimuli presented in complex natural backgrounds. In one situation, a visual fixation task was performed in which the monkey fixated at different distances from the effective stimulus.

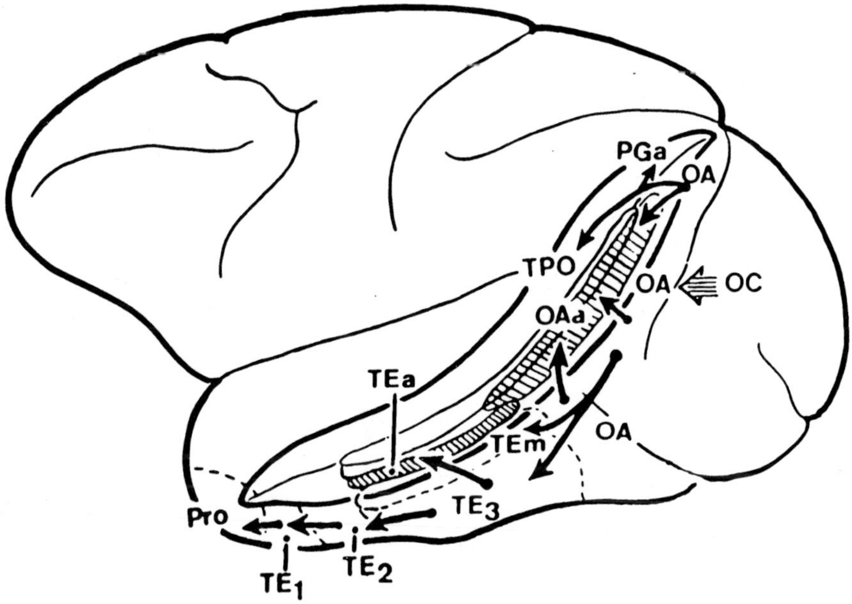

Fig. 4.8 Lateral view of the macaque brain (left hemisphere) showing the different architectonic areas (e.g. TEm, TPO) in and bordering the anterior part of the superior temporal sulcus (STS) of the macaque (see text).

In another situation the monkey had to search for two objects on a screen, and a touch of one object was rewarded with juice, and of another object was punished with saline (see Fig. 4.9). In both situations neuronal responses to the effective stimuli for the neurons were compared when the objects were presented in the natural scene or on a plain background. It was found that the overall response of the neuron to objects was sometimes somewhat reduced when they were presented in natural scenes, though the selectivity of the neurons remained. However, the main finding was that the magnitudes of the responses of the neurons typically became much less in the real scene the further the monkey fixated in the scene away from the object (see Fig. 4.10). Results that are consistent have been described by Sheinberg & Logothetis (2001). It is proposed that this reduced translation invariance in natural scenes helps an unambiguous representation of an object which may be the target for action to be passed to the brain regions that receive from the primate inferior temporal visual cortex. It helps with the binding problem, by reducing in natural scenes the effective receptive field of inferior temporal cortex neurons to approximately the size of an object in the scene. The computational utility and basis for this is considered by Rolls & Deco (2002), Trappenberg, Rolls & Stringer (2002), Deco & Rolls (2004), Aggelopoulos & Rolls (2005) and Rolls & Deco (2006), and includes an advantage for what is at the fovea because of the large cortical magnification of the fovea, and shunting interactions between representations weighted by how far they are from the fovea.

These findings suggest that the principle of providing strong weight to whatever is close to the fovea is an important principle governing the operation of the inferior temporal visual cortex, and in general of the output of the visual system in natural environments. This principle of operation is very important in interfacing the visual system to action systems, because the

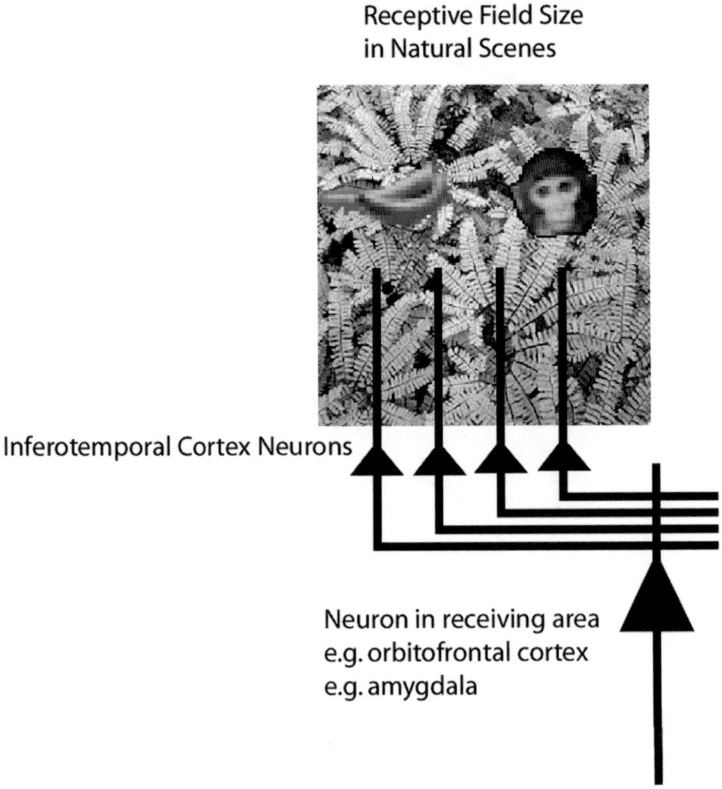

Fig. 4.9 Objects shown in a natural scene, in which the task was to search for and touch one of the stimuli. The objects in the task as run were smaller. The diagram shows that if the receptive fields of inferior temporal cortex neurons are large in natural scenes with multiple objects (in this scene, bananas and a face), then any receiving neuron in structures such as the orbitofrontal cortex and amygdala would receive information from many stimuli in the field of view, and would not be able to provide evidence about each of the stimuli separately.

effective stimulus in making inferior temporal cortex neurons fire is in natural scenes usually on or close to the fovea. This means that the spatial coordinates of where the object is in the scene do not have to be represented in the inferior temporal visual cortex, nor passed from it to the action selection system, as the latter can assume that the object making IT neurons fire is close to the fovea in natural scenes. Thus the position in visual space being fixated provides part of the interface between sensory representations of objects and their coordinates as targets for actions in the world. The small receptive fields of IT neurons in natural scenes make this possible. Moreover, it is now known that asymmetries in the receptive fields of inferior temporal cortex neurons become evident in complex natural cluttered scenes, and this means that there is some information about where a particular object is with respect to the fovea (Aggelopoulos & Rolls 2005, Rolls 2012e). In addition, local, egocentric, processing implemented in the dorsal visual processing stream using e.g. stereodisparity may be used to guide action towards reward-associated objects (Rolls & Deco 2002).

The reduced receptive field size in complex natural scenes also enables emotions to be selective to just what is being fixated, because this is the information that is transmitted by the firing of anterior inferior temporal cortex neurons to structures such as the orbitofrontal cortex and amygdala.

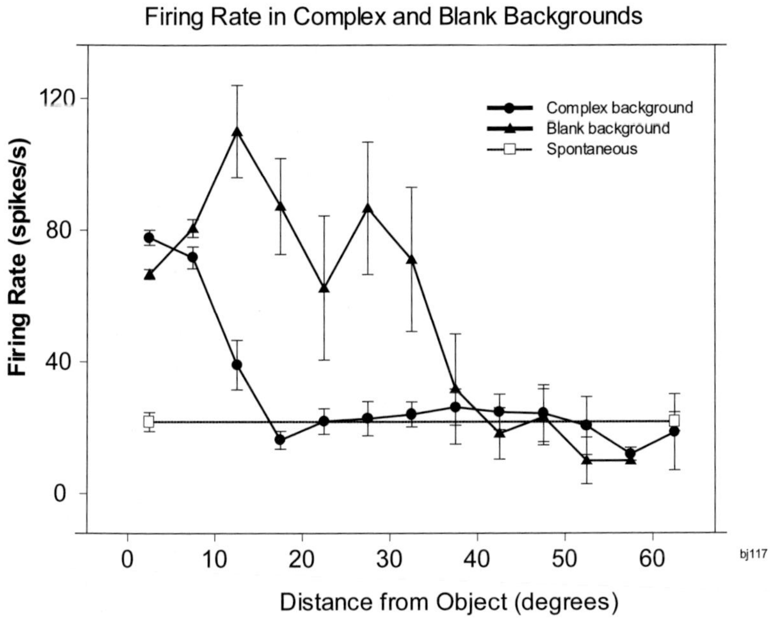

Fig. 4.10 Firing of a temporal cortex neuron to an effective stimulus presented either in a blank background or in a natural scene, as a function of the angle in degrees at which the monkey was fixating away from the effective stimulus. The task was to search for and touch the stimulus. (Reproduced from E. T. Rolls, N. C. Aggelopoulos, and F. Zheng, The receptive fields of inferior temporal cortex neurons in natural scenes, *Journal of Neuroscience* 23, pp. 339–348 ©2003, Society for Neuroscience.)

4.4.4.4 Size and spatial frequency invariance

Some neurons in the inferior temporal visual cortex and cortex in the anterior part of the superior temporal sulcus (IT/STS) respond relatively independently of the size of an effective face stimulus, with a mean size invariance (to a half maximal response) of 12 times (3.5 octaves) (Rolls & Baylis 1986). This is not a property of a simple single-layer network (see Fig. 8.1 of Rolls & Deco (2002)), nor of neurons in V1, which respond best to small stimuli, with a typical size-invariance of 1.5 octaves. (Some neurons in IT/STS also respond to face stimuli that are blurred, or that are line drawn, showing that they can also map the different spatial frequencies with which objects can be represented to the same representation in IT/STS, see Rolls, Baylis & Leonard (1985).)

Some neurons in the temporal cortical visual areas actually represent the absolute size of objects such as faces independently of viewing distance (Rolls & Baylis 1986). The utility of this representation by a small population of neurons is that the absolute size of an object is a useful feature to use as an input to neurons that perform object recognition. Faces only come in certain sizes.

4.4.4.5 Combinations of features in the correct spatial configuration

Many cells in this processing stream respond to combinations of features (including objects), but not to single features presented alone, and the features must have the correct spatial arrangement. This has been shown, for example, with faces, for which it has been shown by masking out or presenting parts of the face (for example eyes, mouth, or hair) in isolation, or by jumbling the features in faces, that some cells in the cortex in IT/STS respond only if two or more features are present, and are in the correct spatial arrangement (Perrett, Rolls &

Caan 1982, Rolls, Tovee, Purcell, Stewart & Azzopardi 1994b, Rolls 2011c). Corresponding evidence has been found for non-face cells. For example, Tanaka, Saito, Fukada & Moriya (1990) showed that some posterior inferior temporal cortex neurons might only respond to the combination of an edge and a small circle if they were in the correct spatial relation to each other. Evidence consistent with the suggestion that neurons are responding to combinations of a few variables represented at the preceding stage of cortical processing is that some neurons in V2 and V4 respond to end-stopped lines, to tongues flanked by inhibitory subregions, or to combinations of colours (Rolls & Deco 2002, Rolls 2008b, Rolls 2012e). Neurons that respond to combinations of features but not to single features indicate that the system is non-linear and can operate using competitive learning (Elliffe, Rolls & Stringer 2002, Rolls 2008b, Rolls 2012e).

4.4.4.6 A view-independent representation

For recognizing and learning about objects (including faces), it is important that an output of the visual system should be not only translation- and size-invariant, but also relatively view-invariant. In an investigation of whether there are such neurons, we found that some temporal cortical neurons reliably responded differently to the faces of two different individuals independently of viewing angle (Hasselmo, Rolls, Baylis & Nalwa 1989b), although in most cases (16/18 neurons) the response was not perfectly view-independent. Mixed together in the same cortical regions there are neurons with view-dependent responses (for example Hasselmo, Rolls, Baylis & Nalwa (1989b) and Rolls & Tovee (1995)). Such neurons might respond, for example, to a view of a profile of a monkey but not to a full-face view of the same monkey (Perrett, Smith, Potter, Mistlin, Head, Milner & Jeeves 1985, Hasselmo et al. 1989b).

These findings, of view-dependent, partially view-independent, and view-independent representations in the same cortical regions are consistent with the hypothesis discussed below that view-independent representations are being built in these regions by associating together the outputs of neurons that respond to different views of the same individual. These findings also provide evidence that one output of the visual system includes representations of what is being seen, in a view-independent way that would be useful for object recognition and for learning associations about objects; and that another output is a view-based representation that would be useful in social interactions to determine whether another individual is looking at one, and for selecting details of motor responses, for which the orientation of the object with respect to the viewer is required (Rolls 2008b).

Further evidence that some neurons in the temporal cortical visual areas have object-based responses comes from a population of neurons that responds to moving faces, for example to a head undergoing ventral flexion, irrespective of whether the view of the head was full face, of either profile, or even of the back of the head, and even of whether the head was inverted which alters the local motion but not the object-based interpretation of the motion (Hasselmo, Rolls, Baylis & Nalwa 1989b, Rolls & Stringer 2007, Rolls 2011c).

There is also evidence that some neurons in the inferior temporal visual cortex have view-independent responses for objects, and these resulted from self-organizing learning occurring during natural experience of the objects without the need for training with rewards (Booth & Rolls 1998).

4.4.4.7 Distributed encoding

An important question for understanding brain function is whether a particular object (or face) is represented in the brain by the firing of one or a few gnostic (or 'grandmother') cells (Barlow 1972), or whether instead the firing of a group or ensemble of cells each with somewhat different responsiveness provides the representation. Advantages of distributed codes include generalization and graceful degradation (fault tolerance), and a potentially very

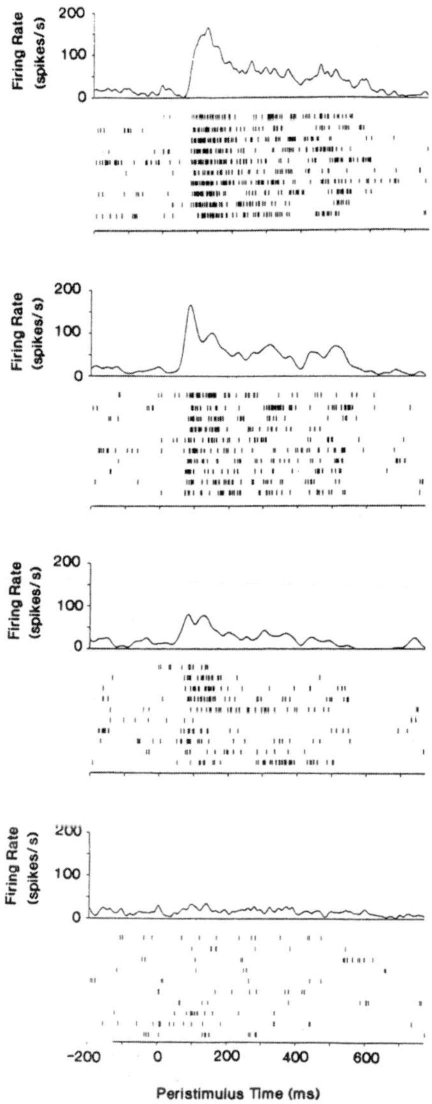

Fig. 4.11 Peristimulus time histograms and rastergrams showing the responses on different trials (originally in random order) of a face-selective neuron in the inferior temporal visual cortex to four different faces. (In the rastergrams each vertical line represents one spike from the neuron, and each row is a separate trial. Each block of the Figure is for a different face.) (Reproduced from *Journal of Neurophysiology*, 70 (2), Information encoding and the responses of single neurons in the primate temporal visual cortex, M. J. Tovee, E. T. Rolls, A. Treves, and R. P. Bellis ©1993, The American Physiological Society.)

high capacity in the number of stimuli that can be represented (that is exponential growth of capacity with the number of neurons in the representation) (Rolls & Treves 1998, Rolls 2008b, Rolls & Treves 2011). If the ensemble encoding is sparse, this provides a good input to an associative memory, for then large numbers of stimuli can be stored (see Appendix A of this book, Chapters 2 and 3 of Rolls & Treves (1998), and Rolls (2008b)). We have shown that in the inferior temporal visual cortex and cortex in the anterior part of the superior temporal sulcus (IT/STS), responses of a group of neurons, but not of a single neuron, provide evidence on which face was shown. We showed, for example, that these neurons typically respond with a graded set of firing to different faces, with firing rates from 100 spikes/s to the most effective face, to no response at all to a number of the least effective faces (Baylis, Rolls & Leonard 1985, Rolls & Tovee 1995, Rolls 2008b, Rolls & Treves 2011). In fact, the firing rate probability distribution of a single neuron to a set of stimuli is approximately exponential (Rolls & Tovee 1995, Treves, Panzeri, Rolls, Booth & Wakeman 1999, Baddeley, Abbott, Booth, Sengpiel, Freeman, Wakeman & Rolls 1997, Franco, Rolls, Aggelopoulos & Jerez 2007, Rolls 2008b, Rolls & Treves 2011). To provide examples, Fig. 4.11 shows typical firing rate changes of a single neuron on different trials to each of several different faces. This makes it clear that from the firing rate on any one trial, information is available about which stimulus was shown, and that the firing rate is graded, with a different firing rate response of the neuron to each stimulus.

The distributed nature of the encoding typical for neurons in the inferior temporal visual cortex is illustrated in Fig. 4.12, which shows that temporal cortical neurons typically responded to several members of a set of five faces, with each neuron having a different profile of responses to each face (Baylis, Rolls & Leonard 1985). It would be difficult for most of these single cells to tell which of even five faces, let alone which of hundreds of faces, had been seen. Yet across a population of such neurons, much information about the particular face that has been seen is provided, as shown below.

The single neuron selectivity or sparseness a^{S} of the activity of inferior temporal cortex neurons was 0.65 over a set of 68 stimuli including 23 faces and 45 non-face natural scenes, and a measure called the response sparseness a^{S}_{r} of the representation, in which the spontaneous rate was subtracted from the firing rate to each stimulus so that the responses of the neuron were being assessed, was 0.38 across the same set of stimuli (Rolls & Tovee 1995). [For the definition of population sparseness see Section A.1.6. For binary neurons (firing for example either at a high rate or not at all), the single neuron sparseness is the proportion of stimuli that a single neuron responds to. These definitions are described further by Franco, Rolls, Aggelopoulos & Jerez (2007), Rolls (2008b), and Rolls & Treves (2011).]

It has been possible to apply information theory to show that each neuron conveys on average approximately 0.4 bits of information about which face in a set of 20 faces has been seen (Tovee & Rolls 1995, Tovee, Rolls, Treves & Bellis 1993, Rolls, Treves, Tovee & Panzeri 1997c). If a neuron responded to only one of the faces in the set of 20, then it could convey (if noiseless) 4.6 bits of information about one of the faces (when that face was shown). If, at the other extreme, it responded to half the faces in the set, it would convey 1 bit of information about which face had been seen on any one trial. In fact, the average maximum information about the best stimulus was 1.8 bits of information. This provides good evidence not only that the representation is distributed, but also that it is a sufficiently reliable representation that useful information can be obtained from it.

The most impressive result obtained so far is that when the information available from a population of neurons about which of 20 faces has been seen is considered, the information increases approximately linearly as the number of cells in the population increases from 1 to 14 (Rolls, Treves & Tovee 1997d, Abbott, Rolls & Tovee 1996) (see Fig. 4.13). Remembering that the information in bits is a logarithmic measure, this shows that the representational capacity of this population of cells increases exponentially (see Fig. 4.14). This is the case both when an optimal, probability estimation, form of decoding of the activity of the neuronal population is used, and also when the neurally plausible dot product type of decoding is used (Fig. 4.13). (The dot product decoding assumes that what reads out the information from the population activity vector is a neuron or a set of neurons that operates just by forming the dot product of the input population vector and its synaptic weight vector – see Rolls, Treves & Tovee (1997d), and Appendix A.) By simulation of further neurons and further stimuli, we have shown that the capacity grows very impressively, approximately as shown in Fig. 4.14 (Abbott, Rolls & Tovee

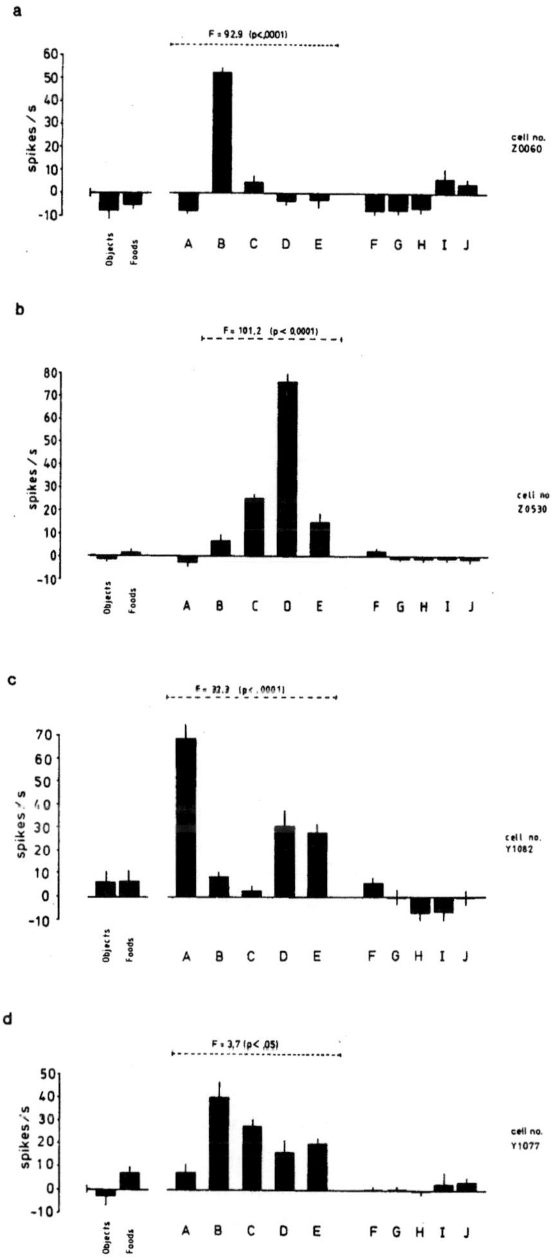

Fig. 4.12 Responses of four different temporal cortex visual neurons to a set of five faces (A–E), and, for comparison, to a wide range of non-face objects and foods. F–J are non-face stimuli. The means and standard errors of the responses computed over 8–10 trials are shown. (Reprinted from *Brain Research*, 342 (1), G. C. Baylis, E. T. Rolls, and C. M. Leonard, Selectivity between faces in the responses of a population of neurons in the cortex in the superior temporal sulcus of the monkey, pp. 91–102, Copyright, 1985, with permission from Elsevier.)

1996). The result has been replicated with simultaneously recorded neurons (Rolls, Franco,

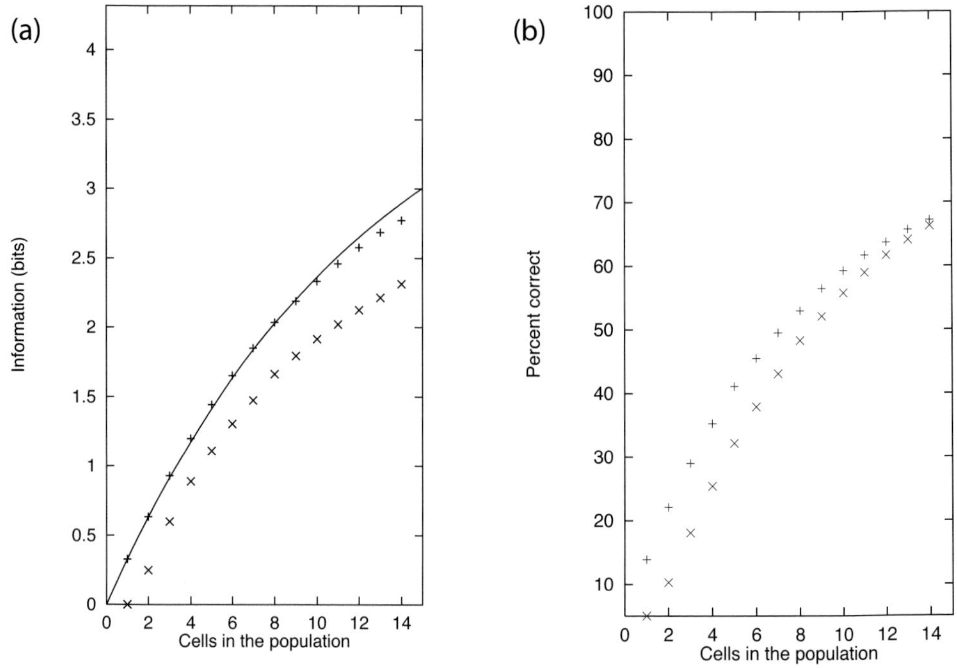

Fig. 4.13 (a) The values for the average information available in the responses of different numbers of these neurons on each trial, about which of a set of 20 face stimuli has been shown. The decoding method was Dot Product (DP, ×) or Probability Estimation (PE, +). The full line indicates the amount of information expected from populations of increasing size, when assuming random correlations within the constraint given by the ceiling (the information in the stimulus set, I = 4.32 bits). (b) The percent correct for the corresponding data to those shown in (a). (Rolls, Treves and Tovee 1997.) (Reproduced from *Experimental Brain Research*, 114 (1) pp. 149–162, The representational capacity of the distributed encoding of information provided by populations of neurons in primate temporal visual cortex, E. T. Rolls, (c) 1997, Springer Science and Business Media. With kind permission from Springer Science and Business Media.)

Aggelopoulos & Reece 2003b, Rolls, Aggelopoulos, Franco & Treves 2004). This result is exactly what would be hoped for from a distributed representation. This result is not what would be expected for local encoding, for which the number of stimuli that could be encoded would increase linearly with the number of cells. (Even if the grandmother cells were noisy, adding more replicates to increase reliability would not lead to more than a linear increase in the number of stimuli that can be encoded as a function of the number of cells.) Moreover, the encoding in the inferior temporal visual cortex about objects remains based on the spike count from each neuron, and not on the relative time of firing of each neuron or stimulus-dependent synchronization, when analysed with simultaneous single neuron recording (Franco, Rolls, Aggelopoulos & Treves 2004, Rolls, Franco, Aggelopoulos & Jerez 2006b) even in natural scenes while an attentional task is being performed (Aggelopoulos, Franco & Rolls 2005). Further, much of the information is available in short times of e.g. 20 or 50 ms (Tovee & Rolls 1995, Rolls, Franco, Aggelopoulos & Jerez 2006b), so that the receiving neuron does not need to integrate over a long time period to estimate a firing rate.

These findings provide very firm evidence that the encoding built at the end of the visual system is distributed, and that part of the power of this representation is that by receiving inputs from relatively small numbers of such neurons, neurons at the next stage of processing (for example in memory structures such as the hippocampus, amygdala, and orbitofrontal

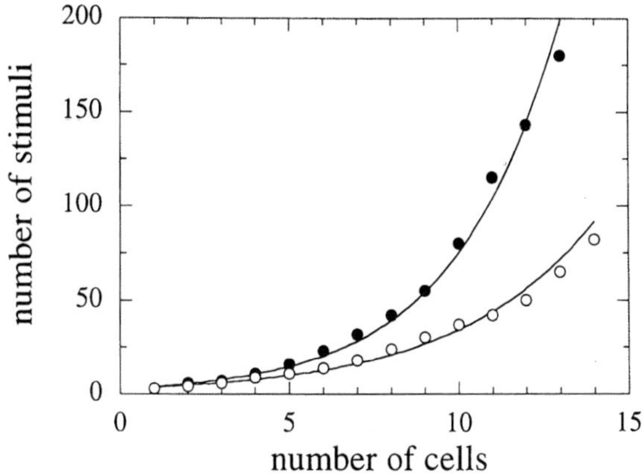

Fig. 4.14 The number of stimuli (in this case from a set of 20 faces) that are encoded in the responses of different numbers of neurons in the temporal lobe visual cortex, based on the results shown in Fig. 4.13. (Data from *Experimental Brain Research*, 114 (1) pp. 149–162, The representational capacity of the distributed encoding of information provided by populations of neurons in primate temporal visual cortex, E. T. Rolls, 1997 and from L. F. Abbott, E. T. Rolls, and M. J. Tovee, (1996). Representational capacity of face coding in monkeys, *Cerebral Cortex*, 6, pp. 498–505.)

cortex) would obtain information about which of a very great number of stimuli had been shown.

This representational capacity of neuronal populations has fundamental implications for the connectivity of the brain, for it shows that neurons need not have hundreds of thousands or millions of inputs to have available to them information about what is represented in another population of cells, but that instead the real numbers of perhaps 8,000–10,000 synapses per neuron would be adequate for them to receive considerable information from the several different sources between which this set of synapses is allocated.

It may be noted that it is unlikely that there are further processing areas beyond those described where ensemble coding changes into grandmother cell encoding. Anatomically, there does not appear to be a whole further set of visual processing areas present in the brain; and outputs from the temporal lobe visual areas such as those described are taken to limbic and related regions such as the amygdala and via the entorhinal cortex to the hippocampus (see Rolls (1994a), Rolls (2000c), Rolls & Treves (1998), Rolls (2008b) and Rolls & Stringer (2005)). Indeed, tracing this pathway onwards, we have found a population of neurons with face-selective responses in the amygdala, and in the majority of these neurons, different responses occur to different faces, with ensemble (not local) coding still being present (Leonard, Rolls, Wilson & Baylis 1985). The amygdala, in turn, projects to another structure that may be important in other behavioural responses to faces, the ventral striatum, and comparable neurons have also been found in the ventral striatum (Williams, Rolls, Leonard & Stern 1993). We have also recorded from face-responding neurons in the part of the orbitofrontal cortex that receives from the IT/STS cortex, and have found that the encoding there is also not local (Rolls, Critchley, Browning & Inoue 2006a).

There are also outputs of the inferior temporal cortex via perirhinal and parahippocampal cortical areas to medial temporal lobe structures such as the hippocampus that are involved in memory and not in emotion. Consistent with the functions of the hippocampus in episodic memory, and the need to maximize the number of memories that can be stored (Rolls 2008b, Rolls 2010b, Rolls 2013c), the representations in the hippocampus are more sparse than in the inferior temporal cortex (Rolls 2008b, Rolls & Treves 2011). In humans, representations in the medial temporal lobe have also been reported to be sparse, with a neuron for example apparently responding to Jennifer Anderson, but here again the representation is sparse distributed rather than like that of a grandmother cell (Quiroga, Kreiman, Koch & Fried 2008).

4.4.5 Face expression, gesture and view represented in a population of neurons in the cortex in the superior temporal sulcus

In addition to the population of neurons that code for face identity, which tend to have object-based representations and are in areas TEa and TEm on the ventral bank of the superior temporal sulcus, there is a separate population in the cortex in the superior temporal sulcus (e.g. area TPO) that conveys information about facial expression (Hasselmo, Rolls & Baylis 1989a) (see e.g. Fig. 4.15).

Some of the neurons in this region tend to have view-based representations (so that information is conveyed for example about whether the face is looking at one, or is looking away), and might respond to moving faces, and to facial gesture (Hasselmo, Rolls, Baylis & Nalwa 1989b). Face expression and motion of parts of the face frequently occur together and are combined to provide important social signals (Hasselmo, Rolls & Baylis 1989a, Hasselmo, Rolls, Baylis & Nalwa 1989b). This combination of face expression and face motion sensitivity in these cortical areas in the superior temporal sulcus has been confirmed (Furl, Hadj-Bouziane, Liu, Averbeck & Ungerleider 2012).

Thus information in cortical areas that project to the amygdala and orbitofrontal cortex is about face identity, and about face expression and gesture. Both types of information are important in social and emotional responses to other primates (including humans), which must be based on who the individual is as well as on the face expression or gesture being made. One output from the amygdala and orbitofrontal cortex face-selective areas (Leonard, Rolls, Wilson & Baylis 1985, Rolls, Critchley, Browning & Inoue 2006a) for this information is probably via the ventral striatum, for a small population of neurons has been found in the ventral striatum with responses selective for faces (Rolls & Williams 1987b, Williams, Rolls, Leonard & Stern 1993).

4.4.6 The brain mechanisms that build the appropriate view-invariant representations of objects required for learning emotional responses to objects, including faces

One of the main goals of this book is advancing understanding of the nature of emotion, of its functions and adaptive value in a Darwinian framework, of how it is implemented in the brain taking mainly a systems-level approach, and how emotion is integrated with decision-making. The main goal of the books by Rolls & Treves (1998), Rolls & Deco (2002), Rolls (2008b) and Rolls & Deco (2010) was to provide some of the foundations for understanding at the computational and neuronal network level how the brain performs its functions. Some of the ways in which the visual system may produce the invariant distributed representations of objects needed for inputs to the emotion-learning systems described in this book have been described by Rolls & Treves (1998), Rolls & Deco (2002), Rolls (2008b) and Rolls (2012e), and include a hierarchical feed-forward series of competitive networks using convergence from stage to stage; and the use of a modified Hebb synaptic learning rule that incorporates a short-term memory trace of previous neuronal activity to help learn the invariant properties of objects from the temporo-spatial statistics produced by the normal viewing of objects (Rolls 2008b, Rolls 2012e, Rolls 2004b, Wallis & Rolls 1997, Rolls & Milward

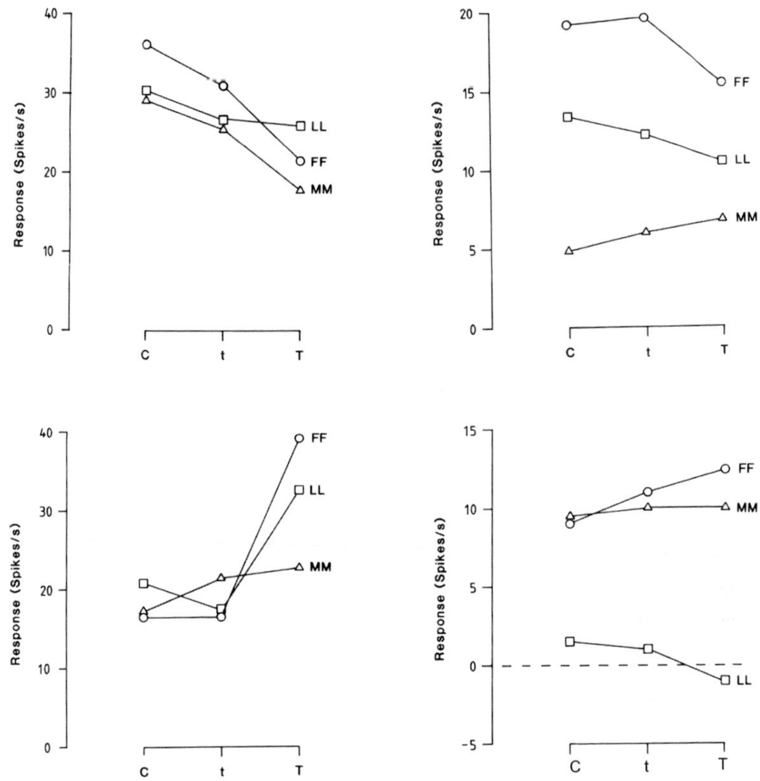

Fig. 4.15 There is a population of neurons in the cortex in the superior temporal sulcus with responses tuned to respond differently to different face expressions. The cells in the two left panels did not discriminate between individuals (faces MM, FF, and MM), but did discriminate between different expressions on the faces of those individuals (C, calm expression; t, mild threat; T, strong threat). In contrast, the cells in the right two panels responded differently to different individuals, and did not discriminate between different expressions. The neurons that discriminated between expressions were found mainly in the cortex in the fundus of the superior temporal sulcus; the neurons that discriminated between identity were in contrast found mainly in the cortex in lateral part of the ventral lip of the superior temporal sulcus (areas TEa and TEm). (Reprinted from *Behavioural Brain Research*, 32 (3), Michael E. Hasselmo, Edmund T. Rolls, and Gordon C. Baylis, The role of expression and identity in the face-selective responses of neurons in the temporal visual cortex of the monkey, pp. 203–218, Copyright, 1989, with permission from Elsevier.)

2000, Stringer & Rolls 2000, Rolls & Stringer 2001a, Elliffe, Rolls & Stringer 2002, Stringer & Rolls 2002, Trappenberg, Rolls & Stringer 2002, Deco & Rolls 2004, Stringer, Perry, Rolls & Proske 2006, Perry, Rolls & Stringer 2006, Perry, Rolls & Stringer 2010, Rolls & Stringer 2007, Stringer & Rolls 2008, Stringer, Rolls & Tromans 2007, Rolls & Stringer 2006).

4.5 The orbitofrontal cortex

4.5.1 Historical background

The prefrontal cortex has for long been implicated in emotion, though it is only relatively recently that there has been a firm scientific foundation for understanding how it functions. Let us look first at some of the background.

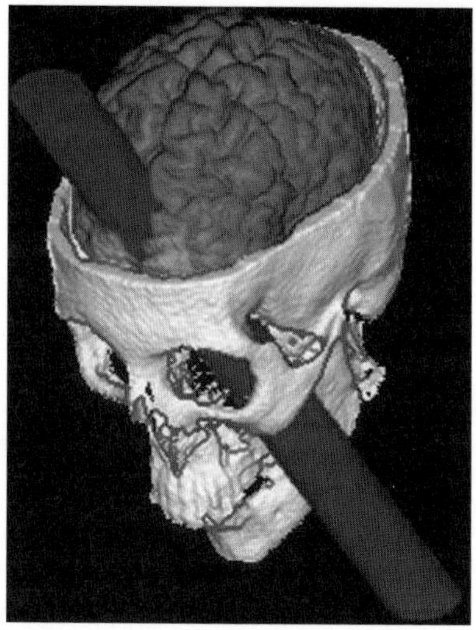

Fig. 4.16 Reconstruction of the possible entry and exit points of the tamping iron that went through Phineas Gage's frontal lobes. (From H Damasio, T Grabowski, R Frank, AM Galaburda, and AR Damasio, The return of Phineas Gage: clues about the brain from the skull of a famous patient, *Science*, 264 (5162), pp. 1102–1105 ©1994, The American Association for the Advancement of Science. Reprinted with permission from AAAS.)

4.5.1.1 Phineas Gage

One of the first indications that the prefrontal cortex is involved in emotion came from the remarkable case of Phineas Gage, who was working as a foreman for a railway development in Vermont in the USA (Harlow 1848). In 1848, he was tamping down explosives with a tamping iron when unexpectedly the tamping detonated the explosive. The tamping iron, a long bar like a crowbar approximately 3 ft 7 inches long, shot into the air and passed upwards through the front of Phineas Gage's brain (see Fig. 4.16) (Damasio, Grabowski, Frank, Galaburda & Damasio 1994). Gage survived but from that time on became a changed person. Formerly he had held responsibility as a foreman, but after the operation he became less reliable, and did not appear to be so concerned about the consequences of his actions. Moreover, in his personal life, he was described as being a changed person ("No longer Gage", short-tempered, capricious and profane). However, these personality and emotional changes took place without other general changes in Phineas Gage's intellectual abilities and intelligence. Hannah and Antonio Damasio and colleagues have reconstructed the site of the brain damage from the fractures found in the skull, and have shown that there would have been considerable damage to the lower (or ventral) part of the frontal cortex, which is where the orbitofrontal cortex is located (Damasio et al. 1994, Damasio 1994)). (It is so-called because it is just above the orbit of the eye.) The case of Phineas Gage suggested that the prefrontal cortex is involved in some way in emotion and personality, and that these functions are dissociable in the brain from many other types of function.

4.5.1.2 Prefrontal leucotomy

Another historical line of evidence implicates the frontal lobes in emotion. During an investigation of the effects of frontal lobe lesions in non-human primates on a short-term spatial memory task, Jacobsen (1936) noted that after the operation one of his animals became calmer and showed less frustration when reward was not given. Hearing of this emotional change, Moniz, a Portuguese neurosurgeon, argued that anxiety, irrational fears, and emotional hyperexcitability in humans might be treated by damage to the frontal lobes. He operated on

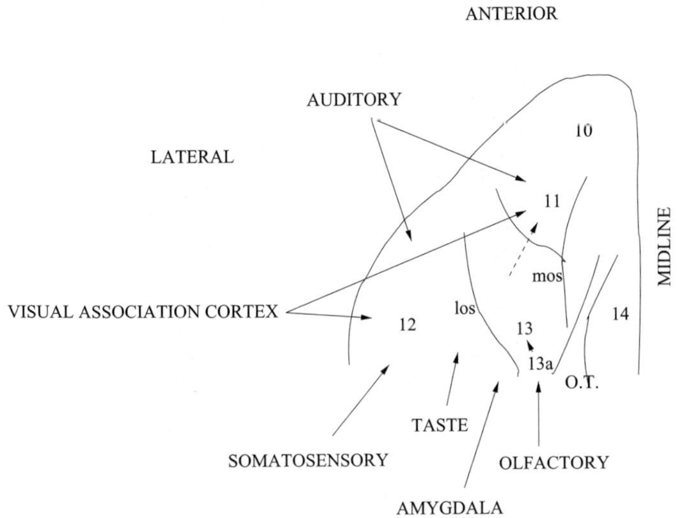

Fig. 4.17 Ventral view of the macaque orbitofrontal cortex. The midline is on the right of the diagram, and the inferior convexity is laterally, on the left. Subdivisions, and some afferents to the orbitofrontal cortex, are shown. mos, medial orbital sulcus; los, lateral orbital sulcus. (Adapted from H. Barbas and D. N. Pandya, Architecture and intrinsic connections of the prefrontal cortex in the rhesus monkey, *Journal of Comparative Neurology*, 286 (3), pp. 353–375, Copyright ©1989, Alan R. Liss, Inc.)

twenty patients and published an enthusiastic report of his findings (Moniz 1936) (see Fulton (1951)). This rapidly led to the widespread use of this surgical procedure, and more than 20,000 patients were subjected to prefrontal 'lobotomies' (in which a part of the frontal lobe was removed) or 'leucotomies' (in which some of the white matter connections of the frontal lobe were cut) of varying extent during the next 15 years. Although irrational anxiety or emotional outbursts were sometimes controlled, it was not clear that the surgery treated effectively the symptoms for which it was intended, side-effects were often apparent, and the effects were irreversible (Rylander 1948, Valenstein 1974). For these reasons these operations have been essentially discontinued. A lesson is that very careful and full assessment and follow-up of patients should be performed when a new neurosurgical (or any medical) procedure is being developed, before it is ever considered for widespread use. In relation to pain, patients who underwent a frontal lobotomy sometimes reported that after the operation they still had pain but that it no longer bothered them affectively (Freeman & Watts 1950, Melzack & Wall 1996).

4.5.2 Topology

Given this historical background, we now turn to a more systematic and fundamental consideration of how some parts of the frontal lobes are involved in emotion. The prefrontal cortex is the region of cortex that receives projections from the mediodorsal nucleus of the thalamus and is situated in front of the motor and premotor cortices (Areas 4 and 6) in the frontal lobe (see Fig. 4.1). Based on the divisions of the mediodorsal nucleus, the prefrontal cortex may be divided into three main regions (Fuster 2008). First, the magnocellular, medial (meaning towards the midline), part of the mediodorsal nucleus projects to the orbital (ventral) surface of the prefrontal cortex (which includes Areas 13 and 12) (see Fig. 4.17). It is called the orbitofrontal cortex, and is the part of the primate prefrontal cortex that appears to be primarily involved in emotion. The orbitofrontal cortex receives information from the part of the visual system concerned with forming representations of objects (the inferior temporal

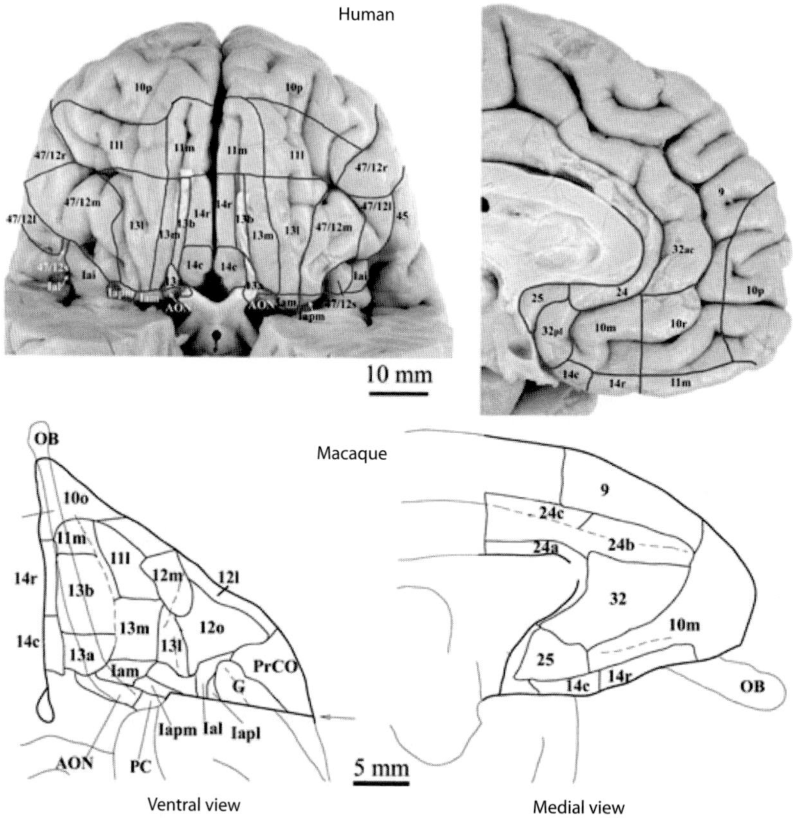

Fig. 4.18 Maps of architectonic areas in the orbitofrontal cortex and medial prefrontal cortex of humans (above) and monkeys (below). Left: ventral view. Right: medial view. The orbitofrontal cortex includes areas 13, 12 (47/12 in humans), and 11. The anterior cingulate cortex includes area 32 and the parts of area 24 shown, with area 25 named the subgenual cingulate cortex. Medial prefrontal cortex area 10 refers to the parts of area 10 shown on the medial views of the brains. AON - anterior olfactory nucleus; G - primary gustatory cortex; lai, lal, lam, lapm - subdivisions of the agranular insular cortex; OB - olfactory bulb; PC - pyriform cortex; PrCO - precentral opercular area. (Above: Adapted from Dost Ongur, Amon T. Ferry, and Joseph L. Price, Architectonic subdivision of the human orbital and medial prefrontal cortex, *Journal of Comparative Neurology*, 460 (3), pp. 425–449, Copyright ©2003, Wiley-Liss, Inc. Below: Adapted from S. T. Carmichael and J. L. Price, Architectonic subdivision of the orbital and medial prefrontal cortex in the macaque monkey, *Journal of Comparative Neurology*, 346 (3), pp. 366–402, Copyright ©1994, Wiley-Liss, Inc.)

visual cortex), and taste, olfactory, and touch (somatosensory, body sensory) inputs (see Figs. 4.1 and 4.2). Second, the parvocellular, lateral, part of the mediodorsal nucleus projects to the dorsolateral prefrontal cortex. This part of the prefrontal cortex receives inputs from the parietal cortex, and is involved in tasks such as spatial short-term memory tasks, attention, and, in humans, functions such as planning (see Fuster (2008), Shallice & Burgess (1996), Rolls & Deco (2002), Deco & Rolls (2003)). Third, the pars paralamellaris (most lateral) part of the mediodorsal nucleus projects to the frontal eye fields (Area 8) in the anterior bank of the arcuate sulcus.

The orbitofrontal cortex is considered in the rest of this section. The cortex on the orbital surface of the frontal lobe includes Area 13 caudally, Area 11 anteriorly, and Area 14 medially, and the cortex on the inferior convexity includes Area 12 (see Figs. 4.17 and 4.18, and

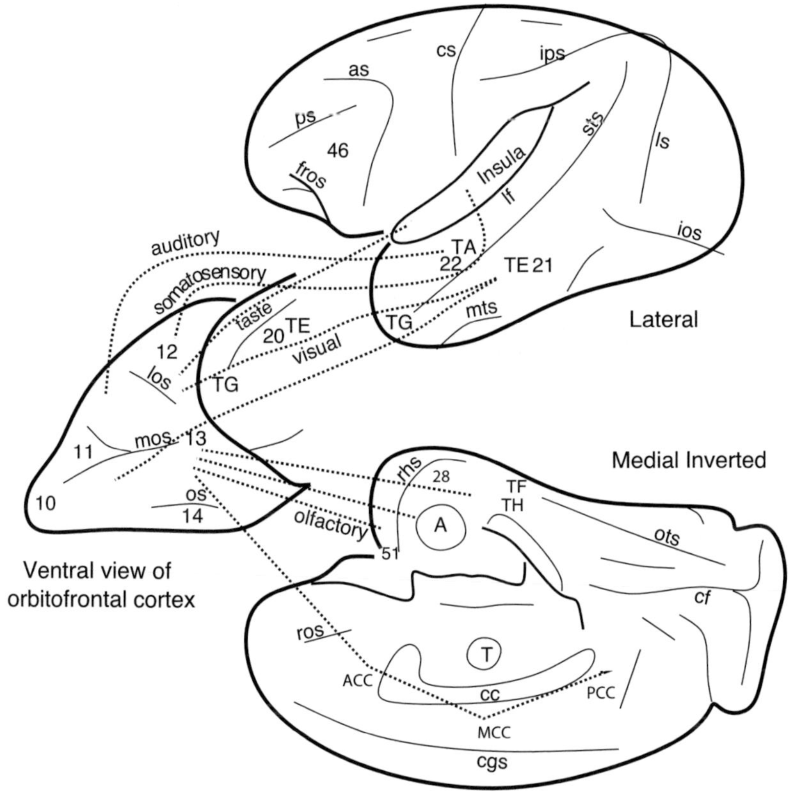

Fig. 4.19 Schematic diagram showing some of the gustatory, olfactory, and visual pathways to the orbitofrontal cortex, and some of the outputs of the orbitofrontal cortex. The secondary taste cortex and the secondary olfactory cortex are within the orbitofrontal cortex. V1, primary visual cortex. V4, visual cortical area V4. Abbreviations: as, arcuate sulcus; cc, corpus callosum; cf, calcarine fissure; cgs, cingulate sulcus; cs, central sulcus; ls, lunate sulcus; ios, inferior occipital sulcus; mos, medial orbital sulcus; os, orbital sulcus; ots, occipito-temporal sulcus; ps, principal sulcus; rhs, rhinal sulcus; sts, superior temporal sulcus; lf, lateral (or Sylvian) fissure (which has been opened to reveal the insula); A, amygdala; ACC, anterior cingulate cortex; INS, insula; MCC, mid-cingulate cortex; PCC, posterior cingulate/retrosplenial cortex; T, thalamus; TE (21), inferior temporal visual cortex; TA (22), superior temporal auditory association cortex; TF and TH, parahippocampal cortex; TG, temporal pole cortex; 12, 13, 11, orbitofrontal cortex; 28, entorhinal cortex; 51, olfactory (prepyriform and periamygdaloid) cortex.

Carmichael & Price (1994), Petrides & Pandya (1994), Ongur & Price (2000), Ongur, Ferry & Price (2003), and Kringelbach & Rolls (2004)). This brain region is poorly developed in rodents, but well developed in primates including humans. To understand the function of this brain region in humans, the majority of the studies described have therefore been performed with macaque monkeys or with humans. There is some variability in the sulcal patterns in the human orbitofrontal cortex (Chiavaras & Petrides 2001), and it is useful to take this into account in imaging studies (Kringelbach & Rolls 2004).

4.5.3 Connections

Some of the connections of the orbitofrontal cortex (Price 2006) are shown schematically in Figs. 4.19, 4.1, 4.2 and 4.17.

Rolls, Yaxley & Sienkiewicz (1990) discovered a taste area in the primate orbitofrontal cortex by showing that neurons in it respond to taste placed into the mouth, and showed that this was the secondary taste cortex in that it receives a major projection from the primary taste cortex (Baylis, Rolls & Baylis 1994). More medially, there is an olfactory area (Rolls & Baylis 1994). Anatomically, there are direct connections from the primary olfactory cortex, pyriform cortex, to area 13a of the posterior orbitofrontal cortex, which in turn has onward projections to a middle part of the orbitofrontal cortex (area 11) (Price, Carmichael, Carnes, Clugnet & Kuroda 1991, Morecraft, Geula & Mesulam 1992, Barbas 1993, Carmichael, Clugnet & Price 1994) (see Figs. 4.17 and 4.19). Visceral inputs may reach the posteromedial and lateral areas from the ventral part of the parvicellular division of the ventroposteromedial nucleus of the thalamus (VPMpc) (Carmichael & Price 1995b). Visual inputs reach the orbitofrontal cortex directly from the inferior temporal visual cortex, the cortex in the superior temporal sulcus, and the temporal pole, especially from areas TEav and the fundus and ventral bank of the superior temporal sulcus (Jones & Powell 1970, Barbas 1988, Barbas 1993, Barbas 1995, Petrides & Pandya 1988, Barbas & Pandya 1989, Seltzer & Pandya 1989, Morecraft et al. 1992, Carmichael & Price 1995b, Saleem, Kondo & Price 2008). There are corresponding auditory inputs (Barbas 1988, Barbas 1993), and somatosensory inputs from somatosensory cortical areas 1, 2 and SII in the frontal and pericentral operculum, and from the dysgranular insula area (Id) (Barbas 1988, Preuss & Goldman-Rakic 1989, Carmichael & Price 1995b, Saleem et al. 2008). The caudal orbitofrontal cortex has strong reciprocal connections with the amygdala (Price et al. 1991, Carmichael & Price 1995a, Barbas 2007). The orbitofrontal cortex also receives inputs via the mediodorsal nucleus of the thalamus, pars magnocellularis, which itself receives afferents from temporal lobe structures such as the prepyriform (olfactory) cortex, amygdala, and inferior temporal cortex (Nauta 1972, Krettek & Price 1974, Krettek & Price 1977).

This orbital network just described is somewhat separate from a medial prefrontal network that includes cingulate cortex areas 24, 32 and 24 and medial prefrontal cortex areas 10 and 14 (Saleem et al. 2008, Carmichael & Price 1995a) (see Section 4.7). This medial prefrontal system is connected with the rostral superior temporal gyrus (STGr) and the dorsal bank of the superior temporal sulcus (STSd), and with the entorhinal, parahippocampal, and cingulate/retrosplenial cortex (Saleem et al. 2008, Insausti, Amaral & Cowan 1987).

The orbitofrontal cortex projects back to temporal lobe areas such as the inferior temporal visual cortex (Saleem et al. 2008), to the amygdala (Barbas 2007) and to the anterior cingulate cortex (Carmichael & Price 1995a, Morecraft & Tanji 2009, Vogt 2009). The orbitofrontal cortex also projects to the preoptic region, lateral hypothalamus and brainstem autonomic areas such as the dorsal motor nucleus of the vagus and the nucleus of the solitary tract, to the ventral tegmental area (Van der Kooy, Koda, McGinty, Gerfen & Bloom 1984, Rempel-Clower & Barbas 1998, Price 2006), and to the head of the caudate nucleus (Kemp & Powell 1970). Further details on the cytoarchitecture and connections of the orbitofrontal cortex including routes via the entorhinal and perirhinal cortex for reward information to reach the hippocampal memory system are available (Petrides & Pandya 1994, Pandya 1996, Carmichael & Price 1994, Carmichael & Price 1995a, Carmichael & Price 1995b, Barbas 1995, Ongur & Price 2000, Ongur et al. 2003, Price 2006, Barbas 2007, Saleem et al. 2008, Mackey & Petrides 2010, Barbas, Zikopoulos & Timbie 2011, Petrides, Tomaiuolo, Yeterian & Pandya 2012, Yeterian, Pandya, Tomaiuolo & Petrides 2012).

4.5.4 Effects of damage to the orbitofrontal cortex

Damage to the caudal orbitofrontal cortex in the monkey produces emotional changes. These include reduced aggression to humans and to stimuli such as a snake and a doll, a reduced tendency to reject foods such as meat (Butter, Snyder & McDonald 1970, Butter & Snyder 1972, Butter, McDonald & Snyder 1969), and a failure to display the normal preference ranking for different foods (Baylis & Gaffan 1991). In the human, euphoria, irresponsibility, lack of affect, and impulsiveness can follow frontal lobe damage (Kolb & Whishaw 2008, Damasio 1994, Eslinger & Damasio 1985), particularly orbitofrontal cortex damage (Rolls, Hornak, Wade & McGrath 1994a, Hornak, Bramham, Rolls, Morris, O'Doherty, Bullock & Polkey 2003, Berlin, Rolls & Kischka 2004, Berlin, Rolls & Iversen 2005).

These changes that follow frontal lobe damage may be related to a failure to react normally to and learn from non-reward in a number of different situations. This failure is evident as a tendency to respond when responses are inappropriate, e.g. no longer rewarded. In particular, macaques with lesions of the orbitofrontal cortex are impaired at tasks that involve learning about which stimuli are rewarding and which are not, and especially in altering behaviour when reinforcement contingencies change. The monkeys may respond when responses are inappropriate, e.g. no longer rewarded, or may respond to a non-rewarded stimulus. For example, monkeys with orbitofrontal cortex damage are impaired on Go/NoGo task performance, in that they Go on the NoGo trials (Iversen & Mishkin 1970)[7], and in an object-reversal task in that they respond to the object that was formerly rewarded with food, and in extinction in that they continue to respond to an object that is no longer rewarded (Butter 1969, Jones & Mishkin 1972, Meunier, Bachevalier & Mishkin 1997)[8].

There is some evidence for dissociation of function within the orbitofrontal cortex, in that lesions to the inferior convexity produced Go/NoGo and object reversal deficits, whereas damage to the caudal orbitofrontal cortex, area 13, produced the extinction deficit (Rosenkilde 1979). The visual discrimination reversal learning deficit shown by monkeys with orbitofrontal cortex damage (Jones & Mishkin 1972, Baylis & Gaffan 1991, Murray & Izquierdo 2007) may be due at least in part to the tendency of these monkeys not to withhold responses to non-rewarded stimuli (Jones & Mishkin 1972) including objects that were previously rewarded during reversal (Rudebeck & Murray 2011), and including foods that are not normally accepted (Butter et al. 1969, Baylis & Gaffan 1991). Consistently, orbitofrontal cortex (but not amygdala lesions) impaired instrumental extinction (Murray & Izquierdo 2007). In a further investigation of possible dissociations, it was found that lesions of areas 11/13 (but not area 14), disrupted

[7] In a Go/NoGo task, on a Go trial one visual stimulus is shown, and a response such as licking a tube can be made to obtain a food reward; and on a NoGo trial, a different visual stimulus is shown, and no response must be made otherwise a punishment, of for example a taste of aversive saline, is obtained (Thorpe, Rolls & Maddison 1983, Rolls, Critchley, Mason & Wakeman 1996a). The task tests for stimulus–reward associations, in that one visual stimulus is associated with food reward, and the other with saline punishment if a response is made. There is a different version of a Go/NoGo task on which on NoGo trials no response must be made in order to obtain reward, and this version of the task with symmetrical reinforcement tests for whether one visual stimulus can be mapped to one behaviour, a response, and another visual stimulus to another behaviour, not responding, in order to obtain reward. Unless otherwise specified, it is the first version of the task that uses asymmetrical reinforcement and that tests for stimulus–reinforcer associations that is referred to in this book.

[8] In a visual discrimination reversal task as run in neurophysiological experiments (Thorpe, Rolls & Maddison 1983, Rolls, Critchley, Mason & Wakeman 1996a), on a trial on which one visual stimulus is shown, the S+ or positive discriminative stimulus S^D, a response such as licking a tube can be made to obtain a food reward; and on a trial on which the other visual stimulus is shown, the S– or negative discriminative stimulus S^{Δ}, no response must be made otherwise a punisher, of for example a taste of aversive saline, is obtained (Thorpe, Rolls & Maddison 1983, Rolls, Critchley, Mason & Wakeman 1996a). After good performance is obtained, the reward association is reversed, so that the visual stimulus that was formerly an S+ becomes an S–, and vice versa. Behaviour typically reverses over a number of trials, so that the new S+ become the stimulus that is worked for. The task tests for the ability to reverse stimulus–reward associations based on a changed of expected value, and if reversal occurs, shows for example that the neuron being recorded encodes the reinforcement association of the visual stimuli, and not the physical identity of visual stimuli. The improvement in reversal learning performance so that after a number of reversal a reversal can take place in as little as one trial (Thorpe, Rolls & Maddison 1983) is referred to as reversal learning set (Deco & Rolls 2005a).

the rapid updating of object value during selective satiation (Rudebeck & Murray 2011). (Selective satiation is a way of measuring reward value that relates to the discovery and much further evidence that reducing the value of a food stimulus by feeding to satiety decreases the responses of orbitofrontal cortex neurons (and activations in humans) selectively to the food with which satiety was produced, providing direct evidence for value representations in the orbitofrontal cortex (Rolls, Sienkiewicz & Yaxley 1989b, Critchley & Rolls 1996a, Kringelbach, O'Doherty, Rolls & Andrews 2003, Rolls & Grabenhorst 2008, Grabenhorst & Rolls 2011).) In contrast, lesions targeting area 14 (the far medial part of the orbitofrontal cortex), but not areas 11/13, impaired the ability of monkeys to learn to stop responding to a previously rewarded object (Rudebeck & Murray 2011). In relation to neuroeconomics, the estimation of predicted reward value as influenced by reward size, and delay to reward, or both, is impaired by orbitofrontal cortex lesions in macaques (Simmons, Minamimoto, Murray & Richmond 2010). Simpler measures, of emotional responses to an artificial snake, are impaired by both orbitofrontal cortex and amygdala lesions (Murray & Izquierdo 2007).

As the rodent appears not to have areas homologous to most areas of the primate orbitofrontal cortex (Wise 2008) (Fig. 1.1) there is little focus on it here, but rat studies are considered and compared with primate studies by Murray, Wise & Rhodes (2011).

Lesions more laterally, in for example the inferior convexity which receives from the inferior temporal visual cortex, can influence tasks in which objects must be remembered for short periods, e.g. delayed matching to sample and delayed matching to non-sample tasks (Passingham 1975, Mishkin & Manning 1978, Kowalska, Bachevalier & Mishkin 1991), and neurons in this region may help to implement this visual object short-term memory by holding the representation active during the delay period (Rosenkilde, Bauer & Fuster 1981, Wilson, O'Sclaidhe & Goldman-Rakic 1993). Whether this inferior convexity area is specifically involved in a short-term object memory is not yet clear (Passingham & Wise 2012), and a medial part of the frontal cortex may also contribute to this function (Kowalska et al. 1991). It should be noted that this short-term memory system for objects (which receives inputs from the temporal lobe visual cortical areas in which objects are represented) is different from the short-term memory system in the dorsolateral part of the prefrontal cortex, which is concerned with spatial short-term memories, consistent with its inputs from the parietal cortex (see, e.g., Williams, Rolls, Leonard & Stern (1993) but see also Deco & Rolls (2003) and Deco, Rolls & Horwitz (2004)). In any case, it is worth noting that the lateral inferior convexity part of the prefrontal cortex could be involved in a function related to short-term memory for objects. This does not exclude this part of the prefrontal cortex from, in addition, being part of the more orbitofrontal system involved in visual to reinforcer association learning and reversal.

The effects of damage to the orbitofrontal cortex in humans are described in Section 4.5.6.

4.5.5 Neurophysiology and functional neuroimaging of the orbitofrontal cortex

The hypothesis that the orbitofrontal cortex is involved in representing reward value and rapidly updating these representations (Rolls 1975, Rolls 1999a, Rolls 2000b, Rolls 2005b) has been investigated by making recordings from single neurons in the orbitofrontal cortex while monkeys performed tasks known to be impaired by damage to the orbitofrontal cortex. It has been shown that some neurons respond to primary reinforcers such as taste and touch, and represent **outcome value**; that others respond to learned secondary reinforcers, such as the sight of a rewarded visual stimulus, and thus encode **expected value**; and that the rapid learning of associations between previously neutral visual stimuli and primary reinforcers to encode expected value is reflected in the responses of orbitofrontal cortex neurons in primates (Rolls 2004c, Rolls 2004e, Rolls 2004f, Rolls 2006b). These types of neuron, and extensions

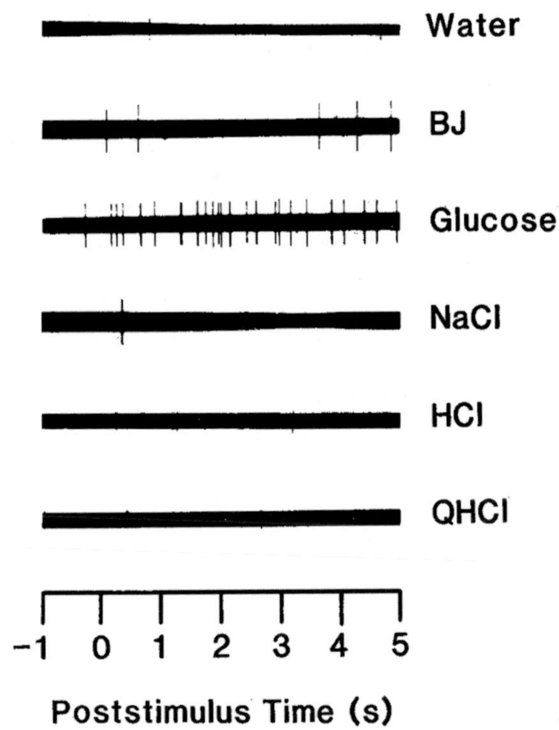

Fig. 4.20 Examples of the responses recorded from one caudolateral orbitofrontal taste cortex neuron to the six taste stimuli, water, 20% blackcurrant juice (BJ), 1 M glucose, 1 M NaCl, 0.01 M HCl, and 0.001 M quinine HCl (QHCl). The stimuli were placed in the mouth at time 0. (Reproduced from *Journal of Neurophysiology*, 64 (4), Gustatory responses of single neurons in the caudolateral orbitofrontal cortex of the macaque monkey, E. T. Rolls, S. Yaxley, Z. J. Sienkiewicz, ©1990, The American Physiological Society.)

of these concepts using functional neuroimaging in humans, are described next.

4.5.5.1 Taste and oral texture: outcome value

One of the discoveries that has helped us to understand the functions of the orbitofrontal cortex in behaviour is that it contains a major cortical representation of taste (Rolls 1997c, Rolls 2005b, Kadohisa, Rolls & Verhagen 2005b, Rolls 2008e, Rolls 2009c, Rolls 2012c, Rolls 2014a) (cf. Fig. 4.2 and Chapter 5). Given that taste can act as a primary reinforcer, that is without learning as a reward or punisher, we now have the start for a fundamental understanding of the functions of the orbitofrontal cortex in stimulus–reinforcer association learning. We now know how one class of primary reinforcer reaches and is represented in the orbitofrontal cortex in terms of its value. A representation of primary reinforcers is essential for a system that is involved in learning associations between previously neutral stimuli and primary reinforcers, e.g. between the sight of an object, and its taste.

The most direct and precise evidence that taste is represented in the primate orbitofrontal cortex comes from recording the activity of single neurons in the macaque monkey orbitofrontal cortex. It has been shown that different single neurons respond differently to the prototypical tastes sweet, salt, bitter, and sour (Rolls, Yaxley & Sienkiewicz 1990), to the 'taste' of water (Rolls, Yaxley & Sienkiewicz 1990), and to the taste of protein or umami (Rolls 2001a, Rolls 2009c) as exemplified by monosodium glutamate (Baylis & Rolls 1991)

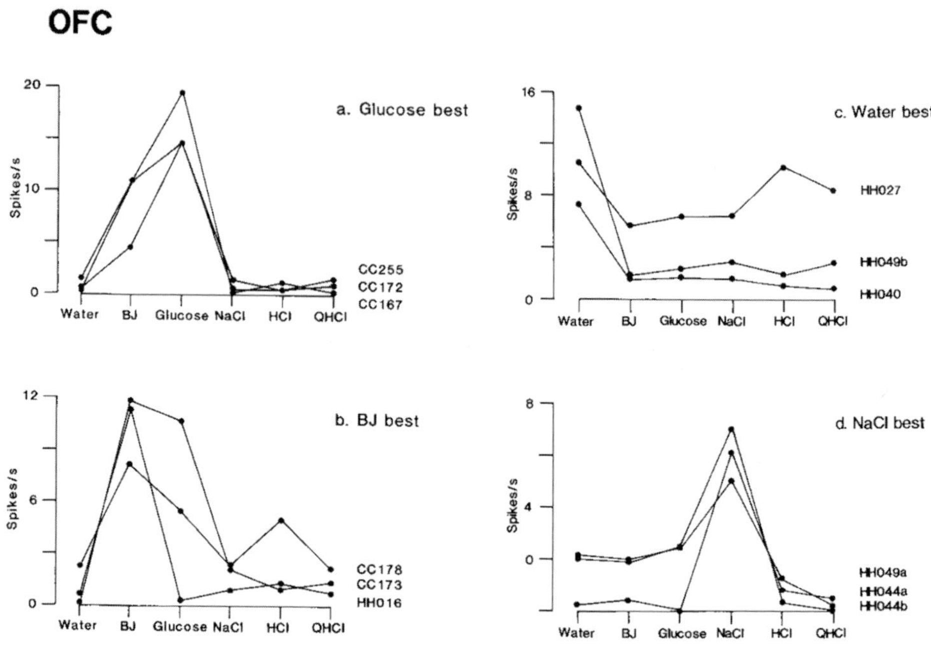

Fig. 4.21 Typical response profiles to different tastes of different orbitofrontal cortex taste neurons. Some responded best to the taste of 1 M glucose (a), to blackcurrant fruit juice (BJ) (b), to water (c), and to 0.1 M sodium chloride (NaCl) (d). HCl, 0.01 M HCl, sour; QHCl, 0.001 M quinine hydrochloride (bitter). (Reproduced from *Journal of Neurophysiology*, 64 (4), Gustatory responses of single neurons in the caudolateral orbitofrontal cortex of the macaque monkey, E. T. Rolls, S. Yaxley, Z. J. Sienkiewicz, ©1990, The American Physiological Society.)

and inosine monophosphate (Rolls, Critchley, Wakeman & Mason 1996c). Each neuron typically responds to more than one taste, as shown in Figs. 4.20 and 4.21, but each taste can be clearly identified by considering the activity of a population of taste cells (Rolls, Critchley, Verhagen & Kadohisa 2010a). This is called population encoding, and it has many very useful properties that are described in Appendix 1 and Section 4.4.4.7, and by Rolls & Treves (1998) and Rolls (2008b). In addition, other neurons are tuned to respond best to astringency (which is a flavour characteristic of tea) as exemplified by tannic acid (Critchley & Rolls 1996a). The input in this case comes through the somatosensory (touch) rather than taste pathways, so astringency is a tactile contribution to flavour. The mouth feel of fat (which contributes to the pleasantness of many foods including chocolate and ice cream) also activates a different population of primate orbitofrontal cortex neurons (see Chapter 5, Rolls, Critchley, Browning, Hernadi & Lenard (1999a), and Verhagen, Rolls & Kadohisa (2003)).

The caudolateral part of the orbitofrontal cortex has been shown anatomically to be the secondary taste cortex, in that it receives connections from the primary taste cortex just behind it in the insular/frontal opercular cortex (see Fig. 4.1) (Baylis, Rolls & Baylis 1994). This caudolateral orbitofrontal cortex region then projects on to other regions in the orbitofrontal cortex (Baylis et al. 1994), and neurons with taste responses (in what can be considered as a tertiary gustatory cortical area) can be found in many regions of the orbitofrontal cortex throughout most of its mediolateral extent (Rolls, Yaxley & Sienkiewicz 1990, Rolls & Baylis 1994, Rolls, Critchley, Wakeman & Mason 1996c, Critchley & Rolls 1996a, Rolls, Verhagen & Kadohisa 2003e, Pritchard, Schwartz & Scott 2007, Rolls 2008e, Rolls 2014a),

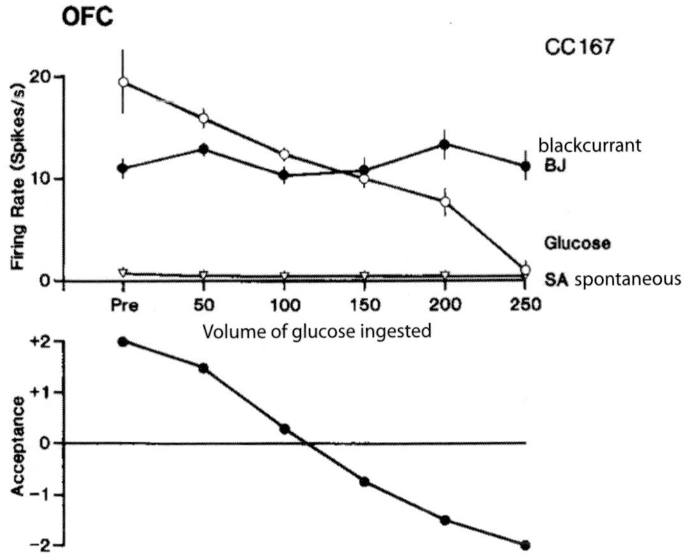

Fig. 4.22 The effect of feeding to satiety with glucose solution on the responses (rate $\pm$ s.e.m.) of a neuron in the secondary taste cortex to the taste of glucose (open circles) and of blackcurrant juice (BJ). The spontaneous firing rate is also indicated (SA). Below the neuronal response data, the behavioural measure of the acceptance or rejection of the solution on a scale from +2 (strong acceptance) to −2 (strong rejection) is shown. The solution used to feed to satiety was 20% glucose. The monkey was fed 50 ml of the solution at each stage of the experiment as indicated along the abscissa, until he was satiated as shown by whether he accepted or rejected the solution. Pre is the firing rate of the neuron before the satiety experiment started. (Reproduced from E. T. Rolls, Z. J. Sienkiewicz, and S. Yaxley, Hunger modulates the responses to gustatory stimuli of single neurons in the caudolateral orbitofrontal cortex of the macaque monkey, *Journal of Neuroscience*, 1 (1) pp. 53–60, Copyright ©1989 Society for Neuroscience.)

with taste neurons in the medial side of mid orbitofrontal cortex illustrated in Fig. 4.28 (Rolls & Baylis 1994).

There is also evidence from functional neuroimaging that taste can activate the human orbitofrontal cortex. For example, Francis, Rolls, Bowtell, McGlone, O'Doherty, Browning, Clare & Smith (1999) showed that the taste of glucose can activate the human orbitofrontal cortex, and O'Doherty, Rolls, Francis, Bowtell & McGlone (2001b) showed that the taste of glucose and salt activate nearby but separate parts of the human orbitofrontal cortex. De Araujo, Kringelbach, Rolls & Hobden (2003a) showed that umami taste (the taste of protein) as exemplified by monosodium glutamate is represented in the human orbitofrontal cortex as well as in the primary taste cortex as shown by functional magnetic resonance imaging (fMRI) (Fig. 5.14). The taste effect of monosodium glutamate (present in e.g. tomato, green vegetables, fish, and human breast milk) was enhanced in an anterior part of the orbitofrontal cortex in particular by combining it with the nucleotide inosine monophosphate (present in e.g. meat and some fish including tuna), and this provides evidence that the activations found in the orbitofrontal cortex are closely related to subjectively reported taste effects (Rolls 2009c, Rolls & Grabenhorst 2008). Small and colleagues have also described activation of the orbitofrontal cortex by taste (Small, Zald, Jones-Gotman, Zatorre, Petrides & Evans 1999, Small, Bender, Veldhuizen, Rudenga, Nachtigal & Felsted 2007).

The nature of the representation of taste in the orbitofrontal cortex is that the reward value of the taste is represented. The evidence for this is that the responses of orbitofrontal

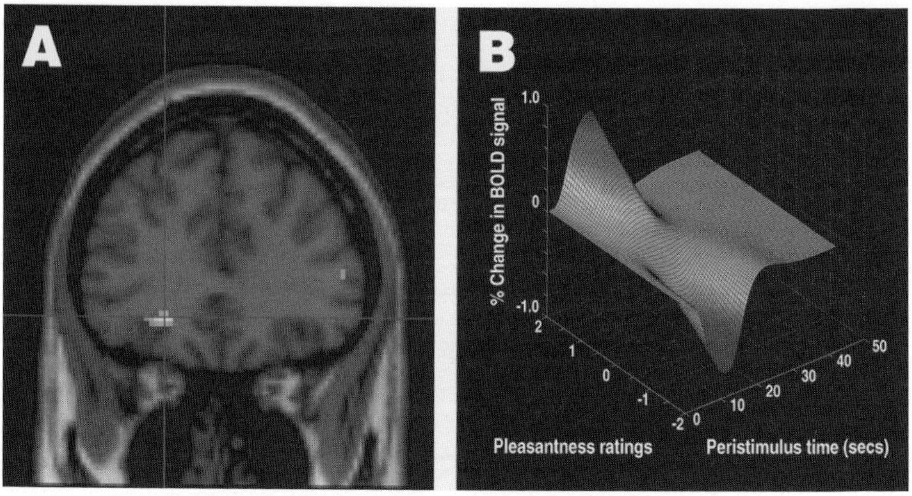

Fig. 4.23 Areas of the human orbitofrontal cortex with activations correlating with pleasantness ratings for food in the mouth. (A) Coronal section through the region of the orbitofrontal cortex from the random effects group analysis showing the peak in the left orbitofrontal cortex (Talairach co-ordinates X,Y,Z=[–22 34 –8], z-score=4.06), in which the BOLD signal in the voxels shown in yellow was significantly correlated with the subjects' subjective pleasantness ratings of the foods throughout an experiment in which the subjects were hungry and found the food pleasant, and were then fed to satiety with the food, after which the pleasantness of the food decreased to neutral or slightly unpleasant. The design was a sensory-specific satiety design, and the pleasantness of the food not eaten in the meal, and the BOLD activation in the orbitofrontal cortex, were not altered by eating the other food to satiety. The two foods were tomato juice and chocolate milk. (B) Plot of the magnitude of the fitted haemodynamic response from a representative single subject against the subjective pleasantness ratings (on a scale from –2 to +2) and peristimulus time in seconds. (See colour plates section.) (This material was originally published in *Cerebral Cortex*, 13 (10) Activation of the Human Orbitofrontal Cortex to a Liquid Food Stimulus is Correlated with its Subjective Pleasantness, pp. 1064–1071 by M.L. Kringelbach, J. O'Doherty, E.T. Rolls, and C. Andrews and has been reproduced by permission of Oxford University Press http://cercor.oxfordjournals.org/content/13/10/1064.full.)

taste neurons are modulated by hunger in just the same way as is the reward value or palatability of a taste. In particular, it has been shown that orbitofrontal cortex taste neurons stop responding to the taste of a food with which the monkey is fed to satiety, and that this parallels the decline in the acceptability of the food (see Fig. 4.22) (Rolls et al. 1989b). In contrast, the representation of taste in the primary taste cortex (Scott, Yaxley, Sienkiewicz & Rolls 1986b, Yaxley, Rolls & Sienkiewicz 1990) is not modulated by hunger (Rolls, Scott, Sienkiewicz & Yaxley 1988, Yaxley, Rolls & Sienkiewicz 1988). Thus in the primary taste cortex of primates (and at earlier stages of taste processing), the reward value of taste is not represented, and instead the identity of the taste is represented (Scott, Yan & Rolls 1995, Rolls & Scott 2003, Rolls 2014a).

Additional evidence that the reward value of food is represented in the orbitofrontal cortex is that monkeys work for electrical stimulation of the orbitofrontal cortex if they are hungry, but not if they are satiated (Mora, Avrith, Phillips & Rolls 1979, Rolls 2005b). Thus the electrical stimulation of this brain region produces reward that is equivalent to food for a hungry animal. Further evidence implicating the firing of neurons in the orbitofrontal cortex in reward is that neurons in the orbitofrontal cortex are activated from many brain-stimulation reward sites (Rolls, Burton & Mora 1980, Mora, Avrith & Rolls 1980, Rolls 2005b). Thus there is clear evidence that it is the reward value of taste that is represented in the orbitofrontal cortex, as shown by devaluation investigations.

In humans, there is evidence that the reward value, and, what can be directly reported in humans, the subjective pleasantness, of food is represented in the orbitofrontal cortex. The evidence comes from an fMRI study in which humans rated the pleasantness of the flavour of chocolate milk and tomato juice, and then ate one of these foods to satiety. It was found that the pleasantness of the flavour of the food eaten to satiety decreased, and that this decrease in pleasantness was reflected in decreased activation in the orbitofrontal cortex (Kringelbach, O'Doherty, Rolls & Andrews 2003) (see Fig. 4.23). (This was measured in a functional magnetic resonance imaging (fMRI) investigation in which the activation is measured by the blood oxygenation-level dependent (BOLD) signal was measured, which reflects increased blood flow due to increased neuronal activity (Stephan, Weiskopf, Drysdale, Robinson & Friston 2007, Rolls, Grabenhorst & Franco 2009).) Further evidence that the pleasantness of flavour is represented here is that the flavour of the food not eaten to satiety showed very little decrease, and correspondingly the activation of the orbitofrontal cortex to this food not eaten in the meal showed little decrease. The phenomenon itself is called sensory-specific satiety, is an important property of reward systems, and is described in more detail in Chapter 5. The experiment of Kringelbach, O'Doherty, Rolls & Andrews (2003) was with a whole food, but further evidence that the pleasantness of taste, or at least a stimulus very closely related to a taste, is represented in the human orbitofrontal cortex is that the orbitofrontal cortex is activated by water in the mouth when thirsty but not when satiated (De Araujo, Kringelbach, Rolls & McGlone 2003b). Thus, the neuroimaging findings with a whole food, and with water when thirsty, provide evidence that the activation to taste *per se* in the human orbitofrontal cortex is related to the subjective pleasantness or affective value of taste and flavour, that is, to *pleasure*. Further evidence on reward value for taste is that in fMRI investigations activations in the human orbitofrontal cortex are linearly related to the subjective pleasantness of the taste (Grabenhorst & Rolls 2008) (Fig. 4.44).

Consistent with these anatomical and neurophysiological findings, damage to the orbitofrontal cortex in the monkey produces altered preferences for foods, including a reduced tendency to reject foods such as meat (Butter et al. 1970, Butter & Snyder 1972, Butter et al. 1969), a failure to display the normal preference ranking for different foods (Baylis & Gaffan 1991), and disrupted the rapid updating of object value during selective satiation (Rudebeck & Murray 2011). In humans there are few published descriptions of changes of affective reactions to foods after selective damage to the orbitofrontal cortex (when damage to the olfactory tract which runs just under the orbitofrontal cortex is excluded). However, of the patients in the groups with damage in the orbitofrontal cortex that we have studied (Rolls, Hornak, Wade & McGrath 1994a, Hornak, Rolls & Wade 1996, Hornak, Bramham, Rolls, Morris, O'Doherty, Bullock & Polkey 2003, Hornak, O'Doherty, Bramham, Rolls, Morris, Bullock & Polkey 2004) and in similar patients, the most common complaint they make to the physician is about the quality of their taste and smell sensations. There are large changes in their emotional behaviour which will be described below (Section 4.5.6), but these patients do not usually actually complain about the emotional changes that others observe. Altered food preferences, often including an increased preference for sweet foods, are common in fronto-temporal dementia (Piguet 2011).

The orbitofrontal cortex also contains neurons that represent oral texture, including viscosity, fat texture, grittiness, capsaicin, and temperature, and some neurons combine this information with taste inputs, as described in Section 5.4.2.2 (Rolls, Critchley, Browning, Hernadi & Lenard 1999a, Verhagen, Rolls & Kadohisa 2003, Rolls, Verhagen & Kadohisa 2003e, Kadohisa, Rolls & Verhagen 2004, Kadohisa, Rolls & Verhagen 2005b, Rolls 2011e). By responding to different combinations of these inputs (e.g. 5.15), and by showing selective effects of reward devaluation by feeding to satiety, these neurons provide evidence about the specific reward outcome value, not about general reward value converted to a common currency, and this is crucial for enabling different actions to be learned to obtain particular goals (outcomes), and for the mechanisms of sensory-specific satiety (Chapters 5 and 9).

In conclusion, the evidence indicates that the reward value of taste is represented in the primate orbitofrontal cortex. There is also evidence that the corresponding subjective evaluation of taste, how pleasant it is, is related to activation of the orbitofrontal cortex. Thus evidence from studies of taste provide evidence that an aspect of affect is represented in the orbitofrontal cortex, and that this is not just general affect, but conveys a detailed representation of taste and its reward value, and is able to implement even the variation in the pleasantness of individual tastes as they vary during a meal, predict choice, and thus represent outcome value.

4.5.5.2 An olfactory representation in the orbitofrontal cortex of expected value

Takagi, Tanabe and colleagues (see Takagi (1991)) described single neurons in the macaque orbitofrontal cortex that were activated by odours. A ventral frontal region has been implicated in olfactory processing in humans in PET[9] and fMRI studies (Jones-Gotman & Zatorre 1988, Zatorre & Jones-Gotman 1991, Zatorre, Jones-Gotman, Evans & Meyer 1992, Rolls, Kringelbach & De Araujo 2003c).

Rolls and colleagues have analysed the rules by which orbitofrontal olfactory representations are formed and operate in primates (Rolls 2001b, Rolls & Grabenhorst 2008, Rolls 2011f). For 65% of neurons in the orbitofrontal olfactory areas, Critchley & Rolls (1996b) showed that the representation of the olfactory stimulus was independent of its association with taste reward (analysed in an olfactory discrimination task with taste reward, as some orbitofrontal cortex olfactory neurons are bimodal, with responses also to taste stimuli (Rolls & Baylis 1994)). For the remaining 35% of the neurons, the odours to which a neuron responded were influenced by the taste (glucose or saline) with which the odour was associated (Critchley & Rolls 1996b). Thus the odour representation for 35% of orbitofrontal neurons appeared to be built by olfactory-to-taste association learning, and thus by learning the neurons come to encode the *expected value* of olfactory stimuli.

This possibility that the odour representation of some primate orbitofrontal cortex olfactory neurons is built by olfactory-to-taste association learning to encode *expected value* was confirmed by reversing the taste with which an odour was associated in the reversal of an olfactory discrimination task. It was found that 73% of the sample of neurons analysed altered the way in which they responded to odour when the taste reinforcer association of the odour was reversed (Rolls, Critchley, Mason & Wakeman 1996a). Reversal was shown by 25% of the neurons (see, for example, Fig. 4.24), and 48% altered their activity in that they no longer discriminated after the reversal. These latter neurons thus respond to a particular odour only if it is associated with a taste reward, and not when it is associated with the taste of salt, a punisher. They do not respond to the other odour in the task when it is associated with reward. Thus they respond to a particular combination of an odour, and its being associated with taste reward and not a taste punisher. They may be described as *conditional olfactory-reward neurons*, and may be important in the mechanism by which stimulus–reinforcer (in this case olfactory-to-taste) reversal learning occurs (Deco & Rolls 2005a), as described in Section 4.5.7.

The olfactory to taste reversal was quite slow, both neurophysiologically and behaviourally, often requiring 20–80 trials, consistent with the need for some stability of flavour (i.e. olfactory and taste combination) representations. The relatively high proportion of olfactory neurons

[9]Positron emission tomography is a method of functional neuroimaging that uses radioactively labelled compounds to measure for example altered blood flow in an area to provide a measure of changing activity.

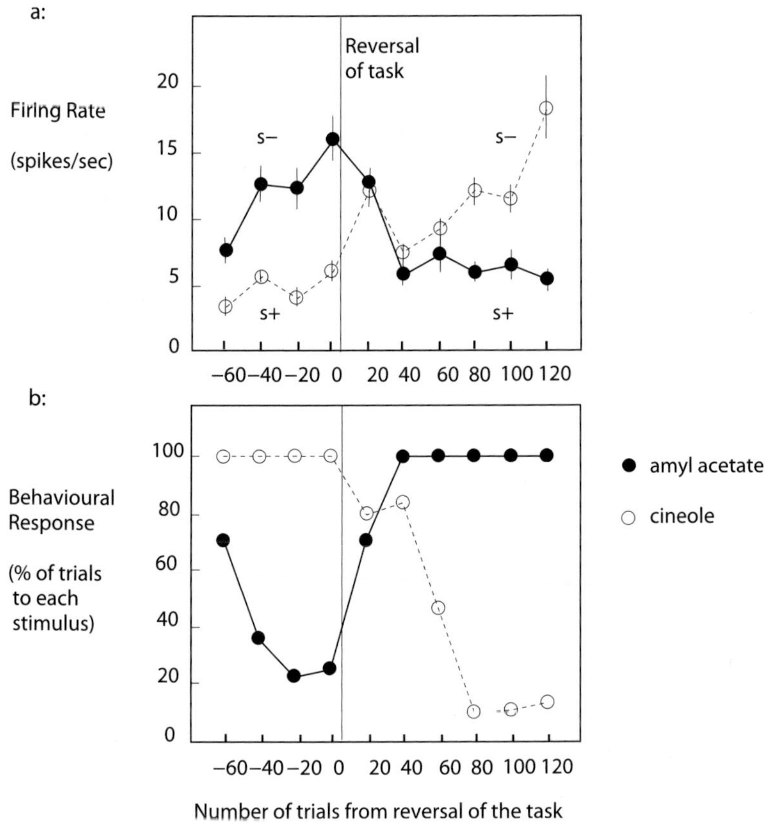

Fig. 4.24 Orbitofrontal cortex: olfactory to taste association reversal. (a) The activity of a single orbitofrontal olfactory neuron during the performance of a two-odour olfactory discrimination task and its reversal is shown. Each point represents the mean poststimulus activity of the neuron in a 500-ms period on approximately 10 trials of the different odourants. The standard errors of these responses are shown. The odourants were amyl acetate (closed circle) (initially S–) and cineole (o) (initially S+). After 80 trials of the task the reward associations of the stimuli were reversed. This neuron reversed its responses to the odourants following the task reversal. (b) The behavioural responses of the monkey during the performance of the olfactory discrimination task. The number of lick responses to each odourant is plotted as a percentage of the number of trials to that odourant in a block of 20 trials of the task. (Reproduced from *Journal of Neurophysiology*, 75 (5), Orbitofrontal cortex neurons: role in olfactory and visual association learning, E. T. Rolls, H. D. Critchley, R. Mason, E. A. Wakeman, pp. 1970–1981, ©1996, The American Physiological Society.)

with modification of responsiveness by taste association in the set of neurons in this experiment was probably related to the fact that the neurons were preselected to show differential responses to the odours associated with different tastes in the olfactory discrimination task. Thus the rule according to which the orbitofrontal olfactory representation was formed was for some neurons by association learning with taste.

The orbitofrontal cortex is likely to be the first stage of processing in humans at which olfactory responses represented expected (reward) value and subjective pleasantness, as activations in primary olfactory cortical areas such as the pyriform cortex are related to the intensity but not the pleasantness of odours (Rolls, Grabenhorst, Margot, da Silva & Velazco 2008a). (In rodents the encoding may be different, in that an influence of reward-association learning on olfactory neuronal responses in the pyriform cortex (a primary olfactory cortical area)

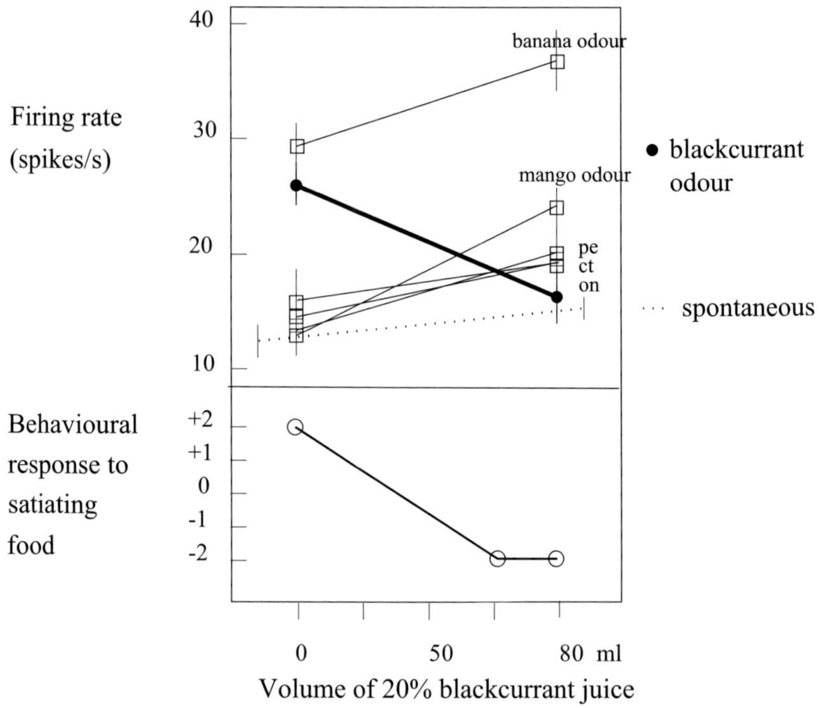

Fig. 4.25 The effect of feeding to satiety on the responses of an olfactory neuron in the orbitofrontal cortex. The monkey was fed to satiety with blackcurrant juice, and the neuronal response to the odour of blackcurrant juice, but not to other odours, decreased as the monkey was being fed to satiety. The neuronal responses reflected the monkey's preference for the blackcurrant juice, as shown in the lower graph. (Reproduced from *Journal of Neurophysiology*, 75 (4), Hunger and satiety modify the responses of olfactory and visual neurons in the primate orbitofrontal cortex, H. D. Critchley and E. T. Rolls pp. 1673–1686, ©1996, The American Physiological Society.)

has been reported (Schoenbaum & Eichenbaum 1995)). In contrast to rodents, the fact that humans can still report accurately the intensity of an odour even when its reward value and pleasantness as influenced by feeding to satiety are decreased to zero (Rolls & Rolls 1997) suggests that modulation of processing to reflect reward value is not a general property of olfactory processing implemented at early stages in primates including humans, as described in Chapter 5 (Section 5.4.4.1).

The olfactory neurons that do not reverse in the reversal of the olfactory–taste reversal task may be carrying information that is in some cases independent of the reinforcer association (i.e. is about olfactory identity). In other cases, the olfactory representation in the orbitofrontal cortex may reflect associations of odours with other primary reinforcers (for example whether sickness has occurred in association with some smells), or may reflect primary reinforcer value provided by some olfactory stimuli. (For example, the smell of flowers may be innately pleasant and attractive and some other odours may be innately unpleasant – see Chapter 3.) In this situation, the olfactory input to some orbitofrontal cortex neurons may represent an unconditioned stimulus input with which other (for example visual) inputs may become associated.

To analyse the nature of the olfactory representation in the orbitofrontal cortex, Critchley & Rolls (1996c) measured the responses of olfactory neurons that responded to food while they fed the monkey to satiety in a reward devaluation experiment. They found that the

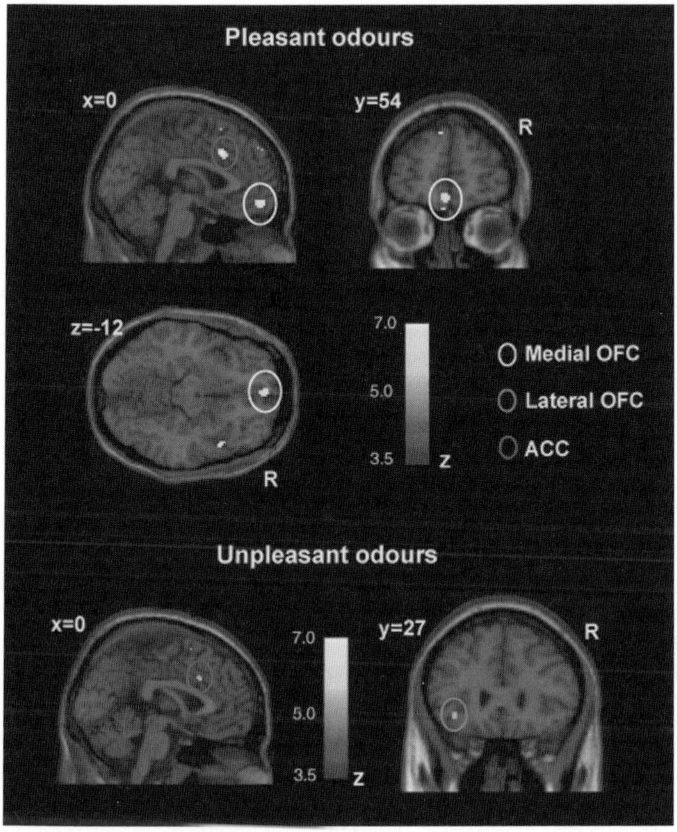

Fig. 4.26 The representation of pleasant and unpleasant odours in the human brain. Above : Group conjunction results for the 3 pleasant odours. Sagittal, horizontal and coronal views are shown at the levels indicated, all including the same activation in the medial orbitofrontal cortex, OFC [0 54 –12] z=5.23). Also shown is activation for the 3 pleasant odours in the anterior cingulate cortex, ACC [2 20 32] z=5.44). These activations were significant at $p<0.05$ fully corrected for multiple comparisons. Below : Group conjunction results for the 3 unpleasant odours. The sagittal view (left) shows an activated region of the anterior cingulate cortex [0 18 36] z=4.42, $p<0.05$, svc). The coronal view (right) shows an activated region of the lateral orbitofrontal cortex [–36 27 –8] z=4.23, $p<0.05$ svc). All the activations were thresholded at $p<0.00001$ to show the extent of the activations. (See colour plates section.) (Reproduced from Edmund T. Rolls, Morten L. Kringelbach, and Ivan E. T. De Araujo, Different representations of pleasant and unpleasant odours in the human brain, *European Journal of Neuroscience*, 18 (3) pp. 695–703, Copyright ©2003, John Wiley and Sons.)

majority of orbitofrontal olfactory neurons reduced their responses to the odour of the food with which the monkey was fed to satiety (see Fig. 4.25). Thus for these neurons, the *expected reward value* of the odour is what is represented in the orbitofrontal cortex.

Consistent with this finding at the neuronal level in non-human primates, activation of a part of the human orbitofrontal cortex is related to the pleasantness and expected value of food odour, in that the activation measured with fMRI produced by one food odour, banana, decreased after banana was eaten for lunch to satiety, but remained strong to another food odour, vanilla, not eaten in the meal (O'Doherty, Rolls, Francis, Bowtell, McGlone, Kobal, Renner & Ahne 2000). Consistent findings were reported by Gottfried, O'Doherty & Dolan (2003).

Further evidence that pleasant odours are represented in the orbitofrontal cortex is that

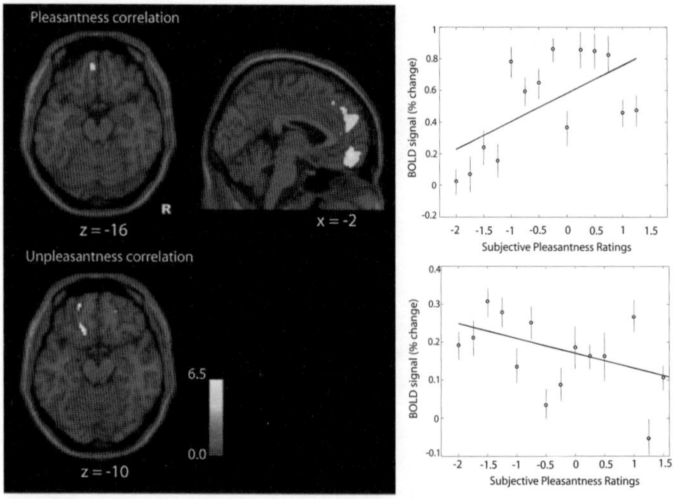

Fig. 4.27 The representation of pleasant and unpleasant odours in the human brain. Random effects group analysis correlation analysis of the BOLD signal with the subjective pleasantness ratings. On the top left is shown the region of the medio-rostral orbitofrontal (peak at [–2 52 –10] z=4.28) correlating positively with pleasantness ratings, as well as the region of the anterior cingulate cortex in the top middle. On the far top-right of the figure is shown the relation between the subjective pleasantness ratings and the BOLD signal from this cluster (in the medial orbitofrontal cortex at Y=52), together with the regression line. The means and s.e.m. across subjects are shown. At the bottom of the figure are shown the regions of left more lateral orbitofrontal cortex (peaks at [–20 54 –14] z=4.26 and [–16 28 –18] z=4.08) correlating negatively with pleasantness ratings. On the far bottom-right of the figure is shown the relation between the subjective pleasantness ratings and the BOLD signal from the first cluster (in the lateral orbitofrontal cortex at Y=54), together with the regression line. The means and s.e.m. across subjects are shown. The activations were thresholded at $p<0.0001$ for extent. (See colour plates section.) (Reproduced from Edmund T. Rolls, Morten L. Kringelbach, and Ivan E. T. De Araujo, Different representations of pleasant and unpleasant odours in the human brain, *European Journal of Neuroscience*, 18 (3) pp. 695–703, Copyright ©2003, John Wiley and Sons.)

3 pleasant odours (linalyl acetate [floral, sweet], geranyl acetate [floral], and alpha-ionone [woody, slightly food-related]) had overlapping activations in the medial orbitofrontal cortex in a region not activated by three unpleasant odours (hexanoic acid, octanol, and isovaleric acid) (Rolls, Kringelbach & De Araujo 2003c) (see Fig. 4.26). Moreover, activation of the medial orbitofrontal cortex was correlated with the subjective pleasantness ratings of the odours, and activation of the lateral orbitofrontal cortex with the subjective unpleasantness ratings of the odours (see Fig. 4.27). Other studies have also shown activation of the human orbitofrontal cortex by odour (Zatorre, Jones-Gotman, Evans & Meyer 1992, Zatorre, Jones-Gotman & Rouby 2000, Royet, Zald, Versace, Costes, Lavenne, Koenig, Gervais, Routtenberg, Gardner & Huang 2000, Anderson, Christoff, Stappen, Panitz, Ghahremani, Glover, Gabrieli & Sobel 2003, Grabenhorst, Rolls, Margot, da Silva & Velazco 2007, Rolls, Grabenhorst, Margot, da Silva & Velazco 2008a).

Although individual neurons do not encode large amounts of information about which of 7–9 odours has been presented, we have shown that the information does increase linearly with the number of neurons in the sample (Rolls, Critchley & Treves 1996b, Rolls, Critchley, Verhagen & Kadohisa 2010a). This ensemble encoding does result in useful amounts of information about which odour has been presented being provided by orbitofrontal olfactory neurons.

The evidence described in this section shows that the positive and negative value of odour

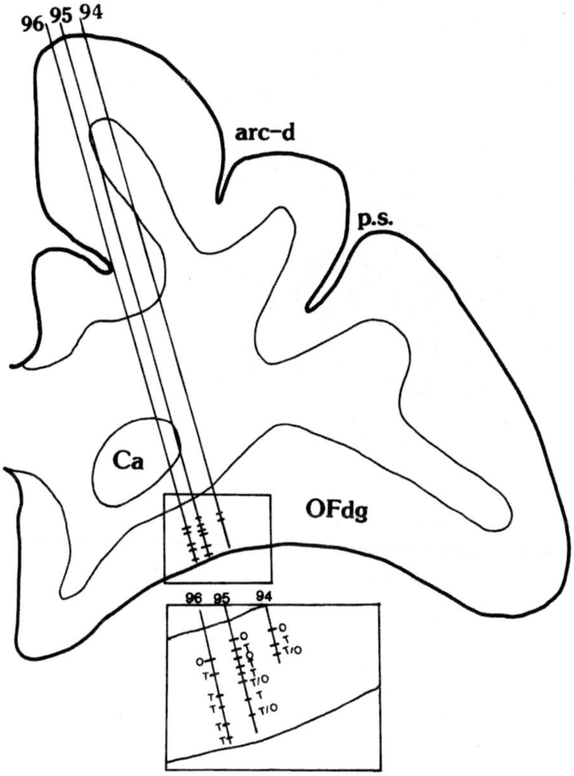

Fig. 4.28 Examples of tracks made into the orbitofrontal cortex in which taste (T) and olfactory (O) neurons were recorded close to each other in the same tracks. Some of the neurons were bimodal (T/O). arc-d, arcuate sulcus; Ca, head of Caudate nucleus; Ofdg, dysgranular part of the Orbitofrontal Cortex; p.s., principal sulcus. (Reproduced from E. T. Rolls and L. L. Baylis, Gustatory, olfactory and visual convergence within the primate orbitofrontal cortex, *Journal of Neuroscience* 14, pp. 5437–5452 ©1994, Society for Neuroscience.)

is represented in the orbitofrontal cortex on a continuous scale. Further evidence for this, and that in contrast a more anterior region that is Tier 3 in Fig. 4.2, the medial prefrontal cortex area 10, is involved in the mechanisms that implement a choice or decision between odours of different value, is described in Chapter 8, including Section 8.7.7.1.

4.5.5.3 Convergence of taste and olfactory inputs in the orbitofrontal cortex: the representation of flavour

In the more medial and anterior parts of the orbitofrontal cortex, not only unimodal taste neurons, but also unimodal olfactory neurons are found (see Fig. 4.28). In addition some single neurons respond to both gustatory and olfactory stimuli, often with correspondence between the two modalities (Rolls & Baylis 1994) (see Fig. 4.29; cf. Fig. 4.2). It is probably here in the orbitofrontal cortex of primates that these two modalities converge to produce the representation of flavour (Rolls & Baylis 1994), and, consistent with this, neurons in the macaque primary taste cortex do not have olfactory responses (Verhagen, Kadohisa & Rolls 2004). Consistently, in a human fMRI investigation of olfactory and taste convergence in the brain, it was shown that there is a part of the human taste insula that is not activated by odour

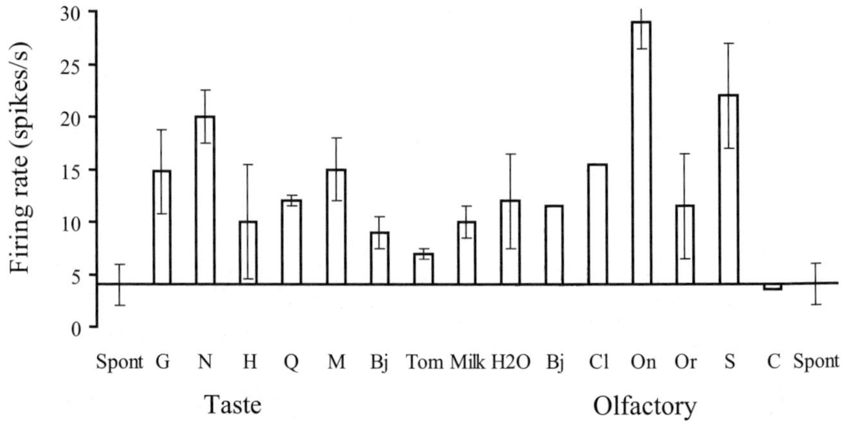

Fig. 4.29 The responses of a bimodal neuron with taste and olfactory responses recorded in the caudolateral orbitofrontal cortex. G, 1 M glucose; N, 0.1 M NaCl; H, 0.01 M HCl; Q, 0.001 M Quinine HCl; M, 0.1 M monosodium glutamate; Bj, 20% blackcurrant juice; Tom, tomato juice; B, banana odour; Cl, clove oil odour; On, onion odour; Or, orange odour; S, salmon odour; C, control no-odour presentation. The mean responses – s.e.m. are shown. The neuron responded best to the savoury tastes of NaCl and monosodium glutamate and to the consonant odours of onion and salmon. (Reproduced from E. T. Rolls and L. L. Baylis, Gustatory, olfactory and visual convergence within the primate orbitofrontal cortex, *Journal of Neuroscience* 14, pp. 5437–5452 ©1994, Society for Neuroscience.)

(De Araujo, Rolls, Kringelbach, McGlone & Phillips 2003c), though if a taste is recalled by an odour the situation could be different because of the role of cortico-cortical backprojections in recall (Rolls 2008b). The evidence described above (Section 4.5.5.2) indicates that these bimodal representations are built by olfactory–gustatory association learning, an example of stimulus–reinforcer association learning.

The human orbitofrontal cortex also reflects the convergence of taste and olfactory inputs, as shown for example by the fact that activations in the human medial orbitofrontal cortex are correlated with both the cross-modal consonance of combined taste and olfactory stimuli (high for example for sweet taste and strawberry odour), as well as for the pleasantness of the combinations, as shown in Fig. 4.30 (De Araujo, Rolls, Kringelbach, McGlone & Phillips 2003c). In addition, the combination of monosodium glutamate taste and a consonant savoury odour produced a supralinear effect in the medial orbitofrontal cortex to produce the rich delicious flavour of umami that makes many foods rich in protein pleasant (McCabe & Rolls 2007, Rolls 2009c).

4.5.5.4 Visual inputs to the orbitofrontal cortex, and visual stimulus–reinforcer association learning and reversal to compute expected value

We have been able to show that there is a major visual input to many neurons in the orbitofrontal cortex, and that what is represented by these neurons is in many cases the reinforcer (reward or punisher) association of visual stimuli. Many of these neurons reflect the relative preference or reward value of different visual stimuli, in that their responses decrease to zero to the sight of one food on which the monkey is being fed to satiety, but remain unchanged to the sight of other food stimuli. In this sense the visual reinforcement-related neurons predict

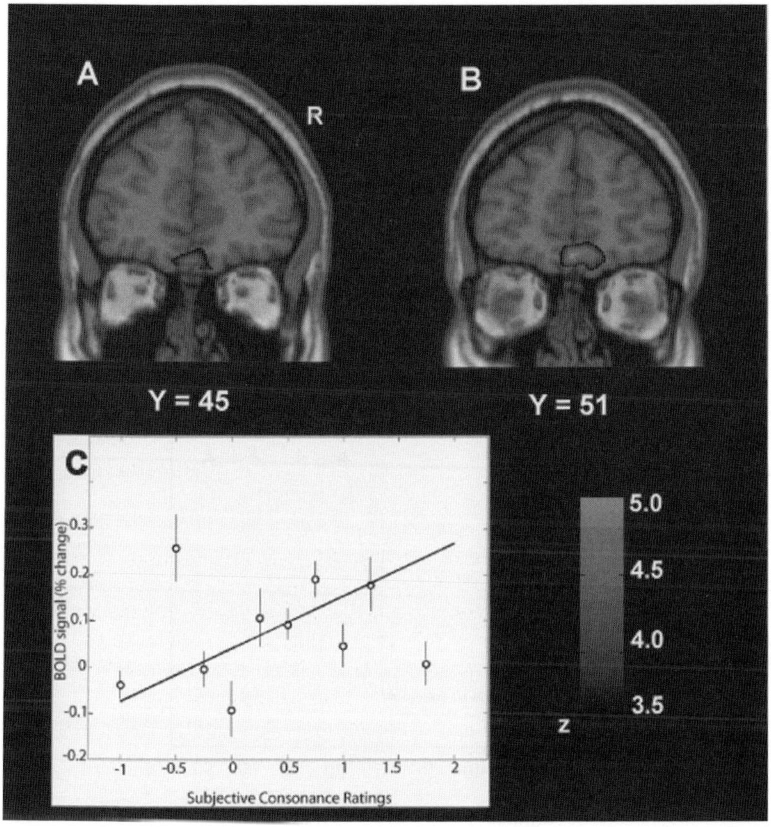

Fig. 4.30 Flavour formation in the human brain, shown by cross-modal olfactory–taste convergence. Brain areas where activations were correlated with the subjective ratings for stimulus (taste–odour) consonance and pleasantness. (A) A second-level, random effects analysis based on individual contrasts (the consonance ratings being the only effect of interest) revealed a significant activation in a medial part of the anterior orbitofrontal cortex. (B) Random effects analysis based on the pleasantness ratings showed a significant cluster of activation located in a (nearby) medial part of the anterior orbitofrontal cortex. The images were thresholded at $p<0.0001$ for illustration. (C) The relation between the BOLD signal from the cluster of voxels in the medial orbitofrontal cortex shown in (A) and the subjective consonance ratings. The analyses shown included all the stimuli included in this investigation. The means and standard errors of the mean across subjects are shown, together with the regression line, for which $r=0.52$. (See colour plates section.) (Reproduced from Ivan E. T. De Araujo, Edmund T. Rolls, Morten L. Kringelbach, Francis McGlone, and Nicola Phillips, Taste-olfactory convergence, and the representation of the pleasantness of flavour, in the human brain, *European Journal of Neuroscience*, 18 (7) pp. 2059–2068 Copyright ©2003, John Wiley and Sons.)

the reward value that is available from the primary reinforcer, the taste. The visual input is from the ventral, temporal lobe, visual stream concerned with 'what' object is being seen, in that orbitofrontal visual neurons frequently respond differentially to objects or images (but depending on their reward association) (Thorpe, Rolls & Maddison 1983, Rolls, Critchley, Mason & Wakeman 1996a). The primary reinforcer that has been used is taste.

The fact that these neurons represent the reinforcer associations of visual stimuli and hence the expected value has been shown to be the case in formal investigations of the activity of orbitofrontal cortex visual neurons, which in many cases reverse their responses to visual stimuli when the taste with which the visual stimulus is associated is reversed by the experimenter (Thorpe, Rolls & Maddison 1983, Rolls, Critchley, Mason & Wakeman 1996a).

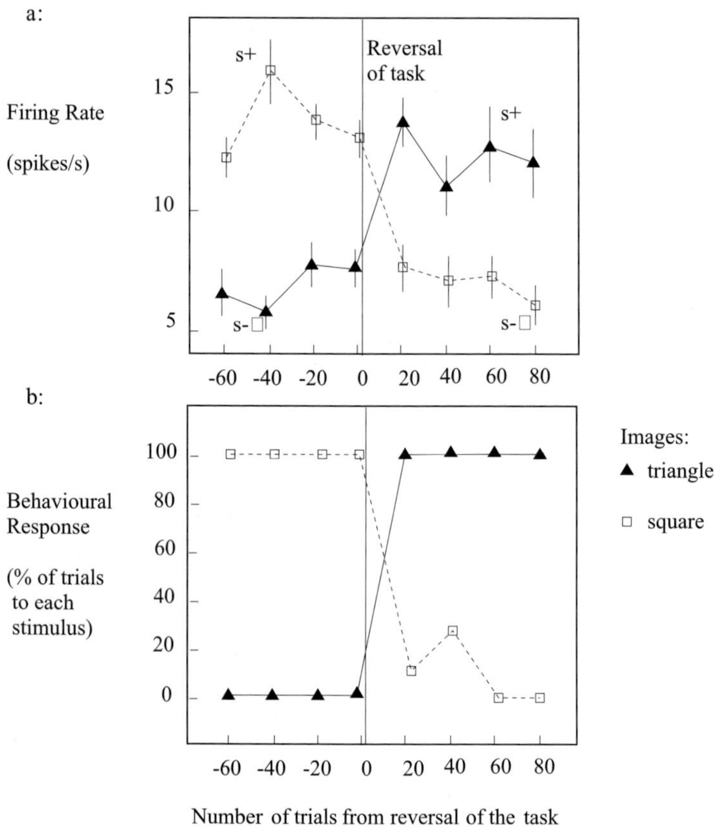

Fig. 4.31 Orbitofrontal cortex: visual discrimination reversal. The activity of an orbitofrontal visual neuron during performance of a visual discrimination task and its reversal. The stimuli were a triangle and a square presented on a video monitor. (a) Each point represents the mean poststimulus activity in a 500 ms period of the neuron based on approximately 10 trials of the different visual stimuli. The standard errors of these responses are shown. After 60 trials of the task the reward associations of the visual stimuli were reversed. s+ indicates that a lick response to that visual stimulus produces fruit juice reward; s– indicates that a lick response to that visual stimulus results in a small drop of aversive tasting saline. This neuron reversed its responses to the visual stimuli following the task reversal. (b) The behavioural response of the monkey to the task. It is shown that the monkey performs well, in that he rapidly learns to lick only to the visual stimulus associated with fruit juice reward. (Reproduced from *Journal of Neurophysiology*, 75 (5), Orbitofrontal cortex neurons: role in olfactory and visual association learning, E. T. Rolls, H. D. Critchley, R. Mason, and E. A. Wakeman, pp. 1970–1981, ©1996, The American Physiological Society.)

An example of the responses of an orbitofrontal cortex neuron that reversed the visual stimulus to which it responded during reward-reversal is shown in Fig. 4.31.

This reversal by orbitofrontal visual neurons can be very fast, in as little as one trial, that is a few seconds (see for example Fig. 4.32). The significance of the visual stimulus, a syringe from which the monkey was fed, was altered during the trials. On trials 1–5, no response of the neuron occurred to the sight of the syringe from which the monkey had been given glucose solution to drink from the syringe on the preceding trials. On trials 6–9, the neuron responded to the sight of the same syringe from which he had been given aversive hypertonic saline drink on the preceding trial. Two more reversals (trials 10–15, and 16–17) were performed. The reversal of the neuron's response when the significance of the visual stimulus was reversed shows that the responses of the neuron only occurred to the stimulus when it was associated

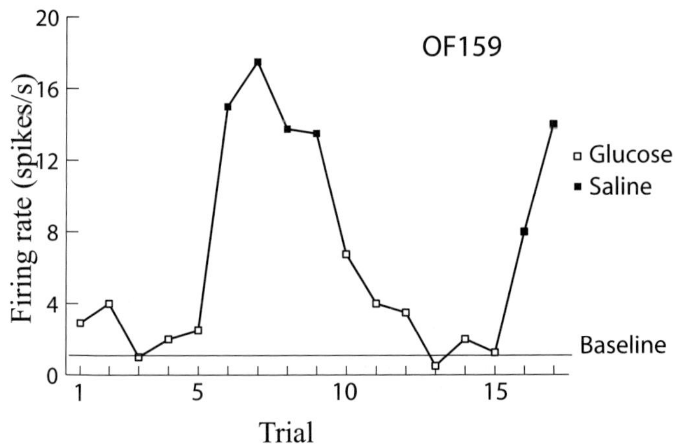

Fig. 4.32 Orbitofrontal cortex: one-trial visual discrimination reversal by a neuron. On trials 1–5, no response of the neuron occurred to the sight of a 2 ml syringe from which the monkey had been given orally glucose solution to drink on the previous trial. On trials 6–9, the neuron responded to the sight of the same syringe from which he had been given aversive hypertonic saline to drink on the previous trial. Two more reversals (trials 10–15, and 16–17) were performed. The reversal of the neuron's response when the significance of the same visual stimulus was reversed shows that the responses of the neuron only occurred to the sight of the visual stimulus when it was associated with a positively reinforcing and not with a negatively reinforcing taste. Moreover, it is shown that the neuronal reversal took only one trial. (Reproduced from *Experimental Brain Research*, 49 (1) pp. 93–115, The orbitofrontal cortex: Neuronal activity in the behaving monkey, S. J. Thorpe, E. T. Rolls, and S. Maddison (c) 1983, Springer Science and Business Media. With kind permission from Springer Science and Business Media.)

with aversive saline and not when it was associated with glucose reward.

These neurons thus reflect the information about which stimulus is currently associated with reward during reversals of visual discrimination tasks – they are reward predicting neurons, that is, they represent *expected value*. If a reversal occurs, then the taste cells provide the information that an unexpected taste reinforcer has been obtained, another group of cells shows a vigorous discharge that reflects the error between the expected reward value and the reward outcome actually obtained (see below), and the visual cells with reinforcer association-related responses reverse the stimulus to which they are responsive. These neurophysiological changes take place rapidly, in as little as 5 s, and are part of the neuronal learning mechanism that enables primates to alter their knowledge of the reinforcer association of visual stimuli so rapidly. This capacity is important whenever behaviour must be corrected when expected reinforcers are not obtained, in, for example, feeding, emotional, and social situations (see Chapters 3 and 5, Rolls (2005b), and Kringelbach & Rolls (2003)). In that these neurons reflect whether a visual stimulus is associated with reward or a punisher, they reflect the relative preference for different stimuli, i.e. the value (Thorpe, Rolls & Maddison 1983, Rolls, Critchley, Mason & Wakeman 1996a) (as found also by Tremblay & Schultz (1999)). Consistent with this evidence that the responses of some orbitofrontal cortex neurons reflect the learned predictive reward value of visual stimuli, Thorpe, Rolls & Maddison (1983) and Tremblay & Schultz (2000) found that orbitofrontal cortex neurons learned to respond differently to new stimuli that did or did not predict reward. Different neurons in the orbitofrontal cortex are tuned to different learned or conditioned reinforcers, with for example approximately 5% responding to visual stimuli associated with taste reward, and 3% to visual stimuli associated with taste punishment (see Table 4.3 on page 125) (Thorpe, Rolls & Maddison 1983, Rolls,

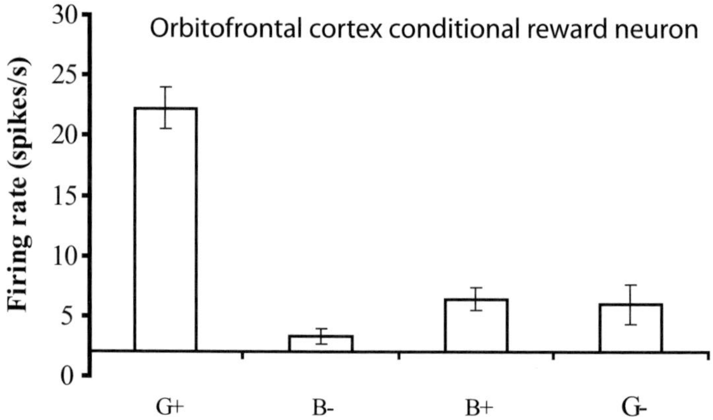

Fig. 4.33 A conditional reward neuron recorded in the orbitofrontal cortex which responded only to the Green stimulus when it was associated with reward (G+), and not to the Blue stimulus when it was associated with Reward (B+), or to either stimuli when they were associated with a punisher, the taste of salt (G– and B–). The mean firing rate ± the s.e.m. is shown. (Reproduced from *Experimental Brain Research*, 49 (1) pp. 93–115, The orbitofrontal cortex: Neuronal activity in the behaving monkey, S. J. Thorpe, E. T. Rolls, and S. Maddison, (c) 1983, Springer Science and Business Media. With kind permission from Springer Science and Business Media.)

Critchley, Mason & Wakeman 1996a).

In the visual discrimination reversal task, a second class of neuron was found that codes for particular stimuli only if they are associated with reward, and not if they are associated with punishment. Such a neuron might respond to a green stimulus associated with reward; after reversal not respond to the green stimulus when it was associated with punishment; and not respond to a blue stimulus irrespective of whether it was associated with reward or punishment (Thorpe, Rolls & Maddison 1983) (see example in Fig. 4.33). They may be described as *conditional visual stimulus-to-taste reward neurons* or *conditional expected value neurons*, and are analogous to their olfactory counterparts described above in Section 4.5.5.2. These neurons are probably important in the mechanisms that implement rapid reversal, as described in Section 4.5.7.

The proportions of neurons showing reversal, or conditional visual stimulus–reinforcer related responses, are shown in Table 4.1. Most visual neurons showed full or conditional reversal, while the proportion of olfactory neurons (see Section 4.5.5.2) was lower (Rolls, Critchley, Mason & Wakeman 1996a).

This reversal learning found in orbitofrontal cortex neurons probably is implemented in the orbitofrontal cortex, for it does not occur one synapse earlier in the visual inferior temporal cortex (Rolls, Judge & Sanghera 1977), and it is in the orbitofrontal cortex that there is convergence of visual and taste pathways on to the same neurons (Thorpe, Rolls & Maddison 1983, Rolls, Critchley, Mason & Wakeman 1996a).

A possible mechanism for this learning is Hebbian modification of synapses conveying visual input on to taste-responsive neurons, implementing a pattern-association network (Rolls & Treves 1998, Rolls 2008b) (see Appendix 1). In this model the unconditioned stimulus forcing the output neurons to respond is the (taste) primary reinforcer, and the (visual or olfactory) conditioned stimulus becomes associated with this by associatively modifiable synapses) (Rolls & Treves 1998, Rolls 1999a, Rolls 2008b). Such a pattern association network could in principle unlearn the association by using associative synapses that incorporate long-

Table 4.1 Proportion of neurons in the primate orbitofrontal cortex showing reversal, or conditional reversal (ceasing to discriminate or ceasing to respond after the reversal), or no change of responses, during visual or olfactory discrimination reversal. (Reproduced from *Journal of Neurophysiology*, 75 (5), Orbitofrontal cortex neurons: role in olfactory and visual association learning, E. T. Rolls, H. D. Critchley, R. Mason, E. A. Wakeman, pp. 1970–81 ©1996, The American Physiological Society.)

	Olfactory Number	cells %	Visual Number	cells %
Reversal	7	25.0	12	70.6
Conditional reversal	12	42.9	4	23.5
No change	9	32.1	1	5.9
Total	28	100.0	17	100.0

term depression (Rolls & Treves 1998, Rolls 2008b). Although reversal might be implemented by having long-term synaptic depression (LTD) for synapses that represented the reward-associated stimulus before the reversal, and long-term potentiation (LTP) of the synapses activated by the new stimulus that after reversal is associated with reward, this would require one-trial LTP and one-trial heterosynaptic LTD to account for one-trial stimulus–reward reversal (Thorpe, Rolls & Maddison 1983, Rolls, Critchley, Mason & Wakeman 1996a, Rolls 2000b) (see Appendix 1). To implement the reversal learning very rapidly, in as little as one trial after a number of reversals when reversal learning set has been acquired, a special switching network the uses a rule in the orbitofrontal cortex may be required, and a model of this is described in Section 4.5.7.

Another way in which it has been shown that the visual neurons in the orbitofrontal cortex reflect the expected value predicted by visual stimuli is by reducing the reward value by feeding to satiety in devaluation experiments. With this sensory-specific satiety (or reward devaluation) paradigm, it has been shown that the visual (as well as the olfactory and taste) responses of orbitofrontal cortex neurons in the macaque decrease to zero as the monkey is fed to satiety with one food, but remain unchanged to another food not eaten in the meal (Critchley & Rolls 1996c) (see example in Fig. 4.34). In that these neurons parallel the changing preference of the monkey for the food being eaten to satiety vs the food not being eaten to satiety, they reflect the relative preference for different visual stimuli, that is the expected value (Thorpe, Rolls & Maddison 1983, Rolls, Critchley, Mason & Wakeman 1996a) (as found also by Tremblay & Schultz (1999) and Wallis & Miller (2003)).

Further evidence that these orbitofrontal cortex neurons encode expected value is that they represent choices made when the 'offers' (the visual stimuli) are different amounts of different qualities of the 'goods' (for example the type of fruit juice that is the reward outcome of the choice) and different probabilities of obtaining reward), as described in Section 9.5 (Padoa-Schioppa & Assad 2006, Padoa-Schioppa 2011).

All this evidence shows that the great majority of neurons in the orbitofrontal cortex encode stimuli, frequently in terms of the (outcome) value or expected value, and do not reflect the actions or responses or spatial responses being performed by the macaques (Thorpe, Rolls & Maddison 1983, Rolls, Critchley, Mason & Wakeman 1996a, Critchley & Rolls 1996c, Rolls & Baylis 1994, Rolls 2005b, Wallis & Miller 2003, Padoa-Schioppa & Assad 2006). These findings are consistent with the hypothesis that expected reward value is represented in the orbitofrontal cortex, reflects stimulus–reinforcer (sensory–sensory) association learning, and that this information is projected to other structures such as the cingulate cortex for action–outcome learning (Section 4.7), or to the basal ganglia for stimulus-response habit learning (Chapter 6). Outputs of the orbitofrontal cortex to the dorsolateral prefrontal cortex may be used in tasks requiring planning, for example where rewarding stimuli must be flexibly linked

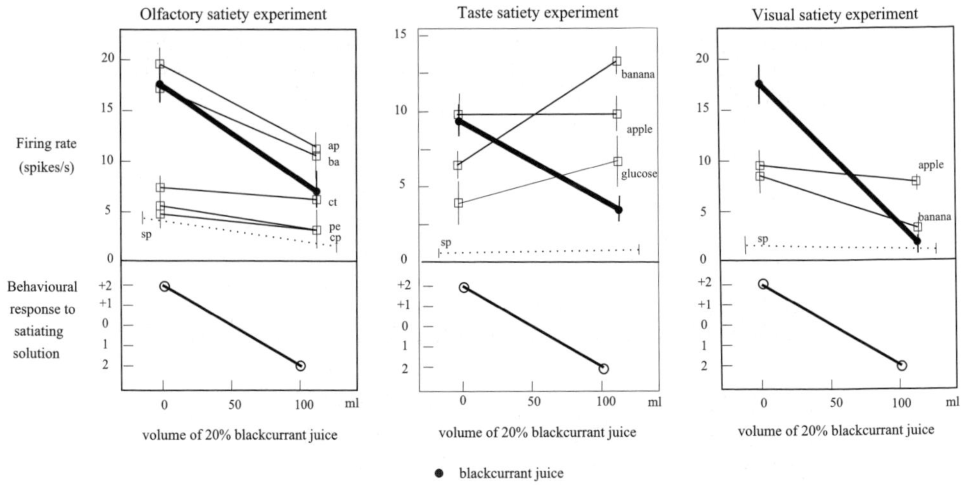

Fig. 4.34 Orbitofrontal cortex neuron with visual, olfactory and taste responses, showing the responses before and after feeding to satiety with blackcurrant juice. The solid circles show the responses to blackcurrant juice. The olfactory stimuli included apple (ap), banana (ba), citral (ct), phenylethanol (pe), and caprylic acid (cp). The spontaneous firing rate of the neuron is shown (sp). (Reproduced from *Journal of Neurophysiology*, 75 (4), Hunger and satiety modify the responses of olfactory and visual neurons in the primate orbitofrontal cortex, H. D. Critchley and E. T. Rolls pp. 1673–1886, ©1996, The American Physiological Society.)

to particular responses, and where delays may be involved, in ways that have been modelled by Deco & Rolls (2003) and Deco & Rolls (2005a).

These studies in macaques provide evidence on the details of the neuronal representations in the primate orbitofrontal cortex which are essential for building a computational understanding for exactly what information is represented in it, how it is represented, how these differ from preceding and succeeding stages, and thus how the orbitofrontal cortex operates computationally (see Appendix 1). However, the types of visual-reward association that have been studied in primates (and confirmed as applying in humans (O'Doherty, Deichmann, Critchley & Dolan 2002)) include objects associated with taste rewards or punishers. It has therefore been useful not only to confirm that these concepts do indeed apply to humans, but also to extend the types of visual conditioned reinforcers to quite abstract reinforcers such as monetary reward. In an fMRI study, O'Doherty, Kringelbach, Rolls, Hornak & Andrews (2001a) used a visual discrimination task in which one stimulus was associated with monetary reward, and a different visual stimulus with monetary loss (punishment). The actual amounts of money won on reward trials and lost on punishment trials were probabilistic. This part of the design, and the fact that unexpected visual discrimination reversals occurred so that there were trials on which money was lost, enabled us to show that the magnitude of the activation of the medial orbitofrontal cortex was correlated with the amount of money won on each trial, and the magnitude of the activation of the lateral orbitofrontal cortex was correlated with the amount of money lost on each trial, as shown in Figs. 4.35 and 4.36.

Consistent with the finding of outcome value and expected value neurons in the same parts of the primate orbitofrontal cortex, the outcome value and the expected value produced activations on the same scale and in the same part of the medial orbitofrontal cortex in humans, when the probability of obtaining the reward was varied to signal different expected values (Rolls, McCabe & Redoute 2008e). This was shown in a probabilistic monetary reward decision task designed to allow variables of interest in neuroeconomics to be measured (Section 9.5). As illustrated in Fig. 4.37a, the subjects could choose either on the right to

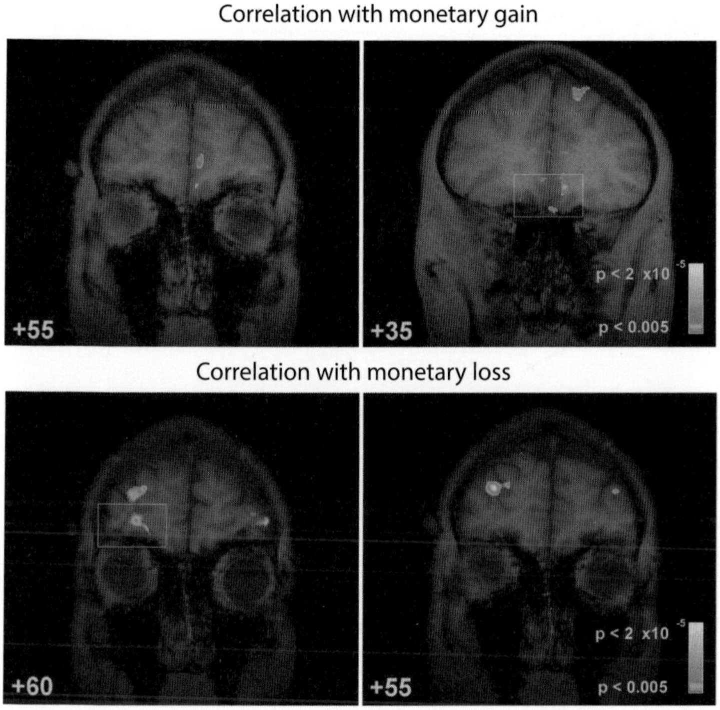

Fig. 4.35 Correlation of brain activations with the amount of money won (upper) or lost (lower) in a visual discrimination reversal task with probabilistic monetary reward and loss. Voxels in the orbitofrontal cortex (upper right, in square box) and pregenual cingulate cortex (upper left) whose activity increased with the amount of money won on each trial. Voxels in an area of left medial orbitofrontal cortex (Talairach coordinates [X,Y,Z] = [–6 34 –28]) correlated positively with Reward Magnitude. Voxels in an area of right lateral orbitofrontal cortex (lower left in square box, Talairach co-ordinates [28 60 –6]) correlated positively with the amount of money lost on each trial. (See colour plates section.) (Reproduced from *Nature Neuroscience*, 4 (1), J. O'Doherty, M. L. Kringelbach, E. T. Rolls, J. Hornak, and C. Andrews, Abstract reward and punishment representations in the human orbitofrontal cortex, pp. 95–102, ©2001, Nature Publishing Group.)

obtain a large reward outcome with a value of 30 pence, or on the left to obtain a smaller reward outcome with a value of 10 pence with a probability of 0.9. On the right, in different trial blocks, the probability of the large reward was 0.9 (making the expected value which approximates probability × reward value = 27 pence); or the probability was 0.33 making the expected value 10 pence; or the probability was 0.16 making the expected value 5 pence. The expected value on the left was 9 pence (p=0.9 of outcome value of 10 pence). The participants learned in the blocks of 30 trials with the different expected values on the right whether to press on the right or the left to maximize their winnings. They took typically less than 10 trials to adjust to the unsignalled change in expected value every 30 trials, and analysis was performed for the last 20 trials of each block when the expected value had been learned. Fig. 4.37b shows the regions of the orbitofrontal / ventromedial prefrontal cortex where the activations were proportional both to the expected value (measured early in the trial) and the outcome value (measured later in each trial, when the reward outcome was made known) (Rolls, McCabe & Redoute 2008e).

Thus in humans and macaques there is evidence that expected value signalled by for example visual as well as olfactory stimuli is represented in the orbitofrontal cortex. This representation of expected value is important in decision-making, as described further in

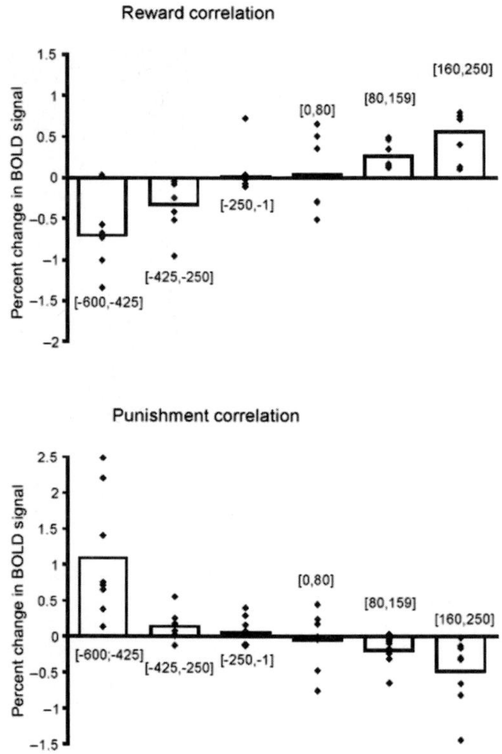

Fig. 4.36 Correlation of brain activations with the amount of money won or lost in a visual discrimination reversal task with probabilistic monetary reward and loss. The mean percent change in the BOLD signal from baseline across subjects for 6 different category ranges of monetary gain or loss plotted along the abscissa. The signal was averaged across a category range within each subject and then the average signal change from each category was averaged across subjects. This is plotted for voxels in the medial OFC that significantly correlated with reward and for voxels in the lateral OFC that significantly correlated with punishment. The ranges of monetary reward and punishment in each category are shown on the chart and were determined by their relative frequencies, which follow from the experimental design. (See colour plates section.) (Reproduced from *Nature Neuroscience*, 4 (1), J. O'Doherty, M. L. Kringelbach, E. T. Rolls, J. Hornak, and C. Andrews, Abstract reward and punishment representations in the human orbitofrontal cortex, pp. 95–102, ©2001, Nature Publishing Group.)

Section 9.5.

4.5.5.5 Negative reward prediction error neurons in the orbitofrontal cortex, and visual stimulus–reinforcer association learning and reversal

In addition to the neurons that encode the reward value of visual stimuli, other neurons (3.5%) in the orbitofrontal cortex detect different types of non-reward, i.e. reward prediction error, the difference between the expected value and the reward outcome value (Thorpe, Rolls & Maddison 1983). For example, some neurons responded in extinction, immediately after a lick had been made to a visual stimulus that had previously been associated with fruit juice reward, and other neurons responded in a reversal task, immediately after the monkey had responded to the previously rewarded visual stimulus, but had obtained the punisher of salt taste rather than reward (see example in Fig. 4.38).

Different populations of such neurons respond to other types of non-reward, including the removal of a formerly approaching taste reward, and the termination of a taste reward (Thorpe,

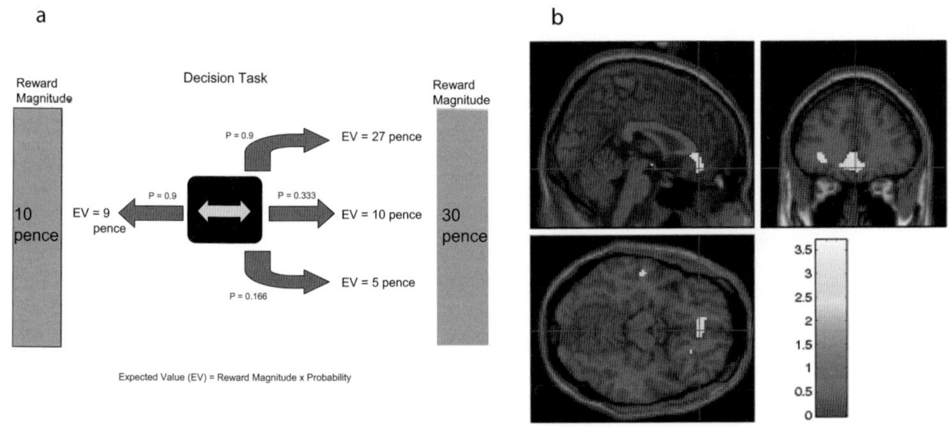

Fig. 4.37 Expected value and outcome value in a probabilistic monetary reward decision task. (a) In the task, subjects could choose either on the right to obtain a large reward with a magnitude of 30 pence, or on the left to obtain a smaller reward with an outcome magnitude of 10 pence with a probability of 0.9 (Expected Value = 9 pence). On the right, in different blocks each 30 trials long, the probability of the large reward was 0.9 (making the Expected Value defined as probability × Reward outcome Magnitude = 27 pence); or the probability was 0.33 (EV=10 pence); or the probability was 0.16 (EV=5 pence). (On the trials on which a reward was not obtained, 0 pence was the Reward outcome Magnitude). (b) Medial orbitofrontal cortex. Conjunction analysis showing brain regions where there were correlations both with Expected Value and with Reward outcome Magnitude (peak MNI coordinates [2 38 -14]). (See colour plates section.) (This material was originally published in *Cerebral Cortex*, 18 (3), Expected Value, Reward Outcome, and Temporal Difference Error Representations in a Probabilistic Decision Task, Edmund T. Rolls, Ciara McCabe, Jerome Redoute, pp. 652–663, ©2008, Oxford University Press and has been reproduced by permission of Oxford University Press http://cercor.oxfordjournals.org/content/15/1.toc.)

Rolls & Maddison 1983) (see Table 4.2). The fact that different non-reward neurons respond to different types of non-reward (e.g. some to the noise of a switch that indicated that extinction of free licking for fruit juice had occurred, and others to the first presentation of a visual stimulus that was not followed by reward in a visual discrimination task) potentially enables context-specific extinction or reversal to occur. Thus the error neurons can be specific to different tasks, and this could provide a mechanism for reversal in one task to be implemented, while at the same time not reversing behaviour in another task. Also, it provides additional evidence to that in Table 4.2 that these neurons did not respond simply as a function of arousal, or just in relation to a general frustrative non-reward/error signal.

The presence of these orbitofrontal cortex non-reward or negative reward prediction error neurons is fully consistent with the hypothesis that they are part of the mechanism by which the orbitofrontal cortex enables very rapid reversal of behaviour by stimulus–reinforcer association relearning when the association of stimuli with reinforcers is altered or reversed (Rolls 1986a, Rolls 1986b, Rolls 1990b, Rolls 1999a, Rolls 2005b). This information appears to be necessary for primates to rapidly alter behavioural responses when reinforcement contingencies are changed, as shown by the effects of damage to the orbitofrontal cortex described above. The existence of neurons in the middle part of the macaque orbitofrontal cortex that respond to non-reward (Thorpe, Rolls & Maddison 1983) (originally described by Thorpe, Maddison & Rolls (1979) and Rolls (1981a)) is confirmed by recordings that revealed 10 such non-reward neurons (of 140 recorded, or approximately 7%) found in delayed match to sample and delayed response tasks by Joaquin Fuster and colleagues (Rosenkilde, Bauer

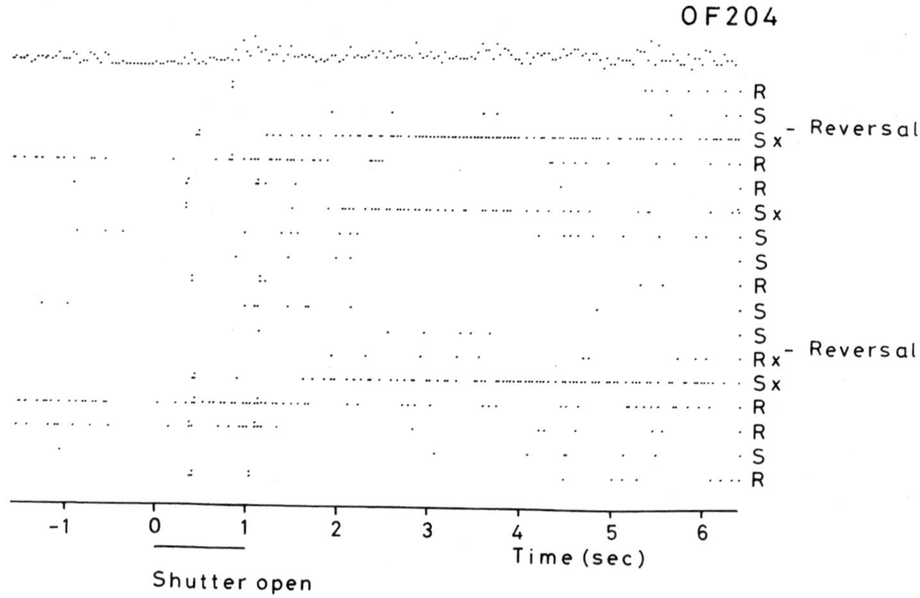

Fig. 4.38 Error neuron: Responses of an orbitofrontal cortex neuron that responded only when the monkey licked to a visual stimulus during reversal, expecting to obtain fruit juice reward, but actually obtaining the taste of aversive saline because it was the first trial of reversal. Each single dot represents an action potential; each vertically arranged double dot represents a lick response. The visual stimulus was shown at time 0 for 1 s. The neuron did not respond on most reward (R) or saline (S) trials, but did respond on the trials marked x, which were the first trials after a reversal of the visual discrimination on which the monkey licked to obtain reward, but actually obtained saline because the task had been reversed. It is notable that after an expected reward was not obtained due to a reversal contingency being applied, on the very next trial the macaque selected the previously non-rewarded stimulus. This shows that rapid reversal can be performed by a non-associative process, and must be rule-based. A model for this is the subject of Section 4.5.7. (Reproduced from *Experimental Brain Research*, 49 (1) pp. 93–115, The orbitofrontal cortex: Neuronal activity in the behaving monkey, S. J. Thorpe, E. T. Rolls, and S. Maddison (c) 1983, Springer Science and Business Media. With kind permission from Springer Science and Business Media.)

& Fuster 1981).

To the extent that the firing of some dopamine neurons may reflect error signals (Waelti, Dickinson & Schultz 2001) (see Section 6.2.4), one might ask where the error information comes from, given that the dopamine neurons themselves may not receive information about expected rewards (e.g. a visual stimulus associated with the sight of food), obtained rewards (e.g. taste), and would have to compute an error from these signals. On the other hand, the orbitofrontal cortex does have all three types of neuron and the required neuroanatomically defined inputs, and this is an important site in the brain for computing error signals.

It is interesting to note the proportions of different types of neuron recorded in the orbitofrontal cortex in relation to what might or might not be seen in a human brain imaging study. The proportions of different types of neuron in the study by Thorpe, Rolls & Maddison (1983) are shown in Table 4.3. It is seen that only a relatively small percentage convey information about, for example, which of two visual stimuli is currently reward-associated in a visual discrimination task. An even smaller proportion (3.5%) responds in relation to non-reward, and in any particular non-reward task, the proportion is very small, that is, just a

Table 4.2 Numbers of orbitofrontal cortex neurons responding in different types of extinction or reversal. The table shows the tasks (rows) in which individual orbitofrontal neurons responded (1), did not respond (0), or were not tested (blank). (Reproduced from *Experimental Brain Research*, 49 (1) pp. 93–115, The orbitofrontal cortex: Neuronal activity in the behaving monkey, S. J. Thorpe, E. T. Rolls, and S. Maddison (c) 1983, Springer Science and Business Media. With kind permission from Springer Science and Business Media.)

Neuron number	1	2	3	4	5	6	7	8	9	10	11	12	13	14	15	16	17	18
Visual discrim: Reversal	1	0	1	0	0	1	1	0						0				
Visual discrim: Extinction	1																	
Ad lib licking: Reversal	1	1		0	0	0		0	1									
Ad lib licking: Extinction	0	0		0	0	0		0	1									
Taste of saline	0		0	0	0	0	0	0	1	0	0	0	0	0	0	0	0	0
Removal of reward	0		1	1	1	0	1	0	1	1	1	1	1	1	1	1	1	1
Visual arousal	1		1	0	0	0	0	0	1	0	0	0	0	0	1	0	0	0

Table 4.3 Proportion of different types of neuron recorded in the macaque orbitofrontal cortex during sensory testing and visual discrimination reversal and related tasks. The number of neurons analysed was 463. (Reproduced from Experimental Brain Research, 49 (1)pp. 93-115, The orbitofrontal cortex: Neuronal activity in the behaving monkey, S. J. Thorpe, E. T. Rolls, and S. Maddison (c) 1983, Springer Science and Business Media. With kind permission from Springer Science and Business Media.)

Sensory testing:	
Visual, non-selective	10.7%
Visual, selective (i.e. responding to some objects or images)	13.2%
Visual, food-selective	5.3%
Visual, aversive objects	3.2%
Taste	7.3%
Visual and taste	2.6%
Removal of a food reward	6.3%
Extinction of ad lib licking for juice reward	7.5%
Visual discrimination reversal task:	
Visual, reversing in the visual discrimination task	5.3%
Visual, conditional discrimination in the visual discrimination task	2.5%
Visual, stimulus-related (not reversing) in the visual discrimination task	0.8%
Non-reward in the visual discrimination task	0.9%
Auditory tone cue signalling the start of a trial of the visual discrimination task	15.1%

fraction of the 3.5%. The implication is that an imaging study might not reveal really what is happening in a brain structure such as the orbitofrontal cortex where quite small proportions of neurons respond to any particular condition; and, especially, one would need to be very careful not to place much weight on a failure to find activation in a particular task, as the proportion of neurons responding may be small, and the time period for which they respond may be small too. For example, non-reward neurons typically respond for 2–8 s on the first two non-reward trials of extinction or reversal (Thorpe, Rolls & Maddison 1983).

In that most neurons in the macaque orbitofrontal cortex respond to reinforcers and punishers, or to stimuli associated with rewards and punishers, and do not respond in relation to responses, the orbitofrontal cortex is closely related to stimulus processing, including the stimuli that give rise to affective states. When it computes errors, it computes mismatches between stimuli that are expected, and stimuli that are obtained, and in this sense the errors are closely related to those required to correct affective states. This type of error representation may thus be different from that represented in the cingulate cortex, in which behavioural responses are represented, where the errors may be more closely related to errors that arise when action–outcome expectations are not met, and where action–outcome rather than stimulus–reinforcer

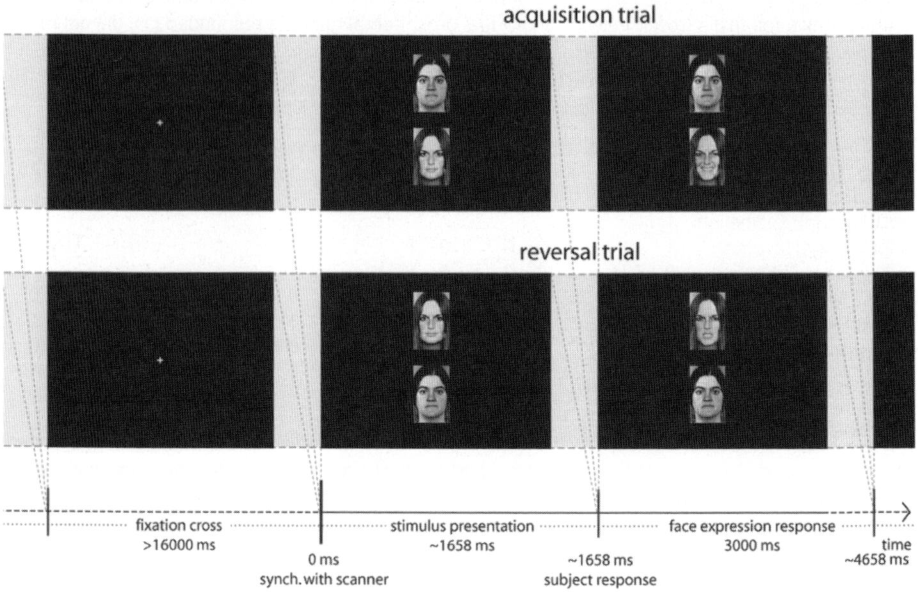

Fig. 4.39 Social reversal task: The trial starts synchronized with the scanner and two people with neutral face expressions are presented to the subject. The subject has to select one of the people by pressing the corresponding button, and the person will then either smile or show an angry face expression for 3000 ms depending on the current mood of the person. The task for the subject is to keep track of the mood of each person and choose the 'happy' person as much as possible (upper row). Over time (after between 4 and 8 correct trials) this will change so that the 'happy' person becomes 'angry' and vice versa, and the subject has to learn to adapt her choices accordingly (bottom row). Randomly intermixed trials with either two men, or two women, were used to control for possible gender and identification effects, and a fixation cross was presented between trials for at least 16000 ms. (Reprinted from *NeuroImage* 20 (2), Morten L. Kringelbach and Edmund T. Rolls, Neural correlates of rapid reversal learning in a simple model of human social interaction, pp. 1371–83, Copyright, 2003, with permission from Elsevier.)

representations need to be corrected (see Section 4.7).

We have also been able to obtain evidence that non-reward used as a signal to reverse behavioural choice is represented in the human orbitofrontal cortex. Kringelbach & Rolls (2003) used the faces of two different people, and if one face was selected then that face smiled, and if the other was selected, the face showed an angry expression. After good performance was acquired, there were repeated reversals of the visual discrimination task (see Fig. 4.39). Kringelbach & Rolls (2003) found that activation of a lateral part of the orbitofrontal cortex in the fMRI study was produced on the error trials, that is when the human chose a face, and did not obtain the expected reward (see Fig. 4.40). Control tasks showed that the response was related to the error, and the mismatch between what was expected and what was obtained, in that just showing an angry face expression did not selectively activate this part of the lateral orbitofrontal cortex. An interesting aspect of this study that makes it relevant to human social behaviour is that the conditioned stimuli were faces of particular individuals, and the unconditioned stimuli were face expressions. Moreover, the study reveals that the human orbitofrontal cortex is very sensitive to social feedback when it must be used to change behaviour (Kringelbach & Rolls 2003, Kringelbach & Rolls 2004).

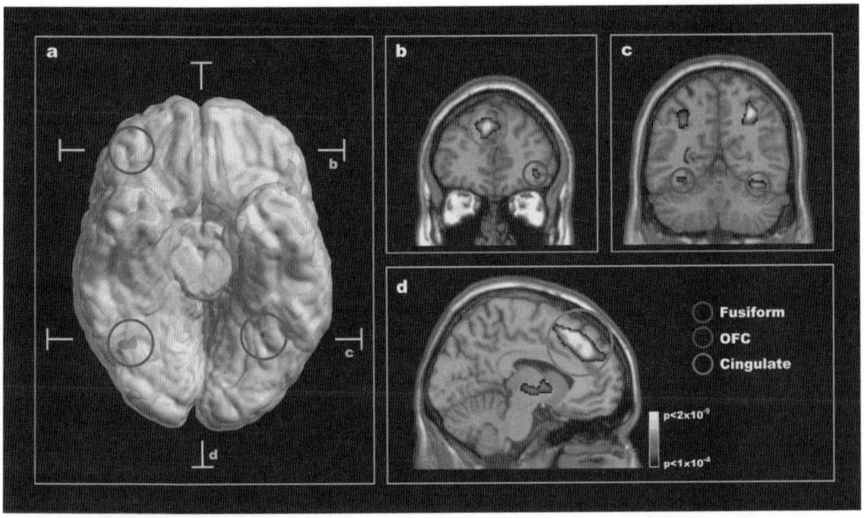

Fig. 4.40 Social reversal: Composite figure showing that changing behaviour based on face expression is correlated with increased brain activity in the human orbitofrontal cortex. a) The figure is based on two different group statistical contrasts from the neuroimaging data which are superimposed on a ventral view of the human brain with the cerebellum removed, and with indication of the location of the two coronal slices (b,c) and the transverse slice (d). The red activations in the orbitofrontal cortex (denoted OFC, maximal activation: z=4.94 [42 42 –8]; and z=5.51 [–46 30 –8] shown on the rendered brain arise from a comparison of reversal events with stable acquisition events, while the blue activations in the fusiform gyrus (denoted Fusiform, maximal activation: z>8 [36 –60 –20] and z=7.80 [–30 –56 –16]) arise from the main effects of face expression. b) The coronal slice through the frontal part of the brain shows the cluster in the right orbitofrontal cortex across all nine subjects when comparing reversal events with stable acquisition events. Significant activity was also seen in an extended area of the anterior cingulate/paracingulate cortex (denoted Cingulate, maximal activation: z=6.88 [–8 22 52]; green circle). c) The coronal slice through the posterior part of the brain shows the brain response to the main effects of face expression with significant activation in the fusiform gyrus and the cortex in the intraparietal sulcus (maximal activation: z>8 [32 –60 46]; and z>8 [–32 –60 44]). d) The transverse slice shows the extent of the activation in the anterior cingulate/paracingulate cortex when comparing reversal events with stable acquisition events. Group statistical results are superimposed on a ventral view of the human brain with the cerebellum removed, and on coronal and transverse slices of the same template brain (activations are thresholded at p=0.0001 for purposes of illustration to show their extent). (See colour plates section.) (Reprinted from *NeuroImage* 20 (2), Morten L. Kringelbach and Edmund T. Rolls, Neural correlates of rapid reversal learning in a simple model of human social interaction, pp. 1371–83, Copyright, 2003, with permission from Elsevier.)

4.5.5.6 A representation of faces in the orbitofrontal cortex

Another type of information represented in the orbitofrontal cortex is information about faces. There is a population of orbitofrontal cortex face-selective neurons that respond in many ways similarly to those in the temporal cortical visual areas (Rolls 1984, Rolls 1992b, Rolls 2000c, Rolls 2007a, Rolls 2008d, Rolls 2011c, Rolls 2012e). The orbitofrontal face-responsive neurons, first observed by Thorpe, Rolls & Maddison (1983), then by Rolls, Critchley, Browning & Inoue (2006a), tend to respond with longer latencies than temporal lobe neurons (140–200 ms typically, compared with 80–100 ms); they also convey information about which face is being seen, by having different responses to different faces (see Fig. 4.41); and are typically rather harder to activate strongly than temporal cortical face-selective neurons, in that many of them respond much better to real faces than to two-dimensional images of faces on a video monitor (cf. Rolls & Baylis (1986)). Some of the orbitofrontal cortex face-selective neurons are responsive to face gesture or movement. The findings are consistent

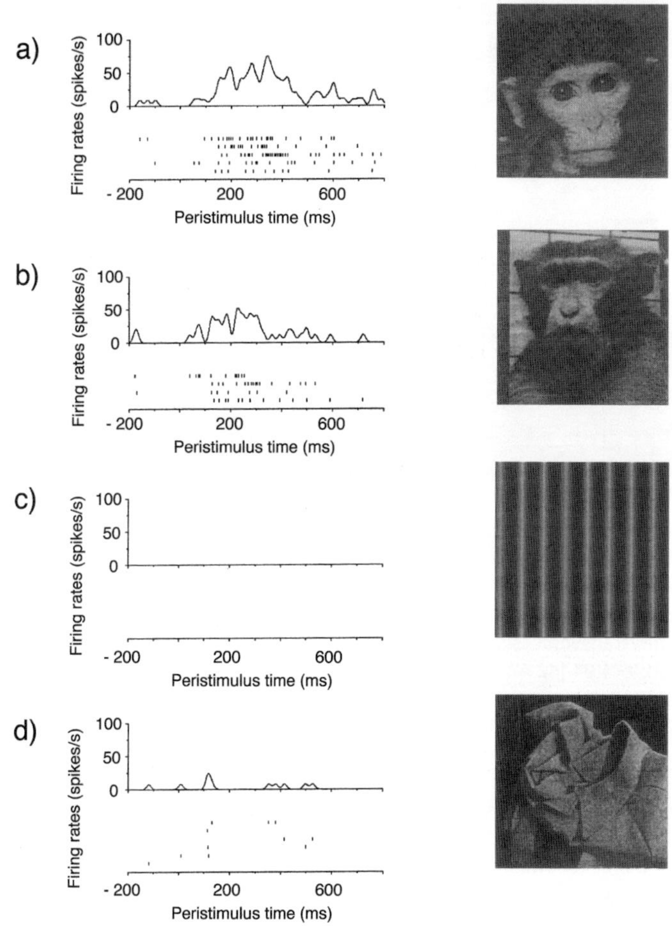

Fig. 4.41 Orbitofrontal cortex face-selective neuron as found in macaques. Peristimulus rastergrams and time histograms are shown. Each trial is a row in the rastergram. Several trials for each stimulus are shown. The ordinate is in spikes/s. The neuron responded best to face (a), also responded, though less to face (b), had different responses to other faces (not shown), and did not respond to non-face stimuli (e.g. (c) and (d)). The stimulus appeared at time 0 on a video monitor. (Reproduced from *Experimental Brain Research*, 170 (1) pp. 743–87, Face-selective and auditory neurons in the primate orbitofrontal cortex, Rolls, E. T., Critchley, H. D., Browning, A. S. and Inoue, K., (c) 2006, Springer Science and Business Media. With kind permission from Springer Science and Business Media.)

with the likelihood that these neurons are activated via the inputs from the temporal cortical visual areas in which face-selective neurons are found (see Fig. 4.2). The significance of the neurons is likely to be related to the fact that faces convey information that is important in social reinforcement, both by conveying face expression (cf. Hasselmo, Rolls & Baylis (1989a)), which can indicate reinforcement, and by encoding information about which individual is present, also important in evaluating and utilizing reinforcing inputs in social situations (Rolls, Critchley, Browning & Inoue 2006a, Rolls 2011c).

Consistent with these findings in macaques, and as described above, in humans, activation of the lateral orbitofrontal cortex occurs when a rewarding smile expression is expected, but an angry face expression is obtained, in a visual discrimination reversal task (Kringelbach & Rolls 2003). This is an example of the operation of a social reinforcer, and, consistent with

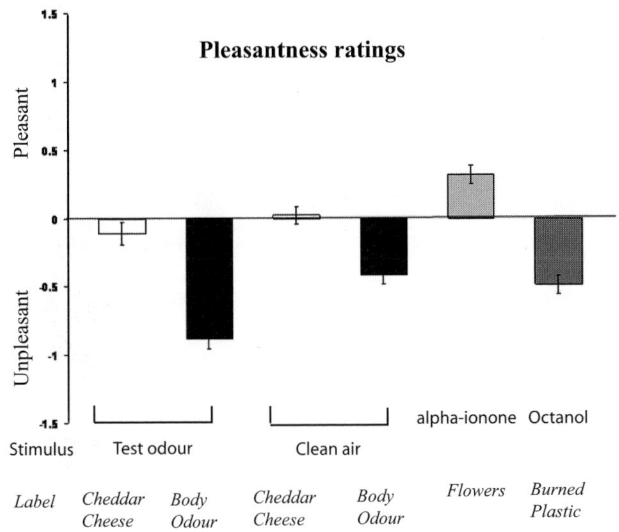

Fig. 4.42 Cognition and emotion. Subjective pleasantness ratings (mean $\pm$ s.e.m. across subjects) to odours labelled with words. The corresponding stimulus and label to each bar are listed in the lower part of the figure. The test odour (isovaleric acid) and clean air were paired in different trials with a label of either 'Cheddar cheese' or 'Body odour'. (Reprinted from *Neuron*, 46 (4), Ivan E. de Araujo, Edmund T. Rolls, Maria Inés Velazco, Christian Margot, and Isabelle Cayeux, Cognitive Modulation of Olfactory Processing, pp. 671–679, Copyright, 2005, with permission from Elsevier.)

these results, Farrow, Zheng, Wilkinson, Spence, Deakin, Tarrier, Griffiths & Woodruff (2001) have found that activation of the orbitofrontal cortex is found when humans are making social judgements. In addition, activation of the medial orbitofrontal cortex is correlated with face attractiveness (O'Doherty et al. 2003b).

Auditory stimuli may have similar representations in the orbitofrontal cortex related to their affective value. For example, Blood et al. (1999) found a correlation between subjective ratings of dissonance and consonance of musical chords and the activations produced in the orbitofrontal cortex (see also Blood & Zatorre (2001) and Frey, Kostopoulos & Petrides (2000)). The transition of harmony towards a pleasant resolution also activates the orbitofrontal cortex (Fujisawa & Cook 2011).

4.5.5.7 Cognitive influences on the orbitofrontal cortex

Affective states, moods, can influence cognitive processing, including perception and memory (see Section 4.12). But cognition can also influence emotional states. This is not only in the sense that cognitively processed events, if decoded as being rewarding or punishing, can produce emotional states (see Section 2.8), but also in the sense described here that a cognitive input can bias emotional states in different directions. The modulation is rather like the top-down effects of attention on perception (Desimone & Duncan 1995, Rolls & Deco 2002, Deco & Rolls 2003, Deco & Rolls 2005c), not only phenomenologically, but also probably computationally. An example of such cognitive influences on the reward/aversive states that are elicited by stimuli was revealed in a study of olfaction described by De Araujo, Rolls, Velazco, Margot & Cayeux (2005).

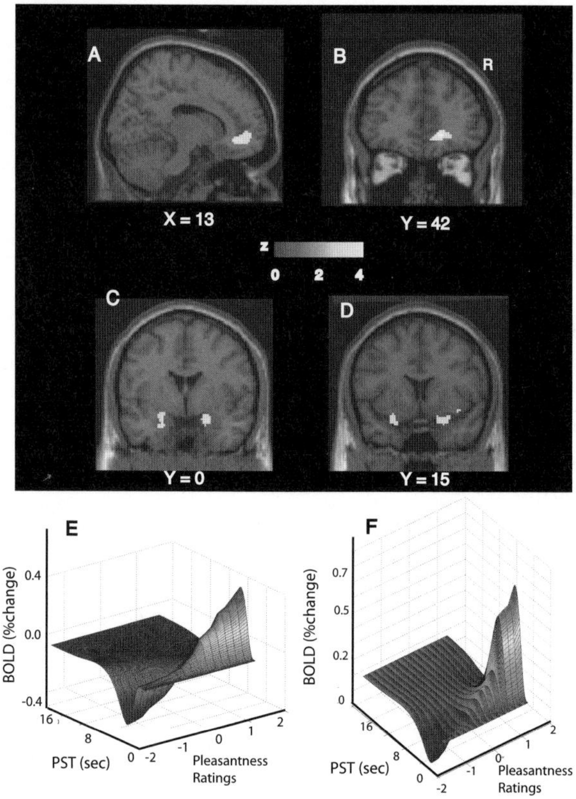

Fig. 4.43 Cognition and emotion. Group (random) effects analysis showing the brain regions where the BOLD signal was correlated with pleasantness ratings given to the test odour. The pleasantness ratings were being modulated by the word labels. (A) Activations in the rostral anterior cingulate cortex, in the region adjoining the medial OFC, shown in a sagittal slice. (B) The same activation shown coronally. (C) Bilateral activations in the amygdala. (D) These activations extended anteriorly to the primary olfactory cortex. The image was thresholded at p<0.0001 uncorrected in order to show the extent of the activation. (E) Parametric plots of the data averaged across all subjects showing that the percentage BOLD change (fitted) correlates with the pleasantness ratings in the region shown in A and B. The parametric plots were very similar for the primary olfactory region shown in D. PST - Post-stimulus time (s). (F) Parametric plots for the amygdala region shown in C. (See colour plates section.) (Reprinted from *Neuron*, 46 (4), Ivan E. de Araujo, Edmund T. Rolls, Maria Inés Velazco, Christian Margot, and Isabelle Cayeux, Cognitive Modulation of Olfactory Processing, pp. 671–679, Copyright, 2005, with permission from Elsevier.)

In this investigation, a standard test odour, isovaleric acid (with a small amount of cheddar cheese flavour added to make it more pleasant), was used as the test olfactory stimulus delivered with an olfactometer during functional neuroimaging with fMRI (De Araujo et al. 2005). This odour is somewhat ambiguous, and might be interpreted as the odour emitted by a cheese-like odour (rather like brie), or might be interpreted as a rather pungent and unpleasant body odour. A word was shown during the 8 s odour delivery. On some trials, the test odour was accompanied by the visually presented word 'Cheddar cheese'. On other trials, the test odour was accompanied by the visually presented word 'Body odour'. A word label was used rather than a picture label to make the modulating input very abstract and cognitive. First, it was found (consistent with psychophysical results of Herz & von Clef (2001)) that the word labels influenced the pleasantness ratings of the test odour, as shown in Fig. 4.42.

However, very interestingly, it was found that the word label modulated the activation to the odour in brain regions activated by odours such as the orbitofrontal cortex (secondary olfactory cortex), cingulate cortex, and amygdala. For example, in the medial orbitofrontal cortex the word label 'Cheddar cheese' caused a larger activation to be produced to the test odour than when the word label 'Body odour' was being presented. In these medial orbitofrontal cortex regions and the amygdala, and even possibly in some parts of the primary olfactory cortical areas, the activations were correlated with the pleasantness ratings, as shown in Fig. 4.43. This is consistent with the finding that the pleasantness of odours is represented in the medial orbitofrontal cortex (Rolls, Kringelbach & De Araujo 2003c).

The effects of the word were smaller when clean air was the stimulus, indicating that the effects being imaged were not just effects of a word to influence representations by a top-down recall process, but were instead cognitive top-down effects on states elicited by odours. This type of modulation is typical of a top-down modulatory process such as has been analysed quantitatively in the case of attention (Deco & Rolls 2005c), and indeed no significant effect of the word was found in the amygdala and earlier olfactory cortical areas. A further implication is that the activations in the human amygdala and primary olfactory cortical areas are more closely bound to the eliciting stimulus and are less influenced by cognition than are activations in the orbitofrontal and cingulate cortices.

These findings show that cognition can influence and indeed modulate reward-related (affective) processing as far down the human olfactory system as the secondary olfactory cortex (in the orbitofrontal cortex), and in the amygdala. This emphasizes the importance of cognitive influences on emotion, and shows how, in situations that might range from enjoying food to a romantic evening, the cognitive top-down influences can play an important role in influencing affective representations in the brain. Indeed, these findings lend support to the hypothesis that an interesting role for cognitive systems in emotion is to help set up the optimal conditions in terms of the reinforcers available and contextual surroundings for reinforcers to produce affective states, as treated further in the dual route hypothesis described in Chapter 10.

In an investigation of top-down cognitive modulation of affective processing in another modality, taste, it was found that activations related to the affective value of umami (delicious savoury) taste and flavor (as shown by correlations with pleasantness ratings) in the orbitofrontal cortex were modulated by word-level descriptors (Grabenhorst, Rolls & Bilderbeck 2008a). Affect-related activations to taste were modulated in a region that receives from the orbitofrontal cortex, the pregenual cingulate cortex, and to taste and flavor in another region that receives from the orbitofrontal cortex, the ventral striatum. Affect-related cognitive modulations were not found in the insular taste cortex, where the intensity but not the pleasantness of the taste was represented. Thus top-down language-level cognitive effects reach far down into the earliest cortical areas that represent the appetitive value of taste and flavor, and this type of modulation may be important in appetite control (Rolls 2012c).

Similar cognitive modulation of affective touch is also found. The cognitive modulation was produced by word labels, 'Rich moisturizing cream' or 'Basic cream', while cream was being applied by slow gentle rubbing to the forearm, or was seen being applied to a forearm. The subjective pleasantness and richness were modulated by the word labels, as were the activations to the sight of touch and also the correlations with pleasantness in the pregenual cingulate/orbitofrontal cortex and ventral striatum (McCabe, Rolls, Bilderbeck & McGlone 2008). Further evidence of how the orbitofrontal cortex is involved in affective aspects of touch was that touch to the forearm [which has C fiber Touch (CT) afferents sensitive to light touch] compared with touch to the glabrous skin of the hand (which does not) revealed activation in the mid-orbitofrontal cortex. This is of interest as previous studies have suggested that the CT system is important in affiliative caress-like touch between individuals (McCabe et al. 2008, Rolls 2010c, Rolls 2013e).

Another example of what could be a similar phenomenon is that colour can have a strong influence on olfactory judgements. This was demonstrated when a white wine was artificially coloured red with an odourless dye, and it was found that participants (undergraduates at the Faculty of Oenology of the University of Bordeaux) described the wine using the descriptors normally used for red wine (Morrot, Brochet & Dubourdieu 2001). In this case it is possible that cognitive states elicited by the sight of what was believed to be red wine modulated the olfactory representation. Another possibility is that in a multimodal region such as the orbitofrontal cortex where the sight, smell, taste and texture are brought together onto individual neurons (see Section 4.5.5), the visual input makes a strong contribution to the convergence, and the resulting representation then is available to cognition for verbal description.

The mechanisms by which cognitive states have top-down effects on emotion are probably similar to the biased competition (Desimone & Duncan 1995, Rolls & Deco 2002, Deco & Rolls 2003, Deco & Rolls 2005c, Rolls & Stringer 2001b, Deco & Rolls 2005b) and biased activation (Rolls 2013a, Grabenhorst & Rolls 2010) mechanisms that subserve top-down attentional effects (see also Section 4.12). In such systems, it is important that the top-down influence does not determine the activity in the system, otherwise stimuli and events would be imagined, and would not represent what was happening in the world. But by having a weak influence, facilitated by the fact that the top-down backprojection connections are relatively weak (Rolls 1989b, Rolls & Treves 1998, Renart, Parga & Rolls 1999a, Renart, Parga & Rolls 1999b, Renart, Moreno, Rocha, Parga & Rolls 2001, Rolls & Stringer 2001b, Rolls & Deco 2002, Deco & Rolls 2005c, Deco & Rolls 2005b, Rolls 2013a), cognition and attention can have beneficial effects in directing sensory and emotional processing towards stimuli and events that the cognitive system has determined are relevant.

Part of the interest and importance of these investigations is that they show that cognitive influences, originating from as high in processing as linguistic representations, can reach down into the first part of the brain in which emotion, affective, hedonic or reward value is made explicit in the representation, the orbitofrontal cortex, to modulate the responses there to affective taste, olfactory, flavour, somatosensory, and visual stimuli. The investigations thus show that linguistic representations can influence how emotional states are represented and thus experienced. It is in this very direct way that cognition can have a powerful effect on emotional states, emotional behaviour, and emotional experience, because the emotional representations in the first cortical area in which affective value is represented, the orbitofrontal cortex, are altered.

4.5.5.8 Attentional modulation of affective vs sensory processing

Attentional instructions at the same, very high, linguistic, level (e.g. 'pay attention to and rate pleasantness' vs 'pay attention to and rate intensity') have a top-down modulatory influence on value representations in the orbitofrontal cortex and anterior cingulate cortex. The attentional instructions can bias processing for a stimulus between a stream through the orbitofrontal and cingulate cortices that processes value and affect, versus a stream involving sensory processing areas such as the insular taste cortex and pyriform primary olfactory cortex.

This modulation of affective processing has been shown for olfactory stimuli (Rolls, Grabenhorst, Margot, da Silva & Velazco 2008a). When subjects were instructed to remember and rate the pleasantness of a jasmin odour, activations in an fMRI investigation were greater in the medial orbitofrontal and pregenual cingulate cortex than when subjects were instructed to remember and rate the intensity of the odour. When the subjects were instructed to remember and rate the intensity, activations were greater in the pyriform primary olfactory cortex and inferior frontal gyrus. Top-down effects of attention occurred not only during odor delivery but started in a preparation period after the instruction before odor delivery, and continued after termination of the odor in a short-term memory period. Thus, depending on the context in

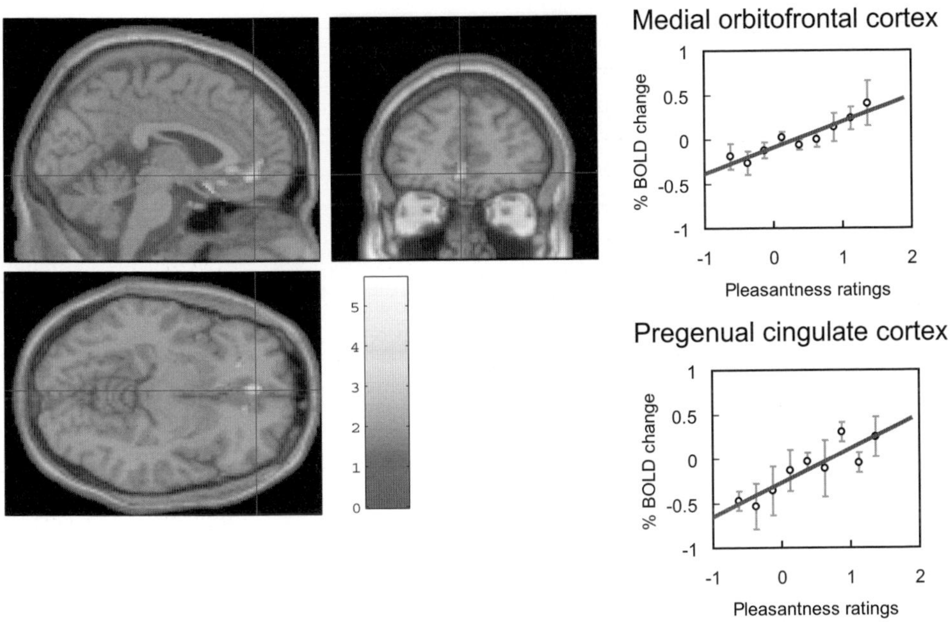

Fig. 4.44 Top-down attention and emotion. Effect of paying attention to the pleasantness of a taste. Left: A significant difference related to the taste period was found in the medial orbitofrontal cortex at [-6 14 -20] z=3.81 p<0.003 (towards the back of the area of activation shown) and in the pregenual cingulate cortex at [-4 46 -8] z=2.90 p<0.04 (at the cursor). Right upper: The correlation between the subjective pleasantness ratings and the activation (% BOLD change) in the orbitofrontal cortex (r=0.94, df=8, p<<0.001). Right lower: The correlation between the pleasantness ratings and the activation (% BOLD change) in the pregenual cingulate cortex r=0.89, df=8, p=0.001). The taste stimulus, monosodium glutamate, was identical on all trials. (See colour plates section.) (Reproduced from Fabian Grabenhorst and Edmund T. Rolls, Selective attention to affective value alters how the brain processes taste stimuli, *European Journal of Neuroscience*, 27 (3) pp. 723–729 Copyright ©2008, John Wiley and Sons.)

which odours are presented and whether affect is relevant, the brain prepares itself, responds to, and remembers an odor differently. These findings show that when attention is paid to affective value, the brain systems engaged to prepare for, represent, and remember a sensory stimulus are different from those engaged when attention is directed to the physical properties of a stimulus such as its intensity.

In an investigation of the effects of selective attention to value and affect vs intensity on taste processing, when subjects were instructed to remember and rate the pleasantness of a savoury taste stimulus, 0.1 M monosodium glutamate, activations were greater in the medial orbitofrontal and pregenual cingulate cortex than when subjects were instructed to remember and rate the intensity of the taste (Grabenhorst & Rolls 2008) (Fig. 4.44). When the subjects were instructed to remember and rate the intensity, activations were greater in the insular taste cortex and a mid-insular cortex region (Fig. 4.45). Thus, depending on the context in which tastes are presented and whether affect is relevant, the brain responds to a taste differently.

The lateral prefrontal cortex, a region implicated in attentional control (Corbetta & Shulman 2002, Bressler, Tang, Sylvester, Shulman & Corbetta 2008, Rolls 2008b), has been shown to be a site of origin for these top-down influences of attention on processing to the affective vs physical properties of stimuli. Grabenhorst & Rolls (2010) have shown with fMRI connectivity analyses (Friston, Buechel, Fink, Morris, Rolls & Dolan 1997) that in the

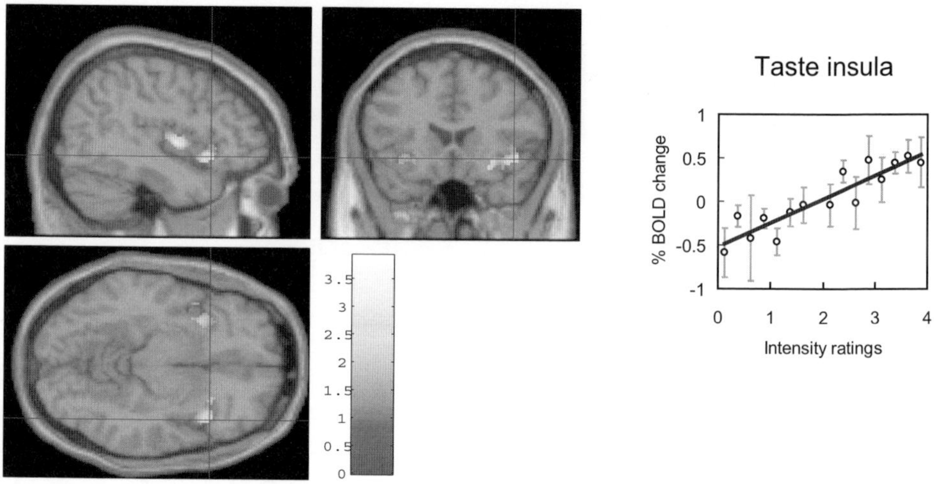

Fig. 4.45 Top-down attention and emotion. Left: Effect of paying attention to the intensity of a taste. Top: A significant difference related to the taste period was found in the taste insula at [42 18 -14] z=2.42 p<0.05 (indicated by the cursor) and in the mid insula at [40 -2 4] z=3.03 p<0.025. Right: The correlation between the intensity ratings and the activation (% BOLD change) in the taste insula (r=0.91, df=14, p<<0.001). The taste stimulus, monosodium glutamate, was identical on all trials. (See colour plates section.) (Reproduced from Fabian Grabenhorst and Edmund T. Rolls, Selective attention to affective value alters how the brain processes taste stimuli, *European Journal of Neuroscience*, 27 (3) pp. 723–729 Copyright ©2008, John Wiley and Sons.)

anterior lateral prefrontal cortex at Y=53 mm the correlation with activity in the orbitofrontal and pregenual cingulate cortex seed regions was greater when attention was to pleasantness compared with when attention was to intensity. Conversely, in a more posterior region of the LPFC at Y=34 mm the correlation with activity in the anterior insula seed region was greater when attention was to intensity compared with when attention was to pleasantness. (These seed regions were chosen as they were the regions where attention to affect or to intensity modulated the effects of the taste stimulus.) Grabenhorst & Rolls (2010) also showed that correlations between areas within each in these separate processing streams were dependent on selective attention to affective value versus physical intensity of the stimulus.

Correlations between signals, including signals at the neuronal or at the functional neuroimaging level, do not reveal the direction of the possible influence of one signal on the other. We extended the previous investigation by introducing and using componential Granger causality analysis, which measures the effect of y (for example a timeseries of activations in one brain area) on x (for example a timeseries of activations in another brain area), and allows interaction effects between y and x to be measured (Ge, Feng, Grabenhorst & Rolls 2012). We showed that there is a top-down attentional effect from the anterior dorsolateral prefrontal cortex to the orbitofrontal cortex when attention is paid to the pleasantness of a taste, and that this effect depends on the activity in the orbitofrontal cortex as shown by the interaction term. Correspondingly there is a top-down attentional effect from the posterior dorsolateral prefrontal cortex to the insular primary taste cortex when attention is paid to the intensity of a taste, and this effect depends on the activity of the insular primary taste cortex as shown by the interaction term. These interaction effects reflect the underlying mechanism, that a weak top-down effect can have a large, non-linear, effect on bottom-up inputs when the bottom-up inputs are weak or ambiguous, as shown by an integrate-and-fire neuronal model of the mechanisms of selective attention (Deco & Rolls 2005c), which describes a mechanism for top-down attention (Desimone & Duncan 1995, Rolls 2008b, Rolls 2013a).

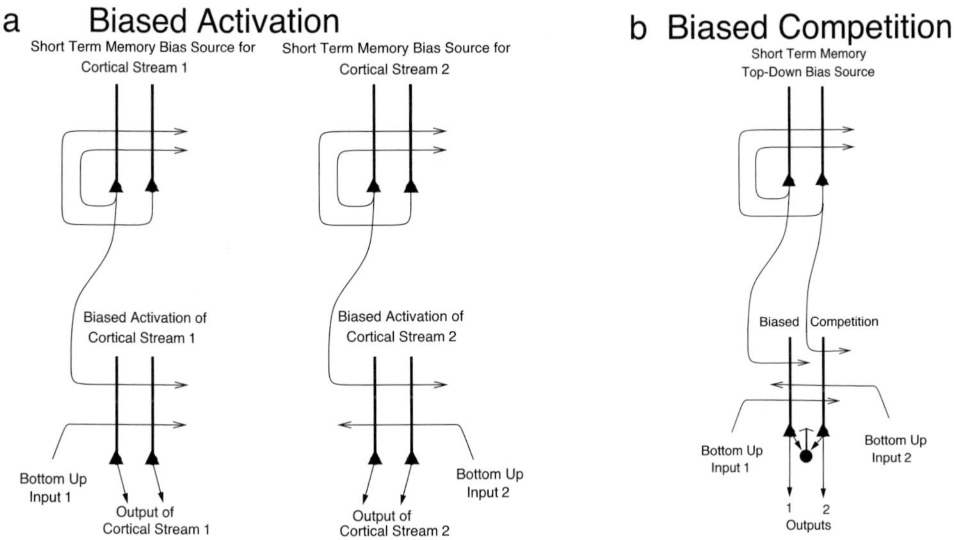

Fig. 4.46 Mechanisms for top-down attention. (a) Biased activation. The short-term memory systems that provide the source of the top-down activations may be separate (as shown), or could be a single network with different attractor states for the different selective attention conditions. The top-down short-term memory systems hold what is being paid attention to active by continuing firing in an attractor state, and bias separately either cortical processing system 1, or cortical processing system 2. This weak top-down bias interacts with the bottom up input to the cortical stream and produces an increase of activity that can be supralinear (Deco and Rolls 2005c). Thus the selective activation of separate cortical processing streams can occur. In the example, stream 1 might process the affective value of a stimulus, and stream 2 might process the intensity and physical properties of the stimulus. The outputs of these separate processing streams then must enter a competition system, which could be for example a cortical attractor decision-making network that makes choices between the two streams, with the choice biased by the activations in the separate streams (see text). (b) Biased competition. There is usually a single attractor network that can enter different attractor states to provide the source of the top-down bias (as shown). If it is a single network, there can be competition within the short-term memory attractor states, implemented through the local GABA inhibitory neurons. The top-down continuing firing of one of the attractor states then biases in a top-down process some of the neurons in a cortical area to respond more to one than the other of the bottom-up inputs, with competition implemented through the GABA inhibitory neurons (symbolized by a filled circle) which make feedback inhibitory connections onto the pyramidal cells (symbolized by a triangle) in the cortical area. The thick vertical lines above the pyramidal cells are the dendrites. The axons are shown with thin lines and the excitatory connections by arrow heads.

The way that one usually thinks of a top-down biased competition mechanism as operating in, for example, visual selective attention (Desimone & Duncan 1995) is that within an area, e.g. a cortical region, some neurons receive a weak top-down input that increases their response to the bottom-up stimuli (Desimone & Duncan 1995), potentially supralinearly if the bottom-up stimuli are weak (Deco & Rolls 2005c, Rolls & Deco 2002, Rolls 2008b). The enhanced firing of the biased neurons then, via the local inhibitory neurons, inhibits the other neurons in the local area from responding to the bottom-up stimuli. This is a local mechanism, in that the inhibition in the neocortex is primarily local, being implemented by cortical inhibitory neurons that typically have inputs and outputs over no more than a few mm (Douglas, Markram & Martin 2004, Rolls 2008b). This model of biased competition is illustrated in Fig. 4.46b.

This type of locally implemented 'biased competition' situation may not apply in the present case, where we have facilitation of processing in a whole cortical area (e.g. orbitofrontal cortex, or pregenual cingulate cortex) or even cortical processing stream (e.g. the linked orbitofrontal and pregenual cingulate cortex) in which any taste neurons may reflect pleasantness and not intensity. So the attentional effect might more accurately be described in this case as biased activation, without local competition being part of the effect. I have therefore proposed a *biased activation theory and model of attention*, illustrated in Fig. 4.46a (Rolls 2013a, Grabenhorst & Rolls 2010), which is a rather different way to implement attention in the brain than biased competition, and each mechanism may apply in different cases, or both mechanisms in some cases. In this case, the short-term memory systems implemented by an attractor network in for example the prefrontal cortex that holds in short-term memory the property to which attention should be paid provides top-down inputs which bias the activations in whole processing streams. The short-term memory in the prefrontal cortex could be implemented in a single attractor network with different attractor states (Rolls 2008b) for the different attentional conditions, or, as suggested by the evidence in this case (Grabenhorst & Rolls 2010), the short-term memory networks may be at least partly physically separate, though close to each other in the prefrontal cortex. The systems being modulated could operate as competitive networks, as attractor networks, or, as I have suggested (Rolls 2008b), as networks that can learn mainly by competitive learning, but can maintain activity in memory using associatively modified recurrent collateral connections to implement attractor dynamics.

The outputs of the separate processing streams showing biased activation (Fig. 4.46a) may need to be compared later to lead to a single behaviour. One way in which this comparison could take place is by both outputs entering a single network cortical attractor model of decision-making, in which positive feedback implemented by the excitatory recurrent collateral connections leads through non-linear dynamics to a single winner, which is ensured by competition between the different possible attractor states produced through inhibitory neurons (Deco & Rolls 2006, Rolls & Deco 2010, Wang 2008, Wang 2002). A second way in which the competition could be implemented is by that usually conceptualized as important in biased competition (Deco & Rolls 2005b, Desimone & Duncan 1995, Rolls & Deco 2002), in which a feedforward competitive network using inhibition through local inhibitory neurons provides a way for a weak top-down signal to bias the output especially if the bottom-up inputs are weak (Deco & Rolls 2005b, Rolls & Deco 2002, Rolls 2008b), and this implementation is what is shown at the bottom of Fig. 4.46b. A third way in which the biased activation reflected in the output of the streams shown in Fig. 4.46a could be taken into account is by a mechanism such as that in the basal ganglia, where in the striatum the different excitatory inputs activate GABA (gamma-amino-butyric acid) neurons, which then directly inhibit each other to make the selection (Rolls 2005b, Rolls 2008b) (Chapter 6).

Biased activation as a mechanism for top-down selective attention may be widespread in the brain, and may be engaged when there is segregated processing of different attributes of stimuli. It may apply not only for affective, value-based vs sensory processing, but also to the dorsal vs ventral visual system in vision, and to the 'what' vs 'where' systems for visual processing (Rolls & Deco 2002, Rolls 2008b, Rolls 2013a).

These findings show that, when attention is paid to affective value, the brain systems engaged to represent stimuli are in part different from those engaged when attention is directed to the physical properties of a stimulus such as its intensity. This has many implications for understanding the effects of many stimuli and recalled memories too, and has many implications for sensory testing. These insights have implications for a number of areas related to neuroeconomics and decision-making, including the design of studies in which attentional instructions may influence which brain systems become engaged, as well as situations in which affective processing may be usefully modulated (for example in the control of the effects of the reward value of food and its role in obesity (Chapter 5), and in addiction (Chapter 6)

(Rolls 2008b, Rolls 2012c).

Another implication is that paying attention to pleasantness, and also cognitive top-down modulation, may be used to enhance pleasant emotional and aesthetic experiences.

4.5.5.9 The topology of the functional neuroimaging activations in the orbitofrontal cortex

Kringelbach & Rolls (2004) have reviewed evidence that the activations found in functional neuroimaging studies by many types of reward appear to involve relatively medial parts of the human orbitofrontal cortex, and unpleasant stimuli or non-reward more lateral parts of the human orbitofrontal cortex. For example, we have obtained evidence from an experiment using pleasant, painful and neutral somatosensory stimulation that there is some spatial segregation of the representation of rewards and punishers, where the effects of pleasant somatosensory stimulation are spatially dissociable from the effects of painful stimulation in the human orbitofrontal cortex (Rolls, O'Doherty, Kringelbach, Francis, Bowtell & McGlone 2003d). Further, pleasant odours activate medial, and unpleasant odours lateral, regions of the human orbitofrontal cortex (Rolls, Kringelbach & De Araujo 2003c). Another example comes from the finding that the administration of amphetamine to naive human subjects activates the orbitofrontal cortex and two regions to which it projects the pregenual cingulate coryex and ventral striatum (Voellm, De Araujo, Cowen, Rolls, Kringelbach, Smith, Jezzard, Heal & Matthews 2004). An indication that a rewarding effect is being produced by the amphetamine in part because of an action in the orbitofrontal cortex is that macaques will self-administer amphetamine to the orbitofrontal cortex (Phillips, Mora & Rolls 1981). A clear indication of a differentiation in function between medial versus lateral areas of the human orbitofrontal cortex was found in our study investigating visual discrimination reversal learning, which showed a clear dissociation between the medial orbitofrontal areas correlating with monetary gain, and the lateral areas correlating with monetary loss (O'Doherty, Kringelbach, Rolls, Hornak & Andrews 2001a). This result, and some of the other studies included in the meta-analysis (Kringelbach & Rolls 2004), can be interpreted as evidence for a difference in humans between medial orbitofrontal cortex areas involved in decoding and monitoring the reward value of reinforcers, and lateral areas involved in evaluating punishers that when detected may lead to a change in current behaviour. A good example of a study showing the latter involved a visual discrimination reversal task in which face identity was associated with a face expression (Kringelbach & Rolls 2003). When the face expression associated with one of the faces reversed and the face expression was being interpreted as a punisher and indicated that behaviour should change, then lateral parts of the orbitofrontal cortex became activated (Fig. 4.40).

At sites where positive value, produced by a reward, are represented, there are, when they are measured, correlations between the conscious, subjective, state of pleasure and the brain activations, where both are measured on every trial. Similarly, at sites where negative value, produced by a punisher or non-reward, are represented, there are correlations between the subjective state of unpleasantness and the brain activations. Fig. 4.47 shows the peaks of the correlations found in many different investigations related to these subjective states of pleasantness (yellow) and of unpleasantness (white) for both the orbitofrontal and the cingulate and ventromedial prefrontal cortices (see also Section 4.7) (Grabenhorst & Rolls 2011). Reference to Fig. 4.18 on page 98 shows the different cytoarchitectonic areas in these regions.

Although our study on abstract reward found that monetary reward and punishment are correlated with activations in different regions of the orbitofrontal cortex (O'Doherty, Kringelbach, Rolls, Hornak & Andrews 2001a), even this evidence does not show that rewards and punishers have totally separate representations in the human brain. In particular, the medial regions of the orbitofrontal cortex that had activations correlating with the magnitude of

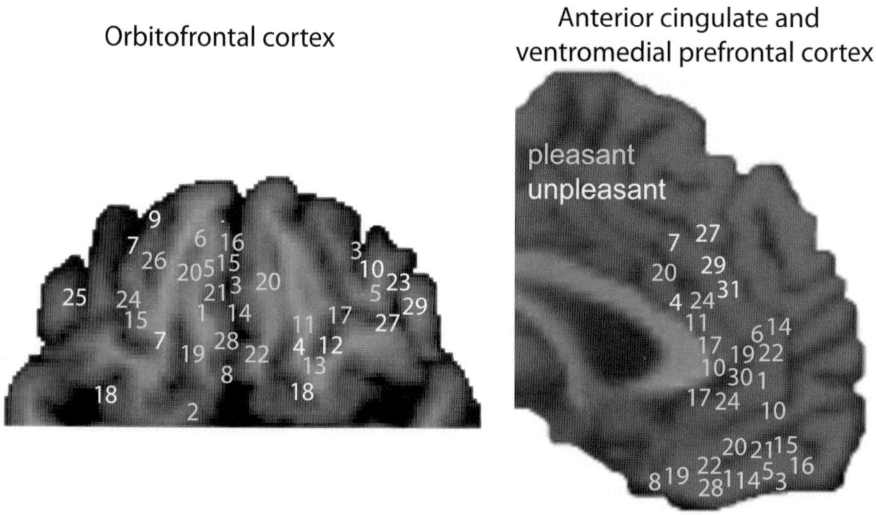

Fig. 4.47 Maps of subjective pleasure in the human orbitofrontal cortex (ventral view) and anterior cingulate and ventromedial prefrontal cortex (sagittal view). Yellow: sites where activations correlate with subjective pleasantness. White: sites where activations correlate with subjective unpleasantness. The numbers refer to effects found in specific studies. Taste: 1, 2; odor: 3-10; flavor: 11-16; oral texture: 17, 18; chocolate: 19; water: 20; wine: 21; oral temperature: 22, 23; somatosensory temperature: 24, 25; the sight of touch: 26, 27; facial attractiveness: 28, 29; erotic pictures: 30; laser-induced pain: 31. (See colour plates section.) (Reprinted from *Trends in Cognitive Sciences*, 15 (2), Fabian Grabenhorst and Edmund T. Rolls, Value, pleasure and choice in the ventral prefrontal cortex, pp. 56–67, Copyright, 2011, with permission from Elsevier.)

monetary reward (area 11) also reflected monetary punishers in the sense that the activations in these medial regions correlated positively with the magnitude of monetary wins and negatively with losses (see Fig. 4.35). Similarly, the more lateral regions (area 10) had activations that correlated negatively with the magnitudes of monetary wins and gains, and positively with monetary loss/punishment. This means that in this experiment the medial and lateral regions were apparently coding for both monetary reward and punishment (albeit in opposite ways). Further evidence for the same principle, but now for pleasant vs unpleasant odours, is illustrated in Fig. 4.27 (Rolls et al. 2003c). The evidence from such experiments would therefore suggest that the segregation between rewards and punishers is not purely spatial but rather encoded in the neuronal responses, which the studies in macaques described above show can be exquisitely tuned differently not only to reinforcers in different sensory modalities (taste, smell, touch etc.), but also to combinations of these, and even within any one modality (e.g. with neurons tuned to different tastes). The functional imaging thus provides a very blurred picture of what is really happening at the neuronal and information representation level in the orbitofrontal cortex. Although it is true that similar neurons may tend to cluster together as a result of a self-organizing competitive network with short range excitatory connections (see Rolls & Treves (1998) and Rolls (2008b)), and this may lead to somewhat localized blobs of activity in the cortex, the presence of such blobs should not be taken as more than a gross reflection of the underlying neuronal representations and computations. Integrating over all this heterogeneous neuronal activity is what leads to an fMRI signal (see Section 8.7.5).

What account might we give for why so many different types of reward are represented in the human medial orbitofrontal cortex? The types of reward include, as described above and in Chapter 5, food reward as shown in sensory-specific satiety experiments (Kringelbach, O'Doherty, Rolls & Andrews 2003), pleasant odours (Rolls, Kringelbach & De Araujo 2003c, Grabenhorst, Rolls, Margot, da Silva & Velazco 2007, Rolls, Grabenhorst, Margot, da Silva & Velazco 2008a), pleasant flavours (McCabe & Rolls 2007, Rolls & McCabe 2007, Grabenhorst et al. 2008a, Grabenhorst & Rolls 2008), pleasant touch (Rolls, O'Doherty, Kringelbach, Francis, Bowtell & McGlone 2003d, McCabe, Rolls, Bilderbeck & McGlone 2008, Rolls, Grabenhorst & Parris 2008b), face attractiveness (O'Doherty et al. 2003b), monetary reward (O'Doherty, Kringelbach, Rolls, Hornak & Andrews 2001a, Rolls, McCabe & Redoute 2008e), conditioned stimuli associated with drug self-administration in addicts (Childress, Mozley, McElgin, Fitzgerald, Reivich & O'Brien 1999), and also the administration of amphetamine to drug-naive human subjects (Voellm, De Araujo, Cowen, Rolls, Kringelbach, Smith, Jezzard, Heal & Matthews 2004). The neuronal recording studies described above in macaques show clearly that there is an exquisite representation of the detailed properties of these different stimuli, with different neurons by virtue of their different tuning to each of these properties and to combinations of these properties providing information about all the individual properties of each particular stimulus. For example, as a population, different orbitofrontal cortex neurons in macaques have different responses to the following properties of oral stimuli, with some neurons encoding each property independently, and others responding to different combinations of them: taste, fat texture, viscosity, astringency, grittiness, capsaicin content, odour, and sight (see above and Chapter 5).

So why are so many of the reward-related properties of stimuli represented in the same medial part of the orbitofrontal cortex? I suggest that part of the functional utility of this is that there can be comparison of the magnitudes of what may be quite different types of reward, implemented by the local lateral inhibition mediated via the inhibitory interneurons.

The architecture required for the implementation is that which is standard for the cerebral cortex: the excitatory pyramidal cells, which are the neurons with the types of often quite selective response just described, connect to inhibitory neurons, which are relatively fewer in number (perhaps 15% of the number of excitatory neurons). The inhibitory neurons receive from random sets of neurons in the vicinity, and project back their summed effects as inhibition to random collections of pyramidal cells. This lateral inhibition system has the effect of controlling the activity of the excitatory neurons, and importantly, the effect of ensuring that the most strongly activated excitatory neurons reduce the activity of less strongly activated excitatory neurons. Contrast enhancement may occur between the competing inputs, and also local scaling of the overall activity of the neurons so that they operate within their working range to reflect in their output firing the inputs being received, in processes that are quantitatively understood and are used in competitive networks (Grossberg 1988, Rolls & Treves 1998, Rolls & Deco 2002, Deco & Rolls 2005c, Rolls 2008b). The result of the mutual inhibition is that the relative magnitude of the different rewards available can be compared, and the most strongly firing neurons after the competition reflect the strongest reward.

This type of comparison would be difficult to implement if each type of reward was represented in a different location in the brain, and may be a useful computational outcome of the fact that different types of reward are represented (by different neurons of course) in the same general brain region, the medial orbitofrontal cortex. This computation would provide scaling of different rewards, both relative to each other when presented simultaneously as in a choice situation, and relative to a fixed maximum if only one reward is present. This would be part of the mechanisms involved in computing relative reward value, and also in adjusting different rewards to be on the same scale of value (see Section 9.5.3).

It may be useful to note that the human medial orbitofrontal cortex region activated by many types of reward may have shifted medially somewhat with respect to its location in macaques. Spurred by the human neuroimaging studies just described, we (Rolls, Kadohisa, Verhagen and Gabbott) have made recordings in the topologically most medial part of the macaque orbitofrontal cortex, and also the nearby anterior cingulate cortex, to determine whether there is a previously undescribed set of reward / taste / olfactory / visual / somatosensory representations in this region (Rolls 2008e). We have not found such neurons in the part of the macaque orbitofrontal cortex that is less than 3–4 mm from the midline (in which area 14 is located). We do find that neurons that respond to the taste, odour, texture, and sight of food start at approximately this laterality, and then extend out laterally from this paramedial orbitofrontal cortex region, through the mid to the far lateral orbitofrontal cortex, at sites shown in Rolls (2008e), which adds to the previous recordings illustrated in a number of other papers (e.g. Rolls & Baylis (1994), Critchley & Rolls (1996a), and Rolls, Critchley, Wakeman & Mason (1996c)). Indeed, some of these more medial sites in which taste neurons are common are illustrated in Fig. 4.28 on page 113 from Rolls & Baylis (1994).

It is quite clear from a retrograde neuronal tracing study with horseradish peroxidase administered to a region containing taste neurons in the macaque lateral orbitofrontal cortex that the lateral part of the orbitofrontal cortex receives direct inputs from the primary taste cortex in the insula (see Fig. 4.48 and Baylis, Rolls & Baylis (1994)). (The location of the macaque primary taste cortex was described by Pritchard, Hamilton, Morse & Norgren (1986).) More medial orbitofrontal cortex areas may also receive inputs directly from the insular and frontal opercular primary taste cortical areas, for, as illustrated in Fig. 4.28, taste neurons are also common in this more medial part of the orbitofrontal cortex (see further Rolls & Baylis (1994) and Critchley & Rolls (1996a)). The same anatomical paper (Baylis, Rolls & Baylis 1994) also showed that a more anterior part of the orbitofrontal cortex is a tertiary taste cortical area, for it receives inputs from the secondary, orbitofrontal, taste cortex, but not from the primary taste cortex. The more middle / medial part of the orbitofrontal cortex (close to the region indicated in Fig. 4.28) also has neurons that decrease their taste responses in relation to sensory-specific satiety, and a few that do not (Critchley & Rolls 1996c). Thus the macaque posterior orbitofrontal cortex contains taste, and also olfactory and visual, neurons throughout its mediolateral extent, apart from the most medial 3–4 mm. In contrast, the taste and olfactory reward areas in humans appear to reach to the midline, and probably do not extend as far lateral as in non-human primates (see e.g. Figs. 4.26, 4.27, 4.30 and 4.43).

I suggest that as the frontal lobes have developed from macaques to humans, more cortex has been added to the dorsolateral prefrontal cortex areas so important in working memory and hence in attention and executive function (Rolls & Deco 2002, Deco & Rolls 2003, Rolls 2008b), thus displacing the inferior convexity prefrontal cortex more medially in humans, and displacing the main orbitofrontal cortex areas of macaques more medially in humans, so that they reach as far as the midline. This would be the same trend that occurs in the temporal lobes of macaques vs humans, in which the enormous development of language areas in the left hemisphere (and corresponding high order processing areas in the right hemisphere) appear to have displaced at least parts of the inferior temporal visual cortex to be much more ventrally and medially represented in for example the human fusiform face and related areas (Rolls & Deco 2002, Baylis, Rolls & Leonard 1987, Dolan, Fink, Rolls, Booth, Holmes, Frackowiak & Friston 1997, Tovee, Rolls & Ramachandran 1996, Kanwisher, McDermott & Chun 1997, Ishai, Ungerleider, Martin & Haxby 2000). The clear mediolateral topology in the orbitofrontal cortex in humans should for this reason not be taken as implying the same topology in monkeys, and this makes comparisons based on topology precarious. Further, from our earliest studies (Thorpe, Rolls & Maddison 1983) we have not seen clear topological segregation of reward, punishment, and error-related neurons in the orbitofrontal cortex of

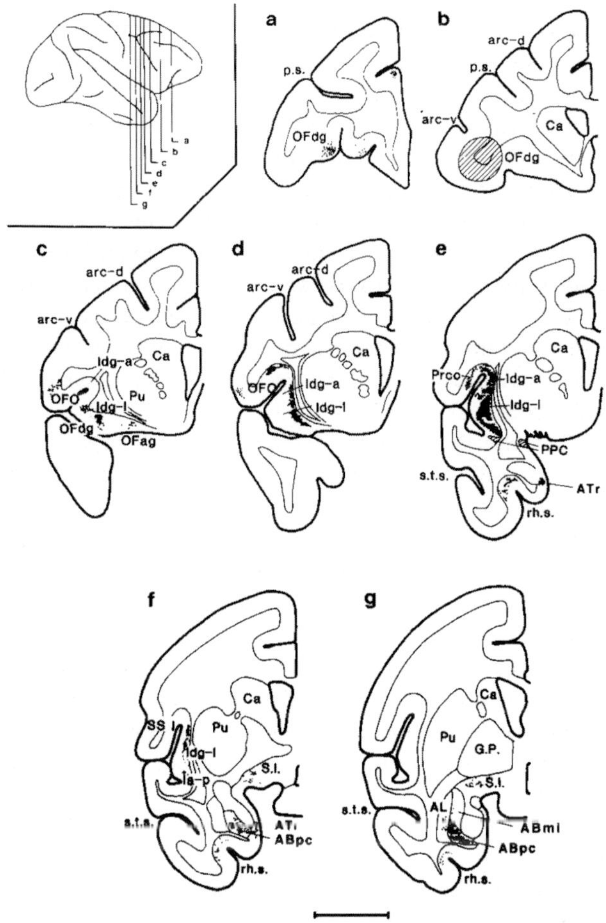

Fig. 4.48 Projections from the primary taste cortex in the upper part of the dysgranular insula and frontal operculum to the orbitofrontal cortex. The horseradish peroxidase injection site into the lateral orbitofrontal cortex where taste neurons were recorded is shown shaded in (b). Filled neurons are shown in e.g.(e) as black circles in the primary taste cortex in the upper part of areas Idg-a (Insula dysgranular area, anterior part: the insular primary taste cortex) and the area labelled Prco in (e) the frontal opercular taste cortex. Abbreviations: AB: basal nucleus of the amygdala with mc magnocellular and pc parvocellular parts; AL: lateral nucleus of the amygdala; arc-d: dorsal limb of the arcuate sulcus; arc-v: ventral limb of the arcuate sulcus; Ca: caudate nucleus; GP: globus pallidus; Idg-l: liminal part of the dysgranular field of the insula; OF: orbitofrontal cortex (with ag agranular and dg dysgranular fields); OFO: orbitofrontal opercular area; PPC: prepyriform cortex (olfactory); Prco: precentral operculum; ps: principal sulcus; Pu: putamen; rh s: rhinal sulcus; SI: substantia innominata; SS 1: primary somaesthetic cortex; sts: superior temporal sulcus. (Reprinted from *Neuroscience*, 64 (3), L. L. Baylis, E. T. Rolls, and G. C. Baylis, Afferent connections of the caudolateral orbitofrontal cortex taste area of the primate, pp. 801–12, Copyright, 1995, with permission from Elsevier.)

monkeys. Moreover, it is important to separate the reward areas of the human orbitofrontal cortex proper as visible from a ventral view in Fig. 4.47 from those in the ventromedial prefrontal / cingulate network visible in the sagittal view in Fig. 4.47. The latter, anterior cingulate networks, receive from the orbitofrontal cortex, and perform different functions, as is made clear in Section 4.7.

Another possible topological trend in the human orbitofrontal cortex may be present in the posterior to anterior direction, with the possibility of some hierarchy (Kringelbach & Rolls 2004). Very abstract reinforcers such as loss of money appear to be represented further anterior towards the frontal pole (e.g. O'Doherty, Kringelbach, Rolls, Hornak & Andrews (2001a)) than in posterior areas representing simple reinforcers such as taste (e.g. De Araujo, Kringelbach, Rolls & Hobden (2003a); De Araujo, Kringelbach, Rolls & McGlone (2003b)) or thermal intensity (Craig, Chen, Bandy & Reiman 2000). This posterior–anterior trend is demonstrated in the statistical results from the meta-analysis (Kringelbach & Rolls 2004) and may reflect some kind of hierarchical processing in the orbitofrontal cortex. Relatively far forward in the orbitofrontal cortex, in area 11, another, memory-related, rather than emotion-related, type of representation is present, for here neurons are activated by novel visual stimuli (Rolls, Browning, Inoue & Hernadi 2005a), and activations in humans are produced by novel visual stimuli (Frey & Petrides 2002).

Another finding is that areas that have supralinear responses to combinations of sensory inputs, for example taste and smell (De Araujo, Rolls, Kringelbach, McGlone & Phillips 2003c), or the umami taste stimuli monosodium glutamate (MSG) and inosine 5′-monophosphate (De Araujo, Kringelbach, Rolls & Hobden 2003a), tend to be more anterior than the areas where the components of the combinations are represented in the orbitofrontal cortex. This could easily reflect hierarchy in the system, with convergence tending to increase from more posterior to more anterior orbitofrontal cortex areas, and thus effects of combinations of inputs becoming more evident anteriorly. This is found in the ventral visual cortical stream (Rolls 2012e). In the ventromedial prefrontal cortex, the highest degree of non-linearity, at the end of the processing stream, may be reflected in the implementation of decision-making between stimuli of different value in medial prefrontal cortex area 10 (see Section 4.8).

4.5.6 The human orbitofrontal cortex

In Section 4.5.5 we have considered evidence from neuroimaging on the functions of the human orbitofrontal cortex in emotion and motivation. In this Section we consider complementary evidence from the effects of damage to the human orbitofrontal cortex.

It is of interest that a number of the symptoms of frontal lobe damage in humans appear to be related to the functions described above of representing primary reinforcers, and of altering behaviour when stimulus–reinforcement associations alter, as described next. Thus, humans with frontal lobe damage can show impairments in a number of tasks in which an alteration of behavioural strategy is required in response to a change in environmental reinforcement contingencies (Goodglass & Kaplan 1979, Jouandet & Gazzaniga 1979, Kolb & Whishaw 2008, Zald & Rauch 2006). For example, Milner (1963) showed that in the Wisconsin card sorting task (in which cards are to be sorted according to the colour, shape, or number of items on each card depending on whether the examiner says 'right' or 'wrong' to each placement), frontal patients either had difficulty in determining the first sorting principle, or in shifting to a second principle when required to. Also, in stylus mazes frontal patients have difficulty in changing direction when a sound indicates that the correct path has been left (Milner 1982). It is of interest that, in both types of test, frontal patients may be able to verbalize the correct rules yet may be unable to correct their behavioural sets or strategies appropriately.

Some of the personality changes that can follow frontal lobe damage may be related to a similar type of dysfunction. For example, the euphoria, irresponsibility, lack of affect, and lack of concern for the present or future that can follow frontal lobe damage (see Zald & Rauch (2006) and Section 4.5.1 on page 95) may also be related to a dysfunction in altering behaviour appropriately in response to a change in reinforcement contingencies. Indeed, in so far as the orbitofrontal cortex is involved in the disconnection of stimulus–reinforcer associations, and such associations are important in learned emotional responses (see above), then it follows that the orbitofrontal cortex is involved in emotional responses by correcting stimulus–reinforcer associations when they become inappropriate (see below). A failure of this process might be reflected in effects such as impulsive behaviour, and a failure to respond appropriately to corrective feedback received from the environment.

The hypotheses about the role of the orbitofrontal cortex in the rapid alteration of stimulus–reinforcer associations, and the functions more generally of the orbitofrontal cortex in human behaviour, have been investigated in recent studies in humans with damage to the ventral parts of the frontal lobe. (The description ventral is given to indicate that there was pathology in the orbitofrontal or related parts of the frontal lobe, and not in the more dorso-lateral parts of the frontal lobe.) A task that was directed at assessing the rapid alteration of stimulus–reinforcer associations was used, because the findings above indicate that the orbitofrontal cortex is involved in this type of learning. This was used instead of the Wisconsin card sorting task, which requires patients to shift from category (or dimension) to category, e.g. from colour to shape. The task used was visual discrimination reversal, in which patients could learn to obtain points by touching one stimulus when it appeared on a video monitor, but had to withhold a response when a different visual stimulus appeared, otherwise a point was lost. After the subjects had acquired the visual discrimination, the reinforcement contingencies unexpectedly reversed. The patients with ventral frontal lesions made more errors in the reversal (or in a similar extinction) task, and completed fewer reversals, than control patients with damage elsewhere in the frontal lobes or in other brain regions (Rolls, Hornak, Wade & McGrath 1994a) (see Fig. 4.49). A reversal deficit in a similar task in patients with ventromedial frontal cortex damage was also reported by Fellows & Farah (2003).

An important aspect of the findings of Rolls, Hornak, Wade & McGrath (1994a) was that the reversal learning impairment correlated highly with the socially inappropriate or disinhibited behaviour of the patients, and also with their subjective evaluation of the changes in their emotional state since the brain damage. The patients were not impaired at other types of memory task, such as paired associate learning. It is of interest that the patients can often verbalize the correct response, yet commit the incorrect action. This is consistent with the hypothesis that the orbitofrontal cortex is normally involved in executing behaviour when the behaviour is performed by evaluating the reinforcement associations of environmental stimuli (see below). The orbitofrontal cortex seems to be involved in this in both humans and non-human primates, when the learning must be performed rapidly, in, for example, acquisition, and during reversal.

To seek positive confirmation that effects on stimulus–reinforcer association learning and reversal were related to orbitofrontal cortex damage rather than to any other associated pathology, a new reversal-learning task was used with a group of patients with discrete, surgically produced, lesions of the orbitofrontal cortex. In the new visual discrimination task (the same as that used in our monetary reward functional neuroimaging task, O'Doherty, Kringelbach, Rolls, Hornak & Andrews (2001a)), two stimuli are always present on the video monitor and the patient obtains 'monetary' reward by touching the correct stimulus, and loses 'money' by touching the incorrect stimulus. This design controls for an effect of the lesion in simply increasing the probability that any response will be made (cf. Aron, Fletcher, Bullmore, Sahakian & Robbins (2003) and Clark, Cools & Robbins (2004)). The task also used probabilistic amounts of reward and punishment on each trial, to make it harder to use a verbal strategy with an explicit rule. The task also had the advantage that it was the same as that used in our human functional neuroimaging study that had showed activation of the orbitofrontal cortex by monetary gain or loss (O'Doherty et al. 2001a). It was found that a group of patients with bilateral orbitofrontal cortex lesions were severely impaired at the

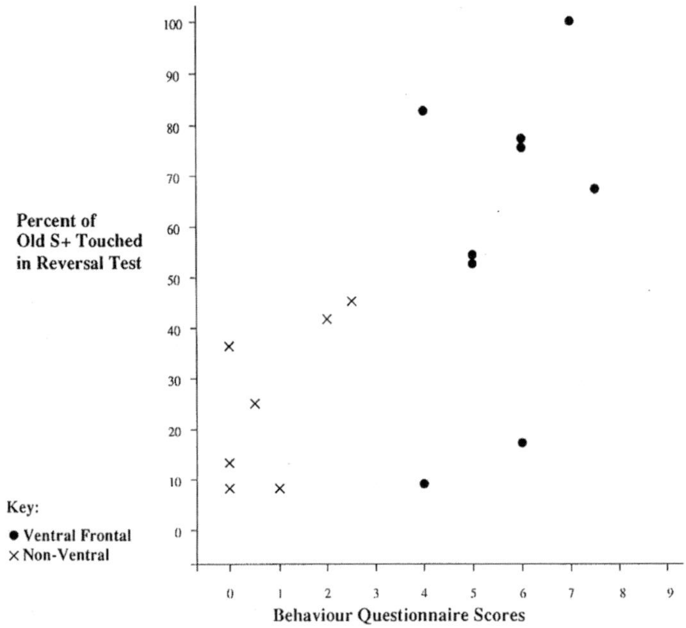

Fig. 4.49 Visual discrimination reversal performance in humans with damage to the ventral part of the frontal lobe. The task was to touch the screen when one image, the S+, was shown in order to obtain a point; and to refrain from touching the screen when a different visual stimulus, the S–, was shown in order to obtain a point. The scattergraph shows that during the reversal the group with ventral damage were more likely to touch the previously rewarded stimulus (Old S+), and that this was related to the score on a Behaviour Questionnaire. Each point represents one patient in the ventral frontal group or in a control group. The Behaviour Questionnaire rating reflected high ratings on at least some of the following: disinhibited or socially inappropriate behaviour; misinterpretation of other people's moods; impulsiveness; unconcern about or underestimation of the seriousness of his condition; and lack of initiative. (Reproduced from *Journal of Neurology, Neurosurgery and Psychiatry*, 57 (2), pp. 1518–25, Emotion-related learning in patients with social and emotional changes associated with frontal lobe damage, E. T. Rolls, J. Hornak, D. Wade, J. McGrath, ©1994, BMJ Publishing Group Ltd. with permission.)

reversal task, in that they accumulated less money (Hornak, O'Doherty, Bramham, Rolls, Morris, Bullock & Polkey 2004) (see Fig. 4.50). These patients often failed to switch their choice of stimulus after a large loss; and often did switch their choice even though they had just received a reward, and this has been quantified in a more recent study (Berlin, Rolls & Kischka 2004). The investigation showed that the impairment was only obtained with bilateral orbitofrontal cortex damage, in that patients with unilateral orbitofrontal cortex (or medial prefrontal cortex) lesions were not impaired in the reversal task (see Fig. 4.50). The importance of the failure to rapidly learn about the value of stimuli from negative feedback has also been described as a critical difficulty for patients with orbitofrontal cortex lesions (Fellows 2007, Wheeler & Fellows 2008, Fellows 2011), and has been contrasted with the effects of lesions to the anterior cingulate cortex which impair the use of feedback to learn about actions (Fellows 2011, Camille, Tsuchida & Fellows 2011) (see Section 4.7).

It is of interest that the patients with bilateral orbitofrontal cortex damage who were impaired at the visual discrimination reversal task had high scores on parts of a Social Behaviour Questionnaire in which the patients were rated on behaviours such as emotion recognition in others (e.g. their sad, angry, or disgusted mood); in interpersonal relationships

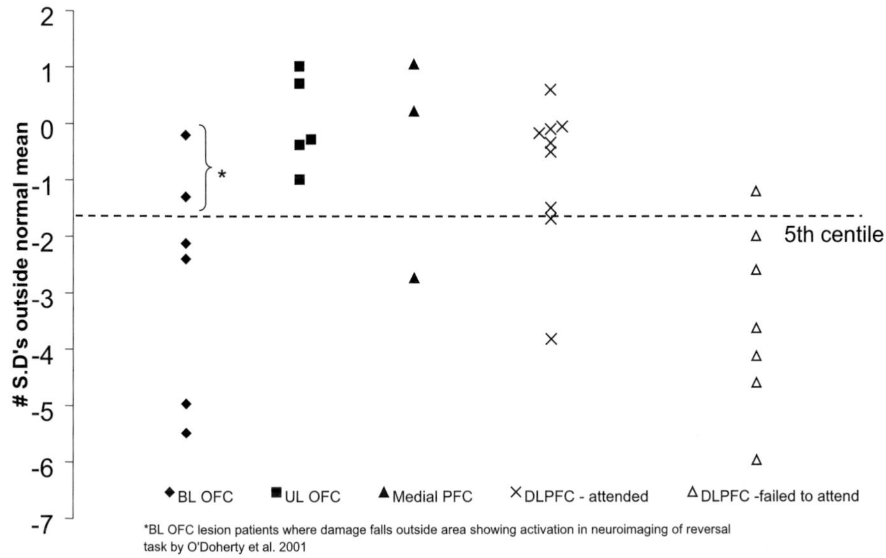

Fig. 4.50 Visual discrimination reversal performance on the probabilistic reversal task in humans with damage to different parts of the ventral part of the frontal lobe. Lesion groups: BL OFC: Bilateral Orbitofrontal cortex; UL OFC: Unilateral Orbitofrontal cortex; Medial PFC: Medial prefrontal cortex; DLPFC: Dorsolateral prefrontal cortex. The patients with bilateral damage to the orbitofrontal cortex performed poorly at the task. Patients with lesions of the dorsolateral prefrontal cortex performed poorly only if they had an attention deficit and failed to pay attention to the part of the display that informed them whether they had won on the current trial of the task. (Attended/Failed to attend: The patient attended/failed to attend to the crucial feedback during the reversal test, namely the amount won or lost on each trial.) (Reproduced from Edmund T. Rolls, J. Hornak, J. O'Doherty, J. Bramham, R. G. Morris, P. R. Bullock, and C. E. Polkey, Reward-related Reversal Learning after Surgical Excisions in Orbital-frontal or Dorsolateral Prefrontal Cortex in Humans, *Journal of Cognitive Neuroscience*, 16 (3), pp. 463–478, ©2004 by the Massachusetts Institute of Technology.)

(such as not caring what others think, and not being close to the family); emotional empathy (e.g. when others are happy, is not happy for them); interpersonal relationships (e.g. does not care what others think, and is not close to his family); public behaviour (is uncooperative); antisocial behaviour (is critical of and impatient with others); impulsivity (does things without thinking); and sociability (is not sociable, and has difficulty making or maintaining close relationships) (Hornak, Bramham, Rolls, Morris, O'Doherty, Bullock & Polkey 2003), all of which could reflect less behavioural sensitivity to different types of punishment and reward. Further, in a Subjective Emotional Change Questionnaire in which the patients reported on any changes in the intensity and/or frequency of their own experience of emotions, the bilateral orbitofrontal cortex lesion patients with deficits in the visual discrimination reversal task reported a number of changes, including changes in sadness, anger, fear and happiness (Hornak et al. 2003).

As described above, these results are complemented by neuroimaging results with fMRI in normal subjects, which showed that in the same task, activation of the medial orbitofrontal cortex was correlated with how much money was won on single trials, and activation of the lateral orbitofrontal cortex was correlated with how much money was lost on single trials (O'Doherty, Kringelbach, Rolls, Hornak & Andrews 2001a). Together, these results on the effects of brain damage to the orbitofrontal cortex, and these and other complementary neuroimaging results described later, provide evidence that at least part of the function of the orbitofrontal cortex in emotion, social behaviour, and decision-making is related to representing reinforcers, detecting changes in the reinforcers being received, using these changes to rapidly reset stimulus–reinforcer associations, and rapidly changing behaviour as a result.

There are likely to be individual differences in all the emotion systems in the brain, and these are likely to be important in personality. For example, and in the context that the lateral orbitofrontal cortex is activated by many non-rewarding and punishing stimuli (Fig. 4.47), the lateral orbitofrontal cortex is recruited more in individuals with problems with 'stop inhibition', that is, in tasks in which a NoGo response must be made occasionally (Somerville, Hare & Casey 2011). Impulsiveness may be related to a relative insensitivity of this system, and not only is the orbitofrontal cortex implicated in this, but one of its output regions, the ventral striatum, is activated more strongly by incentive stimuli (of which examples might be the sight of cookies or of drugs) in people with impulsive/antisocial personalities (Buckholtz, Treadway, Cowan, Woodward, Benning, Li, Ansari, Baldwin, Schwartzman, Shelby, Smith, Cole, Kessler & Zald 2010). Of great interest, in people who are not impulsive and who control their behaviour with the rational system, activations related to signals from the dorsolateral prefrontal cortex, involved in planning, are stronger in the head of the caudate (Buckholtz et al. 2010). An implication is that within the basal ganglia, competition between the emotional system (activating the ventral striatum) and the rational system (activating the head of the caudate) may be one way in which selection of behavioural output between the rational vs the emotional system may be made (see Sections 10.3.1 and 6.3). There are also interesting age-related differences in the sensitivity of these reward and punishment systems. For example, adolescents show increased responsiveness to social cues and monetary rewards than younger people or adults (Somerville et al. 2011).

An idea of how such stimulus–reinforcer learning may play an important role in normal human behaviour, and may be related to the behavioural changes seen clinically in the patients of Rolls, Hornak, Wade & McGrath (1994a) with ventral frontal lobe damage, can be provided by summarizing the behavioural ratings given by the carers of these patients (Rolls et al. 1994a). The patients were rated high on at least some of the following: disinhibition or socially inappropriate behaviour; violence, verbal abusiveness; lack of initiative; misinterpretation of other people's behaviour; anger or irritability; and lack of concern for their own condition. Such behavioural changes correlated with the stimulus–reinforcer reversal and extinction learning impairment (Rolls et al. 1994a). The suggestion thus is that the insensitivity to reinforcement changes in the learning task may be at least part of what produces the changes in behaviour found in these patients with ventral frontal lobe damage.

The more general impact on the behaviour of these patients is that their irresponsibility tended to affect their everyday lives. For example, if such patients had received their brain damage in a road traffic accident, and compensation had been awarded, the patients often tended to spend their money without appropriate concern for the future, sometimes, for example, buying a very expensive car. Such patients often find it difficult to invest in relationships too, and are sometimes described by their family as having changed personalities, in that they care less about a wide range of factors than before the brain damage. The suggestion that follows from this is that the orbitofrontal cortex may normally be involved in much social behaviour, and the ability to respond rapidly and appropriately to social reinforcers is, of course, an important aspect of primate social behaviour. When Goleman (1995) writes about emotional intelligence (see Section 2.7), the functions being performed may be those that we are now discussing, and also those concerned with face-expression decoding which are described in this chapter.

Bechara and colleagues also have findings that are consistent with those described above in patients with frontal lobe damage when they perform a gambling task (Bechara et al.

1994, Bechara et al. 1996, Bechara et al. 1997, Damasio 1994, Bechara et al. 2005, Glascher, Adolphs, Damasio, Bechara, Rudrauf, Calamia, Paul & Tranel 2012). In the Iowa gambling task subjects were asked to select cards from four decks of cards and maximize their winnings. During the task electrodermal activity (Skin Conductance Responses, SCR) of the subject was measured as an index of somatic activation. After each selection of a card, facsimile money is lost or won. Two of the four decks produce large payouts with larger penalties (and can thus be considered high-risk), while the other two decks produce small payouts but smaller penalties (low-risk). The most profitable strategy is therefore to consistently select cards from the two low-risk decks, which is the strategy adopted by normal control subjects. Patients with damage to the ventromedial part of the orbitofrontal cortex, but not the dorsolateral prefrontal cortex, would persistently draw cards from the high-risk packs, and lack anticipatory SCRs while they pondered risky choices. The task was designed to mimic aspects of real-life decision-making that patients with orbitofrontal cortex lesions find difficult. Such decisions typically involve choices between actions associated with differing magnitudes of reward and punishment where the underlying contingencies relating actions to relevant outcomes remain hidden.

Bechara, Damasio, Tranel & Anderson (1998) have reported a dissociation between subjects with different frontal lobe lesions. All subjects with orbitofrontal cortex lesions were impaired on the gambling task, while only those with the most anteriorly placed lesions were normal on working memory tasks. Other subjects with right dorsolateral/high mesial lesions were impaired on working memory tasks but not on the gambling task. Bechara, Damasio, Damasio & Lee (1999) went on to compare subjects with bilateral amygdala but not orbitofrontal cortex lesions, and subjects with orbitofrontal cortex but not amygdala lesions, and found that all subjects were impaired in the gambling task and all failed to develop anticipatory SCRs. However, while subjects with orbitofrontal cortex lesions still, in general, produced SCRs when receiving a monetary reward or punishment, the subjects with bilateral amygdala lesions failed to do so. Fellows & Farah (2005) found that patients with ventromedial prefrontal or with dorsolateral frontal lobe damage were impaired on the Iowa gambling task, yet only the ventromedial frontal damage group had a reversal deficit. (This reversal deficit can be produced in patients with small bilateral lesions of the orbitofrontal cortex, as shown by Hornak, O'Doherty, Bramham, Rolls, Morris, Bullock & Polkey (2004).) Moreover the deficit on the gambling task of the ventromedial prefrontal patients was related to the fact that in the Iowa gambling task the first few choices of a high-risk deck are rewarded, and that later, when a large loss is received from a high-risk deck, an implicit reversal is required. Thus the deficit of patients with orbitofrontal cortex / ventromedial prefrontal cortex damage in the task may be related at least in part to their failure to perform stimulus–reinforcer association reversal learning, rather than for other reasons.

In relation to real-world gambling, impulsive choice measured with a delay-discounting task (and reflecting aversion for a delayed reward) was found in problem gamblers, but impulsive action (measured with the stop-signal task, which requires withholding of a motor response), was especially impaired in pathological gambling (Brevers, Cleeremans, Verbruggen, Bechara, Kornreich, Verbanck & Noel 2012).

Most known cases of human orbitofrontal damage have occurred in adulthood, but two cases of damage acquired in early life were reported by Anderson, Bechara, Damasio, Tranel & Damasio (1999). The two patients showed lifelong behavioural problems, which were resistant to corrective influences. But more importantly, the patients appeared completely to lack knowledge about moral and societal conventions. Interestingly, other patients with late acquired orbitofrontal lesions have retained knowledge of such matters, even if they do not always act in accordance with this explicit knowledge. The lack of this moral knowledge and subsequent reckless behaviour in the two patients with early life damage to the orbitofrontal cortex is consistent with the hypothesis that the orbitofrontal cortex is crucial for stimulus–reinforcer association learning (Rolls 1990b, Rolls 2005b, Rolls 2012c). An implication is that, at least in part because of its importance in utilizing feedback to correct value representations, the orbitofrontal cortex becomes important in moral behaviour (Mendez 2009).

To investigate the possible significance of face-related inputs to orbitofrontal visual neurons described above, we also tested the responses of these patients to faces. We included tests of face (and also voice) expression decoding, because these are ways in which the reinforcing quality of individuals is often indicated. Impairments in the identification of facial and vocal emotional expression were demonstrated in a group of patients with ventral frontal lobe damage who had socially inappropriate behaviour (Hornak, Rolls & Wade 1996, Rolls 1999c) (see Fig. 4.51). The expression identification impairments could occur independently of perceptual impairments in facial recognition, voice discrimination, or environmental sound recognition. The face and voice expression problems did not necessarily occur together in the same patients, providing an indication of separate processing. Poor performance on both expression tests was correlated with the degree of alteration of emotional experience reported by the patients. There was also a strong positive correlation between the degree of altered emotional experience and the severity of the behavioural problems (e.g. disinhibition) found in these patients. A comparison group of patients with brain damage outside the ventral frontal lobe region, without these behavioural problems, was unimpaired on the face expression identification test, was significantly less impaired at vocal expression identification, and reported little subjective emotional change (Hornak et al. 1996, Rolls 1999c). More recent findings confirm that face emotion recognition is impaired following ventromedial, but not dorsal or lateral, prefrontal cortex damage (Heberlein, Padon, Gillihan, Farah & Fellows 2008).

These findings have been extended, and it has been found that patients with face expression decoding problems do not necessarily have impairments at visual discrimination reversal, and vice versa (Hornak, Bramham, Rolls, Morris, O'Doherty, Bullock & Polkey 2003, Hornak, O'Doherty, Bramham, Rolls, Morris, Bullock & Polkey 2004). This is consistent with some topography in the orbitofrontal cortex (see Section 4.5.5.9 and Rolls & Baylis (1994)).

To obtain clear evidence that the changes in face and voice expression identification, emotional behaviour, and subjective emotional state were related to orbitofrontal cortex damage itself, and not to damage to surrounding areas which is present in many closed head injury patients, we performed these assessments in patients with circumscribed lesions made surgically in the course of treatment (Hornak, Bramham, Rolls, Morris, O'Doherty, Bullock & Polkey 2003). This study also enabled us to determine whether there was functional specialization within the orbitofrontal cortex, and whether damage to nearby and connected areas (such as the anterior cingulate cortex) in which some of the patients had lesions could produce similar effects. We found that some patients with bilateral lesions of the orbitofrontal cortex had deficits in voice and face expression identification, and the group had impairments in social behaviour, and significant changes in their subjective emotional state (Hornak et al. 2003). The same group of patients had deficits on the probabilistic monetary reward task (Hornak et al. 2004). Some patients with unilateral damage restricted to the orbitofrontal cortex also had deficits in voice expression identification, and the group did not have significant changes in social behaviour, or in their subjective emotional state. Patients with unilateral lesions of the antero-ventral part of the anterior cingulate cortex and/or medial prefrontal cortex area BA9 were in some cases impaired on voice and face expression identification, had some change in social behaviour, and had significant changes in their subjective emotional state. Patients with dorsolateral prefrontal cortex lesions or with medial lesions outside the anterior cingulate cortex and medial prefrontal BA9 areas were unimpaired on any of these measures of emotion. In all cases in which voice expression identification was impaired, there were no deficits in control tests of the discrimination of unfamiliar voices and the recognition of

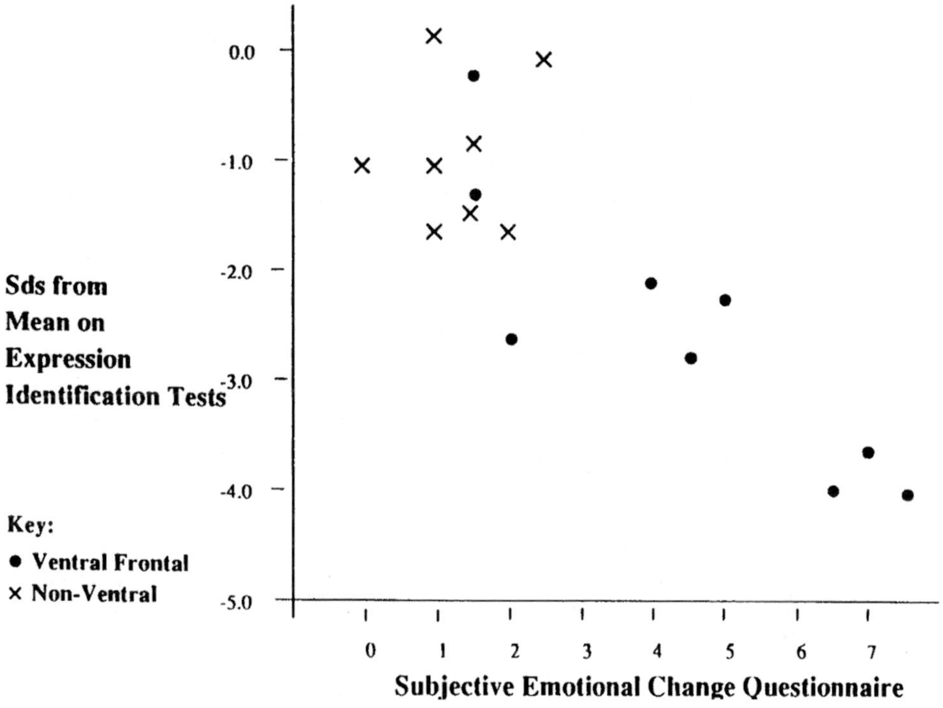

Fig. 4.51 Face expression identification deficit in humans with damage to the ventral part of the frontal lobe, and its relation to the patient's own rating of Subjective Emotional Change since the brain damage, based on sadness (or regret), anger (or frustration), fear (or anxiety), disgust, and excitement or enjoyment. (Reprinted from *Neuropsychologia*, 34 (4), J. Hornak, E.T. Rolls, and D. Wade, Face and voice expression identification in patients with emotional and behavioural changes following ventral frontal lobe damage, pp. 247–61, Copyright, 1996, with permission from Elsevier.)

environmental sounds.

These results (Hornak, Bramham, Rolls, Morris, O'Doherty, Bullock & Polkey 2003) thus confirm that damage restricted to the orbitofrontal cortex can produce impairments in face and voice expression identification, which may be primary reinforcers. The system is sensitive, in that even patients with unilateral orbitofrontal cortex lesions may be impaired. The impairment is not a generic impairment of the ability to recognize any emotions in others, in that frequently voice but not face expression identification was impaired, and vice versa. This implies some functional specialization for visual vs auditory emotion-related processing in the human orbitofrontal cortex. The results also show that the changes in social behaviour can be produced by damage restricted to the orbitofrontal cortex. The patients were particularly likely to be impaired on emotion recognition (they were less likely to notice when others were sad, or happy, or disgusted); on emotional empathy (they were less likely to comfort those who are sad, or afraid, or to feel happy for others who are happy); on interpersonal relationships (not caring what others think, and not being close to his/her family); and were less likely to cooperate with others; were impatient and impulsive; and had difficulty in making and keeping close relationships. The results also show that changes in subjective emotional state (including frequently sadness, anger and happiness) can be produced by damage restricted to the orbitofrontal cortex (Hornak et al. 2003). In addition, the patients with bilateral orbitofrontal cortex lesions were impaired on the probabilistic reversal learning task (Hornak et al. 2004). The findings overall thus make clear the types of deficit found in humans with orbitofrontal cortex damage, and can be easily related to underlying fundamental processes in which the orbitofrontal cortex is involved as described throughout Section 4.5, including decoding and representing primary reinforcers, being sensitive to changes in reinforcers, and rapidly readjusting behaviour to stimuli when the reinforcers available change.

The results (Hornak et al. 2003) also extend these investigations to the anterior cingulate cortex (including some of medial prefrontal cortex area BA9) by showing that lesions in these regions can produce voice and/or face expression identification deficits, and marked changes in subjective emotional state (see Section 4.7).

It is also becoming possible to relate the functions of the orbitofrontal cortex to some psychiatric symptoms. Berlin, Rolls & Kischka (2004), Berlin & Rolls (2004) and Berlin, Rolls & Iversen (2005) compared the symptoms of patients with a personality disorder syndrome, Borderline Personality Disorder (BPD), with those of patients with lesions of the orbitofrontal cortex. The symptoms of the self-harming Borderline Personality Disorder patients include high impulsivity, affective instability, and emotionality; and low extraversion. It was found that orbitofrontal cortex and Borderline Personality Disorder patients performed similarly in that they were more impulsive, reported more inappropriate behaviours in the Frontal Behaviour Questionnaire, and had more Borderline Personality Disorder characteristics, and anger, and less happiness, than control groups (either normals, or patients with lesions outside the orbitofrontal cortex).

One of the measures of impulsiveness was the Matching Familiar Figures Test. In this standard cognitive behavioural measure of impulsivity, created by Kagan (1966), a participant selects (points to), from a set of highly similar pictures, the one that is exactly the same as the standard reference picture. High impulsiveness is reflected in short latencies to make a choice (which are typically 55 s in control subjects), and errors in the choices made. The other measure of impulsiveness was the Barratt Impulsiveness Scale (Patton, Stanford & Barratt 1995) which is a 30-item questionnaire that assesses non-planning impulsivity (attention to details), motor impulsivity (acting without thinking), and cognitive impulsivity (future oriented thinking and coping stability). Both the orbitofrontal and BPD groups were impaired at both measures of impulsiveness.

Both the orbitofrontal and BPD groups also had a faster perception of time (i.e. they underproduced time) than normal controls. This may be one factor underlying their increased impulsiveness, in that they feel that sufficient time has elapsed to initiate action.

It was of considerable interest that the BPD group, as well as the orbitofrontal group, scored highly on the Frontal Behaviour Questionnaire which assessed inappropriate behaviours typical of orbitofrontal cortex patients including disinhibition, social inappropriateness, perseveration, and uncooperativeness. Both groups were also less open to experience (i.e. less open-minded), a personality characteristic.

The orbitofrontal and BPD patients performed differently on other tasks: BPD patients were less extraverted and conscientious, and more neurotic and emotional, than all other groups. Patients with orbitofrontal cortex lesions had more severe deficits in reversing stimulus–reinforcer associations compared to all other groups and had a faster perception of time (overestimated time) than normal controls. These deficits were not related to spatial working memory functions which are impaired by dorsolateral prefrontal cortex damage.

Thus some but not other symptoms of self-harming Borderline Personality Disorder patients are similar to those of patients with orbitofrontal cortex damage. The symptoms the groups have in common include impulsiveness and the inappropriate behaviours typical of 'frontal' patients. This could imply that in BPD patients some aspects of the operation of the orbitofrontal cortex are occurring (whatever their aetiology, which could include innate or acquired changes, and might involve different expression or operation of neurotransmitters) differently to the way they operate in normal control subjects. Part of the interest of this is that it may help to point towards new concepts that may be useful in the treatment of some of the symptoms of patients with Borderline Personality Disorder. On the other hand, other aspects of Borderline Personality Disorder do not appear to be related to orbitofrontal cortex functions, including the more neurotic and more emotional personality characteristics of the BPD group together with their lower extraversion and conscientious (Berlin, Rolls & Kischka 2004, Berlin & Rolls 2004, Berlin, Rolls & Iversen 2005).

Another case in which it is possible to relate psychiatric types of symptom to orbitofrontal cortex function is frontotemporal dementia, which is a progressive neurodegenerative disorder attacking the frontal lobes and producing major and pervasive behavioural changes in personality and social conduct resembling those produced by orbitofrontal lesions (Rahman, Sahakian, Hodges, Rogers & Robbins 1999, Rascovsky, Hodges & al. 2011). Patients appear either socially disinhibited with facetiousness and inappropriate jocularity, or apathetic and withdrawn. Many patients show mental rigidity and inability to appreciate irony or other subtle aspects of language. They tend to engage in ritualistic and stereotypical behaviour, and their planning skills are invariably impaired. The dementia is accompanied by gradual withdrawal from all social interactions. Memory is usually intact but patients have difficulties with working memory and concentration. Interestingly, given the anatomy and physiology of the orbitofrontal cortex, frontotemporal dementia causes profound changes in eating habits, with escalating desire for sweet food coupled with reduced satiety, which is often followed by enormous weight gain (Piguet 2011).

4.5.7 A neurophysiological and computational basis for stimulus–reinforcer association learning and reversal in the orbitofrontal cortex

The neurophysiological and lesion evidence described suggests that one function implemented by the orbitofrontal cortex is rapid stimulus–reinforcer association learning, and the correction of these associations when reinforcement contingencies in the environment change. To implement this, the orbitofrontal cortex has the necessary representation of primary reinforcers, such as taste and somatosensory inputs (see Section 4.3 and Chapter 5). It also receives information about objects, e.g. visual information, and can associate this very rapidly at the neuronal level with primary reinforcers such as taste, and reverse these associations. Another type of stimulus that can be conditioned in this way in the orbitofrontal cortex is olfactory, although here the learning is slower. It is likely that auditory stimuli can be associated with primary reinforcers in the orbitofrontal cortex, though there is less direct evidence on this yet.

The orbitofrontal cortex neurons that detect non-reward in a context-specific manner are likely to be used in behavioural extinction and reversal. Such non-reward neurons may help behaviour in situations in which stimulus–reinforcer associations must be disconnected, not only by helping to reset the reinforcer association of neurons in the orbitofrontal cortex, but also by sending a signal to the striatum which could be routed by the striatum to produce appropriate behaviours for non-reward (Rolls & Johnstone 1992, Williams, Rolls, Leonard & Stern 1993, Rolls 1994a, Rolls 2005b) (see Chapter 6). Indeed, it is via this route, the striatal, as well as by the anterior cingulate cortex, that the orbitofrontal cortex may directly influence behaviour when the orbitofrontal cortex is decoding reinforcement contingencies in the environment, and is altering behaviour in response to altering reinforcement contingencies. Some of the evidence for this is that neurons with responses that reflect these orbitofrontal neuronal responses are found in the ventral part of the head of the caudate nucleus and the ventral striatum, which receive from the orbitofrontal cortex (Rolls, Thorpe & Maddison 1983c, Williams, Rolls, Leonard & Stern 1993); and lesions of the ventral part of the head of the caudate nucleus impair visual discrimination reversal (Divac, Rosvold & Szwarcbart 1967) (see further Chapter 6).

Decoding the reinforcement value of stimuli, which involves for previously neutral (e.g. visual) stimuli learning their association with a primary reinforcer, often rapidly, and which may involve not only rapid learning but also rapid relearning and alteration of responses when reinforcement contingencies change, is then a function proposed for the orbitofrontal cortex. This way of producing behavioural responses would be important in, for example, motivational and emotional behaviour. It would be important in motivational behaviour such as feeding and drinking by enabling primates to learn rapidly about the food reinforcement to be expected from visual stimuli (see Rolls (2005b) and Chapter 5). This is important, for primates frequently eat more than 100 varieties of food; vision by visual-taste association learning can be used to identify when foods are ripe; and during the course of a meal, the pleasantness of the sight of a food eaten in the meal decreases in a sensory-specific way (Rolls, Rolls & Rowe 1983b), a function that is probably implemented by the sensory-specific satiety-related responses of orbitofrontal visual neurons (Critchley & Rolls 1996c).

With regard to emotional behaviour, decoding and rapidly readjusting the reinforcement value of visual signals is likely to be crucial, for emotions can be described as responses elicited by instrumental reinforcing signals (Rolls 1986a, Rolls 1986b, Rolls 1990b, Rolls 1995a, Rolls 1999a, Rolls 2005b) (see Chapter 2). The ability to perform this learning very rapidly is probably very important in social situations in primates, in which reinforcing stimuli are continually being exchanged, and the reinforcement value of these must be continually updated (relearned), based on the actual reinforcers received and given. Although the operation of reinforcers such as taste, smell, and faces are best understood in terms of orbitofrontal cortex operation, there are tactile inputs that are likely to be concerned with reward evaluation, and in humans the rewards processed in the orbitofrontal cortex include quite general rewards such as working for 'points' (Rolls et al. 1994a) or for 'monetary' rewards (O'Doherty, Kringelbach, Rolls, Hornak & Andrews 2001a, Hornak, O'Doherty, Bramham, Rolls, Morris, Bullock & Polkey 2004).

Although the amygdala is concerned with some of the same functions as the orbitofrontal cortex, and receives similar inputs (see Figs. 4.2, 4.19 and 4.55), there is evidence that it may function less effectively in the very rapid learning and reversal of stimulus–reinforcer associations, as indicated by the greater difficulty in obtaining reversal from amygdala neurons (see, e.g., Rolls (2000d)), and by the greater effect of orbitofrontal lesions in leading to continuing behavioural responses to previously rewarded stimuli (see Sections 4.5.4 and 4.5.6). In primates the necessity for very rapid stimulus–reinforcement re-evaluation, and the development of powerful cortical learning systems, may result in the orbitofrontal cortex effectively taking over this aspect of amygdala functions (Rolls 1992a, Rolls 1999a, Rolls 2000d, Rolls 2005b). The mechanism of rapid reversal learning that may be implemented in the orbitofrontal cortex may utilize a working memory of which rule is currently active, which may depend on a highly developed recurrent collateral set of synaptic connections present in the orbitofrontal cortex but not the amygdala, as described by Deco & Rolls (2005a). This offers a more computational account of the different functions of the orbitofrontal cortex and amygdala in emotion than previous accounts (e.g. Pickens, Saddoris, Setlow, Gallagher, Holland & Schoenbaum (2003), and Holland & Gallagher (2004)). The rule-based approach to rapid reversal of value representations requires attractor networks to hold active in short-term memory which rule currently applies, and this mechanism may be part of what evolution provides in the function of the granular orbitofrontal cortex areas that are not present in rodents (see Fig. 1.1 and Section 1.3).

We now consider how stimulus–reinforcer association learning and its reversal may be implemented in the orbitofrontal cortex. The suggested process for the initial association is illustrated in Fig. 4.5 on page 79. If the visual input (e.g. the sight of food) is present at the same time (or just before) the primary reinforcer (e.g. taste) is activating the postsynaptic neuron, then the set of synapses that are driven by the conditioned stimulus become strengthened by the associative process of long-term synaptic potentiation (LTP). The LTP occurs only if the post-synaptic neuron is strongly activated, because the NMDA receptors activated by the presynaptic release of the transmitter glutamate only become unblocked to allow Ca^{2+} entry when the postsynaptic neuron is sufficiently depolarized (see Appendix 1, Rolls & Treves (1998) and Rolls (2008b)). This pattern association learning can learn many associations between conditioned stimuli and primary reinforcers, in fact in the order of the number of synapses per neuron, which is in the order of 5,000–10,000 (see Appendix 1, Rolls & Treves (1998) and Rolls (2008b)). This type of learning also has many other desirable properties, including generalization to similar conditioned stimuli, and graceful degradation (fault tolerance) if the system sustains some damage (see Appendix 1, Rolls & Treves (1998) and Rolls (2008b)). This putative role of NMDA receptors could be tested by using NMDA-receptor blockers applied locally to individual neurons with visual responses in the orbitofrontal cortex during visual discrimination reversal, or by perfusion of the orbitofrontal cortex with an NMDA-receptor blocker to investigate whether this interferes with behavioural visual discrimination reversal.

A first approach to the reversal is as follows, and can be understood by referring to Fig. 4.5 on page 79. Consider a neuron with unconditioned responses to taste in the orbitofrontal cortex. When a particular visual stimulus, say a triangle, was associated with the taste of glucose, the active synaptic connections for this visual (conditioned) stimulus would have shown long-term synaptic potentiation on to the taste neuron, which would respond to the sight of the triangle. During reversal, the same visual stimulus, the triangle, would again activate the same synaptic afferents to the neuron, but that neuron would be inactive when the taste of saline was given. Active presynaptic inputs and a low level of postsynaptic activation is the condition for homosynaptic long-term synaptic depression (LTD, see Fig. A.5 on page 549), which would then occur, resulting in a decline of the response of the neuron to the triangle. At the same time, visual presentation of a square would now be associated with the taste of glucose, which would activate the postsynaptic neuron, leading now to long-term potentiation of afferents on to that neuron made active by the sight of the square.

Although reversal might be implemented in the way just described by having long-term synaptic depression for synapses that represented the reward-associated stimulus before the reversal, and long-term potentiation of the new stimulus that after reversal is associated with reward, this would require one-trial LTP and one-trial homosynaptic LTD to account for one-trial stimulus–reward reversal (Thorpe, Rolls & Maddison 1983, Rolls, Critchley, Mason & Wakeman 1996a, Rolls 2000b). Moreover, the mechanism would not account for reversal learning set, the process by which during repeated reversal learning, performance gradually improves until reversal can occur in one trial. Even more, the mechanism would not account for the fact that after reversal learning set has been acquired, when the contingency is reversed, the animal makes a response to the current S+ expecting to get reward, but instead obtains the punisher. On the very first subsequent trial on which the pre-reversal S– is shown, the animal will perform a response to it expecting now to get reward, *even though the post-reversal S+ has not since the reversal been associated with reward to produce LTP for the post-reversal S+*. (This is in fact illustrated in Fig. 4.38 on page 124.) To implement this very rapid stimulus–reinforcer association reversal, a different mechanism is therefore needed. The mechanism can not rely on associative processes, but instead on a rule-based process, which requires the current rule to be held in mind, in short-term memory. This, and non-reward neurons that maintain their firing for many seconds as illustrated in Fig. 4.38, may be developments provided for by the evolution of granular orbitofrontal cortex areas in primates (see Section

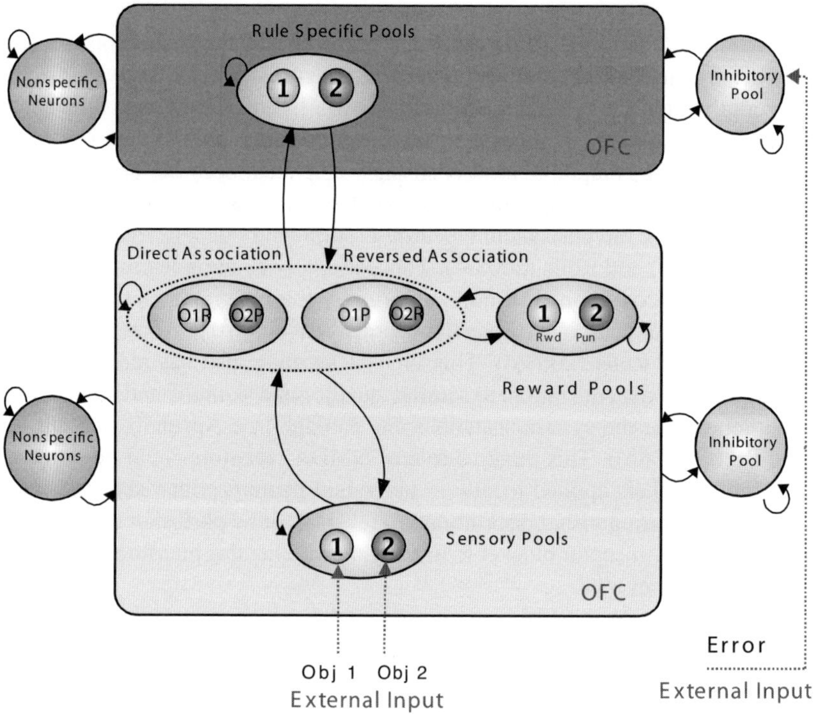

Fig. 4.52 Cortical architecture of the reward reversal model. There is a rule module (top) and a sensory – intermediate neuron – reward module (below). Neurons within each module are fully connected, and form attractor states. The sensory – intermediate neuron – reward module consists of three hierarchically organized levels of attractor network, with stronger synaptic connections in the forward than the backprojection direction. The intermediate level of the sensory – intermediate neuron – reward module contains neurons that respond to combinations of an object and its association with reward or punishment, e.g. object 1–reward (O1R, in the direct association set of pools), and object 1–punishment (O1P in the reversed association set of pools). These intermediate level neurons have the properties of 'conditional reward neurons' described in Section 4.5.5.4 and illustrated in Fig. 4.33, and provide a function for such conditional reward neurons. The rule module acts as a biasing input to bias the competition between the object–reward combination neurons at the intermediate level of the sensory – intermediate neuron – reward module. The whole model is implemented with integrate-and-fire neurons. (This material was originally published in *Cerebral Cortex*, 15 (1), Synaptic and spiking dynamics underlying reward reversal in the orbitofrontal cortex, G. Deco and E. T. Rolls, pp. 15–30 ©2005 Oxford University Press and has been reproduced by permission of Oxford University Press http://cercor.oxfordjournals.org/content/15/1.toc.)

1.3).

A model for how the very rapid, one-trial, reversal could be implemented has now been developed (see Deco & Rolls (2005a) for a full description). The model uses a short-term memory autoassociation attractor network with associatively modifiable synaptic connections to hold the neurons representing the current rule active (see Fig. 4.52). Rule one might correspond to 'stimulus 1 (e.g. a triangle) is associated with reward, and stimulus 2 (e.g. a square) is associated with punishment'. Rule 2 might correspond to the opposite contingency. A small, very biologically plausible, modification of the standard one-layer autoassociation network is that there is a small amount of adaptation in the recurrent collateral synapses that keep the neurons representing the current rule firing. Now consider the case when the neurons representing rule one are firing. How does the rule module reverse? The proposal is that when the non-reward or error neurons described above (Section 4.5.5.5) fire, this additional set of firing neurons destabilizes the rule attractor module, by for example producing extra firing of the inhibitory neurons in the orbitofrontal cortex, which in turn inhibit the excitatory neurons in the rule autoassociation network, thus quenching its attractor state. This error input to the rule attractor network is shown in Fig. 4.52. After neuronal firing in the network has stopped and the error signal, which may last for 10 s as illustrated in Fig. 4.38 on page 124, is no longer present, then firing gradually can build up again in the rule attractor network. (This build-up may be assisted by non-specific inputs from other neurons in the area, as illustrated in Deco & Rolls (2005a).) However, with the competitive processes operating within the rule attractor network between the populations of neurons representing rule 1 and those representing rule 2, and the fact that the neurons or synapses that are part of the rule 1 attractor are partly adapted, the neurons that win the competition and become active are those representing rule 2, and the rule attractor has reversed its state. This process is illustrated in Fig. 4.53, and takes one trial. Reversal learning set takes a number of reversals to acquire because the correct attractors for the relevant rules, and their connections to other 'mapping' neurons, have to be learned.

To achieve the correct 'mapping' from stimuli to their reinforcer association, and thus emotional state, the rule neurons bias the competition in a mapping module, illustrated in Fig. 4.52. The mapping module has sensory input neurons, intermediate 'conditional reward' neurons (of the type described in Section 4.5.5.4 and illustrated in Fig. 4.33) which respond to combinations of stimuli and whether they are currently associated with reward (or for other neurons to a punisher), and output neurons which represent the reinforcement association of the stimulus currently being viewed. (In the case described there are four populations or pools of neurons at the intermediate level, two for the direct rewarding context: object 1-rewarding, object 2-punishing, and two for the reversal condition: object 1-punishing, object 2-rewarding.) These intermediate pools or populations of neurons respond to combinations of the sensory stimuli and the expected reward, e.g. to object 1 and an expected reward (glucose obtained after licking), and are the conditional reward neurons described in Section 4.5.5.4 and illustrated in Fig. 4.33 on page 118. The sensory – intermediate – reward module thus consists of three hierarchically organized levels of attractor network, with stronger synaptic connections in the forward direction from input to output than the backprojection direction. The rule module acts as a biasing input to bias the competition between the object–reward combination neurons at the intermediate level of the sensory – intermediate – reward module. This biasing is achieved because rule 1 has associatively strengthened connections to object 1–rewarding and object 2–punishing neurons. (The whole network could be set up by simple associative learning operating to strengthen connections made with low probability between different neurons that are conjunctively active during the task in the network – see Deco & Rolls (2005a).)

Thus when object 1, e.g. the triangle, is being presented and rule one for direct mapping is in the rule module and biasing the intermediate neurons of the sensory – intermediate – reward module, then the intermediate neurons that fire are the object 1-reward neurons (O1R in Fig. 4.52), and these in turn through associative connections activate the reward neurons (Rwd in Fig. 4.52) at the third, reward/punishment, level of the hierarchy. If on the other hand object 1, e.g. the triangle, is being presented and rule two for reversed mapping is in the rule module and biasing the intermediate neurons of the sensory – intermediate – reward module, then the intermediate neurons that fire are the object 1–punishment (O1P) neurons, and these in turn through associative connections activate the punishment neurons (Pun) at the third, reward/punishment, level of the hierarchy. This model can thus account for one-trial reversal learning, and provides an account for the presence of the conditional reward and conditional punishment neurons found by Thorpe, Rolls & Maddison (1983) and Rolls, Critchley, Mason & Wakeman (1996a) in the orbitofrontal cortex (Section 4.5.5.4).

It is an important part of the architecture that at the intermediate level of the sensory –

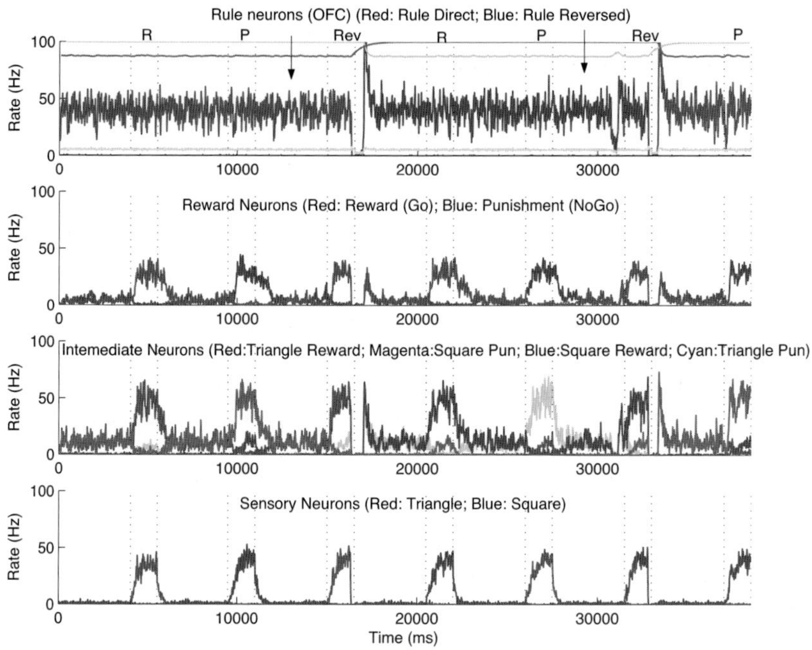

Fig. 4.53 Reward reversal model: Temporal evolution of the averaged population activity for all neural pools (sensory, intermediate (stimulus–reward), and Reward/Punishment) in the stimulus – intermediate – reward module and the rule module, during the execution and the reversal of the Go/NoGo visual discrimination task with a pseudorandom trial sequence after Thorpe, Rolls and Maddison (1983) and Rolls, Critchley, Mason and Wakeman (1996). Bottom row: the sensory neuronal populations, one of which responds to Object 1, a triangle (red), and the other to Object 2, a square (blue). The intermediate conditional stimulus–reward and stimulus–punishment neurons respond to for example Object 1 (Triangle) when it is associated with reward (Rw) (e.g. on trial 1, corresponding to O1R in Fig. 4.52), or to Object 2 (Square) when it is associated with punishment (Pun) (e.g. on trial 2, O2P). The top row shows the firing rate activity in the rule module, with the thin line at the top of this graph showing the mean probability of release $P_{\rm rel}$ of transmitter from the synapses of each population of neurons. The arrows show when the contingencies reversed. R: Reward trial; P: Punishment Trial; Rev: Reversal trial, i.e. the first trial after the reward contingency was reversed when Reward was expected but Punishment was obtained. The intertrial interval was 4 s. The yellow line shows the average activity of the inhibitory neurons. (See text for further details.) (See colour plates section.) (This material was originally published in *Cerebral Cortex*, 15 (1), Synaptic and spiking dynamics underlying reward reversal in the orbitofrontal cortex, G. Deco and E. T. Rolls, pp. 15–30 ©2005 Oxford University Press and has been reproduced by permission of Oxford University Press http://cercor.oxfordjournals.org/content/15/1.toc.)

intermediate – reward module one set of neurons fire if an object being presented is currently associated with reward, and a different set if the object being presented is currently associated with punishment. This representation means that these neurons can be used for different functions, such as the elicitation of emotional or autonomic responses, which can occur for example to particular stimuli associated with particular reinforcers (Rolls 1999a). For example, particular emotions might arise if a particular cognitively processed input such as a particular person is associated with a particular type of reinforcer or reinforcement contingency.

It is also an interesting part of the architecture that associative synaptic modifiability (LTP, and LTD if present) is needed only to set up the functional architecture of the network while the reversal learning set is being acquired. However, once the correct synaptic connections have been set up to implement the architecture illustrated in Fig. 4.52, then no further synaptic modifiability is needed each time reversal occurs, as reversal is achieved just by the error signal quenching the current rule attractor, and the attractor for the other rule then starting up because its synapses are not adapted. This is an interesting prediction of the model. If tested by NMDA receptor blockers, which can block LTP, then it would be important to ensure that non-specific factors produced by the NMDA blockade such as less overall activity in the network, and the stabilizing effects of the long time constants of NMDA receptors, do not contribute to any result obtained. For this reason, use of a procedure for impairing synaptic modifiability other than NMDA receptor blockade would be useful in testing this prediction.

The network just described uses biased competition from a rule module to bias the mapping from sensory stimuli to the representation of a reward vs a punisher. An analogous rule network reversed in the same way by error signals quenching the current rule attractor, can be used to reverse the mapping from stimuli via intermediate stimulus–response neurons to response neurons, and thus to switch the stimulus-to-motor response being mapped in a model of conditional response learning (Deco & Rolls 2003, Deco & Rolls 2005a). While reward rule neurons have not been described yet for the orbitofrontal cortex, neurons which may correspond to stimulus–response rule neurons have been found in the dorsolateral prefrontal cortex (Wallis, Anderson & Miller 2001).

This model also provides a computational account of why the orbitofrontal cortex may play a more important role in rapid reversal learning than the amygdala. The account is based on the fact that a feature of cortical architecture is a highly developed set of local (within 1–2 mm) recurrent collateral excitatory associatively modifiable connections between pyramidal cells (Rolls & Deco 2002, Rolls & Treves 1998). These provide the basis for short-term memory attractor networks, and thus the basis for the rule attractor model which is at the heart of my suggestion for how rapid reversal learning is implemented (Deco & Rolls 2005a). In contrast, the amygdala is thought to have a much less well developed set of recurrent collateral excitatory connections, and thus may not be able to implement rapid reversal learning in the way described using competition biased by a rule module. Instead, the amygdala would need to rely on synaptic relearning as described in the first approach above, and this would be likely to be a slower process, and would certainly not lead to correct choice of the new S+ the first time it is presented after a punishment trial when the reversal contingency changes. Of course, in addition it is possible that the rapidity of LTP, and the efficacy of LTD, both of which would also facilitate rapid reversal, may be enhanced in the orbitofrontal cortex compared to the amygdala. Thus, the cortical neuronal reversal mechanism in the orbitofrontal cortex may be effectively a faster implementation in two ways than what is implemented in the amygdala. The cortical (in this case orbitofrontal cortex) mechanism may have evolved particularly to enable rapid updating by received reinforcers in social and other situations in primates. This hypothesis, that the orbitofrontal cortex, as a rapid learning mechanism, effectively provides an additional route for some of the functions performed by the amygdala, and is very important when this stimulus–reinforcer learning must be rapidly readjusted, has been developed elsewhere (Rolls 1990b, Rolls 1992a, Rolls 1996b, Rolls 1999a, Rolls 2000d, Rolls 2005b).

Another feature of the rule attractor model of rapid reversal learning (Deco & Rolls 2005a) is that it does utilize a set of coupled attractor networks in the orbitofrontal cortex. Consistent with this, Hikosaka & Watanabe (2000) have shown that a short-term memory for reward, such as the flavour of a food, is represented by continuing firing in orbitofrontal cortex neurons in a reward delayed match-to-sample short-term memory task. This could be implemented by associatively modified synaptic connections between taste reward neurons (see Section 4.3) in the orbitofrontal cortex.

Although the mechanism has been described so far for visual-to-taste association learning, this is because neurophysiological experiments on this are most direct. It is likely, given the evidence from the effects of lesions, that taste is only one type of primary reinforcer about which such learning occurs in the orbitofrontal cortex, and is likely to be an example of a much more general type of stimulus–reinforcer learning system. Some of the evidence for this is that humans with orbitofrontal cortex damage are impaired at visual discrimination reversal when working for a reward that consists of points (Rolls, Hornak, Wade & McGrath 1994a) or money (Hornak, Bramham, Rolls, Morris, O'Doherty, Bullock & Polkey 2003) (see Section 4.5.6). Moreover, as described above, there is now evidence that the representation of the affective aspects of touch are represented in the human orbitofrontal cortex (Rolls, O'Doherty, Kringelbach, Francis, Bowtell & McGlone 2003d, McCabe, Rolls, Bilderbeck & McGlone 2008), and learning about what stimuli are associated with this class of primary reinforcer is also likely to be an important aspect of the stimulus–reinforcer association learning performed by the orbitofrontal cortex.

4.5.8 Executive functions of the orbitofrontal cortex

The research described indicates that the orbitofrontal cortex represents the outcome value for many types of reinforcer, computes expected value based in part on associative learning between stimuli and outcome value, and based in part on rule-based reversal of expected value based on unexpected outcomes, that is errors. These representations can influence behaviour, as shown by the effects of lesions of the orbitofrontal cortex, which impair choices when reward predictions are in error, and when punishers should normally control behaviour. The fact that patients with ventromedial prefrontal cortex lesions often can express verbally what the correct choices and actions should be, yet still make the wrong choices, shows that there is a second, reasoning, explicit route to action using language (Section 10.3.1), but that often choices are controlled implicitly by the orbitofrontal cortex.

In that the orbitofrontal cortex may retain as a result of synaptic modification in a pattern associator (see Appendix 1, Rolls & Treves (1990), Rolls & Treves (1998), and Rolls (2008b)) the most recent reinforcer associations for large numbers of different stimuli, it could perhaps be fitted into a view that the frontal cortical areas are in general concerned with different types of executive function, frequently involving working memory (Stuss 2011). However, the term working memory is normally used in neurophysiology to refer to a memory in which the memoranda are held in the memory by continuing neuronal activity, as in an autoassociator or attractor network which has recurrent collateral connections (see, e.g., Rolls & Treves (1998), Rolls (2008b), and Appendix 1). It should be realized that although there may be a functional similarity between such a working memory and the ability of the orbitofrontal cortex to retain the most recent reinforcer association of many stimuli, the implementations are very different. The different implementations do in fact have strong functional consequences: it is difficult to retain more than a few items active in an autoassociative memory, and hence in practice individual items are retained typically only for short periods in such working memories (Deco & Rolls 2005d, Rolls, Dempere-Marco & Deco 2013); whereas in pattern associators, because synaptic modification has taken place, the last reinforcement association of a very large number of stimuli can be stored for long periods, and recalled whenever each stimulus is seen again in the future, without any ongoing neuronal firing to hold the representation active (see, e.g., Rolls & Treves (1998)).

It is useful to note how the orbitofrontal cortex may link to output systems to control behaviour, for the occasions when the orbitofrontal cortex does control behaviour (Fig. 4.2). One route is via the basal ganglia, and this is especially important in setting up habit behaviours (Section 6.3). Another route for actions where the goals are specified by the value representations in the orbitofrontal cortex is the cingulate cortex (Section 4.7). Another set of outputs from the orbitofrontal cortex enables it to influence autonomic function, for example via the connections to the cingulate cortex (Vogt 2009) and to the hypothalamus and amygdala (Rempel-Clower & Barbas 1998, Barbas et al. 2011). The fact that ventral prefrontal lesions block autonomic responses to learned reinforcers (Damasio 1994) [actually known since at least the 1950s, e.g. Elithorn, Piercy & Crosskey (1955) in humans; Grueninger, Kimble, Grueninger & Levine (1965) in macaques], is of course consistent with the hypothesis that learned reinforcers elicit autonomic responses via the orbitofrontal cortex and amygdala (Rolls 1986a, Rolls 1986b, Rolls 1990b, Rolls 2005b). It is worth emphasizing here that this does not prove the hypothesis that behavioural responses elicited by conditioned reinforcers are mediated via peripheral changes, themselves used as 'somatic markers' to determine which response to make. The question of whether there is any returning information from the periphery which is necessary for emotion, as the somatic marker hypothesis postulates, has been considered in Section 2.6.1. The present hypothesis is, in contrast, that somatic markers are not part of the route by which emotions are felt or emotional decisions are taken, but that instead the much more direct neural routes from the orbitofrontal cortex and amygdala to the cingulate cortex and basal ganglia provide pathways that are much more efficient, and are directly implicated in producing, the behavioural responses to learned incentives (see Chapter 6, Section 4.7, and for explicit verbal outputs see Chapter 10).

4.6 The amygdala

Bilateral damage to the amygdala produces a deficit in learning to associate visual and other stimuli with a primary (i.e. unlearned) reward or punisher. For example, monkeys with damage to the amygdala when shown foods and non-foods pick up both and place them in their mouths. When such visual or auditory discrimination learning and learned emotional responses to stimuli are tested more formally, it is found that animals have difficulty in associating the sight or sound of a stimulus with whether it produces a reward, or is noxious and should be avoided (Rolls 1990b, Rolls 1992a, Rolls 2000d, Aggleton 2000, Amaral 2003, Rolls 2005b, Murray & Izquierdo 2007, Murray, Wise & Rhodes 2011)). Similar changes in behaviour have been seen in humans with amygdala damage (Whalen & Phelps 2009). The primate amygdala also contains a population of neurons specialized to respond to faces, and damage to the human amygdala can alter the ability to discriminate between different facial expressions.

Because the amygdala is implicated in some but not other learning processes involved in emotion, Section 4.6.1 provides a description of some of the different associative processes involved in emotion-related learning, as part of the background for considering the functions of the amygdala in emotion, and more generally, for understanding the types of learning that influence decision processes involved in emotional behaviours (see further Section 11.2).

4.6.1 Associative processes involved in emotion-related learning

When a conditioned stimulus (CS) (such as a tone) is paired with a primary reinforcer or unconditioned stimulus (US) (such as a painful stimulus), then there are opportunities for a number of types of association to be formed.

Some of these involve 'classical conditioning' or 'Pavlovian conditioning', in which no action is performed that affects the contingency between the conditioned stimulus and the unconditioned stimulus. Typically an unconditioned response (UR), for example an alteration of heart rate, is produced by the US, and will come to be elicited by the CS as a conditioned response (CR). These responses are typically autonomic (such as the heart beating faster), or endocrine (for example the release of adrenaline (epinephrine in American usage) by the adrenal gland).

In addition, the organism may learn to perform an instrumental response with the skeletal muscles in order to alter the probability that the primary reinforcer will be obtained. In our example, the experimenter might alter the contingencies so that when the tone sounded, if the organism performed an action such as pressing a lever, then the painful stimulus could be avoided. This is confirmed to be instrumental learning if the response learned is arbitrary, for example performing the opposite response, such as raising the lever to avoid the painful stimulus.

In the instrumental learning situation there are still opportunities for many classically conditioned responses including emotional states such as fear to occur, and, as different neural subsystems appear to contribute differently to these different types of learning that occur in emotional situations produced by reinforcers, I will next separate out some of the different associative processes that can occur, to provide a basis for understanding the roles of different neural subsystems in the different emotion-related responses and states, following the general approach reviewed by Cardinal, Parkinson, Hall & Everitt (2002).

4.6.1.1 Pavlovian or classical conditioning

As shown in Fig. 4.54, Pavlovian conditioning has the potential to create multiple associative representations in the brain, as described next (Cardinal et al. 2002, Mackintosh 1983, Gewirtz & Davis 1998, Dickinson 1980, Cardinal & Everitt 2004, Mazur 2012).

Stimulus–Response association. First, the CS may become directly associated with the UR, a simple stimulus–response association that carries no information about the identity of the US (pathway 1 in Fig. 4.54). Such US-elicited responses include preparatory responses which are not specific to the type of US involved (e.g. orienting to a stimulus, or increased arousal), and 'consummatory' responses which are specific to the US such as salivation to food, or blinking to an air puff applied to the eye, or approach to a food. A single US may elicit both preparatory and consummatory responses, and thus the CS may enter into simple S–R associations with several types of response. The nature of the CS can influence which response is evoked; for example if a poorly localized CS such as a tone is paired with food, it may not elicit conditioned approach, while a localized light does. It is notable in this last example that the approach response is skeletal, so that we are going beyond the concept that Pavlovian conditioning applies only to autonomic responses.

A representation of affect, i.e. an emotional state. Second, the CS can evoke a representation of affect, i.e. an emotional state, such as fear or the expectation of reward (pathway 2 in Fig. 4.54). It is demonstrated operationally by the phenomenon of transreinforcer blocking. Blocking is a feature of Pavlovian conditioning in which an animal does not learn about one CS in the presence of another CS that already predicts the same US (Dickinson 1980). In *transreinforcer blocking*, the presence of a CS previously paired with shock can block or prevent conditioning to a CS paired with the absence of otherwise expected food reward (Dickinson & Dearing 1979). These two reinforcers share no common properties other than their aversiveness, and therefore the blocking effect must depend on an association between the CS and affect. Affective states, it is argued (Dickinson & Dearing 1979, Konorski 1967, Cardinal et al. 2002), can therefore be independent of the specific reinforcer and response – they are pure 'value' states. However, I note that, at least in humans, affective states normally have content, that is they are about particular reinforcers (such as feeling happy because I am seeing a friend, or feeling happy because I am receiving a gift), and these states are better described by the third type of association, described next.

Conditioned-Stimulus (CS)–Unconditioned Stimulus (US) associations. Third, the CS

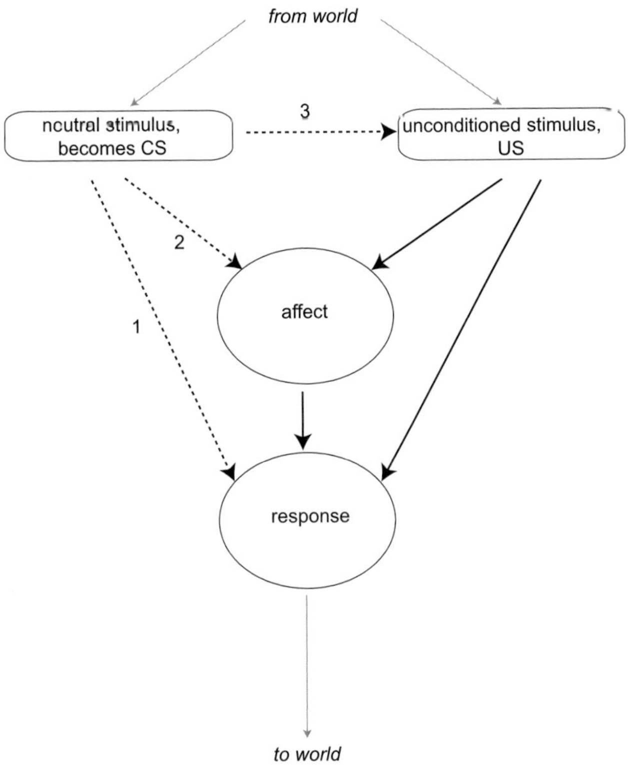

Fig. 4.54 Pavlovian conditioning has the potential to create associations between a conditioned stimulus (CS) and representations of the unconditioned stimulus (US), central affective or emotional states such as fear, and unconditioned responses. Dashed lines represent associatively learned links. Several different types of response may be involved, including preparatory responses which are not specific to the type of US involved (e.g. orienting to a stimulus, or increased arousal), and 'consummatory' responses which are specific to the US such as salivation to food, or blinking to an air puff applied to the eye. (Reprinted from *Neuroscience & Biobehavioral Reviews*, 26 (3), Rudolf N. Cardinal, John A. Parkinson, Jeremy Hall, and Barry J. Everitt, Emotion and motivation: the role of the amygdala, ventral striatum, and prefrontal cortex, pp. 321–352, Copyright, 2002, with permission from Elsevier.)

can become associated with the specific sensory properties of the US including its visual appearance, sound, and smell and its 'consummatory' (primary reinforcing) properties such as its taste, nutritive value, and feel (pathway 3 in Fig. 4.54). An operational demonstration of this type of representation is sensory preconditioning, in which two neutral stimuli are first associated; one neutral stimulus is then paired with a primary reinforcer, and the other stimulus can subsequently evoke a CR (Dickinson 1980). Further evidence for the US specificity of Pavlovian associations comes from the effect of post-conditioning changes in the value of the US. If a CS is paired with a rewarding food, and the food is subsequently devalued by pairing it with a lithium chloride (LiCl) injection to induce nausea, not only does the animal reject the food US, but its reaction to the CS changes (Mackintosh 1983, Holland & Straub 1979). Therefore the CS could not have been associated just with an abstract affective representation, as it was able to retrieve, by association, the new value of the US. As the LiCl pairing does not affect the reaction to a second CS predicting a different food, each CS must have been associated with some specific aspect of its US.

We will see later that different pathways in the brain are involved in the Pavlovian learned autonomic and skeletal responses to a CS, and in the affective representation or state (e.g.

fear), which may itself enter into associations and influence choice.

4.6.1.2 Instrumental learning

In instrumental learning, there is a contingency between the behaviour and the reinforcing outcome. A number of different learning processes may operate during this procedure (Cardinal et al. 2002, Dickinson 1994, Dickinson & Balleine 1994). These learning processes are summarized next as they help to understand some of the different brain mechanisms that become engaged and affect behaviour when emotion-provoking stimuli are delivered. These learning processes are closely related to emotion, for as argued in Chapter 2 emotions are states elicited by instrumental reinforcers. Moreover, as argued in Chapter 3, an important part of the evolutionary adaptive value of emotions is that genes can influence our behaviour efficiently by specifying the goals for our actions, and then instrumental learning in life leads us to learn appropriate behaviours to obtain those gene-specified goals. This of course leads to selection of the genes that specify the goals (rewards and punishers), and thereby promote their own survival into the next generation. Part of the adaptive value of emotional states, as argued in Chapter 3, is that they persist for some time after the reinforcer has gone, and this continuation enables the reinforcers to influence our behaviour (by unconditioned, classically conditioned, and instrumentally learned, processes) for often a considerable time.

An example of a goal-directed behaviour is when an organism presses a lever for food because it knows that lever-pressing produces food and that it wants the food. More formally, behaviour may be said to be goal-directed if it depends on both (1) the instrumental contingency between the action and a particular outcome (A–O contingency), and (2) a representation of the outcome as a goal (Dickinson & Balleine 1994, Cardinal et al. 2002). As two representations must interact, the knowledge required may be called declarative.

Instrumental (Action–Outcome) contingency. Vertebrates, and some invertebrates, can learn the instrumental contingency between an action and its consequence. For example rats can be arbitrarily trained to press a lever down or pull it up in order to obtain a goal. (This is a bidirectional control assay to show that the action is arbitrary.) Not all behaviours can be trained in this way, and in this sense there is some preparedness to learn. For example, locomotor approach to a visual stimulus in rats is predominantly under the control of Pavlovian and not instrumental processes, in that rats could not learn to withhold an approach response to a visual CS in order to be rewarded (Bussey & Everitt 1997).

Incentive value. Rats and monkeys also fulfil the second requirement for instrumental learning: they demonstrate that they want the outcomes for which they work. The goal status (or *incentive value*) of an instrumental outcome can be demonstrated by devaluing it (Dickinson & Balleine 1994, Murray & Izquierdo 2007), and indeed this procedure was used in sensory-specific satiety investigations that reveal value representations in the orbitofrontal cortex (Rolls, Sienkiewicz & Yaxley 1989b, Critchley & Rolls 1996c, Kringelbach, O'Doherty, Rolls & Andrews 2003, Rolls 2008e, Rolls & Grabenhorst 2008) and regions to which it projects including the anterior cingulate cortex (Rolls 2008e) and lateral hypothalamus (Rolls, Murzi, Yaxley, Thorpe & Simpson 1986). For example, if rats are trained to lever-press for food, and then receive pairings of that food with LiCl (lithium chloride, which induces a conditioned taste aversion), they will subsequently work less for that food – even if the test is conducted in extinction, when there is no opportunity to learn a new relationship between a response and the less pleasant outcome (Adams & Dickinson 1981, Colwill & Rescorla 1985). A surprising point is that although after the LiCl conditioning the rats reject the taste of the conditioned food, they may nevertheless initially perform the instrumental response for the food, until they have had the opportunity to re-experience the food by consuming it (Balleine

& Dickinson 1991). Thus the incentive value that controls instrumental performance can be dissociated in a short initial period from the hedonic value that can influence rejection or acceptance of a taste. When the rat re-experiences the food and its new hedonic impact, the instrumental incentive value is updated by a process referred to as *incentive learning* (Balleine & Dickinson 1991, Dickinson & Balleine 1994). A similar phenomenon has been demonstrated for the control of behaviour by motivational state. For example, if a hungry rat is trained to respond for food, and then satiated before being tested in extinction (i.e. with no food available), it will perform the instrumental response as much as a hungry rat, until it experiences the reduced value of the food when satiated (Balleine 1992).

One factor that may lead to this paradoxical behaviour is that if a rat has been highly trained in an instrumental learning task, then that behaviour becomes a stimulus–response habit that is not under normal control by goal availability and even normal stimuli (see below). For example, a rat well trained in a T maze runway task to turn left at the end to obtain food will turn left and bump into the wall if the length of the runway is increased.

Hedonic assessment. Hedonic assessment may be measured directly by questions such as 'How pleasant does the food taste?' (see Section 5.3.1). In monkeys, one can show the monkey a food, and obtain clear evidence on a defined rating scale of how rewarding the food is to the monkey (Burton, Rolls & Mora 1976, Rolls, Judge & Sanghera 1977, Rolls, Sienkiewicz & Yaxley 1989b), by measuring whether he will reach for the food to place it in his mouth (+2), whether he will not reach but will open the mouth readily to accept the food (+1), whether he will swallow the food if it is placed in the mouth (0, neutral), whether he will close his mouth to prevent the food being placed in his mouth (–1), or whether he will use his hand to push away the food to prevent it approaching the mouth (–2). These appear to correspond approximately to the human subjective ratings of very pleasant (+2), pleasant (+1), neutral (0), unpleasant (–1), and very unpleasant (–2) (Rolls, Rolls, Rowe & Sweeney 1981a).

In rodents, it is apparently more difficult to measure hedonic responses to food (Cardinal, Parkinson, Hall & Everitt 2002). The suggestion that orofacial responses such as gaping to a bitter taste placed in the mouth measure hedonics (Cardinal et al. 2002, Garcia 1989) does not appear to be relevant to primates including humans, in that we know from the effects of decerebration that these responses can be reflexes organized in the brain stem (Grill & Norgren 1978) (with consistent evidence from anencephalic humans (Steiner, Glaser, Hawilo & Berridge 2001)). Further, in primates including humans it is found that flavour processing proceeds as far as the primary taste and olfactory cortex without any modulation by hunger, so that hedonics cannot be represented before these primary cortical areas in primates including humans (Rolls, Scott, Sienkiewicz & Yaxley 1988, Yaxley, Rolls & Sienkiewicz 1988, Kringelbach, O'Doherty, Rolls & Andrews 2003, De Araujo, Kringelbach, Rolls & McGlone 2003b, De Araujo, Rolls, Kringelbach, McGlone & Phillips 2003c). In addition, in the secondary but not primary olfactory cortex in humans activations in fMRI experiments are correlated with the pleasantness of the smell, whereas in the primary olfactory cortex activations are correlated with the intensity of the odour (Rolls, Kringelbach & De Araujo 2003c) (see Section 4.5.5.2 and Chapter 5).

Discriminative stimuli. When instrumental responding is rewarded in the presence of a stimulus but not in its absence, that stimulus is established as a discriminative stimulus S^D. For example, in a visual discrimination task, the visual stimulus (e.g. a triangle) that is shown to indicate that a lick response will be rewarded with fruit juice is an S^D. The visual stimulus that indicates that if a response is made it will be punished with salt taste is an S^Δ. This is a Go/NoGo visual discrimination task which we have frequently used to study brain mechanisms involved in processing reward-related visual and olfactory stimuli (Rolls, Judge

& Sanghera 1977, Rolls, Sanghera & Roper-Hall 1979a, Thorpe, Rolls & Maddison 1983, Critchley & Rolls 1996b, Rolls, Critchley, Mason & Wakeman 1996a). Although an S^D can serve as a Pavlovian CS (Colwill & Rescorla 1988), S^Ds have effects that can not be explained in this manner (Holman & Mackintosh 1981): there is a conditional relationship in which an S^D signals the operation of a particular response-reinforcer (instrumental, action–outcome) contingency (Colwill & Rescorla 1990, Rescorla 1990a, Rescorla 1990b).

Stimulus–Response habits. Overtraining in an instrumental task results in instrumental behaviour that becomes performed as a fixed inflexible habit. Under these circumstances, behaviour is under automatic response control, and not under direct control of the goal, in that if the reinforcer is devalued (by for example pairing with LiCl or by satiation), instrumental behaviour may continue for a few trials until the animal obtains the reinforcer, and then the instrumental behaviour stops (Adams 1982, Dickinson 1994, Dickinson 1985, Dickinson, Balleine, Watt, Gonzalez & Boakes 1995, Dickinson, Nicholas & Adams 1983). The interest here is that early on in training the learning and the behaviour are directly guided by the hedonic or reward value of the reinforcer or goal, and if the reinforcer is devalued, the behaviour stops. These processes are implemented in brain regions such as the amygdala and orbitofrontal cortex, as described in this chapter, with reinforcer devaluation studies in primates reviewed by Murray & Izquierdo (2007). During this training period, the conditions are in fact set up for habit, stimulus–response, learned associations, perhaps implemented in the basal ganglia (see Section 6.3), to be learned. Once the stimulus comes automatically and rapidly to produce the response, then behaviour is not being performed in a so literally goal-directed manner.

Pavlovian–instrumental transfer (PIT). If a stimulus that predicts the arrival of sucrose as a result of Pavlovian conditioning is provided during an instrumental task such as working to obtain sucrose, the responding (e.g. lever pressing) can be enhanced (Lovibond 1983, Estes 1948, Dickinson 1994, Dickinson & Balleine 1994). There is an outcome- or response-specific form in which only instrumental performance for sucrose reward is facilitated, and a non-specific form in which performance for other rewards such as food pellets is enhanced (Balleine 1994, Dickinson & Dawson 1987a, Dickinson & Dawson 1987b, Colwill & Rescorla 1988). The effect is sometimes termed conditioned motivation (Rescorla & Solomon 1967), and is an example of the *incentive motivation* effect described by Donald Hebb (Hebb 1949), in which giving a few free salted nuts in a market place will increase the probability that humans will buy some peanuts (the 'salted nut effect'). A similar phenomenon is the release of the pleasant smell of bread cooking near bakeries, which increases motivation to buy bread.

Pavlovian–instrumental transfer is optimal when motivation for the US (e.g. hunger making the taste of bread pleasant) is present, and thus it is argued that the 'Pavlovian value' depends directly on the motivational state in a way in which instrumental incentive value does not (at least when assessed after overtraining using devaluation procedures). It is thus suggested that the Pavlovian CS accesses the US (Cardinal et al. 2002, Dickinson & Dawson 1987a, Dickinson & Dawson 1987b, Dickinson 1986) (in our example, the taste of food), which is a motivation-dependent representation. Pavlovian–instrumental transfer may be involved in cue-induced relapse in drug addiction (Gawin 1991, Tiffany & Drobes 1990, O'Brien, Childress, Ehrman & Robbins 1998).

Summary of instrumental learning. This survey shows that multiple processes, which it turns out may have somewhat different brain implementations as described below, are involved in instrumental learning. One key process is action–outcome learning. The outcome is represented as reward or affective value, such as I suggest is implemented by the firing of orbitofrontal cortex neurons that respond to the taste of food only if hunger is present. The orbitofrontal cortex appears to be involved in the representation of the reward, and in the processes that learn which stimuli are associated with rewards, but not with forming associations between behavioural responses (actions) and rewards (outcomes), in that orbitofrontal cortex neurons in primates do not respond to motor responses or actions.

Other processes influence instrumental learning including Pavlovian processes that can facilitate performance (as in Pavlovian-instrumental transfer, PIT). Further, approach to a food may be under Pavlovian rather than instrumental control. Finally, we must beware of the facts that after overtraining, responses may become inflexibly linked to stimuli, and that the goals, and the reward value of the goals, may no longer be directly influencing behaviour in an ongoing way as shown by devaluation experiments.

4.6.2 Connections of the amygdala

The amygdala is a subcortical region in the anterior part of the temporal lobe. It receives massive projections in the primate from the overlying temporal lobe cortex (Van Hoesen 1981, Amaral, Price, Pitkanen & Carmichael 1992, Ghashghaei & Barbas 2002, Freese & Amaral 2009) (see Fig. 4.55). These come in the monkey to overlapping but partly separate regions of the lateral and basal amygdala from the inferior temporal visual cortex, the superior temporal auditory cortex, the cortex of the temporal pole, and the cortex in the superior temporal sulcus. These inputs thus come from the higher stages of sensory processing in the visual and auditory modalities, and not from early cortical processing areas. Via these inputs, the amygdala receives inputs about objects that could become secondary reinforcers, as a result of pattern association in the amygdala with primary reinforcers. The amygdala also receives inputs that are potentially about primary reinforcers, e.g. taste inputs (from the insula, and from the secondary taste cortex in the orbitofrontal cortex), and somatosensory inputs, potentially about the rewarding or painful aspects of touch (from the somatosensory cortex via the insula) (Mesulam & Mufson 1982a, Mesulam & Mufson 1982b, Friedman, Murray, O'Neill & Mishkin 1986, Freese & Amaral 2009). The amygdala receives strong projections from the posterior orbitofrontal cortex (see Fig. 4.55, areas 12 and 13) where there are value representations, and from the anterior cingulate cortex (Carmichael & Price 1995a, Ghashghaei & Barbas 2002, Freese & Amaral 2009).

Subcortical inputs to the amygdala include projections from the midline thalamic nuclei, the subiculum, and CA1 parts of the hippocampal formation, the hypothalamus and substantia innominata, the nucleus of the solitary tract (which receives gustatory and visceral inputs), and from olfactory structures (Amaral et al. 1992, Pitkanen 2000). Although there are some inputs from early on in some sensory pathways, for example auditory inputs from the medial geniculate nucleus (LeDoux 1987, LeDoux 1992, Pessoa & Adolphs 2010), this route is unlikely to be involved in most emotions, for which cortical analysis of the stimulus is likely to be required. Emotions are usually elicited to environmental stimuli analysed to the object level (including other organisms), and not to retinal arrays of spots or the frequency (tone) of a sound as represented in the cochlea. Consistent with this view (that neural systems involved in emotion in primates generally receive from sensory systems where analysis of the identity of the stimulus as an object is performed), neurons in the inferior temporal visual cortex do not have responses related to the association with reinforcement of visual stimuli (Rolls, Judge & Sanghera 1977); whereas such neurons are found in the amygdala and orbitofrontal cortex (see below; cf. Fig. 4.2). Similarly, processing in the taste system of primates up to and including the primary taste cortex reflects the identity of the tastant, whereas its hedonic value as influenced by hunger is reflected in the responses of neurons in the secondary taste cortex (Rolls 1989a, Rolls 1995b, Rolls & Scott 2003, Rolls 2014a) (see Fig. 4.2).

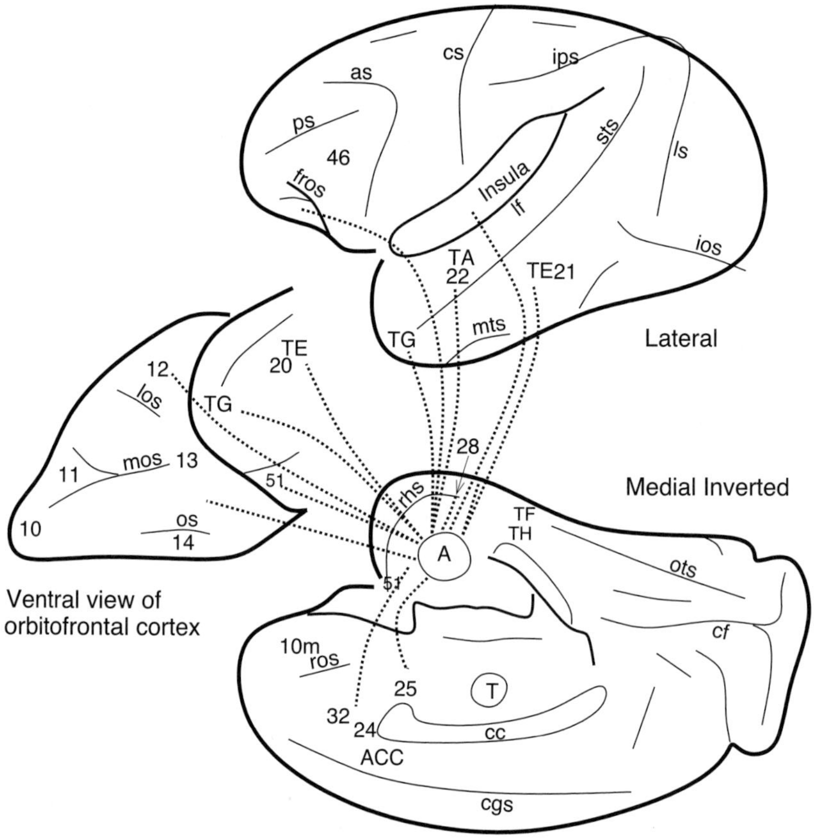

Fig. 4.55 Connections of the amygdala shown on lateral, ventral, and medial inverted views of the monkey brain. Abbreviations: as, arcuate sulcus; cc, corpus callosum; cf, calcarine fissure; cgs, cingulate sulcus; cs, central sulcus; ls, lunate sulcus; ios, inferior occipital sulcus; mos, medial orbital sulcus; os, orbital sulcus; ots, occipito-temporal sulcus; ps, principal sulcus; rhs, rhinal sulcus; sts, superior temporal sulcus; lf, lateral (or Sylvian) fissure (which has been opened to reveal the insula); A, amygdala; ACC, anterior cingulate cortex; INS, insula; T, thalamus; TE (21), inferior temporal visual cortex; TA (22), superior temporal auditory association cortex; TF and TH, parahippocampal cortex; TG, temporal pole cortex; 12, 13, 11, orbitofrontal cortex; 24, 32, parts of the anterior cingulate cortex; 25, subgenual cingulate cortex; 28, entorhinal cortex; 51, olfactory (prepyriform and periamygdaloid) cortex. The cortical connections shown provide afferents to the amygdala, but are reciprocated. (Reproduced from G. W. Van Hoesen, The differential distribution, diversity and sprouting of cortical projections to the amygdala in the rhesus monkey, in Y. Ben-Ari (ed.), *The Amygdaloid Complex*, pp. 77–90 ©1981 Elsevier, with permission.)

The outputs of the amygdala (Amaral et al. 1992, Freese & Amaral 2009) include the well-known projections to the hypothalamus, from the lateral amygdala via the ventral amygdalofugal pathway to the lateral hypothalamus; and from the medial amygdala, which is relatively small in the primate, via the stria terminalis to the medial hypothalamus. The ventral amygdalofugal pathway includes some long descending fibres that project to the autonomic centres in the medulla oblongata, and provides a route for cortically processed signals to reach the brainstem. A further interesting output of the amygdala is to the ventral striatum (Heimer, Switzer & Van Hoesen 1982) including the nucleus accumbens, for via this route information processed in the amygdala could gain access to the basal ganglia and thus influence motor output. (The output of the amygdala also reaches more dorsal parts of the striatum such as the head of the caudate nucleus.) The amygdala also projects to the medial part of the mediodorsal nucleus of the thalamus, which projects to the orbitofrontal cortex, providing another output pathway for the amygdala. In addition, the amygdala has direct projections back to many areas of the temporal, orbitofrontal, and insular cortices from which it receives inputs (Amaral et al. 1992, Freese & Amaral 2009). It is suggested elsewhere (Rolls 1989a, Rolls 1989b, Treves & Rolls 1994, Rolls 1996a, Rolls & Treves 1998, Rolls 2000f, Rolls 2008b) that the functions of these backprojections include the guidance of information representation and storage in the neocortex, and recall (when this is related to reinforcing stimuli). Another interesting set of output pathways of the amygdala are the projections to the entorhinal cortex, which provides the major input to the hippocampus and dentate gyrus, and to the ventral subiculum, which provides a major output of the hippocampus (Amaral et al. 1992). Via these pathways, reward influences may be introduced into the hippocampal memory system, and provide for associations to be formed between viewed places 'out there' and the rewards at those places (Rolls & Xiang 2005, Rolls & Kesner 2006, Rolls 2010b, Rolls 2013c) (see Section 4.12).

These anatomical connections of the amygdala indicate that it is strategically placed to receive highly processed information from the cortex and to influence motor systems, autonomic systems, some of the cortical areas from which it receives inputs, and other limbic areas. The functions mediated through these connections will now be considered, using information available from the effects of damage to the amygdala and from the activity of neurons in the amygdala.

4.6.3 Effects of amygdala lesions

4.6.3.1 Amygdala lesions in primates

Bilateral removal of the amygdala in monkeys produces striking behavioural changes which include tameness, a lack of emotional responsiveness, excessive examination of objects, often with the mouth, and eating of previously rejected items such as meat (Weiskrantz 1956). These behavioural changes comprise much of the Kluver–Bucy syndrome which is produced in monkeys by bilateral anterior temporal lobectomy (Kluver & Bucy 1939). In analyses of the bases of these behavioural changes, it has been observed that there are deficits in some types of learning. For example, Weiskrantz (1956) found that bilateral ablation of the amygdala in the monkey produced a deficit on learning an active avoidance task. The monkeys failed to learn to make a response when a light signalled that shock would follow unless the response was made. He was perhaps the first to suggest that these monkeys had difficulty with forming associations between stimuli and reinforcers, when he suggested that "the effect of amygdalectomy is to make it difficult for reinforcing stimuli, whether positive or negative, to become established or to be recognized as such" (Weiskrantz 1956). In this avoidance task, associations between a stimulus and punishers were impaired.

Evidence soon became available that associations between stimuli and positive reinforcers (reward) were also impaired in, for example, serial reversals of a visual discrimination made to obtain food (Jones & Mishkin 1972, Spiegler & Mishkin 1981). In this task the monkey must learn that food is under one of two objects, and after he has learned this, he must then relearn (reverse) the association as the food is then placed under the other object. Jones & Mishkin (1972) showed that the stages of this task that are particularly affected by damage to this region are those when the monkeys are responding at chance to the two visual stimuli or are starting to respond more to the currently rewarded stimuli, rather than the stage when the monkeys are continuing to make perseverative responses to the previously rewarded visual stimulus. They thus argued that the difficulty produced by this anterior temporal lobe damage is in learning to associate stimuli with reinforcers, in this case with food reward.

However, lesion studies are subject to the criticism that the effects of a lesion could be due to inadvertent damage to other brain structures or pathways close to the intended lesion site. For this reason, many of the older lesion studies are being repeated and extended with lesions in which instead of an ablation (removal) or electrolytic lesion (which can damage axons passing through a brain region), a neurotoxin is used to damage cells in a localized region, but to leave intact fibres of passage. There is evidence from these more selective lesion studies in monkeys that the amygdala is involved in learning associations between visual stimuli and rewards (Murray & Izquierdo 2007). Using such lesions (made with ibotenic acid) in monkeys, impairments in the processing of food reward value were found, in that when the reward value of one set of foods was devalued by feeding it to satiety (i.e. sensory-specific satiety, a reward devaluation procedure, see also Section 4.6.1.2, and used extensively to measure whether neuronal responses are related to value (Rolls, Murzi, Yaxley, Thorpe & Simpson 1986, Rolls, Sienkiewicz & Yaxley 1989b, Critchley & Rolls 1996c, Kringelbach, O'Doherty, Rolls & Andrews 2003, Rolls 2008e)), the monkeys still chose the visual stimuli associated with the foods with which they had been satiated (Malkova, Gaffan & Murray 1997, Baxter & Murray 2000, Murray & Izquierdo 2007). Thus, as with orbitofrontal cortex lesions, damage to the amygdala impairs the linkage of visual stimuli to their value as measured by choices in devaluation paradigms (Murray & Izquierdo 2007).

(Neurophysiologically what is measured in sensory-specific devaluation studies is an effect of devaluing the primary reinforcer, the taste or flavour, on choices of visual or taste stimuli (Rolls et al. 1986, Rolls et al. 1989b, Critchley & Rolls 1996c, Rolls 2008e). It is therefore important to test lesioned animals when the association is directly between a visual stimulus and a primary reinforcer such as taste or flavour.)

Further evidence that neurotoxic lesions of the amygdala in primates affect behaviour to stimuli learned as being reward-related as well as punishment-related is that monkeys with neurotoxic lesions of the amygdala showed abnormal patterns of food choice, picking up and eating foods not normally eaten such as meat, and picking up and placing in their mouths inedible objects (Murray, Gaffan & Flint 1996, Baxter & Murray 2000, Baxter & Murray 2002, Murray & Izquierdo 2007). In addition, neurotoxic amygdala lesions, as well as orbitofrontal cortex lesions, impair emotional responses to snakes and human intruders (Murray & Izquierdo 2007). These symptoms produced by selective amygdala lesions are classical Kluver–Bucy symptoms. Thus in primates, there is evidence that selective amygdala lesions impair some types of behaviour to learned reward-related stimuli as well as to learned punisher-related stimuli. However, we should not conclude that this is the only brain structure involved in this type of learning, for especially when rapid stimulus–reinforcer association learning is performed in primates, the orbitofrontal cortex is involved, as shown in Section 4.5. Further, studies in macaques with neurotoxic (ibotenic acid) lesions of the amygdala reveal relatively mild deficits in social behaviour (Amaral 2003, Amaral, Bauman, Capitanio, Lavenex, Mason, Mauldin-Jourdain & Mendoza 2003, Bauman, Lavenex, Mason, Capitanio & Amaral 2004), and this is consistent with the trend for the orbitofrontal cortex to become relatively more important in emotion and social behaviour in primates including humans. This is shown for example by the findings that damage to the human orbitofrontal cortex does produce large changes in social and emotional behaviour (see Section 4.5.6).

The symptoms of the Kluver–Bucy syndrome, including the emotional changes, could be a result of this type of deficit in learning stimulus–reinforcer associations (Jones & Mishkin 1972, Mishkin & Aggleton 1981, Rolls 1986a, Rolls 1986b, Rolls 1990b, Rolls 1992a, Rolls 2000d). For example, the tameness, the hypoemotionality, the increased orality, and the altered responses to food would arise because of damage to the normal mechanism by which stimuli become associated with a reward or punisher.

Another type of evidence linking the amygdala to reinforcement mechanisms is that monkeys will work in order to obtain electrical stimulation of the amygdala, and that single neurons in the amygdala are activated by brain-stimulation reward of a number of different sites (Rolls 1975, Rolls, Burton & Mora 1980, Rolls 2005b).

A difference between the effects of selective amygdala lesions and orbitofrontal cortex lesions in monkeys is that selective amygdala lesions have no effect on object reversal learning, whereas orbitofrontal cortex lesions do impair object reversal learning (Murray & Izquierdo 2007) (see further Section 4.5.4). Further, and consistently, orbitofrontal but not selective amygdala lesions impair instrumental extinction (i.e. showed a large number of choices of the previously rewarded object when it was no longer rewarded) (Murray & Izquierdo 2007). This is consistent with the evidence described in Section 4.5 that the orbitofrontal cortex is important in rapid, one-trial, learning and reversal between visual stimuli and primary reinforcers using both associative and rule-based mechanisms, and its representations of outcome value, expected value, and negative reward prediction error (Thorpe, Rolls & Maddison 1983, Rolls 2005b, Rolls & Grabenhorst 2008). These contributions of the orbitofrontal cortex are facilitated by its neocortical architecture, which can operate using attractors that are important in many functions including short-term memory, attention, rule-based operation with switching, long-term memory, and decision-making which may help it to compute and utilize non-reward to reset value representations in the orbitofrontal cortex (Rolls 2008b).

4.6.3.2 Amygdala lesions in rats

In rats, there is also evidence that the amygdala is involved in behaviour to stimuli learned as being associated with reward as well as with punishers. We may summarize these investigations in the rat as follows. The central nuclei of the amygdala encode or express Pavlovian S–R (stimulus–response, CS–UR) associations (including conditioned suppression, conditioned orienting, conditioned autonomic and endocrine responses, and Pavlovian–instrumental transfer); and modulate perhaps by arousal the associability of representations stored elsewhere in the brain (Gallagher & Holland 1994, Gallagher & Holland 1992, Holland & Gallagher 1999). In contrast, the basolateral amygdala (BLA) encodes or retrieves the affective value of the predicted US, and can use this to influence action–outcome learning via pathways to brain regions such as the nucleus accumbens and prefrontal cortex including the orbitofrontal cortex (Cardinal et al. 2002). We shall see below that the nucleus accumbens is not involved in action–outcome learning itself, but does allow the affective states retrieved by the BLA to conditioned stimuli to influence instrumental behaviour by for example Pavlovian–instrumental transfer, and facilitating locomotor approach to food which appears to be in rats a Pavlovian process (Cardinal et al. 2002, Cardinal & Everitt 2004). This leaves parts of the prefrontal and cingulate cortices as strong candidates for action–outcome learning.

Some of the evidence on which this summary of the role of the rat amygdala in stimulus-reward associations and emotion is based is described next.

Cador, Robbins & Everitt (1989) obtained evidence consistent with the hypothesis that the learned incentive (conditioned reinforcing) effects of previously neutral stimuli paired with rewards are mediated by the amygdala acting through the ventral striatum, in that amphetamine injections into the ventral striatum enhanced the effects of a conditioned reinforcing stimulus only if the amygdala was intact (Everitt & Robbins 1992, Robbins, Cador, Taylor & Everitt 1989, Everitt, Cardinal, Hall, Parkinson & Robbins 2000, Everitt & Robbins 2013). In another study, Everitt, Cador & Robbins (1989) showed that excitotoxic lesions of the basolateral amygdala disrupted appetitive sexual responses maintained by a visual conditioned reinforcer, but not the behaviour to the primary reinforcer for the male rats, copulation with a female rat in heat (see further Everitt & Robbins (1992)). (The details of the study were that the learned reinforcer or conditioned stimulus was a light for which the male rats worked on a Fixed Ratio 10 schedule (i.e. 10 responses made to obtain a presentation of the light), with access to the female being allowed for the first FR10 completed after a fixed period of 15 min. This is a second-order schedule of reinforcement. For comparison, and this is relevant to Chapter 7, medial preoptic area lesions eliminated the copulatory behaviour of mounting, intromission and ejaculation to the primary reinforcer, the female rat, but did not affect the learned appetitive responding for the conditioned or secondary reinforcing stimulus, the light.) In another study demonstrating the role of the amygdala in responses to learned positive reinforcers in rats, Everitt, Morris, O'Brien & Robbins (1991) showed that a conditioned place preference to a place where rats were given 10% sucrose was abolished by bilateral excitotoxic lesions of the basolateral amygdala. Moreover, the output of the amygdala for this learned reinforcement effect on behaviour appears to be via the ventral striatum, for a unilateral lesion of the amygdala and a contralateral lesion of the nucleus accumbens also impaired the conditioned place preference for the place where sucrose was made available (Everitt et al. 1991, Everitt & Robbins 1992). In another study showing the importance of the basolateral amygdala for effects of learned rewards on behaviour, Whitelaw, Markou, Robbins & Everitt (1996) showed that excitotoxic lesions of the basolateral amygdala in rats impaired behavioural responses to a light associated with intravenous administration of cocaine, but not to the primary reinforcer of the cocaine itself. (A second-order schedule comparable to that described above was used to show the impairment of drug-seeking behaviour, that is responses made to obtain the light associated with delivery of the drug. Self-administration of the drug in a continuous reinforcement schedule was not impaired, showing that the amygdala is not necessary for the primary reinforcing effects of cocaine.)

It has long been known that rats with lesions of the amygdala display altered fear responses. For example, Rolls & Rolls (1973b) showed that rats with amygdala lesions showed less neophobia to new foods. In a model of fear conditioning in the rat, LeDoux and colleagues (see LeDoux (1994), LeDoux (1995), LeDoux (1996); Quirk, Armony, Repa, Li & LeDoux (1996); LeDoux (2000); and Pare, Quirk & LeDoux (2004)) have shown that lesions of the amygdala attenuate fear responses learned when pure tones are associated with footshock. The learned responses include typical classically conditioned responses such as heart-rate changes and freezing to fear-inducing stimuli (see, e.g., LeDoux (1994)), and also operant responses (see, e.g., Gallagher & Holland (1994)). The deficits typically involve particularly the learned (emotional) responses, e.g. fear to the conditioned stimuli, rather than changes in behavioural responses to the unconditioned stimuli such as altered responses to pain per se (but see Hebert, Ardid, Henrie, Tamashiro, Blanchard & Blanchard (1999)). In another type of paradigm, it has been shown that amygdala lesions impair the devaluing effect of pairing a food reward with (aversive) lithium chloride, in that amygdala lesions reduced the classically conditioned responses of the rats to a light previously paired with the food (Hatfield, Han, Conley, Gallagher & Holland 1996).

In a different model of fear-conditioning in the rat, Davis and colleagues (Davis 1992, Davis 1994, Davis, Campeau, Kim & Falls 1995, Davis 2000), have used the fear-potentiated startle test, in which the amplitude of the acoustic startle reflex is increased when elicited in the presence of a stimulus previously paired with shock. The conditioned stimulus can be visual or a low-frequency auditory stimulus. Chemical or electrolytic lesions of either the central nucleus or the lateral and basolateral nuclei of the amygdala block the expression of fear-potentiated startle. These latter amygdala nuclei may be the site of plasticity for fear conditioning, because local infusion of the NMDA (N-methyl-d-aspartate) receptor antagonist AP5 (which blocks long-term potentiation, an index of synaptic plasticity) blocks the acquisition but not the maintenance of fear-potentiated startle (Davis 1992, Davis 1994, Davis et al. 1995, Davis 2000). These investigations have now been extended to primates, in which similar effects are found, with ibotenic acid-induced lesions of the amygdala preventing the acquisition of fear-potentiated startle, though, remarkably, not the expression of fear-potentiated

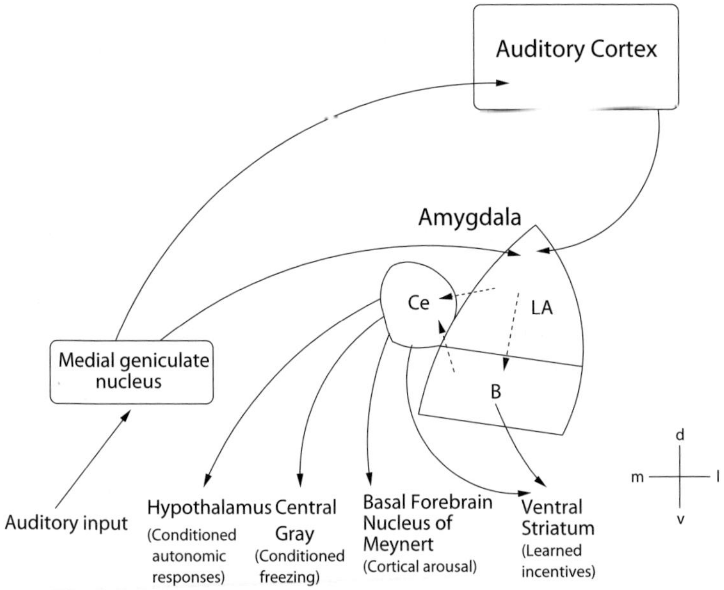

Fig. 4.56 The pathways for fear-conditioning to pure-tone auditory stimuli associated with footshock in the rat. The lateral amygdala (LA) receives auditory information directly from the medial part of the medial geniculate nucleus (the auditory thalamic nucleus), and from the auditory cortex. Intra-amygdala projections (directly and via the basal and basal accessory nuclei, B) end in the central nucleus (Ce) of the amygdala. Different output pathways from the central nucleus and the basal nucleus mediate different conditioned fear-related effects. d, dorsal; v, ventral; m, medial; l, lateral. (Reproduced from G. J. Quirk, J. L. Armony, J. C. Repa, X. F. Li, and J. E. LeDoux, Emotional memory: a search for sites of plasticity, *Cold Spring Harbor Symposia on Quantitative Biology*, 61, pp. 247–257, figure 1b ©1996, Cold Spring Harbor Laboratory Press.)

startle when fear conditioning was carried out prior to the lesion (Davis, Antoniadis, Amaral & Winslow 2008).

Reconsolidation refers to a process in which after a memory has been stored, it may be weakened or lost if recall is performed during the presence of a protein synthesis inhibitor (Debiec, LeDoux & Nader 2002, Debiec, Doyere, Nader & LeDoux 2006). The implication that has been drawn is that whenever a memory is recalled, some reconsolidation process requiring protein synthesis may be needed. The computational utility of reconsolidation is considered by Rolls (2008b). Here, it is of interest that this applies to fear association mechanisms in the amygdala (Doyere, Debiec, Monfils, Schafe & LeDoux 2007), and drug-associated memories in the amygdala (Milton, Lee, Butler, Gardner & Everitt 2008). The findings have interesting implications for the treatment of fear-associated memories. For example, in humans old fear memories can be updated with non-fearful information provided during the reconsolidation window. As a consequence, fear responses are no longer expressed, an effect that can last at least a year and is selective only to reactivated memories without affecting other memories (Schiller, Monfils, Raio, Johnson, LeDoux & Phelps 2010). Procedures that influence the extinction of fear memory may also be useful in the treatment of fear states (Davis 2011).

4.6.3.3 Amygdala output paths

There are separate output pathways for the amygdala for different fear-related responses (see Fig. 4.56). Lesions of the lateral hypothalamus (which receives from the central nucleus of the amygdala) blocked conditioned heart rate (autonomic) responses. Lesions of the central gray of the midbrain (which also receives from the central nucleus of the amygdala) blocked the conditioned freezing but not the conditioned autonomic response (LeDoux, Iwata, Cicchetti & Reis 1988), and lesions of the stria terminalis blocked the neuroendocrine responses (Gray, Piechowski, Yracheta, Rittenhouse, Betha & Van der Kar 1993). In addition, cortical arousal may be produced by the conditioned stimuli via the central nucleus of the amygdala outputs to the cholinergic basal forebrain magnocellular nuclei of Meynert (see Section 4.11.5; Kapp, Whalen, Supple & Pascoe (1992); Wilson & Rolls (1990a), Wilson & Rolls (1990b), Wilson & Rolls (1990c); Rolls & Treves (1998) Section 7.1.5), and Rolls (2008b).

The different output routes for different effects mediated by the amygdala are complemented by separate roles of different nuclei within the amygdala in conditioned fear responses (see Cardinal et al. (2002)). In a study by Killcross, Robbins & Everitt (1997), rats with lesions of the central nucleus exhibited a reduction in the suppression of behaviour (i.e. a reduction in freezing) elicited by a conditioned fear stimulus, but were simultaneously able to direct their actions to avoid further presentations of this aversive stimulus. In contrast, animals with lesions of the basolateral amygdala were unable to avoid the conditioned aversive stimulus by their choice behaviour, but exhibited normal conditioned suppression to this stimulus. This double dissociation indicates separable contributions of different amygdaloid nuclei to different types of conditioned fear behaviour, with the central nuclei especially involved in Pavlovian processes such as conditioned suppression of behaviour, and the basolateral amygdala more involved in instrumental, action–outcome, learning (Cardinal et al. 2002).

Different nuclei of the amygdala correspondingly have different functions in reward-related (or appetitive) learning in rats (Cardinal et al. 2002, Everitt, Cardinal, Parkinson & Robbins 2003, Holland & Gallagher 2003, Holland & Gallagher 2004, Everitt et al. 2000, Gallagher 2000). For example, the basolateral amygdala (BLA) nuclei are involved in some motivational aspects of the classically or Pavlovian conditioned effects of rewards (also known as appetitive reinforcers), in that BLA lesions impair the ability of conditioned stimuli (such as a tone) paired with food in associative learning to influence instrumental behaviour (such as bar pressing to earn food) (Holland & Gallagher 2003), perhaps reflecting impaired outputs to feeding systems in the lateral hypothalamus (see Fig. 4.56). (The BLA lesions also impair the learning of second-order associative conditioning, in that the lesioned rats cannot learn an association of an auditory stimulus with a previously conditioned visual stimulus (Setlow, Gallagher & Holland 2002)). In monkeys (Malkova et al. 1997) as well as rats (Cardinal et al. 2002), BLA lesions also impair reinforcer devaluation effects on actions. *The implication is that BLA lesioned animals cannot use a CS to gain access to the current value of its specific US, and in turn use this US representation as a goal for instrumental action, for freezing, or for fear-potentiated startle.* In this sense, BLA lesions may impair the elicitation of learned affective states used to influence these three types of behaviour. The fact that amygdala lesions do not affect food preferences per se (Rolls & Rolls 1973b, Murray et al. 1996) suggests that affective states elicited by primary reinforcers are not impaired. In contrast, lesions of the central nucleus of the amygdala impaired the ability of conditioned stimuli (such as a tone) paired with food in associative learning to influence food consumption (Holland & Gallagher 2003), which could reflect a reduction in Pavlovian conditioned arousal produced by output pathways from the central nuclei (see Fig. 4.56 and also Everitt, Cardinal, Parkinson & Robbins (2003)).

Another output system of the amygdala is the nucleus accumbens, a part of the striatum (see Section 6.3). The core part of the nucleus accumbens is part of the pathway for approach responses to conditioned stimuli ('autoshaping'), and for Pavlovian–instrumental transfer, but not for the learning of new goal-directed instrumental actions (action–outcome learning) (Cardinal et al. 2002, Cardinal & Everitt 2004). Consistently, dopamine release in the core part of the nucleus accumbens is increased by conditioned emotional stimuli, both appetitive and aversive (Cardinal et al. 2002), and this part of the accumbens may be involved in preparatory aspects of rewarded behaviour, including behaviour when there is a reward delay period (Cardinal, Pennicott, Sugathapala, Robbins & Everitt 2001). In contrast, the release of dopamine in the shell part of the nucleus accumbens is produced by primary (i.e. unconditioned) rewards and punishers such as food, and this part of the accumbens may be involved in consummatory behaviour such as eating (Kelley 1999, Cardinal et al. 2002) (see further Section 6.3). Psychostimulant drugs such as amphetamine may operate in part by sensitizing the process by which non-contingent Pavlovian conditioned stimuli increase the probability of instrumental behaviour and Pavlovian conditioned approach to rewards (Cardinal et al. 2002), an effect related to 'conditioned salience' or 'wanting' (Berridge & Robinson 1998, Robinson & Berridge 1993).

4.6.3.4 Wanting and Liking

This may be an appropriate place to consider the issue of 'wanting' vs 'liking' (or 'desire' vs 'pleasure') discussed by Berridge & Robinson (1998) and Berridge, Robinson & Aldridge (2009). 'Wanting' or conditioned 'incentive salience' effects are used to describe classically conditioned approach behaviours to rewards (Berridge & Robinson 1998, Berridge & Robinson 2003), and this learning is implemented via the amygdala and ventral striatum, is under control of dopamine (Cardinal et al. 2002), and contributes to addiction (Robinson & Berridge 2003). Conditioned 'incentive salience' effects can influence instrumental responses, made for example to obtain food.

A first point is that Berridge & Robinson (1998) suggest that 'liking' can be measured by orofacial reflexes such as ingesting sweet solutions or rejecting bitter solutions. There is evidence that brain opioid systems are involved in influencing the palatability of and hedonic reactions to foods, in that humans report a reduction in the pleasantness of sucrose solution following administration of naltrexone which blocks opiate receptors, but can still discriminate between sucrose solutions (Bertino, Beauchamp & Engelman 1991, Levine & Billington 2004) (see further Section 6.4). One problem here is that orofacial reflexes may reflect brainstem mechanisms that are not at all closely related to the reward value of food as reflected in instrumental actions performed to obtain food. Some of the evidence for this is that these responses occur after decerebration, in which the brainstem is all that remains to control behaviour (Grill & Norgren 1978) (with consistent evidence from anencephalic humans, Steiner et al. (2001)) (see further Section 4.6.1.2 on page 163).

A second point is that normally the rated reward value or pleasantness given in humans to food is closely related to instrumental actions performed to obtain food, as shown by the close relation between pleasantness ratings ('liking') by humans given to a food in a sensory-specific satiety experiment, and whether that food is subsequently eaten in a meal ('wanting') (Rolls, Rowe, Rolls, Kingston, Megson & Gunary 1981b).

Third, a confusion may arise when a stimulus–response habit is formed by overlearning, and persists even when the reward is devalued by for example feeding to satiety. This persistence of stimulus–response habits after reward devaluation should not necessarily be interpreted as 'wanting' when not 'liking', for it may just reflect the operation of a stimulus–response habit system that produces responses after overlearning without any guidance from reward, pleasantness, and liking (see further Section 10.3.1, Cardinal et al. (2002), and Rolls (2013d)). Indeed, I emphasize that after overtraining, responses may become inflexibly linked to stimuli, and the goals, and the reward value of the goals, may no longer be directly influencing behaviour in an ongoing way. If behaviour becomes overlearned and a habit or stimulus-response connection is built up by another brain system (such as the basal ganglia), then animals may make automatic responses that are not goal directed. There has been confusion in the literature caused by overlooking this point (Berridge & Robinson 1998, Berridge, Robinson & Aldridge 2009). The fact that behaviour can become stimulus-response and no longer under the control of the goal need not surprise us. Normally, and certainly during learning before habits set in, we want a goal, and when we get the goal we like it: goal stimuli normally specify what is wanted, and what is liked. Indeed, my theory is that normally we want because we like. This is inherent in my theory, for the genes that make a stimulus (such as a sweet taste) rewarding (i.e. wanted, a goal for action) also make the stimulus liked (i.e. accepted, with a subjective correlate of pleasure, pleasantness, and affective liking) (Chapters 2 and 3).

My approach is that I believe that normally liking, defined by pleasantness ratings of stimuli, is very closely related to wanting, that is being willing to perform behaviours (instrumental actions) to obtain a reward of the pleasant stimulus (Rolls 2005b). Thus motivational behaviour is normally (when not overlearned) controlled by reward stimuli or goals (unless the behaviour is overlearned, see Section 4.6.1.2), and motivational state (e.g. hunger) modulates the reward value of unconditioned and conditioned stimuli such as the taste and sight of food, as described in Chapter 5. Thus normally, liking a goal object and wanting it are different aspects of how reward systems control instrumental behaviour, and this follows from the approach to gene-specified goal or value representations which in a unifying way account for wanting a goal, and liking the goal object when it is obtained, as described in Chapter 2.

Nevertheless, it is possible to dissociate the brain mechanisms involved in 'wanting' and 'liking' experimentally, with the classically conditioned 'incentive salience' stimuli that influence approach and instrumental actions and which influence 'appetitive' behaviour, implemented in part separately from the reward systems that are activated by a primary reinforcer such as the taste of food during 'consummatory' behaviour. In a sense, the 'incentive salience' effects require learning of expected value to predict primary rewards and punishers, and then to influence behaviours, and thus require additional brain mechanisms to those involved in representing primary rewards and punishers.

In summary, there is thus much evidence from the effects of lesions that the amygdala is involved in responses made to stimuli that are associated by learning with primary reinforcers, including rewards as well as punishers. The evidence is consistent with the hypothesis that the amygdala is a brain region for stimulus–reinforcer association learning, and has partly dissociable systems for Pavlovian effects implemented via the central nucleus, and for effects of affective representations implemented via the basolateral amygdala. There is also evidence that it may be involved in whether novel stimuli are approached, for monkeys with amygdala lesions place novel foods and non-food objects in their mouths, and rats with amygdala lesions have decreased neophobia, in that they more quickly accept new foods (Rolls & Rolls 1973b) (see also Dunn & Everitt (1988), Rolls (1992a), Rolls (2000d), and Wilson & Rolls (1993)).

4.6.4 Neuronal activity in the primate amygdala to reinforcing stimuli

There is clear evidence that some neurons in the primate amygdala respond to stimuli that are potentially primary reinforcers. For example, Sanghera, Rolls & Roper-Hall (1979) found some amygdala neurons with taste responses, and these were investigated by Scott, Karadi, Oomura, Nishino, Plata-Salaman, Lenard, Giza & Aou (1993). In an extensive study of 1416 macaque amygdala neurons, Kadohisa, Rolls & Verhagen (2005a) showed that a very rich and detailed representation of the stimulus (such as food) that is in the mouth is provided by neurons that respond to oral stimuli. An example of a macaque single amygdala orally-responsive neuron is shown in Fig. 4.57. The neuron had different responses to different tastes, different temperatures of what was in the mouth, and different viscosities, but had

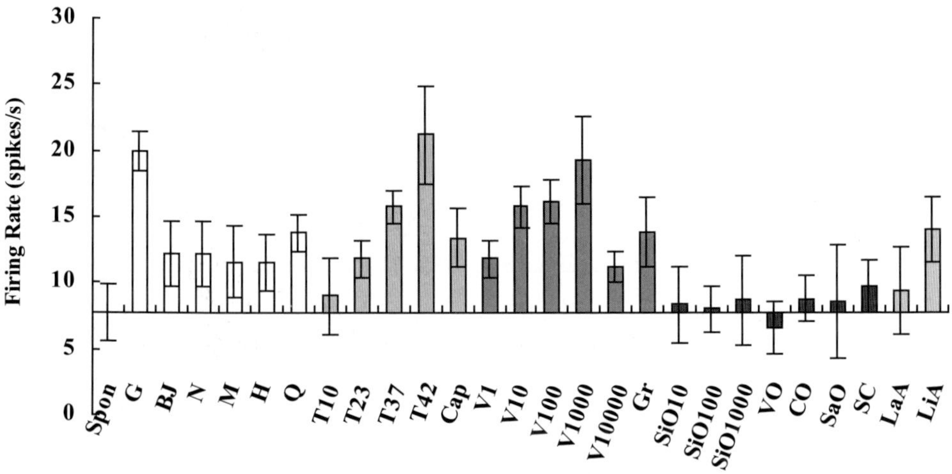

Fig. 4.57 The responses of an amygdala neuron (bo217) with differential responses to taste, temperature and viscosity. The neuron did not respond to fat texture. The mean ($\pm$ the standard error of the mean, sem) firing rate responses to each stimulus calculated in a 1 s period over 4–6 trials are shown. The spontaneous (Spon) firing rate is shown. G, N, M, H and Q are the taste stimuli. T10–T42 are the temperature stimuli. V1 - V10,000 are the CMC viscosity series with the viscosity in cP. The fat texture stimuli were SiO10, SiO100, SiO1000 (silicone oil with the viscosity indicated), vegetable oil (VO), coconut oil (CO) and safflower oil (SaO). BJ is fruit juice; Cap is 10 μM capsaicin; LaA is 0.1 mM lauric acid; LiA is 0.1 mM linoleic acid; Gr is the gritty stimulus. (Reprinted from *Neuroscience*, 132 (1), M. Kadohisa, J. V. Verhagen, and E. T. Rolls, The primate amygdala: Neuronal representations of the viscosity, fat texture, temperature, grittiness and taste of foods, pp. 33–48, Copyright, 2005, with permission from Elsevier.)

no response to the texture of fatty oils. Other amygdala neurons were selective for even one modality, responding for example only to the oral texture of fat (Kadohisa, Rolls & Verhagen 2005a). 3.1% of the recorded amygdala neurons responded to oral stimuli. Of the orally responsive neurons, some (39%) represent the viscosity of oral stimuli, tested using carboxymethyl-cellulose in the range 1–10,000 centiPoise. Other neurons (5%) responded to fat in the mouth by encoding its texture (shown by the responses of these neurons to a range of fats, and also to non-fat oils such as silicone oil ($Si(CH_3)_2O)_n$) and mineral oil (pure hydrocarbon), but no or small responses to the cellulose viscosity series or to the fatty acids linoleic acid and lauric acid). Some neurons (7%) responded to gritty texture (produced by microspheres suspended in carboxymethyl cellulose). Some neurons (41%) responded to the temperature of the liquid in the mouth. Some amygdala neurons responded to capsaicin, and some to fatty acids (but not to fats in the mouth). Some amygdala neurons respond to taste, texture and temperature unimodally, but others combine these inputs. 66% (29/44) had taste responses. An interesting difference is that in terms of best responses to different tastes, 57% of the orbitofrontal cortex taste neurons had their best responses to glucose, whereas 21% of the amygdala neurons had their best response to glucose (χ^2=12.5, df=5, P<0.03) (Kadohisa, Rolls & Verhagen 2005b). (More amygdala neurons had their best responses to sour (HCl) (18%) and monosodium glutamate (14%) (Kadohisa, Rolls & Verhagen 2005b).)

These results show that a very detailed representation of substances in the mouth, which are likely to be primary reinforcers, is present in the primate amygdala (Kadohisa, Rolls

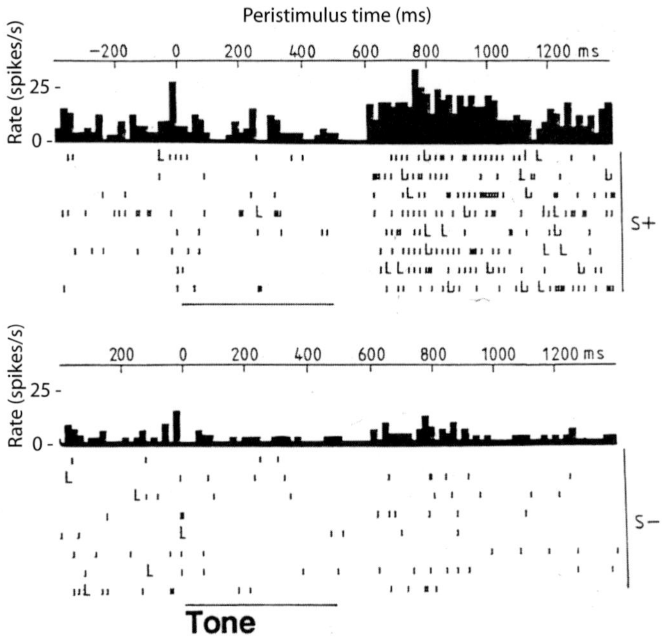

Fig. 4.58 Responses of a primate amygdala neuron in a visual discrimination task. Each tic represents the occurrence of an action potential; each row of tics represents the firing of the neuron on a single trial to the presentation of the S+ visual stimulus (which indicated that a lick could be made to obtain a taste of fruit juice) or of the S– visual stimulus (which indicated that a lick should not be made or (aversive) saline would be delivered. Presentations of the S+ and S- occurred in pseudorandom order but are grouped for clarity. The L indicates the occurrence of the lick response. Bin width = 10 ms. (This material was originally published in E. T. Rolls, Neurophysiology and functions of the primate amygdala, and the neural basis of emotion in J. P. Aggleton (ed.), *The Amygdala*: Second Edition. A Functional Analysis, chapter 13, pp. 447–478 and has been reproduced by permission of Oxford University Press http://ukcatalogue.oup.com/product/9780198505013.do#.Ue5RS6w2FLo and Reprinted from *Neuroscience*, 133 (4), F. A. W. Wilson and E. T. Rolls, The primate amygdala and reinforcement: A dissociation between rule-based and associatively-mediated memory revealed in neuronal activity, pp. 1061–1072, Copyright, 2005, with permission from Elsevier.)

& Verhagen 2005a) (see also Fig. 5.19). Less is known about whether it is though the reinforcer value of the stimuli that is represented. It has previously been shown that satiety produces a rather modest (on average 58%) reduction in the responses of amygdala neurons to taste (Yan & Scott 1996, Rolls & Scott 2003), in comparison to the essentially complete reduction of responsiveness found in orbitofrontal cortex taste neurons (Rolls, Sienkiewicz & Yaxley 1989b). Further, the representation in the amygdala of these oral stimuli does not appear to be on any simple hedonic basis, in that no direction in the multidimensional taste space in Fig. 7 of Kadohisa, Rolls & Verhagen (2005a) reflected the measured preference of the monkeys for the stimuli, nor were the response profiles of the neurons to the set of stimuli closely related to the preferences of the macaques for the stimuli (Kadohisa, Rolls & Verhagen 2005a). The failure to find very strong effects of satiety on the responsiveness of amygdala taste neurons mirrors the earlier finding of Sanghera, Rolls & Roper-Hall (1979) of inconsistent effects of feeding to satiety on the responses of amygdala visual neurons responding to the sight of food.

Recordings from single neurons in the amygdala of the monkey have shown that some neurons do respond to visual stimuli, consistent with the inputs from the temporal lobe visual

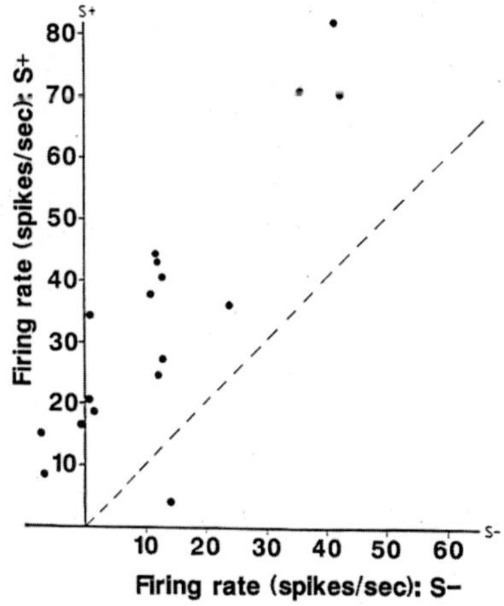

Fig. 4.59 Responses of amygdala neurons that responded more in a visual discrimination task to the reward-related visual stimulus (S+) than to the saline-related visual stimulus (S–). In the task, the macaque monkeys made lick responses to obtain fruit juice when the S+ was the discriminandum, and had to withhold lick responses when the S– was the discriminandum in order to avoid the taste of saline. Each point shows the responses of one neuron to the S+ and to the S– measured in a 0.5 s period starting 100 msec after the visual stimulus was shown. The responses are shown as the change from the spontaneous firing rate. Most of the points lie above the dashed line drawn at 45 degrees, showing that most of these neurons responded more to the S+ than to the S–. (Data from E. T. Rolls, Neurophysiology and functions of the primate amygdala, and the neural basis of emotion in J. P. Aggleton (ed.), *The Amygdala*: Second Edition. A Functional Analysis, chapter 13, pp. 447–478 and from *Neuroscience*, 133 (4), F. A. W. Wilson and E. T. Rolls, The primate amygdala and reinforcement: A dissociation between rule-based and associatively-mediated memory revealed in neuronal activity, pp. 1061–72.)

cortex (Sanghera, Rolls & Roper-Hall 1979). Other neurons responded to auditory, gustatory, olfactory, or somatosensory stimuli, or in relation to movements. In tests of whether the neurons responded on the basis of the association of stimuli with reinforcers, it was found that approximately 20% of the neurons with visual responses had responses that occurred primarily to stimuli associated with reinforcers, for example to food and to a range of stimuli which the monkey had learned signified food in a visual discrimination task (Sanghera, Rolls & Roper-Hall 1979, Rolls 1981c, Wilson & Rolls 1993, Wilson & Rolls 2005, Rolls 2000d) (see example in Fig. 4.58). Many of these neurons responded more to the positive discriminative stimulus (S+) than to the negative visual discriminative stimulus (S–) in the Go/NoGo visual discrimination task, as shown in Fig. 4.59 (Rolls 2000d, Wilson & Rolls 2005). However, none of these neurons (in contrast with some neurons in the hypothalamus and orbitofrontal cortex) responded exclusively to rewarded stimuli, in that all responded at least partly to one or more neutral, novel, or aversive stimuli (see example in Fig. 4.61). Neurons with responses that are probably similar to these have also been described by Ono, Nishino, Sasaki, Fukuda & Muramoto (1980), Nishijo, Ono & Nishino (1988), and by Ono, Tamura, Nishijo, Nakamura & Tabuchi (1989) (see Ono & Nishijo (1992)).

The degree to which the visual responses of these amygdala neurons are associated with reinforcers has been assessed in learning tasks. When the association between a visual stimulus and a reinforcer was altered by reversal (so that the visual stimulus formerly associated with juice reward became associated with aversive saline and vice versa), it was found that 10 of

11 neurons did not reverse their responses (and for the other neuron the evidence was not clear) (Sanghera, Rolls & Roper-Hall 1979, Rolls 1992a, Rolls 2000d). On the other hand, in a rather simpler relearning situation in which salt was added to a piece of food such as a water melon (but it was difficult to be sure that the monkey looked at the stimulus as much after it was salted), the responses of four amygdala neurons to the sight of the water melon diminished (Nishijo et al. 1988). To obtain further evidence on this issue, Wilson & Rolls (2005) tested visual discrimination reversal learning further using a similar procedure to that of Sanghera, Rolls & Roper-Hall (1979) in which two stimuli, one rewarded, and the other associated with punishment, were shown in random order and using an electronic shutter, so that it could be confirmed that the monkey performed a visual discrimination on every trial. The results are illustrated in Fig. 4.60, which shows that the neuron did not reverse its responses when the reinforcement contingency was reversed in the visual discrimination task. This experiment was repeated for two neurons, with identical results. Although more investigations would be useful, the evidence now available indicates that primate amygdala neurons do not alter their activity flexibly and rapidly in relearning visual discrimination reversal learning (see further Rolls (1992a), Rolls (2000d), and Section 5.4.6.3). What has been found in contrast is that neurons in the orbitofrontal cortex do show very rapid, often one-trial, reversal of their responses in visual discrimination reversal, and it therefore seems likely that the orbitofrontal cortex is especially involved when repeated relearning and re-assessment of stimulus–reinforcer associations are required, as described above, rather than initial learning, in which the amygdala may be involved. (It is noted that the amygdala neuron data of Paton, Belova, Morrison & Salzman (2006) do not address the issue convincingly of rapid reversal, for they were not studying rapid reversal, which often took many trials both for the neurons and for the behaviour.)

Evidence that primate amygdala neurons encode reward value is while monkeys chose between saving liquid reward with interest and spending the accumulated reward, some of the neurons reflected the accumulating value (Grabenhorst, Hernadi & Schultz 2012). Overall, there is thus evidence that some amygdala neurons reflect reward value, yet do not reverse their value-related responses rapidly (in the one trial shown by orbitofrontal cortex neurons), and the evidence from the effects of selective amygdala lesions (Murray & Izquierdo 2007) are consistent with this.

LeDoux and colleagues (LeDoux 1995, LeDoux 1996, Quirk et al. 1996, LeDoux 2000, Blair, Tinkelman, Moita & LeDoux 2003, Pare et al. 2004, Johansen, Tarpley, LeDoux & Blair 2010) have made interesting contributions to understanding the role of the amygdala and related systems in fear-conditioning in the rat. They have shown that for some classes of stimulus, such as pure tones, the association between the tone and an aversive unconditioned stimulus (a footshock) is reflected in the responses of neurons in the amygdala. Some of the circuitry involved is shown in Fig. 4.56. The auditory inputs reach the amygdala both from the subcortical, thalamic, auditory nucleus, the medial geniculate (medial part), and from the auditory cortex. These auditory inputs project to the lateral nucleus of the amygdala (LA), which in turn projects to the central nucleus of the amygdala (Ce) both directly and via the basal (B) and accessory basal nuclei of the amygdala. LeDoux has emphasized the role of the subcortical inputs to the amygdala in this type of conditioning, based on the observations that the conditioning to pure tones can take place without the cortex, and that the shortest latencies of the auditory responses in the amygdala are too short to be mediated via the auditory cortex. (Although some conditioning of auditory responses has been found even in the medial geniculate to these pure tones, this conditioning is not of short latency, and LeDoux suggests that it reflects backprojections from the cortex (in which conditioning is also found) to the thalamus.)

The amygdala is well placed anatomically for learning associations between objects and

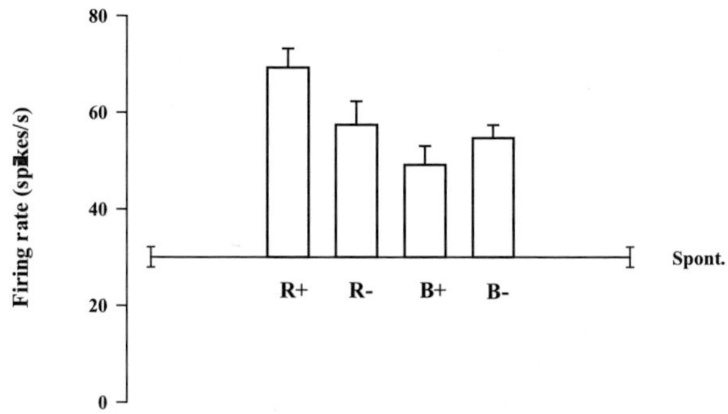

Fig. 4.60 The responses of a macaque amygdala neuron with more activity to a standard rewarded visual stimulus (S+) than to a standard punished visual stimulus (S–) in a Go/NoGo visual discrimination task. The neuron was then tested in a discrimination reversal task with a new pair of stimuli, which were Red and Blue. When the Red stimulus was associated with taste reward (R+), and the blue stimulus was associated with aversive saline if the monkey licked (B–), the neuron did not respond significantly differently to these two stimuli, even though the monkey performed the task correctly. Thus the neuron did not learn the discrimination with the new pair of stimuli. The contingencies were then reversed, and the monkey learned that the Red stimulus was now associated with saline (R–), and the Blue stimulus was associated with taste reward (B+). The neuron did not alter its activity after the reversal. The means and s.e.m. of the neuronal responses based on 4–8 trials for each condition are shown. The spontaneous firing rate of the neuron is also shown (Spont.) (Reprinted from *Neuroscience*, 133 (4), F. A. W. Wilson and E. T. Rolls, The primate amygdala and reinforcement: A dissociation between rule-based and associatively-mediated memory revealed in neuronal activity, pp. 1061–72, Copyright, 2005, with permission from Elsevier.)

primary reinforcers, for it receives inputs from the higher parts of the visual system, and from systems processing primary reinforcers such as taste, smell, and touch (see Fig. 4.2). The association learning in the amygdala may be implemented by Hebb-modifiable synapses from visual and auditory neurons on to neurons receiving inputs from taste, olfactory, or somatosensory primary reinforcers (see Figs. 4.3 and 4.5, Rolls (1986a), Rolls (1986b), Rolls (1990b), and Rolls (1999a)). Consistent with this, Davis and colleagues (Davis 1992, Davis 1994, Davis et al. 1995, Davis 2000) have shown that the stimulus–reinforcer association learning involved in fear-potentiated startle (see Section 4.6.3) is blocked by local application to the lateral amygdala of the NMDA-receptor blocking agent AP5, which blocks long-term potentiation. The hypothesis (see Figs. 4.3 and 4.5, and Appendix 1) thus is that synaptic modification takes place between potential secondary reinforcers and primary reinforcers which project on to the same neurons in the amygdala. One index of synaptic modification is long-term potentiation (see Appendix 1), and consistent with this hypothesis, the potential evoked in the rat amygdala by a pure tone increased (suggesting long-term potentiation) after the tone was paired with footshock as the unconditioned stimulus (Rogan, Staubli & LeDoux 1997). Further, presentation of a tone paired with application of glutamate iontophoretically to activate a single amygdala neuron produced an increased response later to the tone alone, providing evidence that the site of the synaptic modification was on that neuron in the amygdala (Blair, Schafe, Bauer, Rodrigues & LeDoux 2001, LeDoux 2000, Blair, Tinkelman, Moita & LeDoux 2003).

LeDoux (1992, 1995, 1996, 2011) has described a theory of the neural basis of emotion that is conceptually similar to that of Rolls (1975, 1986a, 1986b, 1990b, 1995a, 1999a, 2000a, 2005b) (and this book), except that he focuses mostly on the role of the amygdala in emotion (and not on other brain regions such as the orbitofrontal cortex, which are poorly developed in the rat); except that he focuses mainly on fear (based on his studies of the role of the amygdala and related structures in fear conditioning in the rat); except that he suggests from his neurophysiological findings that an important route for conditioned emotional stimuli to influence behaviour is via the subcortical inputs (especially auditory from the medial part of the medial geniculate nucleus of the thalamus) to the amygdala; and except that he focusses on classically conditioned responses (LeDoux 2011), whereas Rolls' theory is that emotional and motivational states are important intervening states in relation to instrumental actions, as described in Chapters 2 and 3.

The issue of the normal routes for sensory information about potential secondary reinforcers to reach the amygdala via subcortical pathways will now be addressed, because it raises important issues about the stimuli that normally cause emotion, and about brain design. For simple stimuli such as pure tones, there is evidence of subcortical inputs for the conditioned stimuli to the amygdala, and even of the conditioned stimulus–unconditioned stimulus association being learned prior to involvement of the amygdala (see LeDoux (1995), LeDoux (1996), and Quirk et al. (1996)). However, as described above in Section 4.4.3 entitled 'Why reward and punishment associations of stimuli are not represented early in information processing in the primate brain', we humans and other animals do not generally want to learn that a particular pure tone is associated with reward or punishment. Instead, it might be a particular complex pattern of sounds such as a vocalization (or, for example, in vision, a face expression) that carries a reinforcement signal, and this may be independent of the exact pitch at which it is uttered. Thus cases in which some modulation of neuronal responses to pure tones in parts of the brain such as the medial geniculate (the thalamic relay for hearing) where tonotopic tuning is found (LeDoux 1994) may be rather special model systems (i.e. simplified systems on which to perform experiments), and not reflect the way in which auditory-to-reinforcer pattern associations are normally learned. (For discrimination of more complex sounds, such as frequency modulated tone sweeps, the auditory cortex is required.) The same is true for vision, in that we do not normally want to associate particular blobs of light at given positions on our retinae (which is what could be represented at the thalamic level in the lateral geniculate nucleus) with a primary reinforcer, but instead we may want to associate an invariant representation of an object, or of a person's face, or of a facial expression, with a primary reinforcer. Such analysis requires cortical processing, and it is in high-order temporal lobe cortical areas (which provide major afferents to the primate amygdala) that invariant representations of these types of stimulus are found (Rolls 1994b, Wallis & Rolls 1997, Rolls 2000c, Rolls 2008b, Rolls 2012e). Moreover, it is crucial that the representation is invariant (with respect to, for example, position on the retina, size, and, for identity, even viewing angle), so that if an association is learned to the object when in one position on the retina, it can generalize correctly to the same object in different positions on the retina, in different sizes, and even with different viewing angles. For this to occur, the invariant representation must be formed before the object–reinforcer association is learned, otherwise generalization to the same object seen on different occasions would not occur, and different inconsistent associations might even be learned to the same object when seen in slightly different positions on the retina, in slightly different sizes, etc. (Rolls & Treves 1998, Rolls 2008b, Rolls 2012e). Rolls & Treves (1998) and Rolls (2008b) also show that it is not a simple property of neuronal networks that they generalize correctly across variations of position and size; special mechanisms, which happen to take a great deal of cortical visual processing, are required to perform such computations. Similar points may also be made for touch in so far as one considers associations between objects identified by somatosensory input, and primary reinforcers. An example might be selecting a food object by either hand from a whole collection of objects in the dark. These points make it unlikely that the subcortical route for conditioned stimuli to reach the amygdala, suggested by LeDoux (1992, 1995, 1996), is generally relevant to the learning of emotional responses to stimuli (see also Pessoa & Adolphs (2010)).

4.6.5 Responses of these amygdala neurons to novel stimuli that are reinforcing

As described above, some of the amygdala neurons that responded to rewarding visual stimuli also responded to some other stimuli that were not associated with reward. Wilson & Rolls (2005) (see Rolls (2000d)) discovered a possible reason for this. They showed that these neurons with reward-related responses also responded to relatively novel visual stimuli. This was shown in a serial recognition memory task, in which it was found that these neurons responded the first and the second times that visual stimuli were shown in this task (see Fig. 4.61). On the two presentations of each stimulus used in this task, the stimuli were thus either novel or still relatively novel. When the monkeys are given such relatively novel stimuli outside the task, they will reach out for and explore the objects, and in this respect the novel stimuli are reinforcing. Repeated presentation of the stimuli results in habituation of the neuronal response and of behavioural approach, if the stimuli are not associated with a primary reinforcer. It is thus suggested that the amygdala neurons described operate as filters that provide an output if a stimulus is associated with a positive reinforcer, or is positively reinforcing because of relative unfamiliarity, and that provide no output if a stimulus is familiar and has not been associated with a positive primary reinforcer or is associated with a punisher. The functions of this output may be to influence the interest shown in a stimulus, whether it is approached or avoided, whether an affective response occurs to it, and whether a representation of the stimulus is made or maintained via an action mediated through either the basal forebrain nucleus of Meynert or the backprojections to the cerebral cortex (Rolls 1987, Rolls 1989b, Rolls 1990c, Rolls & Treves 1998, Rolls 2000f, Rolls 2008b). It is an important adaptation to the environment to explore relatively novel objects or situations, for in this way advantage due to gene inheritance can become expressed and selected for. This function appears to be implemented in the amygdala in this way. Lesions of the amygdala impair the operation of this mechanism, in that objects are approached and explored indiscriminately, relatively independently of whether they are associated with reinforcers (including punishers), or are novel or familiar.

An interesting observation on the neurons that respond to rewarding and to relatively novel visual stimuli was made in the recognition memory task used by Wilson & Rolls (2005) (see also Rolls (2000d)). It was found that the neurons responded the first time a stimulus was shown, when the monkey had to use the rule 'Do not make a lick response to a stimulus the first time a stimulus is shown, otherwise aversive saline will be obtained', as well as the second time the stimulus was shown when the monkey had to apply the rule 'If a stimulus has been seen before today, lick to it to obtain glucose reward'. Thus these amygdala neurons do not code for reward value when this is based on a rule (e.g. first presentation aversive; second presentation reward), but instead code for reward value when it is decoded on the basis of previous stimulus–reinforcer associations, or when relatively novel stimuli are shown that are treated as rewarding and to be explored.

The details of the neuronal mechanisms that implement the process by which relatively novel stimuli are treated as rewarding in the amygdala are not currently known, but could be as follows. Cortical visual signals which do not show major habituation with repeated visual stimuli, as shown by recordings in the temporal cortical visual areas (Rolls, Judge & Sanghera 1977, Rolls 2008b, Rolls & Treves 2011, Rolls 2012e) reach the amygdala. In the amygdala, neurons respond to these at first, and have the property that they gradually habituate unless the pattern-association mechanism in the amygdala detects co-occurrence of these stimuli with a primary reinforcer, in which case it strengthens the active synapses for that object, so that it continues to produce an output from amygdala neurons that respond to either rewarding or punishing visual stimuli. Neurophysiologically, the habituation condition would correspond in a pattern associator to long-term depression (LTD) of synapses with high

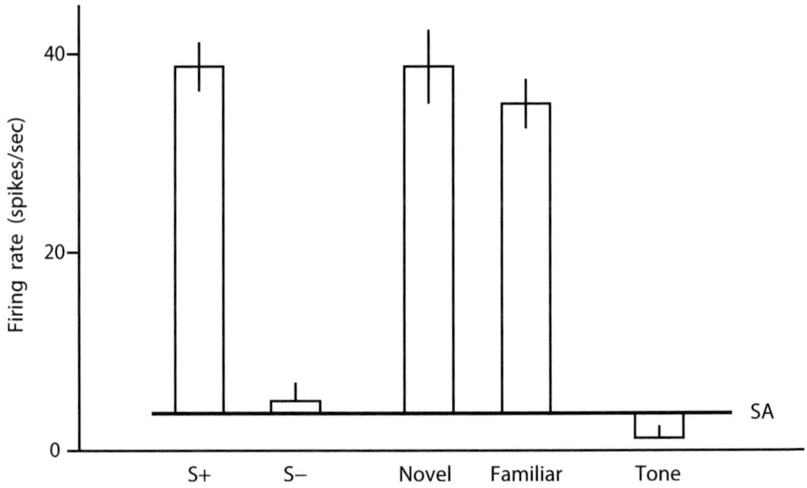

Fig. 4.61 This macaque amygdala neuron responded to the sight of a stimulus associated with food reward (S+), but not to a visual stimulus associated with aversive saline (S–) in a visual discrimination task. The same neuron responded to visual stimuli while they were relatively novel, including here on the first (Novel) and second (Familiar) presentations of new stimuli. The neuron did not respond to the tone that indicated the start of a trial. The visual stimulus appeared when the tone ended, at time=500 ms. SA, spontaneous firing rate of the neuron. The mean responses and the s.e.m. to the different stimuli are shown. (This material has been adapted from Neurophysiology and functions of the primate amygdala and the neural basis of emotion by Edmund T. Rolls, in J. P. Aggleton (ed.), *The Amygdala*: Second Edition. A Functional Analysis, chapter 13, pp. 447–478, ©2000, Oxford University Press and has been reproduced by permission of Oxford University Press http://ukcatalogue.oup.com/product/9780198505013.do.)

presynaptic activity but low postsynaptic activity, that is to homosynaptic LTD (see Rolls & Treves (1998) and Rolls (2008b)).

4.6.6 Neuronal responses in the amygdala to faces

Another interesting group of neurons in the amygdala responds primarily to faces (Rolls 1981c, Leonard, Rolls, Wilson & Baylis 1985). Each of these neurons responds to some but not all of a set of faces, and thus across an ensemble could convey information about the identity of the face (see Fig. 4.62). These neurons are found especially in the basal accessory nucleus of the amygdala (Leonard, Rolls, Wilson & Baylis 1985), a part of the amygdala that develops markedly in primates (Amaral et al. 1992). Similar neurons have been described by Gothard, Battaglia, Erickson, Spitler & Amaral (2007), and, as with face-selective neurons in the orbitofrontal cortex (Rolls, Critchley, Browning & Inoue 2006a), some neurons respond to face identity, some to face expression, and some to combinations of identity and expression. Face-selective neurons have also been found now in the human amygdala (Rutishauser, Tudusciuc, Neumann, Mamelak, Heller, Ross, Philpott, Sutherling & Adolphs 2011). In addition, some neurons in the primate amygdala respond during social interactions (Brothers & Ring 1993).

It is probable that the amygdala neurons responsive to faces (first reported by Sanghera, Rolls & Roper-Hall (1979), see Rolls (2011c)) receive their inputs from the group of neurons in the cortex in the superior temporal sulcus that respond to faces, often on the basis of features present, such as eyes, hair, or mouth, or on the basis of the whole face (Perrett, Rolls & Caan 1982, Rolls 2011c, Rolls 2012e), and consistent with this, the response latencies of the amygdala neurons tend to be longer than those of neurons in the cortex in the superior

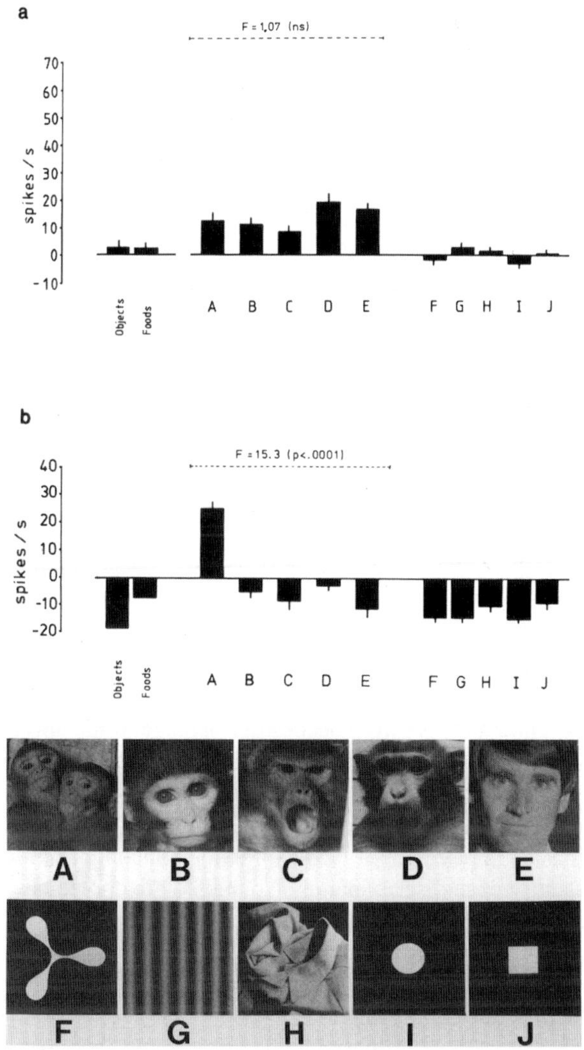

Fig. 4.62 The responses of two neurons (a,b) in the amygdala to a variety of monkey and human face stimuli (A–E), and to non-face stimuli (F–J, objects, and foods). Each bar represents the mean response above baseline with the standard error calculated over 4 to 10 presentations. The F ratio for an analysis of variance calculated over the face sets indicates that the neurons shown range from very selective between faces (neuron b, Y0809) to relatively non-selective (neuron A, Z0264). Some stimuli produced inhibition below the spontaneous firing rate. (Reprinted from *Behavioural Brain Research*, 15 (2), C. M. Leonard, E. T. Rolls, F. A. W. Wilson, and G. C. Baylis, Neurons in the amygdala of the monkey with responses selective for faces, pp. 159–76, Copyright, 1985, with permission from Elsevier.)

temporal sulcus (Leonard, Rolls, Wilson & Baylis 1985, Rolls 1984). It has been suggested that this is part of a system that has evolved for the rapid and reliable identification of individuals from their faces, because of the importance of this in primate social behaviour (Rolls 1981c, Rolls 1984, Rolls 1992a, Rolls 1992b, Rolls 1992c, Leonard, Rolls, Wilson & Baylis 1985, Perrett & Rolls 1983, Leonard, Rolls, Wilson & Baylis 1985, Rolls 2005b, Rolls 2008b). The part of this system in the amygdala may be particularly involved in emotional and social responses to faces. According to one possibility, such emotional and social responses would be 'looked up' (in a pattern associator, see Appendix 1) by a 'key' stimulus, which consisted of the face of a particular individual (Rolls 1984, Rolls 1987, Rolls 1990b, Rolls 1992a, Rolls 1992b, Rolls 1992c, Rolls & Treves 1998, Rolls 1999a). Indeed, it is suggested that the tameness of the Kluver–Bucy syndrome, and the changes in amygdalectomized monkeys in their interactions in a social group (Kling & Steklis 1976, Kling & Brothers 1992) (though these are more subtle after selective amygdala lesions, Amaral (2003) and Murray & Izquierdo (2007)), arise because of damage to this system specialized for processing faces (Rolls 1981a, Rolls 1981c, Rolls 1984, Rolls 1990b, Rolls 1992a, Rolls 1992b, Rolls 1992c, Rolls 2000c, Rolls 2005b, Rolls 2008b, Rolls 2011c, Rolls 2012e). The amygdala may allow neurons that reflect the social significance of faces to be formed using face representations received from the temporal cortical areas, and information about primary reinforcers received from, for example, the somatosensory system (via the insula (Mesulam & Mufson 1982a, Mesulam & Mufson 1982b)), and the gustatory system (via, for example, the orbitofrontal cortex) (see Fig. 4.2).

4.6.7 Evidence from humans

The theory described above about the role of the amygdala in emotion, based largely on research in non-human primates, has been followed up by studies in humans which are producing generally consistent results. One type of evidence comes from the effects of brain damage, which though rarely restricted just to the amygdala, and almost never bilateral, does provide some consistent evidence (Aggleton 1992). For example, in some patients alterations in feeding behaviour and emotion might occur after damage to the amygdala (see Aggleton (1992), Halgren (1992)). In relation to neurons in the macaque amygdala with responses selective for faces and social interactions (Leonard, Rolls, Wilson & Baylis 1985, Brothers & Ring 1993), a patient D. R. has been described who has bilateral damage to or disconnection of the amygdala, and has an impairment of face-expression matching and identification, but not of matching face identity or in discrimination (Young, Aggleton, Hellawell, Johnson, Broks & Hanley 1995, Young, Hellawell, Van de Wal & Johnson 1996). This patient is also impaired at detecting whether someone is gazing at the patient, another important social signal (Perrett et al. 1985). The same patient is also impaired at the auditory recognition of fear and anger (Scott, Young, Calder, Hellawell, Aggleton & Johnson 1997).

Adolphs, Tranel, Damasio & Damasio (1994) also found face expression but not face identity impairments in a patient (SM) with bilateral damage to the amygdala, and extended this to other patients (Adolphs, Tranel & Baron-Cohen 2002, Adolphs, Tranel, Hamann, Young, Calder, Phelps, Anderson, Lee & Damasio 1999) (see also Calder, Young, Rowland, Perrett, Hodges & Etcoff (1996)). A similar impairment was not found in patients with unilateral amygdala damage (Adolphs, Tranel, Damasio & Damasio 1995). The bilateral amygdala patient SM was especially impaired at recognizing the face expression of fear, and also rated expressions of fear, anger, and surprise as less intense than control subjects. It has been shown that SM's impairment stems from an inability to make normal use of information from the eye region of faces when judging emotions, which in turn is related to a lack of spontaneous fixations on the eyes during free viewing of faces (Adolphs, Gosselin, Buchanan, Tranel, Schyns & Damasio 2005), though this is mainly evident just for the first fixation (Kennedy & Adolphs 2011). Although SM fails to look normally at the eye region in all facial expressions, her selective impairment in recognizing fear is explained by the fact that the eyes are the most important feature for identifying this emotion. Indeed, SM's recognition of fearful faces became entirely normal when she was instructed explicitly to look at the eyes. This finding provides a mechanism to explain the amygdala's role in fear recognition, and points to new approaches for the possible rehabilitation of patients with defective emotion perception.

The backprojections to the neocortex from the amygdala may produce larger activations in these cortical areas to visual stimuli which either are fear face expressions, or which occur in association with fear face expressions, for these larger activations are not found in patients with amygdala damage (Phelps 2004, Anderson & Phelps 2001).

The changes in emotion in patients with amygdala lesions are much less marked than those in patients with orbitofrontal cortex damage, and special tests, analogous in some cases to those developed in rodent studies, are necessary to reveal deficits (Phelps & LeDoux 2005). For example, patients with amygdala lesions are impaired at learning conditioned skin conductance responses when a blue square is associated with a shock, and are also impaired in acquiring the same autonomic response to fear by verbally instructed learning or by observational learning (Phelps 2004, Phelps, O'Connor, Gatenby, Gore, Grillon & Davis 2001, Phelps 2006, Whalen & Phelps 2009). The human amygdala appears to be important mainly for some fear responses to some stimuli, such as whether an individual backs off in a social encounter (Adolphs 2003, Adolphs et al. 2005, Phelps 2004, Schiller et al. 2010, Feinstein, Adolphs, Damasio & Tranel 2011). Interestingly, the amygdala was involved during aversive conditioning with primary reinforcers (electric shock) and less so with a secondary reinforcer (money), as suggested by both an fMRI analysis and a follow-up case study with a patient with bilateral amygdala damage (Delgado, Jou & Phelps 2011).

The possibility has been discussed (Blair 2003) that there may be a subcortical pathway to the amygdala which bypasses the temporal cortical visual areas, based partly on evidence that a 'blindsight' patient with a right-sided hemianopia after occipital lobe damage showed some ability to discriminate when guessing between different facial expressions in the blind hemifield (De Gelder, Vroomen, Pourtois & Weiskrantz 1999). Further evidence was that in the same patient activations occurred in the amygdala to fearful vs happy face expressions when these were presented to the blind and seeing hemifields, but only in the fusiform cortex (face) area when the stimuli were presented to the seeing hemifield (Morris, De Gelder, Weiskrantz & Dolan 2001). However, a more relevant cortical area to examine would be the cortex in the anterior part of the superior temporal sulcus, which in macaques as shown by neuronal recording studies (Hasselmo, Rolls & Baylis 1989a) and in human neuroimaging (Haxby, Hoffman & Gobbini 2002) is especially involved in face expression analysis. The evidence from the latency of neuronal responses to faces does not suggest that there is a rapid subcortical pathway for processing faces, for in macaques the latencies of activation of face-selective neurons in the temporal cortex visual areas are typically 80–120 ms (Rolls 1984, Leonard et al. 1985), in the amygdala are typically 110–180 ms (Leonard, Rolls, Wilson & Baylis 1985), and in the orbitofrontal cortex are typically 130–280 ms (Rolls, Critchley, Browning & Inoue 2006a). These latencies are consistent with cortical processing in the temporal cortical visual areas before neurons become activated by faces in the amygdala and orbitofrontal cortex, both of which receive direct inputs from the temporal cortical visual areas as described above.

One potential subcortical route for visual inputs to reach the amygdala via a subcortical pathway involving the superior colliculus and pulvinar has been discussed in the context of blindsight (Tamietto, Pullens, de Gelder, Weiskrantz & Goebel 2012). The arguments described in Section 4.6.4 apply here too, especially as appropriate emotional and social responses to for example faces require information about whose face it is as well as the expression, and the form recognition required for this appears to involves cortical computation (Rolls 2012e). Another argument that applies is that considerable processing in the brain occurs with information that is too low to reach the threshold for interrupting conscious processing, as shown by investigations of the responses of temporal cortex face-selective neurons to brief visual stimuli in the presence of backward masking (Rolls, Tovee, Purcell, Stewart &

Azzopardi 1994b, Rolls & Tovee 1994, Rolls, Tovee & Panzeri 1999b, Rolls 2003, Rolls 2006a).

Deficits produced by amygdala damage may extend beyond face expression recognition deficits and fear conditioning deficits, in that bilateral amygdala patients are impaired not only at 'theory of mind' attributions when these are based on eye gaze, but also when they are related to an inability to recognize 'faux pas' situations in narratives (Stone, Baron-Cohen, Calder, Keane & Young 2003). With respect to autism, in which a 'theory of mind' deficit is a major component (Frith 2001), children with autism have usually been found to be unimpaired in facial affect recognition when the groups are matched on mental age (Baron-Cohen, Wheelwright & Joliffe 1997, Blair 2003). However, some evidence linking the amygdala and autism is that patients with autism or Asperger's syndrome did not activate the amygdala when making mentalistic inferences from the eyes (Baron-Cohen, Ring, Bullmore, Wheelwright, Ashwin & Williams 2000).

There is some evidence that another face expression, disgust, involves special processing by the insula (Section 4.9).

In another system with some apparent specificity, there is some evidence that patients with lesions in the ventral putamen (which does receive inputs from the inferior temporal visual cortex and contains visually responsive neurons (Caan, Perrett & Rolls 1984)) may have impaired anger face recognition (Calder, Keane, Lawrence & Manes 2004), and this was related to evidence that the D2 dopamine receptor blocker sulpiride decreases the identification of angry face expressions (Lawrence, Calder, McGowan & Grasby 2002). Insofar as activation of the ventral putamen may be larger to angry face expressions and of the insula to disgust face expressions, we might note that skeletomotor responses (likely to be involved in anger) are functions of much of the putamen, and that visceral responses (likely to occur in disgust) may be produced in part via the anteroventral insula. Thus the activations of both regions by faces may be related to the responses normally produced by different face expressions.

For comparison, in a much more extensive series of patients it has been shown that damage to the orbitofrontal cortex can produce face expression deficits in the absence of face identification deficits, and that some patients with orbitofrontal cortex damage are impaired at the auditory identification of emotional sounds (Hornak, Rolls & Wade 1996, Hornak, Bramham, Rolls, Morris, O'Doherty, Bullock & Polkey 2003, Rolls 1999c) (see Section 4.5.6). Interestingly, the visual face expression and auditory vocal expression impairments are partly dissociable in these orbitofrontal patients, indicating partially separate processing systems in the orbitofrontal cortex, and indicating that a general emotional impairment produced by these lesions is not the simple explanation of the alterations in face and voice expression processing after damage to the orbitofrontal cortex. I note that the most consistent change after orbitofrontal cortex damage in our series of patients (Rolls, Hornak, Wade & McGrath 1994a, Hornak, Rolls & Wade 1996, Hornak, Bramham, Rolls, Morris, O'Doherty, Bullock & Polkey 2003, Rolls 1999c, Hornak, O'Doherty, Bramham, Rolls, Morris, Bullock & Polkey 2004) is an alteration in voice and face expression decoding, and that the amygdala is strongly connected to the orbitofrontal cortex.

Functional brain imaging studies have also shown activation of the amygdala by face expression. For example, Morris, Frith, Perrett, Rowland, Young, Calder & Dolan (1996) found more activation of the left amygdala by face expressions of fear than of happiness in a PET study. They also reported that the activation increased as the intensity of the fear expression increased, and decreased as the intensity of the happy expression increased. In a metanalysis of 29 neuroimaging studies on the social evaluation of faces, it was found that for negative face evaluations the most consistent activations were in the amygdala, whereas across positive face evaluations the most consistent activations were in the medial prefrontal cortex, pregenual anterior cingulate cortex, and medial orbitofrontal cortex (Mende-Siedlecki,

Said & Todorov 2013).

However, although in studies of the effects of amygdala damage in humans greater impairments have been reported to face expressions of fear than to some other expressions (Adolphs et al. 1994, Scott et al. 1997), and in functional brain imaging studies greater activation may be found to certain classes of emotion-provoking stimuli, e.g. to stimuli that provoke fear compared with those that produce happiness (Morris et al. 1996), or are negatively socially evaluated (Mende-Siedlecki et al. 2013), it is most unlikely that the amygdala is specialized for the decoding of only certain classes of emotional stimulus, such as fear. Indeed, we have recently described a patient with a right amygdala lesion with an impairment of the recognition of disgust face expressions (Gallo, Gamiz, Perez-Garcia, Del Moral & Rolls 2013). The emphasis on fear may be related to the research in rats on the role of the amygdala in fear conditioning (LeDoux 1992, LeDoux 1994, LeDoux 1996, Pare et al. 2004, LeDoux 2011). It is quite clear from single-neuron neurophysiological studies in primates including humans that different amygdala neurons are activated by different classes of both rewarding and punishing stimuli (Sanghera, Rolls & Roper-Hall 1979, Rolls 1992a, Ono & Nishijo 1992, Wilson & Rolls 1993, Wilson & Rolls 2005) and by a wide range of different face stimuli (Leonard, Rolls, Wilson & Baylis 1985, Gothard, Battaglia, Erickson, Spitler & Amaral 2007, Rutishauser, Tudusciuc, Neumann, Mamelak, Heller, Ross, Philpott, Sutherling & Adolphs 2011). Also, lesions of the macaque amygdala impair the learning of both stimulus–reward and stimulus–punisher associations (see Section 4.6.3). Further, electrical stimulation of the macaque and human amygdala at some sites is rewarding, and humans report pleasure from stimulation at such sites (Rolls 1975, Rolls et al. 1980, Sem-Jacobsen 1968, Sem-Jacobsen 1976, Halgren 1992). Further, in a functional neuroimaging study, O'Doherty, Rolls, Francis, Bowtell & McGlone (2001b) showed that activation of the human amygdala was larger and more reliably produced by the pleasant taste of glucose than by the unpleasant taste of salt, both of which are primary reinforcers. Thus any differences in the magnitude of effects between different classes of emotional stimuli that appear in human functional brain imaging studies (Morris et al. 1996, Mende-Siedlecki et al. 2013) or even after amygdala damage (Adolphs et al. 1994, Scott et al. 1997) should not be taken as showing that the human amygdala is involved in only some emotions. Consistent with this view, LaBar, Gitelman, Parrish, Kim, Nobre & Mesulam (2001) showed that both pleasant and unpleasant stimuli produced more activation of the human amygdala than neutral stimuli.

A very interesting clarification is provided by the finding that personality interacts with whether particular stimuli activate the human amygdala. For example, happy face expressions are more likely to activate the human amygdala in extraverts than in introverts (Canli et al. 2002). In addition, positively affective pictures interact with extraversion to produce activation of the amygdala (Canli et al. 2001). This supports the conceptually important point described in section 2.7 that part of the basis of personality may be differential sensitivity to different rewards and punishers, and omission and termination of rewards and punishers. The observations just described are consistent with the hypothesis that part of the basis of extraversion is increased reactivity to positively affective (as compared to negatively affective) face expressions and other positively affective stimuli including pictures. The exact mechanisms involved may be revealed in the future by genetic studies, and these might potentially address for example whether genes control responses to positively affective stimuli; or whether some more general personality trait by altering perhaps mood produces differential top-down biasing of face expression decoding systems in the way outlined in Section 4.12. It has additionally been found that negative pictures interact with neuroticism in producing differential activation of the human amygdala (Canli et al. 2001). Further, FFFS and BIS-related personality traits related to an anxiety-related 'Behavioural Inhibition System', and to a fear-related 'Fight, Flight, Freeze System', are positively correlated to activity in the amygdala in response to negative stimuli (Kennis, Rademaker & Geuze 2013).

Additional factors are that some expressions are much more identifiable than others. For example, we (Hornak, Rolls & Wade 1996, Rolls 1999c) found that happy faces were easier to identify than other face expressions in the Ekman set, and that the orbitofrontal patients we studied were not impaired at identifying the (easy) happy face expression, but showed deficits primarily on the more difficult set of other expressions (fear, surprise, anger, sadness, etc.). Another factor in imaging studies in which the human subjects may be slightly apprehensive is that happy expressions may produce some relaxation in the situation, whereas expressions of fear may do the opposite, and this could contribute to the results found. Thus I suggest caution in interpreting human studies as showing that the amygdala (or orbitofrontal cortex) are involved only in certain emotions. It is much more likely that both are involved in very many emotions, produced to rewarding stimuli as well as to punishers.

4.6.8 Amygdala summary

The evidence described in Section 4.6 implicates the amygdala in the processing of a number of stimuli that are primary reinforcers, including the sight, smell, and taste of food, touch, and pain.

The amygdala also receives information about potential secondary reinforcers, such as visual stimuli, including faces. Many of the deficits produced by amygdala damage are related to impairments in learning associations between stimuli and primary reinforcers, e.g. between visual or auditory stimuli and pain.

The amygdala is not concerned only with aversive reinforcers, in that it receives information about food, and in that amygdala lesions impair the altered behaviour that normally occurs to foods when their reward value is reduced by feeding to satiety.

The associative stimulus–reinforcer learning or conditioning in the amygdala may require NMDA receptor activation for the learning, which appears to occur by a process like long-term potentiation.

We know that autonomic responses learned to conditioned stimuli can depend on outputs from the amygdala to the hypothalamus, and that the effects that learned incentives have on behaviour may involve outputs from the amygdala to the ventral striatum. We also know that there are similar neurons in the ventral striatum to some of those described in the amygdala (Williams, Rolls, Leonard & Stern 1993).

All this evidence is consistent with the hypothesis that there are neuronal networks in the amygdala that perform the required pattern association. Interestingly, there is somewhat of a gap in our knowledge here, for the microcircuitry of the amygdala has been remarkably little studied. It is known from Golgi studies (performed in young rats in which sufficiently few amygdala cells are stained that it is possible to see them individually) that there are pyramidal cells in the amygdala with large dendrites and many synapses (Millhouse & DeOlmos 1983, McDonald 1992, Millhouse 1986). What has not yet been defined is whether visual and taste inputs converge anatomically on to some cells, and whether (as might be predicted) the taste inputs are likely to be strong (e.g. large synapses close to the cell body), whereas the visual inputs are more numerous, and on a part of the dendrite with NMDA receptors. Clearly to bring our understanding fully to the network level, such evidence is required, together with further neurophysiological evidence showing the appropriate convergence at the single neuron level, and evidence that the appropriate synapses on to these single neurons are modifiable by a Hebb-like rule (such as might be implemented using the NMDA receptors, see Appendix 1), in a network of the type shown in Fig. 4.5.

At least part of the importance of the amygdala in emotion appears to be that it is involved in this type of emotional learning. However, the amygdala does not appear to provide such rapid relearning of reward-related emotional responses to stimuli as does the orbitofrontal cortex, as described in Section 4.5. Further, the amygdala does not appear in non-human primates and humans to play such an important role in emotional and social behaviour as the orbitofrontal cortex (see Section 4.5). Further, the deficits described after amygdala damage involve fear conditioning (with classical conditioning of for example autonomic responses and effects on startle especially studied), and somewhat subtle aspects of face expression processing. In evolution, the balance may have moved to the orbitofrontal cortex, which has evolved much more recently, and may allow more powerful computations, such as those involved in rapid reversal learning and rapid correction of behaviour, to be implemented (Rolls 2008b).

4.7 The cingulate cortex

4.7.1 Introduction and overview of the anterior cingulate cortex

The orbitofrontal cortex is involved in representing the value of stimuli. It is in a sense an output region for all the sensory systems, including taste, olfaction, visual, auditory, and somatosensory, that represent 'what' a stimulus is, and uses that information to build what are frequently multimodal representations but in value space rather than 'what' or stimulus identity space. Orbitofrontal cortex neurons focus on value representations for stimuli, and know little about actions.

The anterior cingulate cortex receives inputs from the orbitofrontal cortex about the value of stimuli, that is about goals including the value of outcomes (the reward received) and the expected value. The anterior cingulate cortex in combination with the midcingulate motor area, which contains representations of actions, interfaces actions to outcomes using action–outcome learning, and also takes into account the cost of actions to obtain the goal when selecting actions. The anterior and midcingulate cortical areas are thus relevant to emotion, for they implement the instrumental goal-directed actions that the instrumental reinforcers involved in emotion produce. In the context of its representations of value, damage to the anterior cingulate areas does influence emotion.

The anterior cingulate cortex operates as a system that is aiming to obtain goals, and is taking into account the outcomes received after actions, in that it is sensitive to devaluation of the goal, and will not select an action if the goal has been devalued. This is in contrast to the basal ganglia, which implement a stimulus–motor response mapping which becomes automated as a habit after much learning, and is not sensitive to devaluation of the goal, as described in Chapter 6 and Section 4.6.3.4.

The posterior cingulate cortex has different functions, for it is not activated in the same way as the anterior cingulate cortex by rewards and punishers, and is involved in spatio-topographical and related memory functions with its connections to parietal structures such as the precuneus and with the hippocampus that are involved in these functions (Vogt 2009, Cavanna & Trimble 2006, Pu, Guo, Liua, Yub, Xuea, Rolls, Feng & Liu 2013).

In more detail, the pregenual and the adjoining dorsal anterior cingulate areas can be conceptualized as a relay that allows information about rewards and outcomes to be linked, via longitudinal connections running in the cingulum fibre bundle, to information about actions represented in the mid-cingulate cortex. Bringing together information about specific rewards with information about actions, and the costs associated with actions, is important for associating actions with the value of their outcomes and for selecting the correct action that will lead to a desired reward (Walton, Bannerman, Alterescu & Rushworth 2003, Rushworth, Buckley, Behrens, Walton & Bannerman 2007b, Rolls 2009d, Rushworth, Noonan, Boorman, Walton

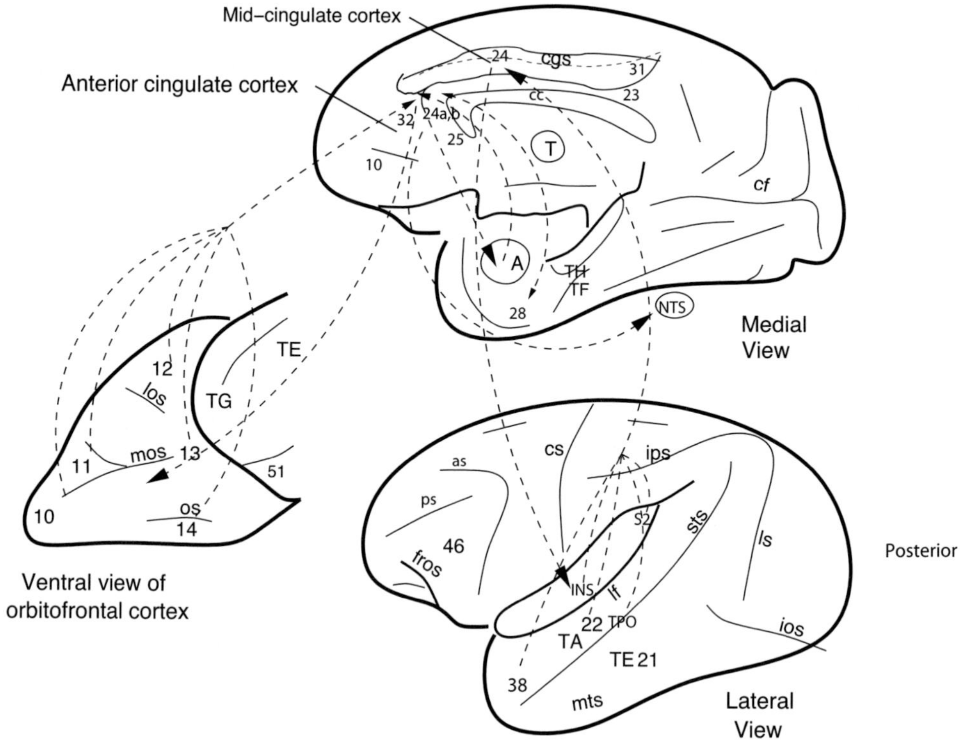

Fig. 4.63 Connections of the anterior cingulate (perigenual) and midcingulate cortical areas (shown on views of the primate brain). The cingulate sulcus (cgs) has been opened to reveal the cortex in the sulcus, with the dashed line indicating the depths (fundus) of the sulcus. The cingulate cortex is in the lower bank of this sulcus, and in the cingulate gyrus which hooks above the corpus callosum and around the corpus callosum at the front and the back. The anterior cingulate cortex extends from cingulate areas 32, 24a and 24b to subgenual cingulate area 25. (The cortex is called subgenual because it is below the genu (knee) formed by the anterior end of the corpus callosum, cc.) The perigenual cingulate cortex tends to have connections with the amygdala and orbitofrontal cortex, whereas area 24c tends to have connections with the somatosensory insula (INS), the auditory association cortex (22, TA), and with the temporal pole cortex (38). The midcingulate areas include area 24d, which is part of the cingulate motor area. Abbreviations: as, arcuate sulcus; cc, corpus callosum; cf, calcarine fissure; cgs, cingulate sulcus; cs, central sulcus; ls, lunate sulcus; ios, inferior occipital sulcus; mos, medial orbital sulcus; os, orbital sulcus; ps, principal sulcus; sts, superior temporal sulcus; lf, lateral (or Sylvian) fissure (which has been opened to reveal the insula); A, amygdala; INS, insula; NTS, autonomic areas in the medulla, including the nucleus of the solitary tract and the dorsal motor nucleus of the vagus; TE (21), inferior temporal visual cortex; TA (22), superior temporal auditory association cortex; TF and TH, parahippocampal cortex; TPO, multimodal cortical area in the superior temporal sulcus; 28, entorhinal cortex; 38, TG, temporal pole cortex; 12, 13, 11, orbitofrontal cortex; 51, olfactory (prepyriform and periamygdaloid) cortex.

& Behrens 2011, Grabenhorst & Rolls 2011). Indeed, consistent with its strong connections to motor areas (Morecraft & Tanji 2009), lesions of the anterior cingulate cortex impair reward-guided action selection (Kennerley, Walton, Behrens, Buckley & Rushworth 2006, Rudebeck, Behrens, Kennerley, Baxter, Buckley, Walton & Rushworth 2008), neuroimaging studies have shown that the anterior cingulate cortex is active when outcome information guides choices (Walton, Devlin & Rushworth 2004), and single neurons in the anterior cingulate cortex encode information about both actions and outcomes including reward prediction errors for actions (Matsumoto, Matsumoto, Abe & Tanaka 2007, Luk & Wallis 2009). For example,

Luk & Wallis (2009) found that in a task where information about three potential outcomes (three types of juice) had to be associated on a trial-by-trial basis with two different responses (two lever movements), many neurons in the anterior cingulate cortex encoded information about both specific outcomes and specific actions.

4.7.2 Anterior cingulate cortex anatomy and connections

The anterior cingulate areas occupy approximately the anterior one third of the cingulate cortex (see Fig. 4.63) and involved in emotion may be distinguished from a mid-cingulate area (i.e. further back than the anterior cingulate region and occupying approximately the middle third of the cingulate cortex) which has been termed the cingulate motor area (Vogt, Derbyshire & Jones 1996, Vogt 2009) and may be involved in action selection (Rushworth, Walton, Kennerley & Bannerman 2004, Rushworth et al. 2011). The anterior cingulate cortex includes area 32 the pregenual (or perigenual, meaning around the genu of the corpus callosum) cingulate cortex, area 25 the subgenual cingulate cortex, and part of area 24 (Figs. 4.63 and 4.18) (Price 2006, Ongur, Ferry & Price 2003, Ongur & Price 2000).

As shown in Fig. 4.63, the anterior cingulate cortex receives strong inputs from the orbitofrontal cortex (Carmichael & Price 1995a, Morecraft & Tanji 2009, Vogt 2009). The anterior cingulate cortex is part of what is described as a 'medial prefrontal network' including all the areas on the medial wall (areas 25, 32, 14r, 14c, 24a and 24b) (which are also interconnected with some areas on the orbital surface, areas 11m, 13a, Iai and 12o) (Price 2006, Ongur & Price 2000). This medial prefrontal network is also connected with the entorhinal, parahippocampal, and cingulate/retrosplenial cortex (Saleem, Kondo & Price 2008). It should be noted that this medial prefrontal network includes area 14 on the most medial part of the orbitofrontal cortex, and that area 14 should not be included in Price and colleagues' 'orbital prefrontal network'. Their 'orbital prefrontal network' includes most of the areas on the posterior, central and lateral orbital surface (agranular insular areas Ial, Iam, Iapl and Iapm, and orbital areas 13b, 13l, 13m, 11l, 12r, 12m and 12l, see Fig. 4.18), which is described as the orbitofrontal cortex here (Section 4.5) and in most previous publications. The term 'ventromedial prefrontal cortex' (vmPFC) is not well defined anatomically, and refers generally to a medial and ventral region of the prefrontal cortex which probably can be taken to include the ventral parts of the 'medial prefrontal network' of Price and colleagues, and also probably medial parts of the orbitofrontal cortex (see further Section 4.8.3).

The outputs of the anterior cingulate cortex reach further back in the cingulate cortex towards the midcingulate cortex, which includes the cingulate motor area (Vogt et al. 1996, Morecraft & Tanji 2009, Vogt 2009). The anterior cingulate cortex also projects forwards to medial prefrontal cortex area 10 (Price 2006, Ongur & Price 2000) (see Section 4.8). Another route for output is via the projections to the striatum / basal ganglia system. The anterior cingulate cortex, including the subgenual cingulate cortex area 25, has outputs that can influence autonomic/visceral function via the hypothalamus, midbrain periaqueductal gray, and insula, as does the orbitofrontal cortex (Rempel-Clower & Barbas 1998, Price 2006, Ongur & Price 2000, Critchley & Harrison 2013).

4.7.3 Anterior cingulate cortex functional neuroimaging and neuronal activity

In early functional neuroimaging investigations, Vogt et al. (1996) showed that pain produced an increase in regional cerebral blood flow (rCBF, measured with positron emission tomography, PET) in an area of perigenual cingulate cortex which included parts of areas 25, 32, 24a, 24b and/or 24c. Vogt et al. suggested that activation of the anterior part of the cingulate area is related to the affective aspect of pain. Lane, Fink, Chau & Dolan (1997a) found increased regional blood flow in a PET study in a far anterior part of the cingulate cortex where it adjoins prefrontal cortex when humans paid attention to the affective aspects of pictures they were being shown which contained pleasant images (e.g. flowers) and unpleasant pictures (e.g. a mangled face and a snake).

Functional magnetic resonance neuroimaging (fMRI) studies are now showing that there are rather separate representations of positively affective, pleasant, stimuli in the anterior/perigenual cingulate cortex (yellow in Fig. 4.47); and of negative, unpleasant, stimuli just posterior to this above the corpus callosum in the anterior cingulate cortex (white in Fig. 4.47) (Rolls 2009d, Grabenhorst & Rolls 2011). The area activated by pain is typically 10–30 mm behind and above the most anterior (i.e. pre- or peri-genual) part of the anterior cingulate cortex (see e.g. Rolls, O'Doherty, Kringelbach, Francis, Bowtell & McGlone (2003d), Fig. 4.4, and Vogt & Sikes (2000)). Pleasant touch was found to activate the most anterior part of the anterior cingulate cortex, just in front of the (genu or knee of the) corpus callosum (i.e. pregenual cingulate cortex) (Rolls, O'Doherty, Kringelbach, Francis, Bowtell & McGlone 2003d, McCabe, Rolls, Bilderbeck & McGlone 2008) (Fig. 4.4). Pleasant temperature applied to the hand also produces a linear activation related to the degree of subjective pleasantness in the pregenual cingulate cortex (Grabenhorst, Rolls & Parris 2008b). Oral somatosensory stimuli such as viscosity and the pleasantness of fat texture also activate this most anterior part of the anterior cingulate cortex (De Araujo & Rolls 2004, Grabenhorst, Rolls, Parris & D'Souza 2010b). More than just somatosensory stimuli are represented, however, in that (pleasant) sweet taste also activates the most anterior part of the anterior cingulate cortex (De Araujo & Rolls 2004, De Araujo, Kringelbach, Rolls & Hobden 2003a) (Fig. 5.14) where attention to pleasantness (Grabenhorst & Rolls 2008) and cognition (Grabenhorst, Rolls & Bilderbeck 2008a) also enhances activations, as do pleasant odours (Rolls, Kringelbach & De Araujo 2003c) (Figs. 4.26 and 4.27), and cognitive inputs that influence the pleasantness of odours (De Araujo et al. 2005) (Fig. 4.43, and also top-down inputs that produce selective attention to odour pleasantness (Rolls, Grabenhorst, Margot, da Silva & Velazco 2008a). Unpleasant odours activate further back in the anterior cingulate cortex (Rolls, Kringelbach & De Araujo 2003c) (Fig. 4.26). Activations in the anterior/perigenual cingulate cortex are also produced by the taste of water when it is rewarding because of thirst (De Araujo, Kringelbach, Rolls & McGlone 2003b), by the flavour of food (Kringelbach, O'Doherty, Rolls & Andrews 2003), and by monetary reward (O'Doherty, Kringelbach, Rolls, Hornak & Andrews 2001a) (Fig. 4.35). Moreover, the outcome value and the expected value of monetary reward activate the pregenual cingulate cortex (Rolls, McCabe & Redoute 2008e). The locations of some of these activations are shown in Fig. 4.47.

In these studies, the anterior cingulate activations were linearly related to the subjective pleasantness or unpleasantness of the stimuli, providing evidence that the anterior cingulate cortex provides a representation of value on a continuous scale. Moreover, evidence was found that there was a common scale of value in the pregenual cingulate cortex, with the affective pleasantness of taste stimuli and of thermal stimuli applied to the hand producing identically scaled BOLD activations (Grabenhorst, D'Souza, Parris, Rolls & Passingham 2010a). The implication is that the anterior cingulate cortex contains a value representation used in decision-making, but that the decision itself may be made elsewhere. Decisions about actions that reflect the outcomes represented in the anterior cingulate cortex may be made further posterior towards the mid-cingulate cortex. Decisions about the value of stimuli may be made in the medial prefrontal cortex area 10 (see Section 4.8), which does receive inputs from the anterior cingulate cortex.

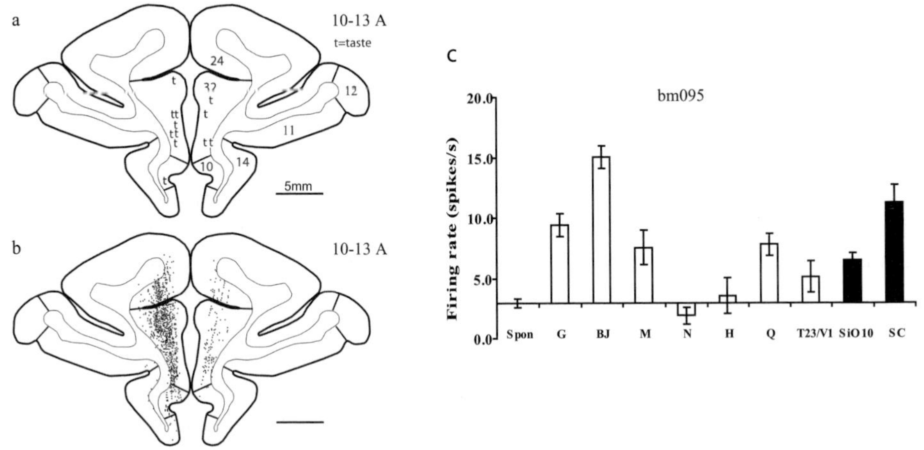

Fig. 4.64 Pregenual cortex taste neurons. The reconstructed positions of the anterior cingulate neurons with taste (t) responses, together with the cytoarchitectonic boundaries determined by Carmichael and Price (1994). Most (11/12) of the taste neurons were in the pregenual cingulate cortex (area 32), as shown. The neurons are shown on a coronal section at 12 mm anterior (A) to the sphenoid reference point. b. The locations of all the 749 neurons recorded in the anterior cingulate region in this study are indicated to show the regions sampled. c. Responses of a pregenual cingulate cortex neuron (bm095) with differential responses to tastes and oral fat texture stimuli. The mean ($\pm$ sem) firing rate responses to each stimulus calculated in a 5 s period over several trials are shown. The spontaneous (Spon) firing rate of 3 spikes/s is shown by the horizontal line, with the responses indicated relative to this line. The taste stimuli were 1 M glucose (G), blackcurrant fruit juice (BJ), 0.1 M NaCl (N), 0.1 M MSG (M), 0.01 M HCl (H) and 0.001 M QuinineHCl (Q); water (T23/V1); single cream (SC); and silicone oil with a viscosity of 10 cP (SiO10). The neuron had significantly different responses to the different stimuli as shown by a one-way ANOVA (F[9,46]=17.7, $p < 10^{10}$). (Data from Rolls, Gabbott, Verhagen, and Kadohisa.) (Reproduced from E. T. Rolls, Functions of the orbitofrontal and pregenual cingulate cortex in taste, olfaction, appetite and emotion, *Acta Physiologica Hungarica*, 95 pp. 131–164, ©2008, Akadémiai Kiadó Zrt.)

In addition to the pregenual cingulate sites that are activated in many of our studies of affective stimuli, it is also frequently found that activation in a region at the intersection of the medial prefrontal cortex, the subgenual cingulate cortex, and the orbitofrontal cortex is activated by positively affective stimuli. The region is well illustrated in Fig. 4.44 which shows regions where paying attention to the pleasantness vs the intensity of a taste increases the activation to the taste (Grabenhorst & Rolls 2008). The region is also illustrated in Figs. 4.26 and 4.27 (lower region) where activations were correlated with the pleasantness of olfactory stimuli (Rolls, Kringelbach & De Araujo 2003c), in Fig. 4.43A and B where cognitive inputs increased activations that were related to the pleasantness of olfactory stimuli (De Araujo, Rolls, Velazco, Margot & Cayeux 2005), in Fig. 5.14 where glucose taste produced activations (De Araujo, Kringelbach, Rolls & Hobden 2003a), and in a similar region in which intraoral fat and sucrose both produced activations (De Araujo & Rolls 2004). This region is also activated by monetary reward (O'Doherty, Kringelbach, Rolls, Hornak & Andrews 2001a) (Fig. 4.35). The region extends from the orbitofrontal cortex to the pregenual cingulate cortex and to a region anterior to this that is probably part of medial prefrontal cortex area 10 (cf. Fig. 4.18). The fact that this region is activated by many rewarding stimuli as just summarized (Fig. 4.47 (Grabenhorst & Rolls 2011)), if lesioned affects emotion (Hornak, Bramham, Rolls, Morris, O'Doherty, Bullock & Polkey 2003), and is connected with the orbitofrontal cortex, indicates that it is important in emotion, perhaps as a region linking the orbitofrontal cortex to outputs.

It is in this context very interesting that chronic electrical stimulation in or close to this region relieves symptoms of treatment-resistant depression in some patients (Mayberg, Lozano, Voon, McNeely, Seminowicz, Hamani, Schwalb & Kennedy 2005, Hamani, Mayberg, Stone, Laxton, Haber & Lozano 2011, Johansen-Berg, Gutman, Behrens, Matthews, Rushworth, Katz, Lozano & Mayberg 2008). The electrical stimulation is likely to be activating not only the neurons in this reward-related region, but also the fibre pathways that connect these regions to each other, to medial prefrontal cortex area 10, and to the ventral striatum (Lujan, Chaturvedi, Choi, Holtzheimer, Gross, Mayberg & McIntyre 2013). Moreover, regional cerebral blood flow may be low (reflecting decreased neural activity) in these medial orbitofrontal and pregenual cingulate regions in depression (Mayberg, Liotti, Brannan, McGinnis, Mahurin, Jerabek, Silva, Tekell, Martin, Lancaster & Fox 1999). It is these regions where activations are linearly related to the reward value and pleasantness of many stimuli (Rolls & Grabenhorst 2008, Grabenhorst & Rolls 2011). This provides a close link between evidence from neuroscience about the functions of this medial region, and the therapeutic potential of these concepts for helping to understand and treat depression (see Section 4.10).

Value representations in the pregenual cingulate cortex are confirmed by recording studies in monkeys (Rolls 2008e, Rolls 2009d). For example, Gabbott, Verhagen, Kadohisa and Rolls found neurons in the pregenual cingulate cortex that respond to taste (see example in Fig. 4.64), and it was demonstrated that the representation is of reward value, for devaluation by feeding to satiety selectively decreased neuronal responses to the food with which the animal was satiated (Rolls 2008e). [It is notable that neurons in area 14, the most ventral part of the 'medial network', were not activated by taste outcome (Rolls 2008e). It is important when designing lesion studies to take into account the locations of reward value neurons, which are found throughout the medio-lateral extent of the orbitofrontal cortex apart from area 14 (Rolls 2008e), which in any case is thought to be part of the medial network (cf Noonan, Kolling, Walton & Rushworth (2012).]

Some single neuron studies indicating encoding of actions and outcomes have often involved rather dorsal recordings above the pregenual cingulate cortex in the dorsal bank of the cingulate sulcus (Matsumoto et al. 2007, Luk & Wallis 2009). In a similar area, action–outcome associations appear to be represented, in that in tasks in which there were different relations between actions and rewards, it was found that even before a response was made, while the monkey was looking at a visual cue, the activity of anterior cingulate cortex neurons depended on the expectation of reward or non-reward (25%), the intention to move or not (25%), or a combination of movement intention and reward expectation (11%) (Matsumoto, Suzuki & Tanaka 2003). Luk & Wallis (2013) described recordings in the same dorsal anterior cingulate cortex area that reflected the outcomes when monkeys made a choice of a left or right lever response to obtain a reward outcome, and also described a weak dissociation for more stimulus-outcome neurons in the orbitofrontal cortex, that is when monkeys had to choose the reward outcome based on which visual stimulus was shown. In the same dorsal anterior cingulate area neurons were more likely to take into account the costs of the actions required to obtain rewards, as well as the probability of obtaining the reward, than were neurons in the orbitofrontal cortex (Kennerley & Wallis 2009, Kennerley, Behrens & Wallis 2011). More ventrally in the anterior cingulate cortex, neurons are more likely to reflect reward outcome rather than primarily actions (Cai & Padoa-Schioppa 2012).

Foraging studies also implicate the anterior cingulate cortex in representing value, and in taking into account costs. Hayden, Pearson & Platt (2011) taught monkeys a simple computerized foraging task in which they could chose to continue foraging in the same patch for diminishing returns, or seek an alternative patch at the expense of paying a cost of a travel delay before foraging could resume. Single neurons in the anterior cingulate cortex that fire to reward receipt did so at an increasing rate as monkeys moved towards leaving a known patch to search for a new one. Patch moving was initiated when the anterior cingulate cortex activity reached a threshold. The threshold firing rate that had to be reached was proportional to the search costs that were to be incurred by switching away from the current foraging patch.

In a neuroimaging study that provides evidence that the anterior cingulate cortex is active when outcome information guides choices made by the individual (Walton et al. 2004), the activations were relatively far back in the anterior cingulate cortex (y=22) towards the midcingulate cortex. This is consistent with the hypothesis that the reward value information in the pregenual cingulate cortex and the negative value representations just behind and dorsal to this in the anterior cingulate cortex are projected posteriorly towards the midcingulate area for interfacing to action. The value representations may also be projected to the dorsal anterior cingulate area in the dorsal bank of the cingulate cortex in which recordings were made from neurons by Wallis and colleagues.

4.7.4 Anterior cingulate cortex lesion effects

Lesion studies in monkeys (Rudebeck et al. 2008) and humans (Camille, Tsuchida & Fellows 2011), have demonstrated a dissociation in the role of the anterior cingulate cortex in action–outcome and of the orbitofrontal cortex in stimulus–outcome associations to guide behaviour (Rushworth, Kolling, Sallet & Mars 2012). Lesions of the anterior cingulate cortex in rats impair he ability to take into account the costs of actions, and this is supported by a neuroimaging study in humans (Croxson, Walton, O'Reilly, Behrens & Rushworth 2009).

An investigation more closely related to the understanding of emotion showed that patients with selective surgical lesions of the antero-ventral part of the anterior cingulate cortex (ACC) and/or medial BA9 were in some cases impaired on voice and face expression identification, had some change in social behaviour, such as inappropriateness, and had significant changes in their subjective emotional state (Hornak, Bramham, Rolls, Morris, O'Doherty, Bullock & Polkey 2003). Unilateral lesions were sufficient to produce these effects, and there were no strong laterality effects. In line with these results in humans, Hadland, Rushworth, Gaffan & Passingham (2003) found diminished social vocalization in monkeys with anterior cingulate lesions, and also emotional and social changes. Consistent with the effects of the anterior cingulate lesions in humans on recognizing voice (and in some cases face) emotional expression (Hornak et al. 2003), neuroimaging studies concerned with vocal expression identification have reported orbital and medial activation. These include a study by Morris et al. (1996) using non-verbal sounds expressing fear, sadness and happiness that, when compared to a neutral condition, activated BA11 (orbital cortex) bilaterally and Medial BA9 on the left. Fear-related increases in activity were also found on the right only in BA11. In another study Phillips, Young, Scott, Calder, Andrew, Giampetro, Williams, Bullmore, Brammer & Gray (1998) found that fearful sounds activated Medial BA32 and BA24 (anterior cingulate at/below the level of the genu of the corpus callosum) - again on the right side only. More extensive studies of facial expression identification have been conducted, and these report activation in a number of sites within both orbital and medial regions, including Medial BA9 and BA32/24 (anterior cingulate) (Blair, Morris, Frith, Perrett & Dolan 1999, Dolan, Fletcher, Morris, Kapur, Deakin & Frith 1996, Nakamura, Kawashima, Ito, Sugiura, Kato, Nakamura, Hatano, Nagumo, Kubota, Fukuda & Kojima 1999).

There is also neuroimaging evidence that complements the effects of lesions (Hornak, Bramham, Rolls, Morris, O'Doherty, Bullock & Polkey 2003) in suggesting a role for certain medial regions in the subjective experience of emotion. In neuroimaging studies with normal human subjects bilateral activations in Medial BA9 were found as subjects viewed emotion-laden stimuli, and in both Medial BA9 as well as in ventral ACC during self-generated emotional experience (i.e., in the absence of a stimulus) as subjects recalled emotions of sadness or happiness (Lane, Reiman, Ahern, Schwartz & Davidson 1997b, Lane, Reiman, Bradley, Lang, Ahern, Davidson & Schwartz 1997c, Lane et al. 1998, Phillips, Drevets, Rauch & Lane 2003a). On the basis of a review of imaging studies which consistently emphasize the importance of anterior and ventral regions of the anterior cingulate cortex for emotion, Bush, Luu & Posner (2000) argue that the anterior cingulate cortex can be divided into a ventral 'affective' division (which includes the subcallosal region and the part anterior to the corpus callosum), and a dorsal 'cognitive' division, a view strengthened by the demonstration of reciprocally inhibitory interactions between these two regions.

The subgenual part (area 25) of the anterior cingulate cortex is, via its outputs to the hypothalamus and brainstem autonomic regions, involved in the autonomic component of emotion (Koski & Paus 2000, Barbas & Pandya 1989, Ongur & Price 2000, Gabbott, Warner, Jays & Bacon 2003, Vogt 2009). The anterior cingulate cortex is also activated in relation to autonomic events, and Nagai, Critchley, Featherstone, Trimble & Dolan (2004) have shown that there is a correlation with skin conductance, a measure of autonomic activity related to sympathetic activation, in the anterior cingulate cortex and related areas. The dorsal anterior and mid-cingulate cortical areas may be especially related to blood pressure, pupil size, heart rate, and electrodermal activity, whereas the subgenual cingulate cortex, with ventromedial prefrontal cortex, appears antisympathetic (and parasympathetic) (Critchley & Harrison 2013).

A current working hypothesis is that the affective part of the anterior cingulate cortex receives inputs about expected rewards and punishers, and about the rewards and punishers received, from the orbitofrontal cortex and amygdala. There is some segregation of the areas that receive these inputs. The anterior cingulate cortex may compare these signals, take into account the cost of actions, and utilize the value representations in action–outcome learning.

4.7.5 Mid-cingulate cortex, the cingulate motor area, and action–outcome learning

The anterior or perigenual cingulate area[10] may be distinguished from a mid-cingulate area (i.e. further back than the perigenual cingulate region and occupying approximately the middle third of the cingulate cortex), which has been termed the cingulate motor area (Vogt et al. 1996, Vogt, Berger & Derbyshire 2003, Vogt 2009). (Both may be included in what anatomically is sometimes designated as the anterior cingulate cortex (Vogt 2009).) This area is also activated by pain but, because this area is also activated in response selection tasks such as divided attention and Stroop tasks (which involve cues that cause conflict such as the word red written in green when the task is to make a response to the green colour), it is suggested that activation of this mid-cingulate area by painful stimuli was related to the response selection processes initiated by painful stimuli (Vogt et al. 1996, Derbyshire, Vogt & Jones 1998). Both the perigenual and the mid-cingulate areas may be activated in functional neuroimaging studies not only by physical pain, but also by social pain, for example being excluded from a social group (Eisenberger & Lieberman 2004).

The mid-cingulate area may be divided into an anterior or rostral cingulate motor area (24c′) concerned with skeletomotor control which may be required in avoidance and fear tasks, and a posterior or caudal cingulate motor area (24d) which may be more involved in skeletomotor orientation (Vogt et al. 2003).

[10]Perigenual cingulate cortex refers to anterior cingulate cortex around the genu of the corpus callosum.

In macaques, lesions of the anterior cingulate cortex that include the midcingulate area do not affect working memory (measured by delayed alternation), and are in this respect different from dorsolateral prefrontal cortex lesions, but may affect task switching (Rushworth, Hadland, Gaffan & Passingham 2003, Rushworth et al. 2004).

In human imaging studies it has been found that the anterior/mid-cingulate cortex is activated when there is a change in response set or when there is conflict between possible responses, but it is not activated when only stimulus selection is at issue (van Veen, Cohen, Botvinick, Stenger & Carter 2001, Rushworth, Hadland, Paus & Sipila 2002).

Some anterior/mid-cingulate neurons respond when errors are made (Niki & Watanabe 1979, Gemba, Sasaki & Brooks 1986), or when rewards are reduced (Shima & Tanji 1998) (and activations are found in corresponding imaging studies, Bush, Vogt, Holmes, Dales, Greve, Jenike & Rosen (2002)). In humans, an event-related potential (ERP), called the error related negativity (ERN), may originate in the area 24c′ (Ullsperger & von Cramon 2001), and many studies provide evidence that errors made in many tasks activate the anterior/mid-cingulate cortex, whereas tasks with response conflict activate the superior frontal gyrus (Rushworth et al. 2004).

Correspondingly, in rodents a part of the medial prefrontal / anterior cingulate cortex termed the prelimbic cortex is involved in learning relations between behavioural responses and reinforcers, that is between actions and outcomes (Balleine & Dickinson 1998, Cardinal et al. 2002, Killcross & Coutureau 2003). Balleine & Dickinson (1998) showed that the sensitivity of instrumental behaviour to whether a particular action was followed by a reward was impaired by prelimbic cortex lesions. When making decisions about actions, it is important to take into account the costs as well as the benefits. There is some evidence implicating the rodent anterior cingulate cortex (prelimbic cortex) in this, in that rats with prelimbic cortex lesions were impaired in a task that required decisions about an action with a large reward but a high barrier to climb, vs an action with a lower reward but no barrier (Walton, Bannerman & Rushworth 2002, Walton et al. 2003).

To perform action–outcome learning, the anterior/mid-cingulate cortical area must contain a representation of the behavioural action just performed, and receive information about rewards and punishers being obtained. The reward-related information may come from structures such as the orbitofrontal cortex and amygdala. In addition, the cortical area involved in action–outcome learning must be able to hold the representation of the action just performed in a type of working memory until the reward or punishment is received (or more probably receive delay-related information from the prefrontal cortex, see Rushworth et al. (2004)), as there may be a delay between the action and the outcome. Attractor networks that maintain a representation of an action that has been made may be a key part of the computation performed in the mid- and anterior cingulate regions, allowing the memory of an action to be associated with the reward outcome, which may be delayed for several seconds.

It should be noted that stimulus–response or habit learning, although instrumental, is separate, in that it involves different associations (between stimuli and responses, not between actions and outcomes), and is implemented in different brain regions such as the basal ganglia (see Section 6.3).

It is useful to place action–outcome learning in the wider context of emotion. When stimuli are presented, they are decoded to determine whether they are primary rewards or punishers by structures such as the orbitofrontal cortex and amygdala. If the stimulus presented has been associated with a primary reward or punisher, this stimulus–stimulus association is also decoded in the orbitofrontal cortex and amygdala. Affective states, and autonomic responses, can be produced by these processes, subjective states are influenced, and choices of stimuli to select are determined. When reinforcer contingencies change, the orbitofrontal cortex is important in reversing the stimulus–stimulus association, and contains appropriate error neurons. It thus seems to be able to implement stimulus selection. The orbitofrontal cortex is involved in this way in decision-making and executive function. On the other hand, if more complex contingencies are operating so that actions that give rise to particular outcomes must be selected, then this clearly requires a representation of actions, and it may be for these situations that the anterior cingulate cortex is especially important. Much affective computation, including the elicitation of affective states, may thus not computationally require the anterior cingulate cortex; but if to obtain the goal particular responses must be selected, then in those affective situations the anterior cingulate cortex may be especially computationally important. We return to the different types of decision-making in Section 11.2.

4.8 Value-related decision-making and medial prefrontal cortex area 10

4.8.1 Decision-making between the value of odours

The evidence described in Section 4.5.5.2 indicates that the primate including human orbitofrontal cortex includes a representation of expected reward value on a continuous scale. Now if we wish to make a decision between the value of two or more stimuli, for example odours, a different representation is needed that is categorical and not continuous, and which identifies which of the two or more stimuli is categorised as more pleasant or rewarding. The categorization requires a choice or decision. To investigate whether there are separate brain regions involved in choices between the value of stimuli, Rolls, Grabenhorst & Parris (2010d) analysed brain responses while humans performed an olfactory decision-making or rating task illustrated in Fig. 4.65.

The olfactory decision-making task was designed (Rolls, Grabenhorst & Parris 2010d) based on the vibrotactile decision-making studies of Romo and colleagues in which vibrotactile stimuli separated by a delay were presented, and a decision had to be made, when the second stimulus was presented, of whether the second frequency was higher than the first (Romo, Hernandez & Zainos 2004). In our design the decision was about whether the second odour was more pleasant than the first, or on other trials was more intense than the first (see Fig. 4.65). To allow a comparison with trials on which choices between stimuli were not made, there were also trials in which only ratings of the continuous affective value and intensity were made, without a choice between stimuli, as described in detail by Rolls et al. (2010d).

The fMRI signals in the medial prefrontal cortex area 10, and in regions to which it projects including the anterior cingulate cortex and insula, were higher when decisions were being made compared to ratings, implicating these regions in decision-making. For comparison, the mid-orbitofrontal cortex had activations related not to decision-making, but to subjective pleasantness ratings, providing a continuous representation of affective value (Rolls et al. 2010d). The medial prefrontal cortex area 10 region activated by the olfactory value decision-making was very close to that illustrated in Fig. 4.66 for thermal value decision-making.

4.8.2 Decision-making between the value of thermal somatosensory stimuli

To further investigate whether representing the affective value of a reward on a continuous scale may occur before and separately from making a binary, for example yes-no, decision about whether to choose the reward, Grabenhorst, Rolls & Parris (2008b) used fMRI in humans to measure activations produced by pleasant warm, unpleasant cold, and affectively complex

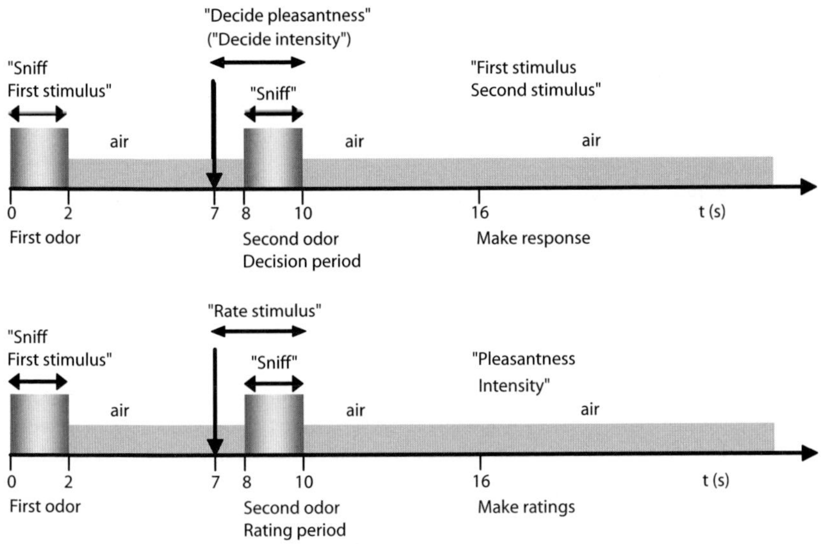

Fig. 4.65 Task design for trials of the olfactory task. On decision trials (upper), the task required a binary choice decision starting during the second odour about which of the two odours was more pleasant, or (on different trials, as indicated by the instruction at t=7 s) more intense. On rating trials (lower), identical stimuli were used, but no decision was required, and instead participants rated the second odour for pleasantness and intensity on continuous analog visual rating scales. The trial types were identical until t=7 s, when the instruction indicated whether the trial type was decide or rate. The second odour was delivered at t=8 s, the subjects were deciding or rating at that time, and the imaging was with respect to this period starting at t=8 s. No responses to indicate the decision made or the rating value could be made until t=16 s. (Reproduced from E.T. Rolls, F. Grabenhorst, and B. A. Parris, Neural systems underlying decisions about affective odors, *Journal of Cognitive Neuroscience*, Volume 22, No. 5, May 2010, pages 1069–1082 ©2010, MIT Press Journals with permission.)

combinations of these stimuli applied to the hand. On some trials the affective value was rated on a continuous scale, and on different trials a Yes-No (binary choice) decision was made about whether the stimulus should be repeated in future. When decision-making was contrasted with just rating the affective stimuli, activations were revealed in the medial prefrontal cortex area 10, implicating this area in choice decision-making (Grabenhorst et al. 2008b) (see Fig. 4.66). Activations that were continuously related to the pleasantness ratings and which were not influenced when a binary (choice) decision was made were found in the orbitofrontal and pregenual cingulate cortex, further implicating these regions in the continuous representation of affective value (Section 4.5).

4.8.3 Value-related decision-making and the medial prefrontal cortex area 10: further evidence

Further evidence implicating medial prefrontal cortex area 10 in value-related decision-making is that activations in this region increase linearly with the easiness of the decision-making task, as is predicted by the model of decision-making in the brain, as described in Chapter 8, and illustrated in Figs. 8.19 on page 404 and Fig. 8.20. The hypothesis is that the orbitofrontal cortex represents value on a continuous scale, and that medial prefrontal cortex area 10, especially in its more anterior part, is involved in the highly nonlinear mechanism of making choices between stimuli or goods of different value. The hypothesis is further that the pregenual cingulate cortex receives from the orbitofrontal cortex, and contains value-based

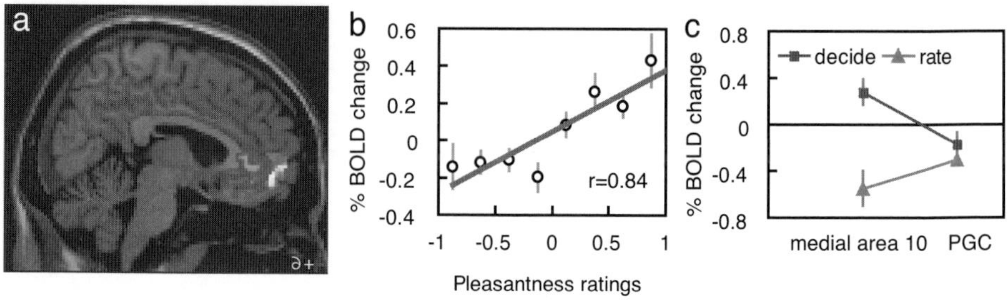

Fig. 4.66 Value-related decision-making and medial prefrontal cortex area 10. (a) A contrast between all trials on which decisions were made and all trials on which ratings were made between thermal stimuli showed a significant effect in the medial prefrontal cortex area 10, as indicated in red ([6 54 -8]). This contrast showed no significant difference in the pregenual cingulate cortex. However, in the pregenual cingulate cortex, as shown in blue, there was a strong and significant correlation with the pleasantness ratings ([4 38 -2]). (b) Shows that the % BOLD signal in the pregenual cingulate cortex was correlated with the pleasantness ratings on the trials on which ratings were made ($r=0.84$, $df=7$, $p=0.005$). (c) Compares the activations (mean $\pm$ sem) in medial area 10 with those in the pregenual cingulate cortex (PGC) for decision and rating trials. There was a significant interaction ($p=0.015$). (See colour plates section.) (Reproduced from Fabian Grabenhorst, Edmund T. Rolls, and Benjamin A. Parris, From affective value to decision-making in the prefrontal cortex, *European Journal of Neuroscience*, 28 (9) pp. 1930–1939, Copyright ©2008, John Wiley and Sons.)

representations used for action–outcome learning. The anterior cingulate cortex also provides a potential route to action from medial prefrontal cortex area 10. Some of the evidence consistent with these hypotheses is that across many different investigations, value based representations tend to be more posterior in the ventromedial prefrontal cortex (VMPFC) (Tier 2 in Fig. 4.2), whereas activations implicated in choice decision-making (Tier 3 in Fig. 4.2) tend to be more anterior, as shown in Fig. 4.67. (The term VMPFC is used to describe a large region of the medial prefrontal cortex that includes parts of the anterior cingulate cortex anterior and ventral to the genu of the corpus callosum, much of the orbitofrontal cortex, and the medial prefrontal cortex area 10. The term VMPFC was used to describe the large region of damage in the patients studied by Bechara, Damasio & Damasio (2000) and illustrated in their Fig. 1. These different areas are indicated in Fig. 4.18.)

Medial prefrontal cortex area 10 is also implicated in decision-making by the criterion used by others (Heekeren, Marrett, Bandettini & Ungerleider 2004, Heekeren, Marrett & Ungerleider 2008) that activation should increase with task easiness, that is with ΔI (Rolls, Grabenhorst & Deco 2010b). Medial area 10 is also implicated in decision-making in that a shopping decision-making task is impaired by medial prefrontal cortex damage (Burgess 2000).

4.9 Insula

There is some evidence that the face expression of disgust involves special processing by the insula. Not only is there some evidence that the insula can be differentially activated by the face expression of disgust (Phillips 2004, Phillips, Williams, Heining, Herba, Russell, Andrew, Bullmore, Brammer, Williams, Morgan, Young & Gray 2004), but also patient NK with an insular lesion is impaired on disgust face and voice expression identification, and on

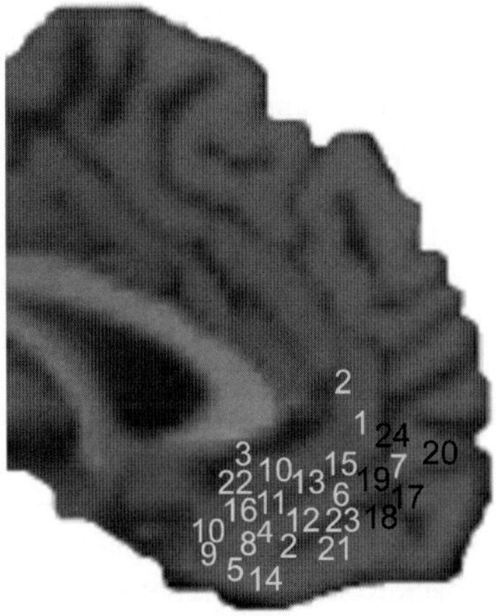

Fig. 4.67 Value-related decision-making and the ventromedial prefrontal cortex. Activations implicated primarily in value-based decision-making (black) or in representing value (yellow) are as follows: 1: (economic) subjective value during intertemporal choice; 2: immediate vs delayed choices; 3: immediate vs delayed primary rewards; 4: expected value during probabilistic decision-making; 5: expected value based on social and experience-based information; 6: expected value of the chosen option; 7: price differential during purchasing decisions; 8: willingness to pay; 9: goal value during decisions about food cues; 10: choice probability during exploitative choices; 11: conjunction of stimulus- and action-based value signals; 12: goal value during decisions about food stimuli; 13: willingness to pay for different goods; 14: willingness to pay for lottery tickets; 15: subjective value of charitable donations; 16: decision value for exchanging monetary against social rewards; 17: binary choice vs valuation of thermal stimuli; 18: binary choice vs valuation of olfactory stimuli; 19: easy vs difficult binary choices about thermal stimuli; 20: easy vs difficult binary choices about olfactory stimuli; 21: value of chosen action; 22: difference in value between choices; 23: prior correct signal during probabilistic reversal learning; 24: free vs forced charitable donation choices. Some of the most anterior activations in the VMPFC area, in medial area 10 (activations 17-20 and 24, shown in blue) were associated with binary choice; the activations related to value tend to be less anterior in the VMPFC. (See supplementary material of Grabenhorst and Rolls 2011 for references to the original studies.) (See colour plates section.) (Reprinted from *Trends in Cognitive Sciences*, 15 (2), Fabian Grabenhorst and Edmund T. Rolls, Value, pleasure and choice in the ventral prefrontal cortex, pp. 56–67, Copyright, 2011, with permission from Elsevier.)

self-experience of disgust (Calder, Keane, Manes, Antoun & Young 2000). However, to place this into perspective, we have recently described a patient with a right amygdala lesion with an impairment of the recognition of disgust face expressions (Gallo, Gamiz, Perez-Garcia, Del Moral & Rolls 2013).

In a neuroeconomics study with monetary reward, it was found that expected value was negatively correlated with activations in the anterior insula [–38 24 16] in a region that has been implicated in disgust, and interestingly, the activations here were also correlated with the uncertainty of the magnitude of the reward that would be obtained (Rolls, McCabe & Redoute 2008e). Effectively there was more insula activation in situations that might be described as aversive. In a bargaining game which is a probe for fairness, the ultimatum game (Montague, King-Casas & Cohen 2006), insula activation was produced by unfair offers (Sanfey, Rilling, Aronson, Nystrom & Cohen 2003). [In the one-round ultimatum game, a pair of players is given an endowment, say $100. The first player proposes a split of the money to the second player, who can respond by either accepting the proposal (take it) or rejecting it (leave it). If the proposal is rejected, neither player receives any money. A rational agent model predicts that proposers should offer as little as possible, and responders should accept whatever they are offered because something is better than nothing. However, responders routinely reject offers less than about 20% of the endowment, and, correspondingly, proposers routinely offer significant amounts. Thus humans routinely act with a sense of 'fairness' in the ultimatum game. While this is not in their short-term interest, it is a strategy or heuristic that may have evolved to promote reciprocation and in the long run mutual benefit for reciprocators.]

Craig has suggested that not only are the human insular cortices involved in processing body feelings (such as pain, pleasure, and temperature) and feelings of emotions (Craig et al. 2000, Damasio, Grabowski, Bechara, Damasio, Ponto, Parvizi & Hichwa 2000), but further, that the insular cortices are the necessary and sufficient platform for feeling states in humans and are, in effect, the sole source of their experience (Craig 2009, Craig 2011).

Damasio has suggested in his somatic marker hypothesis of emotion (Damasio 1996) that the insula and related somatosensory cortical areas play a crucial role in emotion and decision-making, by receiving feedback from the periphery that results in an emotion-related decision being made. A quotation from Damasio (1994) (page 190) follows: "The squirrel did not really think about his various options and calculate the costs and benefits of each. He saw the cat, was jolted by the body state, and ran." Data that appear to support this are that visually based recognition and naming of emotions from face expression was found to be severely impaired by dysfunction in right hemisphere regions that process somatosensory information, even in the absence of damage to visual cortices. Specifically, lesions in right somatosensory-related cortices, notably including SI, SII, anterior supramarginal gyrus, and the insula, were associated with impaired recognition of emotions from human facial expressions (Adolphs, Damasio, Tranel, Cooper & Damasio 2000a).

Menon & Uddin (2010) have suggested that the insula is part of a 'salience' network. They postulate that the insula is sensitive to salient events, and that its core function is to mark such events for additional processing and initiate appropriate control signals.

These observations and thoughts (Berntson, Norman, Bechara, Bruss, Tranel & Cacioppo 2011) lead one to ask whether the insula is a crucial computational centre for emotion, decision-making, and even saliency. The following parsimonious points may be made.

First, the anterior part of the insula contains the primary taste cortex (Fig. 4.2), where neurons fire to tastes independently of hunger, where activations are linearly related to the intensity but not the pleasantness of the taste, and where some neurons respond also to oral viscosity, to oral temperature, and to fat texture in the mouth, but do not respond to visual or olfactory stimuli in discrimination tasks in which a taste or flavour is the reward (Sections 5.4.2.1 and 4.5.5.1, and Chapter 5). Thus the primary taste cortex contains a representation of what the taste is, and not of its outcome value, expected value, or emotional / affective properties. In an even more anterior part of the insula (agranular cortex), there is a region that responds to both taste and odour stimuli (De Araujo, Rolls, Kringelbach, McGlone & Phillips 2003c, McCabe & Rolls 2007).

Second, there is a visceral / autonomic part of the anterior insula that is probably just ventral to the taste insula. This receives visceral inputs from the thalamus (ventral posteromedial nucleus (Carmichael & Price 1995b)), and projects to the orbitofrontal cortex. (The insular cortex neurons are probably the ventral group of insular cortex cells shown in Fig. 4.48 (Baylis, Rolls & Baylis 1994)). Some of the connections of this insular cortical region, including its connections with the anterior cingulate cortex, are shown in Fig. 4.68, which indicates that this part of the anteroventral insula may be thought of as the primary visceral cortex, with important functions on the efferent side in regulating autonomic output via the vagus and sympathetic nerves. This part of the insula has activations that are related to visceral / autonomic function, for example to heart and stomach responses during disgust-associated nausea (Harrison et al. 2010, Critchley & Harrison 2013, Nagai et al. 2004). Further, Krolak-Salmon, Henaff, Isnard, Tallon-Baudry, Guenot, Vighetto, Bertrand & Mauguiere (2003) found that electrical stimulation in the antero-ventral insula produced feelings related to disgust, including viscero-autonomic feelings. Moreover, it is of course to be expected, and is the case, that the autonomic output and the corresponding visceral insular activity will be different for different emotional states, e.g. when eating a food vs when reacting to the disgusting bitter taste of quinine or to pain or the sight of aversive or unpleasant stimuli (Harrison et al. 2010, Critchley & Harrison 2013).

Based on evidence of this type, I make the parsimonious hypothesis that the role of the anterior insula in emotion, disgust including face expressions of disgust, and salience, is that it receives inputs from cortical areas such as the anterior cingulate cortex and orbitofrontal cortex that are involved in the fundamental computations for emotion, and, as the 'head ganglion' of the autonomic nervous system, the anteroventral insula is involved in producing autonomic responses, via pathways of the type illustrated in Fig. 4.68.

Third, the mid- and posterior insula has somatosensory representations of the body (Mufson & Mesulam 1982). A property that may be special about these somatosensory cortical representations is that activations are produced by touch to the body but, in contrast to many other somatosensory cortical areas, not by the sight of touch (McCabe, Rolls, Bilderbeck & McGlone 2008). It was therefore suggested that insular cortex activation thus allows an individual to know that it is touch to the person's body, and not that someone else's body is about to be touched (McCabe, Rolls, Bilderbeck & McGlone 2008). The insular somatosensory cortex may thus provide evidence about what is happening to one's own body (Rolls 2010c). The same might be said of the insular primary taste cortex, which when activated leaves no doubt that one is tasting, and not seeing someone else tasting. So, in a sense, feelings associated with activations of the insular cortex (and they are: the subjective intensity of taste is linearly related to the activation of the primary taste cortex) do inform one about the state of one's own body, and this relates to Craig's suggestions (2009, 2011) about interoceptive feelings. However, this does not mean that the insular cortex is necessary for body feelings, and indeed that seems to be ruled out by the finding that a patient with extensive bilateral damage to the insular cortex reported normal body / emotional feelings (Damasio, Damasio & Tranel 2013).

Finally, the insular somatosensory representations do not appear to be affective, i.e. they do not encode the pleasantness of somatosensory stimuli. In an fMRI investigation in humans, it was found that activations in the somatosensory cortex and ventral posterior insula were correlated with the intensity ratings but not the pleasantness ratings of thermal stimuli, which were warm (41°C), cold (12°C) stimuli, and combinations of warm and cold stimuli, applied to the hand (see Fig. 4.69d-f) (Rolls, Grabenhorst & Parris 2008b). In contrast, the mid-orbitofrontal and pregenual cingulate cortex and a region to which they project, the ventral striatum, had activations that correlated with the subjective pleasantness ratings made to thermal stimuli (Fig. 4.69a-c) (Rolls et al. 2008b).

4.10 Human brain imaging investigations of mood and depression

Brain regions involved in mood and in depression (which has biological and cognitive aspects (Clark & Beck 2010)) have been investigated by mood induction in normal subjects; and by measuring the changes in activity associated with depression, and its treatment by

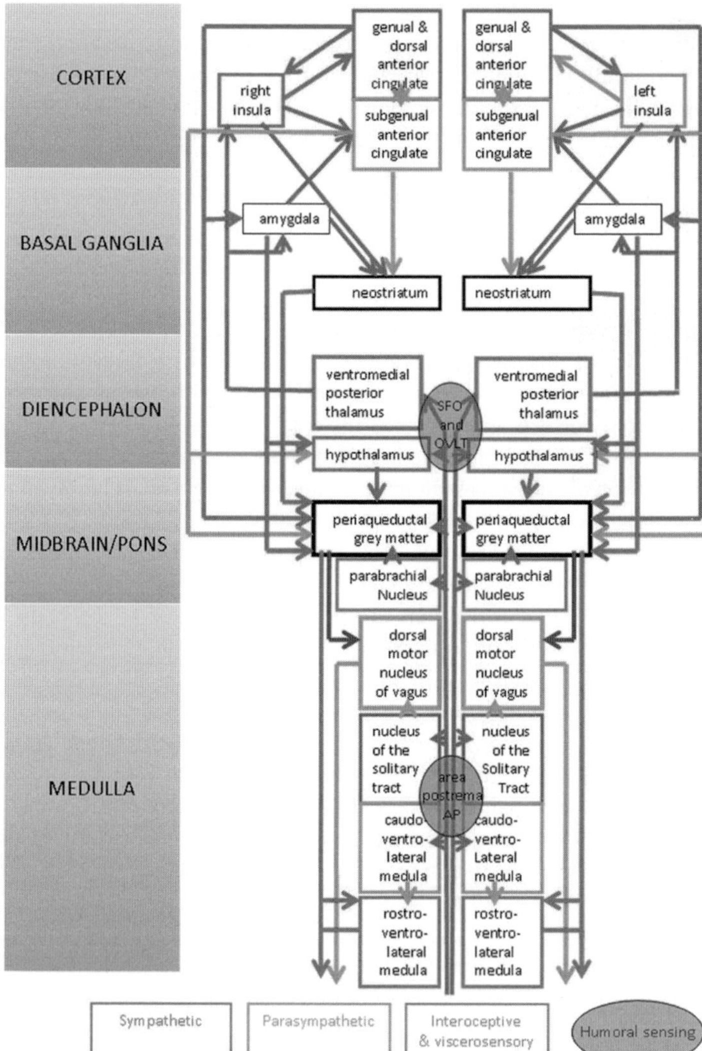

Fig. 4.68 Afferent and efferent neural pathways mediating autonomic system function. Brain regions are linked according to their association with visceral afferent sympathetic and parasympathetic function. SFO: Subfornical organ. OVLT: organum vasculosum of the lamina terminalis. (See colour plates section.) (Reprinted from *Neuron*, 77 (4), Hugo D. Critchley and Neil A. Harrison, Visceral Influences on Brain and Behavior, pp. 624–638, Copyright, 2013, with permission from Elsevier.)

antidepressant drugs (Mayberg 1997, Mayberg et al. 1999, Mayberg 2003, Drevets & Raichle 1992, George, Ketter, Parekh, Herscovitch & Post 1996, Phillips et al. 2003a, Johansen-Berg et al. 2008, Hamani et al. 2011, Lozano, Giacobbe, Hamani, Rizvi, Kennedy, Kolivakis, Debonnel, Sadikot, Lam, Howard, Ilcewicz-Klimek, Honey & Mayberg 2012)).

In PET imaging studies, it has been shown that the induction of a mood of sadness in normal subjects increases glucose metabolism in a subcallosal area of the anterior cingulate cortex (Fig. 4.63 right, with the increase shown in red) (Mayberg 1997, Mayberg, Brannan, Mahurin, Jerabek, Brickman, Tekell, Silva, McGinnis, Glass, Martin & Fox 1997, Mayberg et al. 1999, Mayberg 2003, Mayberg et al. 2005, Hamani et al. 2011). Although this is labelled as Cg25, comparison with Fig. 4.71A shows that the activated area is somewhat anterior to

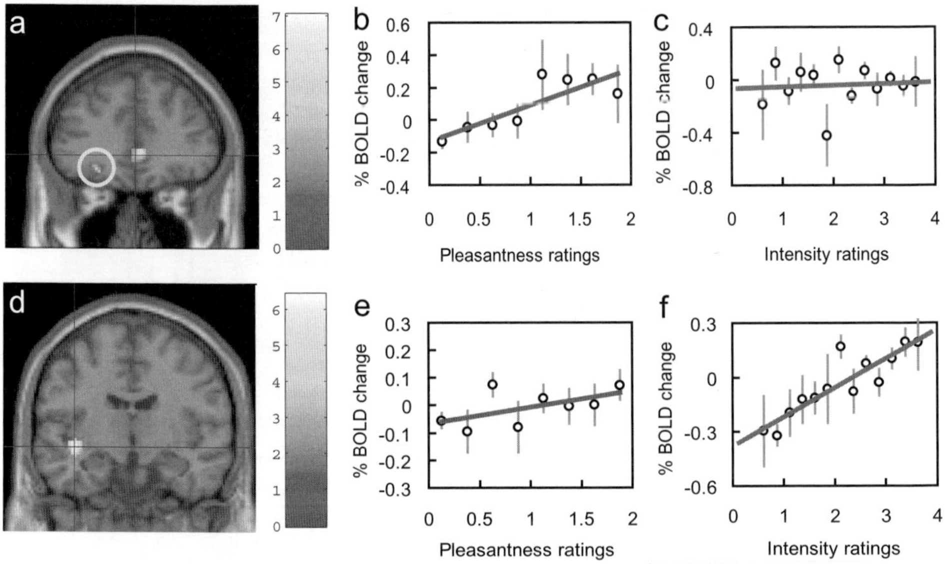

Fig. 4.69 Representation of the pleasantness but not intensity of thermal stimuli in the orbitofrontal cortex (top), and of the intensity but not the pleasantness in the mid ventral (somatosensory) insular cortex (bottom). a. SPM analysis showing a correlation in the mid orbitofrontal cortex (blue circle) at [-26 38 -10] between the BOLD signal and the pleasantness ratings of four thermal stimuli. Correlations are also shown in the pregenual cingulate cortex. For this mid orbitofrontal cortex region, (b) shows the positive correlation between the subjective pleasantness ratings and the BOLD signal ($r=0.84$, $df=7$, $p<0.01$), and (c) shows that there is no correlation between the subjective intensity ratings and the BOLD signal ($r=0.07$, $df=12$, $p=0.8$). d. SPM analysis showing a correlation with intensity in the posterior ventral insula with peak at [-40 -10 -8] between the BOLD signal and the intensity ratings for the four thermal stimuli. For this ventral insula cortex region, (e) shows no correlation between the subjective pleasantness ratings and the BOLD signal ($r=0.56$, $df=7$, $p=0.15$), and (f) shows a positive correlation between the subjective intensity ratings and the BOLD signal ($r=0.89$, $df=12$, $p<0.001$). (See colour plates section.) (Reprinted from *NeuroImage* 41, Edmund T. Rolls, Fabian Grabenhorst and Benjamin A. Parris, Warm pleasant feelings in the brain, pp. 1504–1513, Copyright, 2008 with permission from Elsevier.)

what is area 25 in humans, and could be part of area 24 and may include part of area 10m. I shall therefore refer to it as a subcallosal cingulate area. In this subcallosal area, depression is always associated with increased regional blood flow; and recovery of depression associated with fluoxetine treatment is associated with a decrease of glucose metabolism relative to the metabolism when depressed (as indicated by fluorodeoxyglucose PET) in a corresponding region (Fig. 4.70 left, with the decrease shown in green). This subcallosal area is posterior to the pregenual cingulate regions stretching down into the orbitofrontal cortex where reward value is represented and where activations are linearly related to subjective pleasure. There is now evidence that in the subcallosal area in humans that is activated in depression, single neurons in humans are more likely to respond to negative than to positive stimuli (Laxton, Neimat, Davis, Womelsdorf, Hutchison, Dostrovsky, Hamani, Mayberg & Lozano 2013).

Further evidence on depression is that chronic electrical stimulation in a region that is a little anterior and ventral to the subcallosal depression-related region and that has connections to the orbitofrontal cortex and medial prefrontal cortex area 10 has been found to relieve symptoms of treatment-resistant depression in some patients (Mayberg et al. 2005, Hamani, Mayberg, Snyder, Giacobbe, Kennedy & Lozano 2009, Hamani et al. 2011, Lozano et al.

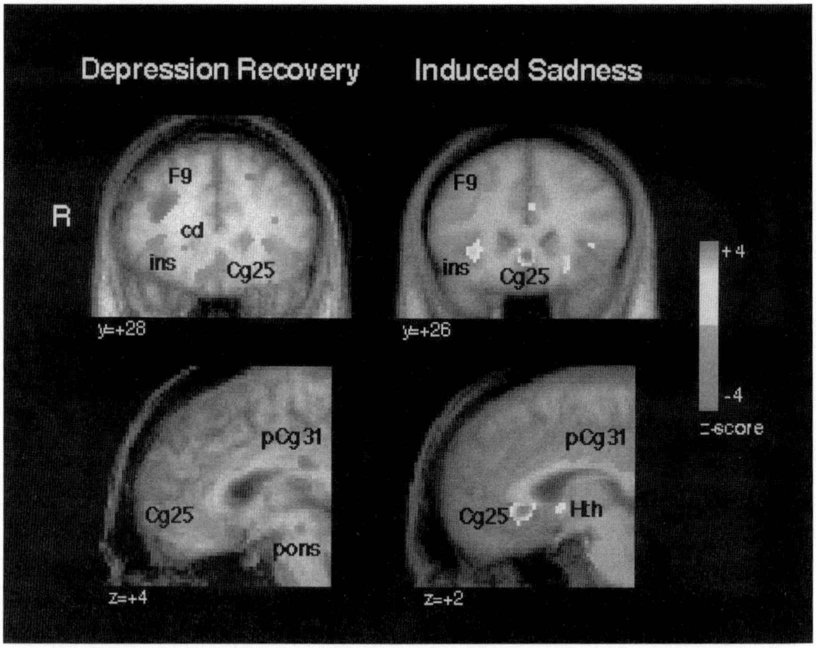

Fig. 4.70 Changes in the subgenual cingulate area (Cg25) associated with the recovery from depression (left), and with the induction of a mood state of sadness (right). Left images: Z-score maps demonstrating changes in regional glucose metabolism (fluorodeoxyglucose PET) in depressed patients following 6 weeks of treatment with the antidepressant fluoxetine. Upper: coronal view; lower, sagittal view). Green indicates that the change is a decrease, and red or yellow an increase (see calibration bar on far right). Right images: changes in regional cerebral blood flow (oxygen-15 water PET) in healthy volunteers 10 min after induction of acute sadness. The recovery from depression and the induction of sadness produce opposite changes in Cg25. Reciprocal changes were seen in a dorsal part of the prefrontal cortex, labelled F9. F, frontal; cd, caudate nucleus; ins, anterior insula; Cg25, subgenual cingulate; Hth, hypothalamus; pCG31, posterior cingulate; R, right. (See colour plates section.) (Reproduced from H. S. Mayberg, M. Liotti, S. K. Brannan, S. McGinnis, R. K. Mahurin, P. A. Jerabek, J. A. Silva, J. L. Tekell, C. C. Martin, J. L. Lancaster, and P. T. Fox, Reciprocal limbic-cortical function and negative mood: converging PET findings in depression and normal sadness, *American Journal of Psychiatry*, 156 (5), pp. 675–682, (c) 1999, American Psychiatric Association.)

2012). Some of the sites where the electrical stimulation was successful are shown by circles in Fig. 4.71B.

In attempts to understand these findings, the following points can be made.

First, there is no great consistency between individuals in exactly where in the anterior cingulate cortex sadness induces activations when measured in fMRI investigations (Smith, Fadok, Purcell, Liu, Stonnington, Spetzler & Baxter 2011), though the subcallosal cingulate cortex is frequently mentioned in this context (Price & Drevets 2012).

Second, anterior and ventral to the subcallosal area there is an extensive region, extending from the medial orbitofrontal cortex to the pregenual cingulate cortex, where rewarding, pleasant, stimuli produce activation (Section 4.5). An example is shown in Fig. 4.44, and a map of sites where activations were related to subjective pleasantness is shown in Fig. 4.47. The implication is that many neurons in this region are normally activated by rewarding, pleasant, stimuli.

Third, when the electrical stimulation is turned on in patients receiving deep brain stimulation for depression, there is within 15 s a feeling of reduced anxiety and tenseness, and within 30 s a feeling that the patient wants to do things, i.e. a reduction of the amotivational

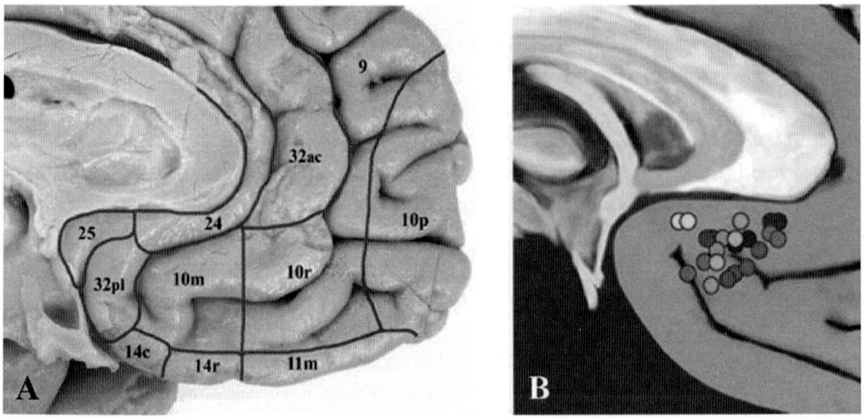

Fig. 4.71 (A) Architectonic subdivision of the medial surface of the human brain according to Ongur, Ferry and Price 2003 (reprinted with permission). (B) Location of deep brain stimulation electrodes in patients with depression who responded to the stimulation. Note that contacts used for chronic stimulation (circles) were clustered in the subcallosal region, not only in cingulate areas 25, 24, and 32pl but also 10m. (Reproduced from *Journal of Neurosurgery*, December, 2009, 111 (6), Deep brain stimulation of the subcallosal cingulate gyrus for depression: anatomical location of active contacts in clinical responders and a suggested guideline for targeting, Hamani, pp. 1209–1215, figure 3, (c) 2009, American Association of Neurological Surgeons http://thejns.org/)

aspect of depression (A.M. Lozano, personal communication, June 2013). The implication is that the electrical stimulation that is useful in the treatment of depression works, at least in part, rapidly, and does not require weeks for some antidepressant effect to develop. The effect of the stimulation is thus at least in part like that in brain-stimulation reward sites in macaques, which has been shown to activate neurons involved in natural rewards (Rolls 2005b, Mora, Avrith, Phillips & Rolls 1979, Rolls, Burton & Mora 1980, Mora, Avrith & Rolls 1980). The positively affective results produced by stimulation in what is a reward-related region antero-ventral to the subcallosal depression-related region in humans does appear to provide a rationale for the treatment of depression by stimulation in this particular region. It would be of interest to know whether similarly therapeutic effects would be found by deep brain stimulation of the orbitofrontal cortex; or of medial prefrontal cortex area 10, which is activated when the stimulation is effective (Lujan et al. 2013). A prediction might even be made that stimulation of the orbitofrontal cortex might be more effective in relieving mood aspects / sadness in depressed patients, whereas stimulation of the pregenual cingulate cortex might be especially effective in treating amotivational aspects of depression, given the role of the anterior cingulate cortex in action–outcome learning. However, what was found with brain-stimulation reward in macaques was that stimulation at any one of several reward sites including the orbitofrontal cortex, nucleus accumbens, amygdala, and lateral hypothalamus / medial forebrain bundle region would activate neurons in the other brain-stimulation reward sites (Rolls et al. 1980).

Fourth, and related to the previous point, tractography (using diffusion tensor imaging) from the sites where deep brain stimulation is effective in relieving depression shows connections to the orbitofrontal cortex, medial prefrontal cortex area 10, nucleus accumbens, amygdala, and hypothalamus (Johansen-Berg et al. 2008, Lujan et al. 2013).

One implication of these points is that the region where the electrical stimulation has been found to be successful in treating depression is that it may be a region in which fibre bundles connecting the orbitofrontal cortex, hypothalamus, pregenual cingulate cortex, medial prefrontal cortex area 10, and amygdala may be being accessed, so that the effects need to be understood in part by taking into account our understanding of the functions of these different areas in emotion; and another implication is that these other sites may also prove fruitful in the treatment of resistant cases of depression.

Further, and in line with the implications just stated, anatomical and functional differences in the orbitofrontal cortex are found in patients with depression (Drevets 2007), in whom anhedonia is a key feature, and the orbitofrontal cortex provides inputs to the anterior cingulate cortex.

Brain networks that may be operating differently in depression have been investigated with functional neuroimaging (Hamilton, Chen & Gotlib 2013). Networks are identified by correlations between the signal levels in sets of cortical areas in the resting state or when different tasks are performed. The signal level referred to may be regional cerebral blood flow (rCBF), or the fMRI BOLD signal. In the default-mode network (DMN, identified by high signal in the resting state when no task is being performed, and which includes the posterior cingulate cortex, the parietal cortex, and the medial prefrontal cortex) depressed patients usually have high resting-state rCBF, consistent with strong ruminating thoughts when not engaged in a task. In an executive network (EN, comprising dorsolateral prefrontal and lateral parietal cortices, in which the signal correlates positively with executive task performance), in depression dorsolateral prefrontal cortex activity is reduced both at rest and in response to negative stimuli. In structures in the salience network (SN, comprising the anterior insula, amygdala, and dorsal anterior cingulate cortex in which the signals correlate positively with ratings of state anxiety), in depression there are larger activations to negative stimuli such as aversive pictures, pain, monetary loss, and sad faces.

Pharmacological investigations of depression and the effects these have on different brain systems are described in Section 6.5.

4.11 Output pathways for emotional responses

4.11.1 The autonomic and endocrine systems

The first output system introduced above in Section 4.2 and indicated in Figs. 4.2 and 4.68 is the autonomic and endocrine system. Through it changes such as increased heart rate and the release of adrenaline, which prepare the body for action, are produced by emotional stimuli. There are brainstem routes through which peripheral stimuli can produce reflex autonomic responses. In addition, there are outputs from the hypothalamus and higher regions to the autonomic brainstem centres (Schwaber, Kapp, Higgins & Rapp 1982, Critchley & Harrison 2013) (Fig. 4.68).

Structures such as the amygdala and orbitofrontal cortex can produce autonomic responses to secondary reinforcing (or classically conditioned) stimuli both directly, for example by direct connections from the amygdala to the dorsal motor nucleus of the vagus (Schwaber et al. 1982), and via the lateral hypothalamus (Rempel-Clower & Barbas 1998). For example, LeDoux et al. (1988) showed that lesions of the lateral hypothalamus (which receives from the central nucleus of the amygdala) blocked conditioned heart rate (autonomic) responses (see also Kapp et al. (1992) (Fig. 4.56)). The outputs of the orbitofrontal cortex are also involved in learned autonomic responses, in that ventral prefrontal lesions block autonomic responses to learned reinforcers (Elithorn, Piercy & Crosskey (1955) and Damasio (1994) in humans; Grueninger, Kimble, Grueninger & Levine (1965) in macaques).

Further, activation of the anterior cingulate and anterior insular cortex in humans is correlated with autonomic states (Nagai et al. 2004, Critchley & Harrison 2013), and the subgenual cingulate cortex has strong projections to brainstem structures that control autonomic activity (Gabbott et al. 2003).

4.11.2 Motor systems for implicit responses, including the basal ganglia

The second type of output is to brain systems concerned with performing actions unconsciously or implicitly, in order to obtain rewards or avoid punishers.

One such system is the cingulate cortex (Fig. 4.2) which is for action–outcome learning, where the actions are being performed in a goal directed and goal-dependent way, in that the actions stop immediately if the goal is devalued. This cingulate system in described in Section 4.7. This system is helped by mechanisms in the dorsolateral and other parts of the medial prefrontal cortex, which using short-term memories enable rules to be implemented and rapidly switched (Miller 2000a, Deco & Rolls 2003, Deco & Rolls 2005b, Rolls 2008b).

Another system is the basal ganglia, with the orbitofrontal cortex, cingulate cortex, and amygdala all having strong outputs to the striatum, especially to the ventral striatum which includes the nucleus accumbens, and the ventromedial part of the head of the caudate nucleus. Other cortical areas, including motor areas, project to other parts of the striatum, and there is the opportunity for convergence in the basal ganglia. This system is especially involved in stimulus-response learning, which is set up by reinforcers, but becomes a habit after considerable training, so no longer depends on goal value, in that just a stimulus-response connection is being made. To be very clear: devaluation of the goal, such as feeding to satiety, does not immediately stop instrumental responses being made to stimuli in this basal ganglia system, in which dopamine plays an important role in setting up the stimulus-response connections, as described in Section 6.3.

4.11.3 Output systems for explicit responses to emotional stimuli

The third type of output is to a system capable of planning many steps ahead and, for example, deferring short-term rewards in order to execute a long-term plan. This system may use syntactic processing in order to perform the planning, and is therefore part of a linguistic system that performs explicit processing. This system, discussed in Chapter 10, is the one in which explicit, declarative, processing occurs. Processing in this system is frequently associated with reason and rationality, in that many of the consequences of possible actions can be taken into account. The actual computation of how rewarding a particular stimulus or situation is, or will be, probably still depends on activity in the orbitofrontal cortex, amygdala, and anterior cingulate cortex, in that the reward value of stimuli is computed and represented in these regions, and in that it is found that verbalized expressions of the reward (or punishment) value of stimuli are dampened by damage to these systems. (For example, damage to the orbitofrontal cortex renders painful input still identifiable as pain, but without the strong affective, 'unpleasant', reaction to it.)

4.11.4 Basal forebrain and hypothalamus

It was suggested above that the hypothalamus and basal forebrain may provide one output system for the amygdala and orbitofrontal cortex for autonomic and other responses to emotional stimuli. Consistent with this, there are neurons in the lateral hypothalamus and basal forebrain of monkeys that respond to visual stimuli associated with rewards such as food (Rolls 1975, Rolls 1981a, Rolls 1981b, Rolls 1982, Rolls 1986a, Rolls 1986b, Rolls 1986c, Rolls 1990b, Rolls 1993, Rolls 1999a, Rolls, Burton & Mora 1976, Burton, Rolls &

Mora 1976, Mora, Rolls & Burton 1976a, Wilson & Rolls 1990b, Wilson & Rolls 1990c). These neurons show rapid reversal of their responses during the reversal of stimulus–reinforcer associations, reflecting inputs from the orbitofrontal cortex. Other neurons in the hypothalamus respond only to stimuli associated with punishment, that is to aversive visual stimuli (Rolls, Sanghera & Roper-Hall 1979a). The responses of these neurons with reinforcement-related activity would be appropriate for producing autonomic responses to emotional stimuli, via pathways that descend from the hypothalamus towards the brainstem autonomic motor nuclei (Saper, Loewy, Swanson & Cowan 1976, Schwaber et al. 1982, Rempel-Clower & Barbas 1998, Critchley & Harrison 2013).

It is also possible that these hypothalamic outputs could influence emotional behaviour (Hahn & Swanson 2010), through, for example, the connections from the hypothalamus to the amygdala (Aggleton, Burton & Passingham 1980), to the substantia nigra (Nauta & Domesick 1978), or even by the connections to the neocortex (Divac 1975, Kievit & Kuypers 1975, Mesulam 1990). Indeed, it is suggested that the latter projection, by releasing acetylcholine in the cerebral cortex when emotional stimuli (including reinforcing and novel stimuli) are seen, provides one way in which emotion can influence the storage of memories in the cerebral cortex (Rolls 1987, Wilson & Rolls 1990a, Wilson & Rolls 1990b, Wilson & Rolls 1990c, Rolls 2005b). In this case, the basal forebrain magnocellular neurons may act as a 'cortical strobe' which facilitates memory storage and processing when the neurons are firing fast, though does not carry a valence-specific signal (see Section 4.11.5).

4.11.5 Basal forebrain cholinergic neurons

Before leaving the learning systems in the amygdala and orbitofrontal cortex, it is useful to consider the role in memory of one of the systems to which they project, the basal forebrain magnocellular nuclei of Meynert. The cells in these nuclei lie just lateral to the lateral hypothalamus in the substantia innominata, and extend forward through the preoptic area into the diagonal band of Broca (Mesulam 1990). These cells, many of which are cholinergic, project directly to the cerebral cortex (Divac 1975, Kievit & Kuypers 1975, Mesulam 1990). These cells provide the major cholinergic input to the cerebral cortex, in that if they are lesioned the cortex is depleted of acetylcholine (Mesulam 1990). Loss of these cells does occur in Alzheimer's disease, and there is consequently a reduction in cortical acetylcholine in this disease (Mesulam 1990, Schliebs & Arendt 2011). This loss of cortical acetylcholine may contribute to the memory loss in Alzheimer's disease, although it may well not be the primary factor in the aetiology (Schliebs & Arendt 2011, Ubhi & Masliah 2013). The cholinergic systems are also important in attention as well as in memory, at least in part by maintaining synaptic transmission, for example by reducing adaptation (Picciotto, Higley & Mineur 2012, Hasselmo & Sarter 2011, Newman, Gupta, Climer, Monaghan & Hasselmo 2012, Deco & Thiele 2011).

In order to investigate the role of the basal forebrain nuclei in memory, Aigner, Mitchell, Aggleton, DeLong, Struble, Price, Wenk, Pettigrew & Mishkin (1991) made neurotoxic lesions of them in monkeys. Some impairments on a simple test of recognition memory, delayed non-match-to-sample, were found. Analysis of the effects of similar lesions in rats showed that performance on memory tasks was impaired, perhaps because of failure to attend properly (Muir, Everitt & Robbins 1994). Damage to the cholinergic neurons in this region in monkeys with a selective neurotoxin was also shown to impair memory (Easton & Gaffan 2000, Easton, Ridley, Baker & Gaffan 2002).

There are quite limited numbers of these basal forebrain neurons (in the order of thousands). Given that there are relatively few of these neurons, it is not likely that they carry the information to be stored in cortical memory circuits, for the number of different patterns that could be represented and stored is so small. (The number of different patterns that could be stored is dependent in a leading way on the number of input connections on to each neuron in a pattern associator, see Appendix 1.) With this few neurons distributed throughout the cerebral cortex, the memory capacity of the whole system would be impractically small. This argument alone indicates that they are unlikely to carry the information to be stored in cortical memory systems. Instead, they could modulate information storage in the cortex of information derived from what provides the numerically major input to cortical neurons, the glutamatergic terminals of other cortical neurons. This modulation may operate by setting thresholds for cortical cells to the appropriate value, or by more directly influencing the cascade of processes involved in long-term potentiation (see Appendix 1). There is indeed evidence that acetylcholine is necessary for cortical synaptic modifiability, as shown by studies in which depletion of acetylcholine and noradrenaline impaired cortical LTP/synaptic modifiability (Bear & Singer 1986). However, non-specific effects of damage to the basal forebrain cholinergic neurons are also likely, with cortical neurons becoming much more sluggish in their responses, and showing much more adaptation, in the absence of cholinergic inputs (Markram & Tsodyks 1996, Abbott, Varela, Sen & Nelson 1997) (see below).

The question then arises of whether the basal forebrain cholinergic neurons tonically release acetylcholine, or whether they release it particularly in response to some external influence. To examine this, recordings have been made from basal forebrain neurons, at least some of which project to the cortex (see Section 5.4.1.2) and will have been the cholinergic neurons just described. It has been found that some of these neurons respond to visual stimuli associated with rewards such as food (Rolls 1975, Rolls 1981a, Rolls 1981b, Rolls 1982, Rolls 1986a, Rolls 1986b, Rolls 1986c, Rolls 1990b, Rolls 1993, Rolls 1999a, Rolls, Burton & Mora 1976, Burton, Rolls & Mora 1976, Mora, Rolls & Burton 1976a, Wilson & Rolls 1990b, Wilson & Rolls 1990c) (see example in Fig. 5.9 on page 238), or with punishment (Rolls, Sanghera & Roper-Hall 1979a); that others respond to novel visual stimuli (Wilson & Rolls 1990a); and that others respond to a range of visual stimuli. For example, in one set of recordings, one group of these neurons (1.5%) responded to novel visual stimuli while monkeys performed recognition or visual discrimination tasks (Wilson & Rolls 1990a). A complementary group of neurons more anteriorly responded to familiar visual stimuli in the same tasks (Rolls, Perrett, Caan & Wilson 1982c, Wilson & Rolls 1990a). A third group of neurons (5.7%) responded to positively reinforcing visual stimuli in visual discrimination and in recognition memory tasks (Wilson & Rolls 1990b, Wilson & Rolls 1990c). In addition, a considerable proportion of these neurons (21.8%) responded to any visual stimuli shown in the tasks, and some (13.1%) responded to the tone cue that preceded the presentation of the visual stimuli in the task, and was provided to enable the monkey to alert to the visual stimuli (Wilson & Rolls 1990a). These neurons did not respond to touch to the leg which induced arousal, so their responses did not simply reflect arousal. Neurons in this region receive inputs from the amygdala (Mesulam 1990, Amaral et al. 1992, Russchen, Amaral & Price 1985) and orbitofrontal cortex, and it is probably via the amygdala and orbitofrontal cortex that the information described here reaches the basal forebrain neurons, for neurons with similar response properties have been found in the amygdala, and the amygdala appears to be involved in decoding visual stimuli that are associated with reinforcers, or are novel (Rolls 1990b, Rolls 1992a, Rolls 2000d, Wilson & Rolls 1993, Wilson & Rolls 2005). Neurons that respond to novel stimuli are also present in the orbitofrontal cortex (Rolls, Browning, Inoue & Hernadi 2005a).

It is therefore suggested that the normal physiological function of these basal forebrain neurons is to send a general activation signal to the cortex when certain classes of environmental stimulus occur. These stimuli are often stimuli to which behavioural activation is appropriate or required, such as positively or negatively reinforcing visual stimuli, or novel visual stimuli. The effect of the firing of these neurons on the cortex is excitatory, and in this way produces activation. This cortical activation may produce behavioural arousal, and may thus facilitate concentration and attention, which are both impaired in Alzheimer's disease. The reduced arousal and concentration may themselves contribute to the memory disorders. But the acetylcholine released from these basal magnocellular neurons may in addition be more directly necessary for memory formation, for Bear & Singer (1986) showed that long-term potentiation, used as an indicator of the synaptic modification which underlies learning, requires the presence in the cortex of acetylcholine as well as noradrenaline. For comparison, acetylcholine in the hippocampus makes it more likely that LTP will occur, probably through activation of an inositol phosphate second messenger cascade (Markram & Siegel 1992, Seigel & Auerbach 1996, Hasselmo & Bower 1993, Hasselmo, Schnell & Barkai 1995).

The adaptive value of the cortical strobe provided by the basal magnocellular neurons may thus be that it facilitates memory storage and attention especially when significant (e.g. reinforcing or novel) environmental stimuli are detected. This means that memory storage is likely to be conserved (new memories are less likely to be laid down) when significant environmental stimuli are not present. In that the basal forebrain projection spreads widely to many areas of the cerebral cortex, and in that there are relatively few basal forebrain neurons (in the order of thousands), the basal forebrain neurons do not determine the actual memories that are stored. Instead the actual memories stored are determined by the active subset of the thousands of cortical afferents on to a strongly activated cortical neuron (Treves & Rolls 1994, Rolls & Treves 1998, Rolls 2008b). The basal forebrain magnocellular neurons would then according to this analysis simply when activated increase the probability that a memory would be stored. Impairment of the normal operation of the basal forebrain magnocellular neurons would be expected to interfere with normal memory by interfering with this function, and this interference could contribute in this way to the memory disorder in Alzheimer's disease.

Another property of cortical neurons (Markram & Tsodyks 1996, Abbott et al. 1997) is that they tend to adapt with repeated input. However, this adaptation is most marked in slices, in which there is no acetylcholine. One effect of acetylcholine is to reduce this adaptation. When recordings are made from single neurons operating in physiological conditions in the awake behaving monkey, peristimulus time histograms of inferior temporal cortex neurons to visual stimuli show only limited adaptation. There is typically an onset of the neuronal response at 80–100 ms after the stimulus, followed within 50 ms by the highest firing rate. There is after that some reduction in the firing rate, but the firing rate is still typically more than half maximal 500 ms later (see example in Fig. 4.11 on page 89). Thus under normal physiological conditions, firing rate adaptation can occur, but does not involve a major adaptation, even when cells are responding fast (at e.g. 100 spikes/s) to a visual stimulus. One of the factors that keeps the response relatively maintained may however be the presence of acetylcholine. Its depletion in some disease states could lead to less sustained neuronal responses (i.e. more adaptation), and this may contribute to the symptoms found.

In summary, the basal forebrain magnocellular neurons may be activated by emotion-related stimuli received through the orbitofrontal cortex and amygdala, and may facilitate the cortex to promote memory storage and attention when emotion-related stimuli are present.

4.11.6 Noradrenergic neurons

The source of the noradrenergic projection to the neocortex is the locus coeruleus (noradrenergic cell group A6) in the pons (Cooper, Bloom & Roth 2003, Sara & Bouret 2012). (Note that noradrenaline is the same as norepinephrine.) There are a few thousand of these neurons that innervate the whole of the cerebral cortex, as well as the amygdala and other structures, so it is unlikely that the noradrenergic neurons convey the specific information stored in synapses that specifies each memory. Instead, to the extent that the noradrenergic neurons are involved in memory (including pattern association), it is likely that they would have a modulatory role on cell excitability, which would influence the extent to which the voltage-dependent NMDA receptors are activated, and thus the likelihood that information carried on specific afferents would be stored (Seigel & Auerbach 1996). Evidence that this may be the case comes from a study in which it was shown that neocortical LTP is impaired if noradrenergic and simultaneously cholinergic inputs to cortical cells are blocked pharmacologically (Bear & Singer 1986).

Further, in a study designed to show whether the noradrenergic modulation is necessary for memory, Borsini & Rolls (1984) showed that intra-amygdaloid injections of noradrenergic receptor blockers did impair the type of learning in which rats gradually learned to accept novel foods.

The function implemented by this noradrenergic input may more be general activation or arousal (Sara & Bouret 2012), rather than a signal that carries information about whether reward vs punishment has been given, for noradrenergic neurons in rats respond to both rewarding and punishing stimuli, and one of the more effective stimuli for producing release of noradrenaline is placing the feet in cool water (McGinty & Szymusiak 1988).

4.12 Effects of emotion on cognitive processing and memory

The analyses above of the neural mechanisms of emotion have been concerned primarily with how stimuli are decoded to produce emotional states, and with how these states can influence behaviour. In addition, current mood state can affect the cognitive evaluation of events or memories (Blaney 1986, Robinson, Watkins & Harmon-Jones 2013). For example, happy memories are more likely to be recalled when happy. Another example is that when people are in a depressed mood, they tend to recall memories that were stored when they were depressed. The recall of depressing memories when depressed can have the effect of perpetuating the depression, and this may be a factor with relevance to the aetiology and treatment of depression. Effectively in humans an attractor state may be set up between the cognitive and mood systems, which activate each other (Rolls & Stringer 2001b), and tend to perpetuate the depressed state.

A normal function of the effects of mood state on memory recall might be to facilitate continuity in the interpretation of the reinforcing value of events in the environment, or in the interpretation of an individual's behaviour by others, or simply to keep behaviour motivated to a particular goal. Another possibility is that the effects of mood on memory do not have adaptive value, but are a consequence of having a general cortical architecture with backprojections (Rolls 2008b). According to the latter hypothesis, the selection pressure is great for leaving the general architecture operational, rather than trying to find a genetic way to switch off backprojections just for the projections of mood systems back to perceptual systems, some of which are illustrated in Fig. 4.72 (cf. Rolls & Stringer (2000)).

How does mood affect memory?

It is suggested that whenever memories are stored, part of the context is stored with the memory. This is very likely to happen in associative neuronal networks such as those in the hippocampus (Rolls 1989b, Rolls 2000e, Rolls 1990c, Rolls 1996a, Treves & Rolls 1994, Rolls & Treves 1998, Rolls, Stringer & Trappenberg 2002, Rolls 2004a, Rolls & Kesner 2006, Rolls & Xiang 2006, Rolls 2008b, Rolls 2010b, Rolls 2013c). The CA3 part of the hippocampus may operate as a single autoassociative memory capable of linking together almost arbitrary co-occurrences of inputs, including inputs about emotional state that reach the entorhinal cortex

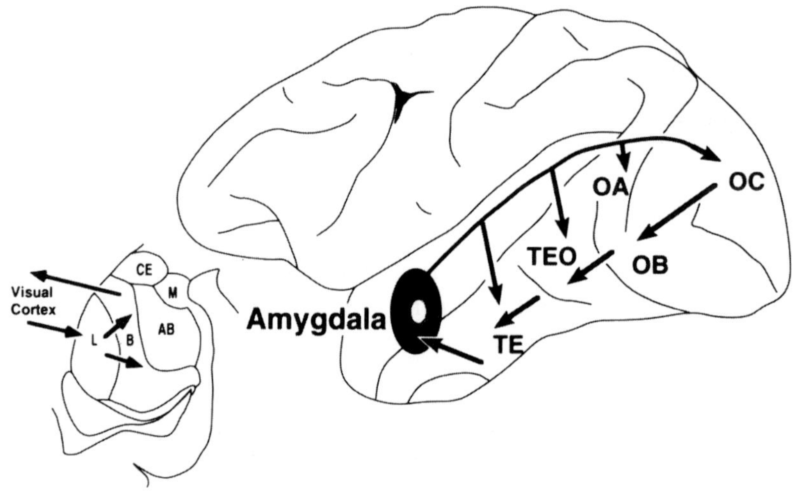

Fig. 4.72 The backprojections from the primate amygdala to the cortex spread more widely than the afferent connections, which for vision come mainly from the inferior temporal visual cortical areas, e.g. area TE. OC, striate cortex; OB, OA, prestriate visual cortical areas; TEO, posterior inferior temporal visual cortex. The insert to the left shows a coronal section of the primate amygdala, with lateral on the left, to indicate that many of the visual cortical afferents reach the lateral nucleus of the amygdala (L), and that many of the backprojections arise from the basal nucleus of the amygdala (B). CE, central nucleus of the amygdala; AB, accessory basal nucleus; M, medial nucleus. (Reproduced from D. G. Amaral, J. L. Price, A. Pitkanen, and S. T. Carmichael, Anatomical organization of the primate amygdaloid complex, in J. P. Aggleton (ed.), *The Amygdala*: Second Edition. A Functional Analysis, pp. 1–66. ©1992, WileyLiss. This material is reproduced with permission of John Wiley & Sons, Inc.)

from, for example, the amygdala. Recall of a memory occurs best in such networks when the input key to the memory is nearest to the original input pattern of activity that was stored (Rolls & Treves 1990, Treves & Rolls 1991, Treves & Rolls 1992, Treves & Rolls 1994, Rolls, Treves, Foster & Perez-Vicente 1997b, Rolls & Treves 1998, Rolls 2008b) (see Appendix 1). It thus follows that a memory of, for example, a happy episode is recalled best when in a happy mood state. This is a special case of a general theory of how context is stored with a memory, and of how context influences recall (Treves & Rolls 1994, Rolls 1996a, Rolls 2008b). The recall itself from the hippocampus is likely to use the highly developed backprojections from the hippocampus to the neocortex shown in Fig. 10.1 on page 485 (Treves & Rolls 1994, Rolls 1996a, Rolls 2008b). The effect of emotional state on cognitive processing and memory is thus suggested to be a particular case of a more general way in which context can affect the storage and retrieval of memories, or can affect cognitive processing.

There is now direct evidence that the hippocampus, which is implicated in the memory for past episodes (Rolls & Treves 1998, Rolls 1999b, Rolls et al. 2002, Rolls 2008b, Rolls 2010b), contains neurons in primates that respond to combinations of spatial information and reward information (Rolls & Xiang 2005), as described next. The ability to form associations between events including where they occur and what is present is a fundamental property of episodic memory (Treves & Rolls 1994, Rolls 1996a, Rolls & Kesner 2006, Rolls 2008b, Rolls 2010b), and this neurophysiological evidence shows that reward-related information, relevant to affect and mood, is associated with other events in the representations in the primate hippocampus (Rolls 2014e). The primate anterior hippocampus (which corresponds to the rodent ventral hippocampus) receives inputs from brain regions involved in reward processing

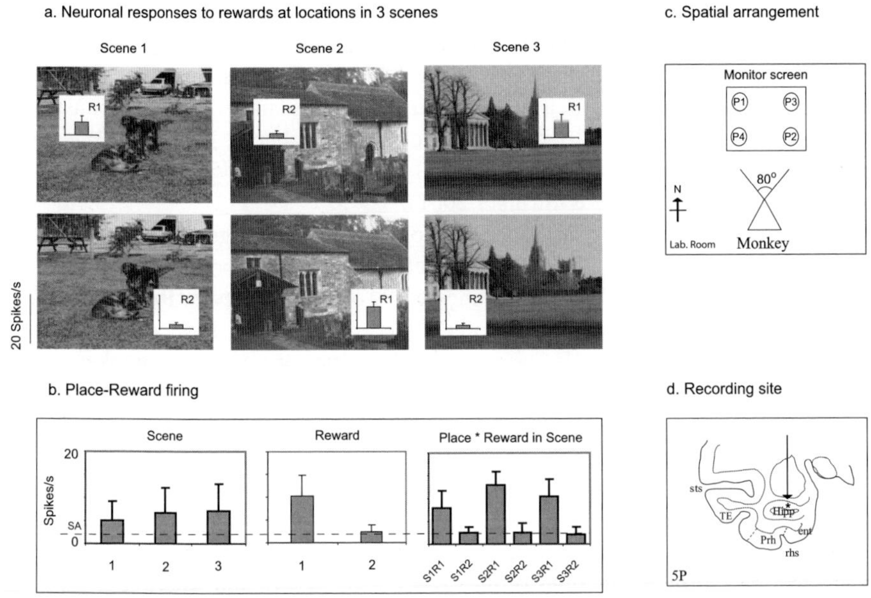

Fig. 4.73 A hippocampal neuron that encoded the particular rewards available at different locations in different scenes. On each trial the monkey could touch a circled location in the scene, and, depending on the location, received either a preferred juice reward or a less preferred juice reward. (a) Firing rate inserts to show the firing in 3 different scenes (S1–S3) of the locations associated with reward 1 (R1, preferred) and reward 2 (R2, less preferred). The mean responses ± s.e.m. are shown. SA, spontaneous firing rate. (b) The firing rates sorted by scene, by reward (1 vs 2), and by scene–reward combinations (e.g. scene 1 reward 1 = S1R1). (c) The spatial arrangement on the screen of the 4 spatial locations (P1–P4). (d) The recording site of the neuron. ent, entorhinal cortex; Hipp, hippocampal pyramidal cell field CA3/CA1 and dentate gyrus; Prh, perirhinal cortex; rhs, rhinal sulcus; sts, superior temporal sulcus; TE, inferior temporal visual cortex. (Reproduced from E. T. Rolls, and J. Z. Xiang, Reward–spatial view representations and learning in the primate hippocampus, *Journal of Neuroscience* 25, pp. 6167–6174 ©2005, Society for Neuroscience.)

such as the amygdala and orbitofrontal cortex via the entorhinal and perirhinal cortex (Amaral et al. 1992, Suzuki & Amaral 1994, Pitkanen, Kelly & Amaral 2002, Stefanacci, Suzuki & Amaral 1996, Ongur & Price 2000, Price 2006).

To investigate how this affective input may be incorporated into primate hippocampal function, Rolls & Xiang (2005) recorded neuronal activity while macaques performed a reward–place association task in which each spatial scene shown on a video monitor had one location that if touched yielded a preferred fruit juice reward, and a second location that yielded a less preferred juice reward. Each scene had different locations for the different rewards. An example of a hippocampal neuron recorded in this task is shown in Fig. 4.73. The neuron responded more to the location in each scene at which the preferred reward was available.

Of 409 neurons analysed, 16% responded more to the location of the preferred reward in different scenes, and 4% to the location of the less preferred reward (Rolls & Xiang 2005). When the locations of the preferred rewards in the scenes were reversed, 70% of 50 neurons tested reversed the location to which they responded, showing that the reward–place associations could be altered by new learning in a few trials. The majority (80%) of these 50 reward–place neurons tested did not respond to object–reward associations in a visual discrimination object–reward association task. Thus the primate hippocampus contains a representation of the reward associations of places 'out there' being viewed, and this is a way in which affective information can be stored as part of an episodic memory, and how the current mood state may influence the retrieval of episodic memories. There is consistent evidence that rewards available in a spatial environment can influence the responsiveness of rodent place neurons (Hölscher, Jacob & Mallot 2003a, Tabuchi, Mulder & Wiener 2003) which respond to the place where the animal is located, not to the view of a place 'out there' (Rolls 1999b, De Araujo, Rolls & Stringer 2001).

This discovery of reward–spatial view neurons built on findings that some hippocampal neurons in primates respond to the place at which the monkey is looking. These spatial view neurons (Rolls, Robertson & Georges-François 1997a, Rolls, Treves, Robertson, Georges-François & Panzeri 1998b, Robertson, Rolls & Georges-François 1998, Rolls 1999b, Rolls & Xiang 2006, Rolls 2010b) code for particular locations at which the monkey is looking in allocentric (world-based rather than egocentric) space, and do not encode the place where the monkey is located (Georges-François, Rolls & Robertson 1999, Rolls, Treves, Robertson, Georges-François & Panzeri 1998b). Part of the interest of spatial view cells is that they could provide the spatial representation required to enable primates to perform object–place memory, for example remembering where they saw a person or object, which is an example of an episodic memory. Consistent with this, some hippocampal neurons respond in object–place memory tasks to combinations of the object being shown and where it is being shown in space (Rolls, Miyashita, Cahusac, Kesner, Niki, Feigenbaum & Bach 1989a, Rolls, Xiang & Franco 2005c). Further evidence for this convergence of spatial and object information in the hippocampus is that in another memory task for which the hippocampus is needed, learning where to make spatial responses conditional on which picture is shown, some primate hippocampal neurons respond to a combination of which picture is shown, and where the response must be made (Miyashita, Rolls, Cahusac, Niki & Feigenbaum 1989, Cahusac, Rolls, Miyashita & Niki 1993). Thus the primate hippocampus contains a representation of places 'out there', and can combine this information by associative learning not only with which object is present at the viewed location (Rolls, Xiang & Franco 2005c, Rolls & Xiang 2006), but also with which reward is present at the viewed location (Rolls & Xiang 2005).

The general principle here then is that the hippocampus may store information about where emotion-related (e.g. rewarding) events happened; may take part in the recall of emotions when particular places are seen again; is part of a hippocampus-related limbic system that is largely independent of limbic structures involved in emotion (Rolls 2014e); and may provide a system in which the current mood can influence which memories are recalled (Rolls & Xiang 2006, Rolls 2008b, Rolls 2010b).

Another brain system where effects of mood on storage and recall could be instantiated is in the backprojection system from structures important in emotion such as the amygdala and orbitofrontal cortex to parts of the cerebral cortex important in the representation of objects, such as the inferior temporal visual cortex (see Fig. 4.72), and more generally, to parts of the cerebral cortex involved in storing memories. It is suggested (Rolls 2008b, Rolls 1989b, Rolls 1989c, Rolls 1990a, Treves & Rolls 1994, Rolls & Treves 1998, Rolls 2000f, Rolls 2008b) that co-activity between forward inputs and backprojecting inputs to strongly activated cortical pyramidal cells would lead to both sets of synapses being modified (see Fig. 4.74). This could result in facilitation or recall of cortical representations (for example of particular faces) that had become associated with emotional states, represented by activity in the amygdala (see further Rolls (1990b)).

Rolls & Stringer (2001b) (see also Rolls (1989b, 2005b, 2008b)) have developed a theory of how the effects of mood on memory and perception could be implemented in the brain. The architecture, shown in Fig. 4.75, uses the massive backprojections from parts of the brain where mood is represented, such as the orbitofrontal cortex and amygdala, to the cortical

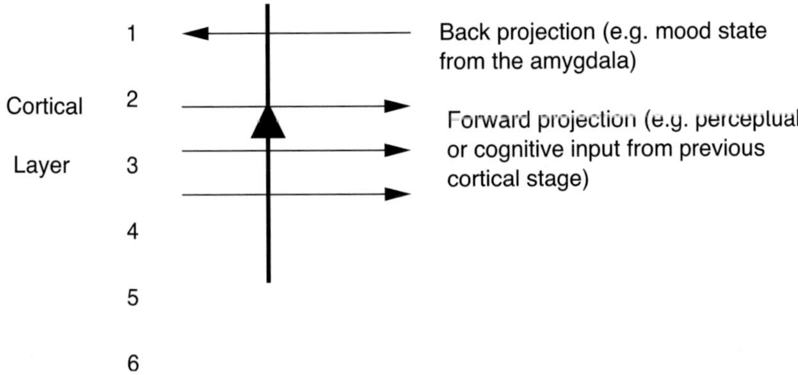

Fig. 4.74 Pyramidal cells in, for example, layers 2 and 3 of the temporal lobe association cortex receive forward inputs from preceding cortical stages of processing, and also backprojections from the amygdala. It is suggested that the backprojections from the amygdala make modifiable synapses on the apical dendrites of cortical pyramidal cells during learning when amygdala neurons are active in relation to a mood state; and that the backprojections from the amygdala via these modified synapses allow mood state to influence later cognitive processing, for example by facilitating some perceptual representations.

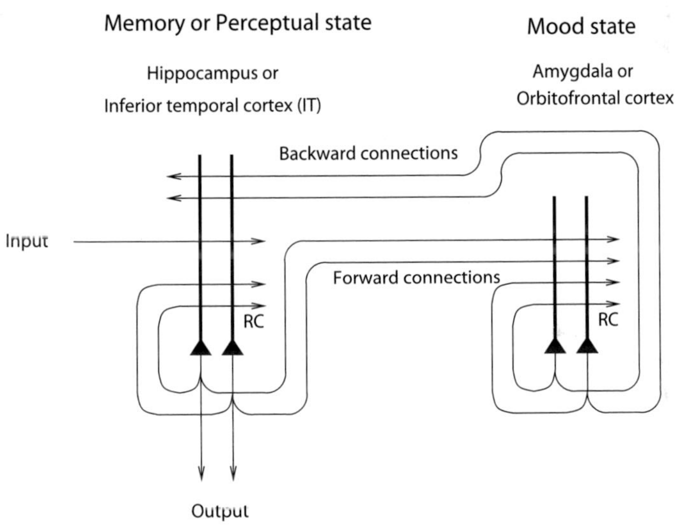

Fig. 4.75 Architecture used to investigate how mood can affect perception and memory. The IT module represents brain areas such as the inferior temporal cortex involved in perception and hippocampus-related cortical areas that have forward connections to regions such as the amygdala and orbitofrontal cortex involved in mood. (Reproduced from E. T. Rolls, and S. M. Stringer, *Network: Computation in Neural Systems*, A model of the interaction between mood and memory, 12 (2) pp. 89 – 109, copyright ©2001, Informa Healthcare. Reproduced with permission of Informa Healthcare.)

areas such as the inferior temporal visual cortex and hippocampus-related areas (labelled IT in Fig. 4.75) that project into these mood-representing areas (Amaral, Price, Pitkanen & Carmichael 1992, Amaral & Price 1984, Price 2006). The model uses an attractor network (see Appendix 1 Section A.3) in the mood module (labelled 'amygdala or orbitofrontal cortex' in Fig. 4.75), which helps the mood to be an enduring state, and also an attractor in the inferior temporal visual cortex (IT) (or any other cortical area that receives backprojections from the amygdala or orbitofrontal cortex). The system is treated as a system of coupled attractors (see

Appendix 1 Section A.4 and Rolls (2008b)), but with an odd twist: many different perceptual states are associated with any one mood state. Overall, there is a large number of perceptual/memory states, and only a few mood states, so that there is a many-to-one relation between perceptual/memory states and the associated mood states. The network displays the properties that one would expect (provided that the coupling parameters g (see Appendix 1, Section A.4 and Rolls (2008b)) are weak). These include the ability of a perceptual input to trigger a mood state in the 'amygdala and orbitofrontal cortex' module if there is not an existing mood, but greater difficulty to induce a new mood if there is already a strong mood attractor present; and the ability of the mood to affect via the backprojections which memories or perceptual states are triggered.

Another interesting finding was that the forward connections to the mood module from the memory module must be relatively strong, if new inputs to the memory module are to alter the firing in the mood module by overcoming an existing mood state being kept active by the recurrent collateral connections. These results are consistent with the general effects needed for forward and backward projections in the brain, namely that forward projections must be relatively strong in order to produce new firing in a module when a new (forward) input is received, and backward projections must be relatively weak, if they are to mildly implement 'top-down' constraints without dominating the activity of earlier modules (Renart, Parga & Rolls 1999a, Renart, Parga & Rolls 1999b, Renart, Moreno, Rocha, Parga & Rolls 2001, Rolls & Deco 2002, Deco & Rolls 2004, Deco & Rolls 2005c, Rolls 2008b). Consistent with this, forward projections terminate on cortical neurons closer to the cell body (where they can have a stronger influence) than long range backprojections (which typically terminate on the distal extremities of the apical dendrite of cortical neurons, in layer 1, the top layer of the cortex (Rolls & Treves 1998, Rolls 2008b, Rockland & Pandya 1979, Markov & Kennedy 2013, Markov, Vezoli, Chameau, Falchier, Quilodran, Huissoud, Lamy, Misery, Giroud, Ullman, Barone, Dehay, Knoblauch & Kennedy 2013).

An interesting property that was revealed by the model is that because of the many-to-few mapping of perceptual to mood states, an effect of a mood was that it tended to make all the perceptual or memory states associated with a particular mood more similar then they would otherwise have been (Rolls & Stringer 2001b). The implication is that the coupling parameter g for the backprojections must be quite weak, as otherwise interference increases in the perceptual/memory module (IT in Fig. 4.75).

In conclusion, emotional states may affect whether or how strongly memories are stored using the basal forebrain memory strobe (see Section 4.11.5); be stored as part of many memories in for example the hippocampus; and may influence both the recall of such memories, and the operation of cognitive processing, using backprojections in the way described in the preceding paragraphs. In turn, cognitive inputs can influence affective states, as described in Chapter 2 and Section 4.5.5.7.

4.13 Laterality effects in human emotional processing

In humans, there is some lateralization of function of emotional processing, with the right hemisphere frequently being implicated in processing face expressions, and perhaps in unconscious emotional processing (Gainotti 2012). Some of the evidence for this is reviewed next.

A first type of evidence comes from the effects of brain damage in humans (Gainotti 2012). Damage to the left hemisphere (in right handed people) is more likely to affect language, and to the right hemisphere is more likely to affect emotional processing. This may be evident, for example, in the greater probability of impairments in recognizing facial expressions after right rather than left hemisphere damage (see Etcoff (1989)). Further, patients are more likely to be depressed by a stroke if it is to the left than to the right hemisphere (see Starkstein & Robinson (1991)). This may indicate that to feel depressed, the right hemisphere is normally involved.

A second type of evidence comes from split brain patients (with the corpus callosum sectioned to prevent epilepsy on one side affecting the other side of the brain). These patients may respond behaviourally to an emotion-provoking stimulus which reaches the right hemisphere, even though they cannot specify verbally (with the left hemisphere) what they saw (Gazzaniga 1988). This is clear evidence for separate processing of implicit information about emotion in humans that can be dissociated from explicit, language-based, systems (see Section 10.3.1).

Third, when faces are flashed rapidly on a screen, there may be better performance in identifying the expression on the face when the stimulus is projected to the right than to the left hemisphere (Strauss & Moscowitsch 1981). These effects on face expression identification are not produced just because face-processing modules are lateralized to the right hemisphere: face identification deficits are not necessarily associated with face expression identification impairments.

Fourth, emotions may be more clearly expressed on the left side than the right side of the face, suggesting some specialization of the right hemisphere in controlling face expression (Nicholls, Ellis, Clement & Yoshino 2004). Consistently, while viewing faces, humans often process more, and also have a gaze bias towards, the left visual field, that is, the right side of the viewee's face is processed, explored and fixated more (Guo, Smith, Powell & Nicholls 2012). This left gaze bias may be a reflection of right hemispheric lateralization in face processing. (This has interesting implications for viewing one's own face in a mirror, where instead of viewing the right side of the face, the same strategy leads to greater fixation of the left of the face. Portrait painters may utilize this effect in making a portrait more acceptable to the portraitee, by emphasizing features in the left side of the face.) There may further be a weak specialization of the right hemisphere for negative emotions, as there is a trend for left-sided face expression to occur more for negative than positive emotions. Further, a left-sided view of the face was judged as being sadder and a right-sided view was rated as being happier (Nicholls et al. 2004). Consistent with a valence effect whereby the right hemisphere may be more related to negative (e.g. sad) emotions, Davidson, Ekman, Saron, Senulis & Friesen (1990) and Davidson (1992) have some evidence from EEG recording that for negative emotional episodes there is more activation of the right side of the brain; and for positive episodes there is more activation of the left side of the brain. However, there may be individual differences in the activation of prefrontal areas that are related to the affective reactivity of the individual (Davidson 2003).

Why should there be some lateralization of emotional processing in humans? One argument is that whenever a function does not need to be represented bilaterally due to the topology of the body (e.g. we have left and right hands, and separate representations of each hand are needed), then it is more efficient to place the group of neurons concerned with that processing close together. One advantage of placing neurons concerned with similar processing close together is that the length of the connections between the neurons will be minimized. This is important for minimizing brain size and weight, which is a significant factor in evolution. If half the neurons concerned with a particular function were on one side of the brain, and the other half were on the contralateral side, then the total length of the connections between the neurons would be large (see further Rolls & Deco (2002) Section 7.4.6, and Rolls (2008b)).

Neurons concerned with the same function are frequently interconnected for a number of reasons. One is that there are recurrent collateral axons between nearby cortical neurons concerned with the same function. One of the functions performed by these excitatory recurrent collaterals is to enable the network to act as a local attractor or autoassociation memory, so that the output of the module can take into account not only the activation produced in any one neuron, but also the activations received by the other connected neurons (see Appendix 1, Section A.3). Another way in which this is performed is by using feedback inhibitory interneurons, which are activated by many of the cortical pyramidal cells in a region. This helps not only autoassociation (and pattern association) networks to remain stable, but also is important for competitive networks, in which categorization of stimuli occurs, by effectively allowing the neurons in a population with the strongest activation by a particular stimulus to remain active (see Rolls & Treves (1998), Chapter 4, and Rolls (2008b).

A second advantage of placing neurons concerned with the same function close together is that this may simplify the wiring rules between neurons which must be implemented genetically (see further Rolls & Deco (2002) Section 7.4.6, and Rolls (2008b)). Given that there are in the order of 35,000 genes in the human genome, and more than 10^{14} synapses, it is clearly impossible for genes to specify all the connections between every neuron. Instead, the genetic rules may specify, for example, that neurons of type y receive approximately 12,000 excitatory synapses with associative long-term potentiation and heterosynaptic long-term depression from other neurons of type y in the surrounding 2 mm (this forms a recurrent collateral pathway); make approximately 12,000 excitatory synapses with associative long-term potentiation and heterosynaptic long-term depression with neurons of type z up to 4 mm away (which might be the next cortical area); receive approximately 500 synapses from neurons of type I within 2 mm (which might be GABA-containing inhibitory feedback neurons); and receive approximately 6000 inputs from neurons of type x up to 4 mm away (which might be the pyramidal cells in the preceding cortical area). This type of specification would build many of the networks found in different brain regions (see Rolls & Stringer (2000) and Rolls (2008b)).

An advantage of this type of genetic specification of connectivity between neuron types, and of keeping neurons concerned with the same computation close together, is that this minimizes the problems of guidance of axons towards their targets. If neurons concerned with the same function were randomly distributed in the brain, then finding the distant correct neurons with which to connect would be an impossible guidance problem. (As it is, some distant parts of the brain that are connected in adults are connected because the connections can be made early in development, before the different brain regions have migrated to become possibly distant.)

All these constraints imply that wherever possible neurons performing the same computation should be close together. Where there is no body-symmetry reason to have separate representations for each side of the body, then the representation would optimally be lateralized. This appears to be the case for certain aspects of emotional processing.

However, it is of interest that this lateralization of function may itself give rise to lateralization of performance. It may be because the brain mechanisms concerned with face expression identification are better represented in the right hemisphere that expression identification is better for the left half of the visual field (which might correspond to the left half of a centrally fixated face). Another possible reason for partial lateralization of human emotion may be that language is predominantly in the left hemisphere (for right-handed people). The result of this may be that although explicit (conscious, verbal) processing related to emotion (see Chapter 10) may take place in the left hemisphere, the implicit type of processing may take place preferentially where there is room in the brain, that is with a bias for the right hemisphere. The suggestion that there are these two types of output route for emotional behaviour is made in Section 4.11, and in Chapter 10. The fact that they are to some extent separate types of output processing may account for the fact that they can be placed in different modules, which happen to be to some extent in different hemispheres.

4.14 Summary

Some of the fundamental architectural and design principles of the brain for sensory, reward, and punishment information processing relevant to emotion in primates *including humans* include the following:

1. For primary reinforcers, the reward value encoding may occur after several stages of processing, as in the primate taste system in which reward is decoded only after the primary taste cortex. The architectural principle here is that in primates there is one main taste information-processing stream in the brain, via the thalamus to the primary taste cortex, and the information about the identity of the taste is not biased with modulation by how good the taste is before this. Thus the taste representation in the primary taste cortex can be used for purposes that are not reward-dependent. For example, it may be important to learn about a particular taste, even if one is not hungry. Even for the primary reinforcers of pleasant touch and pain, although there are different peripheral nerve fibres for pain and touch, it appears that the affective component in primates involves especially the activation of higher cortical areas such as the orbitofrontal cortex, as shown by functional neuroimaging studies and by the effects of damage to the orbitofrontal cortex.

2. For potential secondary reinforcers, analysis is to the stage of invariant object identification in structures such as the inferior temporal visual cortex (Tier 1 in Fig. 4.2) before reward and punisher associations are learned. The reason for this is to enable correct generalization to other instances of the same or similar objects, when a reward or punisher has been associated with as little as one instance (e.g. one view of an object) previously.

3. The representation of the object provided at the end of 'what' processing streams (e.g. the inferior temporal visual cortex) is (appropriately) in a form which is ideal as an input to pattern associators which allow the associations with primary reinforcers to be learned at the next stage of processing. The representations are appropriately encoded in that they can be decoded by dot product decoding of the type that is very neuronally plausible; are distributed so allowing excellent generalization and graceful degradation; have relatively independent information conveyed by different neurons in the ensemble thus allowing very high capacity; and allow much of the information to be read off very quickly, in periods of 20–50 ms.

4. Especially in primates, the visual processing in emotional and social behaviour requires sophisticated representation of individuals using face identity, and for this there are many neurons devoted to face processing. In addition, there is a separate system that encodes face expression, gesture, movement, and view, as all are important in social behaviour, for interpreting whether a particular individual, with his or her own reinforcement associations, is producing threats or appeasements.

5. After mainly unimodal processing to the object level, sensory systems then project into convergence zones. Those especially important for reward and punishment value, and therefore for emotion and motivation, are the orbitofrontal cortex and amygdala, where primary reinforcers are represented in terms of their value. These parts of the brain appear to be especially important in emotion and motivation not only because they are the parts of the brain where in primates the primary (unlearned) reward or punisher value of stimuli is represented, but also because they are the parts of the brain that perform pattern-association learning between potential secondary reinforcers and primary reinforcers to compute expected value. They are thus the parts of the brain involved in learning the emotional and motivational value of stimuli.

6. The value and expected value representations in the orbitofrontal cortex take into account 'risk', i.e. the probability of obtaining a reward outcome, reward magnitude, the temporal discounting of reward value, and the 'intrinsic costs' of stimuli i.e. whether there are positive and negative components, to represent the economic value of stimuli (see further Section 9.5 and Grabenhorst & Rolls (2011)). The value representations are on a common scale, but are not converted into a common single currency, in that different single neurons respond to different rewarding and punishing stimuli (see further Section 9.5). Further evidence that the orbitofrontal cortex provides a value representation is that orbitofrontal cortex neuronal responses and activations selectively decrease to zero during devaluation experiments such as feeding to satiety. The value representations are of stimuli, and actions and responses made are not clearly represented in the orbitofrontal cortex.

7. The activations in the orbitofrontal cortex are linearly related to the subjective value, the subjective consciously reported affective pleasantness or unpleasantness of stimuli, and these representations thus drive the subjective experience of *pleasure* in the explicit system, which is considered further in Chapter 10.

8. The orbitofrontal cortex represents the value of stimuli on a continuous scale. For decisions between stimuli of different value, there is evidence that a more anterior region identified as the *medial prefrontal cortex area 10 is involved in the choice decision-making mechanism*, and that decision confidence is represented in medial area 10, as described further in Chapter 8.

9. The orbitofrontal cortex is involved in the rapid, one-trial, reversal of the value assigned to a stimulus and of emotional behaviour when the instrumental reinforcement contingencies change. This very rapid reversal may be implemented by switching a rule, and is probably one of the developments made possible by the great development of the granular prefrontal cortex including the granular orbitofrontal cortex areas that appear not to be present in rodents. The rapid reversal which is provided by the orbitofrontal cortex much more than the amygdala may be facilitated by the recurrent collateral connections between neurons in the orbitofrontal cortex, which provide for a short-term memory of the current rule. The orbitofrontal cortex thus allows flexibility of emotional behaviour, and rapid sensitivity to the changes in the reinforcers being received. This is very important in primates (including humans), in which it is important in social situations to change behaviour rapidly to what may be subtle cues, such as changes in face expression.

10. Cognitive inputs and states that are decoded as reinforcing and thus lead to emotions are represented in the orbitofrontal cortex. An example is monetary reward or loss. Modulation by cognition of the reinforcement or subjective affective value of stimuli also is expressed in the orbitofrontal cortex. An example is the modulating effect that a word can have on the pleasantness vs unpleasantness value of a test odour, taste, flavour, or touch which is represented in the orbitofrontal cortex.

11. Damage to the orbitofrontal cortex in humans can affect subjective emotional states, can impair emotional behaviour (producing for example some disinhibition and uncooperativeness), can be associated with personality changes including increased impulsiveness, and can impair the ability to identify correctly face and voice expressions.

12. The outputs of the amygdala are involved in many Pavlovian (classically conditioned) effects of stimuli on behaviour, including the elicitation of autonomic responses, and via the ventral striatum of Pavlovian effects on instrumental behaviour, such as Pavlovian-instrumental transfer (PIT).

13. The outputs of the orbitofrontal cortex may be used in structures such as the anterior cingulate cortex for action–outcome learning. As part of this, the pregenual part of the anterior cingulate cortex provides a representation, received from the orbitofrontal cortex, of positive value; and the anterodorsal part of the anterior cingulate cortex provides a representation of negative value. Damage to these anterior cingulate cortex regions does alter emotional behaviour, for example to face expressions, and does alter the subjective experience of emotion. In implementing action–outcome learning, which depends on the value of the goal, the cingulate cortex takes into account the costs of actions required to obtain the rewards (which have been termed extrinsic costs (Grabenhorst & Rolls 2011)).

14. The outputs of the orbitofrontal cortex, amygdala, and anterior cingulate cortex are used in the basal ganglia for stimulus–response (habit) learning (see further Section 6.3).

15. The outputs of the orbitofrontal cortex, amygdala, and anterior cingulate cortex are used, in part via the insula, hypothalamus and brainstem, in autonomic responses to emotion-provoking stimuli that prepare the body. Activations in the anterior insula to emotion-provoking stimuli may reflect the use of these outputs of the orbitofrontal cortex, amygdala, and anterior cingulate cortex in the elicitation of autonomic including visceral, heart-rate, etc. responses.

16. A separate route to action is provided by an explicit, language-based system, for humans can sometimes state verbally what action they should have taken to a reinforcer, even though after orbitofrontal cortex damage they may not have made the appropriate choice when reinforcement contingencies change.

17. A subcallosal anterior cingulate cortex region is implicated in depression, in that it is activated by sadness induction, in that neurons in it respond to negative stimuli, and in that treatments for depression may alter activity in this region. Deep brain stimulation for depression in a nearby area may activate the reward value system that extends from the orbitofrontal cortex through the pregenual cingulate cortex to medial prefrontal cortex area 10.

18. In non-primates including rodents, the design principles may involve less sophisticated design features, partly because the stimuli being processed are simpler. For example, view-invariant object recognition is less developed in non-primates, with the recognition that is possible being based more on physical similarity in terms of texture, colour, simple features, etc. It may be because there is less sophisticated cortical processing of visual stimuli that other sensory systems are also organized more simply, with, for example, some (approximately 30%) modulation of taste processing by hunger early in sensory processing in rodents (Rolls & Scott 2003), and even connectivity of the taste system that allows brainstem taste processing to gain direct access to the amygdala without cortical processing. Further, while it is appropriate usually to have emotional responses to well-processed objects or individuals (e.g. the sight of a particular person), there are instances, such as a loud noise or a pure tone associated with punishment, where it may be possible to tap off a sensory representation early in sensory information processing that can be used to produce emotional responses. This may occur, for example, in rodents, where the subcortical auditory system provides afferents to the amygdala. Another important difference from rodents may be the use of rules that can be rapidly reversed by switching attractor network states, using mechanisms especially developed in the granular prefrontal including orbitofrontal cortical areas of primates and humans (Rolls 2008b).

5 Food reward value, pleasure, hunger, and appetite

5.1 Introduction

In this chapter we consider the rewards and affective states relevant to eating, and those for drinking are described by Rolls (2005b). In these cases there are internal signals which indicate that there is a need for food or water. The food or water are rewards, in that the organism will work to obtain the food or water. The signals that make the food or water rewarding originate internally. In the case of hunger, the internal signals reflect the state of energy balance, reflecting stimuli such as plasma glucose and gastric distension. In the case of thirst, the internal signals reflect the volumes of the cellular and extracellular fluids. In both cases the hunger and thirst operate to maintain the constancy of the internal milieu. The signals operate to alter the reward value that food or water has for the hungry or thirsty organism. The reward signals are conveyed primarily by the taste, texture, smell, and sight of food or water.

In this chapter we will consider where in information processing in these sensory systems the sensory stimulation produced by food is decoded not just as a physical stimulus, but is coded in terms of its reward and affective value. An important aspect of brain organization is that these two aspects of information processing, representing the identity of objects, and representing their affective value, are kept separate, at least in primates including humans. Another important aspect of brain organization for these types of reward is that the learning of which visual stimuli are food or water, or are associated with food or water, takes places in specialized parts of the brain for this type of learning. This learning takes place in the brain after analysis of what the stimulus is.

The study of hunger and thirst allows precise analysis of the relation between motivational states (e.g. hunger and thirst), and emotional states including affective reactions to sensory stimuli such as food. It is also important to understand dysfunctions of the eating control systems that lead to obesity, which is now a major health issue in many countries.

5.2 Peripheral signals for hunger and satiety

To understand how food intake is controlled, we first consider the functions of the different peripheral factors (i.e. factors outside the brain) such as taste, smell, and gastric distension, and the control signals, such as the amount of glucose in the blood. We focus particularly on which sensory inputs produce reward, and on which inputs act as hunger or satiety signals to modulate the reward value of the sensory inputs. Then we consider how the brain integrates these different signals, learns about which stimuli in the environment provide food, and how the brain initiates behaviour to obtain the correct variety and amount of food.

The functions of some different peripheral signals in the control of eating can be revealed with the sham feeding preparation shown in Fig. 5.1. In this situation, the animal can taste, smell, and eat the food normally, but the food drains from the stomach, so that no distension of the stomach occurs, and nor does any food enter the intestine for absorption. It is found

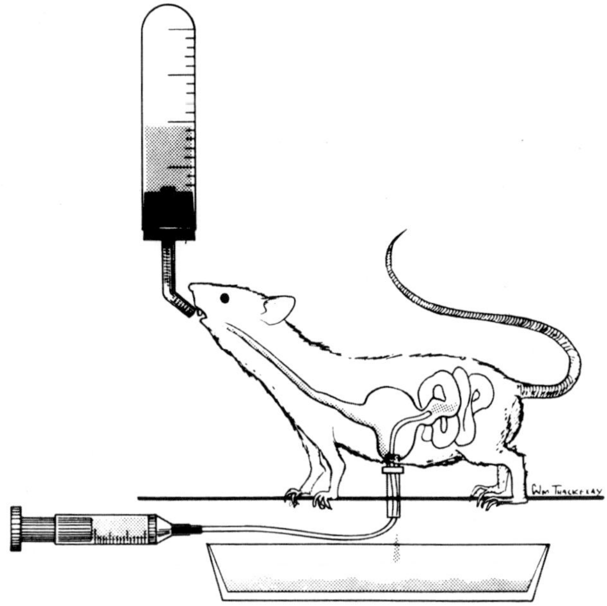

Fig. 5.1 Sham feeding preparation. Food can be tasted, smelled and ingested normally, but then it drains from the stomach so that gastric distension and other gastrointestinal factors are not produced. The diagram also shows a cannula entering the duodenum, so that the role of intestinal factors in eating can be studied by infusions of for example potential satiety-producing substances.

that rats, monkeys, and humans will work to obtain food when they are sham feeding. This finding for primates is demonstrated in Fig. 5.2. This shows that it is the taste and smell of food which provide the immediate reward for food-motivated behaviour. Consistent with this, humans rate the taste and smell of food as being pleasant when they are hungry (see Section 5.3.1).

A second important aspect of sham feeding is that satiety (reduction of appetite) does not occur – instead rats and monkeys continue to eat for often more than an hour when they can taste and smell food normally, but food drains from the stomach, so that it does not accumulate in the stomach and enter the intestine (see e.g. Fig. 5.2, the classical literature reviewed by Grossman (1967), and Gibbs, Maddison & Rolls (1981)). We can conclude that taste and smell, and even swallowing food, do not produce satiety.

There is an important psychological point here – **reward itself does not produce satiety**. Instead, the satiety for feeding is produced by food accumulating in the stomach, and entering the intestine. Evidence that gastric distension is an important satiety signal is that if an animal is allowed to eat to normal satiety, and then the food is drained through a cannula from the stomach, then the animal starts eating again immediately (Gibbs, Maddison & Rolls 1981). Evidence that food entering the intestine can produce satiety is that small infusions of food into the duodenum (the first part of the intestine) reduce sham feeding (Gibbs, Maddison & Rolls 1981). It is also interesting that food delivered directly into the stomach, or even glucose intravenously, is not very rewarding, in that animals learn only with difficulty to perform a response to obtain an intragastric or intravenous infusion of food or fluid (Nicolaidis & Rowland 1976, Nicolaidis & Rowland 1977, Nicolaidis & Rowland 1975).

This evidence, summarized in Table 5.1, emphasizes the point that the taste, smell, and sight of food are what normally provide the reward, and correspondingly the pleasant sensation, associated with eating.

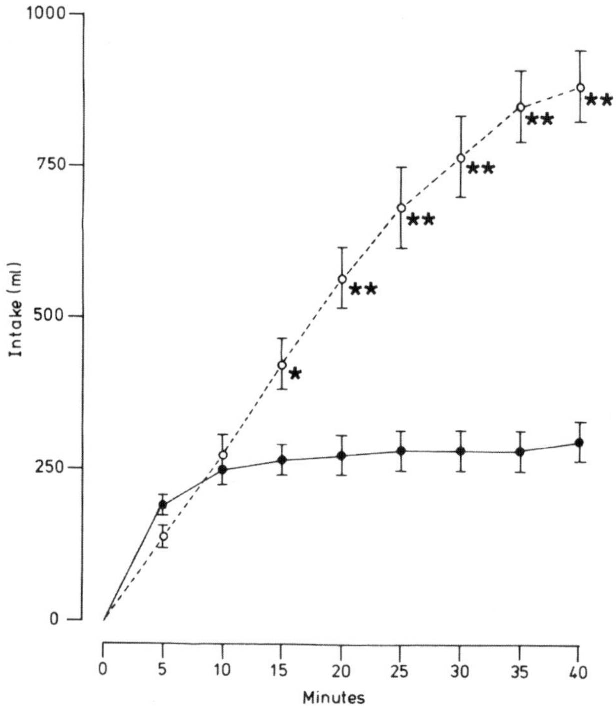

Fig. 5.2 Sham feeding in the monkey. The cumulative intakes of food with normal feeding (gastric cannula closed, closed circles), and with the gastric cannula open (open circles) allowing drainage of food from the stomach, are shown. The stars indicate significant differences between the open and closed gastric cannula conditions. (Reproduced from J. Gibbs, S. P. Maddison, and E. T. Rolls, Satiety role of the small intestine examined in sham-feeding rhesus monkeys, *Journal of Comparative and Physiological Psychology* 95, pp. 1003–1015, ©1981, The Authors.)

Table 5.1 Summary of functions of peripheral signals in feeding

	Reinforcement	**Satiety**
Oropharyngeal factors	Yes	No (though contribute to sensory-specific satiety)
Gastric and intestinal factors	No	Yes

Important conclusions about reward and its relation to hunger and satiety signals follow from what has just been described. First, reward and satiety are different processes. Second, reward is produced by oropharyngeal sensory signals such as the taste and smell of food. Third, satiety is produced by gastric, intestinal, and eventually other signals after the food is absorbed from the intestine. Fourth, hunger and satiety signals modulate the reward value of food (in that the taste and smell of food are rewarding when hunger signals are present and satiety signals are not present). In more general and psychological terminology, motivational state modulates the reward or reinforcement value of sensory stimuli. Fifth, given that reward and satiety are produced by different peripheral signals, one function of brain (i.e. central) processes in the control of feeding is to bring together satiety and reward signals in such a way that satiety modulates the reward value of food.

One of the aims of this chapter is to show how the brain processes sensory stimuli that can produce rewards for animals, where in the brain the reward value of such sensory stimuli is represented, and where and how the motivational signals that reflect hunger modulate this processing as part of the reward-decoding process. Of crucial interest in understanding the rules of operation of this reward system will therefore be where and how in the brain gastric and other satiety signals are brought together with taste and smell signals of food, to produce a taste/smell reward signal that is modulated by satiety.

5.3 The control signals for hunger and satiety

There is a set of different signals that each plays a role in determining the level of hunger vs satiety. These signals must all be integrated by the brain, and must then modulate how rewarding the sensory inputs such as the sight, taste, and smell of food are. These signals that influence hunger and satiety are summarized next, taken to some extent in the order in which they are activated in a meal.

5.3.1 Sensory-specific satiety

During experiments on brain mechanisms of reward and satiety, E. T. Rolls and colleagues observed in 1974 that if a lateral hypothalamic neuron had ceased to respond to a food on which the monkey had been fed to satiety (a discovery described in *The Brain and Reward* (Rolls 1975)), then the neuron might still respond to a different food (see examples in Figs. 5.3 and 5.10, and Section 5.4.1.2). This occurred for neurons with responses associated with the taste (Rolls 1981b, Rolls 1981a, Rolls, Murzi, Yaxley, Thorpe & Simpson 1986) or sight (Rolls 1981b, Rolls & Rolls 1982b, Rolls, Murzi, Yaxley, Thorpe & Simpson 1986) of food. Corresponding to this neuronal specificity of the effects of feeding to satiety, the monkey rejected the food on which he had been fed to satiety, but accepted other foods that he had not been fed. I well remember the occasion on which we discovered sensory-specific satiety in 1974 when we were recording from a lateral hypothalamic neuron in the monkey that responded to the sight of glucose (fed to the monkey from a syringe) and other foods. We fed the monkey to satiety with glucose, and observed the neuronal response to the glucose fall to zero, as illustrated for one such neuron in Fig. 5.3. I then showed the monkey a peanut, and heard a large response of the neuron, which was confirmed by the high firing rate printed out on the teletype (ASR33) by the PDP11 computer. I was disconcerted at first because the monkey was supposed to be satiated, having drunk as much glucose as it wanted. However, I had the presence of mind to offer the peanut to the monkey, and found that the monkey reached out for the peanut, and avidly consumed it. I realized that something interesting was happening in terms of the brain mechanisms that implement satiety, and repeated the observations a number of times, confirming that the lateral hypothalamic neuron did not respond to the sight of the glucose and that the monkey did not accept the glucose, whereas the neuron did respond vigorously to the sight of the peanut, which the monkey avidly reached for and ate. The fact that quantitative firing rates were being printed out on the teletype helped to impress on me the fact that this was a strong effect, which we termed sensory-specific satiety. The neurophysiological finding was published for example in Rolls (1981b) and Rolls et al. (1986). This is now described as a devaluation procedure, and provides evidence that these, and orbitofrontal cortex neurons which provide inputs to the lateral hypothalamus encode **value**.

I lectured on the result to my Oxford undergraduate class, and proposed an experiment to explore the effect in humans. The experiment was performed as an undergraduate practical (with Barbara Rolls as a co-organizer) in which humans rated the pleasantness and intensity of 6 foods, and then ate one of the foods to satiety. Whichever food was eaten to satiety showed a large decrease in the pleasantness rating, whereas other foods that had not been

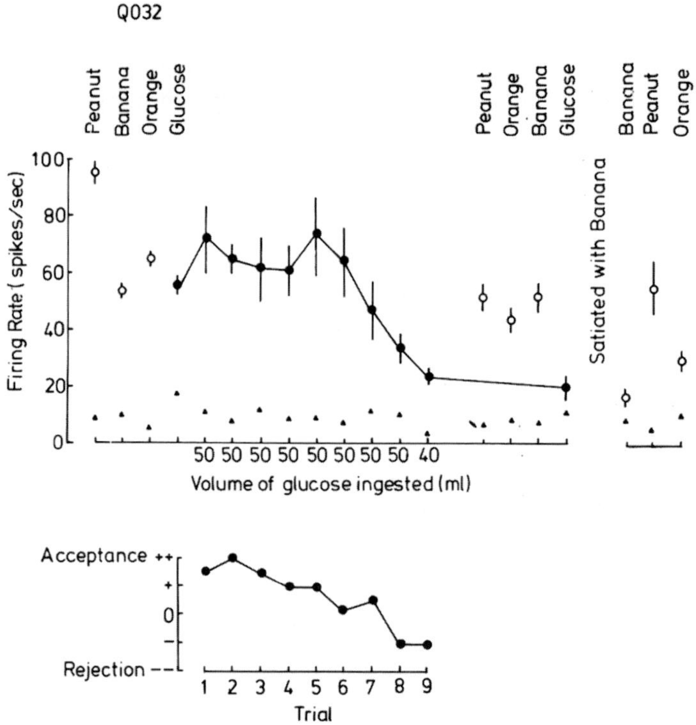

Fig. 5.3 The effect of feeding the monkey to satiety with 20% glucose solution on the responses of a lateral hypothalamic neuron to the sight the glucose (filled circles) and to the sight of other foods (open circles). After the monkey had fed to satiety with glucose, the neuron responded much less to the sight of glucose, but still responded to the other foods. The mean responses of the neuron (± s.e.m.) are shown to the stimuli at different stages of the experiment. The satiety of the monkey, shown below, was measured by whether he accepted or rejected the glucose. After satiety with glucose, a second satiety experiment was performed in which banana was fed to satiety, and after this, the responses of the neuron decreased to the sight of the banana, but remained to the sight of peanut and orange, for which he still had an appetite. (Reprinted from *Brain Research*, 368, E. T. Rolls, E. Murzi, S. Yaxley, S. J. Thorpe and S. Simpson, Sensory-specific satiety: food-specific reduction in responsiveness of ventral forebrain neurons after feeding in the monkey, pp. 79–86. Copyright, 1986, with permission from Elsevier.)

eaten to satiety showed a much smaller decrease, or in some cases even a small increase in pleasantness (e.g. for a sweet food after a savory food had been eaten to satiety), as shown in Fig. 5.4. The result was published by Rolls, Rolls, Rowe & Sweeney (1981a), and led to a series of other investigations on sensory-specific satiety described below.

We performed further experiments to determine whether satiety in humans is specific to foods eaten. These experiments were performed as a result of the neurophysiological and behavioural observations showing the specificity of satiety in the monkey (Rolls 1981b, Rolls 1981a, Rolls, Murzi, Yaxley, Thorpe & Simpson 1986), and the experiment illustrated in Fig. 5.4[11]. In the further experiments, it was found that the pleasantness of the taste of food eaten to satiety decreased more than for foods that had not been eaten (Rolls, Rolls, Rowe & Sweeney 1981a). The results of an experiment of this type are shown in Fig. 5.5.

[11] LeMagnen (1956) had also shown that rats drank more water if several tubes of water each had a different odour added to the water.

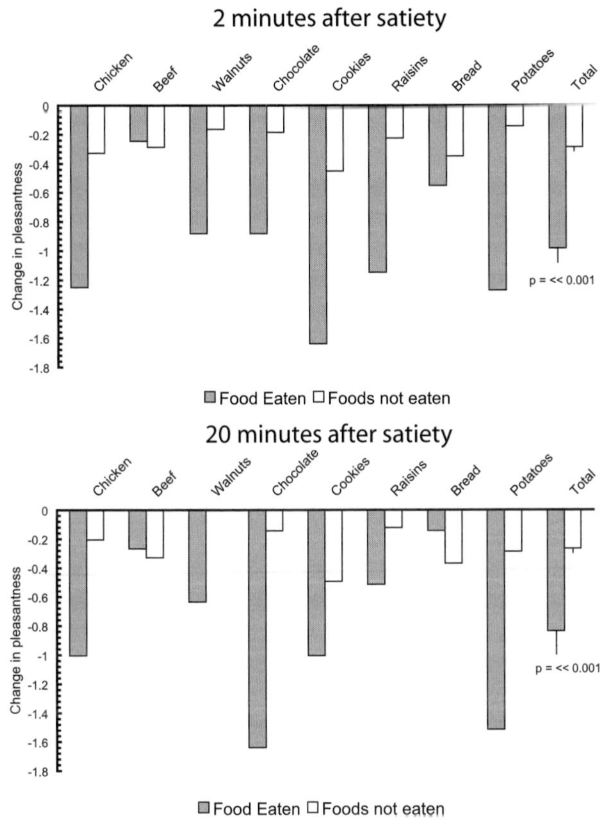

Fig. 5.4 Sensory-specific satiety for the flavour of a food. The change in the pleasantness of the flavour of food after eating one to satiety. For each food, the change of pleasantness after eating that food to satiety is shown (food eaten), compared to the average change of pleasantness of the other foods not eaten in the meal. The ratings are on a scale from +2 very pleasant to –2 very unpleasant, and the change of pleasantness rating from before until after eating one of the foods to satiety is shown. The ratings were made by a group of participants 2 min and 20 min after eating one of the foods to satiety for lunch. (Reprinted from *Physiology and Behavior*, 27 (1), Barbara J. Rolls, Edmund T. Rolls, Edward A. Rowe, and Kevin Sweeney, Sensory specific satiety in man, pp 137–142, Copyright, 1981, with permission from Elsevier.)

One implication of this finding is that if one food is eaten to satiety, appetite reduction for other foods is often incomplete, and this should mean that in humans also at least some of the other foods will be eaten. This has been confirmed by an experiment in which either sausages or cheese with crackers were eaten for lunch. The liking for the food eaten decreased more than for the food not eaten and, when an unexpected second course was offered, more was eaten if a subject had not been given that food in the first course than if he had been given that food in the first course (98% vs 40% of the first course intake eaten in the second courses, $p < 0.01$, Rolls, Rolls, Rowe & Sweeney (1981a)).

A further implication of these findings is that if a variety of foods is available, the total amount consumed will be more than when only one food is offered repeatedly. This prediction has been confirmed in a study in which humans ate more when offered a variety of sandwich fillings than one filling or a variety of types of yoghurt which differed in taste, texture, and colour (Rolls, Rowe, Rolls, Kingston, Megson & Gunary 1981b). It has also been confirmed in a study in which humans were offered a relatively normal meal of four courses, and it was found that the change of food at each course significantly enhanced intake (Rolls, Van Duijenvoorde

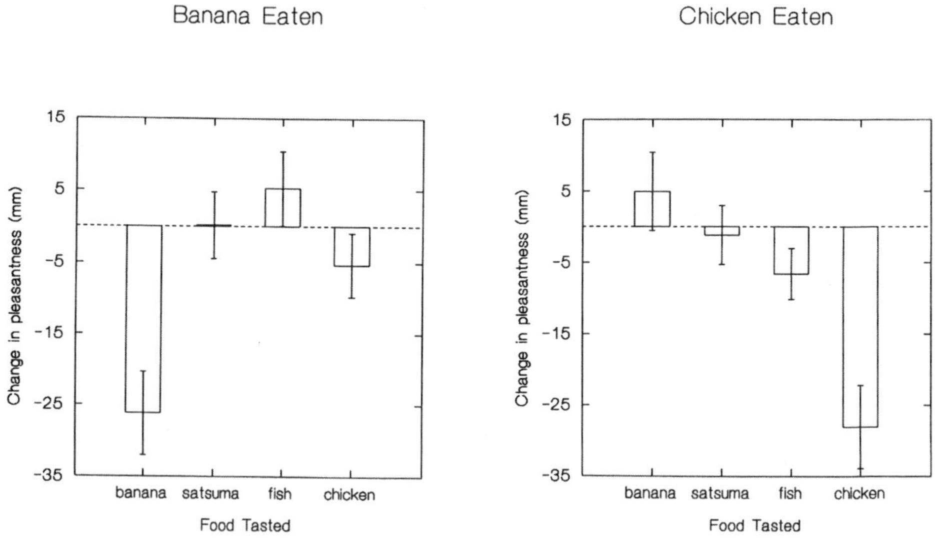

Fig. 5.5 Sensory-specific satiety for the flavour of a food: the changes in the pleasantness of the taste of four different foods after eating banana (left) or chicken (right) to satiety are shown. The change is shown as mm difference (± the standard error of the mean, s.e.m.) on a 100 mm visual analogue rating scale marked at one end 'very pleasant' and at the other end 'very unpleasant'. The decrease of pleasantness of the taste of a food was greater for the food eaten to satiety. (Reprinted from *Physiology and Behavior*, 61 (3), E.T. Rolls and J.H. Rolls, Olfactory Sensory-Specific Satiety in Humans, pp. 461–473, Copyright, 1997, with permission from Elsevier.)

& Rolls 1984a). Because sensory factors such as similarity of colour, shape, flavour, and texture are usually more important than metabolic equivalence in terms of energy, protein, carbohydrate, and fat content in influencing how foods interact in this type of satiety, it has been termed 'sensory-specific satiety' (Rolls & Rolls 1977, Rolls & Rolls 1982b, Rolls, Rolls, Rowe & Sweeney 1981a, Rolls, Rowe, Rolls, Kingston, Megson & Gunary 1981b, Rolls, Rowe & Rolls 1982a, Rolls, Rowe & Rolls 1982b, Rolls & Rolls 1997, Rolls 1999a, Rolls 2005b).

It should be noted that sensory-specific satiety is distinct from alliesthesia, in that alliesthesia is a change in the pleasantness of sensory inputs produced by internal signals (such as glucose in the gut) (Cabanac & Duclaux 1970, Cabanac 1971, Cabanac & Fantino 1977), whereas sensory-specific satiety is a change in the pleasantness of sensory inputs which is accounted for at least partly by the external sensory stimulation received (such as the taste of a particular food), in that as shown above it is at least partly specific to the external sensory stimulation received.

The parallel between these studies of feeding in humans and of the neurophysiology of hypothalamic neurons in the monkey has been extended by the observations that in humans, sensory-specific satiety occurs for the sight (Rolls, Rowe & Rolls 1982a) and smell (Rolls & Rolls 1997) as well as for the taste and even texture (Rolls, Rowe & Rolls 1982a) of food. Further, to complement the finding that in the hypothalamus neurons are found that respond differently to food and to water (see Fig. 5.11, Rolls and colleagues, unpublished observations), and that satiety with water can reduce the responsiveness of hypothalamic neurons that respond to water, it has been shown that in humans motivation-specific satiety can also be detected. For example, satiety with water reduces the pleasantness of the sight and taste of water but not of food (Rolls, Rolls & Rowe 1983b).

Some sensory-specific satiety can be produced just by tasting or even smelling a food

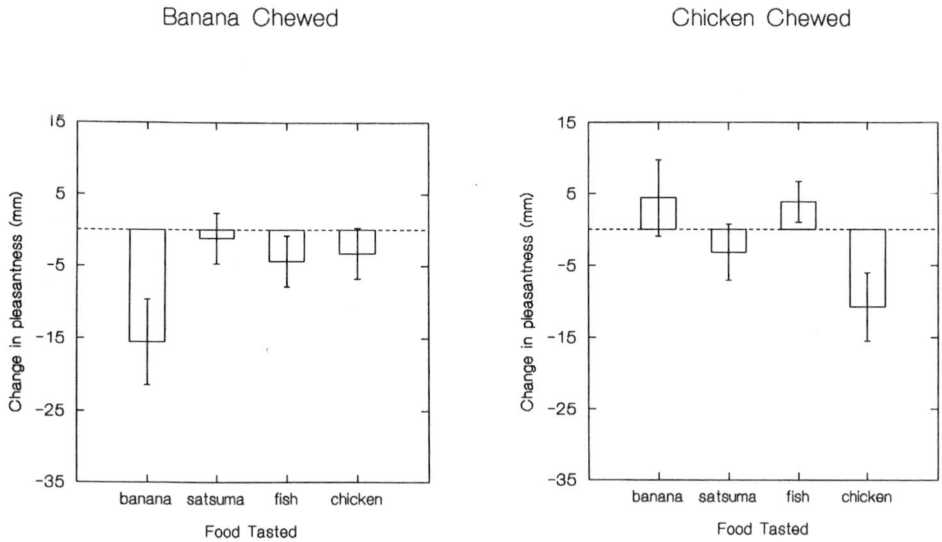

Fig. 5.6 Sensory-specific satiety for the flavour of a food: the change in the pleasantness of the taste of four different foods after chewing but not swallowing banana (left) or chicken (right) for five minutes. Conventions as in Fig. 5.5. The decrease of pleasantness of the taste of a food was greater for the food chewed. (Reprinted from *Physiology and Behavior*, 61 (3), E.T. Rolls and J.H. Rolls, Olfactory Sensory-Specific Satiety in Humans, pp. 461–473, Copyright, 1997, with permission from Elsevier.)

for a few minutes, without swallowing any of it (Rolls & Rolls 1997) (see Fig. 5.6). This shows that just the presence of neuronal activity produced by the taste or the smell of food is sufficient to reduce the firing of neurons which represent the pleasantness of the taste or smell of food. This can occur to some extent even without gastric and post-gastric factors such as gastric distension and intestinal stimulation by food. This indicates that this aspect of sensory-specific satiety can be produced by firing that is sustained for a few minutes in neurons in the pathway. Moreover, the decline in neuronal responsiveness must be at a late stage of the processing of the taste and probably the olfactory signals, in that just smelling the food for several minutes produces much more of a reduction in the pleasantness than in the intensity of the odour, and just tasting the food for several minutes produces much more of a decrease in the pleasantness than in the intensity of the taste (Rolls & Rolls 1997).

It is a general finding with sensory-specific satiety that the decrease is pleasantness is much greater than any decrease in intensity of the food eaten to satiety. Indeed, Rolls, Rolls & Rowe (1983b) specifically addressed this using different concentrations of glucose and salt (NaCl), and showed that the subjective intensity but much less the subjective pleasantness of the tastes was related to the concentrations. Conversely, feeding to satiety produced a much greater decrease in pleasantness than in intensity. The neurophysiological basis for this is that processing as far as the primary taste cortex (Rolls, Scott, Sienkiewicz & Yaxley 1988, Yaxley, Rolls & Sienkiewicz 1988, Grabenhorst & Rolls 2008), the primary olfactory cortex (Rolls, Kringelbach & De Araujo 2003c), and the inferior temporal visual cortex is related to the identity and intensity of the stimulus (Rolls, Judge & Sanghera 1977); whereas in the orbitofrontal cortex it is the pleasantness of the taste (Rolls, Sienkiewicz & Yaxley 1989b, Grabenhorst & Rolls 2008) (Fig. 4.44), smell, and sight of food which is represented (Critchley & Rolls 1996c, Rolls, Kringelbach & De Araujo 2003c, De Araujo, Rolls, Kringelbach, McGlone & Phillips 2003c, Kringelbach, O'Doherty, Rolls & Andrews

2003, De Araujo, Rolls, Velazco, Margot & Cayeux 2005). The adaptive value of this is that it is important that we do not go 'blind' to the taste or sight of food after we have eaten it to satiety, for it is important to be able to learn about the food (e.g. where food has been seen), even when we are not hungry.

It should be noticed that this decrease in the pleasantness of the sensory stimulation produced by a food only occurs if the sensory stimulation is repeated for several minutes. It has the adaptive value of changing the behaviour after a significant amount of that behaviour has been performed. In contrast, the reward value of sensory stimulation may increase over the first short period (of the order of a minute). This is called *incentive motivation* (and the 'salted-nut phenomenon' by Hebb (1949)). It has the adaptive value that once a behaviour has been initiated, it will tend to continue for at least a little while. This is much more adaptive than continually switching behaviour, which has at least some cost in terms of efficiency, and might have a high cost if the different rewards are located far apart. The increase in the rate of behaviour, for example in the rate of feeding in the first part of a meal, probably reflects this effect. It was observed that this typical increase in the rate of working for a reward early on in a meal was not found in rats with amygdala lesions (Rolls & Rolls 1973b), and this implies that part of the mechanism for the increasing hedonic value of a food reward is implemented, at least in the rat, in the amygdala. Associated with this lack of increase in the rate of feeding early on in the meal, in the rat the meal pattern was disturbed. Instead of short rapid meals following by a bout of drinking and then other activity, the rats had long periods in which slow feeding and drinking were interspersed. This emphasizes the suggested function of the reward facilitation normally seen at the start of a period of rewarding sensory stimulation.

The enhanced eating when a variety of foods is available, as a result of the operation of sensory-specific satiety, may have been advantageous in evolution in ensuring that different foods with important different nutrients were consumed, but today in humans, when a wide variety of foods is readily available, it may be a factor which can lead to overeating and obesity. In a test of this in the rat, it has been found that variety itself can lead to obesity (Rolls, Van Duijenvoorde & Rowe 1983a, Rolls & Hetherington 1989).

Advances in understanding the neurophysiological mechanisms of sensory-specific satiety are being made in analyses of information processing in the taste and olfactory systems, as described below.

In addition to the sensory-specific satiety described above which operates primarily during the meal (see above) and during the post-meal period (Rolls, Van Duijenvoorde & Rolls 1984a), there is also evidence for a long-term form of sensory-specific satiety (Rolls & de Waal 1985). This was shown in a study in an Ethiopian refugee camp, in which it was found that refugees who had been in the camp for 6 months found the taste of their three regular foods less pleasant than that of three comparable foods which they had not been eating. The effect was a long-term form of sensory-specific satiety in that it was not found in refugees who had been in the camp and eaten the regular foods for two days (Rolls & de Waal 1985). It is suggested that it is important to recognize the operation of long-term sensory-specific satiety in conditions such as these, for it may enhance malnutrition if the regular foods become less acceptable and so are rejected, exchanged for other less nutritionally effective foods or goods, or are inadequately prepared. It may be advantageous in these circumstances to attempt to minimize the operation of long-term sensory-specific satiety by providing some variety, perhaps even with spices (Rolls & de Waal 1985).

5.3.2 Gastric distension

This is one of the signals that is normally necessary for satiety, as shown by the experiment in which gastric drainage of food after a meal leads to the immediate resumption of eating

(Gibbs, Maddison & Rolls 1981). Gastric distension only builds up if the pyloric sphincter closes. The pyloric sphincter controls the emptying of the stomach into the next part of the gastrointestinal tract, the duodenum. The sphincter closes only when food reaches the duodenum, stimulating chemosensors and osmosensors to regulate the action of the sphincter, by both local neural circuits and by hormones, in what is called the enterogastric loop (Gibbs, Maddison & Rolls 1981, Gibbs, Fauser, Rowe, Rolls, Rolls & Maddison 1979).

5.3.3 Duodenal chemosensors

The duodenum contains receptors sensitive to the chemical composition of the food draining from the stomach. One set of receptors responds to glucose, and can contribute to satiety via the vagus nerve, which carries signals to the brain. The evidence that the vagus is the pathway is that cutting the vagus nerve (vagotomy) abolishes the satiating effects of glucose infusions into the duodenum. Fats infused into the duodenum can also produce satiety, but in this case the link to the brain may be hormonal (a hormone is a blood-borne signal), for vagotomy does not abolish the satiating effect of fat infusions into the duodenum (Greenberg, Smith & Gibbs 1990, Mei 1993).

5.3.4 Glucostatic hypothesis

There are many lines of evidence, summarized next, that one signal that controls appetite is the concentration of glucose circulating in the plasma – we eat in order to maintain glucostasis, i.e. constancy of glucose in the internal milieu (Woods 2012, Begg & Woods 2013a, Begg & Woods 2013b). More accurately, the actual signal appears to be the utilization of glucose by the body and brain – if the arterial minus the venous concentration is low, indicating that the body is not extracting much glucose from the bloodstream, then we feel hungry and eat; and if the utilization measured in this way is high, we feel satiated. Consistent with this correlation between glucose and eating, there is a small reduction in plasma glucose concentration just before the onset of meals in rats, suggesting that the decreasing glucose concentration initiates a meal. At the end of a meal, plasma glucose concentrations (and insulin, which helps the glucose to be used by cells) increase. A second line of evidence is that peripheral injections of insulin, which reduce the concentration of glucose in the plasma (by facilitating its entry to cells and storage as fat), can provoke food intake. Insulin also has direct effects on the brain, where it produces hypophagia (Begg & Woods 2013a). Third, 2-deoxyglucose, a competitive inhibitor of glucose metabolism, elicits feeding. Fourth, infusions of glucose and insulin can reduce feeding. Fifth, one of the brain's monitoring system for glucose availability seems to be in the area postrema in the medulla (part of the brainstem), for infusions there of a competitive inhibitor of glucose, 5-thioglucose, elicit feeding (Ritter, Li, Wang & Dinh 2011, Begg & Woods 2013a).

It is worth noting that in diabetes (that is, diabetes mellitus), the cells can become insulin-resistant, so that in this condition it is difficult to interpret whatever plasma levels of glucose are present in terms of their possible role in hunger and satiety (Begg & Woods 2013a).

5.3.5 Hormonal signals related to hunger and satiety, and their effects on the hypothalamus

There are many peripheral signals including hormonal signals that are produced when food is eaten, and some of these influence hunger and satiety, by their direct or indirect effects on hypothalamic nuclei (Suzuki, Simpson, Minnion, Shillito & Bloom 2010, Begg & Woods 2013b). Some of these effects are now summarized with reference to Fig. 5.7. We start with

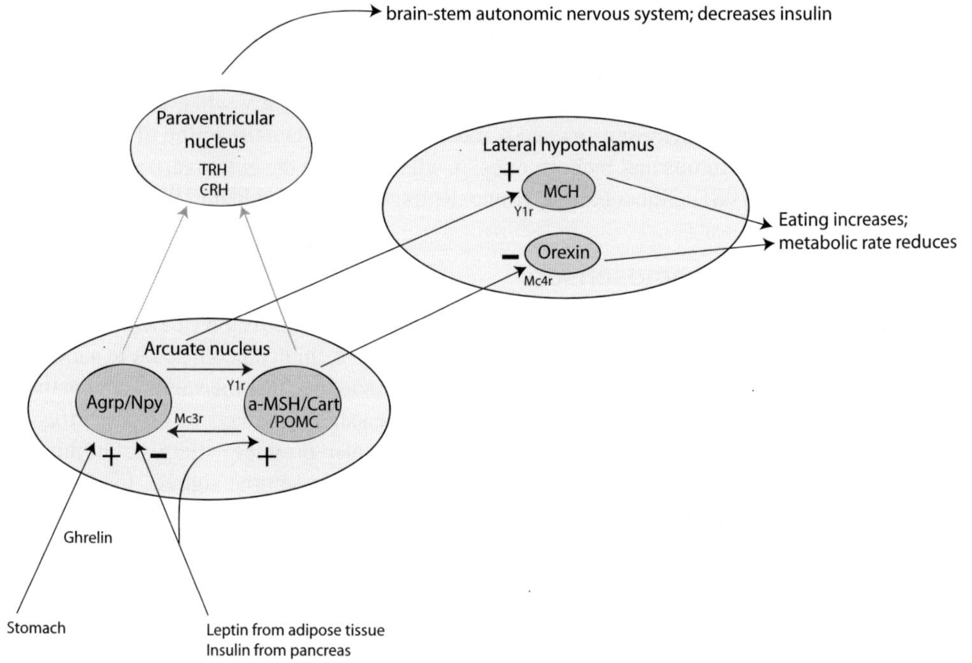

Fig. 5.7 Effects of peripheral hunger and satiety-related signals on some of the neurochemically identified feeding-related neurons of the hypothalamus, including neurons in the arcuate, lateral hypothalamic and paraventricular nuclei (see text for description). Npy/Agrp, neurons containing neuropeptide Y and agouti-related peptide; α-MSH/CART/POMC, neurons containing α-melanocyte-stimulating hormone, cocaine- and amphetamine-regulated transcript, and pro-opiomelanocortin; TRH, thyrotropin-releasing hormone; CRH, corticotrophin-releasing hormone; MCH, melanin-concentrating hormone.

the hormone leptin, with some of the findings as follows (Campfield, Smith, Guisez, Devos & Burn 1995, Cummings & Schwartz 2003, Farooqi & O'Rahilly 2009, Suzuki et al. 2010).

Leptin or OB protein is the hormone encoded by the mouse ob gene (here ob stands for obesity). Genetically obese mice that are double recessive for the ob gene (i.e. obob mice) produce no leptin. Leptin reduces food intake in wild type (lean) mice (who have genes that are OBOB or OBob so that they produce leptin) and in obob mice (showing that obob mice have receptors sensitive to leptin). The satiety effect of leptin can be produced by injections into the brain. Leptin does not produce satiety (reduce food intake) in another type of genetically obese mouse designated dbdb. These mice may be obese because they lack the leptin receptor, or mechanisms associated with it. Leptin has a long time-course: it fluctuates over 24 h, but not in relation to individual meals. Thus it might be appropriate for the longer-term regulation of appetite. Leptin concentration may correlate with body weight/adiposity, consistent with the possibility that it is produced by fat cells, and can signal the total amount of body fat.

A hypothesis consistent with these findings is that leptin is produced in proportion to the amount of body fat, and that this is normally one of the signals that controls how much food is eaten. Although this is an interesting mechanism implicated in the long-term control of body weight, it appears that most obesity in humans cannot be accounted for by malfunction of the leptin system, for even though genetic malfunction of this system can produce obesity in humans, such genetic malfunctions are very rare (Farooqi, Keogh, Kamath, Jones, Gibson, Trussell, Jebb, Lip & O'Rahilly 2001, O'Rahilly 2009) (see Section 5.4.1.2 on page 237). It is found that obese people generally have high levels of leptin, so leptin production is not the problem, and instead leptin resistance (i.e. insensitivity) may be somewhat related to obesity, with the resistance perhaps related in part to smaller effects of leptin on arcuate nucleus Npy/Agrp neurons (Munzberg & Myers 2005), as described below.

We now broaden the approach to include other hormones and signals, and summarize how they influence brain systems involved in appetite control (Suzuki et al. 2010) (Fig. 5.7).

In the lateral hypothalamus (LHA) there are melanin-concentrating hormone (MCH) and orexin producing neurons, and an increase in their activity increases food intake and decreases metabolic rate (see Fig. 5.7). These neurons are activated by neuropeptide Y (Npy), itself a potent stimulator of food intake, produced by neurons in the arcuate nucleus, a hypothalamic nucleus in the ventromedial hypothalamic region. The arcuate Npy neurons also release agouti-related peptide (Agrp), itself a potent stimulator of food intake. One of the signals that activates Npy/Agrp neurons is ghrelin, a hunger-producing hormone produced by the stomach (Cummings, Frayo, Marmonier, Aubert & Chapolet 2004, Suzuki et al. 2010) (see Fig. 5.7). Npy/Agrp neurons increase their firing rates during fasting, and are inhibited by leptin (Cone 2005, Horvath 2005).

Leptin not only inhibits the production of Npy and Agrp by the arcuate Npy/Agrp neurons, but also inhibits the lateral hypothalamic orexin-producing neurons, and these are two ways in which leptin may decrease feeding (Pinto, Roseberry, Liu, Diano, Shanabrough, Cai, Friedman & Horvath 2004). CART (cocaine- and amphetamine-regulated transcript), produced by the α-MSH/CART/POMC neurons in the arcuate nucleus shown in Fig. 5.7, reduces hunger (i.e. is anorexigenic), so does α-melanocyte-stimulating hormone (α-MSH) produced by the same neurons, and these neurons are also activated by leptin, providing more ways in which leptin may act to reduce feeding (Elmquist, Elias & Saper 1999, Cone 2005, Horvath 2005, Carlson 2012) (see Fig. 5.7). Consistent with this, the (very rare) humans with clear genetic dysfunctions of the leptin receptor systems may show overeating and obesity which is treatable by leptin (Farooqi & O'Rahilly 2009), and approximately 4% of obese people have deficient (MC4) receptors for melanocyte stimulating hormone (MSH) (Barsh, Farooqi & O'Rahilly 2000, Cummings & Schwartz 2003, Cone 2005, O'Rahilly 2009). Also consistently, a very rare mutation in the gene encoding POMC in humans results in low MSH levels and obesity (and red hair due to the absence of melanin) (Cone 2005).

The paraventricular nucleus contains the anorectic thyrotropin-releasing hormone (TRH) and corticotrophin-releasing hormone (CRH). Destruction of the paraventricular nucleus causes hyperphagia and obesity. A number of hormones released when food enters the gut also influence food intake, and act via effects on the hypothalamus and on brainstem areas such as the nucleus of the solitary tract, which contains a brainstem relay of afferents from the gut. These hormones include glucagon-like peptide-1 (GLP-1), cholecystokinin (CCK), pancreatic polypeptide (PP), peptide YY (PYY), and oxyntomodulin (Suzuki et al. 2010).

These findings show that many hormones and other signals that influence hunger, satiety, and body weight act on the hypothalamus, but do not address how these effects in the hypothalamus influence the reward value of the sensory stimuli produced by food to influence appetite and food intake. The way in which the reward value of food is represented in the brain to control appetite and obesity, and individual differences in these reward systems, are considered in the rest of this chapter.

5.3.6 Conditioned appetite and satiety

If we eat food containing much energy (e.g. rich in fat) for a few days, we gradually eat less of it. If we eat food containing little energy, we gradually, over days, ingest more of it. This regulation involves learning, learning to associate the sight, taste, smell, texture, etc., of the food with the energy that is released from it in the hours after it is eaten. This form of learning was demonstrated by Booth (1985) who, after several days of offering sandwiches with different energy content and flavours, on a test day offered subjects medium-energy sandwiches (so that the subjects could not select by the amount of energy in the food). The subjects ate few of the sandwiches if they had the flavour of the high-energy sandwiches eaten previously, and many of the sandwiches if they had the flavour of the low-energy sandwiches eaten previously.

5.4 The brain control of eating and reward

5.4.1 The hypothalamus

5.4.1.1 Effects of damage to the hypothalamus

From clinical evidence it has been known since early this century that damage to the base of the brain can influence food intake and body weight. Later it was demonstrated that one critical region is the ventromedial hypothalamus, for bilateral lesions here in animals led to hyperphagia and obesity (Grossman 1967, Grossman 1973). Then Anand & Brobeck (1951) discovered that bilateral lesions of the lateral hypothalamus can produce a reduction in feeding and body weight. Evidence of this type led in the 1950s and 1960s to the view that food intake is controlled by two interacting 'centres', a feeding centre in the lateral hypothalamus and a satiety centre in the ventromedial hypothalamus (Stellar 1954, Woods 2012).

Soon, problems with this evidence for a dual-centre hypothesis of the control of food intake appeared. It appears that lesions of the ventromedial hypothalamus act indirectly to increase feeding. These lesions increase the secretion of insulin by the pancreas, this reduces plasma glucose concentration, and then feeding results. This mechanism is demonstrated by the finding that cutting the vagus nerve, which disconnects the brain from the pancreas, prevents ventromedial hypothalamic lesions from causing hypoglycemia, and also prevents the overeating that otherwise occurs after ventromedial hypothalamic lesions (Bray, Inoue & Nishizawa 1981). More recent studies have implicated melanocortins in the VMH regulation of feeding behaviour: food intake decreases when arcuate nucleus pro-opiomelanocortin (POMC) neurons activate VMH brain-derived neurotrophic factor (BDNF) neurons. Further, hypothalamic obesity can result from damage to either the POMC or BDNF neurons (King 2006).

Damage to cells in the lateral hypothalamus without damaging fibres of passage, using locally injected neurotoxins such as ibotenic acid or N-methyl-D-aspartate (NMDA), produces a lasting decrease in food intake and body weight (Winn, Tarbuck & Dunnett 1984, Dunnett, Lane & Winn 1985, Winn, Clark, Hastings, Clark, Latimer, Rugg & Brownlee 1990, Clark, Clark, Bartle & Winn 1991).

The lesion evidence just described implicates the hypothalamus in the control of food intake and body weight, but does not show what information processing related to the control of food intake is being performed by the hypothalamus and by other brain areas. More direct evidence on the neural processing involved in feeding, based on recordings of the activity of single neurons in the hypothalamus and other brain regions, is described next. These other brain systems include systems that perform sensory analysis involved in the control of feeding such as the taste and olfactory pathways; brain systems that represent the reward value of food, and are influenced by hunger and satiety signals to compute reward value, including the orbitofrontal cortex; brain systems involved in learning about foods including the amygdala and orbitofrontal cortex; and brain systems involved in the initiation of feeding behaviour such as the striatum. Some of the brain regions and pathways described in the text are shown in Fig. 4.1 on a lateral view of the brain of the macaque monkey, and some of the connections are

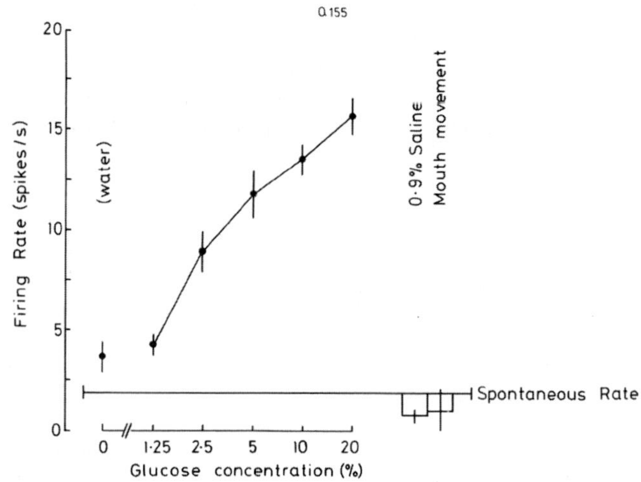

Fig. 5.8 Lateral hypothalamic neuron responding to the taste of food. The firing rate of the neuron depended on the concentration of glucose in the mouth. The neuron did not respond to isotonic saline in the mouth, or in relation to mouth movements. (Reprinted from *Brain Research*, 368 (1), E.T. Rolls, E. Murzi, S. Yaxley, S.J. Thorpe, and S.J. Simpson, Sensory-specific satiety: Food-specific reduction in responsiveness of ventral forebrain neurons after feeding in the monkey, pp. 79–86, Copyright, 1986, with permission from Elsevier.)

shown schematically in Fig. 4.2. Some of the findings described have been made in monkeys, because neuronal activity in non-human primates is especially relevant to understanding brain function and its disorders in humans, and this even includes taste processing (Section 1.3).

5.4.1.2 Neuronal activity in the lateral hypothalamus during feeding

Lateral hypothalamic neurons responsive to the sight, smell, and/or taste of food

It has been found that there is a population of neurons in the lateral hypothalamus and substantia innominata of the monkey with responses that are related to feeding (see Rolls (1981a), Rolls (1981b) and Rolls (1986c)). These neurons, which comprised 13.6% in one sample of 764 hypothalamic neurons, respond to the taste and/or sight of food (Rolls, Burton & Mora 1976). The neurons respond to taste in that they respond only when certain substances, such as glucose solution but not water or saline, are in the mouth, and in that their firing rates are related to the concentration of the substance to which they respond (Rolls, Burton & Mora 1980). These neurons did not respond simply in relation to mouth movements, and comprised 4.3% of the sample of 764 neurons. An example of a primate lateral hypothalamic neuron responding to the taste of food is shown in Fig. 5.8. Similar neurons that respond to palatable tastes have recently been described in the rat lateral hypothalamus (Li, Yoshida, Monk & Katz 2013).

The responses of the neurons associated with the sight of food occurred as soon as the monkey saw the food, before the food was in his mouth, and occurred only to foods and not to non-food objects (Rolls, Sanghera & Roper-Hall 1979a, Mora, Rolls & Burton 1976a) (see example in Fig. 5.9). These neurons comprised 11.8% of the sample of 764 neurons (Rolls, Burton & Mora 1976, Rolls, Burton & Mora 1980). Some of these neurons (2.5% of the total sample) responded to both the sight and taste of food (Rolls, Burton & Mora 1976, Rolls, Burton & Mora 1980). The finding that there are neurons in the lateral hypothalamus of the monkey that respond to the sight of food was confirmed by Ono and colleagues (1980, 1989).

The discovery that there are neurons in the lateral hypothalamus that respond to the sight

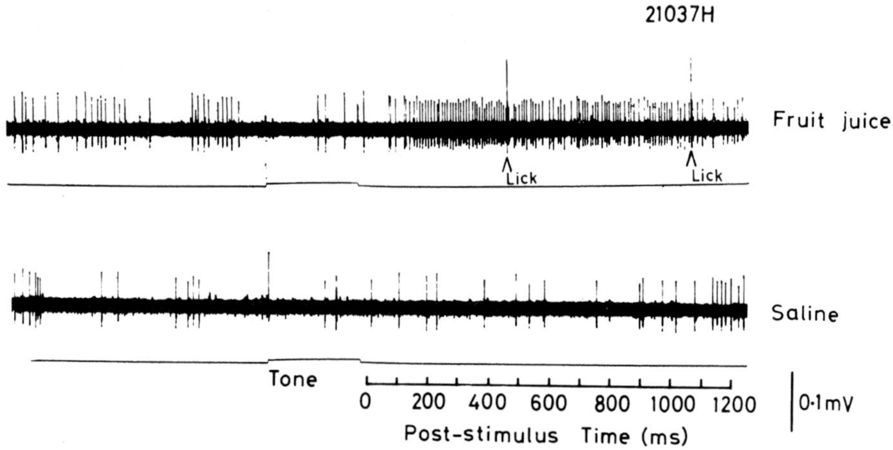

Fig. 5.9 Lateral hypothalamic neuron responding to the sight of food in a visual discrimination task. The neuron increased its firing above the spontaneous rate when a triangle was shown at time 0 which indicated that the monkey could lick a tube in front of his mouth to obtain fruit juice (top trace). The action potentials of the single neuron are the vertical spikes. The neuron did not respond when a square was shown which indicated that if the monkey licked, he would obtain aversive hypertonic saline from the lick tube (bottom trace). The latency of activation of different hypothalamic neurons by the sight of food was 150–200 ms, and compared with a latency of 250–300 ms for the earliest electrical activity associated with the motor responses of a lick made to obtain food when the food-related visual stimulus was shown. (Reprinted from *Brain Research*, 164 (1-2), E.T. Rolls, M.K. Sanghera, and A. Roper-Hall, The latency of activation of neurones in the lateral hypothalamus and substantia innominata during feeding in the monkey, pp. 121–135, Copyright, 1979, with permission from Elsevier.)

of food was an interesting discovery, for it emphasizes the importance in primates of vision, and not just generally, but for motivational behaviour in the selection of a goal object such as food. Indeed, the sight of what we eat conveys important information that can influence not only whether we select the food but also how the food tastes to us (see Section 4.5.5.7). The hypothesis that the lateral hypothalamic neurons were involved in reward effects which the sight and taste of food might produce by activating lateral hypothalamic neurons led to the next experiments, which investigated whether these neurons only responded to the sight and taste of food when it was rewarding. The experiments involved reducing the reward value of the food by feeding as much of the food as was wanted, and then measuring whether the neurons still responded to the sight and taste of the food when it was no longer rewarding.

Effects of devaluation by feeding to satiety show that food reward outcome value and expected value are encoded

When Rolls and colleagues fed monkeys to satiety, they found that gradually the lateral hypothalamic neurons reduced the magnitude of their responses, until when the monkey was satiated the neurons did not respond at all to the sight and taste of food (Burton, Rolls & Mora 1976, Rolls 1981b, Rolls, Murzi, Yaxley, Thorpe & Simpson 1986). An example is shown in Fig. 5.3 of a neuron that stopped responding to the sight of glucose after feeding to satiety with glucose, but which still responded to the sight of other foods. A sensory-specific satiety experiment for a lateral hypothalamic neuron with responses to the taste of food is illustrated in Fig. 5.10. These findings provide evidence that these neurons have activity that is closely related to either or both autonomic responses (such as salivation to the sight of food), and food reward value (leading to approach to and ingestion of a food reward) to the

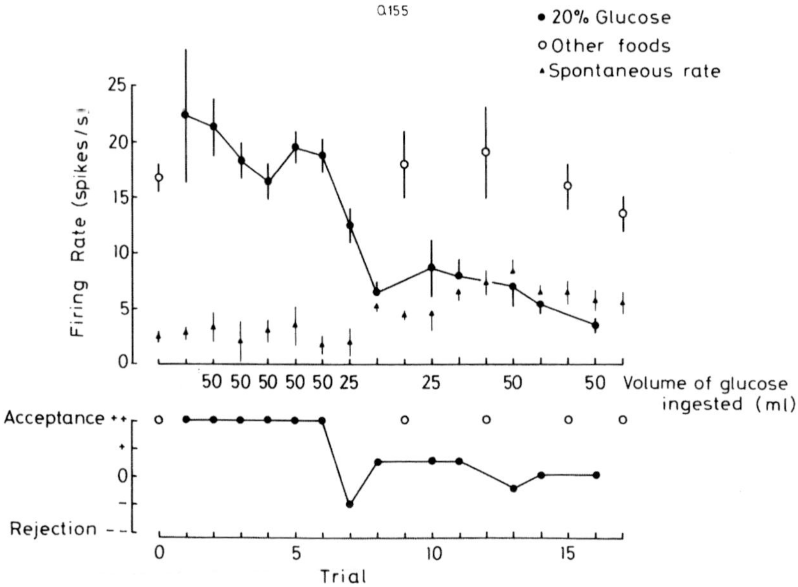

Fig. 5.10 The effect of feeding the monkey to satiety with 20% glucose solution on the responses of a lateral hypothalamic neuron to the taste of the glucose (filled circles) and to the taste of other foods (open circles). After the monkey had fed to satiety with glucose, the neuron responded much less to the taste of glucose, but still responded to the other foods. The mean responses of the neuron ($\pm$ s.e.m.) are shown to the stimuli at different stages of the experiment. The satiety of the monkey, shown below, was measured by whether he accepted or rejected the glucose. (Reprinted from *Brain Research*, 368 (1), E.T. Rolls, E. Murzi, S. Yaxley, S.J. Thorpe, and S.J. Simpson, Sensory-specific satiety: Food-specific reduction in responsiveness of ventral forebrain neurons after feeding in the monkey, pp. 79–86, Copyright (1986), with permission from Elsevier.)

sight and taste of food, which only occur to food if hunger is present.

The signals that reflect the motivational state and perform this modulation probably include many of those described in Section 5.3, such as gastric distension and duodenal stimulation by food (e.g. Gibbs, Maddison & Rolls (1981)), and reach the nucleus of the solitary tract via the vagus nerve as in rats (Ewart 1993, Mei 1993, Mei 1994). The plasma glucose level may be sensed by cells in the hindbrain near the area postrema, and at other sites in the brain (Ritter et al. 2011, Karadi, Oomura, Nishino, Scott, Lenard & Aou 1992, Begg & Woods 2013a). In the monkey there is less evidence about the location of the crucial sites for glucose sensing that control food intake. It is known that there are glucose-sensitive neurons in a number of hindbrain and hypothalamic sites, as shown by micro-electro-osmotic experiments in which glucose is applied locally to a neuron being recorded by using a small current to draw out sodium ion which then drags glucose with it (Oomura & Yoshimatsu 1984, Aou, Oomura, Lenard, Nishino, Inokuchi, Minami & Misaki 1984, Karadi et al. 1992).

The hypothalamus is not necessarily the first stage at which processing of food-related stimuli is modulated by hunger. Evidence on which is the first stage of processing where modulation by hunger occurs in primates is considered for the taste system below. To investigate whether hunger modulates neuronal responses in parts of the visual system through which visual information is likely to reach the hypothalamus (see below), the activity of neurons in the visual inferior temporal cortex was recorded in the same testing situations. It was found that the neuronal responses here to visual stimuli were not dependent on hunger (Rolls, Judge & Sanghera 1977). Nor were the responses of a sample of neurons in the amygdala, which connects the inferior temporal visual cortex to the hypothalamus (see below), found to depend on hunger (Sanghera, Rolls & Roper-Hall 1979, Rolls 1992a). However, in the orbitofrontal cortex, which receives inputs from the inferior temporal visual cortex, and projects into the hypothalamus (Russchen et al. 1985, Rempel-Clower & Barbas 1998, Price 2006), neurons with visual responses to food are found, and neuronal responses to food in this region are modulated by hunger (Thorpe, Rolls & Maddison 1983, Critchley & Rolls 1996c) (see Sections 5.4.2.3, 5.4.4.2 and 5.4.5).

Thus for visual processing, hunger modulates neuronal responsiveness only at late stages of processing (for example in the orbitofrontal cortex) and in the hypothalamus. The adaptive value of modulation of sensory processing only at late stages of processing, which occurs also in the taste system of primates, is discussed when food-related taste processing is described in Section 5.4.2.

Sensory-specific modulation of the responsiveness of lateral hypothalamic neurons and of appetite

During these experiments on satiety it was observed that if a lateral hypothalamic neuron had ceased to respond to a food on which the monkey had been fed to satiety, then the neuron might still respond to a different food (see examples in Figs. 5.3 and 5.10). This occurred for neurons with responses associated with the taste (Rolls 1981b, Rolls, Murzi, Yaxley, Thorpe & Simpson 1986) or sight (Rolls & Rolls 1982b, Rolls 1981b, Rolls, Murzi, Yaxley, Thorpe & Simpson 1986) of food. Corresponding to this neuronal specificity of the effects of feeding to satiety, the monkey rejected the food on which he had been fed to satiety, but accepted other foods which he had not been fed. Thus these neurons encode the value of the food, as shown by the choices made. It was as a result of these neurophysiological discoveries that the experiments on sensory-specific satiety in humans described in Section 5.3.1 were performed.

In addition to sensory-specific satiety, it is also worth noting that the mechanism is motivation-specific, in that some hypothalamic neurons respond more to food, and others more to water, when the monkey is both hungry and thirsty (see Fig. 5.11). Feeding to satiety reduces the responses of neurons that respond to food (see Figs. 5.3, and 5.10), and drinking to satiety reduces the responses of (in this case orbitofrontal cortex) neurons that respond to water (Rolls, Sienkiewicz & Yaxley 1989b).

Effects of learning: expected value in the lateral hypothalamus

The responses of these lateral hypothalamic neurons in the primate become associated with the sight of food as a result of learning. This is shown by experiments in which the neurons come to respond to the sight of a previously neutral stimulus, such as a syringe, from which the monkey is fed orally; in which the neurons cease to respond to a stimulus if it is no longer associated with food (in extinction or passive avoidance); and in which the responses of these neurons remain associated with whichever visual stimulus is associated with food reward in a visual discrimination and its reversals (Mora, Rolls & Burton 1976a, Wilson & Rolls 1990b, Wilson & Rolls 1990c). This type of learning is important for it enables organisms to respond appropriately to environmental stimuli that previous experience has shown are foods. The brain mechanisms for this type of learning are discussed below.

The responses of these neurons suggest that they are involved in representing the expected reward value of food. Further evidence for this is that the responses of these neurons occur with relatively short latencies of 150–200 ms, and thus precede and predict the choice responses of the hungry monkey to food (Rolls, Sanghera & Roper-Hall 1979a) (see Fig. 5.9).

Evidence that the responses of these lateral hypothalamic neurons are related to the reward value of food

Given that these hypothalamic neurons respond to food when it is rewarding, that is when

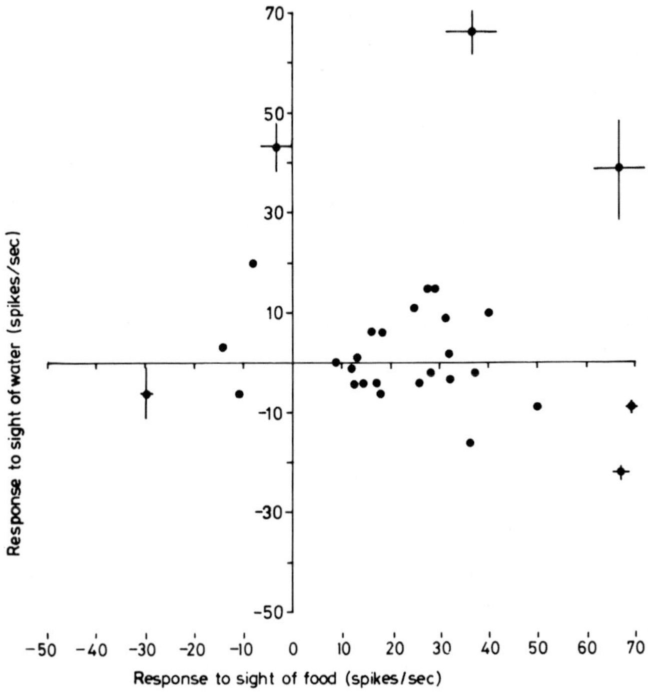

Fig. 5.11 Motivation-specific neuronal responses in the monkey lateral hypothalamus: some neurons responded more to the sight of food, and others to the sight of water, when the monkey was both hungry and thirsty. Each point represents the responses of a different single neuron to the sight of food and to the sight of water. Standard error bars are provided for some of the neurons to provide an indication that the differences in the responses of some of the neurons to the sight of food vs the sight of water were statistically significantly different. (Data of E. T. Rolls and E. Murzi.)

the animal will work to obtain food, it is a possibility that their responses are related to the reward value that food has for the hungry animal. Evidence consistent with this comes from studies with electrical stimulation of the brain. It has been found that electrical stimulation of some brain regions is rewarding in that animals including humans will work to obtain electrical stimulation of some sites in the brain (Olds 1977, Rolls 1975, Rolls 1976, Rolls 1979, Rolls 2005b). At some sites, including the lateral hypothalamus, the electrical stimulation appears to produce a reward that is equivalent to food for the hungry animal, in that the animal will work hard to obtain the stimulation if he is hungry, but will work much less for it if he has been satiated (Olds 1977, Hoebel 1969). There is even evidence that the reward at some sites can mimic food for a hungry animal and at other sites water for a thirsty animal, in that rats chose electrical stimulation at one hypothalamic site when hungry and at a different site when thirsty (Gallistel & Beagley 1971). It was therefore a fascinating discovery when it was found that some of the neurons normally activated by food when the monkey was hungry were also activated by brain-stimulation reward (Rolls 1975, Rolls 1976, Rolls, Burton & Mora 1980). Thus there was convergence of the effects of natural food reward and brain-stimulation reward at some brain sites (e.g. the orbitofrontal cortex and amygdala), on to single hypothalamic neurons. Further, it was shown that self-stimulation occurred through the recording electrode if it was near a region where hypothalamic neurons had been recorded that responded to food, and that this self-stimulation was attenuated by feeding the monkey to satiety (Rolls, Burton & Mora 1980) (see Fig. 5.12).

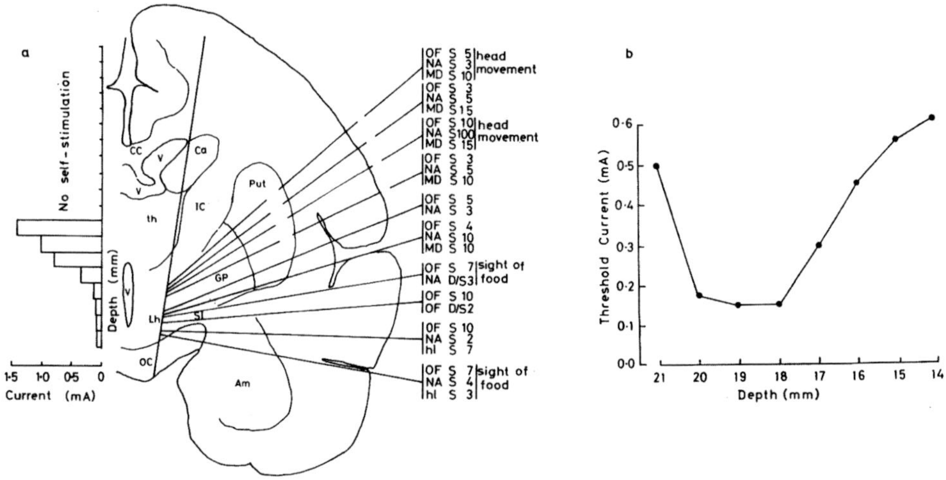

Fig. 5.12 (a) Neurons activated by both brain-stimulation reward and the sight of food were found at the lower end of this microelectrode track in the macaque lateral hypothalamus. Neurons higher up the track in the globus pallidus were activated by brain-stimulation reward and also by head movements. The neurons were trans-synaptically (S) or possibly in some cases directly (D/S) activated with the latencies shown in ms from self-stimulation sites in the orbitofrontal cortex (OF), nucleus accumbens (NA), mediodorsal nucleus of the thalamus (MD), or lateral hypothalamus (hl). (b) Self-stimulation through the recording microelectrode occurred with low currents if the microelectrode was in the hypothalamus close to the neurons activated by the sight of food. (Reprinted from *Brain Research*, 194 (2), E.T. Rolls, M.J. Burton, and F. Mora, Neurophysiological analysis of brain-stimulation reward in the monkey, pp. 339–357, Copyright (1980), with permission from Elsevier.)

The finding that these neurons were activated by brain-stimulation reward is consistent with the hypothesis that their activity is related to reward produced by food, and not to some other effect of food. Indeed, this evidence from the convergence of brain-stimulation reward and food reward on to these hypothalamic neurons, and from the self-stimulation found through the recording electrode, suggests that animals work to obtain activation of these neurons by food, and that this is what makes food rewarding. At the same time this accounts for self-stimulation of some brain sites, which is understood as the animal seeking to activate the neurons that she normally seeks to activate by food when she is hungry. This and other evidence (Rolls 1975, Rolls 2005b) indicates that feeding normally occurs in order to obtain the sensory input produced by food which is rewarding if the animal is hungry.

Sites in the hypothalamus and basal forebrain of neurons that respond to food reward value

These neurons are found as a relatively small proportion of cells in a region which includes the lateral hypothalamus and substantia innominata and extends from the lateral hypothalamus posteriorly through the anterior hypothalamus and lateral preoptic area to a region ventral to and anterior to the anterior commissure (Rolls, Sanghera & Roper-Hall 1979a)) (see Fig. 5.13).

In addition to a role in food reward value and thus in the control of feeding, it seems quite likely that at least some of the hypothalamic feeding-related neurons influence brainstem autonomic motor neurons. Consistent with this, it is known that there are projections from the lateral hypothalamus to the brainstem autonomic motor nuclei, and that lesions of the lateral hypothalamus disrupt conditioned autonomic responses (LeDoux et al. 1988).

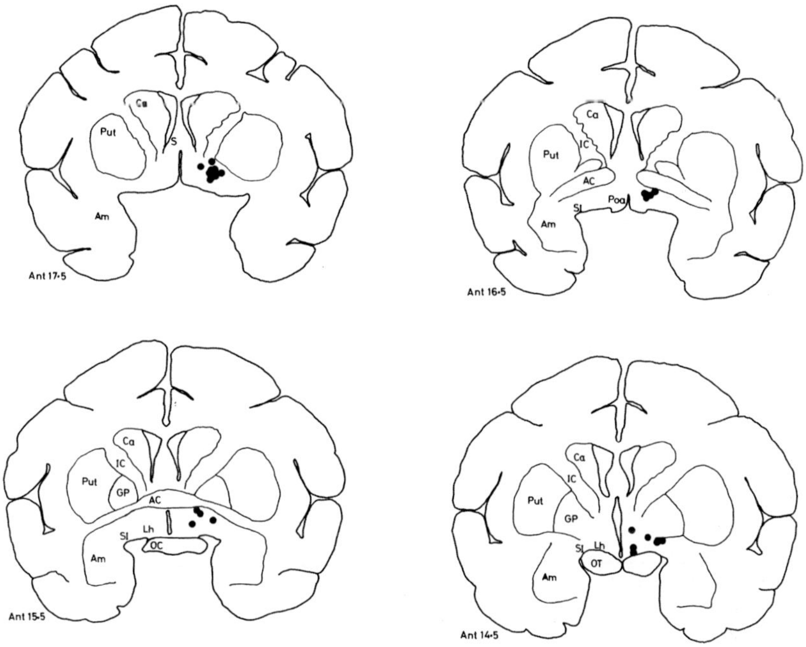

Fig. 5.13 Sites in the lateral hypothalamus and basal forebrain of the macaque at which neurons were recorded that responded to the sight of food. Abbreviations: AC, anterior commissure; Am, amygdala; Ca, caudate nucleus; GP, globus pallidus; IC, internal capsule; Lh, lateral hypothalamus; OC, optic chiasm; OT, optic tract; Poa, preoptic area; Put, putamen; S, septal region; SI, substantia innominata. (Reprinted from *Brain Research*, 164 (1-2), E.T. Rolls, M.K. Sanghera, and A. Roper-Hall, The latency of activation of neurones in the lateral hypothalamus and substantia innominata during feeding in the monkey, pp. 121–135, Copyright, 1979, with permission from Elsevier.)

Functions of the hypothalamus in feeding

The functions of the hypothalamus in feeding are thus related at least in part to the inputs that it receives from forebrain structures such as the orbitofrontal cortex and amygdala, in that it contains neurons that respond to the sight of food, and that are influenced by learning. (Such pattern-specific visual responses, and their modification by learning, require forebrain areas such as the inferior temporal visual cortex and the amygdala, as described below.) This conclusion is consistent with the anatomy of the hypothalamus and substantia innominata, which receive projections from limbic structures such as the orbitofrontal cortex and amygdala which in turn receive projections from the association cortex (Herzog & Van Hoesen 1976, Price 2006). The conclusion is also consistent with the evidence that decerebrate rats retain simple controls of feeding, but do not show normal learning about foods (Grill & Norgren 1978). These rats accept sweet solutions placed in their mouths when hungry and reject them when satiated, so some control of responses to gustatory stimuli which depends on hunger can occur caudal to the level of the hypothalamus. However, these rats are unable to feed themselves, and do not learn to avoid poisoned solutions.

The importance of visual inputs and learning to feeding, in relation to which some hypothalamic neurons respond, is that animals, and especially primates, may eat many foods every day, and must be able to select foods from other visual stimuli, as well as produce appropriate preparative responses to them such as salivation and the release of insulin. They must also be able to initiate appropriate actions in the environment to obtain food. Before any activation of motor neurons, such as those that innervate the masticatory muscles, involved in feeding, it is normally necessary to select which reward in the environment should be selected for action, and then to select an appropriate (arbitrary) action to obtain the selected reward. This indicates that direct connections from food reward systems in the brain directly to motor neurons are likely to be involved only in the lowest level (in the sense of Hughlings Jackson, see Swash (1989)) of the control of behaviour. Instead, food reward systems might be expected to project to an action-control system, and connections therefore from the lateral hypothalamus, amygdala, and orbitofrontal cortex to systems such as the cingulate cortex and basal ganglia are likely to be more important as routes for the initiation of normal feeding (see Section 6.3 on the striatum and basal ganglia).

5.4.2 Brain mechanisms for taste reward value

5.4.2.1 Taste processing up to and including the primary taste cortex of primates is related to the identity of the tastant, and not to its reward value

Given that there are neurons in the hypothalamus that can respond to the taste (and/or sight) of foods but not of non-foods, and that modulation of this sensory input by motivation is seen when recordings are made from these hypothalamic neurons, it may be asked whether these are special properties of hypothalamic neurons which they show because they are specially involved in the control of motivational responses, or whether this degree of specificity and type of modulation are general properties which are evident throughout sensory systems. In one respect it would be inefficient if motivational modulation were present far peripherally, because this would imply that sensory information was being discarded without the possibility for central processing. A subjective correspondent of such a situation might be that it might not be possible to taste food, or even to see food, when satiated! It is perhaps more efficient for most of the system to function similarly whether hungry or satiated, and to have a special system (such as the hypothalamus) following sensory processing where motivational state influences responsiveness. Evidence on the actual state of affairs that exists for visual processing in primates in relation to feeding has been summarized above. In contrast, apparently there is at least some peripheral modulation of taste processing in rats (in the nucleus of the solitary tract) (Scott & Giza 1992, Rolls & Scott 2003). Evidence has now been obtained for primates on the tuning of neurons in the gustatory pathways, and on whether responsiveness at different stages is influenced by motivation, as follows. These investigations on the gustatory pathways have also been able to show where flavour, that is a combination of taste and olfactory input, is computed in the primate brain. The gustatory and olfactory pathways, and some of their onward connections, are shown in Fig. 4.2.

The first central synapse of the gustatory system is in the rostral part of the nucleus of the solitary tract (Beckstead & Norgren 1979, Beckstead, Morse & Norgren 1980, Rolls 2014a). The caudal half of this nucleus receives visceral afferents, and it is a possibility that such visceral information, reflecting, for example, gastric distension, is used to modulate gustatory processing even at this early stage of the gustatory system.

In order to investigate the tuning of neurons in the nucleus of the solitary tract, and whether hunger does influence processing at this first central opportunity in the gustatory system of primates, we recorded the activity of single neurons in the nucleus of the solitary tract. To ensure that our results were relevant to the normal control of feeding (and were not, for example, because of abnormally high levels of artificially administered putative satiety signals), we allowed the monkeys to feed until they were satiated, and determined whether this normal and physiological induction of satiety influenced the responsiveness of neurons in the nucleus of the solitary tract, which were recorded throughout the feeding, until satiety was reached. It was found that in the nucleus of the solitary tract, the first central relay in the gustatory system, neurons are relatively broadly tuned to the prototypical taste stimuli (sweet, salt, bitter, and sour) (Scott, Yaxley, Sienkiewicz & Rolls 1986a). It was also found that neuronal responses in the nucleus of the solitary tract to the taste of food are not influenced by whether the monkey is hungry or satiated (Yaxley, Rolls, Sienkiewicz & Scott 1985).

To investigate whether there are neurons in the primary gustatory cortex in the primate that are more closely tuned to respond to foods as compared to non-foods, and whether hunger modulates the responsiveness of these neurons, we have recorded the activity of single neurons in the primary gustatory cortex during feeding in the monkey. In the primary gustatory cortex in the frontal operculum and insula, neurons are more sharply tuned to gustatory stimuli than in the nucleus of the solitary tract, with some neurons responding primarily, for example, to sweet, and much less to salt, bitter, or sour stimuli (Scott, Yaxley, Sienkiewicz & Rolls 1986b, Yaxley, Rolls & Sienkiewicz 1990). However, here also, hunger does not influence the magnitude of neuronal responses to gustatory stimuli (Rolls, Scott, Sienkiewicz & Yaxley 1988, Yaxley, Rolls & Sienkiewicz 1988). Consistent with this, activations in the human insular primary taste cortex are linearly related to the subjective intensity of the taste and not to the pleasantness rating (Fig. 4.44 (Grabenhorst & Rolls 2008)). Further, activations in the human insular primary taste cortex are related to the concentration of the tastant, for example monosodium glutamate (Grabenhorst, Rolls & Bilderbeck 2008a).

Single neurons in the insular primary taste cortex also represent the viscosity (measured with carboxymethylcellulose) and temperature of stimuli in the mouth, and fat texture, but not the sight and smell of food (Verhagen, Kadohisa & Rolls 2004, Kadohisa, Rolls & Verhagen 2005b). In humans, the insular primary taste cortex is activated not only by taste (Francis, Rolls, Bowtell, McGlone, O'Doherty, Browning, Clare & Smith 1999, Small, Zald, Jones-Gotman, Zatorre, Petrides & Evans 1999, De Araujo, Kringelbach, Rolls & Hobden 2003a, De Araujo & Rolls 2004, De Araujo, Kringelbach, Rolls & McGlone 2003b, Grabenhorst, Rolls & Bilderbeck 2008a, Grabenhorst, Rolls & Bilderbeck 2008a), but also by oral texture including viscosity (with the activation linearly related to the log of the viscosity) and fat texture (De Araujo & Rolls 2004), and temperature (Guest, Grabenhorst, Essick, Chen, Young, McGlone, de Araujo & Rolls 2007). These investigations in humans indicate that there is a taste-related area in the anterior taste insula, in a region typically between Y=10 and Y=20 (see examples in Figs. 5.14 and 4.45), and that activations here are not related to pleasantness, but to intensity (see Fig. 4.45). This is probably the primary taste cortex[12]. Activations posterior to this towards the mid-insula can be produced by oral stimuli including oral texture, chocolate, etc. (De Araujo & Rolls 2004, Small 2010) and any taste where a tasteless control is not subtracted because introducing a tastant into the mouth inevitably produces somatosensory and related effects (Francis, Rolls, Bowtell, McGlone, O'Doherty, Browning, Clare & Smith 1999, De Araujo, Kringelbach, Rolls & Hobden 2003a).

5.4.2.2 Taste and taste-related processing in the orbitofrontal (secondary taste) cortex, including umami taste, astringency, fat, viscosity, temperature and capsaicin

A secondary cortical taste area has been discovered in the caudolateral orbitofrontal taste cortex of the primate in which gustatory neurons can be even more finely tuned to particular

[12] In some different investigations, the [X Y Z] coordinates of the taste cortex in the anterior part of the insular taste cortex were as follows: flavour - rinse [30 18 8] (Grabenhorst & Rolls 2013); [30 12 0] and [32 22 0] (Rolls & McCabe 2007); [34 24 6] (McCabe & Rolls 2007); conjunction of taste - rinse and MSG 0.4M - MSG 0.1 M [34 16 4] (Grabenhorst, Rolls & Bilderbeck 2008a); conjunction of texture - rinse and glucose - rinse [-36 12 6] (De Araujo & Rolls 2004).

taste stimuli (Rolls, Yaxley & Sienkiewicz 1990, Rolls & Treves 1990, Rolls, Sienkiewicz & Yaxley 1989b, Verhagen, Rolls & Kadohisa 2003, Rolls, Verhagen & Kadohisa 2003e, Kadohisa, Rolls & Verhagen 2004, Kadohisa, Rolls & Verhagen 2005b, Rolls, Critchley, Verhagen & Kadohisa 2010a) (see Figs. 4.20, 4.21, 4.22, 4.28, 4.29, 4.34, and 4.48). In addition to representations of the 'prototypical' taste stimuli sweet, salt, bitter, and sour, different neurons in this region respond to other taste and taste-related stimuli that provide information about the reward value of a potential food (Rolls 2008a, Rolls 2006c, Kadohisa, Rolls & Verhagen 2005b). One example of this additional taste information is a set of neurons that respond to umami taste, as described next.

Umami taste. An important food taste which appears to be different from that produced by sweet, salt, bitter, or sour is the taste of protein. At least part of this taste is captured by the Japanese word 'umami', which is a taste common to a diversity of food sources including fish, meats, mushrooms, cheese, some vegetables such as tomatoes, and human mothers' milk. Within these food sources, it is glutamates and $5'$ nucleotides, sometimes in a synergistic combination, that create the umami taste (Ikeda 1909, Yamaguchi 1967, Yamaguchi & Kimizuka 1979, Kawamura & Kare 1992). Monosodium L-glutamate (MSG), and the $5'$ nucleotides guanosine $5'$-monophosphate (GMP), and inosine $5'$-monophosphate (IMP), are examples of umami stimuli.

These findings raise the question of whether umami taste operates through information channels in the primate taste system which are separable from those for the 'prototypical' tastes sweet, salt, bitter, and sour. (Although the concept of four prototypical tastes has been used by tradition, there is increasing discussion about the utility of the concept, and increasing evidence that the taste system is more diverse than this – see, e.g., Kawamura & Kare (1992).) To investigate the neural encoding of glutamate in the primate, Baylis & Rolls (1991) made recordings from 190 taste-responsive neurons in the primary taste cortex and adjoining orbitofrontal cortex taste area in macaques. Single neurons were found that were tuned to respond best to monosodium glutamate (umami taste), just as other cells were found with best responses to glucose (sweet), sodium chloride (salty), HCl (sour), and quinine HCl (bitter). Across the population of neurons, the responsiveness to glutamate was poorly correlated with the responsiveness to NaCl, so that the representation of glutamate was clearly different from that of NaCl. Further, the representation of glutamate was shown to be approximately as different from each of the other four tastants as they are from each other, as shown by multidimensional scaling and cluster analysis. Moreover, it was found that glutamate is approximately as well represented in terms of mean evoked neural activity and the number of cells with best responses to it as the other four stimuli glucose, NaCl, HCl and quinine. It was concluded that in primate taste cortical areas, glutamate, which produces umami taste in humans, is approximately as well represented as are the tastes produced by: glucose (sweet), NaCl (salty), HCl (sour) and quinine HCl (bitter) (Baylis & Rolls 1991).

In a further investigation, these findings have been extended beyond the sodium salt of glutamate to other umami tastants which have the glutamate ion but which do not introduce sodium ion into the experiment; and to a nucleotide umami tastant (Rolls, Critchley, Wakeman & Mason 1996c). In recordings made mainly from neurons in the orbitofrontal cortex taste area, it was shown that single neurons that had their best responses to sodium glutamate also had good responses to glutamic acid. The correlation between the responses to these two tastants was higher than between any other pair which included in addition a prototypical set including glucose (sweet), sodium chloride (salty), HCl (sour), and quinine HCl (bitter). Moreover, the responsiveness to glutamic acid clustered with the response to monosodium glutamate in a cluster analysis with this set of stimuli, and glutamic acid was close to sodium glutamate in a space created by multidimensional scaling. It was also shown that

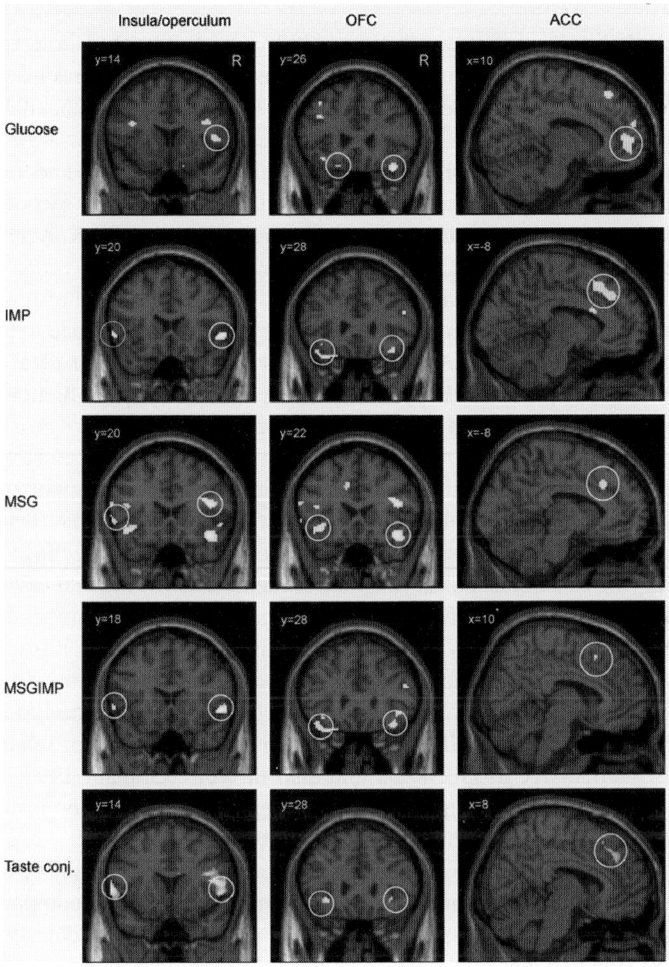

Fig. 5.14 Activation of the human primary taste cortex in the insula/frontal operculum; the orbitofrontal cortex (OFC); and the anterior cingulate cortex (ACC) by taste. The stimuli used included glucose, two umami taste stimuli (monosodium glutamate (MSG) and inosine monophosphate (IMP)), and a mixture of the two umami stimuli. Taste conj. refers to a conjunction analysis over all the taste stimuli. (See colour plates section.) (Reproduced from *Journal of Neurophysiology*, 90 (1), Representation of umami taste in the human brain, I. E. T. De Araujo, M. L. Kringelbach, E. T. Rolls, and P. Hobden, pp. 313–319 ©2003, The American Physiological Society.)

the responses of these neurons to the nucleotide umami tastant inosine 5′-monophosphate were more correlated with their responses to monosodium glutamate than to any prototypical tastant.

Thus neurophysiological evidence in primates does indicate that there is a representation of umami flavour in the cortical areas which is separable from that to the prototypical tastants sweet, salt, bitter, and sour (see further Rolls, Critchley, Browning & Hernadi (1998a)). This representation is probably important in the taste produced by proteins (Chaudhari & Roper 2010, Haid, Widmayer, Voigt, Chaudhari, Boehm & Breer 2013). These neurons are found not only in the orbitofrontal cortex taste areas, but also in the primary taste cortex (Baylis & Rolls 1991).

There is now clear evidence that there are taste receptors on the tongue specialized for umami taste (Chaudhari, Landin & Roper 2000, Zhao, Zhang, Hoon, Chandrashekar, Erlenbach, Ryba & Zucker 2003, Lin, Ogura & Kinnamon 2003, Chandrashekar, Hoon, Ryba & Zuker 2006, Chaudhari & Roper 2010, Haid, Widmayer, Voigt, Chaudhari, Boehm & Breer 2013).

In addition, the umami tastants monosodium glutamate and inosine monophosphate activate the human primary taste cortex in the insula/operculum, the secondary taste cortex in the orbitofrontal cortex, and the cingulate cortex (De Araujo, Kringelbach, Rolls & Hobden 2003a), as shown in Fig. 5.14.

This evidence shows that umami taste, an indicator of the presence of protein, is implemented by neurons in the primary and secondary taste cortex that are tuned to umami stimuli. Umami is a component of many foods which helps to make them taste pleasant, especially when the umami taste is paired with a consonant savoury odour (Rolls, Critchley, Browning & Hernadi 1998a, McCabe & Rolls 2007, Rolls 2009c).

Astringency. Another taste-related stimulus quality that provides important information about the reward value of a potential food source is astringency. In humans, tannic acid elicits a characteristic astringent taste. Oral astringency is perceived as the feeling of long-lasting puckering and drying sensations on the tongue and membranes of the oral cavity. High levels of tannic acid in some potential foods makes them unpalatable without preparative techniques to reduce its presence (Johns & Duquette 1991), yet in small quantities it is commonly used to enhance the flavour of food. In this context tannic acid is a constituent of a large range of spices and condiments, such as ginger, chillies, and black pepper (Uma-Pradeep, Geervani & Eggum 1993). (Tannic acid itself is not present in tea, yet a range of related polyphenol compounds are, particularly in green tea, and also in wine (Graham 1992, Lesschaeve & Noble 2005).) Tannic acid is a natural antioxidant by virtue of its chemical structure (see Critchley & Rolls (1996a)).

The evolutionary adaptive value of the ability to detect astringency may be related to some of the properties of tannic acid. Tannic acid is a member of the class of compounds known as polyphenols, which are present in a wide spectrum of plant matter, particularly in foliage, the skin and husks of fruit and nuts, and the bark of trees. The tannic acid in leaves is produced as a defence against insects. There is less tannic acid in young leaves than in old leaves. Large monkeys cannot obtain the whole of their protein intake from small animals, insects etc., and thus obtain some of their protein from leaves. Tannic acid binds protein (hence its use in tanning) and amino acids, and thus prevents their absorption. Thus it is adaptive for monkeys to be able to taste tannic acid, so that they can select food sources without too much tannic acid (Hladik 1978).

In order to investigate whether astringency is represented in the cortical taste areas concerned with taste, Critchley & Rolls (1996a) recorded from taste-responsive neurons in the orbitofrontal cortex and adjacent insula. Single neurons were found that were tuned to respond to tannic acid (0.001 M), and represented a subpopulation of neurons that was distinct from neurons responsive to the tastes of glucose (sweet), NaCl (salty), HCl (sour), quinine (bitter) and monosodium glutamate (umami). In addition, across the population of taste-responsive neurons, tannic acid was as well represented as the tastes of NaCl, HCl, quinine, or monosodium glutamate. Multidimensional scaling analysis of the neuronal responses to the tastants indicates that tannic acid lies outside the boundaries of the four conventional taste qualities (sweet, sour, bitter, and salty). Taken together these data indicate that the astringent taste of tannic acid should be considered as a distinct 'taste' quality, which receives a separate representation from sweet, salt, bitter, and sour in the primate cortical taste areas. Tannic acid may produce its 'taste' effects not through the taste nerves, but through the somatosensory inputs conveyed through the trigeminal nerve. Astringency is thus strictly not a sixth taste

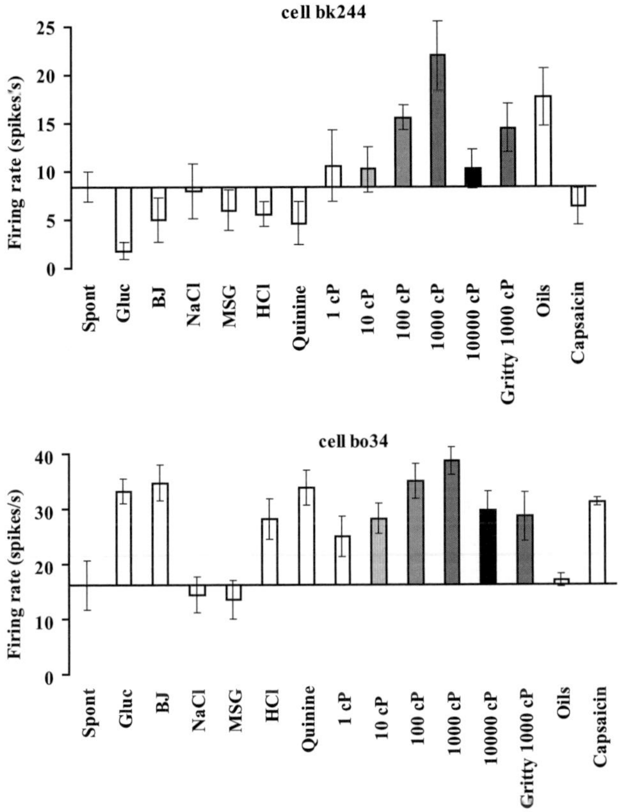

Fig. 5.15 Above. Firing rates (mean ± s.e.m.) of orbitofrontal cortex viscosity-sensitive neuron bk244 which did not have taste responses. The firing rates are shown to the viscosity series (carboxymethylcellulose in the range 1–10,000 centiPoise), to the gritty stimulus (carboxymethylcellulose with Fillite microspheres), to the taste stimuli 1 M glucose (Gluc), 0.1 M NaCl, 0.1 M MSG , 0.01 M HCl and 0.001 M QuinineHCl, and to fruit juice (BJ). Spont = spontaneous firing rate. Below. Firing rates (mean ± s.e.m.) of viscosity-sensitive neuron bo34 which had no response to the oils (mineral oil, vegetable oil, safflower oil and coconut oil, which have viscosities which are all close to 50 cP). The neuron did not respond to the gritty stimulus in a way that was unexpected given the viscosity of the stimulus, was taste tuned, and did respond to capsaicin. (Reproduced from *Journal of Neurophysiology*, 90 (6), Representations of the texture of food in the primate orbitofrontal cortex: neurons responding to viscosity, grittiness, and capsaicin, E. T. Rolls, J. V. Verhagen, and M. Kadohisa, pp. 3711–3724, ©2003, The American Physiological Society.)

in the sense that umami is a fifth taste. However, what has been shown in these studies is that the orosensory, probably somatosensory, sensations produced by tannic acid do converge with effects produced through taste inputs, to result in neurons in the orbitofrontal cortex responding to both taste stimuli and to astringent stimuli.

Food texture: viscosity. Another important type of input to the same region of the orbitofrontal cortex that is concerned with detecting the reward value of a potential food is an input produced by the texture of food in the mouth. We have shown for example that single neurons influenced by taste in this region can in some cases have their responses modulated by the texture of the food (Rolls 2011e). This was shown in experiments in which the texture of food was manipulated by the addition of methyl cellulose or gelatine, or by puréeing a semi-solid food (Rolls 2011e). We have been able to show that some of these neurons respond to the

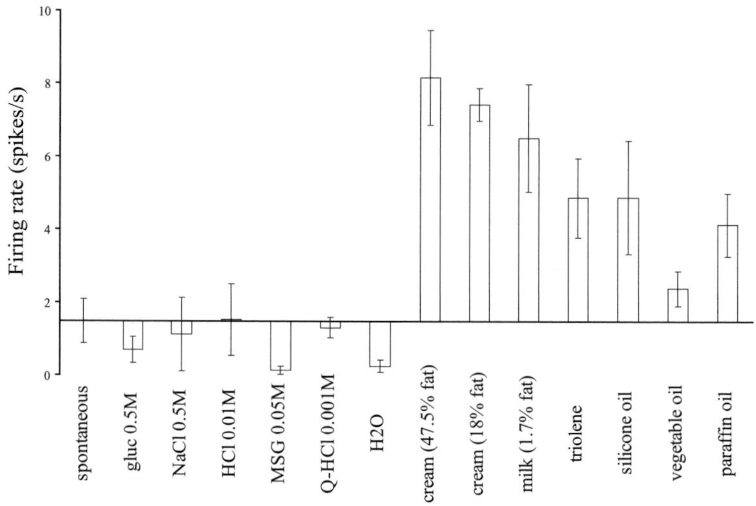

Fig. 5.16 A neuron in the primate orbitofrontal cortex responding to the texture of fat in the mouth. The neuron increased its firing rate to cream (double and single cream, with the fat proportions shown), and responded to texture rather than the chemical structure of the fat in that it also responded to 0.5 ml of silicone oil ($Si(CH_3)_2O)_n$) or paraffin oil (hydrocarbon). The neuron did not have a taste input. Gluc, glucose; NaCl, salt; HCl, sour; Q-HCl, quinine, bitter. The spontaneous firing rate of the cell is also shown. (Reproduced from *Journal of Neuroscience*, 19 (4), Responses to the sensory properties of fat of neurons in the primate orbitofrontal cortex, E. T. Rolls, H. D. Critchley, A. S. Browning, A. Hernadi, and L. Lenard, pp. 1532–1540, ©1999, The Society for Neuroscience.)

viscosity of the food in the mouth, as altered parametrically using the standard food thickening agent carboxymethylcellulose made up in viscosities of 1–10,000 cPoise (Rolls, Verhagen & Kadohisa 2003e). (10,000 cP is approximately the viscosity of toothpaste.) Some of these neurons are unimodal, responding just to texture and not to taste (see Fig. 5.15 upper). Others respond to different combinations of texture and taste, as illustrated in Fig. 5.15 (lower). These recordings provide unique evidence about the texture channels that convey information from the mouth to the cortex, for they show that the system can potentially have responses to texture separately from the other sensory attributes of food, as well as to particular combinations of taste, texture, and other sensory properties of food.

The somatosensory inputs may reach the orbitofrontal cortex via the primary taste cortex in the rostral insula and adjoining frontal operculum, which we have shown does project into this region (Baylis, Rolls & Baylis 1994), and which also contains a representation of the viscosity of what is in the mouth (Verhagen, Kadohisa & Rolls 2004). A number of parts of the insula are known to receive somatosensory inputs (Mesulam & Mufson 1982a, Mesulam & Mufson 1982b, Mufson & Mesulam 1982). The texture of food is an important cue about the quality of the food, for example about the ripeness of fruit.

These findings have been extended to the human, with the finding with fMRI that the activation of the primary taste cortex is proportional to the logarithm of the viscosity of the stimulus in the mouth (De Araujo & Rolls 2004).

Food texture: fat. Texture in the mouth is also an important indicator of whether fat is present in the food, which is important not only as a high value energy source, but also as a potential source of essential fatty acids. In the orbitofrontal cortex, Rolls, Critchley, Browning, Hernadi & Lenard (1999a) have found a population of neurons that responds when fat is in the mouth. An example of such a neuron is shown in Fig. 5.16. This neuron had no response to taste, but some other neurons had convergence of fat texture and taste inputs. The fat-related responses of these neurons are produced at least in part by the texture of the food rather than by chemical receptors sensitive to certain chemicals, in that such neurons typically respond not only to foods such as cream and milk containing fat, but also to paraffin oil (which is a pure hydrocarbon) and to silicone oil (which contains $(Si(CH_3)_2O)_n$).

Some of the fat-related neurons do though have multimodal convergent inputs from the chemical senses, in that in addition to taste inputs some of these neurons respond to the odour associated with a fat, such as the odour of cream (Rolls, Critchley, Browning, Hernadi & Lenard 1999a). The texture-related responses of these oral fat-sensitive neurons are independent of the viscosity of what is in the mouth and of fatty acids in the mouth (Verhagen, Rolls & Kadohisa 2003), so that fat in food can be detected orally by a specialized fat/oil texture channel (Rolls 2011e). Similar neurons have been recorded in the pregenual cingulate cortex (Rolls 2008e).

This type of discovery can be made only at the single neuron level, and paves the way for further studies of the transducing mechanism, understanding of which could be important in the design of foods with pleasant textures which do not bring with them high caloric content with its implications for obesity (Rolls 2011e).

These findings have been extended to the human, with the finding with fMRI that activation of the orbitofrontal cortex and perigenual cingulate cortex is produced by the texture of fat in the mouth (De Araujo & Rolls 2004). Moreover, activations in the orbitofrontal cortex and pregenual cingulate cortex are correlated with the pleasantness of fat texture in the mouth (Grabenhorst, Rolls, Parris & D'Souza 2010b).

5.4.2.3 The reward value of taste is represented in the orbitofrontal cortex

In the primate orbitofrontal cortex, it is found that the responses of taste neurons to the particular food with which a monkey is fed to satiety decrease to zero (Rolls, Sienkiewicz & Yaxley 1989b). An example is shown in Fig. 4.22 on page 105. This neuron reduced its responses to the taste of glucose during the course of feeding as much glucose as the monkey wanted to drink. When the monkey was fully satiated, and did not want to drink any more glucose, the neuron no longer responded to the taste of glucose. Thus the responses of these neurons decrease to zero when the reward value of the food decreases to zero. Interestingly the neuron still responded to other foods, and the monkey chose to eat these other foods. Thus the modulation of the responses of these orbitofrontal cortex taste neurons occurs in a sensory-specific way, and they represent *reward outcome value*.

Another example is shown in Fig. 5.17 (after Rolls, Critchley, Browning, Hernadi & Lenard (1999a)). This neuron decreased its response to the fatty texture of cream when fed to satiety with cream, but still responded to the taste of glucose after feeding to satiety with cream. This indicated sensory-specific satiety for the reward value of the texture of cream in the mouth, and also provides evidence that absolute value and not relative value is represented in the orbitofrontal cortex (Section 9.5.3).

The orbitofrontal cortex is the first stage of the primate taste system in which this modulation of the responses of neurons to the taste of food is affected by hunger, in that this modulation is not found in the nucleus of the solitary tract, or in the frontal opercular or insular primary gustatory cortices (Yaxley, Rolls, Sienkiewicz & Scott 1985, Rolls, Scott, Sienkiewicz & Yaxley 1988, Yaxley, Rolls & Sienkiewicz 1988). It is of course only when hungry that the taste of food is rewarding. This is an indication that the responses of these orbitofrontal cortex taste neurons reflect the reward value of food. The firing of these orbitofrontal neurons may actually implement the reward value of a food. The hypothesis is that primates work to obtain firing of these reward value neurons, by eating food when they are

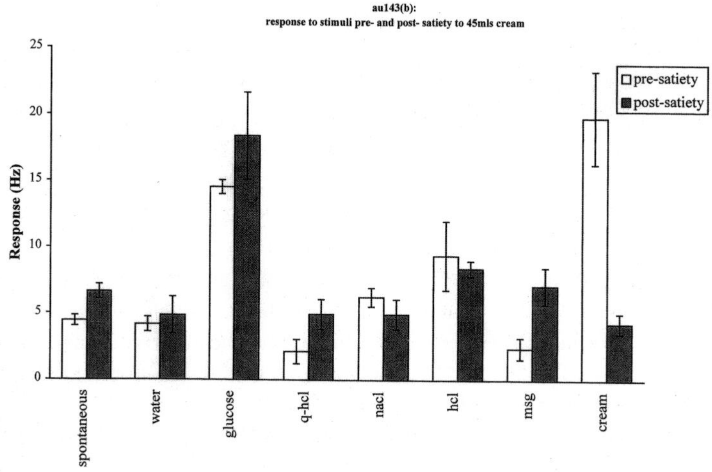

Fig. 5.17 A neuron in the primate orbitofrontal cortex that decreased its response to the texture of fat (cream) in the mouth after feeding to satiety with cream. The neuron did not decrease its response to the taste of glucose after feeding to satiety with fat (single cream). Gluc, 1 M glucose; NaCl 0.1 M, salt; 0.01 M HCl, sour; 0.001 M Q-HCl, quinine, bitter. The spontaneous firing rate of the cell is also shown. (Reproduced from *Journal of Neuroscience*, 19 (4), Responses to the sensory properties of fat of neurons in the primate orbitofrontal cortex, E. T. Rolls, H. D. Critchley, A. S. Browning, A. Hernadi, and L. Lenard, pp. 1532–1540, ©1999, The Society for Neuroscience.)

hungry.

Further evidence that the firing of these orbitofrontal cortex taste neurons does actually implement the primary reward value of food is that in another experiment we showed that monkeys would work to obtain electrical stimulation of this area of the brain (Rolls, Burton & Mora 1980, Mora, Avrith, Phillips & Rolls 1979, Mora, Avrith & Rolls 1980). Moreover, the reward value of the electrical stimulation was dependent on hunger being present. If the monkey was fed to satiety, the monkey no longer found electrical stimulation at this site so rewarding, and stopped working for the electrical stimulation. Indeed, of all the brain sites tested, this orbitofrontal cortex region was the part of the brain in which the reward value of the electrical stimulation was most affected by feeding to satiety (Mora, Avrith, Phillips & Rolls 1979, Mora, Avrith & Rolls 1980, Rolls, Burton & Mora 1980). Thus all this evidence indicates that the reward value of taste is encoded in the secondary taste cortex, and that primates work to obtain food in order to activate these neurons, the activation of which actually mediates reward. This is probably an innate reward system, in that taste can act as a reward in rats without prior training (Berridge, Flynn, Schulkin & Grill 1984).

The neurophysiological discoveries that feeding to satiety reduces the responses of secondary taste cortex neurons, but not neurons earlier in taste processing, are relevant to what normally produces satiety, in that in these experiments the neurons were recorded while the monkeys were fed to normal satiety. It could be that later in satiety there is some modulation of responsiveness earlier in the taste pathways, occurring perhaps as food is absorbed. But even if this does occur, such modulation would not then account for the change in acceptability of food, which of course is seen as the satiety develops, and is used to define satiety. Nor would this modulation be relevant to the decrease in the pleasantness in the taste of a food which occurs when it is eaten to satiety (Cabanac 1971, Rolls, Rolls, Rowe & Sweeney 1981a, Rolls,

Rowe, Rolls, Kingston, Megson & Gunary 1981b, Rolls, Rolls & Rowe 1983b, Rolls & Rolls 1977, Rolls & Rolls 1982b, Rolls 2012c).

Thus it appears that the reduced acceptance of food as satiety develops, and the reduction in its pleasantness, are not produced by a reduction in the responses of neurons in the nucleus of the solitary tract or frontal opercular or insular gustatory cortices to gustatory stimuli. (As described above, the responses of gustatory neurons in these areas do not decrease as satiety develops.) Indeed, after feeding to satiety, humans reported that the taste of the food on which they had been satiated tasted almost as intense as when they were hungry, though much less pleasant (Rolls, Rolls & Rowe 1983b). This comparison is consistent with the possibility that activity in the frontal opercular and insular taste cortices as well as the nucleus of the solitary tract does not reflect the pleasantness of the taste of a food, but rather its sensory qualities independently of motivational state. On the other hand, the responses of the neurons in the orbitofrontal taste area and in the lateral hypothalamus are modulated by satiety, and it is presumably in areas such as these that neuronal activity may be related to whether a food tastes pleasant, and to whether the human or animal will work to obtain and then eat the food, that is to whether the food is rewarding. The situation is not necessarily the same in non-primates, in that in the rat some reduction in the responses of taste neurons in the nucleus of the solitary tract was produced by glucose infusions (Scott & Giza 1992, Scott et al. 1995, Rolls & Scott 2003).

The present results also provide evidence on the nature of the mechanisms that underlie sensory-specific satiety. Sensory-specific satiety, as noted above in Section 5.3.1, is the phenomenon in which the decrease in the palatability and acceptability of a food that has been eaten to satiety are partly specific to the particular food that has been eaten. The results just described suggest that such sensory-specific satiety for taste cannot be largely accounted for by adaptation at the receptor level, in the nucleus of the solitary tract, or in the frontal opercular or insular gustatory cortices, to the food which has been eaten to satiety, otherwise modulation of neuronal responsiveness should have been apparent in the recordings made in these regions. Indeed, the findings suggest that sensory-specific satiety is not represented in the primary gustatory cortex. It is thus of particular interest that a decrease in the response of orbitofrontal cortex neurons occurs which is partly specific to the food that has just been eaten to satiety (Rolls, Sienkiewicz & Yaxley 1989b).

The situation appears to be the same in humans, in whom fMRI investigations show that sensory-specific satiety for food is represented in the orbitofrontal cortex (Kringelbach, O'Doherty, Rolls & Andrews 2003) (see Fig. 4.23 on page 106); that activations in the orbitofrontal cortex and pregenual cingulate cortex are linearly correlated with the subjective pleasantness value of taste (Grabenhorst & Rolls 2008, Rolls 2012c); and in that activations in the insular primary taste cortex are linearly correlated with the subjective intensity of taste (Grabenhorst & Rolls 2008) (Fig. 4.45).

These findings lead to the following proposed neuronal mechanism for sensory-specific satiety (see also Rolls & Treves (1990)). The tuning of neurons becomes more specific for gustatory stimuli through the nucleus of the solitary tract, gustatory thalamus, and frontal opercular taste cortex. Satiety, habituation and adaptation are not features of the responses here. This is what is found in primates (see above). The tuning of neurons becomes even more specific in the orbitofrontal cortex, but here there is some effect of satiety by internal signals such as gastric distension and glucose utilization, and in addition habituation or adaptation with a time course of several minutes which lasts for 1–2 h is a feature of the synapses that are activated. Because of the relative specificity of the tuning of orbitofrontal taste neurons, this results in a decrease in the response to that food, but different foods continue to activate other neurons. This is an important part of the theory, for it accounts for why different orbitofrontal cortex neurons respond to different combinations of sensory inputs, and in this sense as a population encode a *high-dimensional space of reward value* (Rolls 2008b). (For orbitofrontal cortex neurons that respond to two flavours before satiety, it is suggested that the habituation that results in a loss of the response to the taste eaten to satiety (see e.g. Fig. 5.17) occurs because of habituation or adaptation of the afferent neurons or synapses onto these orbitofrontal cortex neurons.) This would result in the orbitofrontal cortex neurons having the required response properties, and it is only then necessary for other parts of the brain to use the activity of the orbitofrontal cortex neurons to reflect the reward value of that particular taste. One output of these neurons may be to the anterior cingulate cortex; and another to the hypothalamic neurons with food-related responses, for their responses to the sight and/or taste of food show a decrease that is partly specific to a food that has just been eaten to satiety (see above). Another output may be to the ventral and adjoining striatum, which may provide an important link between reward systems and action (see Section 6.3).

It is suggested that the computational significance of this architecture is as follows (see also Rolls (1986c), Rolls (1989a), Rolls & Treves (1990), and Rolls (2008b)). If satiety were to operate at an early level of sensory analysis, then because of the broadness of tuning of neurons, responses to non-foods would become attenuated as well as responses to foods (and this could well be dangerous if poisonous non-foods became undetectable). This argument becomes even more compelling when it is realized that satiety typically shows some specificity for the particular food eaten, with others not eaten in the meal remaining relatively pleasant (see above). Unless tuning were relatively fine, this mechanism could not operate, for reduction in neuronal firing after one food had been eaten would inevitably reduce behavioural responsiveness to other foods. Indeed, it is of interest to note that such a sensory-specific satiety mechanism can be built by arranging for tuning to particular foods to become relatively specific at one level of the nervous system (as a result of categorization processing in earlier stages), and then at this stage (but not at prior stages) to allow habituation to be a property of the synapses, as proposed above.

Thus information processing in the taste system illustrates an important principle of higher nervous system function in primates, namely that it is only after several or many stages of sensory information processing (which produce efficient categorization of the stimulus) that there is an interface to motivational systems, to other modalities, or to systems involved in association memory (Rolls & Treves 1990, Rolls & Treves 1998).

The rat may not be a good model for primates (including humans) even for taste information processing, in that in rats there are connections from the nucleus of the solitary tract via a pontine taste area to the amygdala and hypothalamus which bypass the cortex (Norgren 1984), and in that there is some modulation by hunger of taste processing even in the nucleus of the solitary tract (Scott & Giza 1992, Scott et al. 1995, Rolls & Scott 2003). The fact that the connections and operation of even such a phylogenetically old system as the taste system have been reorganized in primates may be related to the importance of cortical processing in primates especially for vision, so that other sensory systems follow suit in order to build multimodal representations of objects, which are motivationally neutral and can be used for many functions, including inputs to systems for recognition, identification, object–place memory and short-term memory as well as for reward value encoding and rapid reversal in stimulus–reinforcer learning systems. Related to this, including the rule-based aspects of the functioning, is, I suggest, the development of the granular prefrontal cortex in primates, including most of the orbitofrontal cortex (Section 1.3.) One value of such organization is that objects can be recognized and learned about even when an object is not rewarding. The system is ideally suited, for example, to learning about where food is located in the environment even when hunger is not present. Modulation of visual and taste processing by hunger early on in sensory processing would mean that one would be blind and ageusic to food when not hungry.

5.4.2.4 Taste processing in rodents

There are major differences in the neural processing of taste in rodents and primates (Rolls & Scott 2003, Small & Scott 2009, Scott & Small 2009, Rolls 2014a). In rodents (and also in primates) taste information is conveyed by cranial nerves 7, 9 and 10 to the rostral part of the nucleus of the solitary tract (NTS) (Norgren 1990, Norgren & Leonard 1971, Norgren & Leonard 1973). However, although in primates the NTS projects to the taste thalamus and thus to the cortex (Fig. 4.2), in rodents the majority of NTS taste neurons responding to stimulation of the taste receptors of the anterior tongue project to the ipsilateral medial aspect of the pontine parabrachial nucleus (PbN), the rodent 'pontine taste area' (Small & Scott 2009, Cho, Li & Smith 2002). The remainder project to adjacent regions of the medulla. From the PbN the rodent gustatory pathway bifurcates into two pathways; 1) a ventral 'affective' projection to the hypothalamus, central gray, ventral striatum, bed nucleus of the stria terminalis and amygdala and 2) a dorsal 'sensory' pathway, which first synapses in the thalamus and then the agranular and dysgranular insular gustatory cortex (Norgren 1990, Norgren & Leonard 1971, Norgren 1974, Norgren 1976, Kosar, Grill & Norgren 1986). These regions, in turn, project back to the PbN to "sculpt the gustatory code" and guide complex feeding behaviours (Norgren 1990, Norgren 1976, Li & Cho 2006, Li, Cho & Smith 2002, Lundy & Norgren 2004, Di Lorenzo 1990, Scott & Small 2009, Small & Scott 2009).

It may be noted that there is strong evidence to indicate that the PbN gustatory relay is absent in the human and the nonhuman primate (Small & Scott 2009, Scott & Small 2009). First, second-order gustatory projections that arise from rostral NTS appear not to synapse in the PbN and instead join the central tegmental tract and project directly to the taste thalamus in primates (Beckstead, Morse & Norgren 1980, Pritchard, Hamilton & Norgren 1989). Second, despite several attempts, no one has successfully isolated taste responses in the monkey PbN (Norgren (1990); Small & Scott (2009) who cite Ralph Norgren, personal communication and Tom Pritchard, personal communication). Third, in monkeys the projection arising from the PbN does not terminate in the region of ventral basal thalamus that contains gustatory responsive neurons (Pritchard et al. 1989).

A further difference of rodent taste processing from that of primates is that physical and chemical signals of satiety have been shown to reduce the taste responsiveness of neurons in the nucleus in the solitary tract, and the pontine taste area, of the rat, with decreases in the order of 30%, as follows (Rolls & Scott 2003, Scott & Small 2009). Gastric distension by air or with 0.3 M NaCl suppress responses in the NTS, with the greatest effect on glucose (Gleen & Erickson 1976). Intravenous infusions of 0.5 g/kg glucose (Giza & Scott 1983), 0.5 U/kg insulin (Giza & Scott 1987a), and 40 μg/kg glucagon (Giza, Deems, Vanderweele & Scott 1993) all cause reductions in taste responsiveness to glucose in the NTS. The intraduodenal infusion of lipids causes a decline in taste responsiveness in the PBN, with the bulk of the suppression borne by glucose cells (Hajnal, Takenouchi & Norgren 1999). The loss of signal that would otherwise be evoked by hedonically positive tastes implies that the pleasure that sustains feeding is reduced, making termination of a meal more likely (Giza, Scott & Vanderweele 1992). Further, if taste activity in NTS is affected by the rat's nutritional state, then intensity judgements in rats should change with satiety. There is evidence that they do. Rats with conditioned aversions to 1.0 M glucose show decreasing acceptance of glucose solutions as their concentrations approach 1.0 M. This acceptance gradient can be compared between euglycemic rats and those made hyperglycemic through intravenous injections (Scott & Giza 1987). Hyperglycemic rats showed greater acceptance at all concentrations from 0.6 to 2.0 M glucose, indicating that they perceived these stimuli to be less intense than did conditioned rats with no glucose load (Giza & Scott 1987b).

The implication is that taste, and the closely related olfactory and visual processing that contribute to food reward value and expected value, are much more difficult to understand in rodents than in primates, partly because there is less segregation of 'what' (identity and intensity) from hedonic processing in rodents, partly because of the more serial hierarchical processing in primates (Fig. 4.2), and partly because in primates there has been great development of the granular orbitofrontal cortex which may help to support the rule-based switching of behaviour important for rapidly reversing stimulus-reward associations and behaviour (Section 1.3).

5.4.3 Convergence between taste and olfactory processing to represent flavour

At some stage in taste processing it is likely that taste representations are brought together with inputs from different modalities, for example with olfactory inputs, to form a representation of flavour. Takagi and his colleagues (Takagi 1991, Tanabe, Yarita, Iino, Ooshima & Takagi 1975b, Tanabe, Iino & Takagi 1975a) found an olfactory area in the medial orbitofrontal cortex. In a mid-mediolateral part of the caudal orbitofrontal cortex is the area investigated by Thorpe, Rolls & Maddison (1983) in which are found many neurons with visual and some with gustatory responses. During our recordings in the caudolateral orbitofrontal cortex taste area our impression was that it was different from the frontal opercular and insular primary taste cortices, in that there were neurons with responses in other modalities within or very close to the caudolateral orbitofrontal taste cortex (Rolls, Yaxley & Sienkiewicz 1990). We therefore investigated systematically whether there are neurons in the secondary taste cortex and adjoining more medial orbitofrontal cortex that respond to stimuli in other modalities, including the olfactory and visual modalities, and whether single neurons in this cortical region in some cases respond to stimuli from more than one modality.

In the resulting investigation of the orbitofrontal cortex taste areas (Rolls & Baylis 1994), we found that of 112 single neurons that responded to any of these modalities, many were unimodal (taste 34%, olfactory 13%, visual 21%), but were found in close proximity to each other. Some single neurons showed convergence, responding, for example, to taste and visual inputs (13%), taste and olfactory inputs (13%), and olfactory and visual inputs (5%). Some of these multimodal single neurons had corresponding sensitivities in the two modalities, in that they responded best to sweet tastes (e.g. 1 M glucose), and responded more in a visual discrimination task to the visual stimulus which signified sweet fruit juice than to that which signified saline; or responded to sweet taste, and in an olfactory discrimination task to fruit odour. An example of one such bimodal neuron is shown in Fig. 4.29 on page 114. The neuron responded best to savoury stimuli: among the tastants best to NaCl (N), and best among the odours to onion odour (On), and well also to salmon (S).

The olfactory input to these neurons was further defined by measuring their responses while the monkey performed an olfactory discrimination task (Critchley & Rolls 1996b, Rolls, Critchley, Mason & Wakeman 1996a). In the task, if one odour was delivered through an olfactometer tube close to the nose, then the monkey could lick to obtain glucose (Reward trials). If a different odour was delivered, the monkey had to avoid licking, otherwise he obtained saline (Saline trials). The neuron shown in Fig. 4.29 responded well to the smell of onion (the discriminative stimulus on saline trials), and much less to the odour of fruit juice (the stimulus on Reward trials). The neuron had a selective and specific response to odour, and did not respond non-specifically in the discrimination task, as shown by the absence of neuronal activity while the monkey performed a visual discrimination task. The different types of neuron (unimodal in different modalities, and multimodal) were frequently found close to one another in tracks made into this region (see Fig. 4.28), consistent with the hypothesis that the multimodal representations are actually being formed from unimodal inputs to this region.

These results show that there are regions in the orbitofrontal cortex of primates where the sensory modalities of taste, vision, and olfaction converge; and that in many cases the neurons have corresponding sensitivities across modalities. It appears to be in these areas that flavour representations are built, where flavour is taken to mean a representation that is evoked best by a combination of gustatory and olfactory input. This orbitofrontal region does appear to be an important region for convergence, for there is only a very low proportion of bimodal taste and olfactory neurons in the primary taste cortex (Rolls & Baylis 1994), and in general primary taste cortex neurons do not respond to olfactory or visual stimuli even if they are associated with the taste of food (Verhagen, Kadohisa & Rolls 2004).

To investigate where flavour is formed in humans by olfactory and taste convergence, De Araujo, Rolls, Kringelbach, McGlone & Phillips (2003c) performed an fMRI investigation with unimodal taste (sucrose), unimodal olfactory (strawberry odour), and a mixture of both. They found that a part of the human insular taste cortex was unimodal for taste, and that both olfactory and taste stimuli activated the orbitofrontal cortex and its posterior extension into the agranular insula. Moreover, supralinear additivity of the olfactory and taste components was found in a part of the orbitofrontal cortex. Further, the consonance and pleasantness subjective ratings of the olfactory and taste mixtures (which included some non-consonant mixtures such as sucrose and savory odour) were correlated with activations in the medial orbitofrontal cortex (see Fig. 4.30).

In an investigation to analyse what makes umami delicious, we found with fMRI that a combination of glutamate taste with a savory odour (vegetable) produced much greater activation of the medial orbitofrontal cortex and pregenual cingulate cortex than the sum of the activations by the taste and olfactory components presented separately (McCabe & Rolls 2007). Supralinear effects were much less (and significantly less) evident for sodium chloride and vegetable odour. Further, activations in these brain regions were correlated with the pleasantness and fullness of the flavor, and with the consonance of the taste and olfactory components. Supralinear effects of glutamate taste and savory odour were not found in the insular primary taste cortex. We thus proposed that glutamate acts by the nonlinear effects it can produce when combined with a consonant odour in multimodal cortical taste-olfactory convergence regions far beyond the taste receptors to produce a delicious flavour of umami (McCabe & Rolls 2007, Rolls 2009c).

Thus the processing that it is possible to analyse in detail at the neuronal level in primates appears to provide a good model for how taste and odour combine to produce pleasant flavour in humans (Rolls 2011f, Rolls 2012c). Further, the anterior insular taste cortex does not normally respond to odour (though if a taste was being recalled by an odour this might happen), though areas just anterior to the anterior insular taste cortex do combine odour and taste, including what may be an agranular area of the insula.

5.4.4 Brain mechanisms for the reward produced by the odour of food

5.4.4.1 The rules underlying the formation of olfactory representations in the primate cortex

A schematic diagram of the olfactory pathways in primates is shown in Fig. 4.2 on page 69. There are direct connections from the olfactory bulb to the primary olfactory cortex, pyriform cortex, and from there a connection to a caudal part of the mid (in terms of medial and lateral) orbitofrontal cortex, area 13a, which in turn has onward projections to the lateral orbitofrontal cortex area which we have shown is secondary taste cortex, and to more rostral parts of the orbitofrontal cortex (area 11) (Price et al. 1991, Carmichael & Price 1994, Carmichael et al. 1994, Ongur & Price 2000, Price 2006) (see Figs. 5.18 and 4.2).

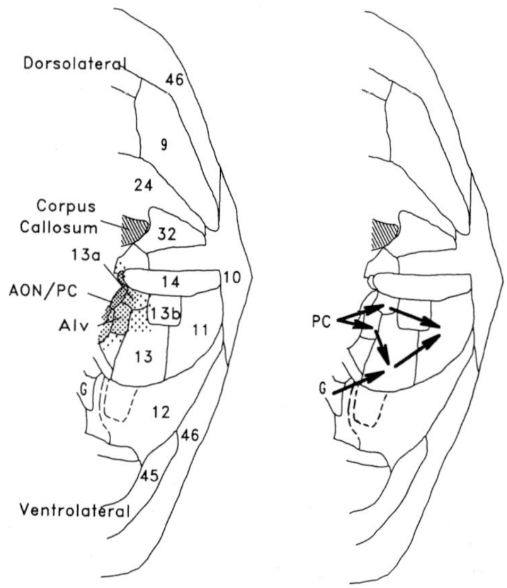

Fig. 5.18 The progression of olfactory inputs to the orbitofrontal cortex in the monkey, drawn on unfolded maps of the frontal lobe. The cortex was unfolded by splitting it along the principal sulcus, which is therefore located at the top and bottom of each map. (Reference to Figs. 4.1 and 4.2 may help to show how the map was constructed.) Left: inputs from the primary olfactory (pyriform) cortex (PC) terminate in the shaded region, that is in the caudal medial part of area 13, i.e. 13a, and in the ventral agranular insular cortex (AIv), which could therefore be termed secondary olfactory cortex. Right: the secondary olfactory cortices then project into the caudolateral orbitofrontal cortex, that is into the secondary taste cortex in that it receives from the primary taste cortex (G); and there are further projections into more anterior and medial parts of the orbitofrontal cortex. (Reproduced from Price, Carmichael, Carnes, Clugnet, and Kuroda, 'Olfactory input to the prefrontal cortex, in Joel L. Davis and Howard Eichenbaum, eds., *Olfaction: A Model System for Computational Neuroscience*, figure from pages 101–120, ©1991 Massachusetts Institute of Technology, by permission of The MIT Press.)

There is evidence that in the olfactory bulb, a coding principle is that in many cases each glomerulus (of which there are approximately 1000) is tuned to respond to its own characteristic hydrocarbon chain length of odourant (Mori, Mataga & Imamura 1992, Imamura, Mataga & Mori 1992, Mori, Nagao & Yoshihara 1999, Mori & Sakano 2011). Evidence for this is that each mitral/tufted cell in the olfactory bulb can be quite sharply tuned, responding for example best to a 5-C length aliphatic odourant (e.g. acid or aldehyde), and being inhibited by nearby hydrocarbon chain-length aliphatic odourants. An effect of this coding might appear to be to spread out the olfactory stimulus space in this early part of the olfactory system, based on the stereochemical structure of the odourant. The code would be spread out in that different parts of chemical space would be relatively evenly represented, in that each part would be represented independently of the presence of other odourants, and in that the code would be relatively sparse, leading to low correlations between the representations of different odours. (Such a coding principle might be facilitated by the presence of in the order of 1000 different genes to code for different olfactory receptor molecules (Buck & Axel 1991, Buck & Bargmann 2013, Mombaerts 2006, Mori & Sakano 2011).)

Is this same coding principle, based on simple physico-chemical properties, used later on in the (primate) olfactory system, or do other principles operate? One example of another coding principle is that representations may be built, for example by competitive learning (Rolls 2008b), that represent the co-occurrence of pairs or groups of odourants, so that particular smells in the environment, which typically are produced by combinations of chemical stimuli, are reflected in the responses of neurons (Wilson & Sullivan 2011). Another coding principle is that olfactory coding might represent in some sense the biological significance of an odour, for example whether it is a food odour that is normally associated with a particular taste. Another principle is that at some stage of olfactory processing the reward or hedonic value of the odourant is represented (whether the odourant smells good), rather than purely the identity of the odourant. For example, whether a food-related odour smells good and encodes expected value depends on hunger, and this hedonic representation of odours must be represented in some part of the olfactory system. To elucidate these issues, and thus to provide principles by which the primate olfactory system may operate, the following investigations were performed.

To investigate how olfactory information is encoded in the orbitofrontal cortex, the responses of single neurons in the orbitofrontal cortex and surrounding areas were recorded during the performance of an olfactory discrimination task (Critchley & Rolls 1996b). The task was designed to show whether there are neurons in this region that categorize odours based on the taste with which the odour is associated. In the task, the delivery of one of eight different odours indicated that the monkey could lick to obtain a taste of sucrose. If one of two other odours was delivered from the olfactometer, the monkey had to refrain from licking, otherwise he received a taste of saline. It was found that 3.1% (48) of the 1580 neurons recorded had olfactory responses, and 34 (2.2%) responded differently to the different odours in the task. The neurons responded with a typical latency of 180 ms from the onset of odourant delivery. 35% of the olfactory neurons with differential responses in the task responded on the basis of the taste reward association of the odourants. Such neurons responded either to all the rewarded stimuli, and to none of the saline-associated stimuli, or vice versa. The remaining 65% of these neurons showed differential selectivity for the stimuli based on the odour quality, and not on the taste reward association of the odour.

The findings thus show that the olfactory representation within the primate orbitofrontal cortex reflects for some neurons (65%) which odour is present independently of its association with taste reward, and that for other neurons (35%), the olfactory response reflects (and encodes) the taste association of the odour (Critchley & Rolls 1996b). The additional finding that some of the odour-responsive neurons were also responsive to taste stimuli supports the hypothesis that odour–taste association learning at the level of single neurons in the orbitofrontal cortex enables such cells to show olfactory responses that reflect the taste association of the odour.

The neurons that classify odours based on the taste with which the odour is associated are likely to respond in this way as a result of learning. Repeated pairing of an odour with a taste (especially if it is a neuron with a taste input) may by pattern-association learning lead it to respond to that odour in future. To investigate whether the responses of neurons to odours could be affected depending on the taste with which the odour was paired, we performed a series of experiments in which the associations of odours and tastes in the olfactory discrimination task were reversed (Rolls, Critchley, Mason & Wakeman 1996a). For example, the monkey might learn that when amyl acetate was delivered, a lick response would result in the delivery of a drop of glucose, and that when cineole was delivered, a lick would result in the delivery of a drop of saline. After this had been learned, the contingency was then reversed, so that cineole might after the reversal be associated with the taste of glucose. Rolls, Critchley, Mason & Wakeman (1996a) found that 68% of the odour-responsive neurons analysed modified their responses following the changes in the taste reward associations of the odourants. Full reversal of the neuronal responses was seen in 25% of the neurons analysed (see example in Fig. 4.24). (In full reversal, the odour to which the neuron responded reversed when the taste with which it was associated reversed.) Extinction of the differential neuronal responses after task reversal was seen in 43% of these neurons. (These neurons simply stopped discriminating between the two odours after the reversal, and are thus conditional olfactory reward neurons analogous to the condition visual reward neurons described in Section 4.5.5.4 and illustrated in Fig. 4.33.)

These findings demonstrate directly a coding principle in primate olfaction whereby the responses of some orbitofrontal cortex olfactory neurons are modified by and depend upon the taste with which the odour is associated. This modification is likely to be important for setting the motivational or reward value of olfactory stimuli for feeding and other rewarded behaviour. It was of interest however that this modification was less complete, and much slower, than the modifications found for orbitofrontal cortex visual neurons during visual-taste reversal (Rolls, Critchley, Mason & Wakeman 1996a). This relative inflexibility of olfactory responses is consistent with the need for some stability in odour–taste associations to facilitate the formation and perception of flavours (Rolls 2011f).

5.4.4.2 The effects of hunger on olfactory processing in the orbitofrontal cortex: evidence that the reward value of odour is represented

It has also been possible to investigate whether the olfactory representation in the orbitofrontal cortex is affected by hunger and reflects reward value in this way too. In satiety devaluation experiments, Critchley & Rolls (1996c) have been able to show that the responses of some olfactory neurons to a food odour are reduced when the monkey is fed to satiety with a food (e.g. fruit juice) with that odour. In particular, seven of nine olfactory neurons that were responsive to the odours of foods, such as blackcurrant juice, were found to reduce their responses to the odour of the satiating food. The decrease was typically at least partly specific to the odour of the food that had been eaten to satiety, potentially providing part of the basis for sensory-specific satiety (Fig. 4.34). (It was also found for eight of nine neurons that had selective responses to the sight of food that they demonstrated a sensory-specific reduction in their visual responses to foods following satiation.) These findings show that the olfactory and visual representations of food, as well as the taste representation of food, in the primate orbitofrontal cortex are modulated by hunger. Usually a component related to sensory-specific satiety can be demonstrated. The findings link at least part of the processing of olfactory and visual information in this brain region to the control of feeding-related behaviour. This is further evidence that part of the olfactory representation in this region is related to the hedonic value of the olfactory stimulus, and in particular that at this level of the olfactory system in primates, the pleasure elicited by the food odour is at least part of what is represented.

To investigate whether the sensory-specific reduction in the responsiveness of the orbitofrontal olfactory neurons might be related to a sensory-specific reduction in the pleasure produced by the odour of a food when it is eaten to satiety, Rolls & Rolls (1997) measured humans' responses to the smell of a food that was eaten to satiety. It was found that the pleasantness of the odour of a food, but much less significantly its intensity, was reduced when the subjects ate it to satiety (Fig. 5.5). It was also found that the pleasantness of the smell of other foods (i.e. not foods eaten in the meal) showed much less decrease. This finding has clear implications for the control of food intake; for ways to keep foods presented in a meal appetitive; and for effects on odour pleasantness ratings that could occur following meals.

In an investigation of the mechanisms of this odour-specific sensory-specific satiety, Rolls & Rolls (1997) allowed humans to chew a food without swallowing, for approximately as long as the food is normally in the mouth during eating. They demonstrated a sensory-specific satiety with this procedure, showing that the sensory-specific satiety does not depend on food reaching the stomach (Fig. 5.6). Thus at least part of the mechanism is likely to be produced by a change in processing in the olfactory pathways. It is not yet known which is the earliest stage of olfactory processing at which this modulation occurs. It is unlikely to be in the receptors of early stages of olfactory processing in the brain, because the change in pleasantness found was much more significant than the change in the intensity (Rolls & Rolls 1997).

In humans, it has been shown that the modulation of the pleasantness of odour by satiety is represented in the orbitofrontal cortex, in that there is a sensory-specific reduction of the fMRI BOLD signal in the orbitofrontal cortex to the odour of a food eaten to satiety, but not to the odour of another food not eaten in a meal (O'Doherty, Rolls, Francis, Bowtell, McGlone, Kobal, Renner & Ahne 2000). In addition, there is evidence in humans that the primary olfactory cortical areas (including the pyriform cortex and cortico-medial amygdala region) represent the identity and intensity of olfactory stimuli, in that in a functional magnetic resonance imaging (fMRI) investigation, activation of these regions was correlated with the subjective intensity ratings but not the subjective pleasantness ratings of six odours (Rolls, Kringelbach & De Araujo 2003c). In contrast, the reward value of odours is represented in the human medial orbitofrontal cortex, in that activation here was correlated with the pleasantness but not intensity ratings of six odours (Rolls, Kringelbach & De Araujo 2003c) (cf. Anderson et al. (2003)), and are increased by paying attention to pleasantness but not intensity (Rolls, Grabenhorst, Margot, da Silva & Velazco 2008a).

In addition to this modulation of neuronal responses to the taste and smell of foods eaten, there will be effects of the energy ingested on taste and smell responses to food. These are likely to depend on factors such as gastric distension, and the concentration of glucose and other indicators including hormonal of hunger/satiety in the systemic circulation which must influence the orbitofrontal cortex, either directly or via the hypothalamus and brainstem (Section 5.3.5) (Karadi, Oomura, Nishino, Scott, Lenard & Aou 1990, Karadi et al. 1992, Oomura, Nishino, Karadi, Aou & Scott 1991, Rolls 2005b).

5.4.4.3 The representation of information about odours by populations of neurons in the orbitofrontal cortex

To investigate how information about odours is represented by the responses of neurons in the primate orbitofrontal cortex, Rolls, Critchley & Treves (1996b) applied information theoretic analyses to the responses of these neurons recorded to 7–9 odours in an olfactory discrimination task. The information reflected by the firing rate of the response accounted for the majority of the information present (86%) when compared with that which was decodable if temporal encoding in the spike train was taken into account. This indicated that temporal encoding had a very minor role in the encoding of olfactory information by orbitofrontal cortex olfactory neurons. The average information about which odourant was presented, averaged across the 38 neurons, was 0.09 bits, a figure that is low when compared with the information values previously published for the responses of temporal lobe face-selective neurons.

In addition, it was shown that the information available from the population as a whole of these neurons increased approximately linearly with the number of neurons in the population (Rolls, Critchley, Verhagen & Kadohisa 2010a). Given that information is a log measure, the number of stimuli that can be encoded increases exponentially with the number of neurons in the sample. Thus the principle of encoding by the populations of neurons is that the combinatorial potential of distributed encoding is used. The significance of this is that with relatively limited numbers of neurons, information about a large number of stimuli can be represented. This means that receiving neurons need only receive from limited numbers of neurons of the type described here, and can nevertheless reflect the information about many stimuli. This type of combinatorial encoding makes brain connectivity possible. The fact that the information can largely be read out from the firing rates of a population of these neurons also makes the decoding of this information (by other neurons) relatively simple (Rolls 2008b, Rolls & Treves 2011).

5.4.5 The responses of orbitofrontal cortex taste and olfactory neurons to the sight of food: expected value neurons

Many of the neurons with visual responses in this region also show olfactory or taste responses (Rolls & Baylis 1994), reverse rapidly in visual discrimination reversal (Rolls, Critchley, Mason & Wakeman 1996a), and only respond to the sight of food if hunger is present (Critchley & Rolls 1996c), and therefore encode expected reward value. This part of the orbitofrontal cortex thus seems to implement mechanisms that can flexibly alter the neuronal responses to visual stimuli depending on the reward (e.g. the taste) associated with the visual stimulus (Thorpe, Rolls & Maddison 1983, Rolls 2000b, Rolls 2004c) (see Section 4.5.5.4). This enables prediction of the taste associated with ingestion of what is seen, and this representation of expected value is related to which stimuli are chosen in these investigations.

The orbitofrontal cortex is implicated more generally in a certain type of learning, namely in extinction and in the reversal of visual discriminations. It is suggested that the taste neurons in this region are important for these functions, for they provide information about whether a reward has been obtained, that is about reward outcome value (Thorpe, Rolls & Maddison 1983, Rolls 2005b, Rolls 2000b, Rolls 2004c). These taste neurons represent a number of important primary reinforcers, others of which include fat texture. The ability of this part of the cortex to perform rapid learning of associations between visual stimuli and primary reinforcers such as taste provides part of the basis for the importance of the orbitofrontal cortex in food-related and emotion-related learning (Rolls 1986b, Rolls 1990b, Rolls 1999a, Rolls 2000b, Rolls 2004c, Rolls 2005b) (see Chapter 4).

The convergence of visual information onto neurons in this region not only enables associations to be learned between the sight of a food and its taste and smell, but also may provide the neural basis for the well-known effect which the sight of a food has on its perceived taste (see Section 4.5.5.7).

5.4.6 Functions of the amygdala and temporal cortex in feeding

5.4.6.1 Effects of lesions

Bilateral damage to the temporal lobes of primates leads to the Kluver-Bucy syndrome, in which lesioned monkeys, for example, select and place in their mouths non-food as well as food items shown to them, and repeatedly fail to avoid noxious stimuli (Kluver & Bucy 1939, Jones & Mishkin 1972, Aggleton & Passingham 1982, Baylis & Gaffan 1991) (see Section 4.6.3). Rats with lesions in the basolateral amygdala also display altered food selection, in that they ingest relatively novel foods (Rolls & Rolls 1973b, Borsini & Rolls 1984), and do not learn normally to avoid to ingest a solution that has previously resulted in sickness (Rolls & Rolls 1973a). (The deficit in learned taste avoidance in rats may be because of damage to the insular taste cortex, which has projections through and to the amygdala (Dunn & Everitt 1988, Scott 2011). The basis for these alterations in food selection and in food-related learning are considered next (see also Rolls (2000d) and Section 4.6.3).

The monkeys with temporal lobe damage have a visual discrimination deficit, in that they are impaired in learning to select one of two objects under which food is found, and thus fail to form correctly an association between the visual stimulus and reinforcement (Jones & Mishkin 1972, Gaffan 1992) (see Section 4.6.3). In the study by Malkova et al. (1997) it was shown that amygdala lesions made with ibotenic acid did impair the processing of reward-related stimuli, in that when the reward value of one set of foods was devalued by feeding it to satiety (i.e. sensory-specific satiety, a reward devaluation procedure, see also Section 4.6.1.2), the monkeys still chose the visual stimuli associated with the foods with which they had been satiated (Malkova et al. 1997, Baxter & Murray 2000, Murray & Izquierdo 2007).

Further evidence that neurotoxic lesions of the amygdala in primates affect behaviour to stimuli learned as being reward-related as well as punishment-related is that monkeys with neurotoxic lesions of the amygdala showed abnormal patterns of food choice, picking up and eating foods not normally eaten such as meat, and picking up and placing in their mouths inedible objects (Murray et al. 1996, Baxter & Murray 2000, Murray & Izquierdo 2007). These symptoms produced by selective amygdala lesions are classical Kluver-Bucy symptoms. Thus in primates, there is evidence that selective amygdala lesions impair some types of behaviour to learned reward-related stimuli such as the sight of food.

Further evidence linking the amygdala to reinforcement mechanisms is that monkeys will work in order to obtain electrical stimulation of the amygdala, and that single neurons in the amygdala are activated by brain-stimulation reward of a number of different sites (Rolls 1975, Rolls et al. 1980) (see Chapter 7 of Rolls (2005b)).

The Kluver-Bucy syndrome is produced by lesions which damage the cortical areas in the anterior part of the temporal lobe and the underlying amygdala (Jones & Mishkin 1972), or by lesions of the amygdala (Weiskrantz 1956, Aggleton & Passingham 1981, Gaffan 1992), or (for the visual aspects) of the temporal lobe neocortex (Akert, Gruesen, Woolsey & Meyer 1961). Lesions to part of the temporal lobe neocortex, damaging the inferior temporal visual cortex and extending into the cortex in the ventral bank of the superior temporal sulcus, produce visual aspects of the syndrome, seen for example as a tendency to select non-food as well as food items (Weiskrantz & Saunders 1984). Anatomically, there are connections from the inferior temporal visual cortex to the amygdala (Herzog & Van Hoesen 1976), which in turn projects to the hypothalamus, thus providing a route for visual information to reach the hypothalamus (Amaral et al. 1992, Pitkanen 2000, Freese & Amaral 2009). This evidence, together with the evidence that damage to the hypothalamus can disrupt feeding (Winn et al. 1984, Dunnett et al. 1985, Winn et al. 1990, Clark et al. 1991), thus indicates that there is a system that includes visual cortex in the temporal lobe, projections to the amygdala, and further connections to structures such as the lateral hypothalamus, which is involved in behavioural responses made on the basis of learned associations between visual stimuli and primary (unlearned) reinforcers such as the taste of food (see Fig. 4.2). Given this evidence from lesion and anatomical studies, the contribution of each of these regions to the visual analysis and learning required for these functions in food selection will be considered using evidence from the activity of single neurons in these regions.

5.4.6.2 Inferior temporal visual cortex

Objects, and not their reward and punishment associations or value, are represented in the inferior temporal visual cortex, as shown by the failure of neurons to reverse and to show devaluation effects, as described in Section 4.4.2 and illustrated in Fig. 4.6 (Rolls, Judge & Sanghera 1977, Rolls, Aggelopoulos & Zheng 2003a, Rolls 2008b, Rolls 2012e).

Nor are reward-related, including food reward-related, representations found in the perirhinal cortex (which anatomically connects the inferior temporal visual cortex to the hippocampus), in that the neurons do not respond differently to the sight of food and non-food objects, and do not respond differently to the visual stimuli in a visual discrimination task (Hölscher & Rolls 2002, Hölscher, Rolls & Xiang 2003b). Instead, perirhinal cortex neurons have activity related to the active resetting of short-term memories required in delayed match to sample tasks (Hölscher & Rolls 2002), and to long-term familiarity memory (Hölscher, Rolls & Xiang 2003b, Rolls, Franco & Stringer 2005b).

A fundamental point about pattern association networks for stimulus–reinforcement association learning can be made from what we have considered (see also Section 4.4.3). It is that sensory processing in the primate brain proceeds as far as the invariant representation of objects independently of reward vs punishment associations. The reason for this systems-level brain design is, I propose, because the visual properties of the world about which reward associations must be learned are generally objects (for example the sight of a banana, or of an orange), and are not just raw pixels or edges, with no invariant properties, which is what is represented in the retina and V1.

The findings described thus indicate that the responses of neurons in the inferior temporal visual cortex do not reflect the association of visual stimuli with reinforcers such as food, or expected reward value. Given these findings, and the lesion evidence described above, it is thus likely that the inferior temporal cortex is an input stage for this process. The next structure on the basis of anatomical connections (see Fig. 4.2) is the amygdala, and this is considered next.

5.4.6.3 Amygdala

The neuronal recordings in the primate amygdala described in Section 4.6.4 show that different populations of amygdala neurons represent what is in the mouth in terms of its taste, texture and temperature (Sanghera, Rolls & Roper-Hall 1979, Ono, Nishino, Sasaki, Fukuda & Muramoto 1980, Ono, Tamura, Nishijo, Nakamura & Tabuchi 1989, Nishijo, Ono & Nishino 1988, Ono & Nishijo 1992, Scott, Karadi, Oomura, Nishino, Plata-Salaman, Lenard, Giza & Aou 1993, Kadohisa, Rolls & Verhagen 2005a) (see example in Fig. 4.57). The multidimensional scaling-based spaces in which the distances reflect the differences between the stimuli encoded by neurons in the insular primary taste cortex, amygdala, and orbitofrontal cortex in primates show that relative to the other two areas, the amygdala emphasizes the representation of oral texture, as indicated in particular by the large part of the space covered by the carboxymethylcellose viscosity (V) series (Fig. 5.19) (Kadohisa, Rolls & Verhagen 2005b, Kadohisa, Rolls & Verhagen 2005a).

The visual representation of foods by amygdala neurons is not completely specific to foods (in that some food-related neurons respond to non-foods or novel stimuli, reversal of neuronal responses when the reward contingencies reverse are not as clear and fast as in the orbitofrontal cortex, and nor are the effects of devaluation by feeding to satiety (Section 4.6.4).

Amygdala neurons with responses that are probably similar to these have also been described by Ono and colleagues (Ono et al. 1980, Ono et al. 1989, Nishijo et al. 1988, Ono & Nishijo 1992). When Nishijo et al. (1988) tested four amygdala neurons in a simpler relearning situation than reversal in which salt was added to a piece of food such as a water melon, the neurons' responses to the sight of the water-melon appeared to diminish. However, in this task it was not clear whether the monkeys continued to look at the stimuli during extinction.

Wilson & Rolls (2005) (see also Rolls (2000d)) extended the analysis of the responses of these amygdala neurons by showing that while they do respond to (some) stimuli associated with primary reinforcement such as food, they do not respond if the reinforcement must be determined on the basis of a rule (such as stimuli when novel are negatively reinforced, and when familiar are positively reinforced). This is consistent with the evidence that the amygdala is involved when reward must be determined, as normally occurs during feeding, by association of a stimulus with a primary reinforcer such as the taste of food, but is not involved when reinforcement must be determined in some other ways (see Rolls (2000d)). In the same study (Wilson & Rolls 2005), it was shown that these amygdala neurons that respond to food can also respond to some other stimuli while they are relatively novel. It is suggested that it is by this mechanism that when relatively novel stimuli are encountered, they are investigated, e.g. by being smelled and then placed in the mouth, to assess whether the new stimuli are foods (Rolls 2000d).

The failure of this population of amygdala neurons to respond only to reinforcing stimuli, and the difficulty in reversing their responses, are in contrast with the responses of certain populations of neurons in the caudal orbitofrontal cortex and in a region to which it projects, the

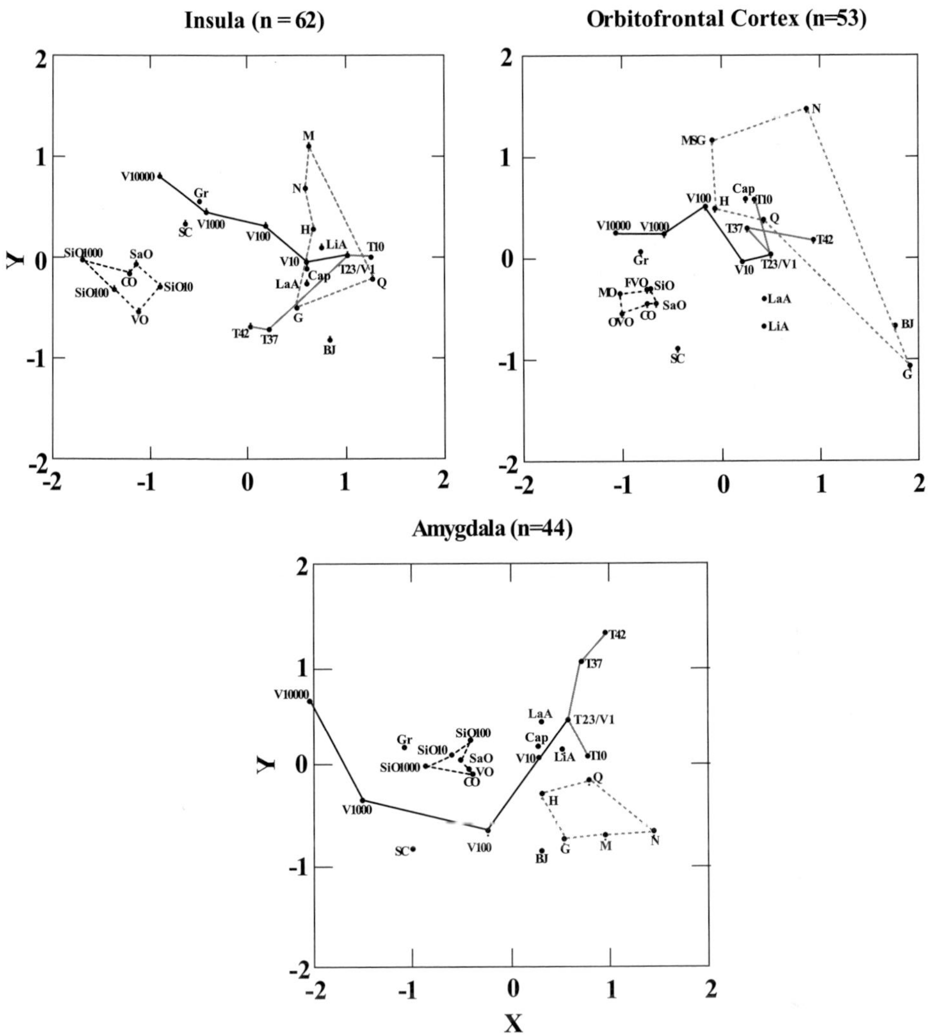

Fig. 5.19 Stimulus space (multidimensional scaling) of the stimulus similarity based on the across-neuron response profiles of insular taste cortex, orbitofrontal cortex, and amygdala neurons. Each space utilizes the interstimulus correlations calculated across the set of neurons analysed in each area. The taste stimuli were 1 M glucose (G), 0.1 M NaCl (N), 0.1 M MSG (M), 0.01 M HCl (H) and 0.001 M QuinineHCl (Q); the temperature stimuli were T10, T23, T37 and T42 where the number indicates the temperature in °C; the viscosity stimuli were V1, V10, V100, V1000 and V10000 where the numeral indicates the viscosity in centiPoise; fat texture stimuli were SiO10, SiO100, SiO1000 (silicone oil with the viscosity indicated),vegetable oil (VO), coconut oil (CO) and safflower oil (SaO). BJ is fruit juice; Cap is 10 μM capsaicin; LaA is 0.1 mM lauric acid; LiA is 0.1 mM linoleic acid; Gr is the gritty stimulus. The solid line joins the members of the viscosity series. Different line styles join the members of the taste, temperature and oil stimuli. The two-dimensional solution for the insula accounted for 95% of the variance, for the OFC for 89% of the variance, and for the amygdala for 90% of the variance. The numbers of neurons in each area with differential responses to oral stimuli tested on the same set of oral stimuli are indicated. (This material was originally published in M. Kadohisa, E. T. Rolls, and J. V. Verhagen, Neuronal representations of stimuli in the mouth: the primate insular taste cortex, orbitofrontal cortex, and amygdala, *Chemical Senses*, 30 (5), pp. 401–419, ©2005 Oxford University Press and has been reproduced by permission of Oxford University Press http://chemse.oxfordjournals.org/content/30/5/401.full.)

basal forebrain, which do show very rapid reversals of their responses in visual discrimination reversal tasks (typically in one or two trials, providing evidence for a rule-based reversal) (Thorpe, Rolls & Maddison 1983, Wilson & Rolls 1990b, Wilson & Rolls 1990c) (see Section 4.5). On the basis of these findings, it is suggested that the orbitofrontal cortex is more involved than the amygdala in the rapid readjustments of behavioural responses made to stimuli such as food when their reinforcement value is repeatedly changing, as in discrimination reversal tasks (Thorpe, Rolls & Maddison 1983, Rolls, Critchley, Mason & Wakeman 1996a, Deco & Rolls 2005a). The ability to flexibly alter responses to stimuli based on their changing reinforcement associations is important in motivated behaviour (such as feeding) and in emotional behaviour, and it is this flexibility that it is suggested the orbitofrontal cortex adds to a more basic capacity which the amygdala implements for stimulus–reinforcement learning (Rolls 1990b, Rolls 2005b, Deco & Rolls 2005a).

These findings thus suggest that the amygdala could be involved in a somewhat inflexible circuit by which visual stimuli are associated with reinforcement. Neuronal responses here do not code uniquely for whether a visual stimulus is associated with reinforcement, partly because the neurons do not reverse rapidly, and partly because the neurons can respond to relatively novel stimuli, which monkeys frequently pick up and place in their mouths for further exploration. Neurons with responses more closely related to reinforcement are found in areas to which the amygdala projects, such as the lateral hypothalamus, substantia innominata, and ventral striatum, and this may be because of the inputs these structures receive from the orbitofrontal cortex. The amygdala may thus be a somewhat slow and inflexible system, compared with the orbitofrontal cortex which has developed greatly in primates, in learning about which visual stimuli have the taste and smell of food.

5.4.7 Functions of the orbitofrontal cortex in feeding

Damage to the orbitofrontal cortex alters food preferences, in that monkeys with damage to the orbitofrontal cortex select and eat foods that are normally rejected (Butter et al. 1969, Baylis & Gaffan 1991). Their food choice behaviour is very similar to that of monkeys with amygdala lesions (Baylis & Gaffan 1991). Lesions of the orbitofrontal cortex also lead to a failure to correct feeding responses when these become inappropriate. Examples of the situations in which these abnormalities in feeding responses are found include: (a) extinction, in that feeding responses continue to be made to the previously reinforced stimulus; (b) reversals of visual discriminations, in that the monkeys make responses to the previously reinforced stimulus or object; (c) Go/Nogo tasks, in that responses are made to the stimulus that is not associated with food reward; and (d) passive avoidance, in that feeding responses are made even when they are punished (Butter 1969, Iversen & Mishkin 1970, Jones & Mishkin 1972, Tanaka 1973, Rosenkilde 1979, Murray & Izquierdo 2007, Fuster 2008) (see Section 4.5.4). Further, lesions of orbitofrontal cortex areas 11/13 disrupt the rapid updating of food object value during selective satiation (Rudebeck & Murray 2011). Changes in the orbitofrontal cortex may be related to some of the changes in eating habits in frontotemporal dementia, in which there may be escalating desire for sweet food coupled with reduced satiety, which is often followed by weight gain (Piguet 2011).

To investigate how the orbitofrontal cortex may be involved in feeding and in the correction of feeding responses when these become inappropriate, recordings have been made of the activity of single neurons in the primate orbitofrontal cortex. The neuronal recordings in the primate orbitofrontal described in Section 4.5.5.1 show that different populations of neurons represent what is in the mouth in terms of its taste, texture and temperature (Kadohisa, Rolls & Verhagen 2005b) (see examples in Figs. 4.20, 4.21, 4.22, 4.29, 4.34, 5.15, and 5.16). The multidimensional scaling-based spaces in which the distances reflect the differences between

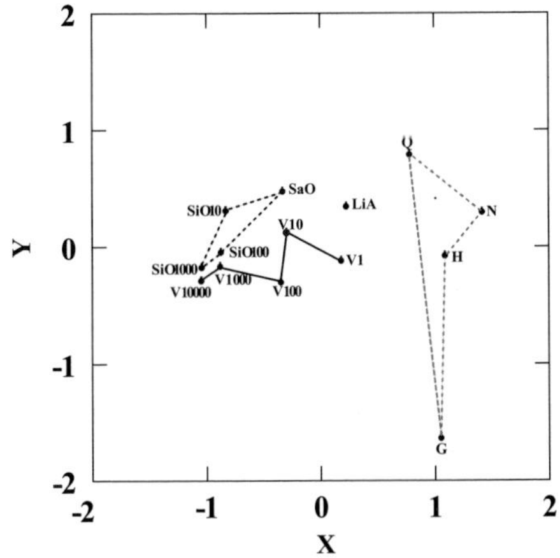

Fig. 5.20 Multidimensional scaling showing the stimulus space based on the human psychophysical ratings of the thickness, taste intensity, taste quality etc. of many of the taste and texture stimuli used in neurophysiological experiments in primates. The stimuli were as described in Fig. 5.19. This 2D space accounted for 97% of the variance. (This material was originally published in M. Kadohisa, E. T. Rolls, and J. V. Verhagen, Neuronal representations of stimuli in the mouth: the primate insular taste cortex, orbitofrontal cortex, and amygdala, *Chemical Senses*, 30 (5), pp. 401–419, ©2005 Oxford University Press and has been reproduced by permission of Oxford University Press http://chemse.oxfordjournals.org/content/30/5/401.full.)

the stimuli encoded by neurons in the insular primary taste cortex, amygdala, and orbitofrontal cortex in primates show that relative to the other two areas, the orbitofrontal cortex emphasizes the representation of taste and its hedonic properties, as indicated in particular by the large part of the space covered by the taste stimuli and the large separation of glucose and fruit juice (BJ) in the space from the other taste stimuli (Fig. 5.19) (Kadohisa, Rolls & Verhagen 2005b). Further it is of considerable interest that the human psychophysical space based on ratings of the magnitude of the following attributes: sweet, salt, bitter, sour, overall taste intensity, odour intensity, oily, slimy, thickness and pleasantness were most similar to the representation provided by neurons in the orbitofrontal cortex, as shown in Fig. 5.20 (Kadohisa, Rolls & Verhagen 2005b). Complementary fMRI investigations in humans show that taste, oral texture, and oral temperature are represented in the human orbitofrontal cortex, and that it is the outcome value that is encoded (O'Doherty, Rolls, Francis, Bowtell, McGlone, Kobal, Renner & Ahne 2000, O'Doherty, Rolls, Francis, Bowtell & McGlone 2001b, De Araujo, Kringelbach, Rolls & Hobden 2003a, Rolls, Kringelbach & De Araujo 2003c, De Araujo, Kringelbach, Rolls & McGlone 2003b, De Araujo, Rolls, Kringelbach, McGlone & Phillips 2003c, De Araujo & Rolls 2004, McCabe & Rolls 2007, Rolls & McCabe 2007, Guest, Grabenhorst, Essick, Chen, Young, McGlone, de Araujo & Rolls 2007, Grabenhorst & Rolls 2008, Grabenhorst, Rolls, Parris & D'Souza 2010b, Grabenhorst, D'Souza, Parris, Rolls & Passingham 2010a, Grabenhorst & Rolls 2010) (Figs. 4.23 and 5.14).

As described in Sections 4.5.5.2–4.5.5.4, other orbitofrontal cortex neurons respond to expected reward value, for example to the sight of food. The evidence described shows that these neurons learn these responses by visual-to-taste association learning, and reverse their responses in one trial, using a rule-based process. These neurons encode expected value in that their responses to the sight of food decrease to zero when the food is devalued by feeding to satiety, and that particular food is no longer chosen to eat. Further evidence that expected value is encoded by these neurons is that the subjective affective state as well as the choices made can be predicted from the activity in the orbitofrontal cortex (Rolls, Grabenhorst &

Franco 2009). Analogous neurons respond to the smell of food, and encode the expected reward value signalled by an odour, as described in Section 4.5.5.2.

As described in Section 4.5.5.5, another population of neurons in the orbitofrontal cortex responds to negative reward prediction error. These neurons can become highly active in feeding situation, and indeed a common feature of these neurons is that they become active if a food that is seen to be approaching the mouth stops approaching, and is slowly moved back away from the monkey (Thorpe, Rolls & Maddison 1983). These neurons are likely to be important in resetting based on a reversal rule the visual stimulus that is treated as indicating that reward can be expected from the visual stimulus currently being seen. But these non-reward neurons also encode very direct information about whether an expected food will be obtained or not, and this plays an important role in feeding behaviour, that is likely to be important in many social situations, including the feeding of an infant which is watching whether food is on its way to the mouth.

Cognition clearly has an important effect on food selection and food intake, and the evidence described in Section 4.5.5.8 shows that this effect is realized by a top-down influence on the activations produced by food in the orbitofrontal cortex.

Similarly, attention to different aspects of a food, its pleasantness vs for example the details of its flavour and the intensity of different components of the flavour, may also have important effects on which parts of the brain process the flavour of the food. Both cognitive and attentional top-down controls are likely to have many applications in treating appetite and feeding disorders, and also in enhancing the pleasure produced by food.

The more rapid reversal of neuronal responses in the orbitofrontal cortex, and in a region to which it projects, the basal forebrain (Thorpe, Rolls & Maddison 1983, Wilson & Rolls 1990b, Wilson & Rolls 1990c), than in the amygdala suggest that the orbitofrontal cortex is more involved than the amygdala in the rapid readjustments of behavioural responses made to stimuli when their reinforcement value is repeatedly changing, as in discrimination reversal tasks (Thorpe, Rolls & Maddison 1983, Rolls 1999a, Deco & Rolls 2005a). The ability to flexibly alter responses to stimuli based on their changing reinforcement associations is important in motivated behaviour (such as feeding) and in emotional behaviour, and it is this flexibility which it is suggested the orbitofrontal cortex adds to a more basic capacity that the amygdala implements for stimulus–reinforcement learning.

The great development of the orbitofrontal cortex in primates, yet the similarity of its connections to those of the amygdala (see Fig. 4.55), and its connections with the amygdala, lead to the suggestion that in evolution, and as part of continuing corticalization of functions, the orbitofrontal cortex has come to be placed hierarchically above the amygdala, and is especially important when rapid readjustment of stimulus–reinforcement associations is required (Rolls 1990b). This suggestion is also consistent with the indication that whereas in rodents subcortical structures such as the amygdala and hypothalamus have access to taste information from the precortical taste system, the same does not occur in primates; and that some precortical processing of taste in relation to the control of feeding occurs in rodents (see above and Scott & Giza (1992) and Rolls & Scott (2003)). In contrast, there is great development and importance of cortical processing of taste in primates, and it is very appropriate that the orbitofrontal cortex area just described is found just medial to the secondary taste cortex, which is in primates in the caudolateral orbitofrontal cortex. It appears that close to this orbitofrontal taste cortex the orbitofrontal cortical area just described develops, and receives inputs from the visual association cortex (inferior temporal cortex), the olfactory (pyriform) cortex, and probably from the somatosensory cortex, so that reward associations between these different modalities can be determined rapidly.

An interesting topic for the future is whether the satiety signals summarized in Sections 5.2 and 5.3 also gain access to the orbitofrontal cortex, and the details of how they modulate there the taste, olfactory and visual neuronal responses to food.

5.4.8 Output pathways for feeding

The orbitofrontal cortex projects to the anterior cingulate cortex, and this provides an output for feeding where action–outcome learning is being or has been performed and the actions are goal-dependent (Section 4.7) (see Fig. 4.2). The orbitofrontal cortex and amygdala project to the striatum, and this basal ganglia route provides an output for feeding, especially for stimulus-response habit controlled feeding (Section 6.3). Autonomic and endocrine functions involved in the control of feeding can be influenced by the hypothalamic and related output connections of the orbitofrontal cortex, amygdala, and anterior cingulate cortex described in Chapter 4 including Sections 4.11 and 4.6.3.3.

5.5 Obesity, bulimia, and anorexia

I conclude this chapter on the brain mechanisms involved in affective responses to food, and appetite control, by considering some of the disturbances in these systems that may contribute to obesity and other eating disorders.

Understanding the mechanisms that control appetite is becoming an increasingly important issue, given the increasing incidence of obesity. Obesity affects approximately one third of adults in the United States (with an additional one third falling into the overweight category). In the UK, there has been a three-fold increase since 1980 to a figure of 20% defined by a Body Mass Index > 30, and there is a realization that it is associated with major health risks (with 1000 deaths each week in the UK attributable to obesity). It is important to understand and thereby be able to minimize and treat obesity because many diseases are associated with a body weight that is much above normal. These diseases include hypertension, cardiovascular disease, hypercholesterolaemia, and gall bladder disease; and in addition obesity is associated with some deficits in reproductive function (e.g. ovulatory failure), and with an excess mortality from certain types of cancer (Schwartz & Porte 2005, O'Rahilly 2009, Guyenet & Schwartz 2012).

There are many factors that can cause or contribute to obesity in humans (Schwartz & Porte 2005, O'Rahilly 2009, Guyenet & Schwartz 2012, Rolls 2007e, Rolls 2011b, Rolls 2012c). Rapid progress is being made in understanding many of these factors at present with the aim of leading to better ways to minimize and treat obesity. These factors include the following (Rolls 2012c):

5.5.1 Genetic factors

Genetic factors are of some importance, with some of the variance in weight and resting metabolic rate in a population of humans attributable to inheritance (Barsh & Schwartz 2002, O'Rahilly 2009). A small proportion of cases of obesity can be related to dysfunctions of the peptide systems in the hypothalamus, with for example 4% of obese people having deficient (MC4) receptors for melanocyte stimulating hormone (Barsh, Farooqi & O'Rahilly 2000, Cummings & Schwartz 2003, Horvath 2005, O'Rahilly 2009). Cases of obesity that can be related to changes in the leptin system are very rare (Farooqi et al. 2001, O'Rahilly 2009). Further, obese people generally have high levels of leptin, so leptin production is not the problem, and instead leptin resistance (i.e. insensitivity) may be somewhat related to obesity, with the resistance perhaps related in part to smaller effects of leptin on arcuate nucleus NPY/AGRP neurons (Munzberg & Myers 2005). However, although there are similarities in fatness within families, these are as strong between spouses as they are between parents and children, so that these similarities cannot be attributed to genetic influences, but presumably reflect the effect of family attitudes to food and weight.

Further, the 'obesity epidemic' that has occurred since 1990 cannot be attributed to genetic changes, for which the time scale is far too short, but instead to factors such as the increased palatability, variety, and availability of food which are some of the crucial drivers of food intake and the amount of food that is eaten in our changed modern environment (Rolls 2005b, Rolls 2007e, Rolls 2011b, Rolls 2012c, Heitmann, Westerterp, Loos, Sorensen, O'Dea, Mc Lean, Jensen, Eisenmann, Speakman, Simpson, Reed & Westerterp-Plantenga 2012) and that are described below. Consistent with this view, food intake has increased in the United States by 20% since 1980 (Guyenet & Schwartz 2012). This view (Rolls 2005b, Rolls 2007e, Rolls 2010d, Rolls 2011b, Rolls 2012c) is becoming increasingly accepted (O'Rahilly 2009).

5.5.2 Brain processing of the sensory properties and pleasantness of food

The way in which the sensory factors produced by the taste, smell, texture and sight of food interact in the brain with satiety signals (such as gastric distension and satiety-related hormones) to determine the pleasantness and palatability of food, and therefore whether and how much food will be eaten, is described above in this chapter. The concept is that convergence of sensory inputs produced by the taste, smell, texture and sight of food occurs in the orbitofrontal cortex to build a representation of food flavour. The orbitofrontal cortex is where the pleasantness and palatability of food are represented, as shown by the discoveries that these representations of food value are only activated if appetite is present and the food is chosen, and correlate with the subjective pleasantness of the food flavour. The orbitofrontal cortex representation of whether food is pleasant (given any satiety signals present) then drives brain areas such as the striatum and cingulate cortex that then lead to eating behaviour.

The fundamental concept this leads to about some of the major causes of obesity is that, over the last 30 years, sensory stimulation produced by the taste, smell, texture and appearance of food, as well as its availability, have increased dramatically, yet the satiety signals produced by stomach distension, satiety hormones etc. summarized in Sections 5.2 and 5.3 have remained essentially unchanged, so that the effect on the brain's control system for appetite is to lead to a net average increase in the reward value and palatability of food which over-rides the satiety signals, and contributes to the tendency to be overstimulated by food and to overeat (Rolls 2005b, Rolls 2007e, Rolls 2011b, Rolls 2012c).

In this scenario, it is important to understand much better the rules used by the brain to produce the representation of the pleasantness of food and how the system is modulated by eating and satiety. This understanding, and how the sensory factors can be designed and controlled so as not to override satiety signals, are important research areas in the understanding, prevention, and treatment of obesity. Advances in understanding the receptors that encode the taste, olfactory, fat texture (Rolls 2011e) and other properties of food, and the processing in the brain of these properties (Rolls 2005b, Rolls 2007e, Rolls 2011b, Rolls 2012c), are also important in providing the potential to produce highly palatable food that is at the same time nutritious and healthy.

An important aspect of this hypothesis is that different humans may have reward systems that are especially strongly driven by the sensory and cognitive factors that make food highly palatable. In a test of this, we showed that activation to the sight and flavor of chocolate in the orbitofrontal and pregenual cingulate cortex were much higher in chocolate cravers than non-cravers (Rolls & McCabe 2007). In more detail, the sight of chocolate produced more activation in chocolate cravers than non-cravers in the medial orbitofrontal cortex and ventral

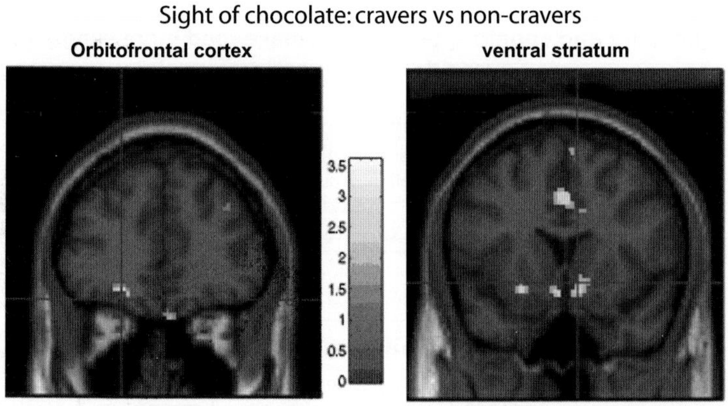

Fig. 5.21 The sight of chocolate produced more activation of mid and medial parts of the orbitofrontal cortex in chocolate cravers than non-cravers (e.g. [-28 42 -10] at the crosshairs), and in the ventral striatum ([-4 16 -12]). (See colour plates section.) (Reproduced from Edmund T. Rolls and Ciara McCabe, Enhanced affective brain representations of chocolate in cravers vs. non-cravers, *European Journal of Neuroscience*, 26 (4) pp. 1067–1076, Copyright ©2007, John Wiley and Sons.)

striatum (Fig. 5.21). For cravers vs non-cravers, a combination of a picture of chocolate with chocolate in the mouth produced a greater effect than the sum of the components (i.e. supralinearity) in the medial orbitofrontal cortex and pregenual cingulate cortex. Furthermore, the pleasantness ratings of the chocolate and chocolate-related stimuli had higher positive correlations with the fMRI signals in the pregenual cingulate cortex and medial orbitofrontal cortex in the cravers than in the non-cravers. Thus there are differences between cravers and non-cravers in their responses to the reward components of a craved food in the orbitofrontal and pregenual cingulate cortex and a region to which they project the ventral striatum that is implicated in addiction (see Chapter 6), and in some of these regions the differences are related to the subjective pleasantness rating value of the craved food (Rolls & McCabe 2007). It was of interest that there were no differences between the cravers and the non-cravers in the activations in the taste insula to the chocolate, so that the differences found were in the tuning of the reward system and not of the purely sensory system (Rolls & McCabe 2007). Individual differences in brain responses to images of food have also been described by Beaver, Lawrence, Ditzhuijzen, Davis, Woods & Calder (2006).

The concept that individual differences in responsiveness to food reward are reflected in brain activations in regions related to the control food intake (Rolls 2005b, Rolls 2007e, Rolls 2011b, Rolls 2012c) may provide a way for understanding and helping to control food intake. In this context, we should remember from Chapters 2 and 3 that individual differences in the reward systems are to be expected given that variation in these systems is an important part of the process of evolution by natural selection. Research in this area with the aim of understanding the relation between the activation of different brain systems by food, and obesity, is developing rapidly (Volkow, Wang, Tomasi & Baler 2013).

5.5.3 Food palatability

A factor in obesity is food palatability, which with modern methods of food production can now be greater than would have been the case during the evolution of our feeding control systems. These brain systems evolved so that internal signals from for example gastric distension and glucose utilization could act to decrease the pleasantness of the sensations produced by feeding sufficiently by the end of a meal to stop further eating. However, the greater palatability of

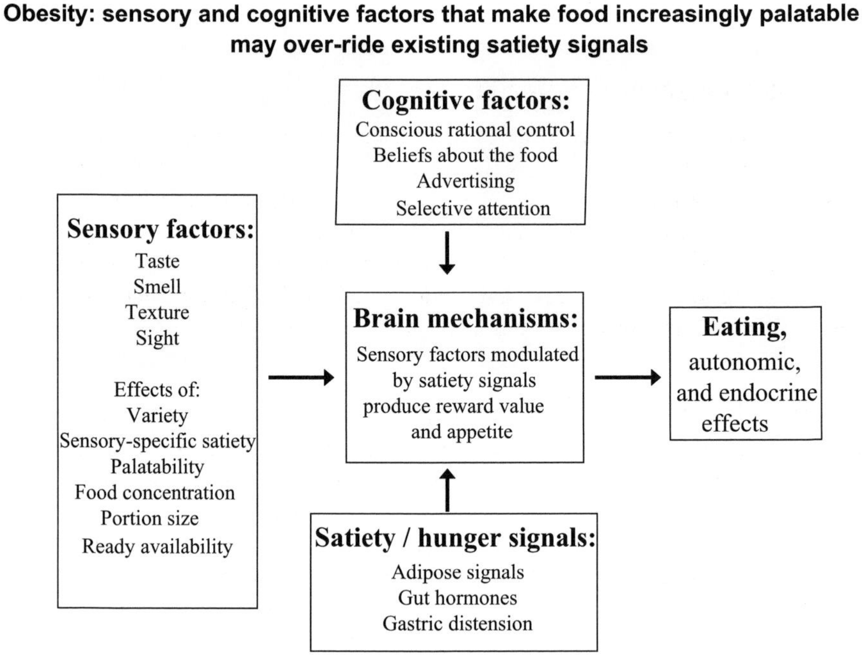

Fig. 5.22 Schematic diagram to show how sensory factors interact in the orbitofrontal cortex with satiety signals to produce the hedonic, rewarding value of food, which leads to appetite and eating. Cognitive and attentional factors directly modulate the reward system in the brain. (Reproduced from Edmund T. Rolls, Taste, olfactory and food texture reward processing in the brain and the control of appetite, *Proceedings of the Nutrition Society*, 71 (4), pp. 488 – 501 ©2012, Cambridge University Press.

modern food may mean that this balance is altered, so that there is a tendency for the greater palatability of food to be insufficiently decreased by a standard amount of food eaten, so that extra food is eaten in a meal (Rolls 2005b, Rolls 2012c) (see Fig. 5.22).

5.5.4 Sensory-specific satiety

Sensory-specific satiety is the decrease in the appetite for a particular food as it is eaten in a meal, without a decrease in the appetite for different foods, as shown above in Chapters 4 and 5. It is an important factor influencing how much of each food is eaten in a meal, and its evolutionary significance may be to encourage eating of a range of different foods, and thus obtaining a range of nutrients. As a result of sensory-specific satiety, if a wide variety of foods is available, overeating in a meal can occur. Given that it is now possible to make available a very wide range of food flavours, textures, and appearances, and that such foods are readily available, this variety effect may be a factor in promoting excess food intake.

5.5.5 Fixed meal times, and the availability of food

Another factor that could contribute to obesity is fixed meal times, in that the normal control of food intake by alterations in inter-meal interval is not readily available in humans, and food may be eaten at a meal-time even if hunger is not present (Rolls 2005b). Even more than this, because of the high and easy availability of food (in the home and workplace) and stimulation by advertising, there is a tendency to start eating again when satiety signals after a previous meal have decreased only a little, and the consequence is that the system again becomes overloaded.

5.5.6 Food saliency, and portion size

Making food salient, for example by placing it on display, may increase food selection particularly in the obese (Schachter 1971, Rodin 1976, Cornell, Rodin & Weingarten 1989), and portion size is a factor, with more being eaten if a large portion of food is presented (Rolls 2012a), though whether this is a factor that can lead to obesity and not just alter test meal size is not yet clear. The driving effects of visual and other stimuli, including the effects of advertising, on the brain systems that are activated by food reward may be different in different individuals, and may contribute to obesity.

5.5.7 Energy density of food

Although gastric emptying rate is slower for high energy density foods, this does not fully compensate for the energy density of the food (Hunt & Stubbs 1975, Hunt 1980). The implication is that eating energy dense foods (e.g. high fat foods) may not allow gastric distension to contribute sufficiently to satiety. Partly at least because of this, the energy density of foods is an important factor that influences how much energy is consumed in a meal (Rolls 2012a). Indeed, it is notable that obese people tend to eat foods with high energy density, and to visit restaurants with high energy density (e.g. high fat) foods. It is also a matter of clinical experience that gastric emptying is faster in obese than in thin individuals, so that gastric distension may play a less effective role in contributing to satiety in the obese. It is also important to remember that the flavour of a food can be conditioned to its energy density, leading over a few days to more eating of low than high energy dense foods, in the phenomena known as conditioned appetite and conditioned satiety (Booth 1985).

5.5.8 Eating rate

A factor related to the above is eating rate, which is typically fast in the obese, and may provide insufficient time for the full effect of satiety signals as food reaches the intestine to operate.

5.5.9 Stress

Another potential factor is stress, which can induce eating and could contribute to a tendency to obesity. (In a rat model of this, mild stress in the presence of food can lead to overeating and obesity. This overeating is reduced by antianxiety drugs.)

5.5.10 Food craving

Binge eating has some parallels to addiction. In one rodent model of binge eating, access to sucrose for several hours each day can lead to binge-like consumption of the sucrose over a period of days (Berner, Bocarsly, Hoebel & Avena 2011). The binge-eating is associated with the release of dopamine. This model brings binge eating close to an addictive process, at least in this model, in that after the binge-eating has become a habit, sucrose withdrawal decreases dopamine release in the ventral striatum (a part of the brain involved in addiction to drugs such as amphetamine), altered binding of dopamine to its receptors in the ventral striatum is produced, and signs of withdrawal from an addiction occur including teeth chattering. In withdrawal, the animals are also hypersensitive to the effects of amphetamine. Another rat model is being used to investigate the binge eating of fat, and whether the reinforcing cues associated with this can be reduced by the GABA-B receptor agonist baclofen (Berner et al. 2011). In humans, there is some overlap of the brain systems activated by food and by cues related to addiction (Volkow et al. 2013).

5.5.11 Energy output

If energy intake is greater than energy output, body weight increases. Energy output is thus an important factor in the equation. However, studies in humans show that although exercise has health benefits, it does not have very significant effects on body weight gain and adiposity in the obese or those who become obese (Wilks, Besson, Lindroos & Ekelund 2011, Thomas, Bouchard, Church, Slentz, Kraus, Redman, Martin, Silva, Vossen, Westerterp & Heymsfield 2012). These findings help to emphasize the importance of understanding the factors that lead to overeating, including factors such as increased responsiveness of the reward system for food in some individuals, and the effects described here that contribute to reward signals produced in modern society being greater than the satiety signals, which have not changed from those in our evolutionary history (Heitmann et al. 2012).

5.5.12 Cognitive factors, and attention

As shown above, cognitive factors, such as preconceptions about the nature of a particular food or odour, can reach down into the olfactory and taste reward value systems in the orbitofrontal cortex that control the palatability of food to influence how pleasant an olfactory, taste, or flavor stimulus is (De Araujo, Rolls, Velazco, Margot & Cayeux 2005, Grabenhorst, Rolls & Bilderbeck 2008a). This has implications for further ways in which food intake can be controlled by cognitive factors, and this needs further investigation. For example, the cognitive factors that have been investigated in these studies are descriptors of the reward value of the food, such as 'rich and delicious'. But it could be that cognitive descriptions of the consequences of eating a particular food, such as 'this food tends to increase body weight', 'this food tends to alter your body shape towards fatness', 'this food tends to make you less attractive', 'this food will reduce the risk of a particular disease', etc., could also modulate the reward value of the food as it is represented in the orbitofrontal cortex. If so, these further types of cognitive modulation could be emphasized in the prevention and treatment of obesity.

In addition, attention to the affective properties of food modulates processing of the reward value of food in the orbitofrontal cortex (Rolls, Grabenhorst, Margot, da Silva & Velazco 2008a, Grabenhorst & Rolls 2008, Ge, Feng, Grabenhorst & Rolls 2012, Luo, Ge, Grabenhorst, Feng & Rolls 2013), and this again suggests that how attention is directed may be important in the extent to which food over-stimulates food intake. Not drawing attention to the reward properties of food, or drawing attention to other properties such as its nutritional value and energy content, could reduce the activation of the brain's reward system by the food, and could be another useful way to help prevent and treat obesity.

5.5.13 Compliance with information about risk factors for obesity

It is important to develop better ways to provide information that will be effective in the long term in decreasing food intake while maintaining a healthy diet, and in promoting an increase in energy expenditure by for example encouraging exercise. In this respect, the individual differences in the brain's response to the reward value of a food, found for example in our study with chocolate cravers and non-cravers (Rolls & McCabe 2007), is one type of factor that may influence whether an individual can comply. But there are individual differences in other factors that may influence compliance, such as impulsiveness, and the orbitofrontal cortex is implicated in this (Berlin, Rolls & Kischka 2004, Berlin, Rolls &

Iversen 2005, Robbins, Gillan, Smith, de Wit & Ersche 2012). It is important to better understand possible individual differences in the ability for an individual to stop, and be influenced by the reasoning system with its long-term interests in comparison to the immediate rewards specified by genes (Chapter 10). It could also be that substances such as alcohol shift this balance, making an individual temporarily or possibly in the long term more impulsive and less under control of the reasoning executive system (Crews & Boettiger 2009), and therefore more likely to eat, and to eat unhealthily. These effects of alcohol on impulsiveness may be complemented by hormonal processes (Barson, Karatayev, Chang, Johnson, Bocarsly, Hoebel & Leibowitz 2009). Understanding these processes, and enabling individuals to benefit from this understanding, may also be useful in the prevention and treatment of obesity.

Overall, I suggest that understanding of all the above processes, and their use in combination rather than purely individually, may provide new avenues to the control of overeating and body weight (Rolls 2012c). I have outlined a number of factors that may tend to promote overeating and obesity in our modern society, for example by increasing the impact of reward signals on the brain's appetite control system, or by making it difficult for individuals to resist the increased hedonic value of food. It is possible that any one of these, or a few in combination, could produce overeating and obesity. In these circumstances, to prevent and treat obesity it is unlikely to be sufficient to reduce and focus on or test just one or a few of these factors. As there are many factors, there may always be others that apply and that tend to promote overeating and obesity. The conclusion I therefore reach is that to prevent and treat obesity, it may be important to address all of the above factors together, given that any one, or a few, could tend to lead to overeating and obesity.

5.6 Conclusions on reward, affective responses to food, and the control of appetite

We have seen in this chapter that the reward value of food, and its subjective complement, the rated affective pleasantness of food, is decoded in primates including humans only after several stages of analysis. First the representation of the taste of the food (its identity and intensity) is made explicit in the primary taste cortex. Only later, in the orbitofrontal cortex, is the reward value made explicit in the representation, for it is here that satiety signals modulate the responses of the taste and flavour neurons. Thus in the control of food intake, the reward value or pleasantness is crucial to the design of how food intake is controlled, and the reward value is represented only in specialized cortical areas. The orbitofrontal cortex is moreover where multimodal representations of food are built, which include taste, texture, olfactory, and visual components. The actual satiety signals are complex, and include sensory-specific satiety, computed in the orbitofrontal cortex, gastric distension, gut satiety signals, plasma glucose, and hormones such as leptin.

The primate orbitofrontal cortex is more closely related to the changing affective value of food than the amygdala, in that the orbitofrontal cortex shows responses that decrease to zero as the reward decreases to zero with satiety, and in that the orbitofrontal cortex tracks (and probably computes) the changing reward value of stimuli as they are altered by stimulus–reinforcer association learning and reversal.

The outputs of the orbitofrontal cortex reach brain regions such as the striatum, cingulate cortex, and dorsolateral prefrontal cortex where behavioural responses to food may be elicited because these structures produce behaviour which makes the orbitofrontal cortex reward neurons fire, as they represent a goal for behaviour. At the same time, outputs from the orbitofrontal cortex, cingulate cortex, and amygdala, in part via the hypothalamus, may provide for appropriate autonomic and endocrine responses to food to be produced, including the release of hormones such as insulin.

6 Pharmacology of emotion, reward, and addiction; the basal ganglia

6.1 Introduction

Dopamine is involved in reward systems in the brain with major dopamine inputs to the orbitofrontal cortex, in addiction, and in the functions of the basal ganglia considered in Section 6.3 which provide one set of outputs from the orbitofrontal cortex, cingulate cortex, and amygdala. We therefore start with an introduction to some of the pharmacology of the dopamine systems in the brain.

Dopamine is normally released from the presynaptic membrane in vesicles when an action potential occurs. The released dopamine travels across the synaptic cleft to activate dopamine receptors (of which there are several types) in the postsynaptic membrane. The pharmacological agents haloperidol, spiroperidol, and pimozide block the DA receptors in the postsynaptic membrane. The drug amphetamine enhances the release of DA from the presynaptic membrane (Fig. 6.1) (Cooper et al. 2003, Iversen, Iversen, Bloom & Roth 2009).

After dopamine is released into the synapse, and some of it activates the postsynaptic receptors, the remaining dopamine is removed from the synapse quickly by a number of mechanisms. One is reuptake into the presynaptic terminal. This process involves dopamine transporter (DAT), and is blocked by amphetamine and by cocaine, which both thus increase the concentration of dopamine in the synapse. Another mechanism for removing DA from

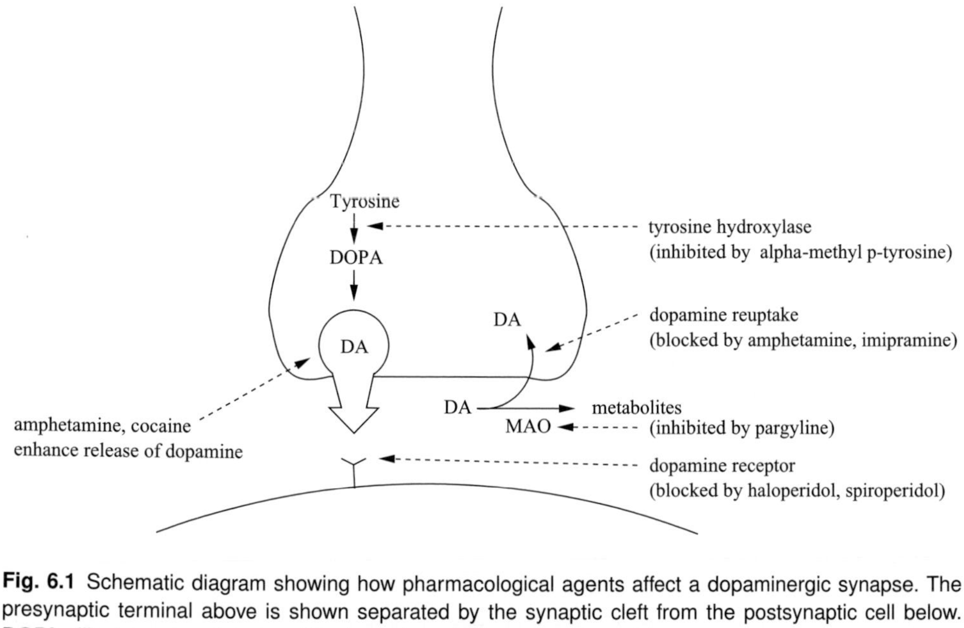

Fig. 6.1 Schematic diagram showing how pharmacological agents affect a dopaminergic synapse. The presynaptic terminal above is shown separated by the synaptic cleft from the postsynaptic cell below. DOPA, dihydroxyphenylalanine; DA, dopamine; MAO, monoamine oxidase.

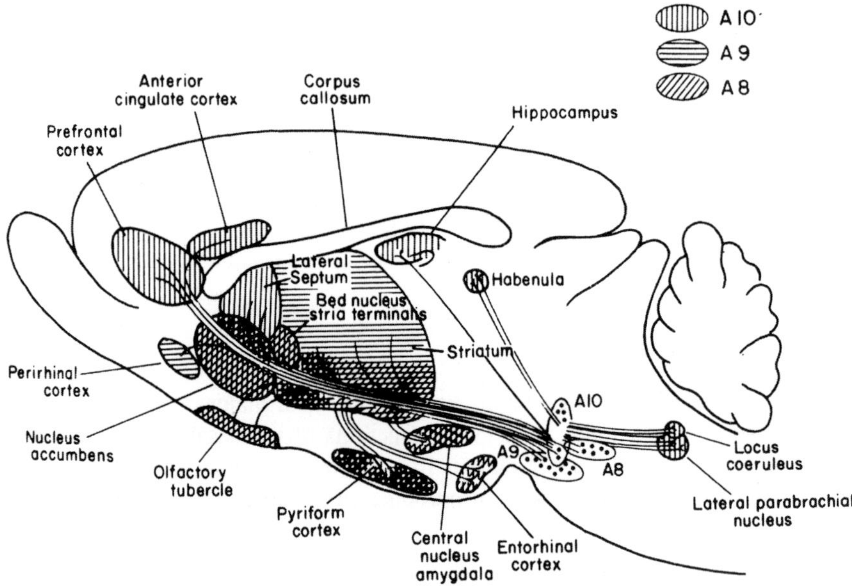

Fig. 6.2 Schematic diagram illustrating the distribution of the main central neuronal pathways containing dopamine. The stippled regions indicate the major nerve-terminal areas and their cell groups of origin. The cell groups in this figure are named according to the nomenclature of Dahlstrom and Fuxe (1965). The A9 cell group in the substantia nigra pars compacta is one of the main DA-containing cell groups, and gives rise mainly to the nigro-striatal dopamine pathway terminating in the striatum. The A10 cell group in the ventral tegmental area is the other main DA-containing cell groups, and gives rise mainly to the meso-limbic DA pathway which terminates in the nucleus accumbens and the olfactory tubercle (together known as the ventral striatum), and the meso-cortical DA pathway which terminates in prefrontal, anterior cingulate, and some other cortical areas. (This material was originally published in *The Biochemical Basis of Neuropharmacology*, 8th edn by J. R. Cooper, F. E. Bloom, and R. H. Roth and has been reproduced by permission of Oxford University Press.)

the synapse is by monoamine oxidase (MAO), which destroys the DA. MAO is present in the synapse, and also in the presynaptic mechanism. MAO inhibitors (MAOI) thus also increase the concentration of DA in the synapse (and also of NA in noradrenergic synapses, and 5-hydroxytryptamine (5-HT, serotonin) in serotonergic synapses). Another mechanism is diffusion out of the synaptic cleft.

The dopaminergic neurons' pathways have been traced using histofluorescence techniques (Dahlström & Fuxe 1965, Ungerstedt 1971, Bjorklund & Lindvall 1986, Cooper, Bloom & Roth 2003). The mesostriatal dopamine projection (see Fig. 6.2) originates mainly (but not exclusively) from the A9 dopamine cell group in the substantia nigra, pars compacta, and projects to the (dorsal or neo-) striatum, in particular the caudate nucleus and putamen. The mesolimbic dopamine system originates mainly from the A10 cell group, and projects to the nucleus accumbens and olfactory tubercle, which together constitute the ventral striatum (see Fig. 6.2). In addition there is a mesocortical dopamine system projecting mainly from the A10 neurons to the frontal cortex, but especially in primates also to other cortical areas, including parts of the temporal cortex. However, these pathways are not completely separate from the mesostriatal projection system, in that the A10 neurons project into the ventromedial part of the striatum, and in that a dorsal and medial set of neurons in the A9 region with horizontally oriented dendrites project into the olfactory tubercle and amygdala (see Phillips & Fibiger (1989)).

6.2 Dopamine and reward

6.2.1 Dopamine and brain-stimulation reward

Rodents, non-human primates, and humans will work to obtain electrical stimulation of some brain regions, including parts of the orbitofrontal cortex, amygdala, lateral hypothalamus, and ventral striatum, as described in Chapter 7 of *Emotion Explained* (Rolls 2005b). This brain-stimulation reward at most brain sites depends on dopamine, as described in Chapter 7 of Rolls (2005b), and summarized briefly here. Dopamine-receptor blockade with spiroperidol which is specific for D2 receptors attenuated hypothalamic self-stimulation without producing arousal or motor deficits (Rolls, Kelly & Shaw 1974a, Rolls, Rolls, Kelly, Shaw & Dale 1974b, Mora, Sanguinetti, Rolls & Shaw 1975) in rodents and monkeys (Mora, Rolls, Burton & Shaw 1976b). Moreover, damage with 6-hydroxydopamine of dopamine pathways at the level of the ventral striatum can abolish brain-stimulation reward from some but not other brain sites.

6.2.2 Self-administration of dopaminergic substances, and addiction

In this section evidence is summarized that a major class of drug, the psychomotor stimulants such as amphetamine and cocaine and both of which stimulate the release of dopamine, can produce their reward by acting on a dopaminergic mechanism in the nucleus accumbens (part of the ventral striatum) (Liebman & Cooper 1989, Phillips & Fibiger 1990, Koob 1992, Koob 1996, Koob & Le Moal 1997, Everitt 1997, Everitt & Robbins 2013), which receives a dopaminergic input from the A10 cell group in the ventral tegmental area. These drugs are addictive, and understanding their mode of action in the brain helps to clarify how these drugs produce their effects. Some of the evidence is as follows:

1. Amphetamine (which increases the release of dopamine and noradrenaline) is self-administered intravenously by humans, monkeys, rats, etc.

2. Amphetamine self-injection intravenously is blocked by dopamine receptor blockers such as pimozide and spiroperidol (Yokel & Wise 1975). The implication is that the psychomotor stimulants produce their reward by causing the release of dopamine which acts on dopamine receptors. The receptor blocker at first increases the rate at which the animal will work for the intravenous injection. The reason for this is that with each lever press for amphetamine, less reward is produced than without the receptor blockade, so the animal works more to obtain the same net amount of reward. This is typical of what happens with low rate operant response behaviour when the magnitude of the reward is reduced. The rate increase is a good control which shows that the dopamine receptor blockade at the doses used does not produce its reward-reducing effect by interfering with motor responses.

3. Apomorphine (which activates D2 dopamine receptors) is self-administered intravenously.

4. Intravenous self-administration of indirect DA agonists such as D-amphetamine and cocaine is much decreased by 6-OHDA lesions of the nucleus accumbens (see Lyness, Friedle & Moore (1980), Roberts, Koob, Klonoff & Fibiger (1980), Koob (1992), and Koob (1996)). In a complementary way, the self-administration of the psychomotor stimulants increases the release of dopamine in the nucleus accumbens (DiChiara, Acquas & Carboni 1992).

5. Rats will learn to self-administer very small quantities of amphetamine to the nucleus accumbens. This effect is abolished by 6-OHDA lesions of the meso-limbic dopamine pathway.

6. Monkeys will learn to self-administer very small quantities of amphetamine to the orbitofrontal cortex (Phillips, Mora & Rolls 1981).

All these points of evidence combine to show that the psychomotor stimulants (though not necessarily all other self-administered drugs) produce their effects by an action on the nucleus accumbens (Koob & Le Moal 1997, Weiss & Koob 2001), or the orbitofrontal cortex, which receives a dopaminergic input. The neurons activated by cocaine in the nucleus accumbens are not in general the same as those activated by water reward (Deadwyler, Hayashizaki, Cheer & Hampson 2004), indicating that there is some continuing specificity of the type of reward encoded that is maintained from the input regions such as the orbitofrontal cortex and amygdala which project to the ventral striatum (see also Section 6.3.3.1). The addictive effects of the dopaminergic drugs implemented via the ventral striatum may be related to 'incentive salience' effects whereby 'wanting' or motivation for the drug-related stimuli is sensitized (Robinson & Berridge 2003, Berridge & Robinson 1998).

In work to understand the factors that influence addiction, Brebner, Childress & Roberts (2002) have found that baclofen, a $GABA_B$ receptor agonist, decreases the reinforcing value of cocaine in rats. (The reinforcement value of the drug is measured by the use of an exponentially increasing ratio schedule of lever presses for each self-injection of cocaine, with rats typically working for as many as approximately 200 lever presses for a single injection of cocaine, but not working beyond this in the ratio. With baclofen, the reinforcing value of the injection is less, in that the animals will work for perhaps only 25 lever presses for each injection. Lever pressing itself can still occur, and some other reinforcers are still effective, in that the baclofen-treated rats will still lever press for food.) The effective site of action of the baclofen appears to be to influence the dopamine-containing neurons, for injections of baclofen into the ventral tegmental area, where the dopamine-containing cell bodies of the A10 group that project to the nucleus accumbens and other areas are located, also disrupt the intravenous self-administration of dopamine, but nucleus accumbens injections of baclofen are much less effective. The possible relevance to binge eating and its possible similarity to addiction is being investigated in a rodent model of binge eating in which rats eat large amounts of fat, and baclofen can influence this (Corwin & Buda-Levin 2004).

In rodents early on in cocaine self-administration the behaviour is under control of an action–outcome system in the nucleus accumbens core and dorsomedial striatum, whereas a dorsolateral striatum-dependent stimulus-response, habit, process controls the behaviour after repeated self-administration over several weeks (Everitt, Belin, Economidou, Pelloux, Dalley & Robbins 2008, Everitt & Robbins 2013).

When humans receive amphetamine, some of the main brain areas that are activated are the medial orbitofrontal cortex, and the rostral part of the anterior cingulate cortex, as well as the ventral striatum (Voellm, De Araujo, Cowen, Rolls, Kringelbach, Smith, Jezzard, Heal & Matthews 2004). This indicates that at least part of the reward and pleasure produced by the psychomotor stimulants may be being produced by activation of the medial orbitofrontal and anterior cingulate cortex, both of which receive dopamine inputs, and in both of which there are neurons and activations produced by natural rewards. Consistently, the orbitofrontal cortex as well as the areas to which it projects such as the ventral striatum are activated in cocaine (another psychomotor stimulant) addicts by exposure to drug-related conditioned stimuli associated with the cocaine (Volkow et al. 2013). Also consistent with the role of the orbitofrontal cortex in the reward value of psychomotor stimulants, amphetamine is self-administered to the orbitofrontal cortex by monkeys (Phillips, Mora & Rolls 1981).

The (Pavlovian) conditioned cues that support addiction and may lead to relapse to addiction by Pavlovian-instrumental transfer (see Section 4.6.1.2 and Cardinal et al. (2002)) may operate in part via the orbitofrontal cortex, for Childress et al. (1999) have shown that cocaine-related cues shown visually in a video to addicts activate the orbitofrontal cortex, and also parts of the anterior cingulate and medial prefrontal cortex. Moreover, the orbitofrontal cortex activation in humans to these drug-conditioned cues can be decreased by baclofen, the GABA-B agonist (Childress et al. 1999). In rodents, cues associated by Pavlovian learning with drug administration also influence the prefrontal and cingulate cortices and related areas (Kelley & Berridge 2002, Kelley 2004a). Presumably dopaminergic substances produce reward in the orbitofrontal cortex by influencing the reward systems known to be present in this region. The reward signals processed in the orbitofrontal cortex include the sight, smell, and taste of food, pleasure produced by touch, the reward value of face expression, social reinforcers, and monetary reinforcers (see Chapters 4 and 5). The orbitofrontal cortex, and also the amygdala, are likely to be the main sources via which these reinforcers gain access to the nucleus accumbens, and thereby may influence dopamine neuron firing (see below).

6.2.3 Behaviours associated with the release of dopamine

The functional role of dopamine can be investigated by determining what factors influence its release. It has been found that the preparatory behaviours for feeding, including foraging for food, food hoarding, and performing instrumental responses to obtain food, are more associated with dopamine release than is the consummatory behaviour of feeding itself (Phillips, Pfaus & Blaha 1991). Also, stimuli conditioned to cocaine delivery may release small amounts of dopamine in the nucleus accumbens (Phillips, Stuber, Heian, Wightman & Carelli 2003b). In another study, Pfaus, Damsma, Nomikos, Wenkstern, Blaha, Phillips & Fibiger (1990) showed that dopamine release in the nucleus accumbens increased in male rats during a 10 min period in which a male and female rat were placed in the same enclosure but were separated by a wire mesh screen, and increased further when the rats were allowed to copulate (see also Phillips et al. (1991)). The dopamine release decreased after the first ejaculation. If a new female was placed behind the mesh screen, the dopamine release increased again, and sexual behaviour was reinstated (Fiorino, Coury & Phillips 1997). (The reinstatement is known as the Coolidge effect.)

In an interesting rat model of binge eating, Colantuoni, Rada, McCarthy, Patten, Avena, Chadeayne & Hoebel (2002) have shown that access to sucrose for several hours each day can lead to binge-like consumption of the sucrose over a period of days. The binge-eating is associated with the release of dopamine. Moreover, the model brings binge eating close to an addictive process, at least in this model, in that after the binge-eating has become a habit, sucrose withdrawal decreases dopamine release in the accumbens, altered binding of dopamine to its receptors in the ventral striatum is produced, and signs of withdrawal from an addiction occur including teeth chattering. In withdrawal, the animals are also hypersensitive to the effects of amphetamine (Avena & Hoebel 2003a, Avena & Hoebel 2003b). An interesting question about this model is whether stressors that increase the release of dopamine such as placing the rats' feet into cold water, if repeated daily, would also cause similar effects. These effects might be similar not only at the pharmacological level, but also at the behavioural level. For example, would animals given such daily repeated stressors show a 'cross-addiction' to sucrose; or to amphetamine? Could this provide a model of the effects of repeated stress on binge eating? In any case, there are interesting implications for the understanding and treatment of binge-eating disorder and bulimia in humans.

Although the majority of the studies have focused on rewarded behaviour, there is also extensive evidence that dopamine can be released by stimuli that are aversive or stressful (Bromberg-Martin, Matsumoto & Hikosaka 2010a). For example, Rada, Mark & Hoebel (1998) showed that dopamine was released in the nucleus accumbens when rats worked to escape from aversive hypothalamic stimulation (see also Hoebel (1997), and Leibowitz & Hoebel (1998)). Also, Gray, Young & Joseph (1997) describe evidence that dopamine can be released in the nucleus accumbens during stress, unavoidable foot-shock, and by a light or a tone associated by Pavlovian conditioning with footshock which produces fear. The necessary condition for the release of dopamine may actually be that an active behavioural response, such as active avoidance of punishment, or working to obtain food, is performed. It may not be just the delivery of reward, or stimuli that signal reward.

Although the most likely process to enhance the release of dopamine in the ventral striatum is an increase in the firing of dopamine neurons, another process is the release of dopamine by a presynaptic influence on the dopamine terminals in the nucleus accumbens. Also consistent with a rather non-specific, activation-related, condition for dopamine release, dopamine release from the meso-cortical dopamine system can be produced by simple manipulations such as stress (Abercrombie, Keefe, DiFrischia & Zigmond 1989, Thierry, Tassin, Blanc & Glowinski 1976).

6.2.4 The activity of dopaminergic neurons and reward

There is extensive evidence that dopamine neurons may signal positive reward prediction error, that is, can respond when a reward is unexpectedly obtained, or when the reward obtained is greater than predicted, or when a stimulus predicting reward is given (Schultz 2013, Glimcher 2011b). This evidence has stimulated the application of reinforcement learning theories in which dopamine-communicated prediction errors are used to train systems in the brain such as the stimulus-response learning system in the basal ganglia. (Reinforcement learning is described in Section A.5.) However, the evidence for this interpretation is not fully consistent, in that some dopamine neurons respond to aversive stimuli, some to rewarding and aversive stimuli, and others to stimuli that may be salient in other ways, for example novel stimuli (Matsumoto & Hikosaka 2009, Bromberg-Martin et al. 2010a). Some of the evidence will now be considered.

Schultz, Romo, Ljunberg, Mirenowicz, Hollerman & Dickinson (1995b) argued from their recordings from dopamine neurons that the firing of these neurons might be involved in reward. For example, dopamine neurons can respond to the taste of a liquid reward in an operant task. However, these neurons may stop responding to such a primary (unlearned) reinforcer quite rapidly as the task is learned, and instead respond only to the earliest indication that a trial of the task is about to begin (Schultz et al. 1995b). **Thus dopamine neurons could not convey information about a primary reward obtained if the trial is successful. They are thus unlike, and could not perform the functions of, the outcome value neurons in the orbitofrontal cortex described in Chapter 4**.

Instead, there is considerable evidence that some dopamine neurons convey a reward prediction error signal (Schultz 2013, Glimcher 2011b), illustrated by the types of response shown in Fig. 6.3A. This type of neuron increases its firing rate to a visual cue that predicts that reward (juice) will be delivered, and decreases its rate to a visual cue that predicts that an aversive stimulus (an air puff) will be delivered (left); and is not activated when a predicted reward is obtained, that is when the juice is delivered (not illustrated in Fig. 6.3A). This type of neuron increases its firing rate to an unpredicted reward outcome, and this is termed a positive reward prediction error response, for the reward outcome is greater than was predicted. This type of neuron decreases its firing if an expected reward stimulus is not received (Fig. 6.3A right), suggesting that it encodes the sign of the prediction error by whether it increases or decreases its firing rate. These neurons encode an accurate prediction error signal, including strong inhibition by omission of rewards and mild excitation by omission of aversive events (Fig. 6.3A right). This is the type of dopamine neuron that is generally discussed (Schultz 2013, Glimcher 2011a). It should be noted that these dopamine neurons are completely different to the negative reward prediction error neurons found in the orbitofrontal cortex, which increase their firing rate when an expected reward is not obtained (see Section 4.5.5.5) and which has never been found for dopamine neurons.

In a further investigation of the function of dopamine neurons, Fiorillo, Tobler & Schultz (2003) found not only the phasic response effects just described, but also that the firing rate of the neurons increased steadily during the 2 s period in which another conditioned stimulus was being shown that predicted that reward would be obtained with a probability

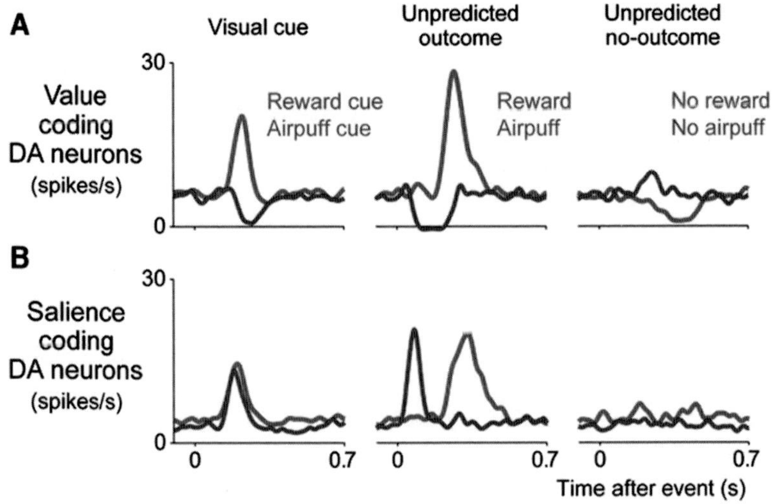

Fig. 6.3 Responses of different types of dopamine neuron. (A) Reward prediction error neurons (see text). (B) Neurons activated by aversive and also by rewarding stimuli, sometime called motivational salience neurons (see text). (See colour plates section.) (Reprinted by permission from Macmillan Publishers Ltd: *Nature*, 459 (7248), Masayuki Matsumoto and Okihide Hikosaka, Two types of dopamine neuron distinctly convey positive and negative motivational signals, copyright, 2009, Nature Publishing Group.)

P of 0.5 (see Fig. 6.4). However, when $P = 0.25$ or $P = 0.75$, the gradually increasing and sustained firing during the conditioned stimulus (CS) was less than when $P = 0.5$. This pattern of results indicates that the tonic, sustained, firing of the dopamine neurons in the delay period reflects reward uncertainty, and not the expected reward, nor the magnitude of the prediction error. Nor could the sustained, tonic, firing indicate expected reward (or expected value, where expected value = probability multiplied by reward value, see Glimcher (2003), Glimcher (2004), and Section 9.5), for this would be highest in the order $P = 1.0, P = 0.75, P = 0.5, P = 0.25, P = 0.0$. Both the phasic and the tonic components were higher for higher reward values (more drops of juice reward). These results are difficult to reconcile with the previously hypothesized (Waelti, Dickinson & Schultz 2001, Dayan & Abbott 2001) 'prediction error' training signal function of the firing of dopamine neurons, for it is difficult to understand how any brain system receiving the phasic ('prediction error') and tonic ('uncertainty of reward') dopamine signals by the same set of neurons could disentangle them and use them for different functions (Shizgal & Arvanitogiannis 2003). However, a possible resolution is that the so-called tonic component arises from averaging across trials, and more importantly from the potential difficulty that there is an asymmetry in the errors that could be conveyed by dopamine neurons, given their low spontaneous firing rate of a few spikes/s (Niv, Duff & Dayan 2005). As a result of this asymmetry, positive prediction errors could be represented by dopamine neurons by firing rates of $\approx$270% above baseline, while negative errors could be represented by a decrease of only $\approx$55% below baseline (see Fig. 6.3). This asymmetry in prediction errors remains a potential problem for the dopamine error hypothesis, but the tonic firing has a possible explanation (Niv et al. 2005).

It has also been shown that dopamine neurons can perform one-trial rule-based reversal (Bromberg-Martin, Matsumoto, Hong & Hikosaka 2010b), and the origin of this I suggest is the orbitofrontal cortex, which performs this function as described in Section 4.5.5.5 and projects via the ventral striatum to the dopamine neurons.

The possibility that dopamine neuron firing may provide an error signal, of the type used

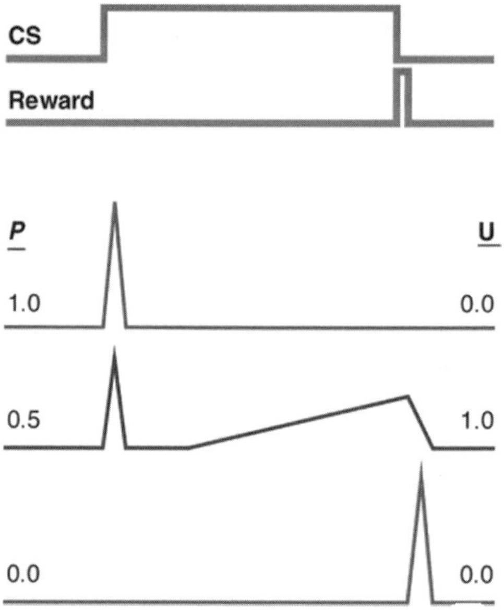

Fig. 6.4 Recordings from midbrain dopamine neurons by Fiorillo, Tobler and Schultz (2003) in a task in which different visual conditioned stimuli (CS) predicted different probabilities P of juice reward after a delay period when the stimulus switched off. The intertrial interval was variable, so that the conditioned stimulus provided information about reward delivery even when $P = 1.0$. When $P = 1.0$, the neurons responded phasically at the onset of the CS, and did not respond to the delivery of the taste reward. When $P = 0.0$, there was no response to the CS, and no response at the end of the CS unless reward was unexpectedly given (as illustrated). However, when $P = 0.5$, the dopamine neurons responded with gradually increasing and sustained firing during the CS. U indicates the uncertainty of reward. (Reproduced from *Science*, 299 (5613), Gambling on dopamine, P. Shizgal and A. Arvanitogiannis, pp. 1856–1858, ©2003, The American Association for the Advancement of Science. Reprinted with permission from AAAS.)

in temporal difference (TD) learning (see Section A.5.3) useful in training neuronal systems to predict reward has continued to be actively studied. The firing of the neurons can be thought of as an error signal about reward prediction (see Section A.5.3), in that the firing occurs in a task when a reward is given, but then moves forward in time when a stimulus is presented that can be used to predict when the taste reward will be obtained (Schultz et al. 1995b). The argument is that there is no prediction error when the taste reward is obtained if it has been signalled by a preceding conditioned stimulus, and that is why the dopamine midbrain neurons do not respond at the time of taste reward delivery, but instead, as least during training, to the onset of the conditioned stimulus (Waelti, Dickinson & Schultz 2001, Schultz 2013, Glimcher 2011b). If a different conditioned stimulus is shown that normally predicts that no taste reward will be given, there is no firing of the dopamine neurons to the onset of that conditioned stimulus. (If after that non-reward conditioned stimulus, a taste reward is unexpectedly given, then the dopamine neurons show a phasic burst of firing, perhaps signalling a reward prediction error.) This hypothesis has been built into models of learning in which the error signal is used to train synaptic connections in dopamine pathway recipient regions (such as presumably the striatum) (Waelti et al. 2001, Dayan & Abbott 2001, Schultz 2013, Glimcher 2011b) (see Section A.5.3). A possible effect of the dopamine to implement TD learning would be for dopamine release to act via D1 receptors in the striatum to facilitate long-term synaptic potentiation (LTP) of the cortical glutamatergic excitatory inputs onto striatal neurons (see Schultz (2013)).

In an application of the temporal difference learning (TD) approach, in a multistep task, monkey dopamine neurons were shown to reflect the TD error quantitatively by reflecting the difference between the sum of multiple future rewards and their prediction (Enomoto, Matsumoto, Nakai, Satoh, Sato, Ueda, Inokawa, Haruno & Kimura 2011). In the task used, the reward probabilities increase towards the end of the multistep sequence, resulting in the highest discounted sum of future reward in the centre of the sequence from which the lower predictions arising from earlier stimuli are subtracted. The dopamine responses match this temporal profile of TD error closely.

A number of difficulties with the dopamine reward prediction error learning hypothesis need to be considered.

One difficulty is the asymmetry of the positive and negative reward prediction error signals that might be available because of the low spontaneous firing rate of dopamine neurons (Fig. 6.3) referred to above.

A second difficulty is that some dopamine neurons appear to reflect at least a positive reward prediction error signal, but it appears to arise with no explanation of how this is computed, or where it comes from (Schultz 2013, Glimcher 2011b). Some suggestions are made below about the source of the inputs that reach dopamine neurons. For example, given that we know that the orbitofrontal cortex contains the necessary signals for this type of computation, including at least reward outcome neurons (taste, flavour, oral texture, etc.), expected reward value neurons, and negative reward prediction error neurons, and novel encoding neurons (see Section 4.5), and that the orbitofrontal cortex provides major inputs to the striatum, it can be suggested that the orbitofrontal cortex, and to some extent the amygdala, provide the source of the inputs to the dopamine neurons via the striatum, even if the striatum or some other as yet unknown part of the brain computes the signals that are reflected in the error signals of some dopamine neurons.

Another point is that reinforcement / temporal difference learning is most applicable to slow learning systems such as those in the basal ganglia for stimulus-response habit learning, and may not be appropriate therefore for most types of learning, many of which can occur in one trial.

A fourth point to be remembered is that there is no evidence that the dopamine neurons reflect different rewards or goals, so they could not be used to direct goal-directed behaviour. In contrast, orbitofrontal cortex neurons encode by their firing many different types of reward value, each appropriate for a different type of goal-directed action. Thus the possible role of some dopamine neurons would seem to be limited to modulating learning in systems where the specific information is in the presynaptic firing of other neurons, whose synaptic connectivity to other neurons may be modulated by dopamine.

A fifth potential problem with the dopamine reward prediction error hypothesis is that there are other types of dopamine neuron, some of which have been studied (Matsumoto & Hikosaka 2009, Bromberg-Martin, Matsumoto & Hikosaka 2010a). These neurons, illustrated in Fig. 6.3B, respond to both rewarding and to aversive stimuli, and could not therefore signal reward prediction error. In more detail, these dopamine neurons increase their firing rate to stimuli predicting reward and to stimuli predicting aversive events (left); and also respond when either an unpredicted reward outcome or an unpredicted aversive stimulus is obtained (middle). These are called 'motivational salience' neurons (Matsumoto & Hikosaka 2009, Bromberg-Martin et al. 2010a), in that they encode something about both positive and negative reinforcers, but not a reward error signal. Another type of dopamine neuron responds only to a cue predicting an aversive stimulus, or to an unpredicted aversive outcome. Another type of dopamine neuron responds to novel stimuli (see Bromberg-Martin et al. (2010a)). Another type of dopamine neuron responds to alerting cues, for example to the first cue in a trial that indicates that a trial is beginning (Bromberg-Martin et al. 2010a, Horvitz 2000, Redgrave,

Prescott & Gurney 1999).

What are we to make of this apparent diversity of dopamine neuron types?

First, the different neuron types seem to reflect the types of neuron found in the primate ventral striatum (including the ventral and medial part of the head of the caudate nucleus) (Rolls & Williams 1987b, Williams, Rolls, Leonard & Stern 1993, Rolls, Thorpe & Maddison 1983c), as described in Section 6.3.3. In these parts of the striatum, there are some neurons that respond to reward-related stimuli, some to punishment-predicting stimuli (e.g. Fig. 6.7), some to novel stimuli (e.g. Fig. 6.8), and many to alerting cues for example as illustrated in Figs. 6.10–6.12. Now this is not surprising: the major inputs to the dopamine neurons (located in the substantia nigra pars compacta) come from the striatum, especially these parts of the striatum (Haber & Knutson 2009). Consistently, salience, rather than reward, is what it has been suggested is encoded in a main region that projects to the dopamine neurons, the striatum, in that head of caudate and accumbens activation in humans occurs to a monetary reward much more when it is made salient by being actively worked for than when it is received passively (Zink, Pagnoni, Martin-Skurski, Chappelow & Berns 2004), and occurs to salient non-rewarding stimuli (Zink, Pagnoni, Martin, Dhamala & Berns 2003).

The implication might be, if between them dopamine neurons reflected all these types of information, that the firing of dopamine neurons might reflect a much more general control over for example the striatum, by facilitating behavioural responses when the dopamine neurons are firing. This could for example facilitate transmission through the striatum and basal ganglia to produce 'go' behaviour to rewarding stimuli, to punishing stimuli (e.g. flee), to novel stimuli (alert and look for more inputs), to cues that indicate that preparations should be made because a cue signal has just arrived, etc.

Somewhat consistent with this, dopamine exerts immediate postsynaptic effects during behavioural performance and approach behaviour. At striatal neurons of the direct pathway (from the striatum directly to the globus pallidus, see Section 6.3), dopamine has excitatory effects via the D1 receptor by eliciting or prolonging glutamate inputs and transitions to the up state (depolarization) of the membrane potential. At striatal neurons in the indirect pathway, (from the striatum via the subthalamic nucleus to the globus pallidus, see Section 6.3) D2 receptor activation has inhibitory effects by reducing glutamate release and prolonging membrane down states (hyperpolarization). Both effects of dopamine tend to promote behavioural output (Gerfen & Surmeier 2011). This is an important effect of dopamine, and depletion of dopamine leads to the akinesia, the lack of voluntary action, in Parkinson's disease.

Indeed, as a whole population, dopamine neurons appear to convey information that would be much better suited to a behaviour preparation or 'Go' role for dopamine release in the striatum. Evidence that is needed on this issue is whether dopamine neurons respond when the animal has to initiate behaviour actively to escape from or avoid aversive (e.g. painful) stimuli (active avoidance), vs to remain still and do nothing to avoid the aversive outcome (passive avoidance).

Some of the evidence reviewed in Section 6.2.3 that the dopamine projection does not convey a specific 'reward' signal is that dopamine release occurs not only to rewards (such as food or brain-stimulation reward, or later in training to an indication that a reward might be given later), but also to aversive stimuli such as aversive stimulation of the medial hypothalamus, foot-shock, and stimuli associated with footshock (Hoebel, Rada, Mark, Parada, Puig de Parada, Pothos & Hernandez 1996, Rada et al. 1998, Hoebel 1997, Leibowitz & Hoebel 1998, Gray et al. 1997, Bromberg-Martin et al. 2010a). (The dopamine release might in this case be related to the firing of dopamine neurons, or to presynaptic terminals on to the dopamine terminals in the nucleus accumbens that cause the release of dopamine.) This evidence argues against the possibility that different populations of dopamine neurons, for example reward prediction error neurons vs all other types of dopamine neuron, are totally separate populations that project to different brain regions (Schultz 2013, Bromberg-Martin, Matsumoto & Hikosaka 2010a).

These findings are consistent with the hypothesis that instead of acting as the reward prediction error signals in a reinforcement learning system, the dopamine projection to the striatum may act as a 'Go' or 'behaviour preparation' signal to set the thresholds of neurons in the striatum, and/or as a general modulatory signal that could help to strengthen synapses of conjunctively active pre- and postsynaptic neurons. In such a system, what is learned would be dependent on the presynaptic firing of all the input axons and the postsynaptic activation of the neuron, and would not be explicitly guided by a dopamine reinforce/teacher signal that would provide feedback after each trial on the degree of success of each trial as in the reinforcement learning algorithm (described in Section A.5). The facts that many of the neurons in the head of the caudate nucleus, and in some other parts of the striatum, respond in relation to signals that indicate that behaviour should be initiated (see Sections 6.3.3 and 6.3.3.4), and that connections from these striatal regions as well as from the hypothalamus reach the dopamine neurons in the substantia nigra, pars compacta, and ventral tegmental area, are fully consistent with the hypothesis that the dopamine neurons are not activated only by reward-related stimuli, but more generally by stimuli including punishing stimuli that can lead to the initiation of behaviour, or at least that dopamine concentrations in brain regions such as the prefrontal cortex reflect the delivery of punishing, non-rewarding, and aversive as well as unexpected rewarding stimuli. Moreover, the dopamine concentrations may remain elevated for periods of many minutes after such stimuli, and are therefore not well suited to a specific teaching signal (Seamans & Yang 2004).

Overall, although there is much evidence that some dopamine neurons encode a reward prediction error signal, there are difficulties with the hypothesis, and an alternative hypothesis is that overall the dopamine neurons together reflect the effects of many salient stimuli, and that dopamine release has the important function of turning on behaviour to such salient stimuli by facilitating information transmission through the basal ganglia. These possibilities can be further evaluated by taking into account the functioning of the basal ganglia, which is considered in Section 6.3.

6.3 The basal ganglia as an output system for emotional and motivational behaviour, and the pharmacology of this system in relation to reward

Now we consider the operation of the basal ganglia, for they provide one of the important output information processing systems in the brain concerned with emotion and motivation. This also provides a foundation for understanding how dopamine in the basal ganglia is related to the operation of reward systems in the brain.

One key issue is the type of information that reaches the basal ganglia from systems such as the amygdala and orbitofrontal cortex, and whether this includes information about rewards and punishers. A second key issue is what the basal ganglia do with the various signals that they receive. A third key issue is whether dopamine inputs to the basal ganglia carry a 'reward prediction error signal', or a more general 'saliency' (e.g. reward, punisher, novel, or cue stimulus for a task) which has the implication of 'prepare' / 'Go') signal to the basal ganglia, and how this input affects the operation of the neuronal systems in the basal ganglia.

The basal ganglia are parts of the brain that include the striatum, globus pallidus, substantia nigra, and subthalamic nucleus, and that are necessary for the normal initiation of movement. For example, depletion of the dopaminergic input to the striatum leads to the lack in the

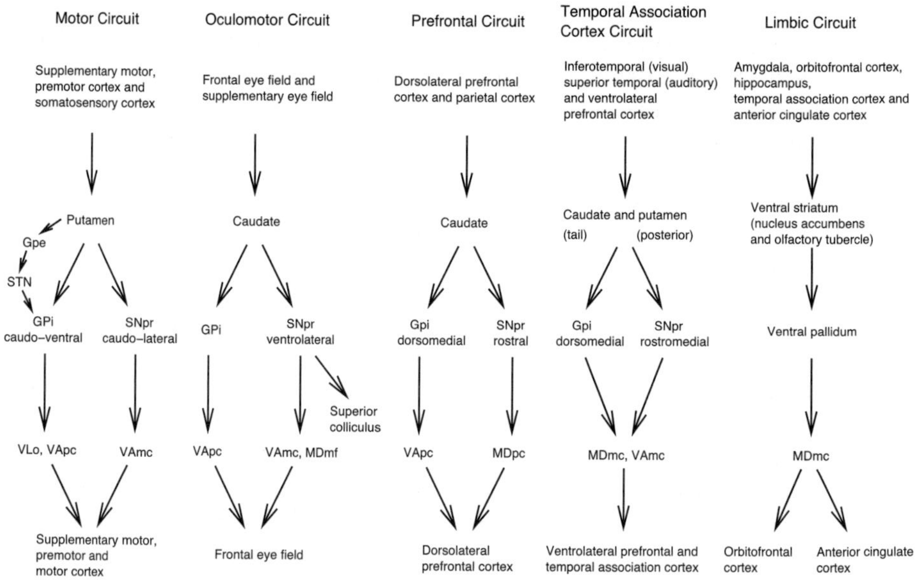

Fig. 6.5 A synthesis of some of the anatomical studies (see text) of the connections of the basal ganglia. GPe, Globus Pallidus, external segment; GPi, Globus Pallidus, internal segment; MD, nucleus medialis dorsalis; SNpr, Substantia Nigra, pars reticulata; VAmc, n. ventralis anterior pars magnocellularis of the thalamus; VApc, n. ventralis anterior pars compacta; VLo, n. ventralis lateralis pars oralis; VLm, n. ventralis pars medialis. An indirect pathway from the striatum via the external segment of the globus pallidus and the subthalamic nucleus (STN) to the internal segment of the globus pallidus is present for the first four circuits (left to right in the figure) of the basal ganglia.

initiation of voluntary movement that occurs in Parkinson's disease. The basal ganglia receive inputs from all parts of the cerebral cortex, including the motor cortex, and have outputs directed strongly towards the premotor and prefrontal cortex via which they could influence movement initiation. There is an interesting organization of the dendrites of the neurons in the basal ganglia which has potentially important implications for understanding how the neuronal network architecture of the basal ganglia enables it to perform its functions (see Rolls & Treves (1998) and Section 6.3.5.1).

6.3.1 Systems-level architecture of the basal ganglia

The point-to-point connectivity of the basal ganglia as shown by experimental anterograde and retrograde neuroanatomical path tracing techniques in the primate is indicated in Figs. 6.5 and 6.6. The general connectivity is for cortical or limbic inputs to reach the striatum, which then projects to the globus pallidus and substantia nigra pars reticulata, which in turn project via the thalamus back to the cerebral cortex (Gurney, Prescott & Redgrave 2001a, Haber & Knutson 2009, DeLong & Wichmann 2010, Gerfen & Surmeier 2011, Buot & Yelnik 2012).) Within this overall scheme, there is a set of at least partially segregated parallel processing streams, as illustrated in Figs. 6.5 and 6.6 (DeLong, Georgopoulos, Crutcher, Mitchell, Richardson & Alexander 1984, Alexander, Crutcher & DeLong 1990, Rolls & Johnstone 1992, Strick, Dum & Picard 1995, Middleton & Strick 1996a, Middleton & Strick 1996b, Middleton & Strick 2000, Kelly & Strick 2004).

First, the motor cortex (area 4) and somatosensory cortex (areas 3, 1, and 2) project somatotopically to the putamen, which has connections through the globus pallidus and substantia nigra to the ventral anterior thalamic nuclei and thus to the supplementary motor cortex. Experiments with a virus transneuronal pathway tracing technique have shown that there might be at least partial segregation within this stream, with different parts of the globus pallidus projecting via different parts of the ventrolateral (VL) thalamic nuclei to the supplementary motor area, the primary motor cortex (area 4), and to the ventral premotor area on the lateral surface of the hemisphere (Middleton & Strick 1996b).

Second, there is an oculomotor circuit (see Fig. 6.5).

Third, the dorsolateral prefrontal and the parietal cortices project to the head and body of the caudate nucleus, which has connections through parts of the globus pallidus and substantia nigra to the ventral anterior group of thalamic nuclei and thus to the dorsolateral prefrontal cortex.

Fourth, the inferior temporal visual cortex and the ventrolateral (inferior convexity) prefrontal cortex to which it is connected project to the posterior and ventral parts of the putamen and the tail of the caudate nucleus (Kemp & Powell 1970, Saint-Cyr, Ungerleider & Desimone 1990, Graybiel & Kimura 1995). Moreover, part of the globus pallidus, perhaps the part influenced by the temporal lobe visual cortex, area TE, may project back (via the thalamus) to area TE (Middleton & Strick 1996a).

Fifth, and of especial interest in the context of reward mechanisms in the brain, limbic and related structures such as the amygdala, orbitofrontal cortex, and hippocampus project to the ventral striatum (which includes the nucleus accumbens), which has connections through the ventral pallidum to the mediodorsal nucleus of the thalamus and thus to the prefrontal and cingulate cortices (Strick et al. 1995, Haber & Knutson 2009, Buot & Yelnik 2012). It is notable that the projections from the amygdala and orbitofrontal cortex are not restricted to the nucleus accumbens, but also occur to the adjacent ventral part of the head of the caudate nucleus (Amaral & Price 1984, Seleman & Goldman-Rakic 1985). These same regions may also project to the striosomes or patches (in for example the head of the caudate nucleus), which are set in the matrix formed by the other cortico-striatal systems (Graybiel & Kimura 1995).

At striatal neurons of the direct pathway (from the striatum directly to the globus pallidus internal segment), dopamine has excitatory effects via the D1 receptor by eliciting or prolonging glutamate excitatory inputs. At striatal neurons in the indirect pathway (from the striatum via the external segment of the globus pallidus via the subthalamic nucleus to the internal segment of the globus pallidus, see Fig. 6.5), D2 receptor activation has inhibitory effects by reducing glutamate release and prolonging membrane down states (hyperpolarization). Both effects of dopamine tend to promote behavioural output (Gerfen & Surmeier 2011).

6.3.2 Systems-level analysis of the basal ganglia: effects of striatal lesions

6.3.2.1 Ventral striatum including nucleus accumbens

There is evidence linking the ventral striatum and its dopamine input to reward, for manipulations of this system alter the incentive effects that learned rewarding stimuli have on behaviour in the rat (Robbins, Cador, Taylor & Everitt 1989, Everitt & Robbins 1992, Everitt & Robbins 2013). The type of task affected is one in which a visual or auditory stimulus is delivered at or just before the delivery of food for which an animal is working. The tone or light becomes associated by learning with the food. Its effects can be measured by whether the rat learns a new operant response to obtain the conditioned reinforcer (the tone or light). This effect in rats is probably produced via the inputs of the amygdala to the ventral striatum, for the effect is abolished by dopamine-depleting lesions of the nucleus accumbens, and amphetamine injections to the nucleus accumbens (which increase the release of dopamine)

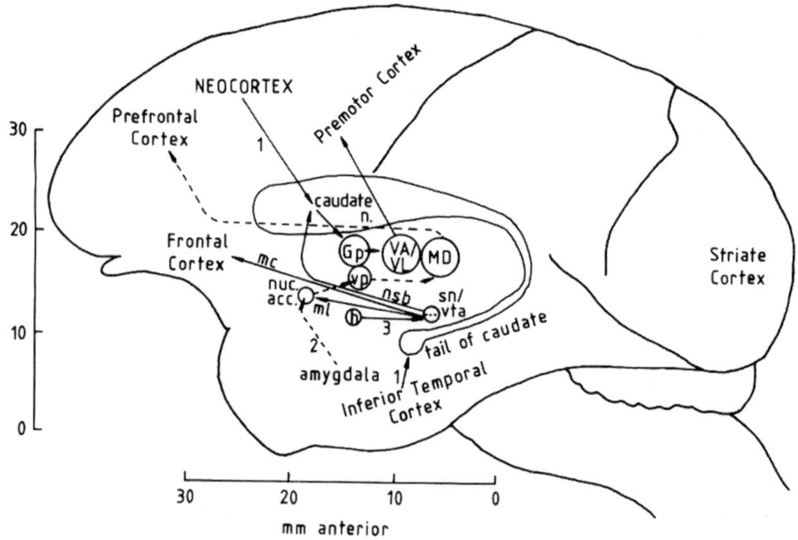

Fig. 6.6 Some of the striatal and connected regions in which the activity of single neurons is described shown on a lateral view of the brain of the macaque monkey. Gp, globus pallidus; h, hypothalamus; sn, substantia nigra, pars compacta (A9 cell group), which gives rise to the nigrostriatal dopaminergic pathway, or nigrostriatal bundle (nsb); vta, ventral tegmental area, containing the A10 cell group, which gives rise to the mesocortical dopamine pathway (mc) projecting to the frontal and cingulate cortices and to the mesolimbic dopamine pathway (ml), which projects to the nucleus accumbens (nuc acc). There is a route from the nucleus accumbens to the ventral pallidum (vp) which then projects to the mediodorsal nucleus of the thalamus (MD) which in turn projects to the prefrontal cortex. Correspondingly, the globus pallidus projects via the ventral anterior and ventrolateral (VA/VL) thalamic nuclei to cortical areas such as the premotor cortex.

increase the effects that these learned or secondary reinforcers have on behaviour (Robbins et al. 1989).

In primates, Stern & Passingham (1996) found that neurotoxic lesions of the ventral striatum produced some changes in emotionality, including increased activity and violent and aggressive behaviour when reward was no longer available during extinction (frustrative non-reward); but some of the changes found in rats were not apparent, perhaps because Stern and Passingham's lesions were small (Stern & Passingham 1995, Stern & Passingham 1996), and in any case in primates the amygdala projects not only to the ventral striatum, but also to the adjoining part of the caudate nucleus.

Further evidence linking the ventral striatum to some types of reward is that rats will self-administer amphetamine into the nucleus accumbens (a part of the ventral striatum), and lesions of the nucleus accumbens attenuate the intravenous self-administration of cocaine (Phillips & Fibiger 1990). Further, opioid receptors in the nucleus accumbens influence the palatability of food (especially fat) in rats, mediating this effect via the lateral hypothalamus (Kelley 2004a).

In addition to this role in reward related probably to inputs to the ventral striatum from the amygdala and orbitofrontal cortex (see Chapter 4), the ventral striatum is also implicated in effects that could be mediated by the hippocampal inputs to the ventral striatum. For example, spatial learning (Schacter, Yang, Innis & Mogenson 1989) and locomotor activity elicited by novel stimuli (Iversen 1984), are influenced by manipulations of the nucleus accumbens.

As described in Chapter 4, the nucleus accumbens may not be involved in action–outcome learning itself, but does allow the affective states retrieved by the basolateral amygdala (BLA) to conditioned stimuli to influence instrumental behaviour by for example Pavlovian-instrumental transfer, and facilitating locomotor approach to food which appears to be in rats a Pavlovian process (Cardinal et al. 2002, Cardinal & Everitt 2004).

6.3.2.2 Dorsal striatum

Damage to other parts of the striatum produces effects that suggest that they are involved in orientation to stimuli, and in the initiation and control of movement. Lesions of the dopamine pathways which deplete the striatum of dopamine lead to a failure to orient to stimuli, a failure to initiate movements, catalepsy, and a failure to eat and drink (Marshall, Richardson & Teitelbaum 1974). In humans, depletion of dopamine in the striatum is found in Parkinson's disease, in which there is akinesia, that is a lack of voluntary movement, bradykinesia (slow movement), rigidity, and tremor (Hornykiewicz 1973). However, consistent with the anatomical evidence, the effects of damage to different regions of the striatum also suggest that there is functional specialization within the striatum (Divac & Oberg 1979, Oberg & Divac 1979). The selective effects may be related to the function of the cortex or limbic structure from which a region of the striatum receives inputs. For example, in the monkey, lesions of the anterodorsal part of the head of the caudate nucleus disrupted delayed spatial alternation performance, a task that requires spatial short-term memory, which is also impaired by lesions of the corresponding cortical region, the dorsolateral prefrontal cortex. Lesions of the ventrolateral part of the head of the caudate nucleus (as of the orbitofrontal cortex which projects to it) impaired object reversal performance, which measures the ability to reverse stimulus–reinforcer associations (see Chapter 4). Lesions of the tail of the caudate nucleus (as of the inferior temporal visual cortex which projects to this part of the caudate) produced a visual pattern discrimination deficit (Divac, Rosvold & Szwarcbart 1967, Iversen 1979). Analogously, in the rat, lesions of the anteromedial head of the caudate nucleus (or of the medial prefrontal cortex, which projects to it) impaired spatial habit reversal, while lesions of the ventrolateral part of the head of the caudate nucleus (or of the orbital prefrontal cortex from which it receives) impaired the withholding of responses in a Go/No-Go task or in extinction (Dunnett & Iversen 1982a, Iversen 1984). Further, in the rat a sensori-motor orientation deficit was produced by damage to a part of the dorsal striatum which receives inputs from lateral cortical areas (Dunnett & Iversen 1982b, Iversen 1984). Similar deficits are produced by selective depletion of dopamine using 6-hydroxydopamine in each of these areas (Dunnett & Iversen 1982a, Dunnett & Iversen 1982b, Iversen 1984).

In rats, the dorsomedial striatum (the equivalent of the primate caudate nucleus) may with its inputs from prelimbic (cingulate) areas be involved in action–outcome learning; the dorsolateral striatum (the equivalent of the primate putamen) with its inputs from sensorimotor cortex in stimulus-response habit behaviour; and the ventral striatum may be involved in some effects of rewards and predicted rewards on both directed behaviour and habits (Balleine, Liljeholm & Ostlund 2009, Balleine & O'Doherty 2010).

6.3.3 Systems-level analysis of the basal ganglia: neuronal activity in different parts of the striatum

We will focus first on neuronal activity in the ventral striatum, because it is particularly relevant to the processing of rewards by the basal ganglia. We again focus on neuronal research in monkeys, because the inputs from the orbitofrontal cortex are so different to those in rodents.

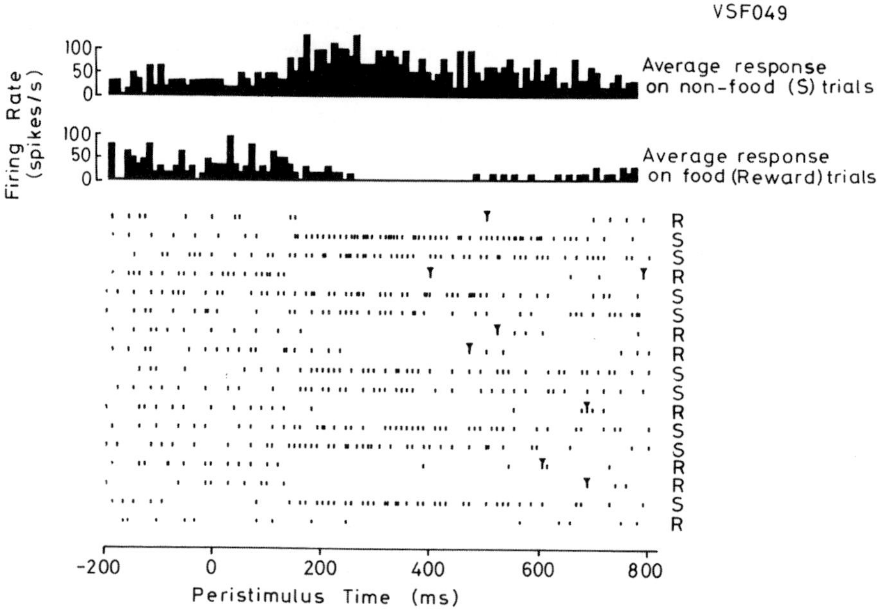

Fig. 6.7 Responses of a ventral striatal neuron in a visual discrimination task. The neuron reduced its firing rate to the S+ on food reward trials (R), and increased its firing rate to the S– on non-food trials (S) on which aversive saline was obtained if a lick was made. Rastergrams and peristimulus time histograms are shown. The inverted triangles show where lick responses were made on the food reward (R) trials. (Reprinted from *Behavioural Brain Research*, 55 (2), Graham V. Williams, Edmund T. Rolls, Christiana M. Leonard, and Chantal Stern, Neuronal responses in the ventral striatum of the behaving macaque, pp. 243–52, Copyright 1993, with permission from Elsevier.)

6.3.3.1 Ventral striatum

To analyse the functions of the ventral striatum, the responses of more than 1000 single neurons were recorded (Rolls & Williams 1987b, Williams, Rolls, Leonard & Stern 1993) in a region that included the nucleus accumbens and olfactory tubercle in five macaque monkeys in test situations in which lesions of the amygdala, hippocampus, and inferior temporal cortex produce deficits, and in which neurons in these structures respond (Rolls 2005b, Rolls & Treves 1998, Rolls 2008b, Rolls 1999b).

One population of ventral striatal neurons was found to respond differently in a visual discrimination task to visual stimuli that indicate that if a lick response is made, the taste of glucose reward will be obtained, and to other visual stimuli that indicate that if a lick response is made, the taste of aversive saline will be obtained. Responses of an example of a neuron of this type are shown in Fig. 6.7. The neuron increased its firing rate to the visual stimulus that indicated that saline would be obtained if a lick was made (the S–), and decreased its firing rate to the visual stimulus that indicated that a response could be made to obtain a taste of glucose (the S+). The differential response latency of this neuron to the reward-related and to the saline-related visual stimulus was approximately 150 ms (see Fig. 6.7), and this value was typical. This neuron thus coded for the valence of the visual stimuli (i.e. whether the visual stimulus was associated with a reward vs a punisher).

Of the neurons that responded to visual stimuli that were rewarding, relatively few responded to all the rewarding stimuli used. That is, only few (1.8%) ventral striatal neurons responded both when food was shown and to the positive discriminative visual stimulus,

Table 6.1 Types of neuronal response found in the macaque ventral striatum (Reprinted from *Behavioural Brain Research*, 55 (2), Graham V. Williams, Edmund T. Rolls, Christiana M. Leonard, and Chantal Stern, Neuronal responses in the ventral striatum of the behaving macaque, pp. 243–52, Copyright 1993, with permission from Elsevier.)

		No./1013	%
1	Visual, recognition-related		
	-novel	39	3.5
	-familiar	11	1.1
2	Visual, association with reinforcement		
	-aversive	14	1.4
	-food	44	4.3
	-food and S+	18/1004	1.8
	-food, context dependent	13	1.3
	-opposite to food/aversive	11	1.1
	-differential to S+ or S– only	44/1112	4.0
3	Visual		
	-general interest	51	5.0
	-non-specific	78/1112	7.0
	-face	17	1.7
4	Movement-related, conditional	50/1112	4.5
5	Somatosensory	76/1112	6.8
6	Cue related	177/1112	15.9
7	Responses to all arousing stimuli	9/1112	0.8
8	Task-related (non-discriminating)	17/1112	1.5
9	During feeding	52/1112	4.7
10	Peripheral visual and auditory stimuli	72/538	13.4
11	Unresponsive	608/1112	54.7

the S+ (e.g. a triangle shown on a video monitor), in a visual discrimination task. Instead, the reward-related neuronal responses were typically more context or stimulus-dependent, responding for example to the sight of food but not to the S+ which signified food (4.3%), differentially to the S+ or S– but not to food (4.0%), or to food if shown in one context but not in another context. Some neurons were classified as having taste or olfactory responses to food (see Table 6.1; Williams, Rolls, Leonard & Stern (1993), Rolls & Williams (1987b)). Some other neurons (1.4%) responded to aversive stimuli. These neurons did not respond simply in relation to arousal, which was produced in control tests by inputs from different modalities, for example by touch of the leg. Thus, as shown in Table 6.1, 13.9% of primate ventral striatal neurons encoded the valence of visual stimuli (Rolls & Williams 1987b, Williams, Rolls, Leonard & Stern 1993). Neurons in the ventral striatum with activity related to the expectation of reward were also found by Schultz, Apicella, Scarnati & Ljungberg (1992).

Another population of ventral striatal neurons responded to novel visual stimuli. An example is shown in Fig. 6.8.

Other ventral striatal neurons responded to faces; to other visual stimuli than discriminative stimuli and faces; in relation to somatosensory stimulation and movement; or to cues that signalled the start of a task (see Table 6.1) (Rolls & Williams 1987b, Williams, Rolls, Leonard & Stern 1993). The cue-related neurons in the ventral striatum were similar to those found in the head of the caudate nucleus (see Section 6.3.3.4), in that they responded to warning cues that signalled the start of a trial, and stopped responding to the cue if it no longer signalled the start of a trial (see example in Fig. 6.10). As shown in Table 6.1, 15.9% of ventral striatal neurons had cue-related responses. These (and other neurons shown in Table 6.1) can thus be described as encoding the salience of stimuli, and respond independently of the valence of the stimuli. Thus valence and salience are represented independently by different populations of neurons in the primate ventral striatum (see Table 6.1).

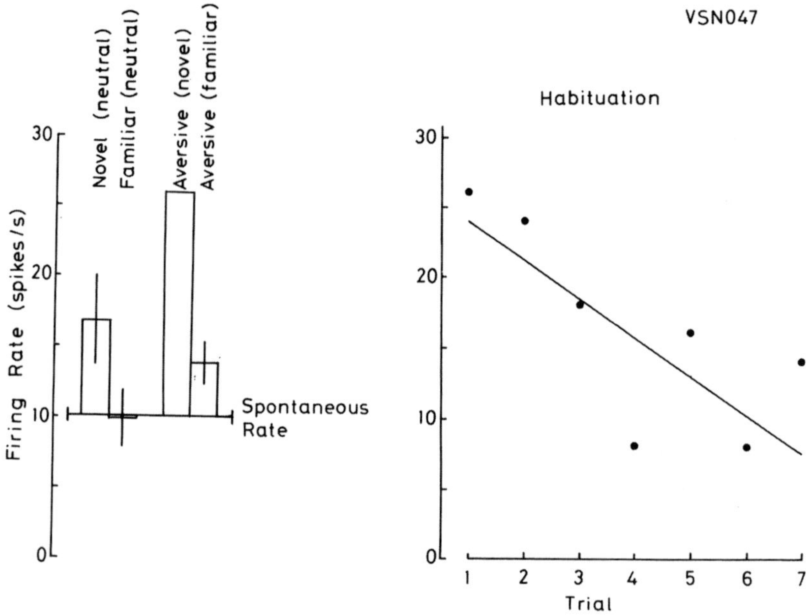

Fig. 6.8 Responses of a ventral striatal neuron to novel visual stimuli. On the right it is shown that the response to novel stimuli, an increase in firing rate to 25 spikes/s from the spontaneous rate of 10 spikes/s, habituated over repeated presentations of the stimulus. The lack of response shown in the left panel to the familiar stimulus was thus only achieved after habituation produced by 4–7 presentations of the stimulus. It is also shown that the neuron responded to aversive stimuli when they had not been seen for more than one day (Aversive (novel)), but did not respond to aversive visual stimuli (such as the sight of a syringe from which the monkey was fed saline, Aversive (familiar)), even though the latter produced arousal. (Reprinted from *Behavioural Brain Research*, 55 (2), Graham V. Williams, Edmund T. Rolls, Christiana M. Leonard, and Chantal Stern, Neuronal responses in the ventral striatum of the behaving macaque, pp. 243–52, Copyright 1993, with permission from Elsevier.)

The neurons with responses to reinforcing or novel visual stimuli may reflect the inputs to the ventral striatum from the amygdala, orbitofrontal cortex, and hippocampus, and are consistent with the hypothesis that the ventral striatum provides a route for learned reinforcing and novel visual stimuli to influence behaviour. It was notable that although some neurons responded to visual stimuli associated with reward (see Table 6.1), 1.4% responded to visual stimuli associated with punishment, and 12% responded to arousing visual stimuli or non-specifically to visual stimuli (see Table 6.1). It was also notable that these neurons were not restricted to the nucleus accumbens, but were found also in the adjacent ventral part of the head of the caudate nucleus (Rolls & Williams 1987b, Williams, Rolls, Leonard & Stern 1993, Rolls, Thorpe & Maddison 1983c), which also receives projections from both the amygdala (Amaral & Price 1984) and orbitofrontal cortex (Seleman & Goldman-Rakic 1985).

A similar influence of reward-related information from the orbitofrontal cortex to the ventral striatum has been described by Simmons, Ravel, Shidara & Richmond (2007).

In human fMRI studies, activations have been described in the ventral striatum that reflect whether monetary rewards can be obtained, and indeed more activation is found for the larger rewards (Knutson, Adams, Fong & Hommer 2001). Interestingly, one of the strongest activations that is found in the ventral striatum is produced by temporal difference reward/punishment prediction errors in Pavlovian (i.e. classical conditioning) tasks (O'Doherty, Dayan, Friston, Critchley & Dolan 2003a, McClure, Berns & Montague 2003,

Seymour, O'Doherty, Dayan, Koltzenburg, Jones, Dolan, Friston & Frackowiak 2004). For example, in a classical conditioning task, a first visual stimulus probabilistically predicted high vs low pain, and a second visual stimulus perfectly predicted whether the pain would be high or low on that trial. Activation of the ventral striatum and a part of the insula was related to the temporal difference error, which arose for example at the transition between the first and second visual stimulus if the first visual stimulus had predicted low pain, but the second informed the subject that the pain would be high (Seymour et al. 2004).

The ventral striatum activations may reflect the operation of a 'critic' in reinforcement learning, in that activations in it are related to temporal difference errors in Pavlovian conditions in which actions are not made (O'Doherty, Dayan, Schultz, Deichmann, Friston & Dolan 2004). In contrast, activation in the dorsal striatum may be closely related to temporal difference prediction errors used to correct an actor, as these activations occurred during an instrumental version of the task in which the subjects had to choose between two stimuli associated with a high probability or low probability of obtaining juice reward (O'Doherty et al. 2004). (The distinction between a 'critic' and an 'actor' in reinforcement learning is described in Appendix 1, Section A.5.3.)

Activations in the ventral striatum related to temporal difference reward/punishment prediction errors in a monetary reward *decision* task are exemplified in the study by Rolls, McCabe & Redoute (2008e). This probabilistic monetary reward decision task is described in Fig. 4.37 on page 123. The design of the task meant that sometimes the participants were expecting a low probability of a high reward of 30 pence, and unexpectedly obtained a high reward value of 30 pence. On these trials, the temporal difference prediction error from the expected value part of the trial to the reward value part of the trial when subjects were informed whether they would obtain the large reward was positive. On other trials when the expected value was high but probabilistically no reward was obtained, the temporal difference prediction error from the expected value part of the trial to the reward value part of the trial was negative. (Temporal difference (TD) errors are described in Appendix 1, Section A.5.3.) It was found that the fMRI BOLD signal in the nucleus accumbens reflected this temporal difference error signal, calculated at the part of the trial when the reward prediction changed from the expected value for that trial block to the actual reward available on that trial, as shown in Fig. 6.9.

Further analyses showed that the activation in the ventral striatum was positively correlated with the reward actually obtained on that trial but not with the expected value. Thus the TD error correlation arose in the nucleus accumbens because at the time that the expected value period ended and the subject was informed about how much reward had been obtained on that trial, the BOLD signal changed to a higher value for large rewards, and to a lower value for low or no reward, from a value that was not a function of the expected value on that trial. A TD error correlation was also found in left cortical area 44 (Broca's area) (as shown in Fig. 6.9), but here the TD correlation arose because the activation became low when the subject was informed that no reward was obtained on a trial, and it appeared that the area was activated especially when the decision was difficult, between two approximately equal values of the expected value. In a part of the midbrain near the dopamine neurons at [14 –20 –16], there was also a correlation with the TD error, but here this was related to a negative correlation between the BOLD signal in the expected value period of each trial and the expected value. (The TD error was thus positive for example whatever reward became available if it was a low expected value trial block, and the TD error was negative if it was a high expected value trial block.) This shows that TD error regressions with functional neuroimaging can arise for a number of different reasons. In this investigation, the reward value on a trial was correlated with the activation in parts of the orbitofrontal cortex, and the expected value was negatively correlated with activations in the anterior insula [–38 24 16], and these cortical areas may be

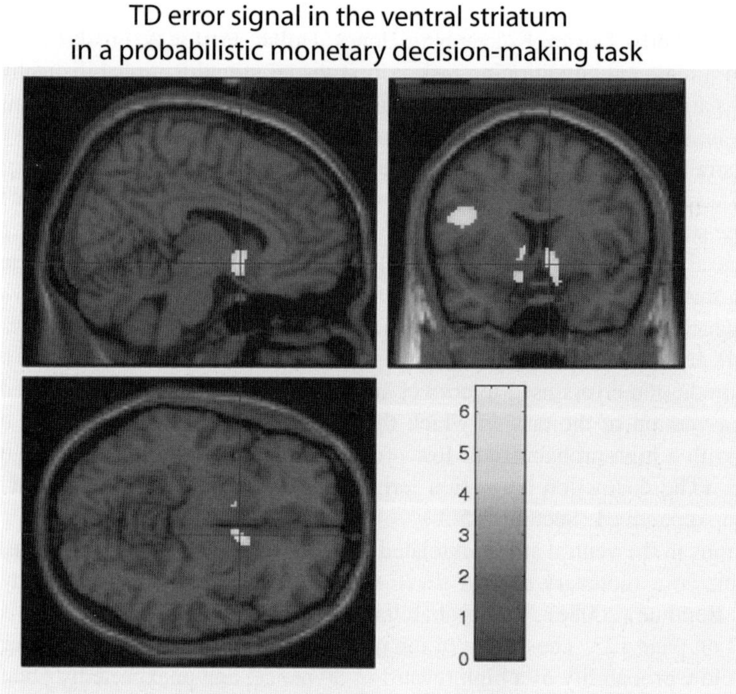

Fig. 6.9 Temporal Difference (TD) error signal in the ventral striatum in a probabilistic monetary decision-making task. The correlation between the TD error and the activation in the nucleus accumbens was significant in a group random effects analysis fully corrected at the cluster level with $p<0.048$ (voxel $z=3.84$) at MNI coordinates [8 8 –8]. The task is illustrated in Fig. 4.37. (See colour plates section.) (This material was originally published in E. T. Rolls, C. McCabe, and J. Redoute, Expected value, reward outcome, and temporal difference error representations in a probabilistic decision task, *Cerebral Cortex*, 18 (3), pp. 652-663, © 2008, Oxford University Press and has been reproduced by permission of Oxford University Press http://cercor.oxfordjournals.org/content/18/3.toc.)

the origins of some of the signals found on other brain areas.

These findings do exemplify the fact that activation of the ventral striatum does reflect the changing expectations of reward (see Appendix 1, Section A.5.3) during the trials of a task, and indeed this is what is illustrated at the neuronal level in Fig. 6.7, where the neuron altered its firing rate within 170 ms of the monkey being shown a visual stimulus that indicated whether reward or saline was available on that trial. Given that ventral striatal neurons of the type illustrated in Fig. 6.7 alter their activity when the visual stimulus is shown informing the macaque about whether reward is available on that trial, it is in fact not surprising that the fMRI correlation analyses do pick up signals during trials that can be interpreted as temporal difference error signals. Whether these fMRI correlations with a temporal difference error reflect more than the activity of single neurons that respond as shown in Fig. 6.7 to the predicted reward value ($\hat{v}$ of Appendix 1, Section A.5.3) rather that the phasic temporal difference error (Δ) will be interesting to examine in future neuronal recordings.

Activations of the ventral striatum that reflect the inputs that it receives from the orbitofrontal cortex and amygdala are commonly reported in functional neuroimaging studies, but it will be important to examine the mechanisms at the neuronal level in the ventral striatum to understand better the exact signals represented by neurons, and exactly what computations the ventral striatum performs using its inputs.

6.3.3.2 Tail of the caudate nucleus, and posteroventral putamen

The projections from the inferior temporal cortex and the prestriate cortex to the striatum arrive mainly, although not exclusively, in the tail (and genu) of the caudate nucleus and in the posteroventral portions of the putamen (Kemp & Powell 1970, Saint-Cyr et al. 1990). The activity of single neurons was analysed in the tail of the caudate nucleus and adjoining part of the ventral putamen by Caan, Perrett & Rolls (1984). Of 195 neurons analysed in two macaque monkeys, 109 (56%) responded to visual stimuli, with latencies of 90–150 ms for the majority of the neurons. The neurons responded to a limited range of complex visual stimuli, and in some cases responded to simpler stimuli such as bars and edges. Typically (for 75% of neurons tested) the neurons habituated rapidly, within 1–8 exposures, to each visual stimulus, but remained responsive to other visual stimuli with a different pattern. This habituation was orientation-specific, in that the neurons responded to the same pattern shown at an orthogonal orientation. The habituation was also relatively short term, in that at least partial dishabituation to one stimulus could be produced by a single intervening presentation of a different visual stimulus. These neurons were relatively unresponsive in a visual discrimination task, having habituated to the discriminative stimuli that had been presented in the task on many previous trials. Consistent findings were obtained by Brown, Desimone & Mishkin (1995).

Given these responses, it may be suggested that these neurons are involved in short-term pattern-specific habituation to visual stimuli. This system would be distinguishable from other habituation systems (involved, for example, in habituation to spots of light) in that it is specialized for patterned visual stimuli that have been highly processed through visual cortical analysis mechanisms, as shown not only by the nature of the neuronal responses, but also by the fact that this system receives inputs from the inferior temporal visual cortex. It may also be suggested that this sensitivity to visual pattern change may have a role in alerting the monkey's attention to new stimuli. This suggestion is consistent with the changes in attention and orientation to stimuli produced by damage to the striatum.

In view of these neurophysiological findings, and the finding that in a visual discrimination task neurons that reflected the reinforcement contingencies of the stimuli were not found, Caan, Perrett & Rolls (1984) suggested that the tail of the caudate nucleus is not directly involved in the development and maintenance of reward or punishment associations to stimuli (and therefore is not closely involved in emotion-related processing), but may aid visual discrimination performance by its sensitivity to change in visual stimuli. Neurons in some other parts of the striatum may, however, be involved in connecting visual stimuli to appropriate motor responses. For example, in the putamen some neurons have early movement-related firing during the performance of a visual discrimination task (Rolls, Thorpe, Boytim, Szabo & Perrett 1984b); and some neurons in the head of the caudate nucleus respond to environmental cues that signal that reward may be obtained (Rolls, Thorpe & Maddison 1983c).

If there are long-term differences over several days, some tail of caudate neurons respond more to the sight of an object with a high reward value, but these neurons do not reverse rapidly during reversals, so do not reflect the current reward value, but a stable longer term bias to look at highly rewarded objects (Yamamoto, Kim & Hikosaka 2013), which may be based on stimulus–response not stimulus–value associations.

6.3.3.3 Postero-ventral putamen

Following these investigations on the caudal striatum which implicated it in visual functions related to a short-term habituation or memory process, a further study was performed to investigate the role of the posterior putamen in visual short-term memory tasks (Johnstone & Rolls 1990, Rolls & Johnstone 1992). Both the inferior temporal visual cortex and the prefrontal cortex project to the posterior ventral parts of the putamen (Goldman & Nauta 1977,

Van Hoesen, Yeterian & Lavizzo-Mourey 1981) and these cortical areas are known to subserve a variety of complex functions, including functions related to memory. For example, cells in both areas respond in a variety of short-term memory tasks (Fuster 1973, Fuster 2008, Fuster & Jervey 1982, Baylis & Rolls 1987, Miyashita & Chang 1988).

Two main groups of neurons with memory-related activity were found in the postero-ventral putamen in a delayed match-to-sample (DMS) task. In the task, the monkey was shown a sample stimulus, and had to remember it during a 2–5 s delay period, after which if a matching stimulus was shown he could make one response, but if a non-matching stimulus was shown he had to make no response (Johnstone & Rolls 1990, Rolls & Johnstone 1992).

First, 11% of the 621 neurons studied responded to the test stimulus which followed the sample stimulus, but did not respond to the sample stimulus. Of these neurons, 43% responded only on non-match trials (test different from sample), 16% only on match trials (test same as the sample), and 41% to the test stimulus irrespective of whether it was the same or different from the sample. These neuronal responses were not related to the licking motor responses since (i) the neurons did not respond in other tasks in which a lick response was required (for example, in an auditory delayed match-to-sample task which was identical to the visual delayed match-to-sample task except that auditory short-term memory rather than visual short-term memory was required; in a serial recognition memory task; or in a visual discrimination task), and (ii) a periresponse time spike-density function indicated that the stimulus onset better predicted neuronal activity.

Second, 9.5% of the neurons responded in the delay period after the sample stimulus, during which the sample was being remembered. These neurons did not respond in the auditory version of the task, indicating that the responses were visual modality-specific (as were the responses of all other neurons in this part of the putamen with activity related to the delayed match-to-sample task). Given that the visual and auditory tasks were very similar apart from the modality of the input stimuli, this suggests that the activity of the neurons was not related to movements, or to rewards or punishers obtained in the tasks (and is thus not closely linked to emotion-related processing), but instead to modality-specific short-term memory-related processing.

In recordings made from pallidal neurons it was found that some responded in both visual and auditory versions of the task (Johnstone & Rolls 1990, Rolls & Johnstone 1992). Of 37 neurons responsive in the visual DMS task that were also tested in the auditory version, seven (19%) responded also in the auditory DMS task. The finding that some of the pallidal neurons active in the DMS task were not modality-specific, whereas only visual modality-specific DMS units were located in the postero-ventral part of the striatum, provides evidence that the pallidum may represent a further stage in information processing in which information from different parts of the striatum can converge.

6.3.3.4 Head of the caudate nucleus

The activity of 394 neurons in the head of the caudate nucleus and most anterior part of the putamen was analysed in three behaving rhesus monkeys (Rolls, Thorpe & Maddison 1983c). Of these neurons, 64.2% had responses related to environmental stimuli, movements, the performance of a visual discrimination task, or eating. However, only relatively small proportions of these neurons had responses that were unconditionally related to visual (9.6%), auditory (3.5%), or gustatory (0.5%) stimuli, or to movements (4.1%). Instead, the majority of the neurons had responses that occurred conditionally in relation to stimuli or movements, in that the responses occurred in only some test situations, *and were often dependent on the performance of a task by the monkeys*. Thus, it was found that in a visual discrimination task 14.5% of the neurons responded during a 0.5 s tone/light cue that signalled the start of each trial (cue-related neurons); 31.1% responded in the period in which the discriminative

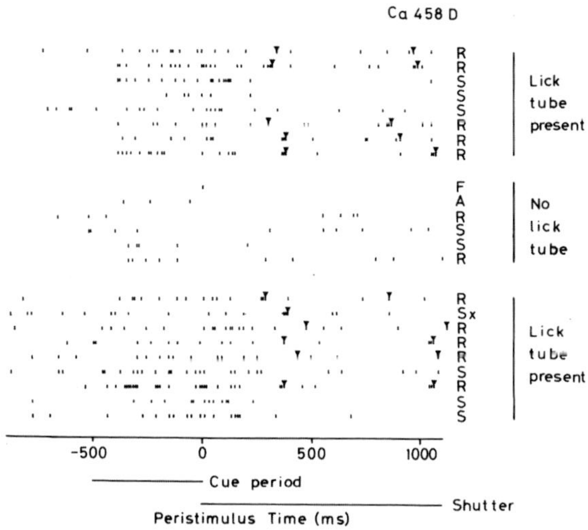

Fig. 6.10 Responses of a cue-related neuron in the head of the caudate nucleus in a Go/NoGo visual discrimination task in which the visual stimulus was presented at time 0. Each trial is a single row of the rastergram, each action potential is represented by a single dot, and a lick made to obtain fruit juice is represented by an inverted triangle. R, Reward trials on which fruit juice was obtained. S, Salt trials on which if a lick was made, a small drop of saline was obtained. Tone and light emitting diode cues were provided starting 500 ms before the visual stimulus was shown. Top set of trials: normal performance of the task with the lick tube close to the mouth. Middle set of trials: the lick tube was removed out of reach, but the tone/LED cue, and discriminative visual stimuli, were still provided. Bottom set of trials: normal performance of the task with the lick tube close to the mouth. F, food reward was shown. A, an aversive visual stimulus was shown. (Reprinted from *Behavioural Brain Research*, 7 (2), E. T Rolls, S. J Thorpe, and S. P Maddison, Responses of striatal neurons in the behaving monkey. 1. Head of the caudate nucleus, pp. 179–210, Copyright 1983, with permission from Elsevier.)

visual stimuli were shown, with 24.3% of these responding more either to the visual stimulus that predicted food reward or to that that predicted punishment (by a taste of saline) (reward prediction neurons); and 6.2% responded in relation to lick responses.

An example of a *cue-related* neuron in the head of the caudate nucleus that started responding as soon as a tone/light-emitting diode (LED) cue was presented indicating that a trial was about to start is shown in Fig. 6.10. At time 0 a discriminative visual stimulus was shown, which indicated if for example it was a triangle that reward could be obtained, or if it was a square that saline would be obtained if a lick was made. The reward trials (R) on which a lick could be made to obtain fruit juice, and saline (S) trials on which a lick should not be made otherwise a drop of aversive saline was obtained, each occurred with probability 0.5. This cue-related neuron stopped responding soon after the visual stimulus appeared, and did not discriminate between reward (R) and punishment (S) trials. It was thus a cue neuron and not a reward-predicting neuron. It could be described as encoding *salience* but not valence. Further evidence that the neuron was not reward or punishment related is that it did not respond on trials on which a food reward was shown (F), or an aversive visual stimulus was shown (A).

If the lick tube was moved away from the lips by a few mm so that juice reward could not be obtained (but the tone/LED still sounded, and was followed by a discriminative visual stimulus), the neuron stopped responding to the tone/LED cue, providing evidence that it was only when the tone/LED cue predicted the start of a trial in the visual discrimination task that the head of caudate neuron responded to the cue. This is shown by the middle set of trials in Fig. 6.10. Approximately half of the cue-related neurons tested showed this learning whereby

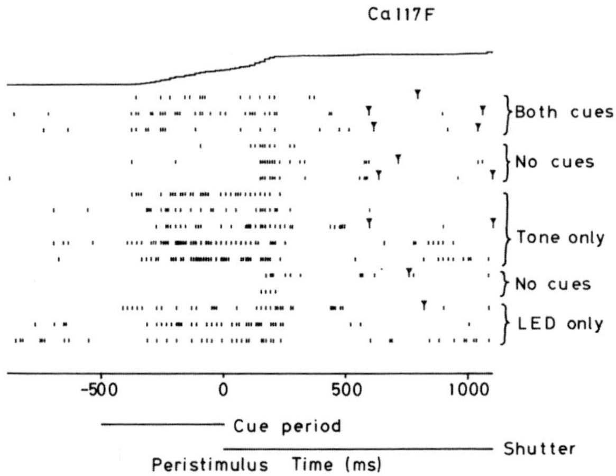

Fig. 6.11 Responses of a cue-related neuron in the head of the caudate nucleus in a Go/NoGo visual discrimination task in which the visual stimulus was presented at time 0, when a mechanical shutter opened to reveal the discriminative stimulus. Each trial is a single row of the rastergram, each action potential is represented by a single dot, and a lick made to obtain fruit juice on Reward trials only is represented by an inverted triangle. Tone and/or light emitting diode (LED) cues were provided starting 500 ms before the visual stimulus was shown. If no 500 ms warning cue was given for the start of a trial, the neuron responded to the first indication that a trial was beginning, the sound of the shutter opening at time 0. The neuron did not predict whether reward would or would not be obtained, in that there was no differential neuronal response on Reward trials (on which licks were made), compared to non-reward trials (on which licks were correctly not made). The line at the top shows the cusum (cumulative sum) statistic. (Reprinted from *Behavioural Brain Research*, 7 (2), E. T Rolls, S. J Thorpe, and S. P Maddison, Responses of striatal neurons in the behaving monkey. 1. Head of the caudate nucleus, pp. 179–210, Copyright 1983, with permission from Elsevier.)

they only responded to a warning cue normally used to start a trial if it actually did signal the start a trial. It typically took just a few trials for this trial predicting effect of a tone/LED cue to be learned and unlearned by these neurons.

Most of these cue-related neurons learned to respond to whichever cue, either a 500 Hz tone, or a light-emitting diode, signalled the start of a trial (see example in Fig. 6.11).

An example of a *reward-predicting* neuron in the head of the caudate nucleus that started responding as soon as a cue was available that a trial was about to start, and which continued firing after a visual stimulus was shown which indicated that a lick response could be made to obtain juice reward (R), but which stopped firing after a visual stimulus was shown that indicated that if a lick response was made, aversive saline (S) would be obtained, is shown in Fig. 6.12. The reward (R) and saline (S) trials each occurred with probability 0.5. This type of neuron, common in the head of the primate caudate nucleus, thus increased its firing as soon as the probability of reward increased at the start of a trial to 0.5, learned to respond to the first cue that signalled the start of a trial, and stopped responding as soon as the probability of reward decreased to 0 on punishment (S) trials. These neurons typically did not respond in relation to the cue stimuli, to the visual stimuli, or to movements, when these occurred independently of the task or performance of the task was prevented, for example by withdrawing the lick tube from which fruit juice could be obtained (Rolls, Thorpe & Maddison 1983c) (as illustrated for a cue-related neuron in Fig. 6.10). That is, the responses of these neurons reflected whether reward would be obtained, and more generally, reflect how much reward will be obtained (Cromwell & Schultz 2003). Similar neurons in the head of the caudate nucleus responded to punishment-predicting stimuli, and indeed approximately as many neurons responded to the saline punishment-associated visual stimulus

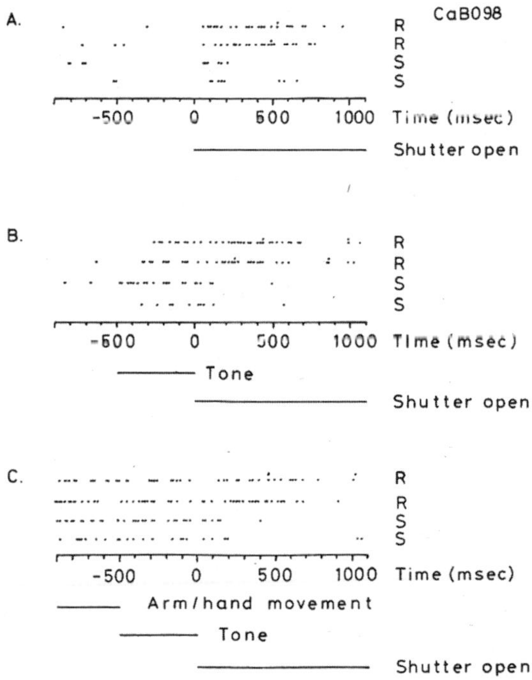

Fig. 6.12 Responses of a reward-predicting neuron in the head of the caudate nucleus in a Go/NoGo visual discrimination task in which the visual stimulus was presented at time 0. Each trial is a single row of the rastergram, each action potential is represented by a single dot, and a lick made to obtain fruit juice is represented by a vertical pair of dots. R, Reward trials on which fruit juice was obtained. S, Salt trials on which if a lick was made, a small drop of saline was obtained. (A) The neuron started to respond approximately 80 ms after the start of the trial when a shutter opened to reveal the discriminative stimulus, continued to respond on reward trials until after the fruit juice was obtained, and stopped responding at approximately 160 ms on trials on which the punisher-related stimulus (S) was shown. (B) The neuron started responding soon after a cue tone sounded indicating the start of a trial. (C) The neuron started responding at the earliest indication that the trial would start, an arm movement made by the macaque to press a button to start the trial. (Reprinted from *Behavioural Brain Research*, 7 (2), E. T Rolls, S. J Thorpe, and S. P Maddison, Responses of striatal neurons in the behaving monkey. 1. Head of the caudate nucleus, pp. 179–210, Copyright 1983, with permission from Elsevier.)

in the Go/NoGo visual discrimination task as to the juice reward-predicting stimulus (Rolls, Thorpe & Maddison 1983c, Rolls, Thorpe, Maddison, Roper-Hall, Puerto & Perrett 1979b, Rolls 1984). Thus some neurons in the head of the caudate nucleus encode the *valence* of visual stimuli. Consistently, Watanabe, Lauwereyns & Hikosaka (2003) have found that one population of neurons in the primate caudate nucleus responds to rewarded eye movements, and a separate population to unrewarded eye movements.

Similar types of response were found when the neurons were tested outside the visual discrimination task, during feeding. Of the neurons tested during feeding, 25.8% responded when the food was seen by the monkey, 6.2% when he tasted it, and 22.4% during a cue given by the experimenter that a food or non-food object was about to be presented. Further evidence on the nature of these neuronal responses was that many of the neurons with cue-related responses only responded to the tone/light cue stimuli when they were cues for the performance of the task or the presentation of food as described above, and some responded to the different cues used in the task (tone/LED) and feeding test (an arm movement made by the experimenter to reach behind a screen to obtain a food or non-food object) situations (Rolls, Thorpe & Maddison 1983c).

The finding that such neurons may respond to environmental stimuli only when they are significant in predicting for example the onset of a trial (a cue neuron), or the delivery of reward (a reward-predicting neuron) (Rolls, Thorpe, Maddison, Roper-Hall, Puerto & Perrett 1979b, Rolls, Thorpe & Maddison 1983c), was confirmed by Evarts and his colleagues. They showed that some neurons in the putamen only responded to the click of a solenoid when it indicated that a fruit juice reward could be obtained (Evarts & Wise 1984). The findings have also been confirmed by Tremblay & Schultz (1998) (see also Schultz, Tremblay & Hollerman (2003)), who reported that macaque caudate neurons come to respond during learning to cues related to the preparation of movement or expectation of reward, and do not respond to cues that do not predict such events.

We have found that this decoding of the significance of environmental events that are signals for the preparation for or initiation of a behavioural response is represented in the firing of a population of neurons in the dorsolateral prefrontal cortex, which projects into the head of the caudate nucleus (E. T. Rolls and G. C. Baylis, unpublished observations 1984). These neurons only respond to the tone cue if it signals the start of a trial of the visual discrimination task, just as do the corresponding population of neurons in the head of the caudate nucleus. The indication that the decoding of significance is performed by the prefrontal cortex, and that the striatum receives only the results of the cortical computation, is considered below and elsewhere (Rolls & Williams 1987a).

These findings indicate that the head of the caudate nucleus and most anterior part of the putamen contain populations of neurons that respond to predictive sensory cues that enable preparation for the performance of tasks such as feeding and tasks in which movements must be initiated, and others that respond during the performance of such tasks in relation to sensory cue that predict reward, and that the majority of these neurons have no unconditional sensory or motor responses. It has therefore been suggested (Rolls, Thorpe, Maddison, Roper-Hall, Puerto & Perrett 1979b, Rolls, Thorpe & Maddison 1983c) that the anterior neostriatum contains neurons that are important for the utilization of environmental cues for the preparation for behavioural responses, and for particular behavioural responses made in particular situations to particular environmental stimuli, that is in stimulus–motor response habit formation. Different neurons in the cue-related group often respond to different subsets of environmentally significant events, and thus convey some information that would be useful in switching behaviour, in preparing to make responses, and in connecting inputs to particular responses (Rolls, Thorpe, Maddison, Roper-Hall, Puerto & Perrett 1979b, Rolls, Thorpe & Maddison 1983c, Rolls 1984). Striatal neurons with similar types of response have also been recorded by Wolfram Schultz and colleagues (Schultz, Apicella, Romo & Scarnati 1995a, Tremblay & Schultz 1998, Cromwell & Schultz 2003, Schultz et al. 2003). Striatal tonically active interneurons (TANs) which have high spontaneous firing rates and respond by decreasing their firing rates may respond to similar cue-predicting and reward-predicting events (Graybiel & Kimura 1995), presumably by receiving inhibitory inputs from the principal striatal neurons described above, the medium spiny neurons.

It is of interest, and just as expected, that some dopamine neurons respond to these cue-related inputs, and other salient including novel and aversive stimuli (Bromberg-Martin, Matsumoto & Hikosaka 2010a) as described in Section 6.2.4, that are found in the head of the caudate nucleus and ventral striatum, for these parts of the striatum provide inputs to the dopamine neurons (Haber & Knutson 2009).

In human fMRI studies, activations have been described in the striatum that reflect whether monetary rewards can be obtained, that is they reflect expected reward value (Delgado, Nystrom, Fissell, Noll & Fiez 2000, Knutson, Adams, Fong & Hommer 2001, Haber &

Knutson 2009, Knutson, Delgado & Phillips 2009, Wu, Sacchet & Knutson 2012) and also reward outcome value (Rolls, McCabe & Redoute 2008e). These activations presumably reflect the activity of the reward-predicting neurons (Rolls, Thorpe, Maddison, Roper-Hall, Puerto & Perrett 1979b, Rolls, Thorpe & Maddison 1983c, Rolls 1984). Activations to monetary reward only if it is being worked for instrumentally (Zink et al. 2004) may reflect the type of task dependence illustrated for a cue-related neuron in Fig. 6.10. Human striatal fMRI activations to non-rewarding but salient stimuli (Zink et al. 2003) may reflect the types of trial-predicting (i.e. cue-related) neurons shown in Figs. 6.10 and 6.11 but not reward-predicting neurons of the type shown in Fig. 6.12.

One would expect human striatal activations also to be demonstrable to punishment-predicting stimuli, given that approximately half of the reward/punishment-predicting neurons respond to punishment-predicting stimuli (Rolls, Thorpe, Maddison, Roper-Hall, Puerto & Perrett 1979b, Rolls, Thorpe & Maddison 1983c, Rolls 1984), and there is some human fMRI evidence for this (Seymour et al. 2004). It is a difficulty (Bromberg-Martin, Matsumoto & Hikosaka 2010a) for the dopamine reward prediction error hypothesis (Schultz et al. 1995b, Schultz, Dayan & Montague 1997, Waelti et al. 2001, Schultz 2004, Schultz 2013) that it cannot account for the formation of striatal neurons that fire to predict punishment. [In particular, if dopamine neurons decrease their firing rate if an expected reward is not received or a punishment is received (Mirenowicz & Schultz 1996, Waelti, Dickinson & Schultz 2001, Tobler, Dickinson & Schultz 2003), then this would not promote learning in the striatum whereby striatal neurons might respond more to the stimulus (e.g. a discriminative stimulus in a visual discrimination task) that predicted punishment.] However, such reward and punisher predicting information is reflected in the firing of orbitofrontal cortex neurons, some of which predict reward, and others of which predict punishment (see Section 4.5), and it is presumably by this orbitofrontal cortex route that punishment-predicting neurons in the head of the caudate nucleus receive this information (rather than being reinforced into this type of firing by a dopamine reward error prediction signal).

It is very interesting that the type of neuron shown in Fig. 6.12 has certain similarities to the midbrain dopamine neurons described by Schultz and colleagues (Schultz et al. 1995b, Mirenowicz & Schultz 1996, Waelti et al. 2001), except that the dopamine neurons respond to the transitions in reward probabilities, rather than the reward probabilities themselves which is what appears to be encoded by the type of head of caudate neuron shown in Fig. 6.12. Thus an alternative to the hypothesis that the dopamine neurons provide a reward-prediction error teaching signal (see Section 6.2.4) is that the firing of the dopamine neurons may reflect feedback connections from these striatal regions as well as from the hypothalamus in which similar neurons are found (see Sections 4.11.4, 4.11.5, and 5.4.1.2) to the dopamine neurons in the substantia nigra, pars compacta, and ventral tegmental area. These feedback connections would then influence the dopamine neurons for short periods primarily when the firing of the striatal neurons changed, implemented by a high-pass filtering effect. This would leave much more open what the functions of the dopamine neurons are (see Sections 6.2.4 and 6.3.7), in that a simple feedback effect might be being implemented (from striatum to the dopamine neurons and back), perhaps to dynamically reset thresholds or gains in the striatum.

6.3.3.5 Anterior putamen

It is clear that the activity of many neurons in the putamen is related to movements (Anderson 1978, Crutcher & DeLong 1984a, Crutcher & DeLong 1984b, DeLong et al. 1984, DeLong & Wichmann 2010). There is a somatotopic organization of neurons in the putamen, with separate areas containing neurons responding to arm, leg, or orofacial movements. Some of these neurons respond only to active movements, and others to active and to passive movements. Some of these neurons respond to somatosensory stimulation, with multiple clusters of neurons responding, for example, to the movement of each joint. Some neurons in the putamen have been shown in experiments in which the arm has been given assisting and opposing loads to respond in relation to the direction of an intended movement, rather than in relation to the muscle forces required to execute the movement (Crutcher & DeLong 1984b). Also, the firing rate of neurons in the putamen tends to be linearly related to the amplitude of movements (Crutcher & DeLong 1984b), and this is of potential clinical relevance, since patients with basal ganglia disease frequently have difficulty in controlling the amplitude of their limb movements.

In order to obtain further evidence on specialization of function within the striatum, the activity of neurons in the putamen has been compared with the activity of neurons recorded in different parts of the striatum in the same tasks (Rolls, Thorpe, Boytim, Szabo & Perrett 1984b). Of 234 neurons recorded in the putamen of two macaque monkeys during the performance of a visual discrimination task and the other tests in which other striatal neurons have been shown to respond (Rolls, Thorpe & Maddison 1983c, Caan, Perrett & Rolls 1984), 68 (29%) had activity that was phasically related to movements (Rolls, Thorpe, Boytim, Szabo & Perrett 1984b). Many of these responded in relation to mouth movements such as licking. Similar neurons were found in the substantia nigra, pars reticulata, to which the putamen projects (Mora, Mogenson & Rolls 1977). The neurons did not have activity related to taste, in that they responded, for example, during tongue protrusion made to a food or non-food object. Some of these neurons responded in relation to the licking mouth movements made in the visual discrimination task, and always also responded when mouth movements were made during clinical testing when a food or non-food object was brought close to the mouth. Their responses were thus unconditionally related to movements, in that they responded in whichever testing situation was used, and were therefore different from the responses of neurons in the head of the caudate nucleus (Rolls, Thorpe & Maddison 1983c).

Of the 68 neurons in the putamen with movement-related activity in these tests, 61 had activity related to mouth movements, and seven had activity related to movements of the body. Of the remaining neurons, 24 (10%) had activity that was task-related in that some change of firing rate associated with the presentation of the tone cue or the opening of the shutter occurred on each trial (Rolls, Thorpe, Boytim, Szabo & Perrett 1984b), four had auditory responses, one responded to environmental stimuli (Rolls, Thorpe & Maddison 1983c), and 137 were not responsive in these test situations.

These findings (Rolls, Thorpe, Boytim, Szabo & Perrett 1984b) provide further evidence that differences between neuronal activity in different regions of the striatum are found even in the same testing situations, and also that the inputs that activate these neurons are derived functionally from the cortex which projects into a particular region of the striatum (in this case sensori-motor cortex, areas 3, 1, 2, 4, and 6).

6.3.4 What computations are performed by the basal ganglia?

The neurophysiological investigations described in Section 6.3.3 indicate that reinforcement-related signals do affect neuronal activity in some parts of the striatum, particularly in the ventral striatum. This finding suggests that pharmacological agents such as dopaminergic drugs that produce reward by acting on the ventral striatum may do so because they are tapping into a system normally involved in providing a route to behavioural output for signals carrying information about learned incentives. Some questions arise. Does the ventral striatum process the inputs in any way before passing them on? Can the ventral striatum be considered as one part of a larger computational system that includes all parts of the basal ganglia, and that operates as a single system with inputs from all parts of the cerebral cortex, allowing selection by competition between all the inputs as well as convergence between them to produce a single behavioural output stream? How do the outputs of the basal ganglia lead to or influence action?

One way to obtain evidence on the information processing being performed by the striatum is to compare neuronal activity in the striatum with that in its corresponding input and output structures. For example, the taste and visual information necessary for the computation that a visual stimulus is no longer associated with taste reward is represented by the activity of different neurons in the orbitofrontal cortex, and the putative result of such a computation, namely neurons that respond in this non-reward situation, are also found in the orbitofrontal cortex (Thorpe, Rolls & Maddison 1983, Rolls 1999a, Rolls 2000b, Rolls 2004c, Rolls & Grabenhorst 2008, Grabenhorst & Rolls 2011) (Section 4.5). However, such neurons that represent the necessary sensory information for this computation, and neurons that respond to the non-reward, were not found in the head of the caudate nucleus or the ventral striatum (Rolls, Thorpe & Maddison 1983c, Williams, Rolls, Leonard & Stern 1993). Instead, in the head of the caudate nucleus, neurons in the same test situation responded in relation to whether the monkey had to make a response on a particular trial, that is many of them responded more on Go than on No-Go trials. This could reflect the output of a cognitive computation performed by the orbitofrontal cortex, indicating whether on the basis of the available sensory information, the current trial should be a Go trial, or a No-Go trial because a visual stimulus previously associated with punishment had been shown.

Similarly, neurons were not found in the ventral striatum that are tuned to all the visual reward, taste reward, olfactory reward, and visual non-reward functions about which macaque orbitofrontal cortex neurons carry information (see Chapter 4). Instead the ventral striatal neurons were usually less easy to classify in these sensory ways, and were especially engaged when tasks were being performed. For example, many of the ventral striatal neurons that respond to visual inputs do so preferentially on the basis of whether the stimuli are recognized, or are associated with reinforcement (Williams, Rolls, Leonard & Stern 1993). Much of the sensory and memory-related processing required to determine whether a stimulus is a face, is recognized, or is associated with reinforcement has been performed in and is evident in neuronal responses in structures such as the amygdala (Leonard, Rolls, Wilson & Baylis 1985, Rolls 2000d), orbitofrontal cortex (Thorpe, Rolls & Maddison 1983, Rolls 2000b, Rolls 2004c, Rolls & Grabenhorst 2008, Grabenhorst & Rolls 2011) and hippocampal system (Rolls & Treves 1998, Rolls 1999b, Rolls & Stringer 2005, Rolls, Franco & Stringer 2005b, Rolls, Xiang & Franco 2005c, Rolls & Xiang 2006, Rolls 2010b).

Similar comparisons can be made for the head and tail of the caudate nucleus, and the posterior putamen (Rolls & Johnstone 1992, Rolls & Treves 1998).

In these four parts of the striatum in which a comparison can be made of processing in the striatum with that in the cortical area that projects to that part of the striatum, it thus appears that the full information represented in the cortex does not reach the striatum, but that rather the striatum receives the output of the computation being performed by a cortical area, and could use this to initiate, switch, or alter behaviour.

The hypothesis arises from these findings that some parts of the striatum, particularly the caudate nucleus, ventral striatum, and posterior putamen, receive the output of these memory-related and cognitive computations, but do not themselves perform them. Instead, on receiving the cortical and limbic outputs, the striatum may be involved in switching behaviour as appropriate as determined by the different, sometimes conflicting, information received from these cortical and limbic areas. On this view, the striatum would be particularly involved in the selection of behavioural responses, and in producing one coherent stream of behavioural output, with the possibility to switch if a higher priority input was received. This process may be achieved by a laterally spreading competitive interaction between striatal or pallidal neurons, which might be implemented by the direct inhibitory connections between nearby neurons in the striatum and globus pallidus. In addition, the inhibitory interneurons within the striatum, the dendrites of which in the striatum may cross the boundary between the matrix and striosomes, may play a part in this interaction between striatal processing streams (Groves 1983, Graybiel & Kimura 1995, Groves, Garcia-Munoz, Linder, Manley, Martone & Young 1995).

Dopamine could play an important role in setting the sensitivity of this response selection function, as suggested by direct iontophoresis of dopamine on to single striatal neurons, which produces a similar decrease in the response of the neuron and in its spontaneous activity in the behaving macaque (Rolls, Thorpe, Boytim, Szabo & Perrett 1984b, Rolls & Williams 1987a). Consistent with dopamine playing an important role of this type, dopamine acting via D1 receptors in the direct pathway, and via D2 receptors in the indirect pathway, promotes behavioural output (Gerfen & Surmeier 2011).

In addition to this response selection function by competition, the basal ganglia may, by the convergence discussed, enable signals originating from non-motor parts of the cerebral cortex to be mapped into motor signals to produce behavioural output. The ways in which these computations might be performed are considered next.

6.3.5 How do the basal ganglia perform their computations?

On the hypothesis just raised, different regions of the striatum, or at least the outputs of such regions, would need to interact. Is there within the striatum the possibility for different regions to interact, and is the partial functional segregation seen within the striatum maintained in processing beyond the striatum? For example, is the segregation maintained throughout the globus pallidus and thalamus with projections to different premotor and even prefrontal regions reached by different regions of the striatum, or is there convergence or the possibility for interaction at some stage during this post-striatal processing?

Given the anatomy of the basal ganglia, interactions between signals reaching the basal ganglia could happen in a number of different ways. One would be for each part of the striatum to receive at least some input from a number of different cortical regions. As discussed above, there is evidence for patches of input from different sources to be brought adjacent to each other in the striatum (Van Hoesen et al. 1981, Seleman & Goldman-Rakic 1985, Graybiel & Kimura 1995). For example, in the caudate nucleus, different regions of association cortex project to adjacent longitudinal strips (Seleman & Goldman-Rakic 1985). Now, the dendrites of striatal neurons have the shape of large plates which lie at right angles to the incoming cortico-striatal fibres (Percheron, Yelnik & François 1984a, Percheron, Yelnik & François 1984b, Percheron, Yelnik, François, Fenelon & Talbi 1994, Yelnik 2002, Buot & Yelnik 2012) (see Figs. 6.13 and 6.14). Thus one way in which interaction may start in the basal ganglia is by virtue of the same striatal neuron receiving inputs on its dendrites from more than just a limited area of the cerebral cortex. This convergence may provide a first level of integration over limited sets of cortico-striatal fibres. The large number of cortical inputs received by each striatal neuron, in the order of 10,000 (Wilson 1995), is consistent with the hypothesis that convergence of inputs carrying different signals is an important aspect of the function of the basal ganglia. The computation that could be performed by this architecture is discussed below for the inputs to the globus pallidus, where the connectivity pattern is comparable.

6.3.5.1 Interaction between neurons and selection of output

The regional segregation of neuronal response types in the striatum described above is consistent with mainly local integration over limited, adjacent sets of cortico-striatal inputs, as suggested by this anatomy. Short-range integration or interactions within the striatum may also be produced by the short length (for example 0.5 mm) of the intra-striatal axons of striatal

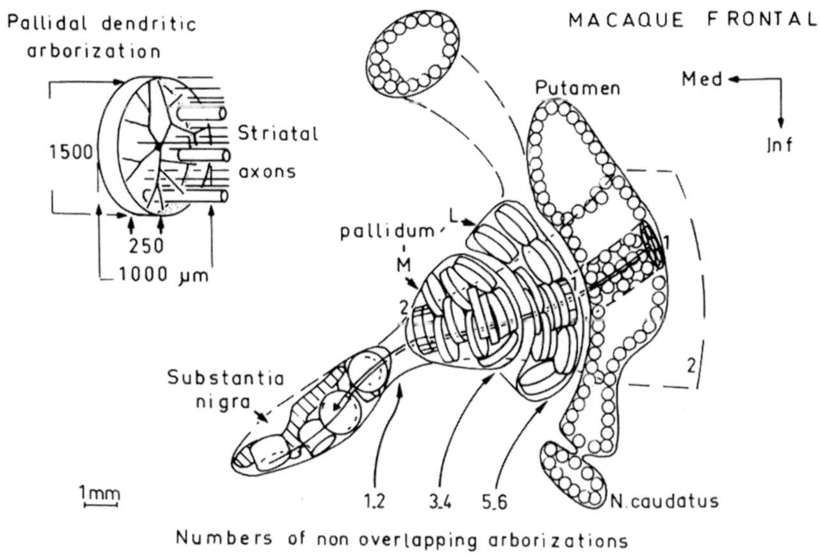

Fig. 6.13 Semi-schematic spatial diagram of the striato-pallido-nigral system (see text). The numbers represent the numbers of non-overlapping arborizations of dendrites in the plane shown. L, lateral or external segment of the globus pallidus; M, medial or internal segment of the globus pallidus. The inserted diagram in the upper left shows the geometry of the dendrites of a typical pallidal neuron, and how the flat dendritic arborization is pierced at right angles by the striatal axons, which make occasional synapses en passage. (Reproduced from Gerard Percheron, Jerome Yelnik, and Chantal Francois, A Golgi analysis of the primate globus pallidus. III. Spatial organization of the striato-pallidal complex, *Journal of Comparative Neurology*, 227 (2) pp. 214–227, Copyright ©2004, John Wiley and Sons.)

neurons. These could produce a more widespread influence if the effect of a strong input to one part of the striatum spread like a lateral competition signal (cf. Groves (1983), Groves et al. (1995)). Such a mechanism could contribute to behavioural response selection in the face of different competing input signals to the striatum. The lateral inhibition could operate, for example, between the striatal principal (that is medium spiny) neurons by direct connections (they receive excitatory connections from the cortex, respond by increasing their firing rates, and could inhibit each other by their local axonal arborizations, which spread in an area as large as their dendritic trees, and which utilize GABA as their inhibitory transmitter). Further lateral inhibition could operate in the pallidum and substantia nigra (see Fig. 6.14). Here again there are local axon collaterals, as widespread as the very large pallidal and nigral dendritic fields. The lateral competition could again operate by direct connections between the neurons.

[Note that pallidal and nigral cells have high spontaneous firing rates (often 25–50 spikes/s), and respond (to their inhibitory striatal inputs) by reducing their firing rates below this high spontaneous rate. Such a decrease in the firing rate of one neuron would release inhibition on nearby neurons, causing them to increase their firing rates, equivalent to responding less. It is very interesting that direct inhibitory connections between the neurons can implement selection, even though at the striatal level the neurons have low spontaneous firing rates and respond by increasing their firing rates, whereas in the globus pallidus and substantia nigra pars reticulata the neurons have a high spontaneous firing rate, and respond by decreasing their firing rate.]

A selection function of this type between processing streams in the basal ganglia, even without any convergence anatomically between the processing streams implemented by feed-

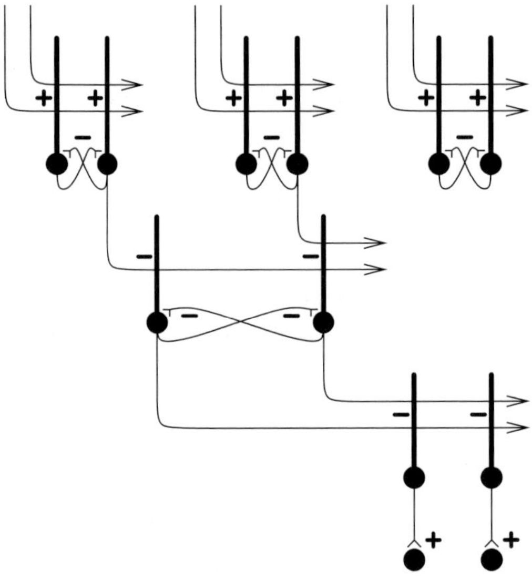

Fig. 6.14 Simple hypothesis of basal ganglia network architecture. A key aspect is that in both the striatum, and in the globus pallidus and substantia nigra pars reticulata, there are direct inhibitory connections (–) between the principal neurons, as shown. These synapses use GABA as a transmitter. Excitatory inputs to the striatum are shown as +. (This material was originally published in *Neural Networks and Brain Function* by E. T. Rolls, and A. Treves, ©1998, Oxford University Press http://ukcatalogue.oup.com/product/9780198524328.do#.Uf9rKKw2FLo.)

forward inputs, might provide an important computational raison d'être for the basal ganglia. The direct inhibitory local connectivity between the principal neurons within the striatum and globus pallidus would seem to provide a simple, and perhaps evolutionarily old, way in which to implement competition between neurons and processing streams. This might even be a primitive design principle that characterizes the basal ganglia. A system such as the basal ganglia with direct inhibitory recurrent collaterals may have evolved easily because it is easier to make stable than architectures such as the cerebral cortex with recurrent excitatory connections. The basal ganglia architecture may have been especially appropriate in motor systems in which instability could produce movement and co-ordination difficulties (Rolls & Treves 1998, Rolls 1999a). Equations that describe the way in which this mutual inhibition between the principal neurons can result in contrast enhancement of neuronal activity in the different competing neurons, and thus selection, are provided by Grossberg (1988), Gurney et al. (2001a), and Gurney, Prescott & Redgrave (2001b).

This hypothesis of lateral competition between the neurons of the basal ganglia can be sketched simply (see also Fig. 6.14 and Rolls & Treves (1998) Chapter 9, where a more detailed neuronal network theory of the operation of the basal ganglia is presented). The inputs from the cortex to the striatum are excitatory, and competition between striatal neurons is implemented by the use of an inhibitory transmitter (GABA), and direct connections between striatal neurons, within an area which is approximately co-extensive with the dendritic arborization. Given that the lateral connections between the striatal neurons are collaterals of the output axons, the output must be inhibitory on to pallidal and nigral neurons. This means that to transmit signals usefully, and in contrast with striatal neurons, the neurons in the globus pallidus and substantia nigra (pars reticulata) must have high spontaneous firing rates, and respond by reducing their firing rates. These pallidal and nigral neurons then repeat the simple scheme for lateral competition between output neurons by having direct lateral inhibitory connections to the other pallidal and nigral neurons. When nigral and pallidal neurons respond by reducing their firing rates, the reduced inhibition through the recurrent collaterals allows the connected pallidal and nigral neurons to fire faster, and also at the same time the main output of the pallidal and nigral neurons allows the thalamic neurons to fire faster. The thalamic neurons then have the standard excitatory influence on their cortical targets.

The simple, and perhaps evolutionarily early, aspect of this basal ganglia architecture is that the striatal, pallidal, and nigral neurons implement competition (for selection) by direct inhibitory recurrent lateral connections of the main output neurons on to other output neurons, with the inputs to each stage of processing (e.g. striatum, globus pallidus) synapsing directly on to the output neurons that inhibit each other (see Fig. 6.14).

Another possible mechanism for interaction within the striatum is provided by the dopaminergic pathway, through which a signal that has descended from, for example, the ventral striatum to the dopamine neurons in the midbrain might thereby influence other parts of the striatum (see Section 6.2.4). Because of the slow conduction speed of the dopaminergic neurons, this latter system would probably not be suitable for rapid switching of behaviour, but only for more tonic, long-term adjustments of sensitivity.

Further levels for integration within the basal ganglia are provided by the striato-pallidal and striato-nigral projections (Percheron, Yelnik & François 1984a, Percheron, Yelnik & François 1984b, Percheron, Yelnik, François, Fenelon & Talbi 1994, Yelnik 2002). The afferent fibres from the striatum again cross at right angles a flat plate or disc formed by the dendrites of the pallidal or nigral neurons (see Fig. 6.13). The discs are approximately 1.5 mm in diameter, and are stacked up one upon the next at right angles to the incoming striatal fibres. The dendritic discs are so large that in the monkey there is room for only perhaps 50 such discs not to overlap in the external pallidal segment, for 10 non-overlapping discs in the medial pallidal segment, and for one overlapping disc in the most medial part of the medial segment of the globus pallidus and in the substantia nigra.

One result of this convergence achieved by this stage of the medial pallidum/substantia nigra is that even if inputs from different cortical regions were kept segregated by specific wiring rules on to different neurons, there might nevertheless well be the possibility for mutual competition between different pallidal neurons, implemented by their mutual inhibitory connections. Given the relatively small number of neurons into which the cortical signals had now been compressed, it would be feasible to have competition (the same effect as lateral inhibition implemented by inhibitory neurons would achieve elsewhere) implemented between the relatively small population of neurons, now all collected into a relatively restricted space, so that the competition could spread widely within these nuclei. This could allow selection by competition between these pathways, that is effectively between information processing in different cortical areas. This could be important in allowing each cortical area to control output when appropriate (depending on the task being performed). Even if full segregation were maintained in the return paths to the cerebral cortex, the return paths could influence each cortical area, allowing it to continue processing if it had the strongest 'call'. Each cortical area on a fully segregated hypothesis might thus have its own non-basal ganglia output routes, but might according to the current suggestion utilize the basal ganglia as a system to select a cortical area or set of areas, depending on how strongly each cortical area is calling for output. The thalamic outputs from the basal ganglia (areas VA and VLo of the thalamus) might according to this hypothesis have to some extent an activity or gain-controlling function on a cortical area (such as might be mediated by diffuse terminals in superficial cortical layers), rather than the strong and selective inputs implemented by a specific thalamic nucleus such as the lateral geniculate.

6.3.5.2 Convergent mapping within the basal ganglia

In addition to this selection function, it is also attractive to at least consider the further hypothesis that there is some convergent mapping achieved by the basal ganglia. This hypothesis is now considered in more detail. The anatomical arrangement just described does provide a possibility for some convergence on to single striatal neurons of cortical input, and on to single pallidal and nigral (pars reticulata) neurons of signals from relatively different parts of the striatum. For what computation might such anatomy provide a structural basis? Within the pallidum, each dendritic disc is flat, is orthogonal to the input fibres that pierce it, but is not filled with dendritic arborizations. Instead, each dendrite typically consists of 4–5 branches that are spread out to occupy only a small part of the surface area of the dendritic disc (see Fig. 6.13). There are thousands of such sparsely populated plates stacked on top of one another. Each pallidal neuron is contacted by a number of the mass of fibres from the striatum that pass it, and given the relatively small collecting area of each pallidal or nigral neuron (4 or 5 dendritic branches in a plane), each such neuron is thus likely to receive a random combination of inputs from different striatal neurons within its collection field. The thinness of the dendritic sheet may help to ensure that each axon does not make more than a few synapses with each dendrite, and that the combinations of inputs received by each dendrite are approximately random. This architecture thus appears to be appropriate for bringing together at random on to single pallidal and nigral neurons, inputs that originate from quite diverse parts of the cerebral cortex. (This is a two-stage process, cortex to striatum, and striatum to pallidum and substantia nigra). By the stage of the medial pallidum and substantia nigra, there is the opportunity for the input field of a single neuron to effectively become very wide, although whether in practice this covers very different cortical areas, or is instead limited to a rather segregated cortex–basal ganglia–cortex loop, remains to be confirmed. However, empirical evidence that convergence does occur from striatum to pallidum is the finding that some of the pallidal neurons active in the delayed match to sample task described in Section 6.3.3.3 were not modality-specific, whereas only visual or auditory modality-specific delayed match to sample neurons were located in the postero-ventral part of the striatum (Johnstone & Rolls 1990, Rolls & Johnstone 1992).

Given then that this architecture could allow individual pallidal and nigral neurons to receive random combinations of inputs from different striatal neurons, the following functional implications arise. Simple associative (Hebbian) learning in the striatum would enable strongly firing striatal neurons to increase the strength of the synapses from the active cortical inputs in what would operate as a competitive network. (Descriptions of competitive networks are provided by Rolls (2008b), Rolls & Treves (1998), and Hertz, Krogh & Palmer (1991).) In a proposal of Nakahara, Amari & Hikosaka (2002), dopamine can influence the firing rates of the striatal neurons, and thus can indirectly affect the Hebbian learning (see further Schultz (2013)). In the pallidum, such conjunctive learning of coactive inputs would be more complex, requiring, for example, a strongly inhibited pallidal neuron to show synaptic strengthening from strongly firing but inhibitory inputs from the striatum. Then, if a particular pallidal or nigral neuron received inputs by chance from striatal neurons that responded to an environmental cue signal that something significant was about to happen, and from striatal neurons that fired because the monkey was making a postural adjustment, this conjunction of events might make that pallidal or nigral neuron become inhibited by (that is respond to) either input alone. Then, in the future, the occurrence of only one of the inputs, for example only the environmental cue, would result in a decrease of firing of that pallidal or nigral neuron, and thus in the appropriate postural adjustment being made by virtue of the output connections of that pallidal or nigral neuron.

This is a proposal that the basal ganglia are able to detect combinations of conjunctively active inputs from quite widespread regions of the cerebral cortex using their combinatorial architecture and a property of synaptic modifiability. In this way it would be possible to trigger any complex pattern of behavioural responses by any complex pattern of environmental inputs, using what is effectively an associative network (operating as a competitive network or pattern associator) to link by learning an antecedent input (for example the environmental salient cue inputs to the striatum) with the succeeding activity (for example a motor signal driving motor responses).

It may be noted that the input events need not include only those from environmental stimuli represented in the caudate nucleus and ventral striatum, but also, if the overlapping properties of the dendrites described above provide sufficient opportunity for convergence, of the context of the movement, provided by inputs via the putamen from sensorimotor cortex. This would then make a system appropriate for triggering an appropriate motor response (learned by trial and error, with the final solution becoming associated with the triggering input events) to any environmental input state. As such, this hypothesis provides a suggested neural basis for 'habit' learning in which the basal ganglia have been implicated (Phillips, Malamut, Bachevalier & Mishkin 1988, Petri & Mishkin 1994, Balleine et al. 2009). The hypothesis could be said to provide a basis for the storage of motor plans in the basal ganglia, which would be instantiated as a series of look-ups of the appropriate motor output pattern to an evolving sequence of input information.

An interesting aspect of this hypothesis is that other parts of the motor system, such as the cortico-cortical pathways, may mediate the control of action in a voluntary, often slow, but goal-directed, action–outcome, way in the early stages of learning. The input context for the movement and the appropriate motor signals (originating during learning from motor cortical areas) could then be learned by the basal ganglia, until after many trials the basal ganglia can perform the required look-up of the correct motor output in an automated, 'habit', or 'stimulus–response', mode. In this sense, the cortico-cortical pathways would set up the conditions, which because of their continuing repetition would be learned by the basal ganglia. The hypothesis introduced above also may provide a basis for the switching between different types of behaviour proposed as a function of the basal ganglia, for if a strong new pattern of inputs was received by the basal ganglia, this would result in a different pattern of outputs being associatively 'looked up' than that currently in progress.

The way in which reinforcement signals present in the ventral striatum could contribute to these functions is that whether reinforcement availability is being indicated by the firing of ventral striatal neurons could be part of the output context being provided by the basal ganglia. If positive reinforcement was being signalled, the implication of the striatal output would be that the animal should make behavioural responses that would lead to approach to the conditioned positive reinforcers, and thus to obtaining primary reinforcement (see Section 6.3.3.1).

6.3.5.3 Learning within the basal ganglia, and the role of dopamine

The outputs of the globus pallidus and substantia nigra directed via the thalamus to motor regions such as the supplementary motor cortex and the premotor cortex potentially provide important output routes for the basal ganglia to produce actions (see Figs. 6.5 and 6.6). However, there are also outputs of the basal ganglia to structures that may not be primarily motor, such as the dorsolateral prefrontal cortex of primates (Middleton & Strick 1994, Middleton & Strick 1996b, Middleton & Strick 2000, Kelly & Strick 2004), and the inferior temporal visual cortex (Middleton & Strick 1996a). The outputs to the dorsolateral prefrontal cortex might be to enable that region to know what response had recently been selected, and thus to remember the response over a delay period (see Rolls & Treves (1998)).

The hypothesis of basal ganglia function just described incorporates associative learning of coactive inputs on to neurons, at both the cortico-striatal stages, and the striato-pallidal and nigral stages. Consistent with this hypothesis (Rolls 1999a, Rolls & Johnstone 1992), it has now been possible to demonstrate long-term potentiation (LTP) in at least some parts of the basal ganglia. For example, Pennartz, Ameerun, Groenewegen & Lopes da Silva (1993) demonstrated LTP of limbic inputs to the nucleus accumbens, and were able to show that such LTP is facilitated by dopamine (see in addition Schultz (2013)). Further, it was shown that coincident cortical input and depolarization in a striatal neuron can induce long-term depression (LTD) of the cortico-striatal synapse if some dopamine is present (Calabresi, Maj, Pisani, Mercuri & Bernardi 1992), and LTP if there is a phasic release of dopamine (Wickens & Kotter 1995, Wickens, Begg & Arbuthnott 1996, Reynolds & Wickens 2002).

Thus one function of dopamine in the basal ganglia may be to set the threshold for learning within the basal ganglia. In what further ways might dopamine come to be important in reward, as indicated by the evidence described in Section 6.2? Given that there are relatively few dopaminergic neurons, it is likely that the information conveyed by the dopamine pathway is relatively general or modulatory, rather than conveying the specific information that must be learned and mapped to the output of the basal ganglia, or the full details of the primary reinforcer obtained (for example which taste, which touch, etc.).

A second possible function, noted above, is that dopamine may play an important role in setting the thresholds of striatal neurons, as suggested by direct iontophoresis of dopamine on to single striatal neurons, which produces a similar decrease in the response of the neuron and in its spontaneous activity in the behaving macaque (Rolls & Williams 1987a, Rolls et al. 1984b). In this way, or perhaps by a different mechanism, the dopamine might also modulate learning in the basal ganglia. A very simple hypothesis is that the modulation of learning is likely to be quite general, making it more likely that information will be stored, that is that conjunctive activity at the inputs to the basal ganglia will become associated.

Another possibility is that activity in the dopamine pathways carries a teaching signal, which might operate as a reinforcer in the type of reinforcement learning system described in Appendix 1, Section A.5 (Houk, Adams & Barto 1995, Schultz 2013). Schultz et al. (1995b) have argued from their recordings from dopamine neurons that this may be the case. For example, dopamine neurons can respond to the taste of a liquid reward in an operant task. However, these neurons may stop responding to such a primary (unlearned) reinforcer quite rapidly as the task is learned, and instead respond only to the earliest indication that a trial of the task is about to begin (Schultz et al. 1995b, Schultz 1998, Schultz 2013). Thus dopamine neurons could not convey information about a primary reward obtained if the trial is successful, in the way that orbitofrontal cortex neurons do, in that the orbitofrontal cortex neurons do respond to the reward obtained on every trial (see Section 4.5). The types of reward to which orbitofrontal cortex neurons respond include food reward, water reward, taste reward, olfactory reward, pleasant touch, and even abstract monetary reward (see Section 4.5). Further evidence that the dopamine projection does not convey a specific ‘reward’ signal is that dopamine release can occur not only to rewards (such as food or brain-stimulation reward, or later in training to an indication that a reward might be given later), but also to aversive stimuli such as aversive stimulation of the medial hypothalamus (see Hoebel et al. (1996) and Gray et al. (1997)), or stress (Seamans & Yang 2004). Further, dopamine neurons may respond to salient stimuli (Horvitz 2000, Redgrave et al. 1999, Bromberg-Martin et al. 2010a). In addition, *salience*, rather than reward, is what it has been suggested is encoded in a main recipient region of the dopamine neurons, the striatum, in that head of caudate and accumbens activation occurs to a monetary reward much more when it is made salient by being actively worked for than when it is received passively (Zink et al. 2004) (a property of the reward-predicting neurons described in Section 6.3.3.4), and occurs to salient non-rewarding stimuli (Zink et al. 2003) (probably reflecting activity of the cue-related neurons described in Section

6.3.3.4). Further, hedonic assessment of rewards, or 'liking', does not depend on dopaminergic processes (Berridge & Robinson 1998).

Given that the dopamine neurons do not appear to encode a signal for the delivery of reward (and this includes the 'hedonic' or 'liking' aspects of reward (Berridge & Robinson 1998)), it is possible that they carry a signal useful in reinforcement learning, by encoding reward prediction error (Houk et al. 1995, Schultz et al. 1995b, Schultz et al. 1997, Tobler et al. 2003, Schultz 2004, Schultz 2013) (see Appendix 1, Section 6.2.4). Presumably this would facilitate long-term synaptic potentiation (LTP) in target areas such as the striatum and parts of the prefrontal cortex where there is conjunctive pre-synaptic input and postsynaptic firing or depolarization, and perhaps produce long-term depression (LTD) if the dopamine became phasically low. This could enable mapping of stimuli that predict reward, through structures such as the basal ganglia, possibly to produce synapses that for each sensory cue would be appropriate for the next part of an action sequence (Suri & Schultz 1998) (see Section A.5.3). However, as noted above, this reinforcement signal would not appear to be appropriate for learning associations to cues that predict punishers.

However, the findings described above on the effects of aversive and salient stimuli on dopaminergic activity (see also Section 6.2.4) suggest an alternative possibility, that dopaminergic activity instead appears to convey information that would be better suited to a preparation or behavioural 'Go' (i.e. prepare to initiate action) role for dopamine release in the striatum. (Consistent with this, high levels of dopamine acting via D1 receptors can facilitate the excitability of striatal neurons (Reynolds & Wickens 2002).) These findings are more consistent with the hypothesis that instead of acting as the reinforce or error signal in a reinforcement learning system (Houk et al. 1995, Schultz et al. 1995b, Schultz et al. 1997, Tobler et al. 2003, Schultz 2004, Schultz 2013), the dopamine projection to the striatum may act as a 'Go' or 'preparation' signal to set the thresholds of neurons in the striatum, and/or as a general modulatory signal that could help to strengthen synapses of conjunctively active pre- and postsynaptic neurons. In such a system, what is learned would be dependent on the presynaptic and postsynaptic terms of striatal neurons, and would not be explicitly guided by a reinforce/reward signal that would provide feedback after each trial on the degree of success of each trial as in the reinforcement learning algorithm (see Appendix 1, Section A.5). The striatum could thus learn associations useful for setting up habit representations, as described in Section 6.3.5.2. On this hypothesis, the crucial aspects of what is learned would depend on conjunctive pre- and postsynaptic activity in the striatum. In this scenario, the dopamine might just reflect activity in the striatum and be used to set thresholds appropriately (based on general behavioural salience) rather than being explicitly forced into a reward prediction error state of firing by unknown inputs. On this hypothesis, a large increase in dopamine release would facilitate Hebbian learning in the corticostriatal system (Reynolds & Wickens 2002) when salient stimuli occurred, and the salience might be produced by for example unexpected or strong rewarding or punishing events, or by novel events, or by events with uncertainty (Seamans & Yang 2004, Shizgal & Arvanitogiannis 2003).

Another view of striatal function is that the striatum might be organized as a set of segregated and independent transmission routes, each one of which would receive from a given region of the cortex, and project finally to separate premotor or prefrontal regions (Strick et al. 1995, Middleton & Strick 1996a, Middleton & Strick 1996b) (though see Kelly & Strick (2004)) (see Figs. 6.5 and 6.6). Even if this is correct, the detection of combinations of conjunctively active inputs, but in this case from limited populations of input axons to the basal ganglia, might still be an important aspect of the function of the basal ganglia.

On all these views of basal ganglia function, the ventral striatum would still be an area allowing convergence of signals from the amygdala, orbitofrontal cortex, and hippocampus. Transmission in this system would be modulated by dopamine. This modulation could influence how much effect reinforcing inputs to the striatum produce on their outputs. Increasing the gain or reducing the threshold could enhance positively reinforcing output if the inputs to the ventral striatum were predominantly indicating positive reinforcement. In a positively reinforcing context, facilitating dopamine transmission in the ventral striatum could lead to a net increase in reward output, and this could be at least part of the mechanism by which dopamine release in the ventral striatum could be rewarding, not especially by facilitating responses to primary reinforcers, but particularly by facilitating responses to conditioned reinforcers (see Section 6.3.3.1).

6.3.6 Synthesis on the role of dopamine in reward and addiction

Dopamine does appear to be involved in the reward produced by stimulation of some brain-stimulation reward sites, notably the ventral tegmental area where the dopamine cell bodies are located. This self-stimulation depends on dopamine release in the nucleus accumbens. Self-stimulation at other sites does not depend on dopamine.

The self-administration of the psychomotor stimulants such as amphetamine and cocaine depends on activation of a dopaminergic system in the nucleus accumbens. Psychostimulant drugs such as amphetamine may operate in part by sensitizing the process by which non-contingent Pavlovian conditioned stimuli increase the probability of instrumental behaviour and Pavlovian conditioned approach to rewards (Cardinal et al. 2002, Cardinal & Everitt 2004), an effect related to 'conditioned salience' or 'wanting' (Berridge & Robinson 1998, Robinson & Berridge 1993, Robinson & Berridge 2003).

The dopamine release produced by these behaviours may be rewarding because it is influencing the activity of an amygdalo-striatal (and in primates also probably orbitofrontal-striatal) system involved in linking the amygdala and orbitofrontal cortex, which can learn stimulus–reinforcer associations, to output systems (see also Section 4.6.3). Effectively, activation of neurons in this system has to be reinforcing if secondary (i.e. conditioned) reinforcers are to influence behaviour. Put very directly, animals must be built to want to activate the neurons in this system which can be activated by stimuli learned to be reinforcers in the amygdala and orbitofrontal cortex. In this system, dopamine release, and the firing of dopamine neurons, may only produce reward if the net input to the ventral striatum from the amygdala and orbitofrontal cortex is positive. The dopamine in this system may just be acting as an input that tends to facilitate transmission through this system, and effectively to help the transmission to produce a 'Go' signal. A particular way to show that the dopamine in this system means 'Go' rather than 'reward' would be to test whether the dopamine neurons fire, and dopamine release occurs and is necessary for, behaviour such as active avoidance to a strong punishing, arousing, salient, stimulus. There is indeed evidence that dopamine is released in the nucleus accumbens by aversive and salient stimuli as well as by rewarding stimuli (see Section 6.2.3, and Horvitz (2000) and Redgrave et al. (1999)).

The pathway from the amygdala to the ventral striatum may, as discussed above, be especially involved in Pavlovian effects that conditioned incentives (secondary reinforcers) have on instrumental action, but not in action–outcome learning. Consistent with this, and in the context of drug seeking behaviour and the role of stimuli associated by stimulus–reinforcer association learning with the reinforcement produced by psychomotor stimulants, Whitelaw et al. (1996) showed that excitotoxic lesions of the basolateral amygdala in rats impaired behavioural responses to a light associated with intravenous administration of cocaine, but not to the primary reinforcer of the cocaine itself (see Section 4.6.3). Part of the function of the ventral striatum in addiction may thus be to draw behaviour towards stimuli associated by conditioning with psychomotor stimulants such as amphetamine and cocaine (Kelley 2004b, Cardinal & Everitt 2004, Everitt & Robbins 2013).

If the psychomotor stimulant drugs produce their rewarding and addictive effects by influencing this amygdalo-striatal transmission, and effectively producing reward by tapping into a system normally involved in secondary as opposed to primary reinforcement, it might be asked why the reward produced by the drug does not extinguish. When no primary reinforcement is being received, the effects that secondary reinforcers have on behaviour normally do decline considerably. Why is the reward apparently in contrast so persistent with the dopaminergic stimulant drugs? Perhaps the following is at least part of the explanation. If the amygdala and orbitofrontal cortex are parts of the brain involved in stimulus–reward association learning and extinction, then the extinction would be expected to be implemented by a reduction in the neuronal responses to a secondary reinforcer during extinction. If the mechanism for extinction (as well as learning) is in the amygdala and orbitofrontal cortex, then tapping into the circuitry after the amygdala and orbitofrontal cortex would not be expected to be subject to the learning and extinction. That is, the firing at the entry into the ventral striatum would have to be interpreted by the system as meaning reward (i.e. that approach should be performed to make these neurons fire), as the stimulus–reward learning system precedes this stage of the amygdalo-striatal circuitry (see Fig. 10.4). Thus, in so far as the psychomotor dopaminergic stimulant drugs of addiction are tapping into a part of the circuitry after stimulus–reward learning and unlearning has been implemented, we would not expect the reward introduced into that part of the system by drugs to extinguish.

A similar argument applies to sensory-specific satiety, which, as it is computed in the orbitofrontal cortex, would not apply to rewarding effects of drugs that have their main effects after the orbitofrontal cortex, in for example the striatum.

6.3.7 Synthesis: emotion, dopamine, reward, punishment, and action selection in the basal ganglia

We have seen that the firing of dopamine neurons does not encode reward. This is the case in that dopamine neuron firing to delivered rewards (such as the taste of food) ceases if the reinforcer is preceded by a predictive cue, and instead the neurons respond to the predictive cue of reward. If that predictive cue is preceded by an earlier cue, the dopamine neuron firing moves forward to the first predictive cue (Schultz et al. 1995b, Schultz et al. 1997, Waelti et al. 2001, Schultz 2004, Schultz 2013). Thus dopamine neuron firing could not be related to the emotions that occur when rewards are delivered, such as pleasant or aversive taste, touch, smell, sounds, visual stimuli such as attractive faces or face expressions, or any other primary reinforcers if they are preceded by a predictive cue that they will be delivered.

Similarly, dopamine neuron firing could not produce the emotions that occur to other stimuli such as the sight or sound of any other emotion-producing stimulus (such as the sight of food or of a loved one or of monetary reward or loss) if it is preceded by a predictive cue.

Further, because dopamine neurons are described as responding phasically (i.e. transiently) only at the time when the probability of reward alters (which is the reward prediction error hypothesis (Schultz et al. 1995b, Schultz et al. 1997, Waelti et al. 2001, Schultz 2004, Schultz 2013)), the dopamine neurons could not implement the emotions that occur throughout the delivery of rewards or punishers (for example throughout a period of pleasant touch), or indeed which may continue after the reinforcing stimulus is no longer present (for example the fear elicited by a stimulus associated with a punisher).

In contrast, the orbitofrontal cortex does contain exquisitely information-rich representations of a very wide range of actual rewards and punishers, including primary reinforcers such as taste, oral texture, temperature, pleasant and painful touch, and face expression; secondary reinforcers such as the sight and smell of stimuli associated with primary reinforcers, and even monetary reward value); implements (together with the amygdala) at the neuronal level the learning of stimulus–reinforcer associations, and their rapid reversal; and moreover has neuronal firing that continues throughout the period in which the reinforcer is being delivered and the emotion is occurring (see Section 4.5). *Thus the primate including human orbitofrontal cortex (and to some extent the amygdala, perhaps more in rodents than primates) is much more closely related to the implementation of emotion than is the activity of dopamine neurons.* The primate orbitofrontal cortex contains the detailed representation of the hedonic value of a very wide range of stimuli that is needed for the details of each emotional state to be differentiated from other emotional states (see Section 4.5). Moreover, fMRI BOLD activations in the orbitofrontal cortex correlate with the reported subjective hedonic experience produced by emotion-provoking stimuli (see Section 4.5).

What role then do the dopamine neurons have in emotion? If their firing is related to 'reward prediction errors', in order to compute this, it is necessary to have a correct prediction or expectancy of reward (e.g. neurons that fire to a visual stimulus that precedes and predicts a reward), and other neurons that indicate whether reward (e.g. the taste of fruit juice) has been obtained. These signals are represented by neurons in the primate orbitofrontal cortex, which also contains error neurons (see Section 4.5). Thus the evidence is that the primate orbitofrontal cortex implements the computation of reward predictions and reward prediction errors. This information from the orbitofrontal cortex appears to reach the ventral striatum, in which reward prediction errors are represented (see Section 6.3.3.1 and Fig. 6.9). This information could then, via the descending projections to the midbrain from the ventral striatum, reach the dopamine neurons.

What role would the dopamine neurons then have? Providing a reward prediction error signal to the orbitofrontal cortex to enable it to learn to predict reinforcers would be simply circular, as the orbitofrontal cortex appears to be important in computing this in the first place, with its direct inputs from sensory systems about primary reinforcers (touch, taste etc.), its direct inputs from sensory systems about potential secondary reinforcers (vision, audition etc.), and its neurons which therefore can perform the relevant computations, which are certainly represented in the orbitofrontal cortex (see Section 4.5). Nor would a dopamine-originating reward prediction error signal appear to be required for the ventral striatum, as it receives inputs from regions such as the orbitofrontal cortex and amygdala. We are left then with the concept that the dopamine neuron firing may be especially important for other parts of the striatum (which do not receive from the orbitofrontal cortex and amygdala), such as for example the putamen, and here a dopaminergic modulation might facilitate appropriate motor habit learning. Whether this process involves explicitly reward prediction error learning, which as described above would not probably be suited to learning associations between sensory inputs and aversive signals (e.g. a visual stimulus followed by pain, cf. Section 6.3.3.1 and Seymour et al. (2004)), or involves instead a more feedback-based influence of striatal activity on dopamine neurons as part of a threshold or gain setting mechanism, remains to be strictly shown. [The reason that a dopamine signal would not be appropriate for learning associations between predictive stimuli and punishers is that if the predictive stimulus is an excitatory cortical input to the striatum, then if this is followed by a decrease of dopamine cell firing which is what is described as being produced by aversive stimuli, then the striatal firing produced by the predictive stimulus would not be potentiated.] On either scenario, the dopamine neurons might be involved in setting up the correct learned mappings in the striatum, but would not then necessarily be involved in the actual implementation of an emotion, apart from maintaining the correct neuronal thresholds in the striatum for processes activated by the emotional state to operate in response to the cortical and amygdala inputs that drive the emotion. Of course, given that the dopamine pathways also project to and influence the orbitofrontal cortex and other parts of the prefrontal cortex, then the threshold-setting function of dopamine will be important, and these cortical areas will not operate correctly without their normal dopamine input. Further, activation of these prefrontal areas by dopaminergic agents will correspondingly be expected to lead to emotional effects, and this is illustrated by the fact that administration of dopamine to normal human participants does increase the fMRI BOLD signal in the orbitofrontal cortex (Voellm, De Araujo, Cowen, Rolls, Kringelbach, Smith, Jezzard, Heal & Matthews 2004).

This synthesis leads to the view that the basal ganglia are very important in the selection of behavioural responses (see Section 6.3.5.1) and in motor habit learning. The role of the ventral striatum in this may be to enable Pavlovian conditioned stimuli to influence the level of instrumental responding by Pavlovian-instrumental transfer (see Sections 4.6.1.2, 4.6.3, 6.3.2 and 6.3.3.1).

6.4 Opiate reward systems, analgesia, and food reward

Electrical stimulation of some regions of the brain can lead to analgesia in animals ranging from rats to humans and can be equivalent in its pain-reducing properties to large doses of morphine (Liebeskind & Paul 1977). These analgesic effects can last for hours after only seconds of stimulation. The analgesia is often for only part of the body, so that a strong pinch to one side but not to the other might be ignored. This shows that the stimulation-produced analgesia is not simply some general interference with the animal's ability to respond to stimulation. The effective stimulation sites are in the medial brainstem, and extend from the rostral medulla (nucleus raphe magnus), through the midbrain central grey matter, towards the hypothalamus. As described by Rolls (2005b), at some sites both analgesia and self-stimulation are found, and at other sites the stimulation is aversive but is followed by analgesia. It has been shown that naloxone, a specific morphine antagonist, reverses, at least partly, stimulation-produced analgesia in both the rat and in humans (Adams 1976, Akil, Mayer & Liebeskind 1976). The endogenous morphine-like peptide enkephalin (Hughes 1975, Hughes, Smith, Kosterlitz, Fothergill, Morgan & Morris 1975) injected intraventricularly yields analgesia (Beluzzi, Grant, Garsky, Sarantakis, Wise & Stein 1976), and central grey matter stimulation releases this substance or a peptide similar to it (Liebeskind, Giesler & Urca 1985). Further, there are stereospecific opiate-binding sites in the central grey matter, and elsewhere in the brain (Kuhar, Pert & Snyder 1973) which mediate the many effects of opioids including pain relief and some types of reward and addiction including that to alcohol (Terenius & Johansson 2010). These findings raise the possibility that stimulation-produced analgesia is effective because it causes the release of a naturally occurring morphine-like substance which acts on opiate receptors in the central grey matter and elsewhere to provide analgesia. The function of this pain-reduction may be, after injury and the initial behavioural reaction to it to prevent further injury, to reduce the on-going effects of continuing severe pain, which could otherwise impair the animal's ability to cope well behaviourally with other needs.

At some of these analgesia-producing sites the electrical stimulation can produce reward (see Koob & Le Moal (1997)). The reward at these sites might be related to the pain-reducing effect of the release of opiates, which can itself be pleasurable and positively reinforcing. However, it is also known that endogenous opiates can be released by behaviours such as grooming (Dunbar 1996), and this may be part of the mechanism by which grooming produces pleasure and relaxation, for blockade of opiate receptors with naloxone greatly reduces grooming interactions.

The food reward system appears to be influenced by opiate systems (Levine & Billington 2004, Gosnell & Levine 2009). For example, peripheral morphine injections increase the intake of a high fat palatable diet more than a high carbohydrate diet in rats, whereas injections of naloxone decreased intake of a preferred diet relative to a nonpreferred diet (see Levine &

Billington (2004)). Ann Kelley and her group showed that injections of a μ-opioid receptor agonist into the nucleus accumbens increase the intake of a high fat diet much more than of a high carbohydrate diet (Zhang, Gosnell & Kelley 1998), and in addition, naltrexone injected into the amygdala decreased the intake of a preferred diet more than of a non-preferred diet (Levine & Billington 2004). Interestingly, humans report a reduction in the pleasantness of sucrose solution following administration of naltrexone, but can still discriminate between sucrose solutions (Bertino et al. 1991, Levine & Billington 2004). Thus there is evidence that brain opioid systems are involved in influencing the palatability of and hedonic reactions to foods, and that in rodents some of these effects are related to actions on the nucleus accumbens and amygdala (see also Berridge & Robinson (2003)). In this context, it is of interest that in humans brain areas influenced by the texture of oral fat include the orbitofrontal cortex, the perigenual cingulate cortex, and also a ventral part of the striatum (De Araujo & Rolls 2004, Grabenhorst, Rolls, Parris & D'Souza 2010b, Rolls 2008e).

6.5 Pharmacology of depression in relation to brain systems involved in emotion

One class of antidepressant drug, the tricyclic antidepressants, of which imipramine is an example, blocks the reuptake of 5-HT (5-hydroxy-tryptamine, serotonin), NA (noradrenaline), and DA (dopamine), in that order of potency. (They inhibit the presynaptic transporters with that order of efficacy.) Another class of drug that has antidepressant properties, the monoamine oxidase inhibitors, blocks the oxidative breakdown of all three of these monoamines. Both types of drug increase the concentration of the catecholamines NA and DA in the synaptic cleft of catecholaminergic neurons, and the catecholamine hypothesis of affective disorders was based on this type of evidence, and also on the concentrations of these monoamines and their metabolites in the brains of depressed patients. The catecholamine hypothesis was that low concentrations of the catecholamines produced depression, and that the antidepressant drugs worked by increasing the concentrations again. However, the catecholamine hypothesis is too simple as it stands, for at least two reasons (Cooper, Bloom & Roth 2003, Iversen, Iversen, Bloom & Roth 2009). First, most of the antidepressant treatments affect 5-HT (which is an indoleamine rather than a catecholamine like DA and NA), and indeed some newer drugs such as fluoxetine (Prozac) are relatively selective 5-HT reuptake inhibitors (SSRIs). Second, when antidepressant drugs are given, the pharmacological effects described take place within hours, whereas the antidepressant effects may take up to 6 weeks to become apparent.

One reason that the rapid increase of concentration of 5-HT produced by most of the antidepressant drugs does not work rapidly appears to be that there are 5-HT$_{1A}$ autoreceptors on the 5-HT cell bodies in the raphe nucleus (and also on the post-synaptic neurons), and when these are activated by the elevated 5-HT, the potassium conductance is increased, producing hyperpolarization of the 5-HT neurons, which decreases their firing, counteracting any influence of the potentially elevated 5-HT concentrations produced by most antidepressant drugs. It may be that this autoreceptor-mediated negative feedback becomes attenuated with a time course of weeks, and then the antidepressant drugs start to influence depression (see e.g. Celada, Puig, Armagos-Bosch, Adell & Artigas (2004)). Also, the blockade of 5-HT$_{2A}$ receptors by some atypical antipsychotic drugs may improve the clinical effects of SSRIs, perhaps by an action on the prefrontal cortex (Celada et al. 2004). Selective noradrenaline reuptake inhibitors (NRIs) such as reboxetine may also be useful in treating depression (Brunello, Mendlewicz, Kasper, Leonard, Montgomery, Craig Nelson, Paykel, Versiani & Racagni 2002).

Overall, the evidence tends to support the hypothesis that central 5-HT is involved in depression, with probably some involvement of NA but much less evidence that DA is involved (Cooper, Bloom & Roth 2003, Iversen, Iversen, Bloom & Roth 2009, Li, Frye & Shelton 2012). The traditional way forward for pharmacological research in this area involves screening a large number of new drugs for potential antidepressant effects. This research has not been closely linked to understanding of the brain systems involved in emotion. It may be hoped that in the future there will be closer links now that progress is being made in understanding the brain mechanisms of emotion.

A notable recent discovery shows that ketamine, a N-methyl-D-aspartate receptor antagonist, produces rapid (within hours) antidepressant responses in patients who are resistant to typical antidepressants, and that the effects may last for two weeks. Basic studies show that ketamine rapidly induces synaptogenesis and reverses the synaptic deficits caused by chronic stress (Duman & Aghajanian 2012). Although this may not be clinically useful, partly due to the potential for misuse of ketamine, it does open up new research concepts.

One potentially fruitful link would be to develop drugs that have potency particularly for some of the brain areas now known to be involved in emotion, such as the orbitofrontal cortex, amygdala, and cingulate cortex. Another potentially fruitful link is to investigate with neuroimaging the brain changes that occur in depression and in its treatment with antidepressants (see, e.g., Fig. 4.72 and Section 4.10), to gain further evidence in humans about the brain systems involved in depression, and potentially, with the use of transmitter-specific techniques available with positron emission tomography (PET), to continue to investigate neuropharmacological and neurochemical aspects of depression in humans, as well as deep brain stimulation (see Section 4.5.6).

6.6 Pharmacology of anxiety in relation to brain systems involved in emotion

One class of antianxiety drug, the benzodiazepines, bind to 'benzodiazepine receptors' in the brain, increasing the frequency of opening of the $GABA_A$ (γ-aminobutyric acid) receptor-activated chloride channels. The influx of chloride through these channels produces hyperpolarization of neurons, and thus a decrease in firing (Cooper, Bloom & Roth 2003, Iversen, Iversen, Bloom & Roth 2009). Barbiturates, which have antianxiety properties, prolong the opening of the same chloride channels. Indeed, many antianxiety treatments facilitate GABA actions, with $GABA_A$ receptors being relevant (Nemeroff 2003).

Given that GABA is the most widespread inhibitory transmitter in the brain, these findings leave open, of course, where the antianxiety drugs work. One early suggestion is that they influence the hippocampus (Gray 1987). However, there is almost no evidence linking the hippocampus to emotion, and instead the evidence indicates that it is involved in memory, often when this has a spatial aspect (including a spatial context), or is episodic, about a particular past event or episode (Rolls & Treves 1998, Rolls 1996a, Rolls 1999b, Rolls & Stringer 2005, Rolls, Franco & Stringer 2005b, Rolls, Stringer & Trappenberg 2002, Rolls, Xiang & Franco 2005c, Rolls & Xiang 2006, Rolls 2010b). Indeed, fornix section, which produces many of the effects of hippocampal and related damage on memory, has no effects on stimulus–reinforcement association learning or reversal (Gaffan, Saunders, Gaffan, Harrison, Shields & Owen 1984, Jones & Mishkin 1972). Further, Rawlins, Winocur & Gray (1983) showed that damage to the hippocampus of rats did not abolish the antianxiety effects of the antianxiety drug chlordiazepoxide in an animal model of anxiety. However, it is possible that if in anxiety states particular episodic memories are retrieved, then the hippocampus may play a role in this memory-related aspect of anxiety.

Evidence is now being sought about the brain states in a number of different clinical anxiety syndromes (Cannistraro & Rauch 2003):

In *post-traumatic stress disorder* (PTSD) there is some evidence for hyperresponsivity of the amygdala, and deficient activation of the ventral/medial prefrontal cortex and hippocampus (Cannistraro & Rauch 2003). It is hypothesized that the low activation of the ventral/medial prefrontal cortex may contribute to difficulty in reversing the learning that led to the anxiety.

In *specific phobias*, there may be abnormal activation produced by phobia-producing stimuli in phobics relative to controls of areas afferent to the amygdala such as the insula (perhaps because tactile imagery is activating somatosensory regions), but not of the amygdala itself; and also abnormal activation of the dorsolateral prefrontal cortex and hippocampus, perhaps related to mnemonic processes being activated during the phobic processing (Cannistraro & Rauch 2003).

In *social phobias* (anxiety states associated with social situations) there may be increased amygdala activation by faces (Cannistraro & Rauch 2003).

In *panic disorder*, there may be increased activation in regions such as the cingulate and orbitofrontal cortex and the hippocampus (Cannistraro & Rauch 2003).

In *obsessive–compulsive disorders* (OCD) there is evidence from PET studies of increased activity in the orbitofrontal cortex, anterior cingulate cortex, and striatum, and activations in these regions are greater in the symptomatic compared to the control neutral state (Cannistraro & Rauch 2003).

In *generalized anxiety disorder* (GAD) cognitive behaviour therapy is frequently used, sometimes in combination with a wide range of types of pharmacological treatment (Hoge, Ivkovic & Fricchione 2012).

As in the case of antidepressant drugs, it may be hoped that future studies will be able to link the effects of antianxiety drugs more closely to areas of the brain known to be involved in emotion, as this may help in the development of better treatments for anxiety, whether by drugs (File 1987) or by other forms of treatment.

6.7 Cannabinoids

Cannabis sativa derivatives (marijuana, hashish etc.) contain substances such as Δ^9-tetra-hydro-cannabinol (Δ^9-THC) that activate a brain cannabinoid receptor (CB1) to influence pain, memory, and cognitive function (Wilson & Nicoll 2002). The brain produces its own (endogenous) cannabinoids such as anandamide, and these may act retrogradely across synapses to influence the release of other transmitters (Wilson & Nicoll 2002). Cannabinoid receptors are widespread in the brain, but those in the hippocampus and neocortex may be related to effects of cannabinoids on memory and cognition, and receptors in the brainstem (e.g. the periaqueductal gray and rostral ventromedial medulla) and spinal cord to effects on pain (Wilson & Nicoll 2002). CB1 receptor agonists produce hyperalgesia, consistent with the hypothesis that endogenous cannabinoids normally regulate nociception. Cannabinoids can also increase appetite and body weight (Di Marzo & Matias 2005).

6.8 Overview of behavioural selection and output systems involved in reward, punishment, emotion, and motivation

Some of the output systems involved in emotion are outlined in Chapter 4. There, output systems from the orbitofrontal cortex and amygdala that project through the hypothalamus and directly to the dorsal motor nucleus of the vagus are described for learned autonomic responses. Output systems involving the striatum and rest of the basal ganglia are implicated in implicit behavioural responses to at least conditioned incentives, and in habit learning. In addition, there are systems for producing explicit emotional responses (Section 10.3.1). In Chapter 3, I consider the fact that a cost–benefit analysis must be performed in order to select an appropriate behavioural response. Here I draw out how reward systems in the brain may act as a suitable interface between sensory and motor systems, and some of the ways in which such interfacing may be implemented in the brain.

In terms of sensory analysis, we have seen in Chapters 4 and 5 how sensory systems set up representations of objects in the world that are without reward/punishment valence, but are suitable as inputs to succeeding stages of processing such as the orbitofrontal cortex and amygdala where the valence can be learned by pattern association with primary reinforcers such as taste and touch. We have seen how the representations are highly appropriate as inputs to pattern-association mechanisms, in that they can be read with a dot product type of decoding that is very neurophysiologically plausible, implemented in the brain by adding in the post-synaptic neuron the contributions of many thousands of inputs each weighted by its synaptic connection strength (see Rolls & Treves (1998) and Rolls (2008b)), and in that each input carries information that is essentially independent (within the limits enforced by the number of stimuli being processed). After this pattern association, we have a representation that is coded in terms of its reward/punishment valence. We also have other sensory stimuli that are decoded by the brain as being primary, that is unlearned, reinforcers, such as the taste of food (Chapter 5), or pleasant touch or pain (Chapter 4), or many others (Table 2.1). We should think of these representations coded in terms of reward and punishment as potential goals for action. Although Milner & Goodale (1995) have characterized the dorsal visual system as being appropriate for the control of action, and the ventral visual system projecting to the primate temporal lobe as being appropriate for perception, the view taken here is that the ventral visual system is also involved in action, indeed is at the heart of action, by providing the representations that are the goals for action. It is precisely because the goals for action are typically objects in the world that the ventral visual system, which is involved in the representation of objects (Rolls 2008b, Rolls 2012e), is an important component of the action system.

We have seen then that reward and punishment decoding systems require certain types of sensory system, so that an important way of understanding much sensory information processing is to realize that it is involved in producing representations suitable as goals for action. The reasons for brain design that have resulted in it using rewards and punishers (including expected rewards and punishers) as goals for actions are considered in Chapter 3. The issue considered here is how, in the brain, reward and punishment systems, which encode goals, are connected to output systems. One feature of the output systems is that they must be built to try to obtain activation of the reward representations in the brain, and to avoid or escape from activation of punishment-related representations in the brain. A second feature is that of response selection, and a third is that of cost–benefit 'analysis' (see Chapter 3).

In Section 6.3, we considered the operation of the basal ganglia in terms of receiving inputs from many reward systems. We showed how they could implement a selection based on competition between inputs, the strongest current reward or punishment (in the common currency, see Chapter 3) winning. Some of the mechanisms for ensuring that one reward does not dominate behaviour for too long include satiety mechanisms, sensory-specific satiety, etc. (see Chapter 5). We showed how the basal ganglia could perhaps also map stimuli to responses, and might include in the association evidence about the reward as represented in the ventral striatum . These other inputs, from the cerebral cortex, include motor and somatosensory systems so that the rewards could produce responses with which they had been associated in the past. This would implement stimulus–response habit learning. The other cortical inputs though come from all areas of cerebral cortex, so effectively the reinforcers could be associated to much more complex actions than just 'responses' of the type represented in primary motor and somatosensory areas (see Rolls & Treves (1998)). The basal ganglia could thus in principle provide one way in which the rewards and punishment representations in the brain could be interfaced to response and action systems. This is an implicit route to action (see Chapter 10), and in line with this, the basal ganglia do not have backprojections to the cortical areas that project into them. This is in contrast with memory systems such as the hippocampus, orbitofrontal cortex, and amygdala, which do have backprojections to the cortical areas from which they receive, potentially allowing retrieval of information from those systems about memories and emotional states (Rolls & Treves 1998, Rolls 2008b). In contrast, the basal ganglia, with no such backprojections, may not allow such explicit retrieval, and indeed we are not aware of how our motor system solves and is processing well-learned problems.

In addition to the basal ganglia route, and the route for explicit reasoning about courses of action to take concerning rewards and punishments (see Section 10.3.1), there are some other possible routes for stimuli that are reinforcers to influence behaviour. There may for example be many brainstem connections between aversive sensory inputs such as the pain-related inputs coming from the C and Aδ fibres, and brainstem response systems. Such systems operate at the reflex level, enabling for example a limb to be pulled away from a noxious stimulus. However, in terms of the definition given in Chapter 1 for reinforcers, which require operant, that is arbitrary, acts to be learnable to the stimuli, such brainstem reflexes would not qualify as being involved in (instrumental) behavioural responses to reinforcers. There may be other sensory-motor routes that also operate at a relatively low level, and that may correspondingly not qualify as reward or punishment systems (cf. Panksepp (1998) and Panksepp (2011a)). To qualify, the systems have to provide a representation of the goals for actions, and allow arbitrary (operant) responses to be learned to obtain such rewards or avoid or escape from such punishers.

Although the basal ganglia are key brain systems involved in this function in terms of habit (stimulus–response) learning, other brain systems, such as the cingulate cortex, may be especially important in action–outcome learning (see Section 4.7). Now that we have clear hypotheses about how and where rewards and punishers are decoded and represented by the brain, it must be an aim of future research to continue to clarify and better understand how the selection is made between the different goals, how the costs of actions are taken into account (perhaps because they are encoded into a common scale as punishers and expected punishers), and how responses for obtaining the selected goals are made (see Section 4.7).

7 Sexual behaviour, reward, and brain function; sexual selection of behaviour

7.1 Introduction

One of the themes of this chapter is the brain control of sexual behaviour, and especially how the brain has evolved to respond to different types of reward to produce sexual behaviour that is adaptive, that is, increases fitness. Part of the chapter is therefore concerned with what is known of the brain mechanisms that underlie sexual behaviour. Understanding the actual neural mechanisms is important not only because this helps to clarify the behaviour itself, but also because this is a foundation for understanding medical and other disorders of these systems, and treatments for them.

However, because there have been many advances recently in understanding and theorizing about the different patterns of sexual behaviour and why they have evolved (Buss 2012), part of the aim of this chapter is to suggest what reward systems could account for this behaviour, and what the properties are of these reward systems. Specific hypotheses are presented about the operation of the neural systems that could implement these reward-related processes. This is intended to be an approach to how the different types of behaviour observed could be produced by particular reward systems designed by natural selection during evolution, and to provide a basis for investigations of the actual neural mechanisms that implement these processes. The aim thus is to link much recent research on sociobiology, evolutionary psychology and the Darwinian adaptive approaches to different types of sexual behaviour (Buss 2012), to new ideas introduced here about how these behaviours could be produced by the sculpting during evolution of systems that are sensitive to different types of reward. The aim is to provide a better understanding of how natural selection may operate in the course of evolution to produce different types of behavioural adaptation by selecting for different types of reward system. The possibility that during evolution a variety of different reward systems could have their sensitivity set differently in different individuals, leading to tendencies towards different types of behaviour in different individuals, each with its own way of being adaptive, is introduced. These new ideas are intended to provide a foundation for future studies of the actual reward systems in the brain that implement these different aspects of sexual behaviour each with its underlying evolutionary 'strategy'[13].

The selection processes that lead to the development of some aspects of sexual behaviour are related to the adaptive value of the function being performed. For example, being healthy

[13] We should note at the outset that there may be two types of evolutionary 'strategy'. A first is to have genetically specified polymorphism, with the two types of individual existing in a mixed evolutionarily stable state (ESS). An example is that some individuals might be 'hawks', and others 'doves', in social situations. The behaviours might be set to occur probabilistically by the genes, and do not necessarily imply a polymorphism (Dawkins 1986a). A second is to have a conditional strategy, in which an individual might change strategy, based on an assessment of the situation. For example, if one's opponent is large, one might not play a hawk. Conditional strategies can also lead to evolutionarily stable states (Maynard Smith 1984). Of the examples that are included in this chapter, some might be polymorphic (mixed) ESSs, e.g. attractiveness (though this can in humans be conditionally modified too!). Probably the majority are conditional ESSs, e.g. the tendency for flirtation, as these are likely to be more effective when information is available on which to base the conditional choice (Maynard Smith 1984, Dawkins 1986a). In many of the cases, the type of strategy that is in operation strictly remains to be determined.

and strong enables a male to survive long enough to reproduce, and to fight off competitors for females. Reward systems built by genes that favour these characteristics evolve by what we can call natural selection, in a use of the term that is close to that of Darwin (1859, 1871). A distinguishing concept here is that the body survives long enough and is healthy enough to reproduce, and when natural selection is used in its narrow sense here it implies 'survival selection'.

However, Darwin (1871) also recognized that evolution can occur by sexual selection, when what is being selected for has no inherent adaptive or survival value for the individual, but is attractive to potential mates (intersexual selection), or helps individuals of the same sex to compete better with each other (intra-sexual selection, for e.g. male–male competition). The most cited example is the peacock's large 'tail', which does not have survival value for the peacock (and indeed it is somewhat of a handicap to have a very long tail), but, because it is attractive to the peahen, becomes prevalent in the population. It turns out that sexual selection may lead to all sorts of behaviours being selected, which have in common that they make the bearer attractive to the opposite sex of the species, and are thus useful in courtship, but which would normally be considered as non-sexual types of behaviour, such as kindness and humour (Miller 2000b). Thus in this chapter we also consider the reward and punishment systems that may be built by sexual selection (see Section 7.7).

There will be primary reinforcers to consider specified by genes, and then in addition the possibility of learning associations between previously neutral stimuli and these primary reinforcers. A major emphasis in this book is that reward and punishment systems are built to guide behaviour efficiently and appropriately for the specifying genes, and in this chapter I show how sexual selection as well as natural ('survival') selection is involved in this process. Insofar as the states elicited by rewards and punishers are emotional states (see Chapters 2 and 3), this chapter thus extends the understanding of emotion to systems shaped by sexual selection.

The intentional stance is adopted in much writing about sociobiology and evolutionary psychology, and is sometimes used here, but should not be taken literally. It is used just as a shorthand. An example is that it might be said that genes are selfish. But this does not mean at all that genes think about whether to be selfish, and then take the decision. Instead it is just shorthand for a statement along the lines 'genes produce behaviour that operates in the context of natural selection to maximize the number of copies of the gene in the next generations'. Much of the behaviour produced is implicit or unconscious, and when the intentional stance is used as a descriptive tool, it should not be taken to mean that there is usually any explicit or conscious processing involved in the behavioural outcome.

Some of the points may seem 'obvious' once they have been made, if the reader is a neo-Darwinian used to the approach taken in evolutionary biology. However, a potential problem of sociobiology is that its stories do seem plausible, given Darwinism – but many stories are plausible. So we must be careful to seek evidence too, not just plausibility; and we need to know how much of the variance of behaviour is accounted for by each sociobiological account of a type of behaviour. In the long term, once sociobiological hypotheses have been presented, they must be tested.

One of the themes of this chapter is how the underlying physiology of reward is related to the sexual behaviour shown by different types of women, and different types of men. One of the key ideas is that reward systems become tuned to biological functions that they serve. For this reason, there will be discussion of the biological functions that could be implemented by different aspects of sexual behaviour.

Sexual behaviour is an interesting type of motivated behaviour to compare with feeding and drinking. For both feeding and drinking, there are internal signals such as plasma glucose or cellular dehydration related to homeostatic control that set the levels of food or water reward in order to produce the appropriate behaviour. In the case of sexual behaviour, there are no similar short-term homeostatic controls. However, the reward value of sexual behaviour has to be set so that it does perhaps occur sufficiently often to lead to successful reproductive behaviour, in terms of passing an individual's genes into the next generation, and helping them to thrive in the offspring. There are several factors that contribute to this, including internal (steroid) hormonal signals that on a seasonal basis, or in relation to the stage of an oestrus cycle, set the relative reward value of sexual behaviour. For example, in rats at the stage of the oestrus cycle when oestrogen is high the appetite for food is suppressed and sexual behaviour is rewarding. The hormonal status can even be set by the environmental stimuli. For example, Lehrman and colleagues (see Lehrman (1965)) described a series of events in ring doves in which seasonal factors lead to bow-cooing in the male, the sight of which stimulates the female to become receptive as a result of hormonal changes. External signals can also adjust the reward value of sexual behaviour. For example, it has been claimed that female macaques release a pheromone (actually produced by bacteria in the vagina under the influence of androgenic hormones in the female) that acts to promote sexual behaviour in males (Baum, Everitt, Herbert & Keverne 1977). (In this example, a 'male' hormone produced in females 'controls' male sexual behaviour through the effect of the pheromone!) Thus both internal and external stimuli can act to influence the reward value of sexual behaviour. In addition, some of the rewards and punishers related to courtship may have no survival or adaptive value for the individual, but have evolved instead by the process of sexual selection (see Section 7.7).

7.2 The ultimate explanation for the reward value of sex

What is the 'ultimate', i.e. evolutionary (see Section 1.3), explanation for the reward value of sex? I show in this Section how it is adaptive for sex to have reward value, because of the advantages of sexual reproduction in searching the high-dimensional complex space in which genotypes evolved by natural selection.

Consider the space shown in Fig. 7.1, generated by the function

$$z = e^{-0.2\sqrt{x^2+y^2}+3(\cos 2x+\sin 2y)}. \tag{7.1}$$

There is a single global maximum, and the aim is to search for it. A local hill-climbing (or gradient descent) search starting at a random position in the space is unlikely to find the global peak, and is likely just to climb one of the smaller local peaks, and get stuck there. For this reason, it would be useful, just occasionally, to make a random jump in the space, and perform local hill-climbing to see if there is a higher peak that can be found from the new starting point. Now this type of search is exactly what sexual reproduction performs. The local hill-climbing is performed by the recombination of gene complexes on one part of a chromosome from one individual with gene complexes on another part of the corresponding chromosome from another individual (which in diploid animals is achieved by crossover at meiosis). If the combination of these two gene complexes in the next generation allows the new individual to perform better, that is to survive and reproduce better so that the new combination gets into the next generation, then a small hill-climb will have been achieved. But after perhaps 20–100 such hill-climbing steps, nothing better may develop, because the peak of the local hill has been reached. In this case, a random jump to somewhere else in the space might be useful, and this is what a mutation achieves. Probabilistically the mutation will not help, but if it does allow the sexual reproduction with its crossover in chromosomes from different individuals to find by hill-climbing a higher peak in the space, then the mutation will have been useful.

In this scenario, the adaptive value of the recombination provided for by crossover, which allows gene complexes on parts of the corresponding chromosome from different

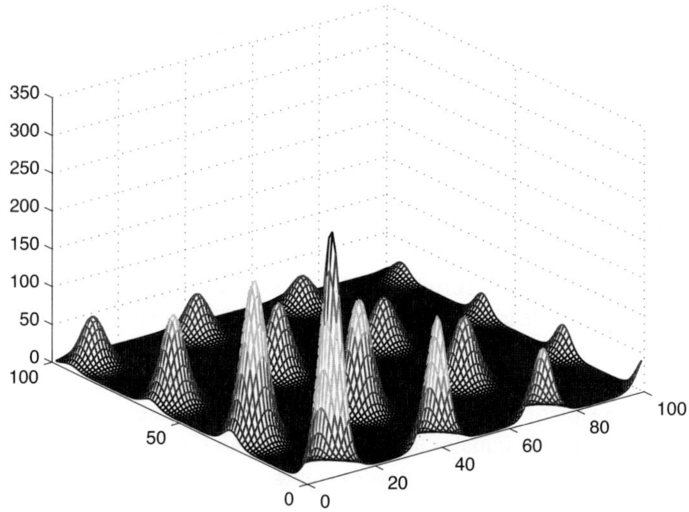

Fig. 7.1 A coarse-textured broadly unimodal space problematic for local search such as hill-climbing or gradient descent, but susceptible to global search methods. Genetics and genetic algorithms use sexual recombination of genes for the local hill-climbing, and occasional mutations to jump to a new part of the search space to search close to that with more sexual reproduction.

individuals to be combined together in the process of sexual reproduction, is an important advantage provided by sexual reproduction. (There may be other advantages too of sexual reproduction with diploidy, in that a gamete could carry chromosomes with a haploid sequence from either grandparent.) Asexual reproduction with mutations alone (with no possibility for recombination) could jump to new locations in the search space, but is very inefficient at finding a peak in the search space, because there is no local hill-climbing, and the process relies much more on happening to jump with a mutation to a very good place in the space. That has a low probability, so produces very slow evolution. Given that evolution is a race against competitor genes, whether from different or the same species, sexual reproduction, which allows rapid evolution, has great adaptive value. My argument is that this adaptive value of sex provides the basis for the evolution brain systems to encode the reward value of sex, which can now be seen as an important goal for individuals to perform actions to obtain. That is my 'ultimate' explanation of the reward value of sex.

Of course, the reward value of sex must be scaled to be not too high, for to optimize sexual reproduction, many other rewards must be sought too, including for example food reward and water reward. Further, each type of reward must be scaled on a common scale to a level at which it is optimal in terms of being selected sufficiently often to maximize the reproductive success of genes. The reward value of food and water should be set such that food and water are selected relatively often, and sex less often. There are frequently factors that influence the value of different rewards to help in this scaling. For example, hunger (which depends on metabolic and many related factors as described in Chapter 5) influences food reward value, thirst (which depends on cellular and extracellular volume (Rolls 2005b)) influences water reward value, and hormones during adolescence start up sex reward value systems as fertility develops. These are some of the processes involved in scaling different rewards to a common scale of value, considered further in Section 9.5.2.

When we simulate on a computer the mathematical search algorithms that are implemented by sexual reproduction, the different individuals that reproduce together to exchange genetic material are of the same type, that is, there are no individuals that one thinks of as female and others as male. The fundamental difference in biological organisms between females and males is that the female has a greater investment in the offspring, for example by providing a nutritive egg, by becoming pregnant and infertile for long periods while the baby grows inside her, and/or by providing breast milk for the offspring. Indeed, it turns out that as soon as any asymmetry in the contributions of the gametes happens, the continuation in evolution of identical types of gamete becomes unstable, and the system evolves to female and male gametes (Parker, Baker & Smith 1972).

My next argument, accordingly, is that because females and males have different interests or goals in terms of what will maximize the reproductive success of their genes (Goetz & Shackelford 2009), females and males have somewhat different reward value systems related to sex. These differences, that is, differences in the reward systems of females vs males, must underlie many of the difference that are described in much of the remainder of this chapter, though environmental factors, upbringing and culture, of course can also influence people. We should remember, in line with one of the themes of this book, that there are many different reward value systems involved in even sexual behaviour, and so many individual differences are to be expected, produced in the evolutionary search by genes for their own success.

I finish this section with a short description, for the more computationally minded, and to amplify the computational arguments above, of how genetic algorithms are often implemented on computers (Holland 1975, Ackley 1987, Goldberg 1989, Rolls & Stringer 2000). The implementation usually involves haploid phenotypes, but the same fundamental principles apply to the more usual diploid phenotypes that are common in biology. The description is of a genetic algorithm that was being used to simulate the evolution of simple, one-layer, neural networks to test whether hypotheses about how genes specify neural architectures in the brain are feasible (Rolls & Stringer 2000).

The processes involve reproduction, ontogenesis followed by tests of how well the offspring can learn to solve particular problems, and natural selection. First, a selection of genes is made for a set of G genotypes in a population, which should be of a certain minimum size for evolution to work correctly. The genes are set out on a chromosome (or chromosomes). (Effects of gene linkage on a chromosome are not considered in simple models.) Each set of genes is a genotype. The selection of individual genotypes from which to breed is made a probabilistic function which increases with the fitness of the genotype, measured by a fitness function that is quantified by how well that genotype builds an individual that can solve the problem that is set. Having chosen two genotypes in this way, two genotypes to specify two new (haploid) offspring for the next generation are made by the genetic processes of sexual reproduction involving both gene recombination and mutation, which occur with specified probabilities. This process is repeated until G genotypes have been produced. Then G individuals are built with the network architectures specified by the G genotypes. The fitness of these individuals is then measured by how well they perform at the computational problem set. In order to solve the computational problem, the networks are trained by presenting the set of input patterns, and adjusting the synaptic weights in the network according to the learning rules specified by the genotype of that individual. In this case, as in biological evolution of the brain, the genes specify design rules for the brain, which then learns from the environment during its lifetime. The individuals then breed again with a probability of being selected for reproduction that is proportional to their fitness relative to that of the whole population. This process is allowed to proceed for many generations, during which the fitness of the best individual in the population, and the average fitness, both increase if evolution is working.

This type of genetic process is an efficient method for searching through a high dimensional space (the space specified by the genes), particularly where the space has many local optima so that simple hill climbing is inefficient, and where there is a single measure of fitness (Holland 1975, Ackley 1987, Goldberg 1989). An additional useful feature of genetic search is that past gene combinations, useful possibly in other contexts, can remain in the population for a number of generations, and can then be reused later on, without the need to search for those gene combinations again. This re-use of past combinations is one of the features of genetic search that can make it powerful, rapid, and show sudden jumps forward.

More detail about the genetic algorithm used (Goldberg 1989) in the investigation of how the evolution of cortical architectures may be implemented (Rolls & Stringer 2000) follows. Each individual genotype was a haploid chromosome of a type that specified classes of neurons, and the possible types of connection within and between them. The values for the genes in the initial chromosome were chosen at random from the possible values. There was a set number of genotypes (and hence individuals) per generation, which was 100 for the simulations described. (Too small a number reduces the amount of diversity in the population sufficiently to lead to poor performance of the genetic evolution.) From each genotype an individual network was constructed, using the specifications for the connectivity contained in the genes for that individual. The actual testing involved presenting the set of patterns to be learned to the network while allowing learning to occur, and then testing the performance of the network by presenting the same, similar, or incomplete test patterns and measuring the output of the network. Then the fitness of the network in solving the problem set was measured.This process was repeated until a fitness measure had been obtained for each of the genotypes.

The next generation of genotypes was then bred by reproduction from the previous genotypes. Two genotypes were selected for reproduction with a probability that was proportional to their fitness relative to the sum of the fitnesses of all individuals in that generation. That is, the probability P_i of an individual i being selected is given by

$$P_i = \frac{F_i}{\sum_j F_j} \tag{7.2}$$

where F_j is the fitness of an individual genotype j, and the sum $\sum_j F_j$ is over all individuals in the population. The genotypes were then bred to produce two offspring genotypes using the processes of recombination and mutation. The probability of recombination was set to 0.4 (so that it occurred with a 40% chance for every breeding pair in every generation), and the probability of mutation of each gene was set to 0.05. The recombination took place with respect to a random point on the chromosome each time it occurred. The mutation also took place at a random place on the chromosome each time it occurred, and the single gene being mutated was altered to a new random value within the range specified for that gene. This reproduction process was repeated until sufficient individual genotypes for the next generation (100) had been produced. The fitness of those genotypes was then measured by building and testing the networks they specified as previously outlined. Then the whole reproduction, ontogenesis, and testing to measure fitness, processes were repeated for many generations, to determine whether the fitness would increase, and if so, what solutions were found for the successful networks (Rolls & Stringer 2000).

We now turn to consider what sex reward value systems have been set up by evolution.

7.3 Mate selection, attractiveness, and love

What factors are decoded by our brains to influence mate attractiveness (reward value) and selection? Many factors are involved in mate selection, and they are not necessarily the same for selection of a short-term vs a long-term partner. The selection of a long-term partner in species with long-term relatively monogamous relationships is influenced for example by parental investment, which is a major evolutionary adaptive factor in promoting long-term relationships. Thus in humans, males choose females because human males do make a parental investment; and females compete for males. Indeed, the selection of a long-term partner in humans is mutual, and this tends to reduce sex differences in partner choice. Consistent with this, David Buss has shown that in contrast, human sex differences in mate selection are more evident in short-term mating (Buss 1989, Buss 1994, Buss 2012).

Species with shared parental investment are primarily those where two parents can help the offspring to survive better than one, and this includes many birds (where one bird must sit on the eggs to incubate them, while the other finds food), and humans (where the human infant is born so immature[14] that care of the offspring for a number of years could, when humans were evolving, make it more likely that the offspring, containing the father's genes, would survive, and then reproduce). Most other mammals are not good models of human pair mate selection and pair bonding, because there is generally less advantage to joint care of the young, and the female, who has made the major investment of the gestation period for the baby, and breast feeding it post-partum (for the whole of which period she will remain relatively infertile), generally assumes most of the responsibility for bringing up her young. In most mammals, females will maximize their reproductive success, given the cost of gestation and lactation, by focussing on the successful rearing of offspring. In contrast, male mammals do not invest by gestation and lactation in their offspring, and the most effective way for males to influence their reproductive success is to maximize the number of fertilizations they achieve, and this is a major factor in mammalian mate selection. This tendency is tempered in humans by the advantage of male investment in the offspring, as ensuring that the immature offspring survive sufficiently long that the chances of their reproductive success is high is an adaptive investment.

7.3.1 Female preferences

Factors that across a range of species influence female selection of male mates include the following.

1. Athleticism. The ability to compete well in mate selection (including being healthy and strong), as this will be useful for her genes when present in her male offspring. Athleticism may be attractive (rewarding) also as an indicator of protection from male marauding (single females are at risk in some species of abuse, and forced copulation, which circumvents female mate choice), from predators, and as an indicator of hunting competency (meat was important in human evolution (Aiello & Wheeler 1995), although the hunt may also have been co-opted by sexual selection as a mating ritual giving the males a chance to show off). Consistent with these points, Buss & Schmitt (1993) showed that women show a strong preference for tall, strong, athletic men.

2. Resources, power and wealth. In species with shared parental investment (which include many birds and humans), having power and wealth may be attractive to the female, because they are indicators of resources that may be provided for her young. Women should desire

[14] Humans are born secondarily altricial (where altricial is the opposite of precocial) because of the narrow female pelvis of humans associated with bipedality, which results in gestation being shortened from an estimated 21 to 9 months (Gould 1985).

men who show willingness to invest resources (which should be defensible, accruable and controllable) in his partner. Women place a greater premium on income or financial prospects than men (Buss 1989). Further, in a cross-cultural study of 37 cultures with 10,047 participants, it was found that irrespective of cultural/political/social background, women consistently placed more value on financial resources (100% more) than men (Buss 1989, Buss 1994, Buss 2012). Women value a man's love as an indicator of resource commitment.

3. Status. Both now and historically, status hierarchies are found in many cultures (and species, for example monkeys' dominance hierarchies, and chickens' pecking order). Status correlates with the control of resources (e.g. alpha male chimpanzees take precedence in feeding), and therefore acts as a good cue for women. Women should therefore find men of high status attractive (e.g. rock stars, politicians, and tribal rulers), and these men should be able to attract the most attractive partners (Betzig 1986). Consistent with this, Buss (1989) showed cross-culturally that women regard high social status as more valuable than do men; and Udry & Eckland (1984) showed that attractive women marry men of high status.

4. Age. Status and higher income are generally only achieved with age, and therefore women should generally find older men attractive. Buss (1989) showed cross-culturally that women prefer older men (3.42 years older on average; and marriage records from 27 countries showed that the average age difference was 2.99 years).

5. Ambition and industriousness, which may be good predictors of future occupational status and income, are attractive. Valued characteristics include those that show a male will work to improve their lot in terms of resources or in terms of rising up in social status (Kyl-Heku & Buss 1996). Cross-culturally, women rated ambition/industriousness as highly desirable (Buss 1989).

6. Testosterone-dependent features may also be attractive. These features include a strong (longer and broader) jaw, a broad chin, strong cheekbones, defined eyebrow ridges, a forward central face, and a lengthened lower face (secondary sexual characteristics which are a result of pubertal hormone levels). High testosterone levels are immuno-suppressing, so these features may be indicators of immuno-competence (and thus honest indicators of fitness). The attractiveness of these masculinized features increases with increased risk of conception across the menstrual cycle (Penton-Voak, Perrett, Castles, Kobayashi, Burt, Murray & Minamisawa 1999, Johnston, Hagel, Franklin, Fink & Grammer 2001). The implication is that the neural mechanism controlling perception of attractiveness must be sensitive to oestrogen/progesterone levels in women.

Another feature thought to depend on prenatal testosterone levels is the 2nd/4th digit ratio. A low ratio reflects a testosterone-rich uterine environment. It has been found that low ratios correlate with female ratings of male dominance and masculinity, although the relationship to attractiveness ratings was less clear (Swaddle & Reierson 2002).

7. Symmetry (in both males and females) may be attractive, in that it may reflect good development in utero, a non-harmful birth, adequate nutrition, and lack of disease and parasitic infections. Fluctuating asymmetry (FA) reflects the degree to which individuals deviate from perfect symmetry on bilateral features (e.g. in humans, both ears, both feet, both hands and arms; in other species, bilateral fins, bilateral tail feathers). Greater asymmetry may reflect deviations in developmental design resulting from the disruptive effects of environmental or genetic abnormalities, and in some species is associated with lower fecundity, slower growth, and poorer survival. A low fluctuating asymmetry may thus be a sign of reproductive fitness (Gangestad & Simpson 2000). In a number of bird species, attractive (symmetric) males employ a strategy of investing more in extra-pair mating than in paternal care, and maximize their reproductive success in this way (Moller & Thornhill 1998). In humans, more symmetrical men reported more lifetime partners (r=0.38), and more extra-pair partners; and women's choice of extra-pair partners was predicted by male symmetry (see Gangestad &

Simpson (2000)). Moreover, women rate men as more attractive if they have high symmetry (low FA). Intellectual ability (which may be attractive to women) is also correlated with symmetry (Gangestad & Thornhill 1999). A further type of evidence here is that the frequency of human female orgasm (which probably results in high sperm retention) correlates with low fluctuating asymmetry (FA) (i.e. being symmetrical) in male partners (Thornhill, Gangestad & Comer 1995).

8. Dependability and faithfulness may be attractive, particularly where there is paternal investment in bringing up the young, as these characteristics may indicate stability of resources (Buss, Abbott, Angeleitner, Asherian, Biaggio, Blancovillasenor, Bruchonschweitzer, Chu, Czapinski, DeRaad, Ekehammar, Ellohamy, Fioravanti, Georgas, Gjerde, Guttman, Hazan, Iwawaki, Janakiramaiah, Khosroshani, Kreitler, Lachenicht, Lee, Liik, Little, Mika, Moadelshahid, Moane, Montero, Mundycastle, Niit, Nsenduluka, Pienkowski, Pirttila-Backman, Deleon, Rousseau, Runco, Safir, Samuels, Sanitioso, Serpell, Smid, Spencer, Tadinac, Todorova, Troland, Vandenbrande, Van Heck, Vanlangenhove & Yang 1990). Emotionally unstable men may also inflict costs on women, and thus women rate emotional stability and maturity as important. For example, jealousy might lead to abuse.

9. Risk-taking by men may be attractive to women, perhaps because it is a form of competitive advertising: surviving the risk may be an honest indicator of high quality genes (Barrett et al. 2002).

10. Characteristics that may not be adaptive in terms of the survival of the male, but that may be attractive because of inter-sexual sexual selection, are common in birds, perhaps less common in most mammals, though present in some primates (Kappeler & van Schaik 2004), and may be present in humans (see Section 7.7). An example of a sexually selected characteristic that may not increase the survival of the individual, but that may be attractive to females and thus increase the fitness of the male in terms of whether his genes are passed on to the next generation by reproduction, is the peacock's tail. These characteristics may in some cases be an honest indicator of health, in the sense that having a large gaudy tail may be a handicap.

11. Odour. The preference by women for the odour of symmetrical men is correlated with the probability of fertility of women as influenced by their cycle (Thornhill & Gangstad 1999). Another way in which odour can influence preference is by pheromones which are related to major histocompatibility complex (MHC) genes, which may provide a molecular mechanism for producing genetic diversity by influencing those who are considered attractive as mates, as described in Section 7.9.

It is important to note that physical factors such as high symmetry and that are indicators of genetic fitness may be especially attractive when women choose short-term partners, and that factors such as resources and faithfulness may be especially important when women choose long-term partners, in what may be termed a conditional mating strategy (Gangestad & Simpson 2000, Buss 2012). This conditionality means that the particular factors that influence preferences alter dynamically, and preferences will often depend on the prevailing circumstances, including the current opportunities and costs.

7.3.2 Male preferences

Males are not always indiscriminate[15]. When a male chooses to invest (for example to produce offspring), there are preferences for the partner with whom they will make the investment. Accurate evaluation of female quality (reproductive value) is therefore important, and a male

[15] In fact, males are probably rarely indiscriminate, in that producing sperm and performing sexual behaviour do have costs, including for example the risk of catching disease.

will need to look out for cues to this, and find these cues attractive (rewarding). The factors that influence attractiveness include the following (see also Barrett et al. (2002)).

1. Youth. As fertility and reproductive value in females is linked to age (reproductive value is higher when younger, and actual fertility in humans peaks in the twenties), males (unlike females) place a special premium on youth. It is not youth per se that men find attractive, but indicators of youth, for example neotenous traits such as blonde hair and wide eyes. An example of this preference is that Buss (1989) showed that male college students preferred an age difference on average of 2.5 years younger. Another indicator of youth might be a small body frame, and it is interesting that this might contribute to the small body frame of some women in this example of sexual dimorphism.

2. Beauty. Features that are most commonly described as the most attractive tend to be those that are oestrogen-dependent, e.g. full lips and cheeks, and short lower facial features. (Oestrogen caps the growth of certain facial bones.) Like testosterone, oestrogen also affects the immune system, and its effects might be seen as 'honest indicators' of genetic fitness.

For example, in one study, Johnston & Franklin (1993) found that when subjects were able to evolve a computer generated image into their ideal standard of female beauty, the beautiful composite had a relatively short lower face, small mouth, and full lips.

In a cross-cultural study, people of different races agreed in their ratings of the attractiveness of faces of Asian, Hispanic, black, and white women (Cunningham, Roberts, Barbee & Druen 1995). In meta-analyses of 11 studies, Langlois, Kalakanis, Rubenstein, Larson, Hallam & Smoot (2000) demonstrated that (a) raters agree about who is and is not attractive, both within and across cultures; (b) attractive children and adults are judged and treated more positively than unattractive children and adults, even by those who know them; and (c) attractive children and adults exhibit more positive behaviours and traits than unattractive children and adults. In an fMRI study, it was found that attractive faces produce more activation of the human medial orbitofrontal cortex than unattractive faces (O'Doherty et al. 2003b).

Further, small babies were even shown to gaze for longer at slides of the more attractive woman when shown pairs of pictures of women that differed in attractiveness (Langlois, Roggman, Casey & Ritter 1987, Langlois, Ritter, Roggman & Vaughn 1991). In another study, 12-month-olds interacted with a stranger. The infants showed more positive affective tone, less withdrawal, and more play involvement with a stranger who wore a professionally constructed attractive than unattractive mask; and played longer with an attractive than an unattractive doll (Langlois, Roggman & Reiser-Danner 1990). These results extend and amplify earlier findings showing that young infants exhibit visual preferences for attractive over unattractive faces. Both visual and behavioural preferences for attractiveness are evidently exhibited much earlier in life than was previously supposed.

Women appear to spend more time on fashion and enhancing beauty than men. Why should this be, when in most mammals it is men who may be gaudy to help in their competition for females, given that females make the larger investment in offspring? In humans, there is of course value to investment by males in their offspring, so women may benefit by attracting a male who will invest time and resources in bring up children together. But nevertheless, women do seem to invest more in bearing and then raising children, so why is the imbalance so marked, with women apparently competing by paying attention to their own beauty and fashion? Perhaps the answer is that males who are willing to make major investments of time and resources in raising the children of a partner are a somewhat limiting resource (as other factors may make it advantageous genetically for men not to invest all their resources in one partner), and because women are competing to obtain and maintain this scarce resource, being beautiful and fashionable is important to women. Faithful men may be a limited resource because there are alternative strategies that may have a low cost, whereas women are essentially committed to a considerable investment in their offspring. These factors lead to greater variability in men's strategies, and thus contribute to making men who invest in their offspring a more limited resource than women who invest in their offspring.

3. Body fat. The face is not the only cue to a woman's reproductive capacity. Although the ideal body weight varies significantly with culture (in cultures with scarcity, obesity is attractive, and relates to status), the ideal distribution of body fat seems to be a universal standard, as measured by the waist-to-hip ratio (which cancels out effects of actual body weight). Consistently, across cultures, men preferred an average ratio of 0.7 (small waist/bigger hips) when rating female figures (line drawings and photographic images) for attractiveness (Singh 1993, Singh 1995, Singh & Young 1995, Singh & Luis 1995). Thornhill & Grammer (1999) also found high correlations between rating of attractiveness of nude females by men of different ethnicity. Long-term health risks (diabetes, hypertension, coronary disease, and stroke) are also associated with a high waist-to-hip ratio, which may therefore be an 'honest indicator' of fitness.

4. Fidelity. The desire for fidelity in females is most obviously related to her concealed ovulation (see next paragraph and Section 7.6), and therefore the degree of paternity certainty males may suffer. Males therefore place a premium on a woman's sexual history. Virginity was a requisite for marriage both historically (before the arrival of contraceptives) and cross-culturally (in non-Westernized societies where virginity is still highly valued) (Buss 1989). Nowadays, female monogamy in previous relationships is a sought after characteristic in future long-term partners (Buss & Schmitt 1993). (Presumably with simple genetic methods now available for identifying the father of a child, the rational thought system (see Chapter 10) might place less value on fidelity with respect to paternity issues as paternity can be established genetically, yet the implicit emotional system may still place high value on fidelity, as during evolution, fidelity was valued as an indicator of paternity probability.) The modern rational emphasis might be especially placed on valuing fidelity because this may indicate less risk of sexually transmitted disease, and perhaps the emotional value of fidelity will be a help in this respect.

5. Attractiveness and the time of ovulation. Although ovulation in some primates and in humans is concealed[16], it would be a premium for men to pick up other cues to ovulation, and find women highly desirable at these times. Possible cues include an increased body temperature reflected in the warm glow of vascularized skin (vandenBerghe & Frost 1986), and pheromonal cues. Indeed, male raters judged the odours of T-shirts worn during the follicular phase as more pleasant and sexy than odours from T-shirts worn during the luteal phase (Singh & Bronstad 2001). In macaques, male interest in females increases during the fertile period, and alpha males more often mate guard females during the fertile phase of the cycle, with possible cues related to the high levels of oestrogen at the time of ovulation (Engelhardt, Pfeifer, Heistermann, Niemitz, Van Hoof & Jodges 2004). Women generally do not know when they are ovulating (and in this sense ovulation may be double blind), but there is a possibility that ovulation could unconsciously affect female behaviour. In fact, Event-Related Potentials (ERPs) were found to be greater to sexual stimuli in ovulating women, and these could reflect increased affective processing of the stimuli (Krug, Plihal, Fehm & Born 2000). This in turn might affect outward behaviour of the female, helping her to attract a mate at this time.

In most species, females invest heavily in the offspring in terms of providing the eggs and providing the care (from gestation until weaning, and far beyond weaning in the case of humans). Females are therefore a 'limited resource' for males allowing the females to

[16] Perhaps so that males may be uncertain who the father is of a baby, and thus not threaten infanticide – see Section 7.4

be the choosier sex during mate choice. This leads therefore to strong levels of male intra-sexual selection, resulting in males typically being the larger and/or more flamboyant sex (an example is the male mandrill's brightly coloured face in comparison to the dull one of the female's). If the sex roles become somewhat reversed, however, this can alter. Dramatic female ornamentation can be seen in the pipefish (a relative of the seahorse). Male pipefish overwhelmingly find the larger, most ornamented females the most attractive (Berglund & Rosenqvist 2001). This stems from the fact that the males of these species have evolved a brood pouch (which, in some species, is vascularized) into which the female can oviposit her eggs. Moreover, the size of the (male) brood pouch (which determines how many embryos a male can store) is also another limiting factor that females compete over. This accounts for why the males are the choosier sex and why females compete in pipefish. Female competition is also found in the spotted sandpiper – a bird with an unusual polyandrous breeding system (i.e. a breeding system with one female with multiple males) (Oring 1986). Here, females arrive on the breeding ground first and must attract males to it. The females must defend from other females the territory that contains the individual territories of their male consorts. The males then provide the important resource of incubating the clutch on their own, and therefore become unavailable as mates. This often leads to a chronic shortage of available males, and thus, female competition is intense, and displays are extremely vigorous and occasionally lead to physical combat. Similar polyandrous tactics are also seen in the jacana (Jenni & Collier 1972).

In humans, male investment in caring for the offspring means that male choice has a strong effect on intrasexual selection in women. Female cosmetic use and designer clothing could be seen as weapons in this competition, and perhaps are reflected in extreme female self-grooming behaviour such as cosmetic surgery, or pathological disorders such as anorexia, bulimia and body dysmorphic disorder. The modern media, by bombarding people with images of beautiful women, may heighten intrasexual selection even further, pushing women's competitive mating mechanisms to a major scale.

Finally in this section, we should note that in addition to the benefits of particular mate choices, the costs also need to be assessed (Kokko, Brooks, McNamara & Houston 2002, Kokko, Brooks, Jennions & Morley 2003), and both the benefits and costs may vary across time.

7.3.3 Pair-bonding, and love

Attachment to a particular partner by pair bonding in a monogamous relationship, which in humans becomes manifest in love between pair-bonded parents, and which occurs in humans because of the advantage to the man of investing in his offspring, may have special mechanisms to facilitate it. Species in which attachment has been investigated include the prairie vole (Young, Gobrogge, Liu & Wang 2011). In monogamous species of prairie voles, mating can increase pair-bonding (as measured by partner preference). Oxytocin, a hormone released from the posterior pituitary, whose other actions include the milk let-down response, is released during mating. Exogenous administration of oxytocin facilitates pair bonding in both female and male prairie voles (Carter 1998). In female prairie voles, antagonists of oxytocin interfere with partner preference formation. In female prairie voles, the endogenous release of oxytocin is thus important in partner preference and attachment. Thus oxytocin has been thought of as the 'hormone of love'. Oxytocin gene knock-out mice fail to recognize familiar conspecifics after repeated social exposures, and injection of oxytocin in the medial amygdala restores social recognition (Ferguson, Aldag, Insel & Young 2001, Winslow & Insel 2004). In males, the effects of oxytocin are facilitated by vasopressin, another posterior pituitary hormone whose other effects include promoting the retention of water by the kidney. In the case of vasopressin, it has been possible to show that the vasopressin V1a receptor (V1aR) is expressed in higher concentration in the ventral forebrain of monogamous prairie voles than in promiscuous (i.e. polygamous) meadow voles, and that viral vector V1aR transfer into the forebrain of the meadow mouse increases its partner preference (i.e. makes it more like a monogamous prairie vole) (Lim, Wang, Olazabal, Ren, Terwilliger & Young 2004, Young & Wang 2004, Young et al. 2011). Thus a single gene may be important in influencing monogamy vs promiscuity in voles. Oxytocin in rodents can affect behaviour in other ways too, for example by facilitating penile erection, reducing the post-ejaculatory refractory period, facilitating receptivity and lordosis in females, and increasing the release of dopamine in the mesolimbic pathway (Argiolas & Melis 2013). Stress, or the administration of the hormone corticosterone which is released during stress, can facilitate the onset of new pair bonds (DeVries, DeVries, Taymans & Carter 1996).

Are similar mechanisms at work in humans to promote pair-bonding and love? There is as yet no definitive evidence, but in humans, oxytocin is released by intercourse, and especially at the time of orgasm, in both women and men (Meston & Frohlich 2000, Kruger, Haake, Chereath, Knapp, Janssen, Exton, Schedlowski & Hartmann 2003). Moreover, although orgasm is thought not to occur in females in most non-human species, it does occur in some female non-human primates (e.g. the Japanese macaque, Macaca fuscata), where it is more likely to occur if the female is mating with a high-ranking male (Troisi & Carosi 1998), and it is possible that this serves as a reward for mating with high-ranking males, and at the same time promotes cryptic choice. (Cryptic female choice is the postcopulatory ability of females to favour the sperm of one male of the same species over another (Thornhill 1983, Ben-Ari 2000, Birkhead & Pizzari 2002, Birkhead 2000)[17]). It has also been reported that women desiring to become pregnant are more likely to have an orgasm after their partner ejaculates (Singh, Meyer, Zambarano & Hurlbert 1998) (see further Section 7.5).

Oxytocin can have many influences on social behaviour, including increasing trust in neuroeconomic games, and presumably between partners too (Churchland & Winkielman 2012).

7.4 Parental attachment, care, and parent–offspring conflict

Many mammal females make strong attachments to their own offspring, and this is also facilitated in many species by oxytocin. One model is the sheep, in which vaginal-cervical stimulation and suckling, which release both oxytocin and endogenous opioids, facilitate maternal bonding (Keverne 1995, Keverne, Nevison & Martel 1997). Oxytocin injections can cause ewes to become attached to an unfamiliar lamb presented at the time oxytocin is released or injected, and oxytocin antagonists can block filial bonding in sheep. Perhaps oxytocin had an initial role in evolution in the milk let-down reflex, and then became appropriate as a hormone that might facilitate mother–infant attachment.

In humans the evidence is much more correlative, but oxytocin release during natural childbirth, and rapid placing of the baby to breast feed and release more oxytocin (Carter

[17] An example of female cryptic choice has been demonstrated by female red junglefowl, Gallus gallus, which reveal postcopulatory selection against related males' sperm that occurs based on major histocompatibilty complex (MHC) similarity. This selection is likely to give the offspring greater disease resistance, by selecting for a diverse immune system in the offspring because of fertilization by an unrelated male with different MHC genes. The effect of MHC similarity was lost following artificial insemination, suggesting that male phenotypic cues, for example the sight or smell of the male, might be required for females to select sperm differentially (Lovlie, Gillingham, Worley, Pizzari & Richardson 2013).

1998, Nissen, Uvnas-Moberg, Svennson, Stock, Widstrom & Winberg 1996, Uvnas-Moberg 1997, Uvnas-Moberg 1998), might facilitate maternal attachment to her baby. This provides an argument in favour (other things being equal) of natural childbirth (Odent 1999). Prolactin, the female hormone that promotes milk production, may also influence maternal attachment. It is certainly a major factor in humans that bonding can change quite suddenly at the time that a child is born, with women having a strong tendency to shift their interests markedly towards the baby as soon as it is born (probably in part under hormonal influences), and this can result in relatively less attachment behaviour to the husband. Understanding the scientific basis for this, and stimulated by this understanding, counselling couples about how their affections and attachments may alter at the time of the birth of a child, may be and should be a very important benefit of this research. In men, oxytocin may also be involved in paternal behaviour (Wynne-Edwards 2001).

Separation from the mother can cause distress (Harlow 1986, Bowlby 1969, Bowlby 1973, Bowlby 1980). In Harlow's studies in monkeys, factors that reduced the effects of separation from the mother included warm soft touch, and the presence of peers. In chicks some auditory signs of distress can be reduced by oxytocin, opioids, and prolactin (Panksepp, Nelson & Bekkedal 1997).

Another aspect of parental care is that there is competition between the mother and child, for example over weaning (Trivers 1974). The mother may wish to devote resources to preparing for her next offspring (by building herself up); and continuing to breast feed delays the onset of fertility and cycling. In contrast, it is to the offspring's genetic advantage to demand milk and attention. The infant's scream can be seen as part of trying to wring resources out of its mother, potentially to an extent that is unfavourable for the mother's genes (Buss 2012).

As described above, females generally have a greater investment in their offspring, and tend to provide more parental care and perhaps become more attached than fathers. This situation is not as extreme in humans as in most other mammals, because human offspring are born relatively immature, and a father who helps to rear the offspring can help to increase the reproductive fitness of his genes.

Lack of parental care in step-fathers is evident in many species, and can be as extreme as the infanticide by a male lion of the pups of another father, so that his new female may come into heat more quickly to have babies by him (Bertram 1975). Infanticide also occurs in non-human primates (Kappeler & van Schaik 2004). In humans, the statistics indicate that step-fathers are much more likely to harm or kill children in the family than are real fathers (Daly & Wilson 1988).

7.5 Sperm competition and its consequences for sexual behaviour: a sociobiological approach

Monogamous primates well spread out over territory have small testes, for example gibbons and some tarsiers. Polygamous primates living in groups with several males in the group have large testes and frequent copulation, e.g. chimpanzees and monkeys (see Ridley (1993a), Harcourt, Purvis & Liles (1995) and Barrett et al. (2002)). The reason for this appears to be sperm warfare – in order to pass his genes on to the next population, a male in a polygamous society with competition between males needs to increase the probability that he will fertilize a female, and the best way to do this is to copulate often, and swamp the female with sperm, so that his sperm have a greater probability of getting to the egg to fertilize it. Therefore in polygamous groups with more than one male, males should have large testes, to produce large numbers of sperm and large quantities of seminal fluid[18]. The largest testis size in relation to body weight is found in chimpanzees, who live in multimale groups, are highly promiscuous, and have on average 13 partners per birth (Wrangham 1993). Sperm competition can be seen as a form of non-combative, non-injurious, male-male intrasexual competition, which has evolved by intrasexual sexual selection (see Section 7.7). Not only testis size, but also seminal vesicle size, is large in species with frequent copulation (Dixson 1998). In monogamous societies, with little competition between sperm, the male should just pick a good partner, produce only enough sperm to fertilize an egg and not enough to compete with others' sperm, stay with her to bring up the children, and guard them because they are his genetic investment (Ridley 1993a).

What about humans? Despite being apparently mainly monogamous, they are intermediate in testis size and penis size – bigger than expected for a monogamous species (Harcourt, Harvey, Larson & Short 1981, Harcourt et al. 1995, Parker, Ball, Stockley & Gage 1997, Barrett et al. 2002, Lynn 2013). Why? Maybe there is some sperm competition? Remember that although humans usually do pair, and are often apparently monogamous, humans do live in groups or colonies. Can we get hints from other animals that are paired, but are also live in colonies?

A problem with comparing humans with most other primates in this respect is that in most primates (and indeed in most mammals), the main parental investment is by the female (in producing the egg, in carrying the foetus, and in feeding the baby until it can become independent). The male does not have to invest in his children for them to have a reasonable chance of surviving. For this reason, the typical pattern in mammals is that the female is choosy in order to obtain healthy and fit males, and to complement this the males compete for females. However, in humans, because the children must be reared for a number of years before they become independent, there is an advantage to paternal investment in helping to bring up the children, in that the paternal resources (e.g. food, shelter, and protection) can increase the chances of the male's genes surviving into the next generation to reproduce again. Part of the reason why investment by both parents is needed in humans is that because of the large final human brain size, at birth the brain is not fully developed, and for this reason the infant needs to be looked after, fed, protected, and helped for a considerable period while the infant's brain develops, favouring pair-bonding between the parents.

A more useful comparison can therefore be made with some birds, such as the swallow, which live in colonies but in which the male and the female pair, and both invest in bringing up the offspring, taking it in turns for example to bring food back to the nest. If checks are made in swallows using DNA techniques for determining paternity, it is found that actually approximately one third of a pair's young are not sired by the 'father', the male of the pair (Birkhead & Moller 1992, Ridley 1993a, Birkhead 2000). What happens is that the female mates sometimes with other males – she commits adultery. She probably does not do this just with a random male either – she may choose an 'attractive' male, in which the signals that attract her are signals that indicate health, strength, and fitness. One well known example of such a signal is the gaudy 'tail' of the male peacock. One argument is that, given that the tail is a real handicap in life, any male that can survive with such a large tail must be very healthy or fit. Another argument is that if his tail is very attractive indeed, then the female should choose him, because her sons with him would probably be attractive too, and also chosen by

[18]Competition between males is the key factor here, for in gorillas which have one male in a polygamous (or strictly polygynous, meaning multiple females) group the testis size is small. The term that describes a multi-male multi-female group is polygynandry, and it is in groups of this type that there are high levels of sperm competition, and the testes are large.

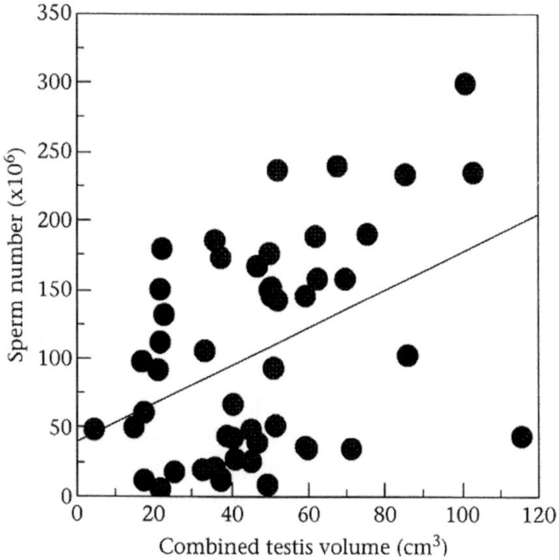

Fig. 7.2 Relation between number of sperm contained in human ejaculate volume and the size of the testes. The relation was significant at P=0.002 in the sample of 50 men. (Reprinted from *Animal Behaviour*, 68 (2), Laight W. Simmons, Renee C. Firman, Gillian Rhodes, and Marianne Peters, Human sperm competition: testis size, sperm production and rates of extrapair copulations, pp. 297–302, Copyright (2004), with permission from Elsevier.)

females[19]. (It is interesting that if a male were popular with females, then even if he had genes that were not better in terms of survival etc., it would be advantageous for a female to have offspring with him, as her sons would be more likely to be attractive to other females, and thus maximize her inclusive fitness. This is an example of Fisherian selection (Fisher 1958), see Section 7.7.)

In such a social system, such as that of the swallow, the wife needs a reliable husband with whom she mates (so that he thinks the offspring are his, which for the system to be stable they must be sometimes) to help provide resources for 'their' offspring. (Remember that a nest must be built, the eggs must be incubated, and the hungry young must be well fed to help them become fit offspring. Here fit means successfully passing on genes into the next generation – see Dawkins (1986b).) But the wife (or at least her genes) also benefits by obtaining as fit genes as possible, by sometimes cheating on her husband. To ensure that her husband does not find out and therefore leave her and stop caring for the young, she deceives the husband by committing her adultery as much as possible secretly, perhaps hiding behind a bush to mate with her lover. So the (swallow) wife maximizes care for her children using her husband, and maximizes her genetic potential by finding a lover with fit genes that are likely to be attractive in her sons to other females (see Ridley (1993a)).

Could anything like the situation just described for birds such as swallows also apply to humans? It appears that it might apply, at least in part, and that similar evolutionary factors might influence human sexual behaviour, and hence make obtaining particular stimuli in the environment rewarding to humans. We need to understand whether this is the case, in

[19]This is an example of the use of the intentional stance in the description, when no real propositional state is likely to occur at all.

order to understand the rewards that drive sexual behaviour in humans. One line of evidence already described is the large testis and penis size of men. In humans, it has been shown that the number of sperm ejaculated is related to testis size (Simmons, Firman, Rhodes & Peters 2004). Fig. 7.2 shows this relation, and also indicates the large variation in both testis size and number of sperm contained in an ejaculate in humans, indicating that there is the potential for variation between humans to play a role in sperm competition. This potential may not be fully realized in modern humans perhaps because of contraceptive practices, in that extrapair paternity rates are estimated at around 4% in modern times (see below), though double paternity in some dizygotic twins does show that conditions for sperm competition in humans can occur (Simmons et al. 2004). (We will get on to the reason for the large penis size soon.) A second line is that some studies in humans of paternity using modern DNA tests suggest that in fact the woman's partner (e.g. husband) is not the father of about 14% of their children. Although surprising, this has been claimed in a study in Liverpool, and in another in the south of England (Baker & Bellis 1995) (see Ridley (1993a)). In other studies, the extrapair paternity rate has been estimated at closer to 2%, although 28% of men and 22% of women did report extrapair copulations (Simmons et al. 2004). Further, an approximate estimate across 53,619 humans in 5 studies yields 24% of men and 20% of women reporting extrapair copulations (estimate made from data in Simmons et al. (2004)). In the data reviewed by Simmons et al. (2004), an approximate estimate of the extra-pair paternity rate is 4%, but there were great variations, with estimates in some traditional cultures of 10–11.8%. The latter estimates are particularly interesting, because estimates of extrapair paternity rates from North American and European cultures, practised in birth control and taught by particular mores, may not reflect the behaviour of our ancestors, selection between whom has shaped the behaviour of modern humans. On balance, these data suggest that while sperm competition may not be a major factor in modern humans, it may be to some extent, and might have been much more important in our ancestors, and have shaped our behaviour to at least some extent. So the possible effects of sperm competition in influencing modern human behaviour are worth exploring further.

So might men produce large amounts of sperm, and have intercourse quite regularly, in order to increase the likelihood that the children produced are theirs, whether by their wife or by their mistress? When women choose men as their lovers, do they choose men who are likely to produce children who are fit, that is children good at passing on their genes, half of which originate from the woman? It appears that women might choose like this, as described below, and that this behaviour may even select genetically for certain characteristics in men, because the woman finds these characteristics rewarding during mate selection. Of course, if such a strategy were employed (presumably mainly unconsciously) all the time in women the system would break down (be unstable), because men would not trust their wives, and the men would not invest in making a home and bringing up their children[20]. So we would not expect this to be the only selective pressure on what women find attractive and rewarding as qualities in men. Pursuing this matter further, we might expect women to find reliability, stability, provision of a home, and help with bringing up her children to be rewarding when selecting a husband; and the likelihood of producing genetically fit children, especially sons who can themselves potentially have many children by a number of women, to be rewarding when selecting a lover (i.e. short-term mate).

What is even more extraordinary is that women may even have evolved ways of influencing whether it is the woman's lover, as opposed to her husband, who fathers her children.

[20]In some tribes, brothers help to bring up their sisters' children, because these children share some of the mother's brother's genes. The brother and sister of course will share some of the same genes, so the behaviour of the brother is appropriate in terms of increasing the fitness of his genes in a promiscuous society.

Apparently she may be able to do this even while deceiving her husband, even to the extent of having regular intercourse with him. The ways in which this might work have been investigated in research described next (Baker & Bellis 1995, Baker 1996). Although much of the research on the sociobiological background of human sexual behaviour, including sperm warfare in humans, is quite new, and many of the hypotheses remain to be fully established and some can now be rejected (Birkhead 2000, Moore, Martin & Birkhead 1999), this research does have interesting potential implications for understanding the rewards that control human behaviour, and for this reason the research, and its potential implications, are considered here.

In the research by Baker & Bellis (1995) and others (see also Ridley (1993a)), it was claimed that if a woman has no orgasm, or if she has an orgasm more than a minute before the male ejaculates, relatively little sperm is retained in the woman. This is a low-retention orgasm. The claim was that if she has an orgasm less that a minute before him or up to 45 min after him, then much more of the sperm stays in the woman, and some of it is essentially sucked up by the cervix during and just following the later stages of her perceived orgasm. This is a high-retention orgasm. [This effect, known as upsuck, does not literally mean that seminal fluid is sucked up physically into the womb, with a resulting low volume of fluid lost during the outflow from the woman 30–45 min later. Instead, the mechanism of sperm retention claimed was that in a high-retention orgasm, more sperm enter the channels in the cervical mucus, and either swim right through them into the womb, or stay in the cervical mucus. In both high- and low-retention orgasms, the volume of the outflow, which includes more than sperm, was claimed to be similar (see Baker & Bellis (1995), p. 237).] After a high-retention orgasm, it was claimed (Baker & Bellis 1995) that the woman is more likely to conceive (by that intercourse) even if she already has sperm in her reproductive tract left from intercourse in the previous 4 or so days. Baker & Bellis (1995) then (using a questionnaire) found that in women who were faithful (having intercourse only with their husbands) about 55% of the orgasms were of the high-retention (i.e. most fertile) type. By contrast, in unfaithful women having intercourse with their husbands, only 45% of the copulations were high-retention, but 70% of the copulations with the lover were of the high-retention type. Moreover, the unfaithful women were having sex with their lovers at times of the month when they were most fertile, that is when they were just about to ovulate. The result in the research sample was that an unfaithful woman could have sex twice as often with her husband as with her lover, but was still slightly more likely to conceive a child by the lover than by the husband. Put another way, the women in this sample would be more than twice as likely to conceive during sex with their lover than with their partner[21]. Thus women appear to be able to influence to some extent who is the father of their children, not only by having intercourse with lovers, but also by influencing whether they will become pregnant by their lover. The ways in which reward mechanisms might help this process are described later in this chapter. Some evidence for such selection is that domestic fowls (hens) appear to select which sperm fertilize their eggs, in that when inseminated with sperm of different cocks, the fertilization was non-random (Birkhead, Chaline, Biggins, Burke & Pizzari 2004).

These data are at present quite controversial, although there is evidence that women have orgasms more frequently after their partner has ejaculated when they desire to become pregnant (Singh et al. 1998), and this might be a mechanism for cryptic choice (Birkhead & Pizzari 2002) when mating with an attractive lover, in that a woman is more likely to have an orgasm with an attractive (symmetric) partner (Thornhill et al. 1995). If female orgasm

[21] Given that 14% of children are not the children of the male partner according to Baker and Bellis, this suggests (and not taking into account fertility factors such as the time of month, whether the woman is more likely to synchronize ovulation with a lover, and possible differences in contraceptives used) that the average across the whole population of the number of copulations women have with lovers rather than their partners could be in the order of 7.5%. When effects of fertility etc. are taken into account, it will be less than 7.5%.

is involved in influencing who the father is of a baby, then it might be expected that female orgasm might be somewhat variable in whether it occurs, as part of a putative selection process. Another possible contributory factor in the evolution of female orgasm is that it provides motivation to solicit multiple partners, for example if she does not have an orgasm with one partner, or if she has an orgasm with one partner who then enters a refractory state after ejaculation (cf. Hrdy (1999) and Hrdy (1996)). Indeed, polyandrous mating situations make it adaptive (in order to conceal paternity) for a female to be able to have orgasms without a long refractory period between each, that is to be able to have multiple orgasms. Although a similar argument might be applied to men, a refractory period might nevertheless be adaptive in men in part because of limited sperm resources, and the utility of competing with adequate sperm numbers when insemination does occur. Indeed, dominant males may release limited sperm because of their multiple matings, and this indeed is a factor cited as accounting for females competing for the first mating (Wedell, Gage & Parker 2002).

Another finding by Baker & Bellis (1995) indicates that men have evolved strategies to optimize the chances of their genes in this sperm selection process. One is that men were reported to ejaculate more sperm if they have not been for some time with the woman with whom they are having intercourse. An effect consistent with this is that a man who spends a greater (relative to a man who spends a lesser) proportion of time apart from the partner since the couple's last copulation report (a) that his partner is more attractive, (b) that other men find his partner more attractive, (c) greater interest in copulating with the partner, and (d) that his partner is more sexually interested in him (Shackelford, Le Blanc, Weekes-Shackelford, Bleske-Rechek, Euler & Hoier 2002, Shackelford & Goetz 2007). (This effect is not just dependent on the time since he has last inseminated his partner, but is related to the time the couple have been apart, so the effects may be interpreted as being related to possible insemination of the partner while away, and not just to sexual frustration (Shackelford et al. 2002).) The (evolutionary, adaptive) function of this may be for the man to increase the chances of his sperm in what could be a sperm war with the sperm of another man. The aim would be to outnumber the other sperm. Moreover, the man should do this as quickly as possible after returning from an absence, as time could be of the essence in determining which sperm get to the egg first if the woman has had intercourse with another man recently. The implication of this for reward mechanisms in men is that after an absence, having intercourse quite soon with the woman from whom the man has been absent should be very rewarding (and this is what is reported (Shackelford et al. 2002)). Possible neural mechanisms for this are considered later. There is good evidence that processes of this type do occur in some species. For example, Pizzari, Cornwallis, Lovlie, Jakobsson & Birkhead (2003) found in domestic fowl that males show status-dependent investment in female according to the level of female promiscuity: they progressively reduce sperm investment in a particular female but, on encountering a new female, instantaneously increase their sperm investment; and they preferentially allocate sperm to females with large sexual ornaments signalling superior maternal investment. These results indicate that female promiscuity leads to the evolution of sophisticated male sexual behaviour.

It even appears that there should be some reward value in having intercourse very soon with the woman after an absence, because the action of the glans penis, with its groove behind the head, may be to pull sperm already in the vagina out of it using repeated thrusting and pulling back (Baker & Bellis 1995) (at least in some ancestors, Birkhead (2000)). The potential advantage to this in the sperm warfare may be the biological function that, as a result of evolution, leads to thrusting and withdrawal of the penis during intercourse being rewarding (perhaps to both men and women). Such thrusting and withdrawal of the penis during intercourse should occur especially vigorously (and should therefore have evolved to become especially rewarding) after an absence by the man. The possible advantage in the sperm warfare that shaped our evolution could also result in its being rewarding for a man to have intercourse with a woman if he has just seen her having intercourse with another man. (This could be part of the biological background of why some men find videos showing sex involving women rewarding.) However, large numbers of sperm from a previous man usually remain in the vagina for only up to 45 min after intercourse, after which a flowback of sperm and other fluids (the discharge of semen and other secretions) from the vagina usually occurs. Thus the evolutionary shaping of the glans penis, and the rewards produced by thrusting and withdrawing it and the shaft of the penis in the vagina, are likely to have adaptive value more in our ancestors than in us.

Baker & Bellis (1995) proposed that a second human male strategy might be to ejaculate not only sperm that can potentially fertilize an egg, but also killer (or kamikaze) sperm that kill the sperm of another male, and blocker sperm that remain in the mucus at the entrance to the cervix blocking access through the channels in the mucus to other sperm. However, this hypothesis of different sperm types in humans is now strongly criticized, and there is little evidence for different sperm types in humans, and for kamikaze-like effects (Moore et al. 1999, Birkhead 2000, Short 1998). (Nevertheless, there are many interesting sperm adaptations for competition in other species. For example, in the wood mouse the sperm from one individual form 'trains' that increase the motility of the sperm twofold, thus facilitating fertilization by that individual's sperm (Moore, Dvorakova, Jenkins & Breed 2002).) Independently of this argument, given that (the majority of) sperm remain viable once out of the vagina and in the uterus or Fallopian tubes for up to about four days, it becomes important (read adaptive) for a man to have intercourse with his partner at least as often as say twice per week. This would ensure that at least some of the male partner's sperm were present to compete with any other sperm that might arrive as a result of an extra-pair copulation. So because of this function of sperm warfare, the brain should be built to make male intercourse with his partner rewarding at least approximately twice per week.

A third argument of Baker & Bellis (1995) (see also Smith (1984) and Baker & Bellis (1993)) is that it is important (in the fitness sense) that a male should help his lover to have an orgasm, which should occur only just before or for 45 min after he has ejaculated for the upsuck effect to operate. [The orgasm was proposed to cause the upsuck effect of sperm into the uterus. This might give the woman some control over whether she will accept new sperm, even when she has had intercourse and has blocking sperm in her. The operation of this female 'strategy' is facilitated by the facts that sperm remain in the vagina only for a short time because of the flowback, and because the acidity of the vagina makes sperm viable in the vagina for less than 12 h. The result is that the upsuck effect with a lover can operate preferentially on his (recently ejaculated) sperm, because many of the sperm from previous intercourse will be ejected within 45 min in the flowback, and the majority in the vagina will be dead within 12 h. Whether female orgasm does facilitate sperm retention and the likelihood of fertilization is not yet clear (Levin 2002).] For this reason, men should find intercourse with a lover very exciting and rewarding if this tends to increase the likelihood that their lover will have an orgasm. This biological function of an orgasm in women provides a general reason why men should find it rewarding when a woman has an orgasm (and should therefore try to produce orgasms in women, and be disappointed when they do not occur). This process might be helped if one factor that tended to produce ejaculation in men was knowledge that the woman was having an orgasm. Of course, the reverse may occur – a woman may be triggered to orgasm especially just after she receives an ejaculation, especially if it is from a male with whom (presumably mainly subconsciously) she wishes to conceive. (Indeed, there is evidence that women have orgasms more frequently when they desire to become pregnant (Singh et al. 1998), and with men with an index of healthy genes, low asymmetry (Thornhill et al. 1995, Thornhill & Gangestad 1996).) If she does not have an orgasm, she may fake an orgasm (as this is rewarding to the male), and this may be part of her deception mechanism.

While some of these findings do require careful assessment, there is an interesting report that does underlie the importance of factors related to sperm motility in the outcome of sexual behaviour. It was found that the sex bias of a man's siblings is associated with his sperm speed; men with female-biased siblings (i.e. men with relatively many sisters) had significantly slower sperm than men with male-biased siblings (Mossman, Slate, Birkhead, Moore & Pacey 2013). This is consistent with the hypothesis that offspring sex may be adaptively manipulated to maximize the offspring's reproductive fitness (e.g., parents with genes for good male fertility traits, such as high sperm speed, would produce primarily sons and fewer daughters because the offspring will inherit advantageous male fertility genes). Conversely, parents with poor male fertility genes would produce primarily daughters (Mossman et al. 2013).

Having now outlined some of the functions at play in sexual behaviour we are in a better position later in this chapter to consider the brain processes that implement rewards to produce these different types of behaviour.

7.6 Concealed ovulation and its consequences for sexual behaviour

Women, and a few non-human primate species, have concealed ovulation. It is not clear to males, or to themselves, when they are fertile. Why do women conceal their ovulation? Diamond (1997) considers evidence that a first process that occurs in evolution is that promiscuity or harems in the mating system give rise to concealed ovulation. This is the 'many fathers' theory. The concealed ovulation (concealed even from the woman, so that she can deceive better – what might be termed 'deceiving conceiving') – makes sure that men do not know who the father is (because they do not know when ovulation has occurred), and thus will not attack the young. (It frequently occurs in the animal kingdom that males kill their female's children if they have been born of other males, a process that enables genes to maximize their own reproductive potential. This occurs because the female will stop lactating and will come back into a reproductive state so that the new male can reproduce. Moreover, it will minimize potential use of his resources in helping to bring up children without his genes.)

A second process can then occur in evolution: monogamy evolves. Monogamy, Diamond (1997) argues, has never evolved in species that have bold advertisement of ovulation. It usually evolved in species with (i.e. that already have) concealed ovulation – the 'daddy-at-home' theory. The concealed ovulation means that fathers stay at home all the time (and help), because they want to be assured of their paternity; and because they think that they are the father, because they have been at home (Simmen-Tulberg & Moller 1993). Thus the consequences of concealed ovulation may be that fathers find it rewarding (and have emotions about) staying at home with their partner to guard a primarily monogamous relationship. Indeed, monogamy can be thought of as a form of mate guarding.

Consistent with these hypotheses, it has been found that free-living Hanuman langur females do have long periods of receptivity during which the time of ovulation is variable, that there is the opportunity for paternity confusion in that ovulation is concealed from the males, that there is a dominant male who tries to monopolize the females, and that nevertheless non-dominant males father a substantial proportion of the offspring (Heistermann, Ziegler, van Schaik, Launhardt, Winkler & Hodges 2001). This is direct evidence that extended periods of sexual receptivity in catarrhine primates may have evolved as a female strategy to confuse paternity.

Concealed ovulation could also play a role in combination with female orgasm to enable female cryptic choice, which would it has been suggested (see Section 7.5) occur if a woman has an orgasm with a man who she wants to be the father of her children. The contribution of the concealed ovulation would be to promote male–male competition.

Thus the interests of females and males may not be consistent, and this leads to the development of measures and countermeasures. Concealed ovulation can be seen as a protection against infanticide. Concealed ovulation promotes polyandry, and this results in multiple matings, and sperm competition and sperm allocation as a response to this. Females may then counter with mechanisms for cryptic choice, such as for example selective orgasms.

7.7 Sexual selection of sexual and non-sexual behaviour

7.7.1 Sexual selection and natural selection

Darwin (1871) distinguished natural selection from sexual selection, and this distinction has been consolidated and developed (Fisher 1930, Fisher 1958, Zahavi 1975, Hamilton 1964, Hamilton 1996, Dawkins 1986b, Grafen 1990a, Grafen 1990b, Dawkins 1995, Miller 2000b). Natural selection can be used in a narrow sense to refer to selection processes that lead to the development of characteristics that have a function of providing adaptive or survival value to an individual so that the individual can reproduce, and pass on its genes. In its narrow sense, natural selection can be thought of as 'survival or adaptation selection'. An example might be a gene or genes that specify that the sensory properties of food should be rewarding (and should taste pleasant) when we are in a physiological need state for food. Many of the reward and punishment systems described in this book deal with this type of reward and punishment decoding that has evolved to enable genes to influence behaviour in directions in a high-dimensional space of rewards and punishments that are adaptive for survival and health of the individual, and thus promote reproductive success or fitness of the genes that build such adaptive functionality. We can include kin-related altruistic behaviours (see Chapter 3) because the behaviour is adaptive in promoting the survival of kin, and thus promoting the likelihood that the kin (who contain one's genes) survive and reproduce. Resources and wealth are also understood as making males attractive and being selected by natural selection, in that the wealth and resources may be useful to the female in bringing up her children.

Darwin (1871) also recognized that evolution can occur by sexual selection, when what is being selected for has no inherent adaptive or survival value, but is attractive to potential mates (inter-sexual selection), or helps in competing with others of the same sex (intra-sexual selection). The most cited example is the peacock's large tail, which does not have survival value for the peacock (and indeed it is somewhat of a handicap to have a very long tail), but, because it is attractive to the peahen, becomes prevalent in the population. Indeed, part of the reason for the long tail being attractive may be that it is an honest signal of phenotypic fitness (or 'fitness indicator'), in that having a very long tail is a handicap to survival (Zahavi 1975), though the signalling system that reveals this only operates correctly if certain conditions apply (Grafen 1990a, Grafen 1990b, Maynard Smith & Harper 2003)[22]. The inherited genes for a long tail may be expressed in the female's sons, and they will accordingly be attractive to females in the next generation. Although the female offspring of the mating will not express the male father's attractive long-tail genes, these genes are likely to be expressed in her sons. The female has to evolve to find the characteristic being selected for in males attractive for this situation to lead to a runaway explosion of the characteristic being selected for by the choosiness of females. Indeed, the fact that the female who chose a long-tailed male has

[22]The conditions under which a handicap signalling system can lead to sexual selection are i: the female can correctly infer a male's quality from his advertisement (honesty); ii: signals are costly; and iii: a given signal is more costly for a male of low quality.

children following her mating with genes for liking long-tailed males, and for generating long tails, is part of what leads to the runaway process that can occur with sexual selection. The fact that the long tail is actually a handicap for the peacock, and so is a signal of general physical fitness in the male, may be one way in which sexual selection can occur stably (Zahavi 1975, Grafen 1990a, Grafen 1990b). The peacock tail example is categorized as sexual selection because the long tail is not adaptive to the individual with the long tail, though of course it is adaptive to have a long tail if females are choosing it because it indicates general physical fitness. However, sexual selection can occur when a revealing or index signal or fitness indicator is not associated with a handicap, but is hard to fake, so that it is necessarily an honest fitness indicator (Maynard Smith & Harper 2003). An example occurs in birds that may show bare skin as part of their courtship, providing a sign that they are parasite resistant (Hamilton & Zuk 1982). Handicaps are costly to produce, and should reduce fitness in contexts other than mating. If the signal is an index signal, it is relatively cost-free, cannot be easily faked, and should correlate with some trait that contributes to fitness in contexts other than mating (Maynard Smith & Harper 2003).

Some characteristics of sexual selection that help to separate it from natural or survival selection are as follows:

First, the sexually selected characteristic is sexually dimorphic, with the male typically showing the characteristic. (For example the peacock but not the peahen has the long tail.) This occurs because it is the female who is being choosy, and is selecting males. The female is the choosy one because she has a considerable investment in her offspring, whom she may need to nurture until birth, and then rear until independent, and for this reason has a much more limited reproductive potential than the male, who could in principle father large numbers of offspring to optimize his genetic potential. This is an example of a sexual dimorphism selected by inter-sexual selection. An example of a sexual dimorphism selected by intra-sexual selection is the deer's antlers.

Second, sexually selected characteristics are typically species-specific (consistent with choice by the female of the species of a relatively arbitrary feature in males that may not itself have survival value), whereas naturally selected characteristics may, because they have survival value for individuals, be found in many species within a genus, and even across genera.

Third, and accordingly, the competition is within a species for sexual selection, whereas competition may be across as well as within species for natural (survival) selection.

Fourth, sexual selection operates most efficiently in polygynous species, that is species where some (attractive) males must mate with two or more females, and unattractive males must be more likely to be childless. Polygyny does seem to have been present to at least some extent in our ancestors, as shown for example by body size differences, with males larger than females. This situation is selected because males compete hard with each other in polygynous species compared to monogamous, where there is less competition. In humans, the male is 10% taller, 20% heavier, 50% stronger in the upper body muscles, and 100% stronger in the hand grip strength than the average female (Miller 2000b).

Fifth, the sexually selected characteristics are likely to be apparent after but not before puberty. In humans, one possible example is the deep male voice.

Sixth, there may be marked differences between individuals, as it is these differences that are being used for mate choice. In contrast, when natural or survival selection is operating efficiently, there may be little variation between individuals.

Seventh, the fitness indicator should be costly or difficult to produce, as in this way it can reflect real fitness, and be kept honest.

Overall, Darwinian natural or survival selection increases health, strength, and potentially resources, and survival of the individual, and thus ability to mate and reproduce. Inter-sexual

sexual selection does not make the individual healthier, but does make the individual more attractive as a mate, as in female choice, an example of intersexual selection. Intrasexual sexual selection does not necessarily help survival of the individual, but does help in competition for a mate, for example in intimidation of one male by another (Darwin 1871, Kappeler & van Schaik 2004). The behaviours and characteristics involved in sperm competition described in this chapter are produced by intrasexual sexual selection.

It turns out that many of the best examples of inter-sexual sexual selection are in birds (for example the peacock's tail, and the male lyre bird's tail). Some of the examples in birds may be related to the visual system of birds, which is good at identifying sign stimuli and innate releasing stimuli, and this may facilitate the evolution of elaborate displays. (Is the rhesus macaque's red posterior an exception?) In contrast, mammals have a more general-purpose visual system that can recognize objects invariantly, and does not therefore need to specialize in analysing particular low-level sensory features of stimuli (Rolls & Deco 2002). In mammals, including primates, the selection is often by size, strength, physical prowess, and aggressiveness, which provide for direct physical competition, and are examples of intra-sexual selection (Kappeler & van Schaik 2004).

It has been suggested that sexual selection is important for further types of characteristic in humans. For example, it has been suggested that human mental abilities that may be important in courtship such as kindness, humour, and telling stories, are the type of characteristic that may be sexually selected in humans (Miller 2000b). Before assessing this (in Section 7.7.2), and illuminating thus some of what may be sexually selected rewards and punishers that therefore contribute to human affective states, we should note a twist in how sexual selection may operate in humans.

In humans, because babies are born relatively immature and may take years of demanding care before they can look after themselves, there is some advantage to male genes of providing at least some parental care for the children. That is, the father may invest in his offspring. In this situation, where there is a male investment, the male may optimize the chance of his genes faring well by being choosy about his wife. The implication is that in humans, sexual selection may be of female characteristics (by males), as well as of male characteristics (by females). This may mean that the differences between the sexes may not be as large as can often be the case with inter-sexual sexual selection, where the female is the main chooser. One example of how sexual selection may affect female characteristics is in the selection for large breasts. These may be selected to be larger in humans than is really necessary for milk production, by the incorporation of additional fat. This characteristic may be attractive to males (and hence produce affective responses in males) because it is a symbol relating to fertility and child rearing potential, and not because large breasts have any particular adaptive value. It has even been suggested that the large breast size makes them useful to males as a sign of reproductive potential, for their pertness is maximal when a (young) woman's fertility and reproductive potential is at its highest. Although large breasts may be less pert with age, and it might thus be thought to be an advantage for women not to have large breasts, it may be possible that this is offset by the advantageous signal of a pert but large breast when fertility and reproductive potential is at its maximal when young, as this may attract high status males (even though there may be disadvantages later) (Miller 2000b). Thus it is possible that inter-sexual selection contributes to the large breast size of some women. The fact that the variation is quite large is consistent with this being a sexually selected, not survival-selected, characteristic. Thus sexual selection of characteristics may occur in women as well as in men.

We may also note that the term 'natural selection' encompasses in its broad sense both 'survival or adaptation selection', and sexual selection. Both are processes now understood to be driven by the selection of genes, and it is gene competition and replication into the next generation that is the driving force of biological evolution (Dawkins 1989, Dawkins 1986b).

The distinction can be made that with 'survival or adaptation selection', the genes being selected for make the individual animal stronger, healthier, and more likely to survive and reproduce, whereas sexual selection operates by sexual choice selecting for genes that may have little survival value to the individual, but enable the individual to be selected as a mate or to compete for a mate in intra-sexual selection, and thus pass on the genes selected by intra-sexual or inter-sexual selection.

Insofar as the states elicited by rewards and punishers are emotional states (see Chapters 2 and 3), this chapter thus extends the understanding of emotion to systems shaped by sexual selection. For example, sexual selection may select symmetric and thus attractive faces which may produce emotional states.

7.7.2 Non-sexual characteristics may be sexually selected for courtship

Miller (2000b) has developed the hypothesis that courtship provides an opportunity for sexual selection to select non-sexual mental characteristics such as kindness, humour, the ability to tell stories, creativity, art, and even language. He postulates that these are "courtship tools, evolved to attract and entertain sexual partners". Sexual selection views organisms as advertisers of their phenotypic fitness, and Miller sees these characteristics as such signals. From this perspective, hunting is seen as a costly and inefficient exercise (in comparison with food gathering) undertaken by men to obtain small gifts of meat for women, but at the same time to show how competitive and fit the successful hunter is in relation to other men. Conspicuous waste, and conspicuous consumption, are often signs in nature that sexual selection is at work, with high costs for behaviours that seem maladaptive in terms of survival and natural selection in the narrow sense. The mental characteristics described above are not only costly in terms of time, but may rely on many genes operating efficiently for these characteristics to be expressed well, and so, Miller suggests, may be 'fitness indicators'. Consistent with sexual selection, there is also great individual variability in these characteristics, providing a basis for choice.

One mental characteristic that Miller suggests could have evolved in this way is kindness, which is very highly valued by both sexes (Buss 2012, Buss 1994). In human evolution, being kind to the mother's children may have been seen as an attractive characteristic in men during courtship, especially when relationships may not have lasted for many years, and the children might not be those of the courting male. Kindness may also be used as an indicator of future cooperation. In a sense kindness thus may indicate potential useful benefits, consistent with the fact that across cultures human females tend to prefer males who have high social status, good income, ambition, intelligence, and energy (Buss 2012, Buss 1994). Kindness may also be related to kin altruism (Hamilton 1964) or to reciprocal altruism (Trivers 1971), both of which are genetically adaptive strategies (see Chapter 2)[23]. Although the simple interpretation of all these characteristics is that they indicate a good provider and potential material and genetic benefits (and thus would be subject to natural or survival selection), Miller (2000b) argues that at least kindness is being used in addition as a fitness indicator and is being sexually selected. Although morality can be related in part to kin and reciprocal altruism (Ridley 1996) (see Section 11.3), moral behaviour may bring reproductive benefits through the social status that it inspires (Zahavi & Zahavi 1997) or by direct mate choice for moralistic displays during courtship (Tessman 1995, Miller 2000b). The suggestion made by Miller (2000b) is that the status of moral behaviour helps to attract mates, because it may

[23] Interestingly, the etymology of kindness is Old English cynd, kin, hence looking after kin, relations.

reflect fitness as the moral behaviour may have costs. He suggests that "*Morality is a system of sexually selected handicaps*".

Miller (2000b) (page 258 ff) also suggests that art, language and creativity can be explained by sexual selection, and that they are difficult to account for by survival selection. He suggests that art develops from courtship ornamentation, and uses bowerbirds as an evolutionary example. Male bowerbirds ornament their often enormous and structurally elaborate nests or bowers with mosses, ferns, shells, berries and bark to attract female bowerbirds. The nests are used just to attract females, and after insemination the females go off and build their own cup-shaped nests, lay their eggs, and raise their offspring by themselves with no male support. Darwin himself viewed human ornamentation and clothing as outcomes of sexual selection. Sexual selection for artistic ability does not mean of course that the art itself needs to be about sex. This example helps to show that sexual selection can lead to changes in what is valued and found attractive, in areas that might be precursors to art in humans. Miller (2000b) suggests that language evolved as a courtship device in males to attract females. Miller (2000b) also suggests that creativity may be related to systems that can explore random new ideas, and also is a courtship device in males to attract females.

One potential problem with this approach is that sexual selection favours fast runaway evolution, because sexual preferences are genetically correlated with the ornaments they favour (as described in section 7.7). Why does mental capacity not develop more rapidly, and with larger sex differences, in humans, if Miller (2000) is right? Why is there not a faster runaway? Miller suggests a number of possible reasons.

1. There is a high genetic correlation between human males and females, with 22/23 chromosomes the same.

2. The female's brain must evolve to be able to appreciate the male's mental adornment – and might even be one step ahead to judge effectively. Further, similar or partly overlapping brain mechanisms may be used to produce (in males) and perceive (in females). In addition, male self-monitoring (and female practice) may help appraisal. Males may even internalize female's appreciation systems, to predict their responses.

3. There is mutual choice in humans: males choose females because human males do make a parental investment; and females compete for males. Indeed, the selection of a long-term partner is mutual, and this tends to reduce sex differences. Consistent with this, David Buss has shown that, in contrast, human sex differences are more evident in short-term mating (Buss 1989, Buss 1994, Buss 2012). It is likely in fact that sexual selection works mainly through long-term relationships, because of concealed ovulation in women. This means that only in a relatively long-term relationship is it likely that a man will become the father of a woman's child, because only if he mates with her regularly is there a reasonable probability that he will hit her fertile time.

Another criticism of the approach of Miller (2000b) is that many of these characteristics may have survival value, and are not purely sexually selected. For example, language has many uses in problem solving, planning ahead, and correcting multiple step plans which are likely to be very important to enable immediate rewards to be deferred, and longer term goals to be achieved (see Chapter 10, and Pinker (1997)).

7.8 Individual differences in sexual rewards

Before considering how biological reward systems might have evolved in order to implement the types of behaviours just described, we first consider possible individual differences in these types of sexual behaviour, because these have implications for how the reward systems may differ in different individuals to produce these differences in sexual behaviour. We remind ourselves that genetic specification of different reward mechanisms could produce a polymorphic, fixed, evolutionarily stable strategy, as described in the first footnote of this chapter on page 323. An alternative mechanism is a conditional strategy (see the same footnote), which can also be evolutionarily stable (Maynard Smith 1984). In many of the examples discussed here, it is not clear which is the more likely. We should also note that many factors are likely to produce differences between the emotional behaviour of males and females. For example, in many species, females are attracted to dominant males, thus further favouring male competitiveness. Further, females may be attracted to males favoured by other women. Both might be accounted for by their predictive relation to producing genetically successful male offspring.

In addition, when considering individual differences in sexual behaviour, it is important to remember that conditional mating strategies may be employed (Gangestad & Simpson 2000, Buss 2012). For example, physical factors such as high symmetry that are indicators of genetic fitness may be especially attractive when women choose short-term partners, and factors such as resources and faithfulness may be especially important when women choose long-term partners. Indeed, because of conditional strategies, the choices made in different situations or contexts may be quite dynamical. To a considerable extent differences between individuals may reflect different weightings given to different rewards (benefits) and punishers (costs) by different individuals, so that the behaviour on any one occasion (e.g. promiscuous vs faithful) may reflect how each of these rewards and punishers operate in a given context. Thus different individuals might tend to act in the different ways described below based on the values of a number of reward and punishment factors in a multidimensional (partly gene-specified) space, but should not be thought of as being simply of one type or another.

7.8.1 Overview

Is the range of stimuli and situations related to sexual behaviour that different people find rewarding different, and can any differences be related to a biological function such as sperm warfare? It is plausible that there are such differences, and that they could be related to sperm warfare. Although experimental data on this issue in relation to an underlying function such as sperm competition are not yet available, the possibilities are sufficiently plausible that they are worth elaborating, in part as a guide to stimulating further concepts and experimental research in this area.

A hypothesis that seems plausible is that some individuals might be of the type that would specialize in sperm warfare. Such individuals might find especially rewarding the types of stimuli that would make them especially successful in sperm warfare, and their resulting behaviour might reflect the stimuli they find most rewarding. If men, they might be built to find variety in sexual partners especially rewarding, and to be ambitious and competitive. This could increase their fitness, by enabling them potentially to have many children with different women. A risk of this 'unfaithful' strategy, which would tend to keep it in check, is that the man might make insufficient investment in helping any of his lovers and her children by him to ensure that the children flourish and themselves reproduce successfully. Women might avoid such men if they were not already in receipt of sufficient resources to provide for their children, and the partners of such women might require that they be faithful, even to the extent of guarding them. Such 'unfaithful' individuals, who would be likely to specialize in sperm warfare, if women, might be unfaithful and as a result be fit if they had a tendency to choose genetically fit men to be the father of their children, while at the same time having as a partner to help bring up the children another man who was not necessarily as genetically fit as their lover, but would help to bring up the children. For this to be an evolutionarily stable strategy, it might be expected that at least some of the children would be children of the partner, otherwise the deception might be too obvious. Part of the risk of this strategy, which keeps it in balance with others in the population, is that if her deception is discovered, the woman risks losing the resources being provided for her and her children by her partner. Too great a tendency to unfaithfulness would also be unstable because of the associated risks of sexually transmitted disease.

Other individuals in the population might be genetically predisposed to use a different strategy, of being faithful to their partner. This could benefit a faithful woman's genes, because her children would have a partner who could be relied on to help bring up the children, and put all his resources into this (because he would be sure that his genes were in the children, and because he would not be tempted by other women). (In addition, he might not be very attractive or successful in life, and might not have the opportunity to be tempted away.) Her fitness would be increased by the fact that her children would be likely to survive, but reduced by the fact that the genes with which she has mated would not be as advantageous, and nor would she benefit from the effect of pure variety of genes with which to combine her own, which is part of the advantage of sexual reproduction. There could also be an advantage to a man's genes for him to be faithful, because in being faithful he would be less likely to catch a disease, and would be more likely to put sufficient resources into his children to ensure that they have a good start in life; and would be more likely to attract a faithful woman as his partner, so that the children in whom he invested would be more likely to be his. The cost of this strategy would be that he might have fewer children than if he were unfaithful, and his children might, if the behaviour is controlled genetically, be less likely themselves to have large numbers of children, because they would not be likely to be the unfaithful type.

It is suggested that these different strategies, because each has associated advantages and costs, could be retained in a stable balance in populations in which genetic factors at least partly predisposed the individual to be of the unfaithful or faithful type[24]. Of course, in a real human population it might be expected that there would be continuous variation between individuals in the tendency to be faithful or unfaithful, and for the actual range of differences found in a population to be being constantly adjusted depending on the fitness of the different types of strategy, and on the environment too, such as the availability of resources (see the first footnote of this chapter on page 323). (The availability of resources could affect the balance. For example, if food and other resources were readily available, so that the advantage of care by both parents was less than in more harsh environments in which perhaps the man might be specialized for hunting, then the relative advantages of unfaithfulness in the population would be higher.)

The two contrasted phenotypes might be kept in stable balance by the advantages of extra-pair copulations such as more reproductive success for males and more fit genes for females, and the advantages of not having extra-pair copulations such as being less likely to be cheated on oneself while one is away not mateguarding (if a male) and of losing resources if detected (if a female) (Simmons et al. 2004).

Evidence that genetic factors do actually influence the likelihood of infidelity comes from the finding of what might be called a 'promiscuity gene' (Hamer & Copeland 1998). The research (conducted at the National Institutes of Cancer in Washington) has so far been conducted in men, but there could be a parallel in women. Very interestingly in relation to the points made about dopamine and reward in this book, the gene affects the D4 dopamine receptor (DRD4), and in particular it comes in a long form or a short form. Approximately 30% of men in the study carried the long form of the gene, and they were likely to have 20% more sexual partners than those with the short form. Men with the long form were

[24]Richard Dawkins (1976) described a stable situation of this type with faithful and philanderer males, and coy and fast females.

likely to have an average of 10 sexual partners in their lifetime, whereas those with the short form were less likely to have sought such variety. Further, it was found that two aspects of novelty seeking, exploratory excitability and impulsiveness, were higher in humans with the long form of the DRD4 gene (Keltikangas-Jarvinen, Elovainio, Kivimaki, Lichtermann, Ekelund & Peltonen 2003), though it must be noted that this effect was not substantiated in a meta-analysis (Kluger, Siegfried & Ebstein 2002), and in any case is infrequent and would not account for much of the variation found overall in the population. Further evidence that the human dopamine D4 receptor gene (DRD4) is related to promiscuity and infidelity is that individuals with at least one 7-repeat allele on this gene report a greater categorical rate of promiscuous sexual behaviour (i.e., having ever had a 'one-night stand') and report a more than 50% increase in instances of sexual infidelity (Garcia, MacKillop, Aller, Merriwether, Wilson & Lum 2010).

Hamer and colleagues also described a gene that influences sex drive that is different to that for promiscuity. This is a serotonin (i.e. 5-hydroxytryptamine)-related gene which influences anxiety (Greenberg, Li, Lucas, Hu, Sirota, Benjamin, Lesch, Hamer & Murphy 2000). Men with the high anxiety form of this gene had more frequent sex, and those with the calm, happy and optimistic form had less sex. These findings are starting to show that genetic approaches may provide an important type of support for the suggestion made in this chapter that different strategies for sexual behaviour, and in particular a strategy to be faithful vs a strategy to be unfaithful, could be influenced at least in part by genes.

Next we will consider how natural selection (in the broad sense, including sexual selection) might make different types of stimuli differently rewarding to different people in order to produce these different types of behaviour. This will just be a possible scenario, because I know of little actual evidence on this. Then we will consider what such evidence might look like when it does become available.

7.8.2 How might different types of behaviour be produced by natural selection altering the relative reward value of different stimuli in different individuals?

We will consider what could occur hypothetically in different types of women, predisposed to be unfaithful and faithful, and in different types of men, predisposed to be unfaithful and faithful, for clarity. We remember that in practice there would be likely to be a continuous distribution of these differences in a human population. (We note that in addition to the two types of evolutionarily stable strategy outlined in the first footnote of this chapter on page 323, the different behaviours do not have to be equally successful. One type of behaviour might just be 'making the best of a bad job'.)

First we consider women who might be genetically predisposed to be unfaithful and promote sperm warfare. (Sometimes the shorthand used for this is 'unfaithful woman', but this should always be taken to mean 'genetically predisposed to be an unfaithful woman'.) We might suppose that they should be especially attractive to men, and may therefore tend to be youthful-looking and thin, to indicate that they are at a fertile period of their lives, and are not already pregnant. They should not be shy, might be extravert, and might be flirtatious in order to attract men. They should like (sexually) aggressive men (because this is an indicator that her sons with him would pass on her genes to women that they were able to take as lovers). They might even like a man aggressive to other men as in war, because in war his genes (potentially in his children with her) will tend to survive and to be passed on, and he will be a potential protection in war. Women with genes predisposing them to be unfaithful might be attracted to men with a 'reputation' – because this also indicates that they will produce sons who are good at passing on (her) genes; should be good at finding a partner for stability, to bring up her children, but also good at deceiving him; should like men with large testes (which could correlate with testosterone levels, and thus perhaps be indicated by secondary sexual characteristics such as body hair); should like men with a large penis (because this would be good at sperm warfare by sucking out other men's sperm, and thus is an indicator of genetic fitness in sperm warfare); should be able to assess men for sexual fitness, not necessarily fast but by evaluating his position in society, power, wealth, and bodily fitness (one index of which is the shape of the buttocks which may reflect running ability). She might herself be sexually aggressive, because it is important (in terms of fitness) that when she takes risks and is unfaithful, she chooses the right man, with genes that will make her children fit, and does not choose just any man. She might also be likely to control sexual behaviour, rather than be passive – she wants to control whether and when (in relation to whether she is fertile) a man impregnates her, and if and when in relation to his ejaculation she has an orgasm. (She might, for example, choose to have intercourse with a fit lover especially when she is most fertile, and to orgasm soon after him. She might choose to have intercourse with her partner at other times, and either not to have an orgasm, or to orgasm before he does, to prevent upsuck. For this reason, and partly to please her partner, she might fake her orgasms.) She might be especially attracted to novel men, and indeed might need some element of novelty to make her have an orgasm and thus be likely to conceive. In this respect, she should be built to be continually searching for something better. She might also for this reason, because it is advantageous to her to control when and with whom she has orgasms, appear to need more stimulation to have an orgasm, and be especially likely to have orgasms with novel men or in novel situations. She may also tend to reproduce young, because of the risk of disease. Such an unfaithful woman, because of the risk that her deception might be discovered, might use her attractiveness to make relationships with a number of men, and have backup policies with several men, as insurance and support for her young.

Second, we consider women whose genes might have built them to be faithful. She might be less attractive, and once with a partner might take fewer steps to be attractive (she might not be thin, and might be less worried about her weight; she might be less concerned with cosmetics and might dress sensibly rather than provocatively). She might be reliable, looking for domestic security (to provide reliable resources for her and her children, as she has chosen to put her resources into bringing up her children well, rather than taking risks and possibly having genetically more fit children with a lover but risking the support for all her children). She might be relatively passive during intercourse, and not try to control sex (because with only one male, she does not need to control whether/when a male ejaculates in her, and if/when she orgasms). Partly for this reason, she might find it relatively easy to have orgasms, because she does not need to control who fertilizes her, and because orgasms (associated with oxytocin release, see Section 7.3) might promote attachment to the (same) partner. Multiple orgasms in this situation could help, though they might be especially useful if the woman was 'trying' to conceive. The main prediction here is that orgasms would be much more consistent (either present or not) than in women genetically predisposed to be unfaithful. The woman genetically predisposed to be faithful might tend to reproduce older, because she has less risk of disease. She might be shy, could be introvert, and might be expected not to be a flirtatious type. She should make very stable relationships with friends in a supporting society (to ensure care of her young, a high priority to her, and to listen to gossip, to learn of potentially threatening males or females). She should disapprove of women with a reputation, as they are a threat to her security, e.g. by attracting her partner and thus threatening her resources.

Some evidence consistent with these hypotheses is that promiscuity is correlated with personality, in particular with extraversion, and with low conscientiousness and agreeableness (Schmitt 2004). These findings were made in a study involving 16,362 participants from 52 nations whose personality was measured by questionnaire on the Big Five personality dimensions, and on Relationship Exclusivity, which has two sub-components, Relationship Infidelity (identified by the items 'adulterous', 'not devoted', 'not faithful', 'not monogamous', 'polygamous', and 'unfaithful'), and Sexual Promiscuity (identified by the items 'loose' and 'promiscuous'). Impulsiveness may be an underlying characteristic, as impulsive sensation seeking is most closely related within the Big Five to low conscientiousness and agreeableness, and the strongest correlate of risky sexual behaviour is impulsive sensation-seeking (Zuckerman 1994, Hoyle, Fejfar & Miller 2000, Zuckerman & Kuhlman 2000). In a link to brain mechanisms, it has been found that humans with orbitofrontal cortex damage are impulsive (Berlin, Rolls & Kischka 2004, Berlin & Rolls 2004, Berlin, Rolls & Iversen 2005). Relationship infidelity was associated with low conscientiousness and agreeableness, that is, again with impulsive sensation seeking.

Men genetically predisposed to be unfaithful and to participate in sperm warfare might be built by their genes as follows. First, at the simple physical level, they might have large testes and a large penis, both good in sperm warfare (see above). Second, they should be successful with other women, as this indicates how well a woman's sons with them would pass her genes on to future generations. (This could be 'why' some women are interested in a man's reputation, and why this could help to make a man attractive.) These men could be competitive and aggressive (both sexually and in war, see above); have high testosterone (possibly indicated by bodily hair and other secondary sexual characteristics); be ambitious, wealthy, successful and powerful (because these indicate potential to provide resources); possibly creative, intellectual, musical, etc. because these may be ways to keep women interested, and may be used in courtship. (There is the suggestion that women are selecting men's brains to be good at courtship, so that a man's brain would parallel a peacock's 'tail', see Ridley (1993a) and Miller (2000b); and if so, this selection might be particularly evident in unfaithful men.) Such men might also be good at deceit, as this would be an advantage in deception of their partner and their lover's partner.

Men genetically predisposed to be faithful might have smaller testes and penes on average; and have lower concentrations of testosterone and be less aggressive, and even possibly less ambitious. They should be less interested in and attracted by women other than their partner, that is they should be built less to keep searching for novelty; they should be stable, reliable, good at providing a home, and truthful, all of which would appeal to a woman genetically predisposed to be faithful. He should denounce men (or women) with a reputation, because they, and that type of behaviour, are a threat to him, given that he is inclined to make his major investment in one woman, and it is to his genes' advantage that the children he helps to bring up are his.

7.8.3 How being tuned to different types of reward could help to produce individual differences in sexual behaviour

Given the hypotheses discussed in Section 7.8.2 [and they are of course only hypotheses, although personality and genetic differences related to promiscuity are now being identified (Schmitt 2004, Garcia et al. 2010)], it is now possible to ask how differences in sexual behaviour might be produced by genes influencing the different types of stimulation and situation that different individuals find rewarding. (We remember that an alternative to a polymorphic fixed ESS is a conditional strategy, see first footnote of this chapter on page 323. A conditional strategy might not alter what would be found inherently rewarding, but might alter how different types of reward were perceived.) As above, when the term 'unfaithful man or woman' is used, it is simply shorthand for the description 'man or woman predisposed to be unfaithful'.

1. Unfaithful women could be built to find external (relative to internal) stimulation of the genitals particularly necessary for reward, because this helps them to control impregnation.

2. Unfaithful women could be built to need much (external and sometimes adventurous and novel) stimulation to produce enough reward/pleasure for them to orgasm. (This would be part of the control of the impregnation process, making it particularly likely that they would have an orgasm and facilitate fertilization with a lover, who would probably be more novel than a regular partner. It would also be part of the mechanism that would encourage them to keep searching for something better, because some novelty would tend to be arousing.)

3. It is possible that sensory-specific satiety, a reduction in sexual desire for a particular person with whom intercourse has just taken place, relative to other men, would be more pronounced in unfaithful women, as a mechanism to facilitate searching for new genes, and sperm competition.

4. Unfaithful women could be built to like control, both of whether and when sex occurs with a particular man, and during sex, partly by requiring particular types of stimulation (novel and external), and perhaps partly by making control per se rewarding and important to them.

5. Unfaithful women could be built to find social interactions, sometimes flirtatious and provocative, including clothes, cosmetics etc., with men (and with novel men perhaps especially), particularly rewarding, as a mechanism to attract and obtain potential lovers.

6. Unfaithful women could tend to be smaller, with oestrogen-dependent features such as wide eyes and a small lower face, to keep their bodies in trim, and to age less than faithful women, in order to attract males with fit genes. In fact, sexual dimorphism should be especially pronounced in those predisposed to be unfaithful.

7. In a complementary way, women predisposed to be faithful could be tuned to internal vs external stimulation during intercourse, to need less stimulation and particularly less novel stimulation to have an orgasm, to show less sensory-specific satiety for the partner, to be more passive rather than controlling before and during sex, and to be less socially provocative.

8. In a corresponding way, men predisposed to be unfaithful might be tuned to find it rewarding to produce an orgasm in women (because this is a way to facilitate the chances of their sperm in a sperm war), and therefore be willing to work hard for this; to find vigorous thrusting during intercourse particularly rewarding (to serve the biological function of increasing their chances in sperm competition); to be especially attracted to attractive, novel, and interactive women (to serve the biological function of finding genes able to produce fit daughters who will themselves attract males); and to not be satisfied for long with the same situation, but continually be searching for new relationships and lovers.

9. Partial reinforcement (i.e. only sometimes giving a reinforcer or reward) by an unfaithful woman should be greatly reinforcing to an unfaithful man (beyond the normal partial reinforcement effect, which itself increases the amount a person will work for a reward), because this is a test of how motivated and successful the man is to pass on his genes, a quality that the unfaithful woman will value for her sons. The unfaithful woman may even titrate the partial reinforcement level to see just how persistent, and thus potentially fit, the man is.

It may be emphasized that the reward processes that have just been described might be those to which different people are predisposed, and probably operate primarily through an implicit or unconscious system for rewards. In addition to this implicit system with its predispositions, humans have an explicit processing system which can of course influence the actual choice that is made (see Chapter 10).

7.9 The neural reward mechanisms that might mediate some aspects of sexual behaviour

In Section 7.5 sociobiological research on sexual behaviour was described. In Section 7.8 we speculated about possible individual differences in such sexual behaviour. In both these sections we produced hypotheses about how genes might influence sexual behaviour by building particular reward systems and mechanisms into animals. We now consider how the brain might implement these different reward processes. Might there be a few principles of operation of the brain reward systems that could help to account for the quite complex sexual behaviour that is apparent in humans? How are these mechanisms implemented neurophysiologically in the brain? We consider what is known on these issues in this Section. Although the actual brain mechanisms are not fully worked out, the intention of the approach being taken here is to suggest what could be implemented in the brain mechanisms that provide the rewards for sexual behaviour, to guide future research and thinking.

Examples of quite simple neurophysiological rules and processes that could govern the operation of reward mechanisms for sexual behaviour and that could account for many of the effects discussed above are given next.

1. Olfactory rewards and pheromones. Pheromones, which are typically olfactory stimuli, can trigger a number of different types of sexual behaviour, and thus either affect what is rewarding, or in some cases can act as rewards (Dulac & Torello 2003, Beauchamp & Yamazaki 2003, Dulac & Kimchi 2007).

First, pheromones can produce slow and long-lasting effects by influencing hormones, affecting for example reproductive cycles. They produce the Lee-Boot effect, in which the oestrous cycles of female mice housed together without a male slow down and eventually stop. They act in the Whitten effect, in which the mice start cycling again if they are exposed to the odour of a male or his urine. They act in the Vandenbergh effect, the acceleration in the onset of puberty in a female rodent caused by the odour of a male. They act in the Bruce effect, in which if a recently impregnated female mouse encounters a male mouse other than the one with which she mated, the pregnancy is very likely to fail. The new male can then mate with her. This form of genetic warfare happening after the sperm-warfare stage is clearly to the advantage of the new male's genes, and presumably to the advantage of the female's genes, because it means that her pregnancies will tend to be with males who are not only able to oust other males, but are with males who are with her, so that her offspring will not be harmed by the new male, and may even be protected. The pheromones that produce these effects are produced in males under the influence of testosterone (see Carlson (2012)). These effects depend on an accessory olfactory system, the vomeronasal organ and its projections to the accessory olfactory bulb. The accessory olfactory bulb in turn projects to the medial nucleus of the amygdala, which in turn projects to the preoptic area, anterior hypothalamus, and ventromedial hypothalamus, and these pheromonal effects are produced by influences on hormones such as luteinizing hormone (LH) and prolactin (PRL) (Dulac & Torello 2003). Pheromones can cause groups of women housed together to start cycling together. The evolutionary significance of the synchronized cycling might be to increase male–male competition and selection. In addition, shared care may be facilitated by synchronized breeding, and this could increase the survival of the offspring.

Second, pheromones can act as attracting or rewarding signals, and rapidly influence behaviour. For example, pheromones present in the vaginal secretions of hamsters attract males. In some monkeys, bacteria in the vagina produce more of a pheromone under the influence of an androgen (male sex hormone) produced in small quantities in the adrenal glands, and this pheromone increases the attractiveness of the female to the male (Baum et al. 1977). (In this case, male sexual behaviour is induced by a male hormone produced in females.) Male rats also produce pheromones, which are attractive to females. In humans, body odours are not generally described as attractive, but there is a whole industry based on perfume, the odour of a mate may become attractive by conditioning, and there is some evidence that androstenol, a substance found in the underarm sweat of males especially, may increase the number of social interactions that women have with men (Cowley & Brooksbank 1991). In humans, it has been reported that a putative female pheromone oestra-1,3,5,(10),16-tetraen-3ol-acetate (EST) activates the male anterior medial thalamus and right inferior frontal gyrus at concentrations that cannot be detected consciously (Sobel, Prabhakaran, Hartley, Desmond, Glover, Sullivan & Gabrieli 1999). It has also been reported that androstadien-3-one, a putative male pheromone, activates the preoptic area in women. Conversely, EST activates the hypothalamus in men. Both activate cortical olfactory areas in both men and women (Savic 2002, Savic 2001, Savic, Berglund, Gulyas & Roland 2001).

There is interesting research showing that pheromones act through the vomeronasal system, though this system appears to be vestigial and disconnected in humans and Old World monkeys (such as macaques) (Dulac & Torello 2003, Meredith 2001, Dulac & Kimchi 2007). The vomeronasal system in rodents includes receptors in a specialized organ in the nose that connect to the accessory olfactory bulb, and utilize a set of genes that specify approximately 293 types of V1R and 100 types of V2R olfactory pheromone receptor (Dulac & Torello 2003). Pheromones that activate these receptors are involved in behaviours in rodents such as (with the pheromone 2-sec-butyl-4,5-dihydrothiazole produced by male mice) inducing oestrus in females, intermale aggression, and attracting females (Dulac & Torello 2003). Monti-Bloch and colleagues (Monti-Bloch, Jennings-White, Dolberg & Berliner 1994, Monti-Bloch, Jennings-White & Berliner 1998, Berliner, Monti-Bloch, Jennings-White & Diaz-Sanchez 1996) applied what they termed 'vomeropherins' to the vomeronasal system while they recorded negative potentials from the (probably vestigial) human vomeronasal organ. They found vomeropherins that activated the vomeronasal organ but not the olfactory epithelium. Conversely, conventional odourants activated the olfactory epithelium but not the vomeronasal organ. Interestingly, males and females were sensitive to different vomeropherins. In men, the vomeropherin pregna-4,20-diene-3,6-dione (PDD) in concentrations of 5×10^{-9} M activated the vomeronasal organ and reduced luteinizing-hormone pulsatility and levels, and follicle-stimulating hormone (FSH) pulsatility. The pheromone also reduced respiratory frequency, increased cardiac frequency, and produced changes in electrodermal activity and the EEG (electroencephalogram). No significant effects of this pheromone were produced in women. In women (but not in men) the vomeropherins PH56 and PH94B activated the vomeronasal organ, and increased electrodermal activity, skin temperature, and alpha-cortical (EEG) activity. These findings raise interesting possibilities requiring much further exploration about the function of the human vomeronasal organ and accessory olfactory system, including potential roles in acting as a reward, or in influencing reward systems. One factor though is that in humans the vomeronasal organ may be vestigial and not connected to the brain (Dulac & Torello 2003). Another is that most of the genes in humans that should produce accessory olfactory system pheromone receptors are pseudogenes[25], so that no receptors can be produced,

[25] A pseudogene is a DNA sequence that is related to a functional gene but cannot be transcribed owing to mutational changes or the lack of regulatory sequences.

with only 5 of the V1R pheromone genes believed not to be inactivated in humans (Dulac & Torello 2003). It appears that pheromonal effects in humans may be produced through the main olfactory system.

In a different line of research, it has been suggested that another way in which animals including humans respond to some pheromones as rewards or as aversive stimuli could be a molecular mechanism for producing genetic diversity by influencing those who are considered attractive as mates (Dulac & Torello 2003, Jacob, McClintock, Zelano & Ober 2002, Potts 2002, Beauchamp & Yamazaki 2003). In particular, major histocompatibility complex (MHC)-dependent abortion and mate choice, based on olfaction, can maintain MHC diversity, and probably functions both to avoid genome-wide inbreeding and produce MHC-heterozygous offspring with increased immune responsiveness (Eggert, Holler, Luszyk, Muller-Ruchholtz & Ferstl 1996, Apanius, Penn, Slev, Ruff & Potts 1997, Potts 2002, Penn & Potts 1998, Potts, Manning & Wakeland 1991, Beauchamp & Yamazaki 2003, Jacob et al. 2002). Each individual has approximately 50 MHC genes, each with 500 alleles (different possible types, one instance of which is provided by each parent). These genes are involved in the process by which a cell infected with an antigen (from a virus or bacterium) displays short peptide sequences of it at the cell surface, and the T lymphocytes of the immune system then recognize the fragment, and build an antibody to it. This MHC gene system must maintain great diversity to help detect uncommon antigens, with an advantage arising from mating with an individual with different MHC genes. At least some of the MHC genes are very closely associated with gene-specified pheromone receptors, with individual pheromone receptor cells often expressing one or a few MHC genes in a complex with specific V2R-specified receptors (Dulac & Torello 2003). In addition, for this system to work, the MHC-linked pheromone receptor must be linked to a genetically coded pathway that passes through the brain as far as the stage at which behavioural preferences are generated; and the MHC genes must specify the odours being produced. The system is very sensitive, in that if a mutation occurs in one of the MHC genes, this produces a discriminably different odour to a mouse (Schaefer, Yamazaki, Osada, Restrepo & Beauchamp 2002). In another example, the MHC type of a foetus is evident in the smell emanating from the (mouse) mother by half term (Beauchamp & Yamazaki 2003). It has been speculated that this may help a male to know whether he is the father of the baby, which can be useful to the male in a mixed mating situation. In an example from humans, odourl 'pheromones' from T shirts are rated as pleasant by Hutterite women if one or more (compared to the more typical zero) of the MHC genes of the stranger who produced the odour on the T shirt matches a paternal MHC gene of the woman making the rating (Jacob et al. 2002). This is in contrast to most studies in rodents, in which diversity was preferred. However, in the rodent studies, what was being preferred was some diversity against a background of many similar MHC genes. Putting the different studies together, the rule may be to have a preference to avoid mating with individuals with very similar MHC profiles (to help produce diverse MHC immune systems), but to prefer some similarity compared to none (to help minimize outbreeding costs (Bateson 1983, Ochoa & Jaffe 1999) and to preserve immunocompetence (Penn & Potts 1998)). It may be that these pheromone-like effects in humans are produced by receptors in the main olfactory system (Schaefer, Young & Restrepo 2001).

2. The attractiveness, reward value, and beauty of women to men is determined by a number of factors to which the brain must be sensitive (Buss 1989, Buss 2012, Barrett et al. 2002, Thornhill & Gangestad 1996, Betzig 1997). One factor is a low waist-to-hip ratio. Waist-to-hip ratio in women correlates negatively with oestrogen, age, fertility, and health, and positively with age. Low waist-to-hip ratios (0.6–0.7) in women are maximally attractive to men. One of the obvious ways in which a low ratio indicates fertility is that it will reflect whether the woman is pregnant. It may be partly because of the biologically relevant signals given by a low

waist-to-hip ratio that thinness and dieting are rewarding, and this may even be selecting for a small body build in women. Other indicators with similar biological signalling functions that are therefore rewarding to men and make women attractive include a youthful face (sometimes almost a baby face, with a small nose); slow ageing; symmetry (because symmetry is reduced by environmental insults, e.g. parasites and toxins, and genetic disruptions such as mutations and inbreeding, and so reflects fitness); smooth unblemished skin; etc. All these signals of attractiveness and beauty might be selected for particularly in women predisposed to be unfaithful (because they must attract genetically fit men as lovers, even if they cannot have them as partners). Sexual restraint in women could make them attractive to men because this implies chastity and thus protection of the potential investment of a man in bringing up putatively his children with that woman. In addition, the relative reward value of different signals may vary as a function of the environment. Women who perceive that they are in an environment where men are not likely to invest, act and dress in a more sexually provocative manner, and use copulation to attract desirable men. That is, women may be designed to show sexual restraint (thus giving cues of paternity reliability) when investing males may be accessible, and less sexual restraint (to access material benefits) when each male can or will invest little.

An implication for brain mechanisms is that all these factors that reflect attractiveness, which include information from face analysis, must be used in the brain to determine reward value. Part of this process is reflected in the greater activation found to attractive than unattractive faces in the medial orbitofrontal cortex (O'Doherty et al. 2003b). Another example is that low (i.e. attractive) waist-to-hip ratios in women activate the orbitofrontal and anterior cingulate cortices in men (Platek & Singh 2010).

3. The attractiveness of men is influenced by their power, status in society, wealth, and ambition as a predictor of these (Buss 2012). These factors are rewarding and attractive to women because they are an indication of the resources that can be provided by the man for the woman, to help bring up her children to maturity and reproduction. Aggressiveness and competitiveness with other men, and domination and success with other women, may be attractive because they indicate fitness (in terms of genetic potential) of the man's genes, and thus of hers in their children. (Aggression and competitiveness in men can thus be ascribed to women's choice.) Physical factors such as symmetry, firm buttocks and a muscular build also make men attractive to women because they serve as biological signals of health and fertility, and also possibly because they indicate that such men can cope well despite the 'handicap' of a high level of testosterone, which suppresses the immune system. These factors are reviewed by Buss (2012), Buss (1989), Barrett et al. (2002), Thornhill & Gangestad (1996), and in the articles in Betzig (1997). To a woman predisposed to be faithful, indicators of a man's potential parental investment in her children as indicated by caring, stability, and lack of reputation should make a man attractive.

The operation of some of these factors can be understood in terms of a parental investment model. The parental investment model implies that the sex investing more (most commonly the female) will be most choosy; whereas the sex investing least (most commonly the male) should be most competitive (Kenrick, DaSadalla, Groth & Trost 1990). High male parental investment in humans contrasts with most other mammalian species. So the above may be less true of humans. The result is that when one measures patterns for what makes a stranger attractive, they are like those of other mammals; whereas when one measures what makes a long-term partner attractive, more similar selectivity should be found between males and females – that is, the requirements for marriage (high investment) are much more stringent than for dating (low investment), and the balance may shift under these conditions from males selecting females mainly on attractiveness to males selecting females as partners who will be faithful and protect their investment (Kenrick et al. 1990).

4. Repeated thrusting and withdrawal of the penis during intercourse should be rewarding to the man (and possibly also to the woman), because it serves the biological function (in sperm warfare) of helping to remove from the vagina sperm that could remain from previous intercourse, possibly with another male, for up to 12 h. If the only aim was to deposit semen in the vagina, then there would be little point in this repeated thrusting and withdrawal, which typically occurs in males 100–500 times during intercourse in humans (see Baker & Bellis (1995)). An implication for brain reward systems is that stimulation of the glans and of the shaft of the penis should be rewarding, but should only bring the man to ejaculate after a reasonable number of thrust and withdrawal cycles have been completed. Humans may emphasize this design feature, in that many more cycles are completed before ejaculation than in many other species such as macaques (and rats, an example of a species in which the male will ejaculate as soon as the hard cervical plug from previous copulation is removed).

5. Correspondingly, if the woman is to take advantage of the sperm retention effect she can use with a new lover, she should not be brought to orgasm by the first thrust or two, but only after the greater part of the thrusting has been completed should she be likely to be brought to orgasm. The woman may actually facilitate this process, by tightening her vagina during most of the thrusting (which would help the potential sperm-removal effect of the thrusting and withdrawal), and relaxing it later on during intercourse, soon before she has an orgasm. If she does have this relaxation later on, this would make it less likely that when the male ejaculates he would remove his own sperm if he keeps moving for a short time, or that she would expel his sperm by muscular contractions.

6. After ejaculation in a woman, a man's thrusting movements should no longer be rewarding (or he would tend to suck out his own sperm), and the penis should shrink quite soon and withdraw slowly so as not to suck out sperm. Moreover, he should not feel like intercourse with that woman for 30–45 min (as that is the time period within which significant amounts of his sperm remain in the vagina, before the flowback). Thus when it occurs after ejaculation, satiety should be rapid, strong, and last for at least the next 30–45 min in men. The reward that rubbing the penis has before ejaculation is described as turning rapidly to being unpleasant or even painful after ejaculation, and this switch from pleasure to pain is what would be predicted by the biological function being performed. That this switch may not be a simple switch controlled only by whether the neural circuitry has recently produced ejaculation is that introduction of a new female (in many animals and in humans) may enable the whole circuitry to be reset, resulting in rapid re-erection, re-initiation of thrusting movements, and the reward or pleasure associated with rubbing the penis, and eventually in ejaculation again in the new female. The adaptive value of this novelty effect (sometimes known as the Coolidge effect after a remark made by President Coolidge of the United States[26]) in potentially enhancing fitness is clear. The sperm competition hypothesis might predict that intercourse with the man's partner would only need to become very rewarding again within about four days, as by this time the woman would need 'topping up' with his sperm (Baker & Bellis 1995).

7. The rapid speed of a first ejaculation by a man into a woman, and the slow last one (which could be useful in conditions such as promiscuous mating, see Baker (1996)) could be due to the satiety mechanism having a longer time-course each time it is successively activated,

[26]The story is that Calvin Coolidge and his wife were touring a farm when Mrs Coolidge asked the farmer whether the continuous and vigorous sexual activity among the flock of hens was the work of only one rooster. The reply was yes."You might point that out to Mr Coolidge", she said. The President then asked the farmer whether a different hen was involved each time. The answer, again, was yes. "You might point that out to Mrs Coolidge", he said.

perhaps as a result of some neural adaptation of the reward relative to the aversive aspects of the stimulation. This could be related to a sensory-specific satiety effect, which would need to be specific to the mate, and to the mating opportunities available.

8. We would predict that it should be rewarding to a man to induce an orgasm in a woman, because of its (probably not consciously realized or intended) biological function of increasing the likelihood, at least under conditions of sperm warfare, that conception of his child would occur. (Such an unconscious function could be a factor that might contribute to the reward value in both men and women of sex without a condom.)

9. In women, orgasm should be particularly likely to occur under conditions when they 'want' (perhaps subconsciously) to conceive, and this does appear to be the case (Singh et al. 1998). For this biological function, particularly in women predisposed to be unfaithful and therefore possibly trying to manipulate using sperm warfare which person they are impregnated by, orgasm might generally be difficult; might not always be stimulated to occur with the regular partner; might be more likely to occur with the lover; and with the lover might be especially stimulated by his ejaculation so that the upsuck effect for his sperm occurs optimally. Neurophysiological predictions are that the reward systems in unfaithful women might (relative to those in faithful women) be less easily activated, but particularly stimulated by novelty, especially by a novel man with genes perceived to be fit. Indeed, women predisposed to be unfaithful may find variety in sex, and sexual adventurousness, especially rewarding. They may always need something new, because they are built to always be looking for better sexual and related stimulation – because this predicts how fit their sons will be. This may extend to the courtship battle, which some believe may have played a role in the rapid evolution of the human brain (see Ridley (1993a)). The argument is that the most creative brains intellectually, musically, and artistically will be successful in having many children with women, because they can provide the variety that unfaithful women are predisposed to want – the variety of all sorts of stimulation is needed to keep an unfaithful woman interested in continuing her relationship with him, and thus in passing his genes into the next generation. The suggestion by G. F. Miller (Miller 1992, Miller 2000b, Ridley 1993a) that brain size has evolved for courtship might be extended to be important also beyond initial courtship, to keeping a partner interested while children are raised.

10. In women, we might expect that refractoriness after orgasm might be stronger for unfaithful women, and to be at least partly sensory-specific (for the male with whom she has just had intercourse), because there may (at least in the past) have been an advantage to females to allow sperm competition to occur, implying intercourse with another male in the not too distant future. This would be less important for women predisposed to be faithful, in whom even multiple orgasms might occur, helping to reward her and her partner (see above) in the mutual relationship.

11. A neurophysiological mechanism operating in a man that made sex with a woman more rewarding if she was relatively novel could contribute to a number of phenomena. It could contribute to make the reward value of a particular woman for a man higher if he has not seen her for some time. The biological function of this is that then the chance is greater that she has had intercourse with another man, and a sperm competition situation, in which speed is of the essence, could be necessary. Evidence that men do have appropriate behaviour for this situation is that the volume a man ejaculates into a particular woman increases with the length of the time since he has last seen her (Baker & Bellis 1995). The same neurophysiological mechanism could contribute to a form of sensory-specific satiety in which even after intercourse and ejaculation with one woman, a man may be quickly aroused again

by another woman. (Possibly it is partly because of this arousing effect of a novel potential lover that the sight of others having intercourse, e.g. in a video, might be arousing. Also possibly related is that the sperm warfare hypothesis might predict that if a man saw someone else having intercourse with his partner, a fit response might be to have intercourse with her too, to promote sperm warfare. However, this would not be an adaptive response if the woman had not yet had an orgasm, and did subsequently have one as a result of the second intercourse.) A similar neurophysiological mechanism could also contribute to making a man wish to have intercourse perhaps every four days, or sooner if he suspects infidelity.

12. There should be at least a small tendency to become attached to (find more rewarding) a person with whom intercourse has occurred (especially if it leads to orgasm in the woman, as described in Section 7.3 on oxytocin). For the woman this is one way of seeking resources for her potential child, by becoming attached to a person who may now be disposed to provide resources to help his genes. For the man such an attachment mechanism is one way of increasing the probability that he will provide for his potential offspring with her, and thus for the success of his genes.

13. The rewards produced by tactile stimulation are such that touch can be rewarding and feel pleasant, and this can occur in situations that are not explicitly sexual as well as in more sexual episodes. One example is grooming in monkeys, which may be rewarding because it serves a number of functions, including removing skin parasites, indicating commitment to another by the investment of time, or by trusting another to touch one, as a preliminary to more sexual touch, etc. Where in the brain is the pleasantness of touch made explicit? Is it in or before the somatosensory cortex of primates, or primarily after this in some of the connected areas such as the insula, orbitofrontal cortex, or amygdala (see Figs. 4.1 and 4.2)? As shown in Chapter 4, one area of the brain in which the pleasantness of touch is made explicit is in a part of the orbitofrontal cortex. The area of the orbitofrontal cortex in which pleasant touch is represented was different from the area in which taste and odour are represented (see Chapter 4). This is an early indication that there may be brain mechanisms specialized for processing the affective or rewarding aspects of touch in humans. Doubtless there will be a number of brain regions in addition to the orbitofrontal cortex where such information is represented. Perhaps one function of the representation in the orbitofrontal cortex is to act as a representation of touch as a primary reinforcer or unconditioned stimulus in stimulus–reinforcement association learning (see Chapter 4). The orbitofrontal representation of pleasant touch may also be involved in the subjective affective feeling produced by the touch, for orbitofrontal cortex damage in humans does blunt the affective component of other affective stimuli such as pain (Melzack & Wall 1996). Aspects of touch that may make it particularly pleasant include slight unpredictability, and a psychological component that reflects what it is one believes is providing the touch, and who is performing the touching. It will be of interest to determine where in the somatosensory system such cognitive influences converge with inputs originating from touch receptors to alter the affective component of the touch.

With regard to tactile stimulation that women may find rewarding in the early stages of a relationship or sexual episode, gentle touch, hugging, and kissing on any part of the body may be rewarding, perhaps as an indicator of caring, protection, and investment of time offered by a man. Because of the importance to a woman of indicators of investment by a man, women also have fantasies and prefer literature that emphasizes romance, commitment, and attachment rather than explicit details of sexual encounters and the physical stimulation being exchanged (Ellis & Symons 1990). Stimulation of the nipples may be rewarding partly to promote the biological function of breast-feeding and attachment. Its sexually arousing effects might be related to the fact that such stimulation may cause the release of the hormone oxytocin, which stimulates movements or contractions of the uterus. The movements might have a biological function in relation to later orgasm and the upsuck effect.

With regard to more explicitly sexual genital stimulation in women, both external (clitoral and vulval) and internal (vaginal, including the G spot on the anterior wall of the vagina) stimulation can be rewarding and pleasant. The possibility that women predisposed to be unfaithful might require more such stimulation to produce an orgasm, might be especially stimulated by a novel lover with fit genes and by novelty in the situation, and might be biased towards finding external as compared with internal stimulation more rewarding has been introduced above, together with the biological functions that might be served by being made differentially sensitive to these different types of reward.

The active control of a sexual episode may be rewarding not only to men (because being in control of sex is likely to make his genes fit), but also particularly to women predisposed to be unfaithful, because they can then determine whether they proceed to intercourse with that particular man, and also whether they receive the right stimulation to have an orgasm with that particular man, with its biological function of controlling the likelihood of conception with that particular man. It is also possible that a lack of control could act as a reward sometimes in some women, because the feeling of being dominated by a particular man could indicate potential fitness in her sons with him (who might be likely to dominate other women).

The reward value that oral sex can have (in both males and females) could be related to the biological function of determining whether the other person is disease-free (using sight, smell, and taste), and, if performed randomly, of detecting infidelity in a partner (by smell, possibly reduced volume of ejaculate from a male, etc.) (Ridley 1993a).

7.10 Brain regions involved in the control of sexual behaviour, and especially in the rewards produced by sexual behaviour

In males, the preoptic area (see Fig. 7.3) is involved in the control of sexual behaviour (Hull, Meisel & Sachs 2002). Lesions of this region permanently abolish male sexual behaviour; electrical stimulation can elicit copulatory activity; metabolic activity is induced (as shown by c-fos) in the preoptic area during copulation; and small implants of testosterone into the preoptic area restore sexual behaviour in castrated rats (Hull et al. 2002, Carlson 2012, Everitt et al. 1989, Everitt 1990, Everitt & Robbins 1992). This region appears to have neurons in it that respond to sex-related rewards in primates, in that Aou, Oomura, Lenard, Nishino, Inokuchi, Minami & Misaki (1984) described some preoptic neurons in the male macaque that increased their firing rates when he could see a female macaque seated on a chair that he could pull towards him. The same neurons did not respond to the sight of food (Y. Oomura, personal communication), and so reflected information about the specific type of reward available. They also described neuronal activity changes in the medial preoptic area of the male monkey that were related to the commencement of sexual behaviour, penile erection, and the refractory period following ejaculation. Similarly, neuronal activity changes in the female medial preoptic area were related to the commencement of sexual behaviour and presentation. Increased neuronal activity in the dorsomedial hypothalamic nucleus in the male monkey and in the ventromedial hypothalamic nucleus in the female monkey were synchronized to each mating act. These findings, and studies using local electrical stimulation, suggested the involvement of medial preoptic area neurons in sexual arousal, and of male dorsomedial hypothalamic and female ventromedial hypothalamic neurons in copulation (Aou, Oomura, Lenard, Nishino, Inokuchi, Minami & Misaki 1984). Further evidence that these brain areas

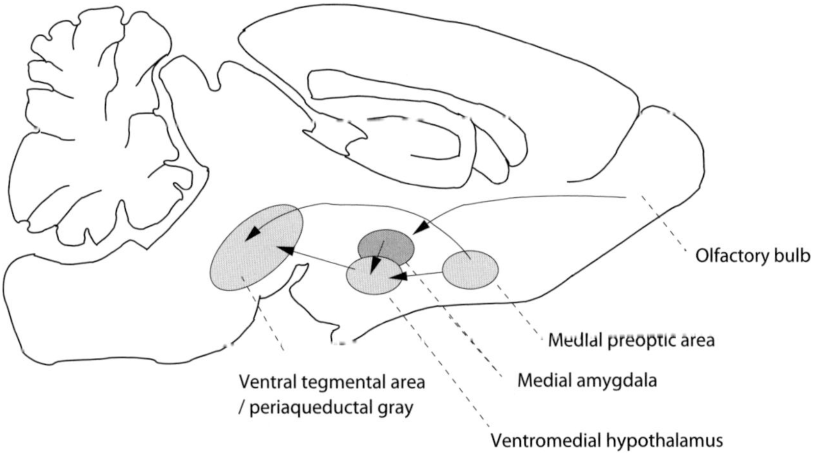

Fig. 7.3 Some of the brain regions implicated in sexual behaviour, shown on a midline view of a rat brain.

are involved in sex-related rewards is that the hormone testosterone affects brain-stimulation reward at some sites in this general region (e.g. in the posterior hypothalamus), but not at sites in, for example, the lateral hypothalamus (Caggiula 1970), where hunger modulates brain-stimulation reward (see Chapter 5).

In females, the medial preoptic area is involved in the control of reproductive cycles. It is probably also involved in controlling sexual behaviour directly (Blaustein & Erskine 2002). Neurons in it and connected areas respond to vagino-cervical stimulation in a hormone-dependent way (Blaustein & Erskine 2002). The ventromedial nucleus of the hypothalamus (VMH) is involved in some aspects of sexual behaviour, including lordosis (standing still in a receptive position) in rodents, and this behaviour can be reinstated in ovariectomized female rats by injections of oestradiol and progesterone into the ventromedial nucleus (Blaustein & Erskine 2002). Outputs from the VMH project to the periaqueductal gray of the midbrain, which is also necessary for female sexual behaviour such as lordosis in rodents (see Carlson (2012)), via descending influences on spinal cord reflexes implemented via the reticular formation neurons and the reticulospinal tracts (Pfaff 1980, Pfaff 1982, Priest & Pfaff 1995) (see Fig. 7.4). The VMH receives inputs from regions such as the medial amygdala.

The preoptic area receives inputs from the amygdala and orbitofrontal cortex, and thus receives information from the inferior temporal visual cortex (including information about face identity and expression), from the superior temporal auditory association cortex, from the olfactory system, and from the somatosensory system. The operation of these circuits has been described in Chapters 4 and 5. In one example described in Section 4.6.3, Everitt et al. (1989) showed that excitotoxic lesions of the basolateral amygdala disrupted appetitive sexual responses maintained by a visual conditioned reinforcer, but not the behaviour to the primary reinforcer for the male rats, copulation with a female rat in heat (see further Everitt (1990) and Everitt & Robbins (1992)). (The details of the study were that the learned reinforcer or conditioned stimulus was a light for which the male rats worked on a FR10 schedule (i.e. 10 responses made to obtain a presentation of the light), with access to the female being allowed for the first FR10 completed after a fixed period of 15 min. This is a second-order schedule of reinforcement.) For comparison, medial preoptic area lesions eliminated the copulatory behaviour of mounting, intromission and ejaculation to the primary reinforcer, the female rat, but did not affect the learned appetitive responding for the conditioned or secondary reinforcing stimulus, the light. The conclusion from such studies is that the amygdala is involved in

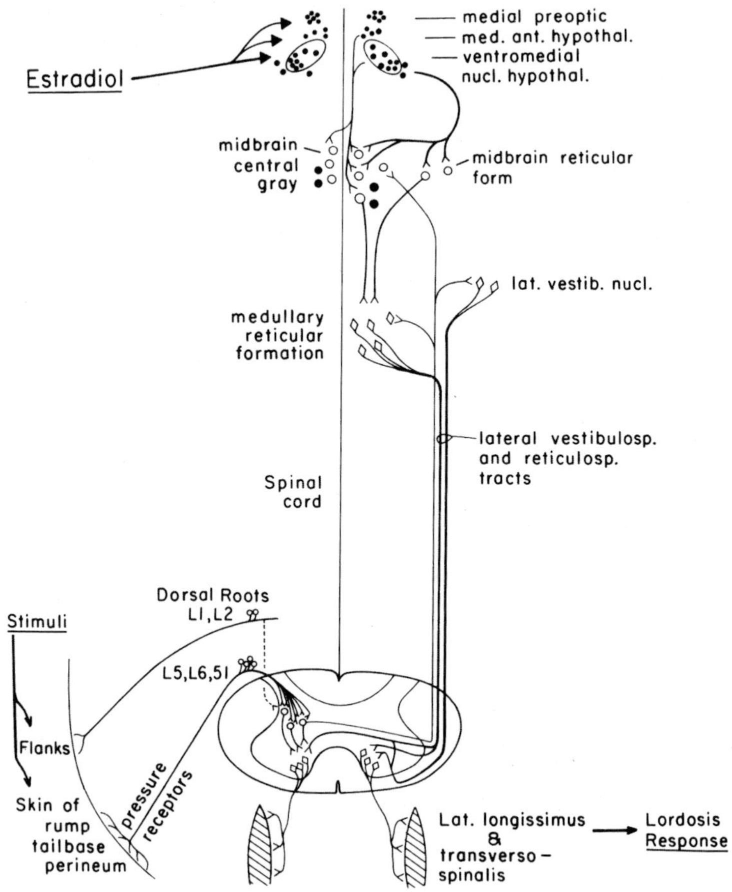

Fig. 7.4 Neural circuitry involved in the lordosis response of the female rat to flank, rump, and perineal stimulation by male rats after she is made sexually receptive by oestrogen (estradiol) in the hypothalamus. (Reproduced from D.W. Pfaff 1980 *Estrogens and Brain Function*, figure 13.1. ©1980, Springer Science and Business Media with kind permission.)

stimulus–reinforcement association learning when the primary reinforcer is a sexual reward. On the other hand, the preoptic area is not involved in such stimulus–reinforcement association learning, but is involved in the rewarding effects of primary sexual rewards. Olfactory inputs reach the medial preoptic area via the medial amygdala and bed nucleus of the stria terminalis, and this pathway provides a route for olfactory stimuli to influence sexual behaviour (Hull et al. 2002). Somatosensory inputs from the genitals also reach the medial preoptic area, via the central tegmental field of the midbrain (Hull et al. 2002).

In an example illustrating part of the importance of the orbitofrontal cortex and of somatosensory reinforcers, evidence from fMRI indicates that the pleasantness of touch is represented especially in the orbitofrontal cortex (see Fig. 4.4). Presumably the pleasant effects of sexual touch are also represented in this and connected brain areas (see, e.g., Tiihonen, Kuikka, Kupila, Partanen, Vainio, Airaksinen, Eronen, Hallikainen, Paanila, Kinnunen & Huttunen (1994)). It is presumably by these neural circuits in the orbitofrontal cortex and amygdala that the effects related to the control of sexual behaviour described above are implemented, and much of the decoding of the relevant stimuli, and then their interpretation as primary reinforcers, or learning about their reinforcing properties by stimulus–reinforcement association learning, occurs. A number of the effects described in Section 7.9 are related to a diminution over time of the reward value produced by the same stimulus or individual, and the enhancement of behaviour produced by novel stimuli or individuals. It is also presumably in regions such as the orbitofrontal cortex and amygdala that such effects, which require a representation of individuals, and systems that can show a form of learning with stimulus repetition to implement sensory-specific satiety and novelty effects, are implemented.

The outputs of the preoptic area include connections to the lateral tegmental field in the midbrain, and in this region neurons are found that respond in relation to different aspects of male sexual behaviour (Shimura & Shimokochi 1990). However, it is likely that only some outputs of the orbitofrontal cortex and amygdala that control sexual behaviour act through the preoptic area. The preoptic area route may be necessary for computationally simple aspects of sexual behaviour such as copulation in males, but the attractive effect of sexual stimuli may survive damage to the medial preoptic area (see Carlson (2012)), suggesting that, as for feeding, outputs of the amygdala and orbitofrontal cortex can influence behaviour through the striatum (see Chapters 4 and 5).

In functional neuroimaging studies in humans (Georgiadis & Kringelbach 2012), a distinction has been suggested between brain areas activated by 'wanting' sexual stimuli, and by 'liking' sexual stimuli, following the distinction suggested by Berridge (1996). First, we can note that 'wanting' corresponds to states related to the expected value of stimuli, and to the conditioned incentive and secondary reinforcing effects of stimuli; and that 'liking' corresponds to the outcome value of stimuli, the more primary rewards. Second, we can note that during the 'anticipatory' or 'wanting' phase, the body is preparing itself physiologically and in terms of actions to obtain the goals of sexual behaviour, and so it is not surprising that the emphasis is on conditioned reinforcers and actions to obtain those conditioned reinforcers, whereas during the consummatory phase, the behavioural responses being made, and the brain regions activated, are different. Third, we can note that although the behaviour required for the anticipatory phase is necessarily different from the behaviour required in the value outcome (or consummatory) phase, the actual goals, the reward value being specified by the genes, may be similar (see Section 4.6.3.4).

In functional neuroimaging studies, activations are sometimes described as being different for sexual arousing stimuli compared to other stimuli in high order areas of the visual cortex (Georgiadis & Kringelbach 2012). However, this does not mean that individual neurons encode the reward value of these sexual stimuli, as the neuroimaging studies could just reflect greater arousal associated with such stimuli modulating activations. For visual stimuli associated with food reward, it has been shown that visual cortex neurons do not encode reward value, in that their responses do not reverse during vidual discrimination reversal (Rolls, Judge & Sanghera 1977). The neuroimaging studies can not address this issue, so must not be over-interpreted. Single neuron studies do show that there are sex anticipation or expected reward value neurons in the primate preoptic area (Aou et al. 1984), which receives from the orbitofrontal cortex and amygdala, and that these neurons do not respond to the sight of food, so in line with other specific reward representations described in Chapter 4, there are also sex reward value specific neurons in primates, and on that basis they are likely to be present in humans too. In the neuroimaging studies, activations to these expected sex reward value or anticipatory stimuli are found in the orbitofrontal cortex (including in men strong activation to women with biologically optimal waist-to-hip ratios), anterior cingulate cortex, and amygdala, and regions to which they project as outputs such as the ventral striatum and hypothalamus (Georgiadis & Kringelbach 2012), but the neuroimaging studies do not address the specificity of the sex-related reward vs other reward-related responses, as the activity of thousands of neurons is imaged in any voxel, and the coding of reward specificity is at the neuronal level (which is the computationally relevant level), as shown in Chapter 4. In the pregenual cingulate cortex activations are more related to erotic images including images of single nudes (probably reflecting its expected reward value inputs from the orbitofrontal cortex), whereas responses more posteriorly towards the midcingulate cortex tended to be associated with penile responses or long blocks of explicit video-type sexual visual stimuli (reviewed by Georgiadis & Kringelbach (2012)), consistent with it being a more action or motor related area (Section 4.7). Dopamine pathways project into the ventral striatum, and interestingly variations in dopamine-related genes both predict ventral striatum responsivity and sexual motivation, the latter indicated by reports about the number of sexual partners and age of first sexual intercourse (see review by Georgiadis & Kringelbach (2012)).

Also interestingly, when women look at male faces this leads to an increase in activity in the medial orbitofrontal cortex/ventromedial prefrontal cortex during the late follicular phase (when women are fertile) relative to the luteal phase. This activity is correlated with the perceived attractiveness as well as individual estradiol to progesterone ratio (Rupp & Wallen 2009), suggesting a key role for the orbitofrontal cortex in mate selection.

During orgasm (which might be thought of as the reward outcome phase of sexual behaviour), there is in women a strong activation of the orbitofrontal cortex, which correlates with the subjective pleasure (Georgiadis, Kortekaas, Kuipers, Nieuwenburg, Pruim, Reinders & Holstege 2006) (see also Georgiadis & Kringelbach (2012)). This is consistent with the representation of the outcome value of other specific rewards in the orbitofrontal cortex, but by different neurons (Chapter 4).

During early development in males, the steroid hormone testosterone masculinizes the brain, and the effects produced include sexual dimorphism in a part of the preoptic area, which is larger in males than females (Morris, Jordan & Breedlove 2004). Before birth, boys and girls already differ hormonally. At about week 7 of human gestation, the testes begin to produce hormones, resulting in a substantial sex difference in testosterone concentrations (Hines 2010). This sex difference appears to be maximal between approximately weeks 8 and 24 of gestation. In regard to children's play, evidence from studies of genetic disorders, of maternal treatment with hormones, and of normal variability in hormones all point to the same conclusion: testosterone concentrations prenatally influence children's subsequent sex-typed toy, playmate and activity preferences (Hines 2010). A consistent finding is that girls exposed to unusually high levels of androgens prenatally, owing to congenital adrenal hyperplasia, show increased male-typical play and reduced female-typical play. Similarly, children whose mothers took androgenic progestins during pregnancy show increased male-typical toy and activity preferences, whereas the opposite is the case for children whose mothers took anti-androgenic progestins (Hines 2010). The effects of the early hormone environment also extend to personality characteristics that show sex differences. Probably the best-established links in this area involve empathy, which is typically higher in females, and physical aggression, which is typically higher in males (Hines 2010).

During puberty there are many changes in sexual behaviour, and associated with these some changes in brain connectivity and function occur, in for example the amygdala, prefrontal cortex, and striatum, but much remains to be understood, including to what extent these changes are steroid-dependent (Sisk & Foster 2004).

Much research remains to be performed to understand the details of the implementation of the rewards underlying sexual behaviour described earlier in this chapter in brain regions such as the amygdala, orbitofrontal cortex, preoptic area, and hypothalamus.

7.11 Conclusion

We can conclude this chapter by remembering that there is some evidence on how the brain produces sexual behaviour by being sensitive to certain rewards, and that reward systems for rewards of the type described in Section 7.9 may have been built in the brain by genes as their way of increasing their fitness. It will be interesting to know how these different reward systems actually operate in the brain. In any case, the overall conclusion is that genes do appear to build reward systems that will lead to behaviour that will enhance their own survival in future generations. The issue of the role of reward (and punishment) systems in brain design by genetic variation and natural selection is described in Chapter 3.

8 Decision-making mechanisms

8.1 Introduction

We have seen in Chapter 4 how the reward value of stimuli is represented on a continuous scale in the orbitofrontal cortex. For example, the firing rate of orbitofrontal cortex neurons with food-related responses decreases steadily as monkeys are fed to satiety, and similarly, activations in the medial orbitofrontal cortex to food become smaller as humans are fed to satiety, and indeed the activations are linearly related to the subjective pleasure (measured by the pleasantness rating on every trial) produced by the taste or flavour of food. Similarly, activations in the human orbitofrontal cortex are correlated with how much money is won on a trial.

However, we almost always need to choose between different rewards that may be available, that is between different stimuli that produce different emotional states. How do we compare the reward values, and take a decision for one of the rewards on each occasion? It is very important that we make a real choice on a particular occasion, for the medieval tale told by Duns Scotus was of a donkey situated between two equidistant delicious food rewards that might never make a decision and might starve. The implication is that on each particular occasion, even if the rewards are almost equal, there has to be a mechanism in the brain to make a definite and fast choice on one trial, and then stay with that choice until the reward is obtained. Staying with a choice is adaptive, for if we took a decision and then changed our minds and kept dithering, we might never get the reward, which might disappear, or be gained by others. That also underlines that there is often adaptive value in having a decision-making mechanism that operates fast. Another desirable property of the decision-making process might be that some probabilistic component to the decision-making might be advantageous, for if we occasionally sample an option that on average has not paid off as well as another, we would be able to discover whether the rewards available for different choices had changed, which is likely to apply often in the real world [27]. Another desirable property of the decision mechanism is that it should be separate from the system that represents the reward value on a continuous scale, for at the same time that we can report on the continuous value of two rewards, we can make a decision on an individual trial to choose one or the other. This implies separate representations. Separate representations may also be useful because the inhibitory neurons need to respond differently for these two types of process. Another desirable property is that once a decision has been made about the goal that is chosen, it is likely to be useful to maintain that decision as a short-term memory, as it is then the goal for actions that need to be organized and performed over time to obtain the chosen goal. We will see that all of these are properties of the biologically plausible approach to decision-making described here.

In this chapter, a biologically plausible model of decision-making is described, and it is shown how it can be used to help understand decision-making mechanisms in the brain. Section 8.7 considers confidence in decisions that have been made, even before feedback about the decision is provided in a particular trial, and how decisions may be corrected if decision

[27]To the extent that decision-making by other individuals is probabilistic, then checking options that may not have worked earlier is likely to be another part of the adaptive value of sometimes, probabilistically, choosing the less favoured option.

confidence is low. Other, phenomenal, models of decision-making that provide mathematical models that attempt to capture the phenomena but without a biological implementation of the mechanisms are described in Section B.1.1. Rate models that move towards a firing rate description of decision-making are described in Section B.1.2. Section B.1.3 contains a more advanced discussion of the more biologically plausible integrate-and-fire model described in this chapter. The equations for its integrate-and fire implementation are provided in Section B.4 (see also Wang (2002), Deco & Rolls (2006); and *The Noisy Brain* (Rolls & Deco 2010) for a fuller treatment of stochastic neurodynamics. Sections B.5 and B.6 describe the mean-field implementation. The role of synaptic facilitation in sequential decision-making is considered in Section B.2. Decision-making where the responses must be postponed after the evidence for the decision has been made available is considered in Section B.3.

8.2 Decision-making in an attractor network

8.2.1 An attractor decision-making network

Consider the architecture shown in Fig. 8.1a. A set of cortical neurons has recurrent collateral excitatory synaptic connections w_{ij} from the other neurons. The evidence for decision 1 is applied via the λ_1 inputs, and for decision 2 via the λ_2 inputs. The synaptic weights w_{ij} have been associatively modified during training in the presence of λ_1 and at a different time of λ_2. The Hebbian or associative synaptic modification is such that if the presynaptic terminal and the postsynaptic neuron are simultaneously active, the synaptic connections become stronger. There are inhibitory neurons (not shown in Fig. 8.1a) which keep the total firing in the network within bounds, and in fact implement competition between the neuronal populations. As a result of the associative synaptic modification (specified in Equation A.13), there are strong connections within the set of neurons activated by λ_1, and strong connections within the set of neurons activated by λ_2. These strengthened synapses provide positive feedback, so that if the whole or part of λ_1 is applied, that set of neurons becomes active, and maintains its activity for a long period even when the input λ_1 is removed. The neurons activated by λ_1 if firing inhibit the neurons activated by λ_2 through the inhibitory interneurons, so that just one population wins the competition and maintains its activity. This thus provides a model of memory, and its retrieval. This is called an attractor network, because a subset of the neurons within either population is sufficient to attract the system into a state in which all the neurons in that population are active, by using the strengthened recurrent collateral connections. The properties of attractor or autoassociation networks are described in Section A.3 and elsewhere (Hertz et al. 1991, Rolls 2008b, Hopfield 1982).

For decision-making, when λ_1 and λ_2 are applied simultaneously, each attractor competes through the inhibitory interneurons (not shown), until one wins the competition, and the network falls into one of the high firing rate attractors that represents the decision. When the network starts from a state of spontaneous firing, the biasing inputs encourage one of the attractors to gradually win the competition, but this process is influenced by the Poisson-like firing (spiking) of the neurons, so that which attractor wins is probabilistic. (Poisson-like indicates that the firing times are random for a given mean firing rate.) If the evidence in favour of the two decisions is equal, the network chooses each decision probabilistically on 50% of the trials. The model shows how probabilistic decision-making could be implemented in the brain. The model also shows how the evidence can be accumulated over long periods of time because of the integrating action of the attractor short-term memory network, with the recurrent collaterals feeding back information to be combined with the continuing inputs λ_1 and λ_2. The model produces shorter reaction or decision times as a function of the magnitude

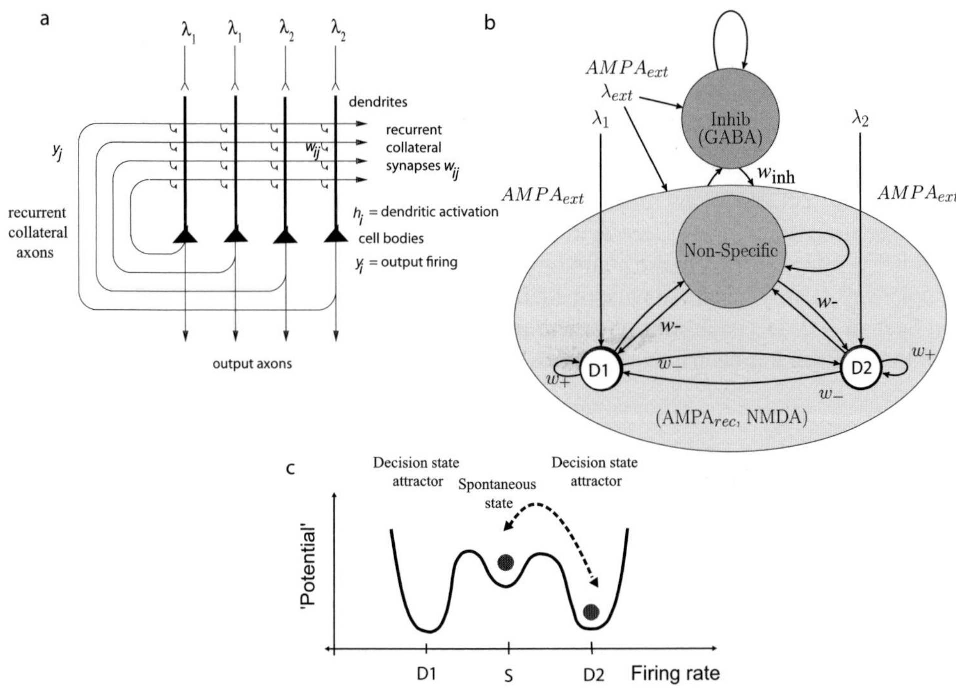

Fig. 8.1 (a) Attractor or autoassociation single network architecture for decision-making. The cell body of each neuron is shown as a triangle (like a cortical pyramidal cell), the dendrite is vertical, and receives recurrent collateral synaptic connections $w_{\rm ij}$ from the other neurons. The evidence for decision 1 is applied via the λ_1 inputs, and for decision 2 via the λ_2 inputs. The synaptic weights w_{ij} have been associatively modified during training in the presence of λ_1 and at a different time of λ_2. When λ_1 and λ_2 are applied, each attractor competes through the inhibitory interneurons (not shown), until one wins the competition, and the network falls into one of the high firing rate attractors that represents the decision. The noise in the network caused by the random spiking times of the neurons (for a given mean rate) means that on some trials, for given inputs, the neurons in the decision 1 (D1) attractor are more likely to win, and on other trials the neurons in the decision 2 (D2) attractor are more likely to win. This makes the decision-making probabilistic, for, as shown in (c), the noise influences when the system will jump out of the spontaneous firing stable (low energy) state S, and whether it jumps into the high firing state for decision 1 (D1) or decision 2 (D2). (b) The architecture of the integrate-and-fire network used to model decision-making (see text). The synaptic weights between the neural populations (decision pools D1 and D2, the nos-specific pool, and the inhibitory pool are 1 except where indicated. In particular, the recurrent weights, indicated by a recurrent arrow, between the neurons within an attractor decision-making pool have strong weights w_+, and between the different pools have the weak strength w_-. (c) A multistable 'effective energy landscape' for decision-making with stable states shown as low 'potential' basins. Even when the inputs are being applied to the network, the spontaneous firing rate state is stable, and noise provokes transitions from the low firing rate spontaneous state S into the high firing rate decision attractor state D1 or D2. If the noise is greater, the escaping time to a decision state, and thus the decision or reaction time, will be shorter (see Rolls and Deco 2010). (See colour plates section.)

of the difference between the evidence for the two decisions: difficult decisions take longer, partly because the firing rates take longer to reach a decision threshold if the difference between the inputs is small.

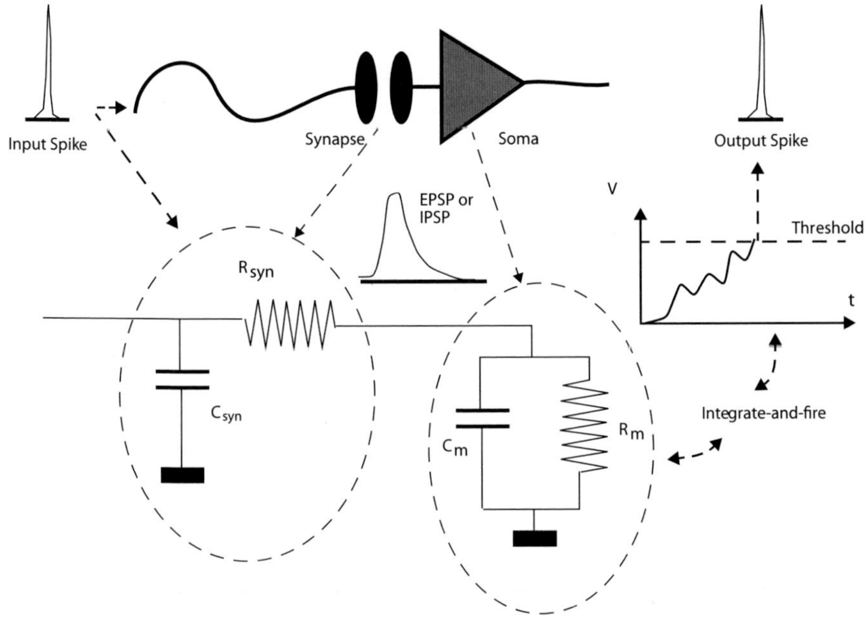

Fig. 8.2 Integrate-and-fire neuron. The basic circuit of an integrate-and-fire model consists of the neuron's membrane capacitance C_m in parallel with the membrane's resistance R_m (the reciprocal of the membrane conductance $g_{\rm m}$) driven by a synaptic current with a conductance and time constant determined by the synaptic resistance $R_{\rm syn}$ (the reciprocal of the synaptic conductance g_j) and capacitance $C_{\rm syn}$ shown in the figure. These effects produce excitatory or inhibitory postsynaptic potentials, EPSPs or IPSPs. These potentials are integrated by the cell, and if a threshold $V_{\rm thr}$ is reached a δ-pulse (spike) is fired and transmitted to other neurons, and the membrane potential is reset. (Reproduced from Gustavo Deco and Edmund T. Rolls, Attention and working memory: a dynamical model of neuronal activity in the prefrontal cortex, *European Journal of Neuroscience*, 18 (8) pp. 2374–2390, Copyright ©2003, John Wiley and Sons.)

8.2.2 An integrate-and-fire implementation of the attractor network for probabilistic decision-making

Because cortical neurons have almost random firing times for a given mean firing rate, i.e. the firing times follow approximately a Poisson distribution (Rolls & Treves 2011), the mean firing rates over short periods (e.g. 20–100 ms) of all the neurons in one of the decision-making populations may be higher than in the other population. These are referred to as statistical fluctuations. These fluctuations can result in the mean rate of one decision population increasing more than the other on a single trial, and influencing which decision is taken on that trial. To model these neuronal spiking time related fluctuations, we need an implementation of the decision-making network that incorporates spiking times. A simple such model is an integrate-and-fire model, which models the synapses and the membrane potentials as dynamical variables, and then produces a spike (not itself modelled to keep the implementation simple) which is then transmitted to the other neurons.

A leaky integrate-and-fire neuron along the lines just introduced can be modelled as shown schematically in Fig. 8.2. The model describes the depolarization of the membrane potential V (which typically is dynamically changing as a result of the synaptic effects described below between approximately –70 and –50 mV) until threshold $V_{\rm thr}$ (typically –50 mV) is reached when a spike is emitted and the potential is reset to $V_{\rm reset}$ (typically –55 mV). The membrane time constant $\tau_{\rm m}$ is set by the membrane capacitance $C_{\rm m}$ and the membrane leakage conductance $g_{\rm m}$ where $\tau_{\rm m} = C_{\rm m}/g_{\rm m}$. Changes in the membrane potential V (see right of Fig. 8.2) are produced by the input spikes operating through the dynamically modelled synapses (left of Fig. 8.2). There are very many such synapses, and the input currents produced from all these synapses result in excitatory postsynaptic potentials (EPSPs) and inhibitory postsynaptic potentials (IPSPs) that are summed by the integrate-and-fire neuron. When the threshold for firing is reached by the membrane potential V, a spike is emitted. The equations for the implementation are given in Section B.4.

An attractor network model of decision-making using integrate-and-fire neurons was developed by Wang (2002), based on a neurodynamical model introduced by Brunel & Wang (2001). The model has been extended and successfully applied to several experimental paradigms including attention and short-term memory as well as decision-making (Rolls & Deco 2002, Deco & Rolls 2002, Deco & Rolls 2003, Deco & Rolls 2004, Deco, Rolls & Horwitz 2004, Szabo, Almeida, Deco & Stetter 2004, Deco & Rolls 2005c, Deco & Rolls 2006, Wang 2008, Rolls, Grabenhorst & Deco 2010b, Rolls, Grabenhorst & Deco 2010c, Rolls & Deco 2010, Smerieri, Rolls & Feng 2010, Deco, Rolls & Romo 2010, Rolls & Deco 2011b, Rolls 2012b, Martinez-Garcia, Rolls, Deco & Romo 2011, Rolls, Dempere-Marco & Deco 2013). In this framework, probabilistic decision-making is modelled by an attractor single network organized into a discrete set of neuronal populations or pools, as illustrated in Fig. 8.1b. The network contains $N_{\rm E}$ (excitatory) pyramidal cells and $N_{\rm I}$ inhibitory interneurons. In the simulations, we often use $N_{\rm E} = 800$ and $N_{\rm I} = 200$, consistent with the neurophysiologically observed proportion of 80% pyramidal cells versus 20% interneurons (Abeles 1991, Rolls & Deco 2002) for a network with 1000 neurons, but effects of the number of neurons N in the network can be investigated. The neurons are fully connected (with synaptic strengths that are 1.0 unless specified otherwise). In the network illustrated in Fig. 8.1b, there are two decision-making populations, D1 and D2, each with 10% of the excitatory neurons, but the number of decision populations can be altered as needed. The recurrent synaptic connections within a decision population (indicated by the recurrent arrows in Fig. 8.1b) have a high strength of w_+ (typically 2.1), so that the population is self-sustaining in its activity, once started, and is at a biologically realistic firing rate. The remainder of the excitatory neurons are in a non-specific pool (NS), which represent other neurons in the cortex that are not involved in the particular task but fire spontaneously and contribute to the background noise (randomness) caused by the Poisson-like firing of the integrate-and-fire neurons. Their connections to the decision-making pools and the connections between the different decision-making pools are set to a value w_- which is calculated as a fraction of w_+ to make the total excitation in the network constant so that it balances the inhibition and produces a mean spontaneous firing rate for all the excitatory neurons of 3 spikes/s when no inputs λ_1 etc. have been applied (Brunel & Wang 2001, Wang 2002, Deco & Rolls 2006). A typical value for w_- is 0.86. These synaptic connection strengths are prescribed, but are generally consistent with a Hebbian associative learning process, in which synapses are strengthened when there is both presynaptic and postsynaptic activity (Equation A.13). In this way, the synapses between neurons within a decision-making pool, which tend to be firing at the same time due to the λ inputs, are strong, and the synapses between neurons in different pools, which tend to be active at different times, are weaker.

All the excitatory synapses between the excitatory neurons use glutamate as a transmitter and have short time constant ($\tau_{\rm AMPA}$=10 ms) receptors that open ion channels, and long time constant ($\tau_{\rm NMDA}$=100 ms) receptors that open voltage-dependent ion channels, both of which inject currents into a neuron and produce depolarization in the direction of the firing threshold. (Details are provided in Section B.4, and further background to these networks is provided by Rolls (2008b) and Rolls & Deco (2010).) The inclusion of the long time constant NMDA receptors in the model helps to maintain the persistence of the high firing rate attractor state (Wang 1999), and also prevents gamma oscillations, which arise only if the NMDA receptor contribution is insufficient (Brunel & Wang 2003, Rolls, Webb & Deco 2012, Wang 2010). [I hypothesize that in evolution the NMDA to AMPA channel conductance ratios have been set to a level that minimizes gamma oscillations consistent with the need to allow AMPA to be sufficiently strong to ensure rapid processing into attractor states (Battaglia & Treves 1998, Panzeri, Rolls, Battaglia & Lavis 2001).] The inhibitory neurons use GABA as a transmitter which hyperpolarizes the neurons, with the strength of w_{inh} typically 1.0 (Fig. 8.1b).

The evidence λ_1 for decision 1 is applied to pool D1 through 800 synapses onto each neuron, and the evidence λ_2 for decision 2 is applied to pool D2 in the same way (Fig. 8.1b). The same sets of 800 synapses on every neuron in the network also receive external inputs at a rate λ_{ext}=3 spikes/s, a typical firing rate for the spontaneous activity of cortical neurons, to reflect background activity from other cortical areas. The distribution of these inputs onto each neuron over time is what would be produced by Poisson spikes trains at 3 spikes/s on each of the 800 externally connected synapses onto each neuron, and this is one of the sources of noise in the network. Another of the sources of noise (randomness) in the network is the almost Poisson distributed spike times of the neurons in the network. As the network become larger and approaches an infinite number of neurons, the statistical fluctuations caused by this source of noise in the network become smoothed out and disappear, as described in more detail later.

8.3 Mean-field analysis of the attractor decision-making network

An advantage of this integrate-and-fire model is that it has a mean-field equivalent (Wang 2002, Brunel & Wang 2001, Rolls & Deco 2010). This approach used in theoretical physics applies to an infinite size system (i.e. an infinite number of neurons) in which the statistical fluctuations due to the randomness in the firing times of individual neurons have averaged out. (The statistical fluctuations in a finite size system are referred to as finite size noise, and increase as the system becomes smaller.) One advantage of analysing the system with this mean field analysis is that the effects of the parameters in the system on the steady states that it can reach (its fixed points), and where changes in the parameters make it change from one state to another (the phase boundaries) can be determined. This is very useful to for example select the synaptic weight values in the system that will produce the required stable states, for example a maintenance of a decision in short-term memory once the decision has been taken. The mean field analysis can show this without any noise due to the statistical fluctuations, and this allows a fast and accurate investigation of the effects of different parameter values. The mean field analysis does not describe the dynamics of the system, just the states that it can reach from different starting points, whether those states are stable, the firing rates of the neurons when in these states, etc. The details of the mean field analysis are provided in Sections B.5 and B.6. Extensions of the mean field analysis to help analyse a system with noise are developed in the Appendix of *The Noisy Brain* (Rolls & Deco 2010).

The essence of the mean-field approximation is to simplify the integrate-and-fire equations by replacing after the diffusion approximation (Tuckwell 1988, Amit & Brunel 1997, Brunel & Wang 2001), the sums of the synaptic components by the average D.C. component and a fluctuation term. The stationary dynamics of each population can be described by the *population transfer function*, which provides the average population rate as a function of the average input current. The set of stationary, self-reproducing rates ν_i for the different populations i in the network can be found by solving a set of coupled self-consistency equations using the formulation derived by Brunel & Wang (2001) (see Section B.5). The

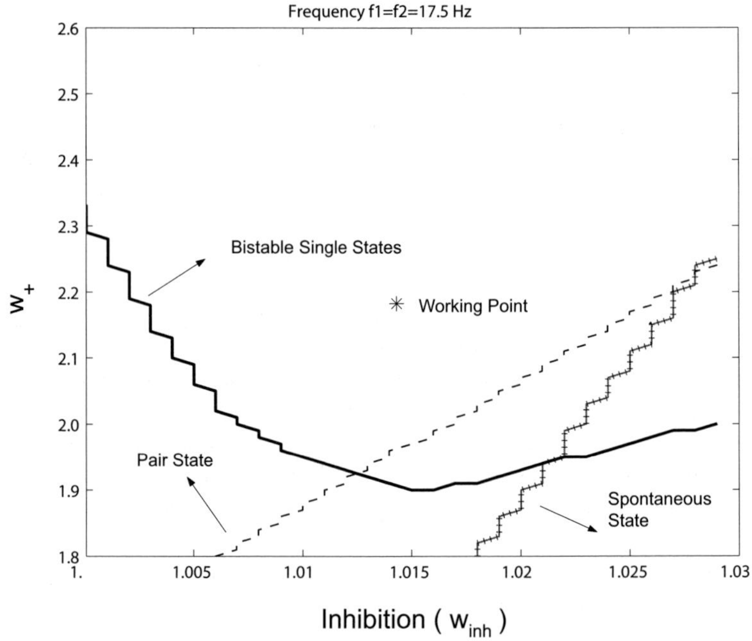

Fig. 8.3 Mean-field analysis to determine suitable values of the synaptic weights for the decision-making network. The bifurcation diagram is for the particular case where the behavioural decision-making is at chance due to λ_1 and λ_2 being equal and low. The diagram shows how the stable states of the average firing rate vary as a function of the synaptic strengths w_+ and w_{inh}. (The label f1=f2=17.5 Hz refers to the low frequency of vibrotactile stimulation being modelled.) The different regions where single states, a pair state, and a spontaneous firing rate state are stable are shown, as described in the text. 'Bistable Single State' refers to the region of the space where the system can maintain one of the possible two high firing rate states active, but not both, so is in a decision-making regime. The working point for the separate integrate-and-fire simulations was chosen as the working point in this diagram, with a connectivity in the network given by w_+=2.2 and w_{inh}=1.015. (Reproduced from Gustavo Deco and Edmund T. Rolls, Decision-making and Weber's law: a neurophysiological model, *European Journal of Neuroscience*, 24 (3) pp. 901–916, Copyright ©2006, John Wiley and Sons.)

equations governing the activities in the mean-field approximation can hence be studied by standard methods of dynamical systems. The formulation departs from the equations describing the dynamics of one neuron to reach a stochastic analysis of the mean-first passage time of the membrane potentials, which results in a description of the population spiking rates as functions of the model parameters, in the limit of very large N, the number of neurons in the network.

To investigate how the stable states depend on the connection parameters w_+ and w_{inh}, Deco & Rolls (2006) solved the mean-field equations for particular values of these parameters starting at different initial conditions. For example, to investigate the stability of the state described by population D1 being in an active state and all other populations inactive, we initialized the system with that population at 10 Hz, all other excitatory populations (including the non-specific ones) at 3 Hz, and the inhibitory population at 9 Hz. If and only if, after solving the equations numerically, the population D1 is still active (meaning that they have a firing rate $\geq$10 Hz) but no other excitatory population is active, we conclude that the state is stable. This procedure is then repeated for all other combinations of w_+ and w_{inh} to find the region where the active population D1 is stable. The stable regions of the other states are found in the same way.

An example of the use of a mean-field analysis to determine the operating regime of the decision-making network is provided in Fig. 8.3. This presents the bifurcation diagrams for a particular case where the behavioural decision-making is hardest and is in fact purely random (i.e. at chance) because λ_1 (here f1) and λ_2 (here f2) are equal and small. Figure 8.3 shows how the stable states of average firing vary as a function of the strength of w_+ and w_{inh} for the case: f1=f2=17.5 Hz of vibrotactile stimulation in the study by Deco & Rolls (2006). To the lower right of the red zig-zag line in Fig. 8.3 is a region labelled 'Spontaneous State' where only the spontaneous firing rate state was stable, and no high firing rate attractor state was possible, because w_+ was too low and w_{inh} was too high. In the region of the space above all the lines that is labelled 'Bistable Single State', the system can maintain one of the possible two high firing rate states active, but not both, so is in a decision-making regime. 'Bistable' in this context refers to the fact that the spontaneous firing rate state was also a stable state, even when the decision cues λ_1 and λ_2 were being applied. Because this was the decision-making region of the parameter space, the values for w_+ and for w_{inh} that were chosen were those indicated by the * labelled 'Working Point'. These values were chosen in the sense that they were used in the later integrate-and-fire simulations performed as part of the same investigation (Deco & Rolls 2006). The integrate-and-fire simulations were necessary, because it was only with these that the probabilistic decision-making could be investigated, because the probabilistic behaviour on a single trial was the result of the statistical fluctuations in a finite size network of, for example, 1000 neurons. The regions of the space in the lower left of Fig. 8.3 labelled 'Pair State' is where both of the decision pools D1 and D2 could be simultaneously active because the inhibition was low. As this was not a true decision-making system between D1 and D2, the 'Working Point' was not chosen in this region.

Figure 8.3 also shows very large regions of stability around the working point, so that the network behaviour described here is very robust.

8.4 Stability, energy landscapes, and noise

In the previous section, I discussed regions of the parameter space where the system is stable. Physicists have developed an analysis of stability in terms of energy landscapes, in which a low energy valley in an energy landscape is a stable state: there is no where further to fall.

The energy analogy was formalized by Hopfield (1982), and can be introduced as follows, with a more detailed treatment provided in *The Noisy Brain* by Rolls & Deco (2010). The stable points of an attractor network can be visualized in an energy landscape (see Fig. 8.1c). The area in the energy landscape within which the system will move to a stable attractor state is called its basin of attraction. The attractor dynamics can be pictured by energy landscapes, which indicate the basins of attraction by valleys, and the attractor states or fixed points by the bottom of the valleys.

The stability of an attractor is characterized by the average time in which the system stays in the basin of attraction under the influence of noise. The noise provokes transitions to other attractor states. One source of noise results from the interplay between the Poissonian character of the spikes and the finite-size effect due to the limited number of neurons in the network (Rolls & Deco 2010).

Two factors determine the stability. First, if the depths of the attractors are shallow (as in the Spontaneous compared to the D1 and D2 valleys in Fig. 8.1c), then less force is needed to move a ball from one valley to the next. Second, high noise will make it more likely that the system will jump over an energy boundary from one state to another. The noise could arise not only from the probabilistic spiking of the neurons which has significant effects in finite size integrate-and-fire networks (Rolls & Deco 2010) including networks with diluted connectivity (Rolls & Webb 2012) and graded firing rates (Webb, Rolls, Deco & Feng 2011), but also from any other source of noise in the brain or the environment (Faisal, Selen & Wolpert 2008), including noise in the stimuli, variations in attention and alertness, the effects of distractors, etc.

Hopfield (1982) defined the energy at a given point in time as being a function of the synaptic weights and the current firing rates as follows

$$E = -\frac{1}{2}\sum_{i,j} w_{ij}(y_i - <y>)(y_j - <y>). \tag{8.1}$$

where y_i is the firing rate of the postsynaptic neuron, y_j is the firing rate of the presynaptic neuron, w_{ij} is the strength of the synapse connecting them, and $<y>$ is the mean firing rate of the neurons. The important concept here is that if two neurons are in the same attractor population and are therefore connected by strong positive synaptic weights, and have high firing rates, then that implies stability, for they excite each other. The system can be described as being in harmony, and without frustration. If that is true for all the neurons within a population, then the energy will be low, which is the effect of the negative sign in Equation 8.1. Hopfield (1982) showed that in the system that he studied, recall can be thought of as moving towards an energy minimum. A decision-making network is effectively performing memory recall with competing inputs, and the same analysis applies. (I note that the system defined by Hopfield had an energy function, in that the neurons were connected by symmetric synaptic weights (produced for example by associative synaptic modification of the recurrent collateral synapses) and there was no self-coupling (Hertz, Krogh & Palmer 1991, Moreno-Bote, Rinzel & Rubin 2007, Hopfield & Herz 1995).[28])

In an attractor network in which a retrieval cue is provided to initiate recall but then removed, a landscape can be defined in terms of the synaptic weights. The retrieval cues of decision variables λ can be thought of as modifying the shape of the energy landscape, as described by Rolls & Deco (2010) in their section 2.3.

The way in which we conceptualize the operation of an attractor network used for noise-driven stochastic decision-making, stimulus detection, etc., is as follows. The noise in the system (caused for example by statistical fluctuations produced by the Poisson-like neuronal firing in a finite-sized system (Rolls & Deco 2010)) produces changes in neuronal firing. These changes may accumulate stochastically, and eventually may become sufficiently large that the firing is sufficient to produce energy to cause the system to jump over an energy barrier (see Fig. 8.1c). Opposing this noise-driven fluctuation will be the flow being caused by the shape and depth of the fixed energy landscape defined by the synaptic weights and the applied external input bias or biases. The noisy statistical fluctuation is a diffusion-like process. If the spontaneous firing rate state is stable with the decision cues applied (see Fig.

[28]The situation is more complicated in an attractor network if it does not have a formal energy function. One such condition is when the connectivity is randomly diluted, for then the synaptic weights between pairs of neurons will not be symmetric. Indeed, in general, neuronal systems do not admit such an energy function. (This is the case in that it is not in general possible to define the flow in terms of the gradient of an energy function. Hopfield defined first an energy function, and from there derived dynamics.) However, such diluted connectivity systems can still operate as attractor systems (Treves 1993, Treves 1991b, Treves 1991a, Treves & Rolls 1991, Treves, Rolls & Simmen 1997, Rolls & Treves 1998, Battaglia & Treves 1998, Rolls & Webb 2012), and the concept of an energy function and landscape is useful for discussion purposes. In practice, a Lyapunov function can be used to prove analytically that there is a stable fixed point such as an attractor basin (Khalil 1996), and even in systems where this can not be proved analytically, it may still be possible to show numerically that there are stable fixed points, to measure the flow towards those fixed points which describes the depth of the attractor basin as we have done for this type of network (Loh, Rolls & Deco 2007a), and to use the concept of energy or potential landscapes to help visualize the properties of the system.

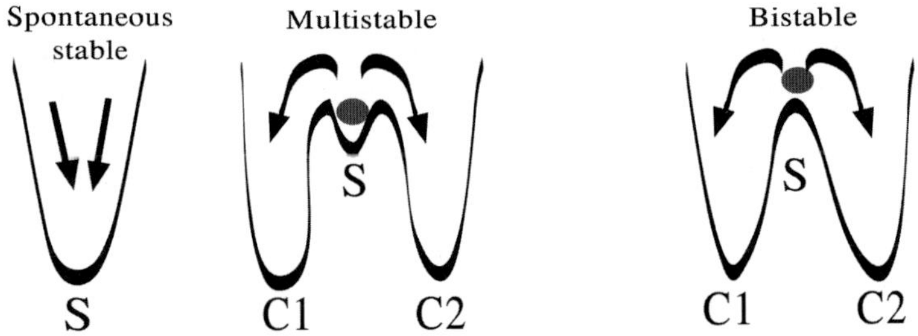

Fig. 8.4 Computational principles underlying the different dynamical regimes of the decision-making attractor network (see text). The x-axis represents the neuronal activity of one of the populations (ν_i) and the landscape represents an energy landscape regulating the evolution of the system. S is a stable state of spontaneous activity, C2 is a high firing rate state of this neuronal population corresponding to the choice implemented by this population, and C1 is a low firing rate state present when the other population wins the competition. Left: a situation in which only the spontaneous state S is stable. This might occur if the external inputs λ_1 and λ_2 are weak. Middle: the population may be either in C1, or in C2, or in a spontaneous state of firing S when no population has won the competition. This can be a scenario even when the decision cues λ_1 and λ_2 are being applied during the decision-making period. This may occur especially if λ_1 and λ_2 are weak. Right: the neuronal population is either in a high firing rate stable state C2, or in a low firing rate state C1 because another population is firing fast and inhibiting our neuronal population. There is no stable spontaneous state. This may occur especially if λ_1 and λ_2 are strong.

8.4), eventually the noise may provoke a transition over the energy barrier in an escaping time, and the system will drop, again noisily, down the valley on the other side of the hill. The rate of change of the firing rate is again measured by the flow, and is influenced by the synaptic weights and applied biases, and by the statistical fluctuations. In this scenario, the reaction times will depend on the amount of noise, influenced by the size of the network, and by the fixed 'effective energy landscape' as determined by the synaptic weights and applied biasing inputs λ, which will produce an escaping time as defined further in the Appendix of Rolls & Deco (2010). We frequently refer to a system in which the spontaneous state as well as a decision state is stable in the absence of noise even when the decision cues are being applied as a 'multistable system'. While in a spontaneous stable state, the system may be thought of as being driven by the noise, and it is primarily when the system has reached a ridge at the edge of the spontaneous valley and the system is close to a bifurcation point into a high firing rate close to the ridge that the attractor system can be thought of as accumulating evidence from the input stimuli (Deco, Scarano & Soto-Faraco 2007). The noise-driven escaping time from the stable spontaneous state is important in understanding long and variable reaction times, and such reaction times are present primarily in the scenario when the parameters make the spontaneous state stable, as described further by Marti, Deco, Mattia, Gigante & Del Giudice (2008) and in Section B.1.3.1.

If the spontaneous state is not stable (see Fig. 8.4 right, the situation mainly analyzed by Wang (2002, 2008)), the reaction times will be influenced primarily by the flow as influenced by the gradient of the energy landscape, and by the noise caused by the random neuronal firings. An escaping time from a stable spontaneous state attractor will not in this situation contribute to the reaction times (Section B.1.3.1).

8.5 Neurophysiology of vibrotactile decision-making

The link between perception and action can be conceptualized by a chain of neural operations, which leads a stimulus to guide behaviour to make a decision to choose a particular action or motor response. For example, when subjects discriminate two stimuli separated by a time interval, the chain of neural operations encompasses mechanisms from the encoding of sensory stimuli, the attentional filtering of relevant features, their maintenance in working memory, to the comparison or decision, which in turn leads to a motor response (Romo & Salinas 2001, Romo & Salinas 2003). A number of neurophysiological experiments on decision-making are providing information on the neural mechanisms involved, by analysing the responses of neurons that correlate with the animal's behaviour (Werner & Mountcastle 1965, Talbot, Darian-Smith, Kornhuber & Mountcastle 1968, Salzman, Britten & Newsome 1990, Kim & Shadlen 1999, Gold & Shadlen 2000, Schall 2001, Hernandez, Zainos & Romo 2002, Romo, Hernandez, Zainos, Lemus & Brody 2002, Romo, Hernandez, Zainos & Salinas 2003, Glimcher 2003, Glimcher 2004, Romo et al. 2004, Smith & Ratcliff 2004, Sugrue, Corrado & Newsome 2005, Gold & Shadlen 2007, Churchland, Kiani & Shadlen 2008, Churchland, Kiani, Chaudhuri, Wang, Pouget & Shadlen 2011).

In this section, I briefly describe a paradigm for studying the mechanisms of decision-making, the vibrotactile sequential discrimination task, because evidence on the neuronal basis is available, and because this has been modelled with the integrate-and-fire attractor model of decision-making described earlier in this chapter (Deco & Rolls 2006). This therefore provides a useful way to introduce the neurophysiological and computational bases of decision-making.

The neuronal substrate of the ability to discriminate two sequential vibrotactile stimuli has been investigated by Romo and colleagues (Romo & Salinas 2001, Hernandez, Zainos & Romo 2002, Romo, Hernandez, Zainos, Lemus & Brody 2002, Romo, Hernandez, Zainos & Salinas 2003, Romo & Salinas 2003, Romo, Hernandez & Zainos 2004, de Lafuente & Romo 2005). They used a task where trained macaques must decide and report which of two mechanical vibrations applied sequentially to their fingertips has the higher frequency of vibration by pressing one of two pushbuttons. This decision-making paradigm requires therefore the following processes: (1) the perception of the first stimulus, a 500 ms long vibration at frequency f1; (2) the storing of a trace of the f1 stimulus in short-term memory during a delay of typically 3 s; (3) the perception of the second stimulus, a 500 ms long vibration at frequency f2; and (4) the comparison of the second stimulus f2 to the trace of f1, and choosing a motor act based on this comparison (f2-f1). The vibrotactile stimuli f1 and f2 utilized were in the range of frequencies called *flutter*, i.e. within approximately 5–50 Hz.

Single neuron recordings in the ventral premotor cortex (VPC) of macaques reveal neurons whose firing rate is dependent only on the difference between the two applied frequencies, the sign of that difference being the determining factor for correct task performance (Romo, Hernandez & Zainos 2004, de Lafuente & Romo 2005). These neurons are only activated during the presentation of f2, with some responding to the condition f1<f2, and others to the condition f1>f2. These neurons, which are shown in figure 2(G, H, I) of Romo, Hernandez & Zainos (2004) (see example in Fig. 8.5), reflect the decision-making step of the comparison. Other VPC neurons encode f1 during both the stimulus presentation and the delay period.

Earlier brain areas provide inputs useful to the VPC. In the primary somatosensory area S1 the average firing rates of neurons in S1 convey information about the vibrotactile frequency f1 or f2 during the stimulation period. (The neuronal responses stop reflecting information about the stimuli immediately after the end of the stimulus.) The firing rates increase monotonically with stimulus frequency (Romo & Salinas 2003). Neurons in the secondary somatosensory area S2 respond to f1 and show significant delay activity for a few hundred milliseconds after the end of the f1 stimulus (Romo et al. 2002). Some neurons have positive and others negative monotonic relationships between their firing rate and the vibrotactile stimulus frequency. During the initial part of f2 (ca. 200 ms) the firing rate reflects either f1 or f2; later, during the last 300 ms, the firing rate reflects the comparison (f2-f1), and therefore the result of the decision. Prefrontal cortex (PFC) neurons (Brody, Hernandez, Zainos & Romo 2003)

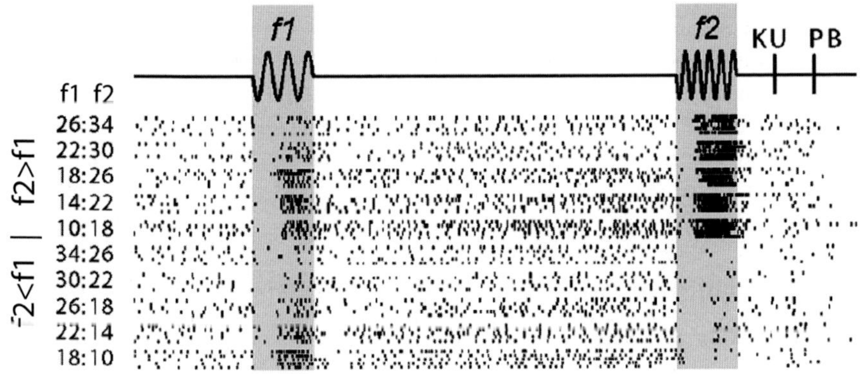

Fig. 8.5 A neuron in the ventral premotor cortex that responded to a vibrotactile stimulus during the f1 stimulation and during the delay period. However, the strongest response was for condition f2 > f1 during the f2 period. In the raster plot, each row of ticks is a trial, and each tick is an action potential. Trials were delivered in random order with 5 trials per stimulus pair shown. The labels on the left show the f1, f2 stimulus pairs for each set of 5 trials illustrated. At KU (key up) the monkey releases the key and presses either a lateral or a medial push button (PB) to indicate whether the comparison frequency (f2) was higher or lower than the base frequency (f1). (Reprinted from *Neuron*, 41 (1), Ranulfo Romo, Adrian Hernandez, and Antonio Zainos, Neuronal Correlates of a Perceptual Decision in Ventral Premotor Cortex, pp. 165–173, Copyright 2004, with permission from Elsevier.)

also have a positive or negative monotonic firing rate relationship with f1. Furthermore, PFC neurons convey information about f1 into the delay period, with some neurons carrying it only during the early part of the delay period (*early neurons*), others only during the late part of the delay period (*late neurons*), and others persistently throughout the entire delay period (*persistent neurons*). During the presentation of the second stimulus f2, PFC neurons also respond like S2 neurons. Some PFC neurons respond as a function of f2 during the initial part of the comparison period, whereas other neurons show a firing rate dependency only on f1 before and at the onset of the second stimulus. In the latter part of the comparison, the firing rate reflects the comparison f2-f1. Medial premotor cortex (MPC) neurons respond similarly to PFC neurons, i.e. MPC neurons respond during f1 itself, with either positive or negative monotonic firing rate relationships, during the late part of the delay period in an f1-dependent manner in the same way as the *late* PFC neurons, and during the comparison period reflecting the comparison f2-f1 (Hernandez et al. 2002).

In summary, in the sequential vibrotactile discrimination task, S1 is predominantly sensory and the primary motor cortex (M1) is predominantly motor. A number of other cortical areas have activity that reflects the encoding, short-term memory, and comparison functions involved, perhaps as a result of information exchange between these cortical areas: the differences between S2, MPC and VPC are reflected mainly in their different latencies. VPC (and MPC) neurons seem to reflect the core of the processing that links sensory information with action, and therefore they may represent the decision-making process itself, rather than the representation of the stimulus. Consequently VPC neurons are excellent candidates for encoding also the probabilistic behavioural response as expressed in Weber's law.

Key questions are how ventral premotor cortex (VPC) neurons (or neurons with similar activity in connected areas such as MPC) implement the decision-making process. What are the principles by which the probabilistic decisions are taken? How is the processing implemented by the neurons? I now show how the model can account for many aspects of the decision-making. The description shows the properties of the decision-making model, and how it can be used to understand decision-making processes in the brain.

Although this is not an example of decision-making between rewards of two different values, the mechanism for different types of decision-making is thought to be generic, and so this example is used to illustrate the generic mechanisms involved in decision-making, with the mechanism being implemented in different cortical areas, in each of which a different type of decision, or for that matter memory recall, or stimulus categorization, is performed.

8.6 Probabilistic decision-making by the integrate-and-fire attractor model

8.6.1 Integrate-and-fire simulations of decision-making

Deco & Rolls (2006) aimed to model the behaviour of the VPC neurons as shown in Fig. 8.5 from Romo, Hernandez & Zainos (2004) which reflect the decision-making performed during the comparison period. Therefore, Deco & Rolls (2006) studied the non-stationary probabilistic behaviour of the spiking network defined in Fig. 8.1, during this comparison period (during the presentation of f2), by stimulating the network simultaneously with f1 and f2. The decision was about whether the frequency of stimulus f1 was greater than f2, for which the decision pool corresponding to D1 in Fig. 8.1b was termed pool (f1>f2), and if stimulus f1 was less than f2 in frequency, then the decision pool corresponding to D2 in Fig. 8.1b was termed (f1<f2). The two stimuli f1 and f2 to be compared were coded into λ_1 and λ_2, respectively, as these encode the two vibrotactile stimuli to be compared.

8.6.2 Decision-making on single trials

Figure 8.6 shows for a single trial a typical time course of the network of VPC neurons during the decision period when the two stimuli are being compared for the case of f1=35 Hz and f2=25 Hz. The top part of Fig. 8.6 plots the time course of the mean firing rate of the populations (f1>f2), (f1<f2), and the inhibitory population. The bin widths used for the simulations were 20 ms. The transition shown corresponds to a correct trial, i.e. a transition to the correct final attractor encoding the result of the discrimination f1>f2. We observe that after 200 ms the populations (f1>f2) and (f1<f2) start to separate in such a way that the population (f1>f2) wins the competition and the network performs a transition to a single-state final attractor corresponding to a correct discrimination (i.e. high activity in the population (f1>f2) and low activity in the population (f1<f2)). The bottom part of Fig. 8.6 plots the corresponding rastergrams of 10 randomly selected neurons for each pool in the network. Each vertical line corresponds to the generation of a spike. The spiking activity shows how the firing makes the transition to the correct final single-state attractor. Further examples of the neuronal decision-making process on individual trials are shown in Figs. 8.7 and 8.14.

Romo et al. (2004) analysed the responses of VPC neurons performing the comparison as a function of both f1 and f2 (and showed the neurophysiological findings in their Figure 2G,H,I, see Fig. 8.5). Figure 8.7 shows the simulation results that correspond to those cases. Figure 8.7A shows rastergrams of a single neuron of the population (f1<f2) during the decision period starting when the f1 and f2 stimuli are applied at time = 0 ms. (The neuron should thus fire at a high rate only on trials when f2 is greater than f1, and data are shown only for correct trials.) The labels on the left indicate the vibrotactile frequencies of the f1, f2 stimulus pairs between which a decision was being made. Each row of ticks is a trial (with 10 trials of the single neuron shown for each case), and each tick is a spike. All neurons were tested with 10 trials per stimulus pair, selecting only trials where the network performed correctly.

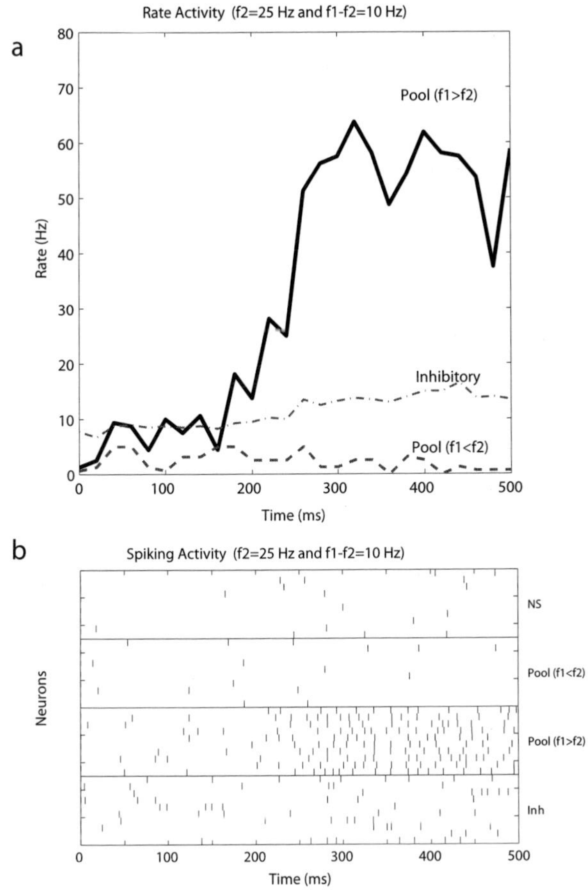

Fig. 8.6 The time course of a decision. The activity of the simulated ventral premotor cortex (VPC) neurons is shown during the decision period for the case of f1=35 Hz and f2=25 Hz. The stimuli were applied continuously starting at time = 0 ms. (a) The time course of the average spiking rate of the populations (f1>f2), (f1<f2), and the inhibitory population. The bin widths used for the simulations were 20 ms. (b) The corresponding rastergrams of 10 randomly selected neurons for each pool in the network. Each vertical line corresponds to the generation of a spike. In the rastergram, NS refers to neurons in the non-specific population, and Inh to neurons in the inhibitory population. The spiking activity shows the transition to the correct final single-state attractor, i.e. a transition to the correct final attractor encoding the result of the discrimination (f1>f2) (see text). (Reproduced from Gustavo Deco and Edmund T. Rolls, Decision-making and Weber's law: a neurophysiological model, *European Journal of Neuroscience*, 24 (3) pp. 901–916, Copyright ©2006, John Wiley and Sons.)

The top 5 cases correspond to a situation where f1<f2 and therefore the population (f1<f2) is highly activated after 100–200 ms. The lower 5 cases correspond to a situation where f1>f2 and therefore the population (f1<f2) is not activated. (The population (f1>f2), not shown in Fig. 8.7, won the competition in the lower 5 cases shown in Fig. 8.7, and therefore inhibited the (f1<f2) population in the correctly discriminated trials selected for this Figure.) Figure 8.7 shows that the firing rate at the end of the simulation period shown, at 250 ms, is high only when f2 is greater than f1, and that the final firing rate on these correct trials is relatively independent of the exact values of f1 and f2 (including the difference between f2 and f1), and responds just depending on the sign of the difference between f2 and f1, reaching a high rate only when f2 is greater than f1.

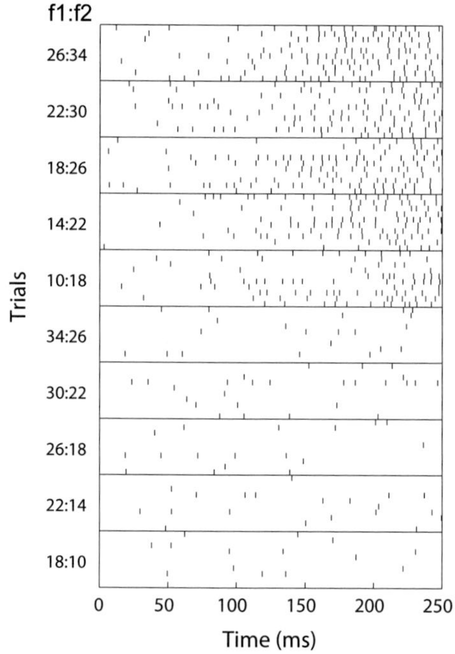

Fig. 8.7 Responses of a single neuron of the population (f1<f2) during the decision period between f1 and f2. The simulations corresponds to the experimental cases measured and studied by Romo et al. (2004) (see figure 2G,H,I of that paper, and Fig. 8.5). The different stimulation cases labelled on the left indicate f1, f2 pairs of the vibrotactile stimulation frequencies. In the rastergrams, each row of ticks is a trial, and each tick is a spike. Ten correct trials are shown for each stimulus pair case. (Reproduced from Gustavo Deco and Edmund T. Rolls, Decision-making and Weber's law: a neurophysiological model, *European Journal of Neuroscience*, 24 (3) pp. 901–916, Copyright ©2006, John Wiley and Sons.))

8.6.3 The probabilistic nature of the decision-making

The decision-making implemented by this attractor model is probabilistic, as can be seen by assessing the performance over many trials.

Figure 8.8 shows the probability of correct discrimination as a function of the difference between the two presented vibrotactile frequencies to be compared. We assume that f1>f2 by a Δ-value, i.e. f1=f2+Δ. (In Fig. 8.8 this value is called 'Delta frequency (f1-f2)'.) Each diamond-point in the Figure corresponds to the result calculated by averaging 200 trials of the full spiking simulations. The criterion for a correct decision was that during the 500 ms comparison period, the network evolved to a 'single-state' attractor that showed a high level of spiking activity (larger than 10 Hz) for the population (f1>f2), and simultaneously a low level of spiking activity for the population (f1<f2) (at the level of the spontaneous activity).

Figure 8.8 shows that the decision-making is probabilistic, and that the probability of a correct discrimination increases as Δf, the difference between the two stimuli being compared, increases. When Δf is 0, the network performs at chance, and its choices are 50% correct. The second panel of Fig. 8.8 shows a good fit between the actual neuronal data described by Romo & Salinas (2003) for the f2=20 Hz condition (indicated by *), and the results obtained with the model (Deco & Rolls 2006).

Figure 8.8 shows in its different panels that correspond to different base vibrotactile frequencies f2, that to reach a threshold of correct classification of for example 85% correct (horizontal dashed line in Fig. 8.8), the difference between f1 and f2 must become larger as

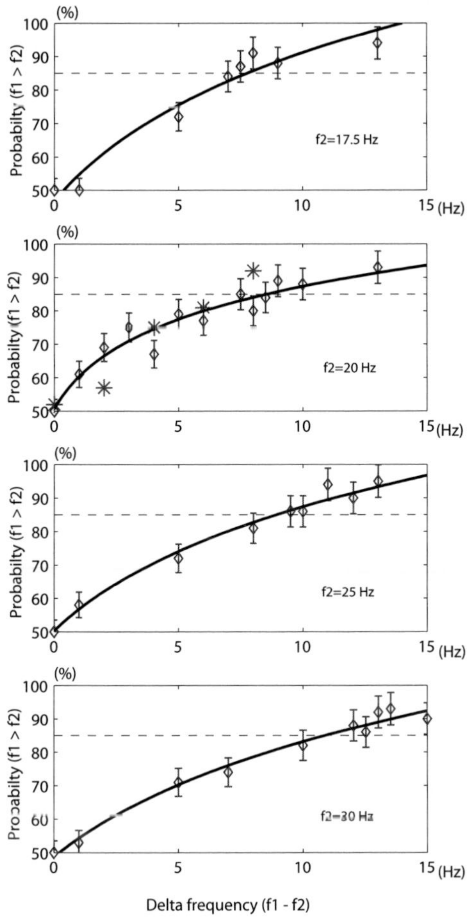

Fig. 8.8 Probability of correct discrimination (± sd) as a function of the difference between the two presented vibrotactile frequencies to be compared. In the simulations, we assume that f1>f2 by a Δ-value (labelled 'Delta frequency (f1-f2)'), i.e. f1=f2+Δ. The points correspond to the trial averaged spiking simulations. The line interpolates the points with a logarithmic function. The horizontal dashed line represents the threshold of correct classification for a performance of 85% correct discrimination. The second panel down includes actual neuronal data (indicated by *) described by Romo and Salinas (2003) for the f2=20 Hz condition. (Reproduced from Gustavo Deco and Edmund T. Rolls, Decision-making and Weber's law: a neurophysiological model, *European Journal of Neuroscience*, 24 (3) pp. 901–916, Copyright ©2006, John Wiley and Sons.)

the base frequency f2 increases.

8.6.4 Probabilistic decision-making and Weber's law

The finding just described, that the difference between the two inputs, λ_1 and λ_2, which we can term $\Delta\lambda$ (sometimes referred to as ΔI when we are considering decisions about stimulus intensity, and also known as the 'difference-threshold' or 'just-noticeable difference' (jnd)), for correct discrimination increases as the stimulus magnitude increases is very interesting, for this reminds one of Weber's Law, a fundamental observation about decision-making. Indeed, Weber's law (enunciated by Ernst Heinrich Weber 1795–1878) states that the ratio of the difference-threshold to the background intensity is a constant. Weber's law is often expressed

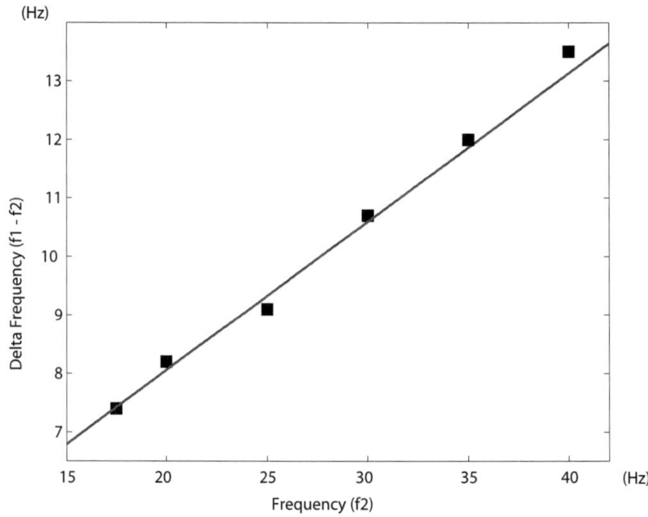

Fig. 8.9 Weber's law for the vibrotactile discrimination task decision-making simulation. The critical discrimination Δ-value ('difference-threshold') is shown corresponding to an 85% correct performance level as a function of the base frequency f2. The 'difference-threshold' increases linearly as a function of the base frequency. (Reproduced from Gustavo Deco and Edmund T. Rolls, Decision-making and Weber's law: a neurophysiological model, *European Journal of Neuroscience*, 24 (3) pp. 901–916, Copyright ©2006, John Wiley and Sons.)

as $\Delta I/I$ is a constant, where I stands for stimulus intensity, and ΔI for the smallest difference of intensity that can just be discriminated.

To assess whether the integrate-and-fire attractor decision-making model can provide an account of Weber's law, Fig. 8.9 plots the critical discrimination Δ-value corresponding to an 85% correct performance level (the 'difference threshold') as a function of the base frequency f2. The 'difference threshold' increases linearly as a function of the base frequency, that is, Δf/f is a constant (Deco & Rolls 2006). This corresponds to Weber's law for the vibrotactile discrimination task. (In the case simulated, the stimuli were vibrotactile frequencies, hence the use of f to denote the frequencies of the stimuli.)

The firing rates of the winning attractor are almost independent of Weber's law, which is not encoded in the firing rates (Deco & Rolls 2006). What is found is just a small increase in the firing rate of the winning attractor as Δf increases, and it is shown in Section 8.7 that this is related to decision confidence.

The model provides insights into the mechanisms by which Weber's law is implemented. We hypothesized that because Δf/f is practically constant in the model, the difference of frequencies Δf required to push the single attractor network towards an attractor basin might increase with f because as f increases, shunting (divisive) inhibition produced by inhibitory feedback inputs (from the inhibitory interneurons) might act divisively on the pyramidal cells in the attractor network to shunt the excitatory inputs f1 and f2. In more detail, as the base frequency f increases, more excitation will be provided to the network by the inputs λ_1 and λ_2, this will tend to increase the firing rates of the pyramidal cells which will in turn provide a larger excitatory input to the inhibitory neurons. This will tend to make the inhibitory neurons fire faster, and their GABA synapses onto the pyramidal cells will be more active. Because these GABA synapses open chloride channels and act with a driving potential $V_I = -70$ mV which is relatively close to the membrane potential (which will be in the range $V_L = -70$ mV to $V_{\rm thr} = -50$ mV), a large part of the GABA synaptic input to the pyramidal cells will

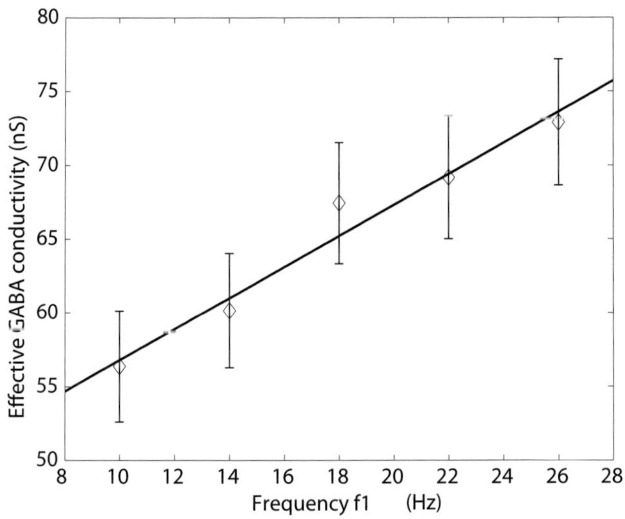

Fig. 8.10 The conductance in nS (mean $\pm$ sd) produced by the GABA inputs to the pyramidal cells as a function of the base frequency f1. The effective conductance produced through the GABA synapses (i.e. $I_{\text{GABA}}/(V - V_{\text{I}})$) was averaged over the time window in which the stimuli were presented in one of the excitatory neuron pools, when the base frequency was f1, and f2-f1 was set to 8 Hz. (Reproduced from Gustavo Deco and Edmund T. Rolls, Decision-making and Weber's law: a neurophysiological model, *European Journal of Neuroscience*, 24 (3) pp. 901–916, Copyright ©2006, John Wiley and Sons.)

tend to shunt, that is to act divisively upon, the excitatory inputs to the pyramidal cells from the vibrotactile biasing inputs λ_1 and λ_2. To compensate for this current shunting effect, f1 and f2 are likely to need to increase in proportion to the base frequency f in order to maintain the efficacy of their biasing effect. To assess this hypothesis, we measured the change in conductance produced by the GABA inputs as a function of the base frequency. Figure 8.10 shows that the conductance increases linearly with the base frequency (as does the firing rate of the GABA neurons, not illustrated). The shunting effect does appear therefore to be dividing the excitatory inputs to the pyramidal cells in the linear way as a function of f that we hypothesized. The inhibitory feedback is mainly divisive because the GABA-activated channels operate primarily as a current shunt, and do not produce much hyperpolarization, given that V_I is relatively close to the membrane potential. After the division implemented by the feedback inhibition, the differential bias required to push the network reliably into one of the attractors must then be larger, and effectively the driving force ($\lambda_1 - \lambda_2$ or $\Delta\lambda$) must get larger in proportion to the inhibition. As the inhibition is proportional to λ, this produces the result that $\Delta\lambda/\lambda$ is approximately a constant. We thus propose that Weber's law, $\Delta I/I$ is a constant, is implemented in part by shunting effects acting on pyramidal cells that are produced by inhibitory neuron inputs which increase linearly as the baseline input I increases, so that the difference of intensities ΔI required to push the network reliably into one of its attractors must increase in proportion to the base input I. Deco & Rolls (2006) therefore proposed that Weber's law is implemented by shunting effects acting on pyramidal cells that are produced by inhibitory neuron inputs which increase linearly as the base frequency increases, so that the difference of frequencies Δf required to push the network reliably into one of its decision attractors must increase in proportion to the base frequency. We checked the excitatory inputs to the pyramidal cells (for which $V_E = 0$ mV), and found that their conductances were much smaller (in the order of 5 nS for the AMPA and 15 nS for the NMDA receptors) than those produced by the GABA receptors, so that it is the GABA-induced conductance changes that

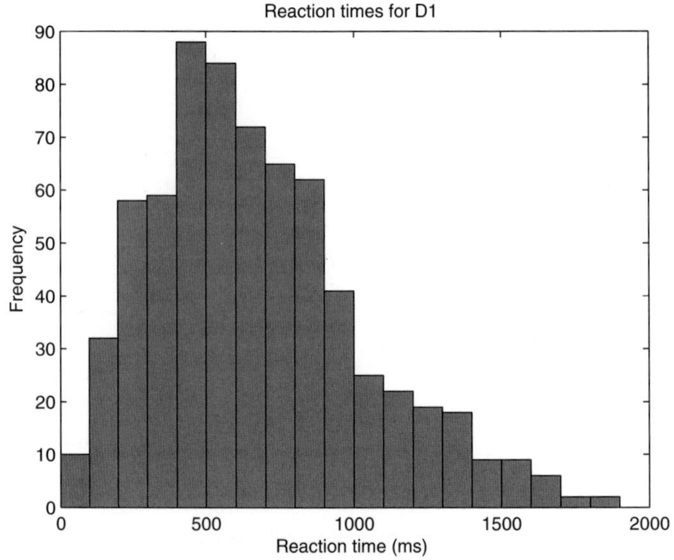

Fig. 8.11 Reaction time distribution for the decision-making attractor network described in Section 8.7. The difference between the two stimuli was relatively small (ΔI=16 Hz, though sufficient to produce 81% correct choices). The criterion for the reaction time was the time after application of both stimuli at which the firing rate of the neurons in the correct attractor became 25 Hz or more greater than that of the neurons in the incorrect attractor, and remained in that state for the remainder of the trial.

dominate, and that produce the shunting inhibition.

Further properties of the attractor network model of decision-making that enable it to implement Weber's law include stability of the spontaneous firing rate condition, even when the decision cues are applied, so that the system depends on the noise to escape this starting state (Deco & Rolls 2006, Rolls & Deco 2010). In addition, behavioural evidence in humans showing Weber's law like behaviour for the decision-making involved in the discrimination of two vibrotactile stimuli suggests that the neurodynamical mechanisms and computational principle underlying this process are consistent with a fluctuation-driven scenario in a multistable regime (Deco et al. 2007).

Weber's law holds in most though not all discrimination situations, and to the extent that Weber's law does generally hold, the model described here provides a computational neuroscience-based account of how it arises. This is the first time when the implementation of a psychophysical law is not the firing rate of the neurons, nor the spike timing, nor is single neuron based, but instead is based on the synaptic connectivity of the network and on statistical fluctuations due to the spiking activity in the network.

8.6.5 Decision times

Because of the noise-driven stochastic nature of the decision-making, the reaction (or decision) times even for one set of parameters vary from trial to trial. An example of the distribution of reaction times of the attractor network is shown in Fig. 8.11. This distribution is for a case when the difference between the two stimuli is relatively small (ΔI = 16 Hz for the simulations described in Section 8.7, though sufficient to produce 81% correct choices). The considerable variability of the reaction times across trials, and the long tail of the probability distribution, provide a very useful basis for understanding the variability from trial to trial that is evident in human choice reaction times (Welford 1980). Indeed, human studies commonly report skewed reaction time distributions with a long right tail (Luce 1986, Ratcliff & Rouder 1998, Ratcliff, Zandt & McKoon 1999, Usher & McClelland 2001, Marti, Deco, Mattia, Gigante & Del Giudice 2008).

The reaction or decision time distribution depends very much on whether the spontaneous state is stable when the decision cues are being applied (Section B.1.3.1). In the 'multistable regime', with a stable spontaneous state apart from the noise, the reaction time is dominated by the statistical fluctuations, and has to wait until the noise causes the system to jump out of the spontaneous state, helped perhaps by some drift caused by unequal λs. In this case, the decision times will be very variable, and will have a long right tail of very long decision times, as illustrated in Fig. B.7 (right) on page 603.

On the other hand, in the 'bistable' regime (with two decision pools) in which the spontaneous state is not stable, the system starts moving immediately towards one of the decision states, and although the noise can influence the decision, the system cannot wait in the spontaneous state for long just for a statistical fluctuation to cause a decision. In this regime, the decision times will be faster, and much less variable, as illustrated in Fig. B.7 (left, red).

It is a strength of this attractor model of decision-making that it can account for these two types of decision time distributions, and can provide a clear account of how they arise (Marti, Deco, Mattia, Gigante & Del Giudice 2008) (Section B.1.3.1).

The reaction times of this model of decision-making become faster as the discrimination becomes easier, that is as $\Delta\lambda$ (or equivalently ΔI) increases. An example is provided in Fig. 8.15. The effects can be understood by the biasing effect of the $\Delta\lambda$ to alter the shape of the energy function, and thus to increase the flow towards one of the attractors (see Sections B.1.3.1, 8.4, and Rolls & Deco (2010)).

8.6.6 Finite-size noise effects

8.6.6.1 The effects of increasing the size of the network

The results described earlier indicate that the probabilistic settling of the system is related to the finite size noise effects of the spiking dynamics of the individual neurons with their Poisson-like spike trains in a network of limited size. The concept here is that the smaller the network, the greater will be the statistical fluctuations (i.e. the noise) caused by the random spiking times of the individual neurons in the network. In an infinitely large system, the statistical fluctuations would be smoothed out, and reach zero. To investigate this further, and to show what sizes of network are in practice influenced by these finite-size related statistical fluctuations, an important issue when considering the operation of real neuronal networks in the brain, Deco & Rolls (2006) simulated networks with different numbers of neurons, N. The noise due to the finite size effects is expected to increase as the network becomes smaller, and indeed to be proportional to $1/\sqrt{N}$.

Figure 8.12 shows the effects of altering N on the operation of the network, where $N = N_{\mathrm{E}} + N_{\mathrm{I}}$, and $N_{\mathrm{E}} : N_{\mathrm{I}}$, was held at 4:1 as in the simulations shown earlier. The simulations were for f1=30 Hz and f2=22 Hz. Figure 8.12 shows overall that when N is larger than approximately 1,000, the network shows the expected settling to the (f1 $>$ f2) attractor state on a proportion of occasions that is in the range 85–93%, increasing only a little as the number of neurons reaches 4,000 (top panel). The settling remains probabilistic, as shown by the standard deviations in the probability that the (f1 $>$ f2) attractor state will be reached (top panel). When N is less than approximately 1,000, the finite size noise effects become very marked, as shown by the fact that the network reaches the correct attractor state (f1$>$f2) much less frequently, and in that the time for a decision to be reached can be premature and fast, as the large fluctuations in the stochastic noise can cause the system to reach the criterion [in

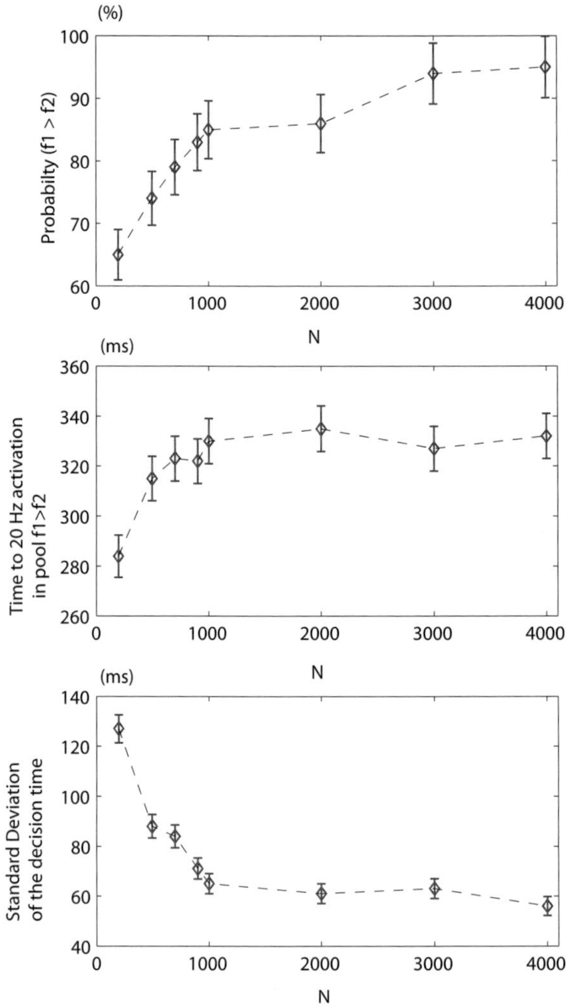

Fig. 8.12 The effects of altering N, the number of neurons in the network, on the operation of the decision-making network. The simulations were for f1=30 Hz and f2=22 Hz. The top panel shows the probability that the network will settle into the correct (f1>f2) attractor state. The mean $\pm$ the standard deviation is shown. The middle panel shows the time for a decision to be reached, that is for the system to reach a criterion of a firing rate of 20 Hz in the pool (f1>f2). The mean $\pm$ the standard deviation of the sampled mean is shown. The bottom panel shows the standard deviation of the reaction time. (Reproduced from Gustavo Deco and Edmund T. Rolls, Decision-making and Weber's law: a neurophysiological model, *European Journal of Neuroscience*, 24 (3) pp. 901–916, Copyright ©2006, John Wiley and Sons.)

this case of a firing rate of 20 Hz in the pool (f1>f2)] too quickly.

The overall conclusion of the results shown in Fig. 8.12 is that the size of the network, N, does influence the probabilistic settling of the network to the decision state. None of these probabilistic attractor and decision-related settling effects would of course be found in a mean-field or purely rate simulation, without spiking activity. The size of N in the brain is likely to be greater than 1,000 (and probably in the neocortex in the range 4,000–12,000) (Rolls 2008b, Rolls & Deco 2010).

Networks in the brain have graded firing rate representations, and diluted connectivity between the neurons. We have performed investigations to determine whether in biologically realistic networks with graded firing rate representations, and with diluted connectivity, and with a realistic size of several thousand synapses onto each neuron, noise is still a significant factor in the operation of these networks. This is important to assess, as the mechanisms that these attractor networks incorporate do appear to provide a firm foundation for understanding the brain mechanisms of decision-making. [The results shown in Fig. 8.12 are for a sparseness of 0.1, and a binary firing rate probability distribution (i.e. one in which all the neurons in the winning attractor have the same average high firing rate, and the other neurons in the network have a low firing rate).]

8.6.6.2 Graded firing rate representations increase noise in decision-making networks

Representations in the cortex are often distributed with graded firing rates in the neuronal populations (Rolls 2008b, Rolls & Treves 2011). The firing rate probability distribution of each neuron to a set of stimuli is often exponential or gamma. In processes in the brain such as decision-making that are influenced by the noise produced by the close to random spike timings of each neuron for a given mean rate, the noise with this graded type of representation may be larger than with the binary firing rate distribution that is usually investigated.

In integrate-and-fire simulations of an attractor decision-making network, we showed that the noise is indeed greater for a given sparseness of the representation for graded, exponential, than for binary firing rate distributions (Webb, Rolls, Deco & Feng 2011). The greater noise was measured by faster escaping times from the spontaneous firing rate state when the decision cues are applied, and this corresponds to faster decision or reaction times. The greater noise was also evident as less stability of the spontaneous firing state before the decision cues are applied. The underlying cause may be the large noise contributed by the few neurons with rather high firing rates, given that for a Poisson distribution the variance increases with (and is equal to) the mean rate.

The implication is that spiking-related noise will continue to be a factor that influences processes such as decision-making, signal detection, short-term memory, and memory recall even with the quite large networks found in the cerebral cortex. In these networks there are several thousand recurrent collateral synapses onto each neuron. The greater noise with graded firing rate distributions has the advantage that it can increase the speed of operation of cortical circuitry (Webb, Rolls, Deco & Feng 2011).

8.6.6.3 Diluted network connectivity decreases the noise in decision-making networks

The connectivity of the cerebral cortex is diluted, with the probability of excitatory connections between even nearby pyramidal cells rarely more than 0.1, and in the hippocampus 0.04 (Rolls 2008b).

To investigate the extent to which this diluted connectivity affects the dynamics of attractor networks in the cerebral cortex, we simulated an integrate-and-fire attractor network taking decisions between competing inputs with diluted connectivity of 0.25 or 0.1, and with the same number of synaptic connections per neuron for the recurrent collateral synapses within an attractor population as for full connectivity (Rolls & Webb 2012).

The results indicated that there was less spiking-related noise with the diluted connectivity in that the stability of the network when in the spontaneous state of firing increased, and the accuracy of the correct decisions increased. The decision times were a little slower with diluted than with complete connectivity (Rolls & Webb 2012).

Given that the capacity of the network is set by the number of recurrent collateral synaptic connections per neuron (Rolls 2008b), on which there is a biological limit, the findings indicate that the stability of cortical networks, and the accuracy of their correct decisions or memory recall operations, can be increased by utilizing diluted connectivity and correspondingly increasing the number of neurons in the network, with little impact on the speed of processing of the cortex. Thus diluted connectivity can decrease cortical spiking-related noise, when the number of connections per neuron is held constant as the dilution, and hence the number of excitatory neurons, is increased.

Quite large integrate-and-fire networks were simulated in this investigation, with 1600 recurrent collateral synapses onto each neuron, and 4480 excitatory neurons, and we were able to show that with diluted networks this large, moving towards the size of cortical networks, the statistical fluctuations caused by the spiking-related noise still produced probabilistic decision-making.

In addition, we showed that in this decision-making network the Fano factor (the variance/mean) for the trial-to-trial variability of the neuronal firing decreases from the spontaneous firing state value when the attractor network makes a decision (Rolls & Webb 2012), providing a neuronal network account of this change in variability found in many cortical regions when they are activated (Churchland, Yu, Cunningham, Sugrue, Cohen, Corrado, Newsome, Clark, Hosseini, Scott, Bradley, Smith, Kohn, Movshon, Armstrong, Moore, Chang, Snyder, Lisberger, Priebe, Finn, Ferster, Ryu, Santhanam, Sahani & Shenoy 2010).

It turns out that the diluted connectivity that is a feature of cortical recurrent collateral connectivity may have a fundamental basis in the design of cortical networks by genes. If the specification is that neurons of a given class should make connections with other neurons in a given class with an element of randomness in the selection, then dilution provides the property that there will rarely be more than one synapse between a pair of neurons that are within this recurrent connectivity. This has been shown to be highly advantageous, for multiple synapses between some pairs of neurons in an attractor network have been shown to distort the energy landscape so much that the memory capacity, the number of patterns that can be stored and correctly retrieved, is greatly reduced (Rolls 2012f).

8.7 Confidence in decisions

In this Section I consider how probabilistic decision-making is influenced by the easiness vs the difficulty of the decision, and how confidence in a decision emerges as a property of the neuronal attractor network decision-making process that is described earlier in this Chapter (8). Indeed, it has been shown how the difficulty of the decision, set quantitatively by the magnitude of the difference between the stimuli ΔI, influences the decision-making network. Here we extend this approach considerably. A link from discriminability to confidence can be made, for it is well established that subjective decision confidence increases with discriminability, ΔI (Vickers 1979, Vickers & Packer 1982, Jonsson, Olsson & Olsson 2005). This confidence can be reported before any feedback about whether the decision was correct is provided to the subject. The process is adaptive, for it may enable poor decisions to be corrected before the outcome of the decision is even known.

Given that confidence in a decision is higher after a correct decision than after an incorrect decision has been made (Vickers & Packer 1982), I show how this emerges as a property of the neuronal attractor network decision-making process. In more detail, if one makes a correct decision, consistent with the evidence, then one's confidence is higher than when one makes an incorrect decision (as shown by confidence ratings) (Vickers & Packer 1982), and consistent with this the probability that a rat will abort a trial is higher if a decision just made is incorrect (Kepecs, Uchida, Zariwala & Mainen 2008). It is also shown (in Section

8.7.8) how being correct vs making an error influences, as different functions of ΔI, the neuronal activity involved in making the choice, and also the fMRI BOLD (functional magnetic resonance imaging blood oxygenation level) signals that are associated with choice decision-making. This leads to the conclusion that decision confidence is an *emergent property* of the 'mechanistic' (i.e. biologically plausible at the integrate-and-fire level) model of decision-making described. Next it is shown how fMRI experiments can be used to test the predictions from the model.

Then in Section 8.8 I show how if a decision must be made based on one's confidence about a decision just made, a second decision-making network can read the information encoded in the firing rates of the first decision-making network to make a decision based on confidence.

A fundamental issue in understanding how the brain takes decisions is to identify a neural signature for decision-making processes and to explain how this signature arises as a result of the operation of dynamic cortical neural networks. Evidence from single neuron recordings in monkeys (Kim & Shadlen 1999) shows that neuronal responses in a motion decision-making task occur earlier on easy vs difficult trials in a decision-related brain region, the dorsolateral prefrontal cortex.

In the human dorsolateral prefrontal cortex, higher fMRI BOLD signals can be observed on easy trials vs difficult trials in a similar decision-making task (Heekeren, Marrett, Bandettini & Ungerleider 2004). On the basis of these findings it has been suggested (Heekeren et al. 2004) that the dorsolateral prefrontal cortex implements a general mechanism for decision-making in the brain which is thought to involve the comparison of sensory input signals until a decision criterion is reached and a choice is made. Thus a neural signature of decision-making seems to involve higher levels of activity when an easy compared to a difficult decision is taken. However, the fact that some areas of the brain thought to be involved in decision-making show earlier or larger neuronal responses on easy trials (Kim & Shadlen 1999) and reflect decision confidence (Kiani & Shadlen 2009) does not by itself provide a theoretical understanding about what is special about this effect as an indicator of decision-making, or lead to an understanding of how confidence is computed.

To address these issues, we simulated integrate-and-fire models of attractor-based choice decision-making, and predicted from them the neuronal firing rates in the decision attractor populations and the fMRI BOLD signals on easy vs difficult trials (Rolls, Grabenhorst & Deco 2010b). We then performed two fMRI investigations of decision-making about the reward value and subjective pleasantness of thermal and olfactory stimuli, and showed that areas implicated by other analyses of the same datasets in decision-making (Rolls & Grabenhorst 2008, Grabenhorst, Rolls & Parris 2008b, Rolls, Grabenhorst & Parris 2010d) do show the predicted difference between activations on easy vs difficult trials (Rolls, Grabenhorst & Deco 2010b), found also by other investigators (Heekeren et al. 2004, Heekeren et al. 2008).

The model makes detailed predictions about the neuronal activity that underlies the decision-making. This provides a fundamental and unifying approach to decision-making in the brain that specifies how probabilistic decisions influenced by neuronal noise are taken, and how activity at the synaptic, neuronal, network, neuroimaging, behavioural choice, and subjective confidence levels of investigation are related to the decision-making process so that further predictions can be tested.

8.7.1 The model of decision-making

The theoretical framework of the model used here (Rolls, Grabenhorst & Deco 2010b, Rolls, Grabenhorst & Deco 2010c) was that described earlier in this chapter. In this framework, we model probabilistic decision-making by a network of interacting neurons organized into a discrete set of populations, as depicted in Fig. 8.13.

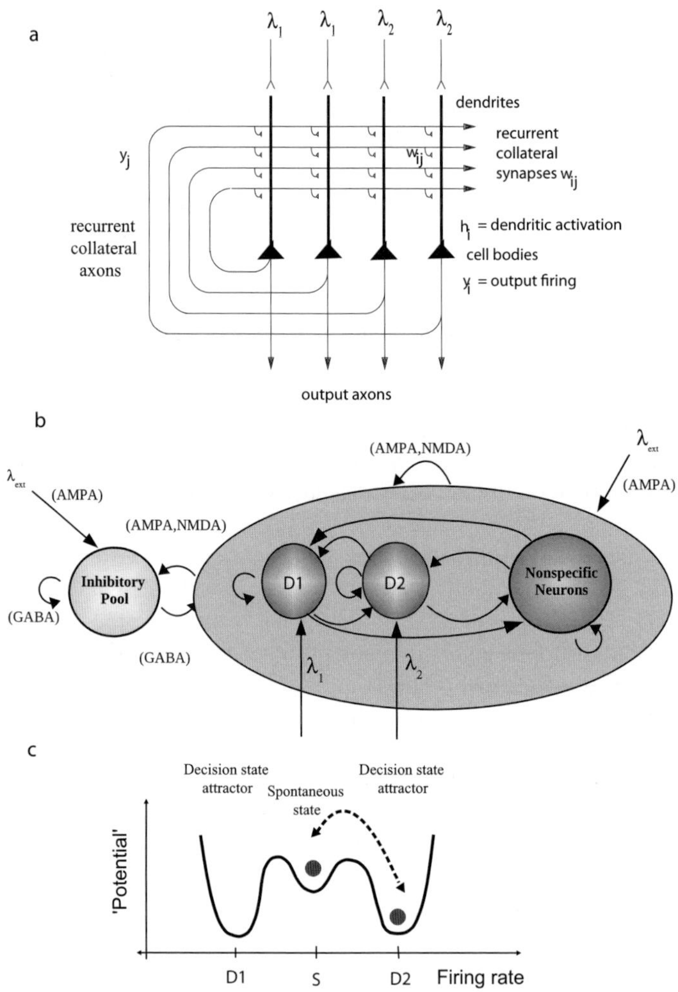

Fig. 8.13 (a) Attractor or autoassociation single network architecture for decision-making. The evidence for decision 1 is applied via the λ_1 inputs, and for decision 2 via the λ_2 inputs. The synaptic weights w_{ij} have been associatively modified during training in the presence of λ_1 and at a different time of λ_2. When λ_1 and λ_2 are applied, each attractor competes through the inhibitory interneurons (not shown), until one wins the competition, and the network falls into one of the high firing rate attractors that represents the decision. The noise in the network caused by the random spiking times of the neurons (for a given mean rate) means that on some trials, for given inputs, the neurons in the decision 1 (D1) attractor are more likely to win, and on other trials the neurons in the decision 2 (D2) attractor are more likely to win. This makes the decision-making probabilistic, for, as shown in (c), the noise influences when the system will jump out of the spontaneous firing stable (low energy) state S, and whether it jumps into the high firing state for decision 1 (D1) or decision 2 (D2). (b) The architecture of the integrate-and-fire network used to model decision-making (see text). (c) A multistable 'effective energy landscape' for decision-making with stable states shown as low 'potential' basins. Even when the inputs are being applied to the network, the spontaneous firing rate state is stable, and noise provokes transitions from the low firing rate spontaneous state S into the high firing rate decision attractor state D1 or D2.

The model simulated for the investigations described in this Section was similar to that described in Section 8.2.2, and the description here focusses on the differences. The network contains N_{E} (excitatory) pyramidal cells and N_{I} inhibitory interneurons. In the simulations, we used N_E=400 and N_I=100, consistent with the neurophysiologically observed proportion of 80% pyramidal cells versus 20% interneurons (Abeles 1991, Rolls & Deco 2002). There were two decision populations of neurons, D1 and D2, each comprising 0.1 of the excitatory neurons in the network, with the remaining excitatory neurons in the non-specific pool. The neurons in the two specific (i.e. decision) populations receive (in addition to the noise input at 3 Hz per external synaptic input) added firing to the external inputs that encodes the evidence for the decision to be made. When applying the decision evidence, the rate of the Poisson train to the neurons of the specific population D1 is increased by an extra value of λ_1, and to population D2 increased by λ_2, as these encode the two stimuli to be compared. The simulations were run for 2 s of spontaneous activity, and then for a further 2 s while the stimuli were being applied.

During the spontaneous period, the stimuli applied to D1 and D2 (and to all the other neurons in the network) had a value of 3 Hz. (This 3 Hz is the firing rate being applied by Poisson spikes to all 800 external synaptic inputs of each neuron in the network, so the total synaptic bombardment on each neuron is 2400 spikes/s.) During the decision period, the mean input to each external synapse of each neuron of D1 and D2 was increased to 3.04 Hz per synapse (an extra 32 Hz per neuron). For ΔI=0, 32 extra Hz to the spontaneous was applied to each neuron of both D1 and D2. For ΔI=16, 32 + 8 Hz was the extra applied to D1 and corresponds to λ_1 in Fig. 8.13, and 32 − 8 Hz was the extra applied to D2, etc. The firing rates, and the absolute value of the sum of the synaptic currents (AMPA, NMDA, and GABA, defined in Section B.4), in all four populations of neurons were saved every 50 ms for later analysis (Rolls, Grabenhorst & Deco 2010b, Rolls, Grabenhorst & Deco 2010c).

The criterion for which population won, that is for which decision was taken, was a mean rate for one population for the last second of the simulation that was 10 Hz greater than that of the other population. (This is in the context that the spontaneous rate was typically close to 3 spikes/s, and that the winning population typically had a mean firing rate of 35–40 Hz, as will be shown.)

The latency of a decision was measured by the time of the first 50 ms bin of three consecutive bins at which the mean rate of one population was more than 25 Hz higher than that of the other population.

The parameters for the synaptic weights and input currents were chosen using the mean-field equivalent of this network (Brunel & Wang 2001, Deco & Rolls 2006) so that in the absence of noise when the input stimuli are being applied there were three stable states, the spontaneous firing rate state (with a mean firing for the pyramidal cells of approximately 3 spikes/s), and two high firing rate attractor states (with a mean firing for the pyramidal cells of approximately 40 spikes/s), with one neuronal population (D1) representing decision 1, and the other population (D2) decision 2. In particular, w_+ was set to 2.1 (Rolls, Grabenhorst & Deco 2010b, Rolls, Grabenhorst & Deco 2010c). We describe this as a multistable system, and show its 'effective energy landscape' in Fig. 8.13 and discuss it in Section 8.4.

8.7.2 Neuronal responses on difficult vs easy trials, and decision confidence

Figure 8.14a and e show the mean firing rates of the two neuronal populations D1 and D2 for two trial types, easy trials (ΔI=160 Hz) and difficult trials (ΔI=0) (where ΔI is the difference in spikes/s summed across all synapses to each neuron between the two inputs, λ_1 to population D1, and λ_2 to population D2). The results are shown for correct trials, that is, trials on which the D1 population won the competition and fired with a rate of > 10 spikes/s more than the rate of D2 for the last 1000 ms of the simulation runs. Figure 8.14b shows the mean firing rates of the four populations of neurons on a difficult trial, and Fig. 8.14c

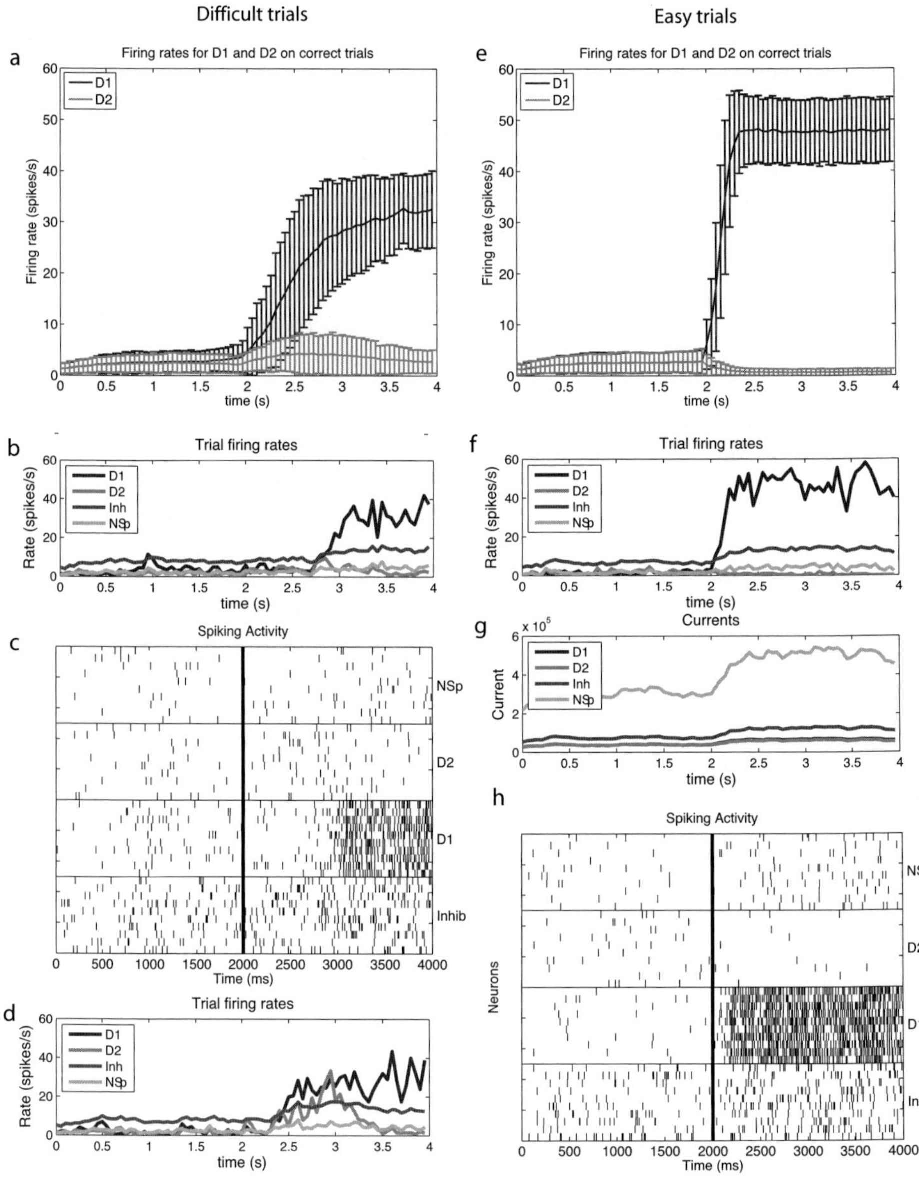

Fig. 8.14 (a) and (e) Firing rates (mean $\pm$ sd) for difficult (ΔI=0) and easy (ΔI=160) trials. The period 0–2 s is the spontaneous firing, and the decision cues were turned on at time = 2 s. D1: firing rate of the D1 population of neurons on correct trials on which the D1 population won. D2: firing rate of the D2 population of neurons on the correct trials on which the D1 population won. A correct trial was one in which in which the mean rate of the D1 attractor averaged > 10 spikes/s for the last 1000 ms of the simulation runs. (b) The mean firing rates of the four populations of neurons on a difficult trial. Inh is the inhibitory population that uses GABA as a transmitter. NSp is the non-specific population of neurons (see Fig. 8.13). (c) Rastergrams for the trial shown in b. 10 neurons from each of the four pools of neurons are shown. (d) The firing rates on another difficult trial (ΔI=0) showing prolonged competition between the D1 and D2 attractors until the D1 attractor finally wins after approximately 1100 ms. (f) Firing rate plots for the 4 neuronal populations on a single easy trial (ΔI=160). (g) The synaptic currents in the four neuronal populations on the trial shown in f. (h) Rastergrams for the easy trial shown in f and g. 10 neurons from each of the four pools of neurons are shown. (See colour plates section.) (Reprinted from *NeuroImage*, 33 (2), Edmund T. Rolls, Fabian Grabenhorst, and Gustavo Deco, Choice, difficulty, and confidence in the brain, pp. 694–706, Copyright 2010, with permission from Elsevier.)

shows the rastergrams for the same trial, for which the energy landscape is also shown in Fig. 8.13d. Figure 8.14d shows the firing rates on another difficult trial (ΔI=0) to illustrate the variability shown from trial to trial, with on this trial prolonged competition between the D1 and D2 attractors until the D1 attractor finally won after approximately 1100 ms. Figure 8.14f shows firing rate plots for the four neuronal populations on an example of a single easy trial (ΔI=160), Fig. 8.14g shows the synaptic currents in the four neuronal populations on the same trial, and Fig. 8.14h shows rastergrams for the same trial (Rolls, Grabenhorst & Deco 2010b).

Three important points are made by the results shown in Fig. 8.14. First, the network falls into its decision attractor faster on easy trials than on difficult trials. We would accordingly expect reaction times to be shorter on easy than on difficult trials. We might also expect the BOLD signal related to the activity of the network to be higher on easy than on difficult trials because it starts sooner on easy trials.

Second, the mean firing rate after the network has settled into the correct decision attractor is higher on easy than on difficult trials. We might therefore expect the BOLD signal related to the activity of the network to be higher on easy than on difficult trials because the maintained activity in the attractor is higher on easy trials. This shows that the exact firing rate in the attractor is a result not only of the internal recurrent collateral effect, but also of the external input to the neurons, which in Fig. 8.14a is 32 Hz to each neuron (summed across all synapses) of D1 and D2, but in Fig. 8.14e is increased by a further 80 Hz to D1, and decreased (from the 32 Hz added) by 80 Hz to D2 (i.e. the total external input to the network is the same, but ΔI=0 for Fig. 8.14a, and ΔI=160 for Fig. 8.14b).

Third, the variability of the firing rate is high, with the standard deviations of the mean firing rate calculated in 50 ms epochs indicated in order to quantify the variability. The large standard deviations on difficult trials for the first second after the decision cues are applied at t=2 s reflects the fact that on some trials the network has entered an attractor state after 1000 ms, but on other trials it has not yet reached the attractor, although it does so later. This trial by trial variability is indicated by the firing rates on individual trials and the rastergrams in the lower part of Fig. 8.14. The effects evident in Fig. 8.14 are quantified, and elucidated over a range of values for ΔI, next.

Figure 8.15a shows the firing rates (mean $\pm$ sd) on correct trials when in the D1 attractor as a function of ΔI. ΔI=0 corresponds to the most difficult decision, and ΔI=160 corresponds to easy. The firing rates for both the winning population D1 and for the losing population D2 are shown. The firing rates were measured in the last 1 s of firing, i.e. between t=3 and t=4 s. It is clear that the mean firing rate of the winning population increases monotonically as ΔI increases, and interestingly, the increase is approximately linear (Pearson $r = 0.995$, p<10^{-6}). The higher mean firing rates as ΔI increases are due not only to higher peak firing, but also to the fact that the variability becomes less as ΔI increases ($r = -0.95$, p<10^{-4}), reflecting the fact that the system is more noisy and unstable with low ΔI, whereas the firing rate in the attractor is maintained more stably with smaller statistical fluctuations against the Poisson effects of the random spike timings at high ΔI. (The measure of variation indicated in the figure is the standard deviation, and this is shown here unless otherwise stated to quantify the degree of variation, which is a fundamental aspect of the operation of these neuronal decision-making networks.)

As shown in Fig. 8.15a, the firing rates of the losing population decrease as ΔI increases. The decrease of firing rate of the losing population is due in part to feedback inhibition through the inhibitory neurons by the winning population. Thus the difference of firing rates between the winning and losing populations, as well as the firing rate of the winning population D1, both clearly reflect ΔI, and in a sense the confidence in the decision.

The increase of the firing rate when in the D1 attractor (upper thick line) as ΔI increases

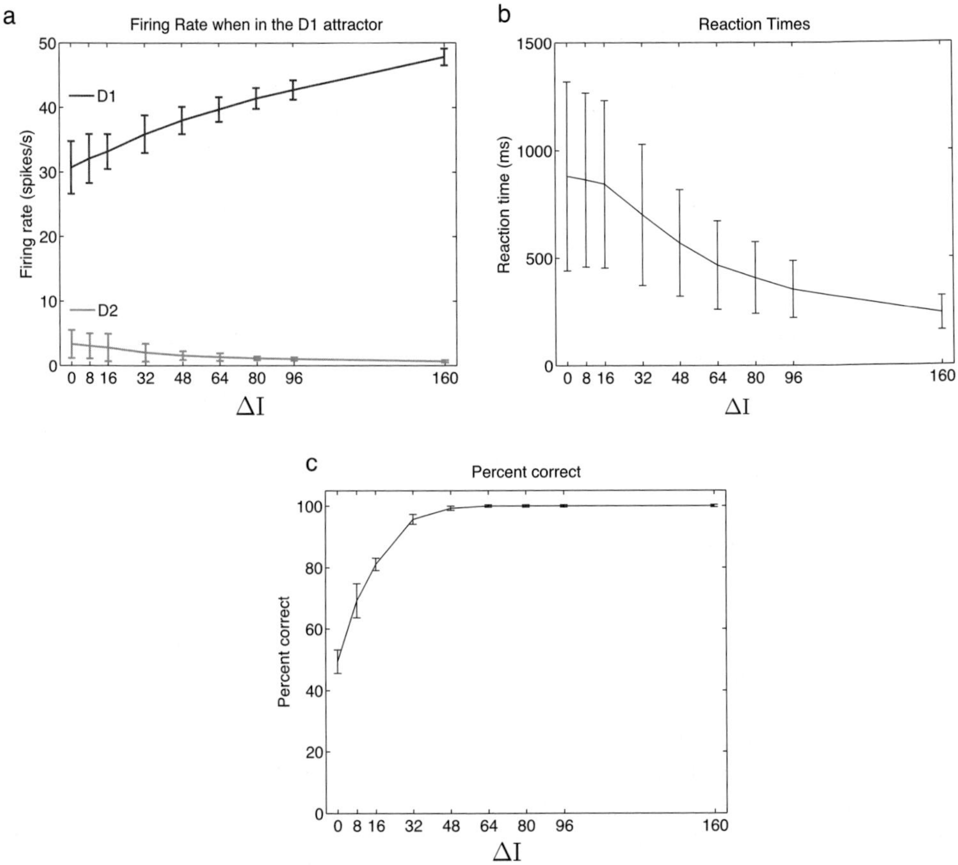

Fig. 8.15 (a) Firing rates (mean $\pm$ sd) on correct trials when in the D1 attractor as a function of ΔI. ΔI=0 corresponds to difficult, and ΔI=160 spikes/s corresponds to easy. The firing rates for both the winning population D1 and for the losing population D2 are shown for correct trials by thick lines. All the results are for 1000 simulation trials for each parameter value, and all the results shown are statistically highly significant. (b) Reaction times (mean $\pm$ sd) for the D1 population to win on correct trials as a function of the difference in inputs ΔI to D1 and D2. (c) Per cent correct performance, i.e. the percentage of trials on which the D1 population won, as a function of the difference in inputs ΔI to D1 and D2. The mean was calculated over 1000 trials, and the standard deviation was estimated by the variation in 10 groups each of 100 trials. (See colour plates section.) (Reprinted from *NeuroImage*, 33 (2), Edmund T. Rolls, Fabian Grabenhorst, and Gustavo Deco, Choice, difficulty, and confidence in the brain, pp. 694–706, Copyright 2010, with permission from Elsevier.)

thus can be related to the confidence in the decision, and, as will be shown next in Fig. 8.15b, the performance as shown by the percentage of correct choices. The firing rate of the losing attractor (D2, lower thick line) decreases as ΔI increases, due to feedback inhibition from the winning D1 attractor, and thus the difference in the firing rates of the two attractors also reflects well the decision confidence.

I emphasize from these findings (Rolls, Grabenhorst & Deco 2010b) that the firing rate of the winning attractor reflects ΔI, and thus the confidence in the decision which is closely related to ΔI.

8.7.3 Decision times of the neuronal responses

The time for the network to reach the correct D1 attractor, i.e. the reaction or decision time of the network, is shown as a function of ΔI in Fig. 8.15b (mean $\pm$ sd). Interestingly, the reaction time continues to decrease ($r = -0.95$, p<10^{-4}) over a wide range of ΔI, even when as shown in Fig. 8.15c the network is starting to perform at 100% correct. The decreasing reaction time as ΔI increases is attributable to the altered 'effective energy landscape' (see Section 8.4): a larger input to D1 tends to produce occasionally higher firing rates, and these statistically are more likely to induce a significant depression in the landscape towards which the network flows sooner than with low ΔI. Correspondingly, the variability (quantified by the standard deviation) of the reaction times is greatest at low ΔI, and decreases as ΔI increases ($r = -0.95$, p<10^{-4}). This variability would not be found with a deterministic system (i.e. the standard deviations would be 0 throughout, and such systems include those investigated with mean-field analyses), and is entirely due to the random statistical fluctuations caused by the random spiking of the neurons in the integrate-and-fire network.

8.7.4 Percentage correct

At ΔI=0, there is no influence on the network to fall more into attractor D1 representing decision 1 than attractor D2 representing decision 2, and its decisions are at chance, with approximately 50% of decisions being for D1. As ΔI increases, the proportion of trials on which D1 is reached increases. The relation between ΔI and percentage correct is shown in Fig. 8.15c. Interestingly, the performance becomes 100% correct with ΔI=64, whereas as shown in Figs. 8.15a and b the firing rates while in the D1 attractor (and therefore potentially the BOLD signal), continue to increase as ΔI increases further, and the reaction times continue to decrease as ΔI increases further. It is a clear prediction for neurophysiological and behavioural measures that the firing rates with decisions made by this attractor process continue to increase as ΔI is increased beyond the level for very good performance as indicated by the percentage of correct decisions, and the neuronal and behavioural reaction times continue to decrease as ΔI is increased beyond the level for very good performance. Figure 8.15c also shows that the variability in the percentage correct (in this case measured over blocks of 100 trials) is large with ΔI=0, and decreases as ΔI increases. This is consistent with unbiased effects of the noise producing very variable effects in the energy landscape at ΔI=0, but in the external inputs biasing the energy landscape more and more as ΔI increases, so that the flow is much more likely to be towards the D1 attractor.

8.7.5 Simulation of fMRI signals: haemodynamic convolution of synaptic activity

The links between neural and synaptic activity, and functional magnetic resonance neuroimaging (fMRI) measurements, are still not fully understood. The fMRI signal is unfortunately strongly filtered and perturbed by the haemodynamic delay inherent in the blood oxygen level-dependent (BOLD) contrast mechanism (Buxton & Frank 1997). The fMRI signal is only a secondary consequence of neuronal activity, and yields therefore a blurred distortion of the temporal development of the underlying brain processes. Regionally, increased oxidative metabolism causes a transient decrease in oxyhaemoglobin and increase in deoxyhaemoglobin, as well as an increase in CO_2 and NO. This provokes over several seconds a local dilatation and increased blood flow in the affected regions that leads by overcompensation to a relative decrease in the concentration of deoxyhaemoglobin in the venules draining the activated region, and the alteration of deoxyhaemoglobin, which is paramagnetic, can be detected by changes in T2 or T2* in the MRI signal as a result of the decreased sus-

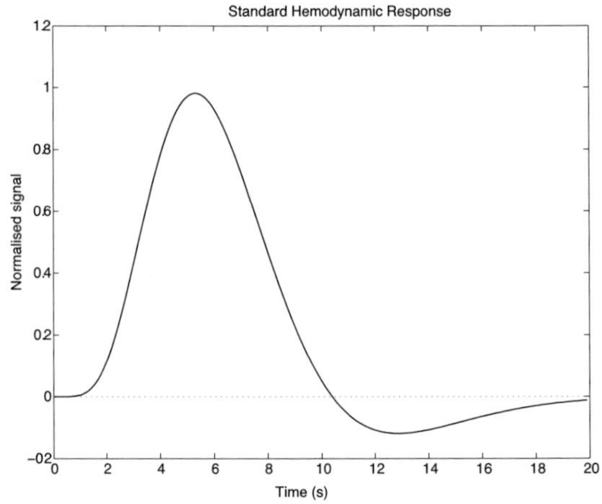

Fig. 8.16 The standard haemodynamic response function $h(t)$ (see text).

ceptibility and thus decreased local inhomogeneity which increases the MR intensity value (Glover 1999, Buxton & Frank 1997, Buxton, Wong & Frank 1998).

The fMRI BOLD (blood oxygen level-dependent) signal may reflect the total synaptic activity in an area (as ions need to be pumped back across the cell membrane) (perhaps, it has been suggested, better than the spiking neuronal activity (Logothetis, Pauls, Augath, Trinath & Oeltermann 2001)), and is spatially and temporally filtered. The filtering reflects the inherent spatial resolution with which the blood flow changes, as well as the resolution of the scanner, and spatial filtering which may be applied for statistical purposes, and the slow temporal response of the blood flow changes (Glover 1999, Buxton & Frank 1997, Buxton et al. 1998). Glover (1999) demonstrated that a good fit of the haemodynamical response $h(t)$ can be achieved by the following analytic function:

$$h(t) = c_1 t^{n_1} e^{-\frac{t}{t_1}} - a_2 c_2 t^{n_2} e^{-\frac{t}{t_2}}$$

$$c_i = \max(t^{n_i} e^{-\frac{t}{t_i}})$$

where t is the time, and c_1, c_2, a_2, n_1, and n_2 are parameters that are adjusted to fit the experimentally measured haemodynamical response. Figure 8.16 plots the haemodynamic standard response $h(t)$ for a biologically realistic set of parameters (see Deco, Rolls & Horwitz (2004)).

The temporal evolution of fMRI signals can be simulated from an integrate-and-fire population of neurons by convolving the total synaptic activity in the simulated population of neurons with the standard haemodynamic response formulation of Glover (1999) (Deco, Rolls & Horwitz 2004, Horwitz & Tagamets 1999). The rationale for this is that the major metabolic expenditure in neural activity is the energy required to pump back against the electrochemical gradient the ions that have entered neurons as a result of the ion channels opened by synaptic activity, and that mechanisms have evolved to increase local blood flow in order to help this increased metabolic demand to be met. (In fact, the increased blood flow overcompensates, and the blood oxygenation level-dependent (BOLD) signal by reflecting the consequent alteration of deoxyhaemoglobin which is paramagnetic reflects this.)

The total synaptic current ($I_{\rm syn}$) is given by the sum of the absolute values of the glutamatergic excitatory components (implemented through NMDA and AMPA receptors) and inhibitory components (GABA) (Tagamets & Horwitz 1998, Horwitz, Tagamets & McIntosh 1999, Rolls & Deco 2002, Deco, Rolls & Horwitz 2004). In our integrate-and-fire simulations the external excitatory contributions are produced through AMPA receptors ($I_{\mathrm{AMPA,ext}}$), while the excitatory recurrent synaptic currents are produced through AMPA and NMDA receptors ($I_{\mathrm{AMPA,rec}}$ and $I_{\mathrm{NMDA,rec}}$). The GABA inhibitory currents are denoted by I_{GABA}. Consequently, the simulated fMRI signal activity S_{fMRI} is calculated by the following convolution equation:

$$S_{\mathrm{fMRI}}(t) = \int_0^{\infty} h(t-t')I_{\mathrm{syn}}(t')\,dt'.$$

Deco, Rolls & Horwitz (2004) applied this approach to predicting fMRI BOLD signals based on activity simulated at the integrate-and-fire level of neuronal activity in the dorsolateral prefrontal cortex. They showed that differences in the fMRI BOLD signal from the dorsal as compared to the ventral prefrontal cortex in working memory tasks may reflect a higher level of inhibition in the dorsolateral prefrontal cortex. In their simulation the convolution was calculated numerically by sampling the total synaptic activity every 0.1 s and introducing a cut-off at a delay of 25 s. The parameters utilized for the haemodynamic standard response $h(t)$ were taken from the paper of Glover (1999), and were: $n_1 = 6.0$, $t_1 = 0.9$s, $n_2 = 12.0$, $t_2 = 0.9$s, and $a_2 = 0.2$.

8.7.6 Prediction of the BOLD signals on difficult vs easy decision-making trials

We now show how this model makes predictions for the fMRI BOLD signals that would occur in brain areas in which decision-making processing of the type described is taking place. The BOLD signals were predicted from the firing rates of the neurons in the network (or from the synaptic currents flowing in the neurons as described later) by convolving the neuronal activity with the haemodynamic response function in a realistic period, the two seconds after the decision cues are applied. This is a reasonable period to take, as decisions will be taken within this time, and the attractor state may not necessarily be maintained for longer than this. (The attractor states might be maintained for longer if the response that can be made is not known until later, as in some fMRI tasks with delays, and then the effects described might be expected to be larger, given the mean firing rate effects shown in Fig. 8.14.)

In more detail, the haemodynamic signal associated with the decision was calculated by convolving the neuronal activity or the synaptic currents of the neurons with the haemodynamic response function used with SPM5 (Statistical Parametric Mapping, Wellcome Department of Imaging Neuroscience, London) (as this was the function also used in the analyses by SPM of the experimental fMRI data) (Rolls, Grabenhorst & Deco 2010b). For the convolution, the pre-decision period of spontaneous activity was padded out so that it lasted for 30 s, and after the 2 s period of decision-making activity, each trial was padded out for a further 18 s with spontaneous activity, so that the effects found in a 2 s period of decision-making could be measured against a steady background. The predicted BOLD signals are shown with t=0 corresponding to the time when the decision stimuli were turned on, just as in related analyses of the experimental fMRI data, to enable direct comparisons (Rolls, Grabenhorst & Deco 2010b).

As shown in Fig. 8.17a, the predicted fMRI response is larger for easy ($\Delta I = 160$ spikes/s) than for difficult trials (ΔI=0), with intermediate trials (ΔI=80) producing an intermediate fMRI response. The difference in the peak response for ΔI=0 and ΔI=160 is highly significant ($p \ll 0.001$). Importantly, the BOLD response is inherently variable from brain regions associated with this type of decision-making process, and this is nothing to do with the noise arising in the measurement of the BOLD response with a scanner. If the system

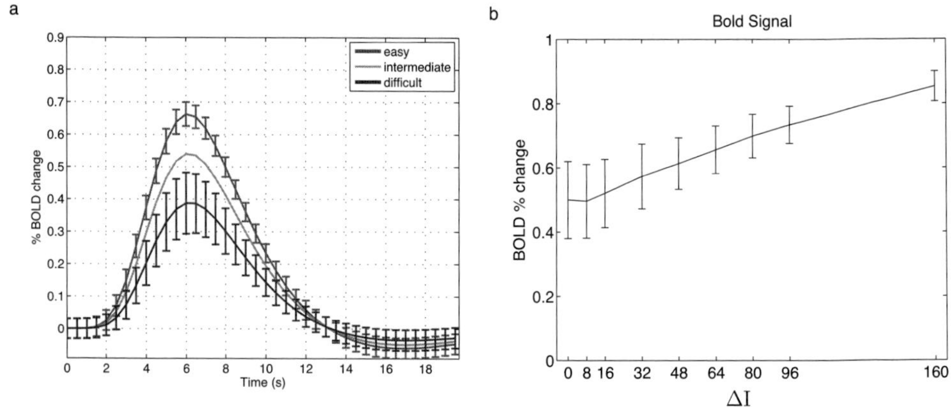

Fig. 8.17 (a) The percentage change in the simulated BOLD signal on easy trials (ΔI=160 spikes/s), on intermediate trials (ΔI=80), and on difficult trials (ΔI=0). The mean $\pm$ sd are shown for the easy and difficult trials. The percentage change in the BOLD signal was calculated from the firing rates of the D1 and D2 populations, and analogous effects were found with calculation from the synaptic currents averaged for example across all 4 populations of neurons. (b) The percentage change in the BOLD signal (peak mean $\pm$ sd) averaged across correct and incorrect trials as a function of ΔI. ΔI=0 corresponds to difficult, and ΔI=160 corresponds to easy. The percent change was measured as the change from the level of activity in a period of 1 s immediately before the decision cues were applied at t=0 s, and was calculated from the firing rates of the neurons in the D1 and D2 populations. The BOLD per cent change scaling is arbitrary, and is set so that the lowest value for the peak of a BOLD response is 0.5%. (See colour plates section.) (Reprinted from *NeuroImage*, 33 (2), Edmund T. Rolls, Fabian Grabenhorst, and Gustavo Deco, Choice, difficulty, and confidence in the brain, pp. 694–706, Copyright 2010, with permission from Elsevier.)

were deterministic, the standard deviations, shown as a measure of the variability in Fig. 8.17a, would be 0. It is the statistical fluctuations caused by the noisy (random) spike timings of the neurons that account for the variability in the BOLD signals in Fig. 8.17a. Interestingly, the variability is larger on the difficult trials (ΔI=0) than on the easy trials (ΔI=160), as shown in Fig. 8.17a, and indeed this also can be taken as an indicator that attractor decision-making processes of the type described here are taking place in a brain region.

Figure 8.17b shows that the percentage change in the BOLD signal (peak mean $\pm$ sd) averaged across correct and incorrect trials increases monotonically as a function of ΔI. This again can be taken as an indicator (provided that fMRI signal saturation effects are minimized) that attractor decision-making processes of the type described here are taking place in a brain region. The percentage change in Fig. 8.17b was calculated by convolution of the firing rates of the neurons in the D1 and D2 populations with the haemodynamic response function. Interestingly, the percentage change in the BOLD signal is approximately linearly related throughout this range to ΔI (r=0.995, p<10^{-7}). The effects shown in Figs. 8.17a and b can be related to the earlier onset of a high firing rate attractor state when ΔI is larger (see Figs. 8.14 and 8.15b), and to a higher firing rate when in the attractor state (as shown in Figs. 8.14 and 8.15a). As expected from the decrease in the variability of the neuronal activity as ΔI increases (Fig. 8.15a), the variability (standard deviation) in the predicted BOLD signal also decreases as ΔI increases, as shown in Fig. 8.17b (r=0.955, p<10^{-4}).

Similar effects, though smaller in degree, were found when the percentage change of the BOLD signal was calculated from the synaptic activity in all populations of neurons in the network (D1, D2, GABA, and non-specific, see Fig. 8.13), as shown in Fig. 8.18a. The percentage change in the BOLD signal is approximately linearly related throughout this range

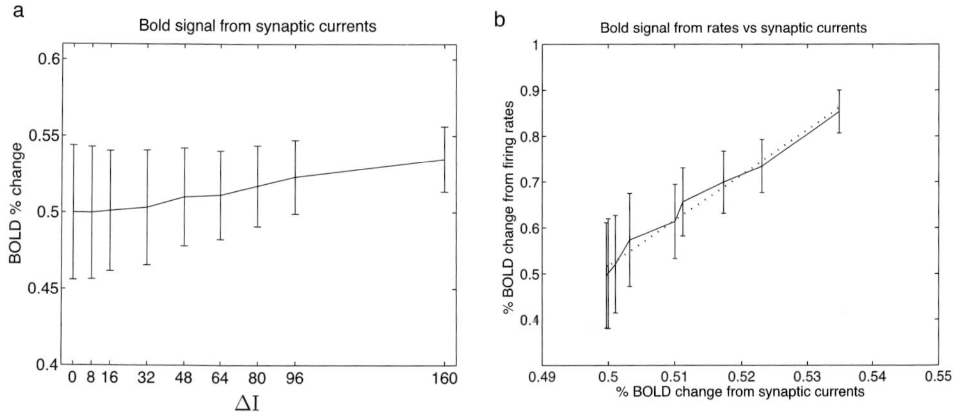

Fig. 8.18 (a) The percentage change of the BOLD signal (mean $\pm$ sd) calculated from the synaptic currents in all populations of neurons in the network (D1, D2, GABA, and non-specific, see Fig. 8.13). (Analogous results were found when the currents were calculated from the D1 and D2 populations; or from the D1, D2 and GABA populations.) (b) The relation between the BOLD current predicted from the firing rates and from the synaptic currents (r=0.99, p<10^{-6}) for values of ΔI between 0 and 160. The fitted linear regression line is shown. The BOLD per cent change scaling is arbitrary, and is set so that the lowest value is 0.5%. (Reprinted from *NeuroImage*, 33 (2), Edmund T. Rolls, Fabian Grabenhorst, and Gustavo Deco, Choice, difficulty, and confidence in the brain, pp. 694–706, Copyright 2010, with permission from Elsevier.)

to ΔI (r=0.991, p<10^{-6}). Fig. 8.18b shows the relation in the model between the BOLD signal predicted from the firing rates and from the synaptic currents for values of ΔI between 0 and 160 Hz. The fitted linear regression line is shown (r=0.99, p<10^{-6}).

The findings shown in Fig. 8.18b are of interest when considering how the fMRI BOLD signal is generated in the cortex. The fMRI BOLD signal is produced by an alteration of blood flow in response to activity in a brain region. The BOLD signal, derived from the magnetic susceptibility of deoxyhaemoglobin, reflects an overcompensation in the blood flow, resulting in more deoxyhaemoglobin in active areas. The coupling of the activity in a brain region to the altered blood flow is complex (Logothetis et al. 2001, Logothetis 2008, Mangia, Giove, Tkac, Logothetis, Henry, Olman, Maraviglia, Di Salle & Ugurbil 2009), but may reflect the energy needed to pump ions that have crossed the cell membrane as a result of synaptic activity to be pumped back against the electrochemical gradient. In Fig. 8.17 predicted BOLD effects are shown related to the firing rate of the two populations D1 and D2 of neurons in the attractor network. In Fig. 8.18 are shown predicted BOLD effects related to the sum of the synaptic currents in all the neurons in the network, with analogous results found with the synaptic currents in only the D1 and D2 neurons, or in the D1, D2, and GABA neurons in the network. Although it has been suggested that synaptic activity is better coupled to the blood flow and hence the BOLD signal than the firing rates (Logothetis et al. 2001, Logothetis 2008, Mangia et al. 2009), in the neocortex these might be expected to be quite closely related, and indeed the integrate-and-fire model shows a linear relation between the BOLD signal predicted from the firing rates and from the synaptic currents (r=0.99, p<10^{-6}, Fig. 8.18b), providing an indication that at least in the cerebral cortex the BOLD signal may be related to the firing rates of the neurons as well as to the synaptic currents.

8.7.7 Neuroimaging investigations of task difficulty, and confidence

Two functional neuroimaging investigations were performed to test the predictions of the model just described. Task difficulty was altered parametrically to determine whether there was a close relation between the BOLD signal and task difficulty (Rolls, Grabenhorst & Deco 2010b), and whether this was present especially in brain areas implicated in choice decision-making by other criteria (Grabenhorst, Rolls & Parris 2008b, Rolls, Grabenhorst & Parris 2010d). The decisions were about the pleasantness of olfactory (Rolls, Grabenhorst & Parris 2010d) or thermal (Grabenhorst, Rolls & Parris 2008b) stimuli.

8.7.7.1 Olfactory pleasantness decision task

The olfactory decision-making task illustrated in Fig. 4.65 was used (Rolls, Grabenhorst & Parris 2010d). ΔI, the difference in pleasantness of the two stimuli between which a decision was being made, was obtained for each trial by the absolute value of the difference in the (average) rated pleasantness of that pair of stimuli for each subject. Thus, two odours of similar pleasantness would have a small ΔI, and two odours of different pleasantness would have a large ΔI. This measure thus reflects the difficulty of the decision, and is independent of whether the second odour happened to be pleasant or unpleasant. This value for ΔI on every trial was used to investigate whether at brain sites where there was more activation on easy vs difficult trials (as shown by a contrast analysis), the BOLD signal was related to ΔI. Because the stimuli were randomized, the analysis did not reflect the pleasantness or unpleasantness of the second odour, but only how different it was in pleasantness from the first odour, independently of the sign of the difference. The regressor was thus decision difficulty.

8.7.7.2 Temperature pleasantness decision task

Warm and cool thermal stimuli, and mixtures of them, were applied to the hand. In a previous investigation of the same dataset, we compared brain responses when participants were taking decisions about whether they would select a thermal stimulus (yes vs no), with activations to the same stimuli on different trials when only affective ratings were required and there was no decision about whether the participants would say yes or no to the stimuli if they were available in the future (Grabenhorst, Rolls & Parris 2008b). In the investigation on task difficulty, we analysed data only on decision trials, and the analyses were about how activations with the stimuli were related to the difficulty of the decision (Rolls, Grabenhorst & Deco 2010b), which was not investigated previously. Both the decision and rating trials were identical from the start of each trial at t=0 s until t=5 s when a visual stimulus was shown for 1 s stating 'decide' or 'rate' the thermal stimulus being applied, and at t=6 s a green cross appeared until t=10 s. On decide trials from t=6 until t=10 s the participants had to decide whether yes or no was the decision on that trial. At t=10 s a visual stimulus with yes above no or vice versa in random order was shown for 2 s, and the participant had to press the upper or lower button on the button box as appropriate to indicate the response. On rating trials from t=6 until t=10 s the participants had to encode the pleasantness and intensity of the thermal stimulus being applied, so that the ratings could be made later. On rating trials at t=10 s the pleasantness rating could be made using the same button box, and then the intensity rating was made. The thermal stimuli were a warm pleasant stimulus (41°C) applied to the hand ('warm2'), a cool unpleasant stimulus (12°C) applied to the hand ('cold'), a combined warm and cold stimulus ('warm2+cold'), and a second combination designed to be less pleasant (39°C + 12°C) ('warm1+cold'), delivered with Peltier devices as described previously (Grabenhorst, Rolls & Parris 2008b).

ΔI for the thermal stimuli was the absolute value of the pleasantness rating, based on the concept that it is more difficult to choose whether a stimulus should be repeated in future if it is close to neutral (0) in rated pleasantness, versus is rated as being pleasant (with the maximum pleasantness being +2), or as being unpleasant (with the most unpleasant being −2).

8.7.7.3 fMRI analyses

The criteria used to identify regions involved in choice decision-making in earlier investigations with the same data set were that a brain region should show more brain activity with identical stimuli on trials on which a choice decision was being made than when the continuous affective value of the stimuli were being rated, but no choice was being made between stimuli, or about whether the stimulus would be chosen again (Grabenhorst, Rolls & Parris 2008b, Rolls, Grabenhorst & Parris 2010d, Rolls & Grabenhorst 2008). For the olfactory task, a contrast of decision vs rating trials showed activations in the medial prefrontal cortex medial area 10 at [2 50 −12] z=3.78 p<0.001 (Rolls, Grabenhorst & Parris 2010d). For the thermal task, a contrast of decision vs rating trials showed activations in the medial prefrontal cortex medial area 10, at [6 54 −8] z=3.24 p=0.022 (Grabenhorst, Rolls & Parris 2008b).

8.7.7.4 Brain areas with activations related to easiness and confidence

Figure 8.19 shows experimental data with the fMRI BOLD signal measured on easy and difficult trials of the olfactory affective decision task (left) and the thermal affective decision task (right) (Rolls, Grabenhorst & Deco 2010b). The upper records are for prefrontal cortex medial area 10 in a region identified by the following criterion as being involved in choice decision-making. The criterion was that a brain region for identical stimuli should show more activity when a choice decision was being made than when a rating on a continuous scale of affective value was being made. Figure 8.19 shows for medial prefrontal cortex area 10 that there is a larger BOLD signal on easy than on difficult trials. The top diagram shows the medial prefrontal area activated in this contrast for decisions about which olfactory stimulus was more pleasant (yellow), and for decisions about whether the thermal stimulus would be chosen in future based on whether it was pleasant or unpleasant (red).

In more detail, for the thermal stimuli, the contrast was the warm2 and the cold trials (which were both easy in that the percentage of the choices were far from the chance value of 50%, and in particular were 96±1% (mean±sem) for the warm, and 18±6% for the cold), versus the mixed stimulus of warm2+cold (which was difficult in that the percentage of choices of 'Yes, it would be chosen in future' was 64+9%). For the temperature easy vs difficult decisions about pleasantness, the activation in medial area 10 had peaks at [4 42 −4] z=3.59 p=0.020 and [6 52 −4] z=3.09 p=0.045.

For the olfactory decision task, the activations in medial area 10 for easy vs difficult choices were at [−4 62 −2] z=2.84 p=0.046, confirmed in a finite impulse response (FIR) analysis with a peak at 6–8 s after the decision time at [−4 54 −6] z=3.50 p=0.002. (In the olfactory task, the easy trials were those in which one of the pair of odours was from the pleasant set, and the other from the unpleasant set. The mean difference in pleasantness, corresponding to ΔI, was 1.76±0.25 (mean±sem). The difficult trials were those in which both odours on a trial were from the pleasant set, or from the unpleasant set. The mean difference in pleasantness, corresponding to ΔI, was 0.72±0.16. For easy trials, the percentage correct was 90±2, and for difficult trials was 59±8.) No other significant effects in the a priori regions of interest (Grabenhorst, Rolls & Parris 2008b, Rolls, Grabenhorst & Parris 2010d) were found for the easy vs difficult trial contrast in either the thermal or olfactory reward decision task (Rolls, Grabenhorst & Deco 2010b).

The lower records in Fig. 8.19 are for the same easy and difficult trials, but in parts of the pregenual cingulate and mid-orbitofrontal cortex implicated by the same criteria in representing the subjective reward value of the stimuli, but not in making choice decisions

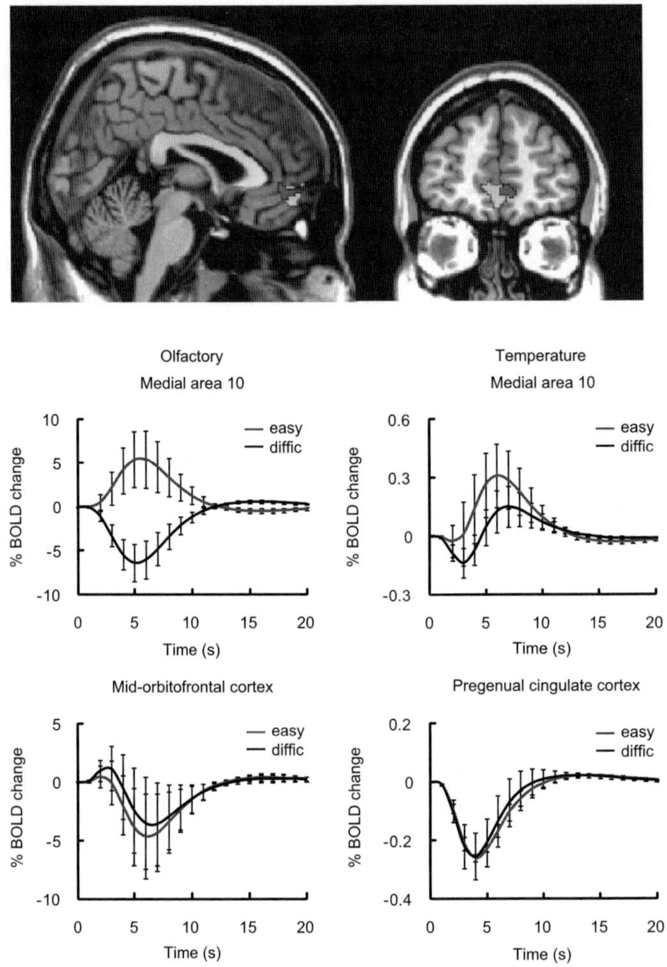

Fig. 8.19 Top: Medial prefrontal cortex area 10 activated on easy vs difficult trials in the olfactory pleasantness decision task (yellow) and the thermal pleasantness decision task (red). Middle: experimental data showing the BOLD signal in medial area 10 on easy and difficult trials of the olfactory affective decision task (left) and the thermal affective decision task (right). This medial area 10 was a region identified by other criteria (see text) as being involved in choice decision-making. Bottom: The BOLD signal for the same easy and difficult trials, but in parts of the pregenual cingulate and mid-orbitofrontal cortex implicated by other criteria (see text) in representing the subjective reward value of the stimuli on a continuous scale, but not in making choice decisions between the stimuli, or about whether to choose the stimulus in future. (See colour plates section.) (Reprinted from *NeuroImage*, 33 (2), Edmund T. Rolls, Fabian Grabenhorst, and Gustavo Deco, Choice, difficulty, and confidence in the brain, pp. 694–706, Copyright 2010, with permission from Elsevier.)

between the stimuli. [For the pregenual cingulate cortex, there was a correlation of the activations with the subjective ratings of pleasantness of the thermal stimuli at [4 38 −2] z=4.24 p=0.001. For the mid-orbitofrontal cortex, there was a correlation of the activations with the subjective ratings of pleasantness of the thermal stimuli at [40 36 −12] z=3.13 p=0.024.] The BOLD signal was similar in these brain regions for easy and difficult trials, as shown in Fig. 8.19, and there was no effect in the contrast between easy and difficult trials.

Figure 8.20 shows the experimental fMRI data with the change in the BOLD signal for medial prefrontal cortex area 10 indicated as a function of ΔI, the difference in pleasantness of

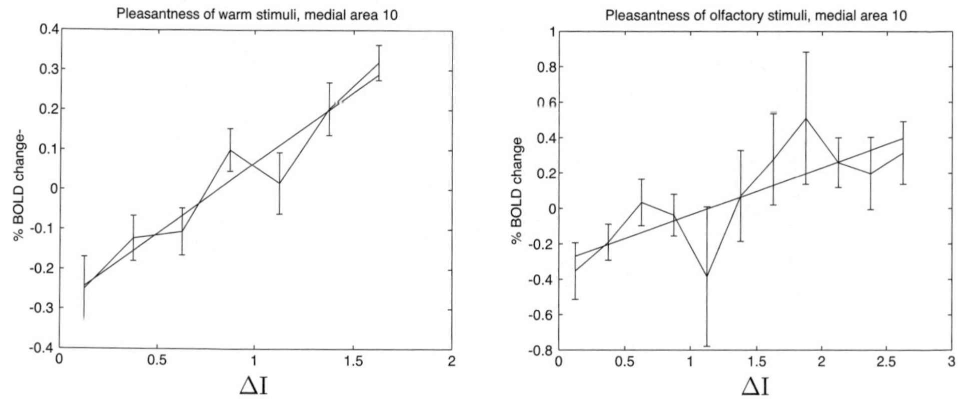

Fig. 8.20 Experimental fMRI data showing the change in the BOLD signal (mean±sem, with the fitted linear regression line shown) as a function of ΔI, the difference in pleasantness of warm stimuli or olfactory stimuli about which decision was being made, for medial prefrontal cortex area 10. (Reprinted from *NeuroImage*, 33 (2), Edmund T. Rolls, Fabian Grabenhorst, and Gustavo Deco, Choice, difficulty, and confidence in the brain, pp. 694–706, Copyright 2010, with permission from Elsevier.)

warm stimuli or olfactory stimuli about which decision was being made, and thus the easiness of the decision. For the olfactory decision task, ΔI was the difference in pleasantness (for a given subject) between the mean pleasantness of the first odour and the mean pleasantness of the second odour between which decision was being taken, about which was more pleasant (Rolls et al. 2010b). It is shown in Fig. 8.20 (right) that there was a clear and approximately linear relation between the BOLD signal and ΔI for the olfactory pleasantness decision-making task ($r = 0.77, p = 0.005$). The coordinates for these data were as given for Fig. 8.19.

For the warm decision task, ΔI was the difference in mean pleasantness for a given subject from 0 for a given thermal stimulus about which a decision was being made about whether it should or should not be repeated in future (Grabenhorst et al. 2008b). It is shown in Fig. 8.20 (left) that there was a clear and approximately linear relation between the BOLD signal and ΔI for the thermal pleasantness decision-making task ($r = 0.96, p < 0.001$). The coordinates for these data were as given for Fig. 8.19.

These experimental findings are thus consistent with the predictions made from the model, and provide strong support for the type of model of decision-making described in this book. Moreover, they show that decision confidence, which increases with ΔI, can be read off from fMRI BOLD signals in parts of the brain involved in making choices, as shown in this unifying theory.

8.7.8 Correct decisions vs errors, and confidence

If one makes a correct decision, consistent with the evidence, then one's confidence is higher than when one makes an incorrect decision (as shown by confidence ratings) (Vickers 1979, Vickers & Packer 1982). Consistent with this, the probability that a rat will abort a trial to try again is higher if a decision just made is incorrect (Kepecs et al. 2008). This occurs before the outcome of the choice is made known to the subject.

Why does this occur, and in which brain regions is the underlying processing implemented? It is shown in this Section (8.7.8) that the integrate-and-fire attractor decision-making network described in this book predicts higher and shorter latency neuronal responses, and higher

BOLD signals, in brain areas involved in making choices, on correct than on error trials, and how these changes vary with ΔI and thus compute decision confidence. The reason for this behaviour of the choice attractor network is that on correct trials, when the network influenced by the spiking noise has reached an attractor state supported by the recurrent connections between the neurons, the external inputs to the network that provide the evidence for the decision will have firing rates that are consistent with the decision, so the firing rate of the winning attractor will be higher when the correct attractor (given the evidence) wins the competition than when the incorrect attractor wins the competition. For this effect to remain present after the choice, the decision stimuli, or a short-term memory of them, need of course to be present, providing an on-going bias to the decision-making network that is consistent (on correct trials) or inconsistent (on error trials) with the decision just taken.

It is then shown in an experimental fMRI investigation that this BOLD signature of correct vs incorrect decisions, which reflects confidence in whether a decision just taken is correct, is found in the medial prefrontal cortex area 10, the posterior and subgenual cingulate cortex, and the dorsolateral prefrontal cortex, but not in the mid-orbitofrontal cortex, where activations instead reflect the pleasantness or subjective affective value of the stimuli used as inputs to the choice decision-making process (Rolls, Grabenhorst & Deco 2010c). This approach to decision-making, in contrast to phenomenal mathematical models of decision-making as an accumulation or diffusion process (Vickers 1979, Vickers & Packer 1982, Ratcliff & Rouder 1998, Ratcliff, Zandt & McKoon 1999, Usher & McClelland 2001), thus makes testable predictions about how correct vs error performance is implemented in the brain, and these predictions are supported by experimental results showing that areas involved in choice decision-making (or that receive from them) have activity consistent with these predictions, and that other areas not involved in the choice-making part of the process do not.

8.7.8.1 Operation of the attractor network model on correct vs error trials

The attractor network model of decision-making is the same as that described in the first part of this chapter, and the simulations are from the same test runs as those described earlier.

Figure 8.21a and d show the mean firing rates of the two neuronal populations D1 and D2 for correct trials (a) and incorrect trials (b) for an intermediate level of task difficulty (ΔI=32 Hz) (where ΔI is the difference in spikes/s summed across all synapses to each neuron between the two inputs, λ_1 to population D1, and λ_2 to population D2) (Rolls, Grabenhorst & Deco 2010c). In the correct trials, the population D1 won, and on incorrect trials, the population D2 won. The winning population was defined as that which fired with a rate of $>$ 10 spikes/s for the last 1000 ms of the simulation runs. (This provided a clear criterion for which attractor won the competition as shown by the binary distribution of the rates of the two attractors found over 1000 simulation trials, and as exemplified by the single trials in Fig. 8.21.) Figures 8.21a and d show that the winning population had higher firing rates on correct than on incorrect trials. Figure 8.21b shows the firing rates of the four populations of neurons on a single trial for a correct decision, and Fig. 8.21c shows the rastergrams for the same trial. Figure 8.21e shows the firing rates of the four populations of neurons on a single trial for a incorrect decision, and Fig. 8.21f shows the rastergrams for the same trial. From Figs. 8.21a and d it is clear that the variability of the firing rate is high from trial to trial, with the standard deviations of the mean firing rate calculated in 50 ms epochs indicated in order to quantify the variability. This is due to the spiking noise in the network, which influences the decision taken, resulting in probabilistic decision-making, and incorrect choices on some trials. The effects evident in Fig. 8.21 are quantified, and elucidated over a range of values for ΔI, next.

Figure 8.22a shows the firing rates (mean $\pm$ sd) on correct and error trials of the winning and losing attractors as a function of ΔI. ΔI=0 corresponds to the most difficult decision, and ΔI=160 corresponds to easy. The firing rates were measured in the last 1 s of firing,

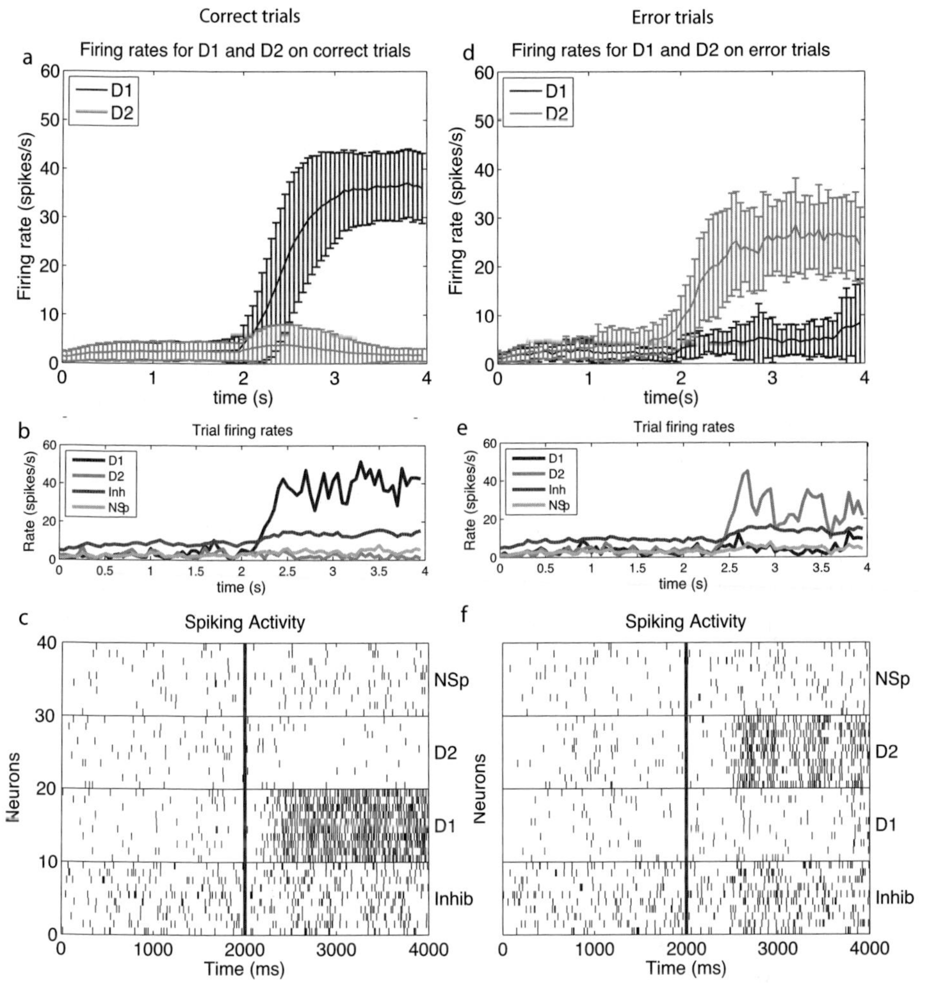

Fig. 8.21 (a and d) Firing rates (mean $\pm$ sd) for correct and error trials for an intermediate level of difficulty (ΔI=32). The period 0–2 s is the spontaneous firing, and the decision cues were turned on at time = 2 s. The means were calculated over 1000 trials. D1: firing rate of the D1 population of neurons, which is the correct population. D2: firing rate of the D2 population of neurons, which is the incorrect population. A correct trial was one in which in which the mean rate of the D1 attractor averaged $>$ 10 spikes/s for the last 1000 ms of the simulation runs. (Given the attractor nature of the network and the parameters used, the network reached one of the attractors on $>$90% of the 1000 trials, and this criterion clearly separated these trials, as indicated by the mean rates and standard deviations for the last 1 s of the simulation as shown.) (b and e) The firing rates of the four populations of neurons on a single trial for a correct (b) and incorrect (e) decision. Inh is the inhibitory population that uses GABA as a transmitter. NSp is the non-specific population of neurons. (c and f) Rastergrams for the trials shown in (b) and (e). 10 neurons from each of the four pools of neurons are shown. (See colour plates Appendix D.) (Reproduced from *Journal of Neurophysiology*, 104 (5), Decision-making, errors, and confidence in the brain, E.T. Rolls, F. Grabenhorst, and G. Deco, pp. 2359–2374 ©2010, The American Physiological Society.)

i.e. between t=3 and t=4 s. It is clear that the mean firing rate of the winning attractor D1 on correct trials increases monotonically as ΔI increases, and interestingly, the increase is approximately linear (Pearson $r = 0.995, p < 10^{-6}$). The higher mean firing rates of the winning D1 attractor on correct trials as ΔI increases are due not only to higher peak firing,

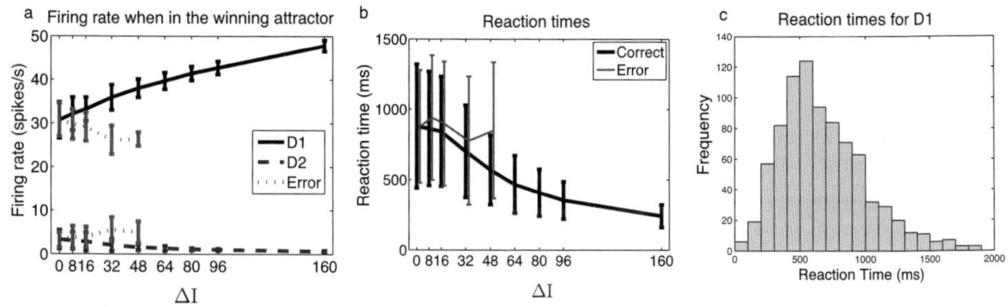

Fig. 8.22 (a) Firing rates (mean ± sd) on correct and error trials when in the winning attractor as a function of ΔI. ΔI=0 corresponds to difficult, and ΔI=160 corresponds to easy. The firing rates on correct trials for the winning population D1 are shown by solid lines, and for the losing population D2 by dashed lines. All the results are for 1000 simulation trials for each parameter value, and all the results shown are statistically highly significant. The results on error trials are shown by the dotted red lines, and in this case the D2 attractor wins, and the D1 attractor loses the competition. (There were no error trials for values of ΔI=64 Hz or above.) (b) Reaction times (mean ± sd) for the D1 population to win on correct trials (thick line), and for D2 to win on error trials (thin line), as a function of the difference in inputs ΔI to D1 and D2. The plot for the error trials has been offset by a small amount so that its values can be seen clearly. ΔI=0 corresponds to difficult, and ΔI=160 corresponds to easy. (c) The distribution of reaction times for the model for ΔI=32 illustrating the long tail of slow responses. Reaction times are shown for 837 correct trials, the level of performance was 95.7% correct, and the mean reaction time was 701 ms. (See colour plates Appendix D.) (Reproduced from *Journal of Neurophysiology*, 104 (5), Decision-making, errors, and confidence in the brain, E.T. Rolls, F. Grabenhorst, and G. Deco, pp. 2359–2374 ©2010, The American Physiological Society.)

but also to the fact that the variability becomes less as ΔI increases ($r = -0.95, p < 10^{-4}$), reflecting the fact that the system is more noisy and unstable with low ΔI, whereas the firing rate in the correctly winning D1 attractor is maintained more stably with smaller statistical fluctuations against the Poisson effects of the random spike timings at high ΔI. (The measure of variation indicated in the Figure is the standard deviation, and this is shown throughout unless otherwise stated to quantify the degree of variation, which is a fundamental aspect of the operation of these neuronal decision-making networks.) The increase of the firing rate when in the D1 attractor on correct trials (solid black line) as ΔI increases thus reflects the confidence in the decision, and, as is shown in Fig. 8.15c, the performance as shown by the percentage of correct choices. On correct trials, the firing rate of the losing attractor (D2, dashed blue line) is of course low, and decreases further as ΔI increases on correct trials, due to feedback inhibition from the winning D1 attractor, and thus the difference in the firing rates of the two attractors also reflects well the decision confidence.

When we make an incorrect choice, our confidence in our decision is likely to be low (Vickers 1979, Vickers & Packer 1982). Exactly this is represented in the firing rates of the neurons on incorrect trials, for as shown in dotted red lines in Fig. 8.22a, when an incorrect choice is made (and D2 wins the competition because of noise), the firing rate of the D2 attractor when winning decreases as ΔI increases (upper dotted red line starting at 31 spikes/s). The reason for this is that the external inputs, the evidence for the decision, are now working against the internal recurrent attractor dynamics, which have reached the wrong decision because of the noise in the network. Thus on error trials, the confidence in a decision is also reflected in the firing rates of the attractors (Rolls, Grabenhorst & Deco 2010c).

Conversely, the firing rate of the losing attractor (D1) on incorrect trials, which is low with ΔI=0 (approximately 3 spikes/s), increases by a few spikes/s as ΔI increases (lower dotted red line in Fig. 8.22a). The reason for this is that the noise has contributed to the D1 attractor losing, and there is more external input against this decision being applied to the D1 neurons as ΔI increases, tending to increase their firing rate from the low value. At the same time, the D1 neurons receive less feedback inhibition from the incorrectly winning population D2 via the inhibitory neurons as ΔI increases.

The time for the network to reach the correct D1 attractor, i.e. the reaction time of the network, is shown as a function of ΔI for correct and incorrect trials in Fig. 8.22b (mean $\pm$ sd). Interestingly, the reaction time continues to decrease ($r = -0.95, p < 10^{-4}$) over a wide range of ΔI, even when as shown in Fig. 8.22c the network is starting to perform at 100% correct. The decreasing reaction time as ΔI increases is attributable to the altered 'effective energy landscape' (see Section 8.4): a larger input to D1 tends to produce occasionally higher firing rates, and these statistically are more likely to induce a significant depression in the landscape towards which the network flows sooner than with low ΔI. Correspondingly, the variability (quantified by the standard deviation) of the reaction times is greatest at low ΔI, and decreases as ΔI increases ($r = -0.95, p < 10^{-4}$). This variability would not be found with a deterministic system (i.e. the standard deviations would be 0 throughout, and such systems include those investigated with mean-field analyses), and is entirely due to the random statistical fluctuations caused by the random spiking of the neurons in the integrate-and-fire network.

Very interestingly, the reaction times of the network are longer for incorrect (error) than for correct decisions, as shown by the thin graph in Fig. 8.22b (Rolls, Grabenhorst & Deco 2010c). This difference, though not large, was statistically significant. (The effect was found for the means of the 4 non-zero values of ΔI for which there were errors ($p < 0.05$), and for ΔI=8 for example, the reaction time distribution was longer for error compared to correct trials, $p < 0.01$ and confirmed by the non-parametric Mann-Whitney test.) This models effects that are found in human performance (Vickers & Packer 1982), especially with difficult decisions (Luce 1986, Welford 1980), and that have also been found in lateral intraparietal (LIP) cortex neurons in a motion coherence discrimination task (Roitman & Shadlen 2002) and in a related attractor model of this (Wong, Huk, Shadlen & Wang 2007). The actual mechanism for this in this biologically plausible attractor decision-making network is that on error trials, the noise is fighting the effects of the difference in the inputs λ_1 and λ_2 that bias the decision-making, and it takes on average relatively long for the noise, on error trials, to become by chance sufficiently large to overcome the effects of this input bias (Rolls, Grabenhorst & Deco 2010c). This effect will contribute to the smaller BOLD signal on error than on correct trials described below.

The distribution of reaction times for the model has a long tail of slow responses, as shown in Fig. 8.22c for ΔI=32, capturing this characteristic of human reaction time distributions (Luce 1986, Welford 1980, Ratcliff & Rouder 1998, Ratcliff, Zandt & McKoon 1999, Usher & McClelland 2001, Marti, Deco, Mattia, Gigante & Del Giudice 2008).

The relation between ΔI and percentage correct is shown in Fig. 8.15c on page 396, and described in Section 8.7.4.

8.7.8.2 Predictions of fMRI BOLD signals from the model

We now show how this model makes predictions for the fMRI BOLD signals that would occur on correct vs incorrect trials in brain areas in which decision-making processing of the type described is taking place. The BOLD signals were predicted from the firing rates of the neurons in the network (or from the synaptic currents flowing in the neurons as described later) by convolving the neuronal activity with the haemodynamic response function in a realistic period, the two seconds after the decision cues are applied. This is a reasonable period to take, as decisions will be taken within this time, and the attractor state may not necessarily be maintained for longer than this. (The attractor states might be maintained for

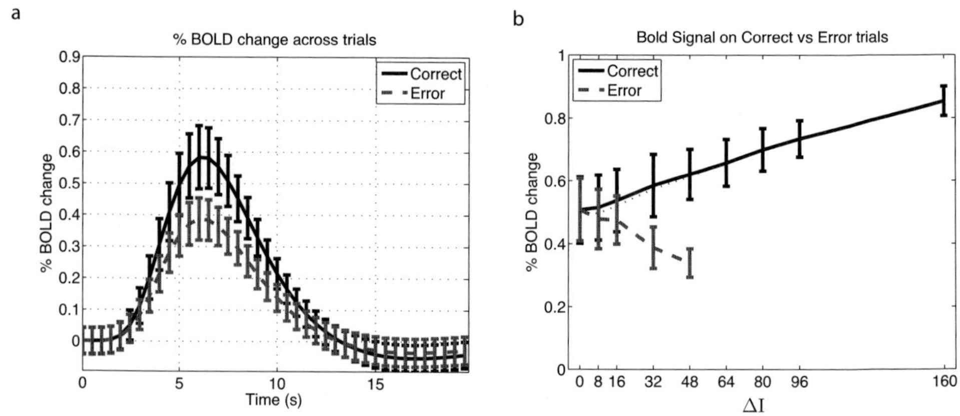

Fig. 8.23 (a) The predicted percentage change (mean $\pm$ sd) in the BOLD signal on correct and error trials for $\Delta I = 32$. The percentage change in the BOLD signal was calculated from the firing rates of the D1 and D2 populations, and analogous effects were found with calculation from the synaptic currents averaged for example across all 4 populations of neurons. (b) The percentage change in the BOLD signal (peak mean $\pm$ sd) computed separately for correct and error trials as a function of ΔI. ΔI=0 corresponds to difficult, and ΔI=160 corresponds to easy. The percentage change was measured as the change from the level of activity in the simulation period 1–2 s, before the decision cues were applied at t=2 s, and was calculated from the firing rates of the neurons in the D1 and D2 populations. The BOLD percentage change scaling is arbitrary, and is set so that the lowest value on correct trials is 0.5%. The thin dotted line just below the line for the predicted response on correct trials shows the predicted response from all trials, that is correct and error trials. (Reproduced from *Journal of Neurophysiology*, 104 (5), Decision-making, errors, and confidence in the brain, E.T. Rolls, F. Grabenhorst, and G. Deco, pp. 2359–2374 ©2010, The American Physiological Society.)

longer if the response that can be made is not known until later, as in some fMRI tasks with delays including that described here, and then the effects described might be expected to be larger, given the mean firing rate effects shown in Fig. 8.21. Indeed, it is an advantage of the type of model described here that it is a short-term memory attractor network that can maintain its firing whether or not the decision cues remain, as this continuing firing enables the decision state to be maintained until a response based on it can be guided and made.) As shown in Fig. 8.23a, the predicted fMRI response is larger for correct vs incorrect trials in the decision-making network (Rolls, Grabenhorst & Deco 2010c). The results are shown for a level of difficulty in which there is a reasonable proportion of error trials (ΔI=32).

Figure 8.23b shows that the difference between the BOLD signal on correct vs incorrect trials increases with ΔI. The reason for this is that on correct trials, with increasing ΔI the external evidence adds more strongly to the firing produced by the internal recurrent collateral attractor effect in the winning attractor (Fig. 8.22a), and thus the BOLD signal increases with ΔI (Fig. 8.23b). On the other hand, on incorrect trials, the external evidence adds less than on correct trials to the winning attractor, and also adds more than on correct trials to the firing rates in the losing attractor, the firing rate of which through the inhibitory interneurons decreases the firing in the winning attractor, as shown in Fig. 8.22a. Because on incorrect trials the firing of the winning attractor decreases with ΔI (Fig. 8.22a), the BOLD signal decreases with ΔI on incorrect trials (Fig. 8.23b). An important result of the simulations is that it is the firing rate of the winning attractor that dominates the predicted BOLD signals, not the smaller effects seen in the losing attractor (Rolls, Grabenhorst & Deco 2010c). Although it is largely the higher overall neural activity on correct trials that results in the larger predicted BOLD signal on correct than error trials (Fig. 8.22a), an additional contributor is the shorter decision

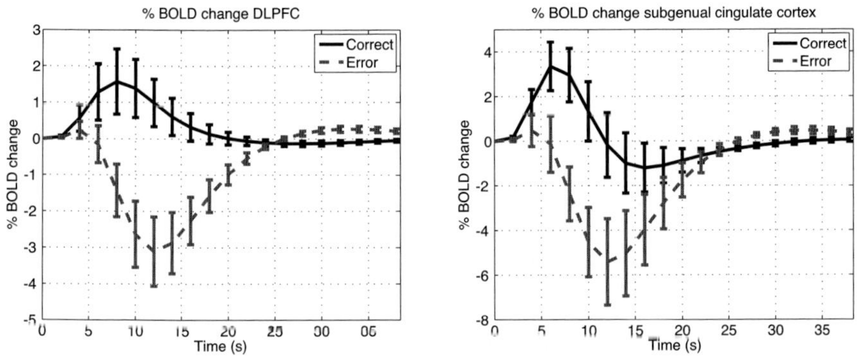

Fig. 8.24 The timecourses of the activations on correct and on error trials for the dorsolateral prefrontal cortex (left) and subgenual cingulate cortex (right), at sites where the contrast correct − error was significant. (Reproduced from *Journal of Neurophysiology*, 104 (5), Decision-making, errors, and confidence in the brain, E.T. Rolls, F. Grabenhorst, and G. Deco, pp. 2359–2374 ©2010, The American Physiological Society.)

latency for correct than error trials illustrated in Fig. 8.22b.

Figure 8.23b also shows with the thin dotted line (just below the line for the predicted response on correct trials) the predicted response from all trials, that is correct and error trials. The prediction of the BOLD signal for all trials is relatively close to the prediction for the correct trials because with low ΔI the predictions for correct and error trials are close as indicated in Fig. 8.22b, and with larger values of ΔI there are fewer error trials.

8.7.8.3 fMRI BOLD signals that are larger on correct than error trials

The model predicts that the BOLD signal will be larger in at least some brain areas involved in choice decision-making on correct than on incorrect trials. We tested this by performing a contrast analysis on correct vs incorrect trials in the olfactory decision-making task described in Section 8.7.7.1, in which the participants had to decide whether the second odour was more pleasant than the first. Error trials were defined as choices that do not reflect the mean pleasantness ratings (Rolls, Grabenhorst & Deco 2010c). (The rationale for this was that noise in the system might influence the binary choice made on an individual trial, and each participant's estimate of what was the more pleasant of each pair was given by the mean pleasantness rating across all trials for each odour being compared on a particular trial.) For example, if citral was rated on average for pleasantness as +1.5 and vanillin as +1.0, and the subject chose vanillin over citral, this was classified as an error trial. At the single subject level, contrasts between correct vs error trials were computed within each odour pair. At the group level, these odour-specific contrast maps were combined across subjects.

Four brain regions had significant effects in the correct vs error contrast (Rolls, Grabenhorst & Deco 2010c). They were the medial prefrontal cortex area 10 [2 50 −12]; the posterior cingulate cortex [−18 −32 34]; the subgenual cingulate cortex [10 24 −8]; and the dorsolateral prefrontal cortex (DLPFC) [24 14 34]). Figure 8.24 shows the timecourses of the activations on correct and on error trials for the dorsolateral prefrontal cortex (left) and subgenual cingulate cortex (right). The brain regions where these activations were found are close to those illustrated in Fig. 8.25 (top).

To investigate whether correct vs error effects are more likely to be found in areas that are implicated in decision-making by an earlier study that showed significant differences for trials on which decisions were made vs trials when only rating and no binary choices were made (Rolls, Grabenhorst & Parris 2010d), we performed ANOVAs on the parameter estimates for correct − incorrect decision contrasts vs the correlations with the pleasantness ratings. (In the previous investigation, brain areas implicated in decision-making included medial area 10, and in pleasantness ratings the orbitofrontal cortex.) We found that the posterior cingulate cortex, subgenual cingulate cortex, dorsolateral prefrontal cortex, and medial prefrontal cortex area 10 had considerable parameter estimates from the general linear model implemented in SPM for correct – error trials, and low for correlations with pleasantness; whereas the orbitofrontal cortex showed high parameter estimates for correlations with pleasantness, but low for correct – incorrect contrasts (Rolls, Grabenhorst & Deco 2010c). ANOVAs on these effects showed very significant interactions which indicated that activations in the medial prefrontal cortex area 10, the posterior and subgenual cingulate cortex, and the dorsolateral prefrontal cortex were related more to whether a choice decision was correct or incorrect and less to pleasantness, whereas activations in a control region the mid-orbitofrontal were related more to pleasantness and less to whether the choice was correct or incorrect (Rolls, Grabenhorst & Deco 2010c).

8.7.8.4 fMRI signals linearly related to choice easiness with correct vs incorrect choices

Another prediction of the model is that in decision-making areas of the brain, the magnitude of the BOLD signal should increase with ΔI on correct trials, and decrease with ΔI on error trials (Fig. 8.23b). To investigate this, we performed separate SPM regression analyses for correct and error trials in which the regressor for this was ΔI, the mean absolute difference in pleasantness between the two odours presented on a given trial. The analyses showed that for correct trials, positive correlations of the BOLD signal with ΔI were found in the posterior cingulate cortex [-8 -40 32], and on error trials, negative correlations of the BOLD signal with ΔI were found. These analyses also showed that on error trials, negative correlations of the BOLD signal with ΔI were found in the subgenual cingulate cortex [10 16 -4]. This effect is illustrated in Fig. 8.25 which shows the BOLD signal as a function of (discretized values of) ΔI for correct and incorrect trials. The signs of the correlations ($r = 0.55$ on correct trials, and $r = -0.81$ on error trials) are as predicted for a decision-making area of the brain, and are significantly different (p<0.003). These analyses also showed that on error trials, negative correlations of the BOLD signal with ΔI were found in the dorsolateral prefrontal cortex [30 18 28], and again the signs of the correlations ($r = 0.65$ on correct trials, and $r = -0.95$ on error trials) are as predicted for a decision-making area of the brain, and are significantly different ($p < 0.001$) (Fig. 8.25). Similarly, in medial prefrontal cortex area 10 the signs of the correlations ($r = 0.53$ on correct trials, and $r = -0.62$ on error trials) are as predicted for a decision-making area of the brain, and are significantly different ($p = 0.032$) (Fig. 8.25) (Rolls, Grabenhorst & Deco 2010c).

For comparison, we also show in Fig. 8.25 the analyses of the percentage change in the BOLD signal for correct and for error trials for the mid-orbitofrontal cortex, chosen as a control brain region. Activations in this area did not have a significant relation to decision-making vs rating (Rolls, Grabenhorst & Parris 2010d), and were not correlated with trial easiness as indexed by ΔI (Rolls, Grabenhorst & Deco 2010b), but did have a correlation with the pleasantness of the odour that was presented (Rolls, Grabenhorst & Parris 2010d). In this mid-orbitofrontal cortex region the correlation between the BOLD signal and ΔI was $r = 0.22$ on correct trials, and $r = -0.19$ on error trials, and these are not significantly different ($p = 0.46$). Thus this brain area that is not implicated in the binary choice decision-making, but does represent information relevant to the decision, the pleasantness of the stimuli, did not have significantly different activations on correct – error trials, and did not have significantly different correlations with the BOLD signal on correct and incorrect trials. This is a useful control condition. Thus a difference in the correlations of the BOLD signal with ΔI for correct vs error trials appears to be a sensitive measure for a brain area involved in decision-making.

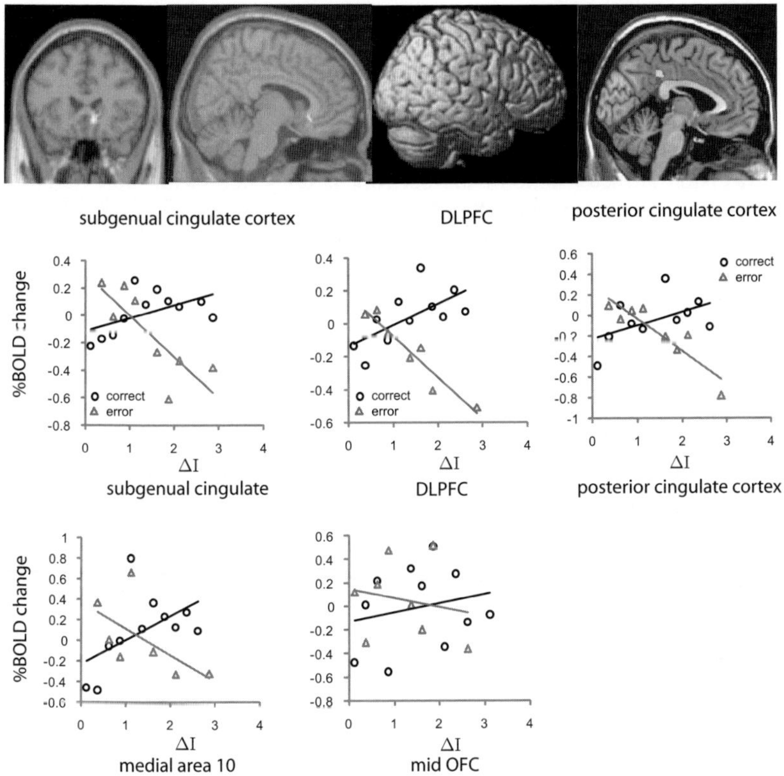

Fig. 8.25 Above: The subgenual cingulate cortex (with coronal and parasagittal slices), dorsolateral prefrontal cortex (DLPFC) and posterior cingulate cortex regions with the percentage change in the BOLD signal positively correlated with ΔI on correct trials, and negatively correlated on error trials. Below: Separate regression plots for the relation between the BOLD signal and ΔI on correct and on error trials for these regions and for the medial prefrontal cortex area 10, and for a control region, the mid-orbitofrontal cortex (mid OFC) in which effects were not found. The regression plots show for discretized values of ΔI (averaged across subjects) the BOLD signal as a function of ΔI for correct and incorrect trials. For example, for the posterior cingulate cortex the signs of the correlations ($r = 0.51$ on correct trials, and $r = -0.91$ on error trials) are as predicted for a decision-making area of the brain, and are significantly different ($p<0.001$). The medial prefrontal cortex coordinates used for extracting the data were [−4 54 −6] with a 10 mm sphere around this location, the site in the same subjects for the peak of the contrast for easy − difficult trials (Rolls, Grabenhorst and Deco 2010b). The same region [2 50 −12] showed more activity when binary decisions were made compared to when ratings were made in the same subjects (Rolls, Grabenhorst and Deco 2010b). (See colour plates Appendix D.) (Reproduced from *Journal of Neurophysiology*, 104 (5), Decision-making, errors, and confidence in the brain, E.T. Rolls, F. Grabenhorst, and G. Deco, pp. 2359–2374 ©2010, The American Physiological Society.)

An implication is that a sensitive criterion for identifying areas of the brain involved in decision-making is a higher activation on easy than on difficult trials, and that this will be especially evident when only correct trials are included in the analysis. A further signature is that the activations are expected to increase with ΔI on correct trials, and to decrease on error trials with ΔI (Rolls, Grabenhorst & Deco 2010c). Part of the reason that activations are higher with larger ΔI with all trials included is that these trials will mostly be correct, whereas difficult trials, with lower values of ΔI, will include more error trials.

8.7.8.5 Evaluation of the model: a basis for understanding brain processes and confidence for correct vs incorrect decisions

The spiking network model predicts probabilistic decision-making with larger neuronal responses in the winning attractor on correct than on error trials, because the spiking noise-influenced decision attractor state of the network is consistent with the external evidence, and this neuronal activity in turn predicts larger BOLD responses on correct than error trials in brain regions involved in making choices. Moreover, the model predicts that the neuronal activity in the winning attractor and the BOLD response will become larger on correct trials as ΔI increases and confidence increases; and will become smaller in the winning attractor as confidence decreases on error trials as ΔI increases. These effects can be understood in that on an individual trial the spiking-related and other noise will influence the decision made and therefore which attractor is firing, that for the correct or the incorrect choice. If the winner is that for the correct choice, then the firing rate will be higher with increasing ΔI as then the external evidence, the incoming firing rates, will be higher for this attractor than for the losing attractor, and as ΔI increases, will increase the firing rates more and more for the winning attractor. On the other hand, if the incorrect attractor wins on a particular trial, then the incoming evidence will provide weak support for the winning (incorrect) attractor, and will instead tend to increase the relatively low firing rates of the losing (correct) attractor, which in turn through the inhibitory interneurons will tend to decrease the firing rates further as ΔI increases in the winning but incorrect attractor. These results with these effects are shown in Fig. 8.22a.

In this situation, the model is very useful, for because it includes synaptic currents and firing rates, it is possible to predict from these the BOLD signal by convolution with the haemodynamic response function. However, on correct trials as ΔI increases, the firing rate of the winning (correct) population increases, but of the losing (incorrect) population decreases, as shown in Fig. 8.22a, so the model is needed to show which effect dominates the BOLD response, and it is found quantitatively to be the increase in the high firing rate attractor state that dominates the BOLD signal, rather than the decrease in the low firing rate state in the losing attractor, as shown in Fig. 8.23b. Similarly, on incorrect trials as ΔI increases, the firing rate of the high firing rate incorrect attractor will decrease, and of the low firing rate correct attractor will increase, but the net effect predicted for the BOLD signal is a decrease as ΔI increases (see Fig. 8.23b). The model makes qualitatively similar predictions from the synaptic currents.

A fascinating and important property of this biologically based model of decision-making is that decision confidence on correct vs error trials is an *emergent property* of the neuronal decision-making mechanism, and is represented by the firing rates of the winning attractor on correct vs error trials, which also alter in the same way as decision confidence as a function of ΔI. This was shown for the first time by Rolls, Grabenhorst & Deco (2010c). It is also an emergent property of the neuronal theory of decision-making, yet elegantly simple, that the firing rates of the neurons in the winning attractor on correct trials increase with ΔI, and that the firing rates of the neurons in the winning attractor on error trials decrease with ΔI (Rolls, Grabenhorst & Deco 2010c).

I note that the way we infer confidence from the ΔI of the ratings given is not only based on previous research in which confidence ratings and/or behaviour are related to ΔI (Vickers & Packer 1982, Jonsson et al. 2005, Kepecs et al. 2008), but is also not unlike the way in which 'decision utility' (Kahneman, Wakker & Sarin 1997), often referred to as 'subjective value' (Kable & Glimcher 2007), is usually inferred from choices or from neural activity (Kable & Glimcher 2007). In more detail, not only does decision confidence increase with ΔI, but also decision confidence is lower on error than on correct trials (Vickers & Packer 1982, Jonsson et al. 2005). The theory of decision-making described here indicates that in addition decision confidence on error trials decreases as ΔI increases, and shows how noise in the brain is related to these decision-related effects.

Kepecs, Uchida, Zariwala & Mainen (2008) have described a model of confidence estimation in which each stimulus, and a memory for the category boundary, is encoded as a distribution of values, and a choice is made by comparing each sample with the decision boundary, and a confidence value is estimated by calculating the absolute value of the distance from the decision boundary. This is unlike the present model, which instead is a plausible neuronal network model in which confidence emerges from the firing rates in the decision-making neuronal mechanism.

The fMRI results described here provide powerful support for this model of decision-making (Deco & Rolls 2006, Rolls & Deco 2010, Rolls, Grabenhorst & Deco 2010b, Rolls, Grabenhorst & Deco 2010c), in that not only does the BOLD signal in brain areas implicated in decision-making increase with ΔI when all trials are considered, but also the BOLD signal decreases on error trials as ΔI increases, and increases on correct trials as ΔI increases. In an attractor model of the activity of lateral intraparietal (LIP) cortex neurons in a motion coherence discrimination task (Roitman & Shadlen 2002), Wong et al. (2007) have also found longer reaction times on error than on correct trials, but have not related this to confidence or to ΔI, and also have not shown how the firing rates and the predicted BOLD signal from the process are influenced by ΔI and are related to decision confidence.

In another comparison, the accumulator, counter, or race models of decision-making in which the noisy evidence for different choices accumulates until some criterion is reached (Vickers 1979, Vickers & Packer 1982, Ratcliff & Rouder 1998, Ratcliff et al. 1999, Usher & McClelland 2001) (see Appendix B) do not describe a neurobiological mechanism, do not make specific predictions about how neuronal firing rates, synaptic currents, or BOLD signals will alter as decisions become easier, and do not make specific predictions about confidence in a decision, but do account for behavioural performance. In this context, it is thus of interest that the integrate-and-fire attractor approach as well as the other approaches can both be analysed as diffusion processes (Roxin & Ledberg 2008), and that our approach is not inconsistent with these accumulator or with Bayesian (Ma, Beck, Latham & Pouget 2006, Beck, Ma, Kiani, Hanks, Churchland, Roitman, Shadlen, Latham & Pouget 2008, Ma, Beck & Pouget 2008) approaches to decision-making. However, while accumulator models implement a linear diffusion process operation with noisy inputs, the attractor model implements a non-linear diffusion process once it has left the boundary peak between two valleys in the energy landscape, which becomes faster due to the recurrent positive feedback in the network between the population of co-active neurons. Once the attractor has reached the new valley it may be relatively stable (see Fig. 8.13). Consistent with this analysis of a non-linear diffusion process for decision-making, it is harder to move the decision away from the way it is going by electrical stimulation if the stimulation is applied later rather than earlier in a trial in the lateral intraparietal area (LIP) during a motion discrimination task (Wong, Huk, Shadlen & Wang 2007).

In the fMRI study of the olfactory decision-making task, we found that neural activity was larger on correct than on error trials in the medial prefrontal cortex area 10, the posterior cingulate cortex, the subgenual cingulate cortex, and the dorsolateral prefrontal cortex. We also showed that in the same brain regions the BOLD signal increases with ΔI on correct trials, and decreases with ΔI on error trials, showing that decision confidence is represented in neural activity in these areas (Rolls, Grabenhorst & Deco 2010c). These effects are predicted from the model for brain areas involved in taking the decision, which in making the choice falls into a high firing rate attractor state. Medial prefrontal cortex area 10 is implicated in decision-making in that the BOLD signal is larger on trials on which choices must be made about which of the two stimuli presented is more pleasant, compared to trials on which the same stimuli are presented but a rating must be made on a continuous scale of the pleasantness of the (second) odour with no choice between the two odours (Rolls, Grabenhorst & Parris 2010d). Medial prefrontal cortex area 10 is also implicated in decision-making by the criterion used by others (Heekeren, Marrett, Bandettini & Ungerleider 2004, Heekeren, Marrett & Ungerleider 2008) that activation should increase with task easiness, that is with ΔI (Rolls, Grabenhorst & Deco 2010b). Medial area 10 is also implicated in decision-making in that a shopping decision-making task is impaired by medial prefrontal cortex damage (Burgess 2000).

The posterior cingulate cortex is implicated in decision-making in that some neurons there respond when risky, uncertain choices are made (McCoy & Platt 2005b); and some neurons respond more when an expected large reward is not obtained, maintaining that firing until the next trial (Hayden, Nair, McCoy & Platt 2008) (probably reflecting input from orbitofrontal cortex error neurons that have attractor state-like persistent firing that encodes and maintains a negative reward prediction error signal (Thorpe, Rolls & Maddison 1983, Rolls & Grabenhorst 2008, Rolls 2009b)).

The subgenual cingulate cortex is connected with the ventromedial prefrontal cortical areas (Johansen-Berg et al. 2008), and the activations we found there in the subgenual cingulate cortex may reflect inputs from the ventromedial prefrontal cortex. Further, neural activity in the subgenual cingulate cortex has been implicated in representing relative chosen value in an uncertain decision environment (Boorman, Behrens, Woolrich & Rushworth 2009).

The dorsolateral prefrontal cortex region activated in the present study has been implicated by earlier studies in decision-making, including decision-making about visual and vibrotactile stimuli (Heekeren et al. 2004, Kim & Shadlen 1999, Preuschhof, Heekeren, Taskin, Schubert & Villringer 2006).

An important control point is that activity in the mid-orbitofrontal cortex (which was not implicated in choices between the odours but that did have activations related to the pleasantness of the odours (Rolls, Grabenhorst & Parris 2010d)) did not show different activations on correct vs incorrect trials, and did not have activations that increased with ΔI on correct trials, and decreased with ΔI on error trials (Rolls, Grabenhorst & Deco 2010c). This is what is predicted for a brain area not involved in binary choice decision-making, but in representing pleasantness on a continuous scale, which is an important input to the decision-making system, providing the values of λ in Fig. 8.13. As shown earlier, there were significant dissociations between the decision-making areas and the mid-orbitofrontal cortex in terms of whether the activity was different on correct vs error trials, or was correlated on a continuous scale with subjective pleasantness, a representation that is likely to be a precursor and prerequisite for choice decisions about pleasantness (Rolls & Grabenhorst 2008, Grabenhorst, Rolls & Parris 2008b, Rolls, Grabenhorst & Parris 2010d, Rolls, Grabenhorst & Deco 2010b, Rolls, Grabenhorst & Deco 2010c). I note that ΔI is not related in any simple way to the pleasantness of the second odour, presented at the onset time for the fMRI analyses described here. Instead, ΔI is the absolute value of the difference in the pleasantness of the first and second odours, and this could be high if the second odour is much less pleasant than the first.

It is a fundamentally important aspect of our theory of decision-making that the evidence for the decision-making, the values of λ in Fig. 8.13, are continuous-valued representations, and require a separate representation from the choice itself, which takes place in a separate network. It is this that enables us to simultaneously report the exact value on a continuous scale of two perhaps quite similar discriminanda, such as the pleasantness, motion or frequency of two stimuli, and at the same time make a binary choice between the stimuli using a different network in the brain.

8.8 Decisions based on confidence in one's decisions: self-monitoring

8.8.1 Decisions about confidence estimates

We have seen that after a binary decision there is nevertheless a continuous-valued representation of decision confidence encoded in the firing rates of the neurons in a decision-making integrate-and-fire attractor neuronal network (Fig. 8.22). What happens if instead of having to report or assess the continuous-valued representation of confidence in a decision one has taken, one needs to take a decision based on one's (partly) continuous-valued confidence estimate that one has just made a correct or incorrect decision? One might for example wait for a reward if one thinks one's decision was correct, or alternatively stop waiting on that trial and start another trial or action. We propose that in this case, one needs a second decision-making network, which takes decisions based on one's decision confidence (Insabato, Pannunzi, Rolls & Deco 2010).

8.8.2 A theory for decisions about confidence estimates

The architecture has a decision-making network, and a separate confidence decision network that receives inputs from the decision-making network, as shown in Fig. 8.26. The decision-making network has two main pools or populations of neurons, DA which becomes active for decision A, and DB which becomes active for decision B. Pool DA receives sensory information about stimulus A, and Pool DB receives sensory information about stimulus B. (I sometimes refer to stimulus A as odour A, and to stimulus B as odour B, as A and B were used in a neurophysiological investigation of odour decision-making to categorize an odour as A or B when there were different odour proportions in the mixture (Kepecs et al. 2008), as described in Section 8.8.3.) Each of these pools has strong recurrent collateral connections between its own neurons of strength w_+, so that each operates as an attractor population. There are inhibitory neurons with global connectivity to implement the competition between the attractor subpopulations. When stimulus A is applied, pool DA will usually win the competition and end up with high firing indicating that decision A has been reached. When stimulus B is applied, pool DB will usually win the competition and end up with high firing indicating that decision B has been reached. If a mixture of stimuli A and B is applied, the decision-making network will probabilistically choose decision A or B influenced by the proportion of stimuli A and B in the mixture.

First I describe the operation of the decision-making (first) network, and show how the firing rates of its neurons reflect decision confidence. This part of the system operates in the same way as described earlier in this chapter. Figure 8.27c shows the proportion of correct decisions as a function of the proportion of stimulus A and stimulus B in the mixture. The decision-making is probabilistic because of the spiking-related randomness in the network (Wang 2002, Deco & Rolls 2006, Deco, Rolls & Romo 2009b, Deco & Marti 2007, Marti, Deco, Mattia, Gigante & Del Giudice 2008, Rolls & Deco 2010). Figure 8.27a shows that on trials when the DA neuronal population which represents decision A correctly wins and has a high firing rate, the firing rate increases further with the discriminability of the stimuli $\Delta\lambda$, and thus encodes increasing confidence. ($\Delta\lambda$ is defined as (A−B)/((A+B)/2). $\Delta\lambda$ is thus large and positive if only A is present, is large and negative if only B is present, and is 0 if A and B are present in equal proportions. $\Delta\lambda$ is another notation for ΔI.) The reason for the increase of firing rate with $\Delta\lambda$ on correct trials is that the external inputs from the stimuli A or B then support the (noise-influenced) winning attractor (pool DA) and add to the firing rates being produced by the recurrent collateral connections in the winning attractor. On the other hand, on error trials the firing rates of the winning pool (now DB, which represents decision

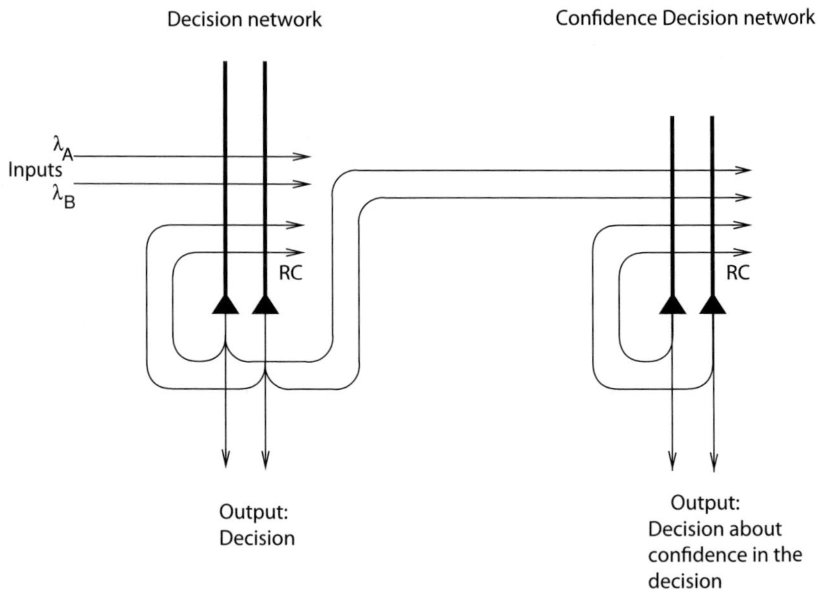

Fig. 8.26 Network architecture for decisions about confidence estimates. The first network is a decision-making network, and its outputs are sent to a second network that makes decisions based on the firing rates from the first network, which reflect the decision confidence. In the first network, high firing of neuronal population (or pool) DA represents decision A, and high firing of population DB represents decision B. Pools DA and DB receive a stimulus-related input (respectively λ_A and λ_B), the evidence for each of the decisions, and these bias the attractor networks, which have internal positive feedback produced by the recurrent excitatory connections (RC). Pools DA and DB compete through inhibitory interneurons. The neurons are integrate-and-fire spiking neurons with random spiking times (for a given mean firing rate) which introduce noise into the network and influence the decision-making, making it probabilistic. The second network is a confidence decision attractor network, and receives inputs from the first network. The confidence decision network has two selective pools of neurons, one of which (C) responds to represent confidence in the decision, and the other of which responds when there is little or a lack of confidence in the decision (LC). The C neurons receive the outputs from the selective pools of the (first) decision-making network, and the LC neurons receive $\lambda_{\mathrm{Reference}}$ which is from the same source but saturates at 40 spikes/s, a rate that is close to the rates averaged across correct and error trials of the sum of the firing in the selective pools in the (first) decision-making network. (Reproduced from *Journal of Neurophysiology*, 104 (1), Confidence-related decision-making, A. Insabato, M. Pannunzi, E. T. Rolls, and G. Deco, pp. 539–547 ©2010, The American Physiological Society.)

B and wins despite the evidence because of noisy firing in the network) become lower as $\Delta\lambda$ increases, because then the external sensory inputs are inconsistent with the decision that has been taken, and do not support and increase the firing rate of the winning pool (Rolls, Grabenhorst & Deco 2010c). Confidence, which increases with $\Delta\lambda$ on correct trials and decreases with $\Delta\lambda$ on error trials (Vickers 1979, Vickers & Packer 1982, Jonsson, Olsson & Olsson 2005, Kepecs, Uchida, Zariwala & Mainen 2008, Rolls, Grabenhorst & Deco 2010c), is thus encoded in the firing rates of the winning attractor, and is an emergent property of the decision-making network. Moreover, the sum of the activity of the winning and losing populations also represents decision confidence on correct and error trials, as shown in Fig. 8.27b. It is this total firing from pools DA and DB of the first, decision-making, network, which reflects decision confidence, that is provided as the input to the confidence (second) network.

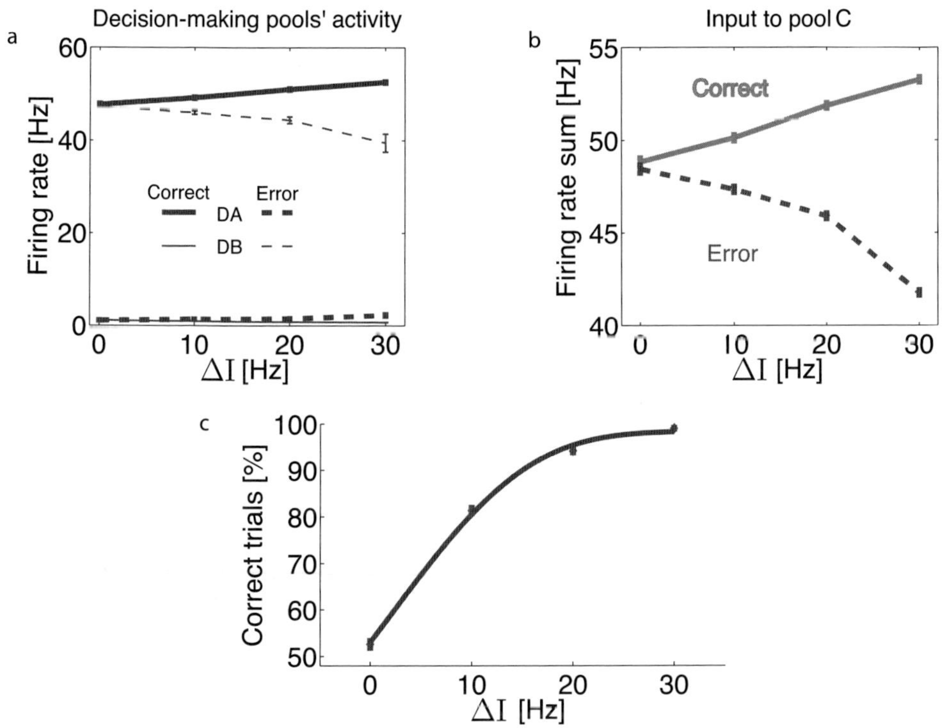

Fig. 8.27 Performance of the decision-making (first) network. (a) When pool DA correctly wins the competition, its firing rates are high and increase as a function of $\Delta\lambda$. When pool DB incorrectly wins making an error due to the noise and has a high firing rate, its firing rate decreases as a function of $\Delta\lambda$. The low firing rates when DB loses the competition on correct trials, and when DA loses the competition on error trials, are also shown. The error bars represent the sem. Confidence is thus encoded in the firing rates of the winning attractor, and is an emergent property of the decision-making network. (b) Sum of the firing rates from the DA and DB populations as a function of $\Delta\lambda$. This provides the input to the confidence (second) network selective pool C. The error bars show the sem. (c) The percentage correct performance of the decision-making network as a function of $\Delta\lambda$. (The error bars were estimated from the binomial distribution, and were small. The points are fitted by a Weibull function.) (Reproduced from *Journal of Neurophysiology*, 104 (1), Confidence related decision-making, A. Insabato, M. Pannunzi, E. T. Rolls, and G. Deco, pp. 539–547 ©2010, The American Physiological Society.)

I now consider the operation of the confidence decision (second) network. The confidence network has two selective pools of neurons, one of which (C) responds to represent confidence in the decision, and the other of which responds when there is little or a lack of confidence in the decision (LC). (In the experiment of Kepecs et al. (2008), C corresponds to a decision to stay and wait for a reward, i.e. what they call the positive outcome population, though it really represents confidence or a prediction that the decision just taken will have a positive outcome. LC corresponds to a decision to abort a trial and not wait for a possible reward, i.e. what they call the negative outcome population, though it really represents lack of confidence that the decision just taken will have a positive outcome, equivalent to confidence that the decision just taken *will have* a negative outcome.) If the output firing of the winning attractor of the first, decision-making, network (whether DA or DB, reflected in their sum, as shown in Fig. 8.27b) is high because the decision just taken has sensory inputs consonant with the decision, then the confidence decision network acting as a second level network takes the decision, probabilistically as before, to have confidence in the decision, and the C population

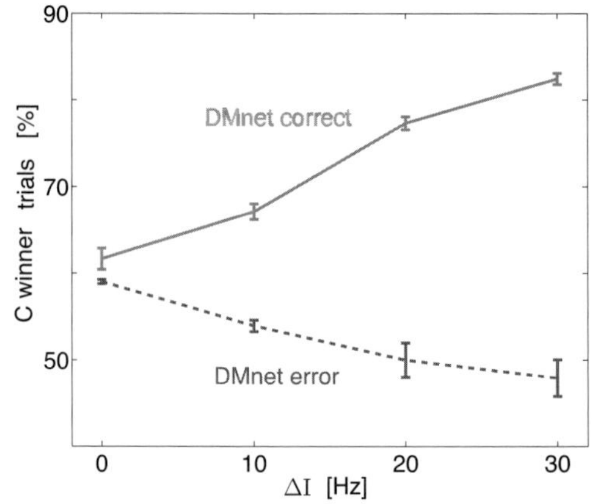

Fig. 8.28 Performance of the confidence decision (second) network. The percentage of trials on which in the second network the Confidence (C) population won the competition as a function of $\Delta\lambda$ for trials on which the decision-making (first) network (DMnet) was correct or incorrect. The performance of the LC population was the complement of this. (The parameters were set so that with $\Delta\lambda$ close to 0, approximately 60% of the trials were C trials, to be qualitatively in the same direction as in the experimental findings of Kepecs et al. 2008.) (Reproduced from *Journal of Neurophysiology*, 104 (1), Confidence-related decision-making, A. Insabato, M. Pannunzi, E. T. Rolls, and G. Deco, pp. 539–547 ©2010, The American Physiological Society.)

probabilistically wins the competition. If the output firing of DA and DB (reflected in their sum) is low because the decision just taken has sensory inputs that are not consonant with the decision, then with weaker driving inputs to the C network, it loses the competition with LC. The confidence network in this case takes the decision, probabilistically as before, to have a lack of confidence in the decision, in that the LC population wins the competition. The confidence decision network thus acts as a decision-making network to make confident decisions if the firing rates from the first, decision-making, network are high, and to make lack of confidence decisions if the firing rates from the first, decision-making, network are low.

As a result of the competition between the inputs to the C population and the inputs saturating at 40 Hz to the LC population, on trials when the (first) decision network is correct, the C population tends to win the competition more frequently as $\Delta\lambda$ increases, as shown in Fig. 8.28. Thus a decision to act confidently about one's first decision is more likely to be made as $\Delta\lambda$ increases on correct trials. On the other hand, when the first network makes an error, the C population tends to win the competition less frequently as $\Delta\lambda$ increases, as shown in Fig. 8.28, and correspondingly on error trials the proportion of trials on which the LC population wins increases with $\Delta\lambda$. (The percentage correct of the LC population is the complement of that shown in Fig. 8.28.) Thus a decision to lack confidence about one's first decision is more likely to be made as $\Delta\lambda$ increases on error trials, and this might make one abort such a trial, as in the experiment of Kepecs et al. (2008).

The general time structure of the neuronal activity in the model is in good accordance with the experimental results (Kepecs et al. 2008): as shown in Fig. 8.29, the confidence decision takes place after the first decision, and separation of the firing rates of the two selective populations C and LC occurs after the (first) decision-making network has reached a decision state, as in Fig. 3a-d of Kepecs et al. (2008).

It is important to examine the firing rates in the C and the LC attractor neuronal populations as a function of $\Delta\lambda$ on correct and incorrect trials, for they provide an account for neuronal responses recorded during decision-making (Kepecs et al. 2008), and those neurophysiological

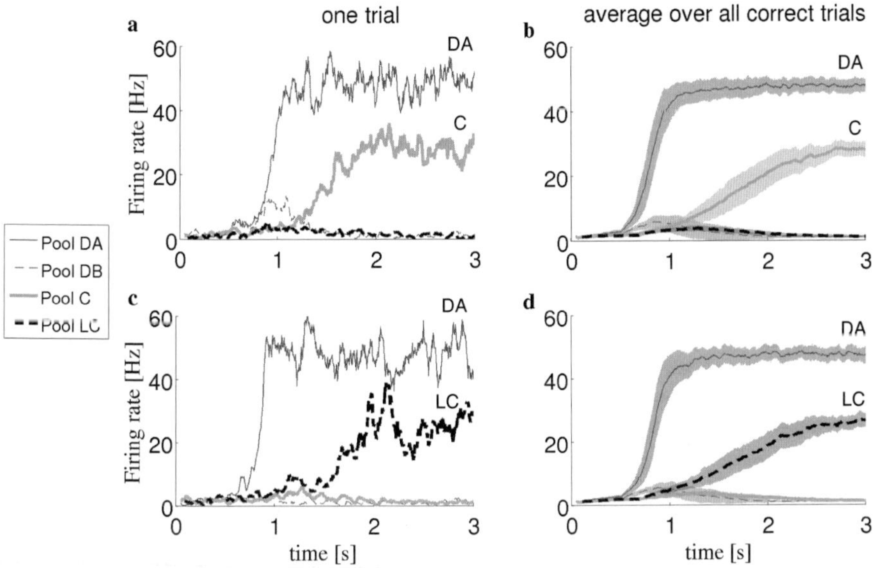

Fig. 8.29 Examples of the firing rate time courses of the selective pools in the decision-making (first) network and in the confidence decision (second) network. Each plot shows the activity in time of selective pools in the decision-making network in which pool DA won, and in the confidence network, for a difficult decision ($\Delta\lambda$=0). On 60% of trials the confidence network selective pool C won the competition as shown in the first row: (a) single trial, (b) average over all correct trials. On 40% of trials pool LC won the competition: (c) single trial, (d) average over all correct trials. The separation of the firing rates begins after the decision is taken and the general temporal structure of the network is in accordance with the experimental results of Kepecs et al. (2008). (Reproduced from *Journal of Neurophysiology*, 104 (1), Confidence-related decision-making, A. Insabato, M. Pannunzi, E. T. Rolls, and G. Deco, pp. 539–547 ©2010, The American Physiological Society.)

results in turn validate the model. We find for the confidence decision-making network that on correct trials with high $\Delta\lambda$=30 (easy decisions), C has a high firing rate, whereas it has a lower rate for $\Delta\lambda$=10, that is difficult decisions, as shown in Fig. 8.30. Conversely, on error trials when the firing rates in the first level, decision-making, network are lower, the confidence neurons C lose the competition and have relatively low firing rates, which decrease even further as the magnitude of $\Delta\lambda$ increases.

The firing rates (mean) in the confidence decision-making network of the C (confident, 'positive outcome') and LC (lack of confidence, 'negative outcome') populations of neurons for trials when the first decision-making network is correct or incorrect as a function of $\Delta\lambda$ are shown in Fig. 8.31. The thick lines show the mean firing rates for the C and LC pools for all trials on which the first network was correct, and separately for those in which the first network was in error. (We identify the LC population of neurons with the negative outcome population of neurons described by Kepecs et al. (2008), which have similar properties, as shown in Fig. 8.32. Further, we identify the C population of neurons with the positive outcome population of neurons described by Kepecs et al. (2008), which have similar properties, as shown in Fig. 8.32.)

However, as shown in Fig. 8.28, the confidence decision-making network was itself increasingly incorrect (i.e. took a confidence decision that was inconsistent with the decision taken by the (first) decision-making network) as $\Delta\lambda$ approached 0, and the firing rates in the thick lines of Fig. 8.31 reflect the fact that on some trials the C network won the competition, and on some trials it lost. This is effectively how Kepecs et al. (2008) presented their data (for

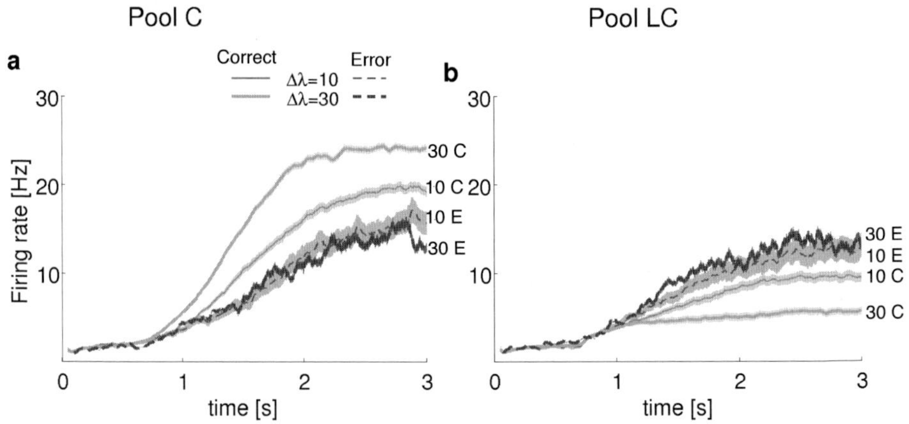

Fig. 8.30 Firing rates in the confidence decision-making network of the C (confident) and LC (lack of confidence) populations of neurons for trials when the first decision-making network is correct or incorrect for easy decisions ($\Delta\lambda$=30) and difficult ($\Delta\lambda$=10) decisions. Key: 30C–$\Delta\lambda$=30 first network correct; 10C–$\Delta\lambda$=10 first network correct; 10E–$\Delta\lambda$=10 first network error; 30E–$\Delta\lambda$=30 first network error. The firing rates are averaged across trials independently of which attractor the C / LC populations reached, and correspond to the firing rates in the thick box in Fig. 8.31. (The shaded areas represent the sem). The decision cues were turned on at t=500 ms. (Reproduced from *Journal of Neurophysiology*, 104 (1), Confidence-related decision-making, A. Insabato, M. Pannunzi, E. T. Rolls, and G. Deco, pp. 539–547 ©2010, The American Physiological Society.)

they knew only whether the decision itself was correct, and did not measure while recording whether the rat took a confidence-related decision to stay with or abort a trial), and there is good correspondence, as can be seen by comparing Fig. 8.32 with Fig. 8.28.

If instead of taking the mean firing rate of the C neurons based only on whether the first decision was correct, we take just the trials on which the C (confidence) pool won the competition, the thin lines of Fig. 8.31 show for the C pool an average rate of close to 28 spikes/s that tends to increase with $\Delta\lambda$ when the first network is correct, and tends to decrease with $\Delta\lambda$ when the first network is in error. (This is supported by the data shown in Fig. 8.30.) If we take just the trials on which the C population lost the competition, the thin lines show for the C pool an average rate of close to 2 spikes/s. Conversely, for the LC pool of neurons, if we take just the trials on which the LC population won the competition, the thin lines show for the LC pool an average rate of close to 26 spikes/s. If we take just the trials on which the LC population lost the competition, the thin lines show for this LC pool an average rate of close to 2 spikes/s. These firing rates shown in the thin lines in Fig. 8.31 are generally as expected, and the differences with $\Delta\lambda$ are due to whether the output of the decision-making (first) network shown in Fig. 8.27b are consistent or inconsistent with the decision taken by the confidence decision (second) network, which is of course influenced by the spiking noise in the confidence decision network, which can take the wrong decision given the evidence it receives from the decision-making network shown in Fig. 8.27b.

The fact that the changes of firing rates found in the rat by Kepecs et al. (2008) as shown in Fig. 8.32 as a function of $\Delta\lambda$ are comparable with those shown in the thick lines in Fig. 8.31 provides good support for the present model. However, Kepecs et al. (2008) did not distinguish trials in which a second-layer confidence decision network was in error or not

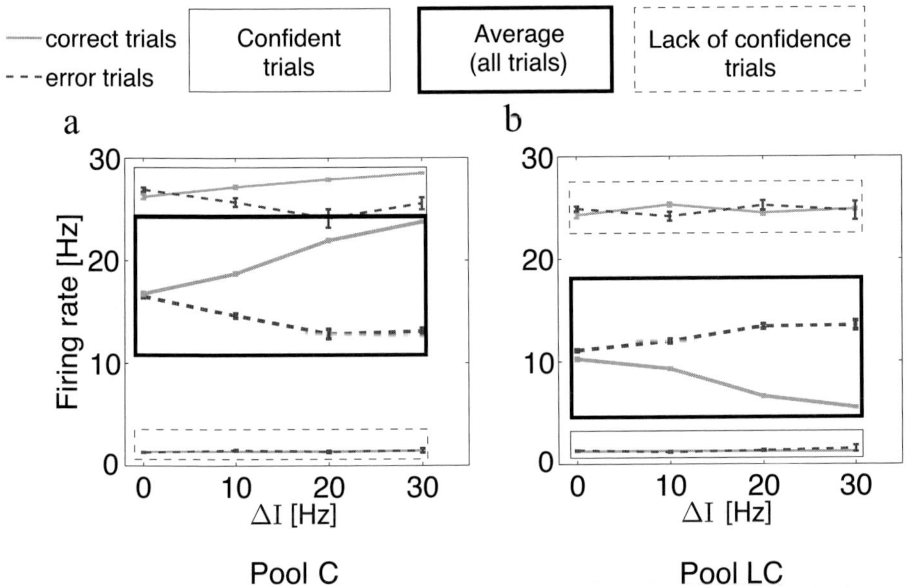

Fig. 8.31 Firing rates (mean $\pm$ s.e.m.) in the confidence decision-making network of the C (confident, 'positive outcome') (a), and LC (lack of confidence, 'negative outcome') (b) populations of neurons. In the solid thin boxes the firing rates of the C (left panel) and LC (right panel) pools are shown on trials on which the C (confidence) population won the competition. The lines in the solid thin boxes show for the C pool an average rate of close to 28 spikes/s which tends to increase with $\Delta\lambda$ when the first network is correct, and tends to decrease with $\Delta\lambda$ when the first network is in error. In the dashed thin boxes the firing rates of the C (left panel) and LC (right panel) pools are shown on trials on which the LC (lack of confidence) population won the competition. Again for the C population, if we take just the trials on which the C population lost the competition, the lines in the dashed thin boxes show for the C pool an average rate of close to 2 spikes/s. The activities of the C and LC populations of neurons, averaged over all trials, confident and lack of confidence, are shown in the thick boxes. As shown in Fig. 8.28, the confidence decision-making network was itself increasingly incorrect as $\Delta\lambda$ approached 0, and the firing rates in the thick lines reflect the fact that on some trials the C population won the competition, and on some trials it lost. (Reproduced from *Journal of Neurophysiology*, 104 (1), Confidence-related decision-making, A. Insabato, M. Pannunzi, E. T. Rolls, and G. Deco, pp. 539–547 ©2010, The American Physiological Society.)

as they did not record neuronal activity when they could examine whether the rat aborted a trial, and we suggest that it would now be interesting to do this. Further, it is notable that the change of firing rate with $\Delta\lambda$ found in the rat matches only that of the thick lines in Fig. 8.31 which includes all trials irrespective of the decision taken by the confidence decision (second) network, and not by the thin lines in Fig. 8.31 which reflect the decision taken by the confidence network. This leads to the novel prediction that different results will be found to those presented by Kepecs et al. (2008) if in a future experiment the responses of similar neurons are separated according to whether each trial is aborted or not. We predict in particular that the neurons will have activity like that shown in the thin lines in Fig. 8.31, and will be of two types (Insabato, Pannunzi, Rolls & Deco 2010).

One type will be similar to that of the C (confidence in the prior decision) neurons shown in Fig. 8.31 in which the firing rate is high on trials on which the confidence decision is to stay with the first decision, and low if the confidence (second) decision is to abort the trial. The prediction further is that the firing rates of these confidence neurons will change with $\Delta\lambda$ as shown by the thin lines in Fig. 8.31a, that is these high firing rates will tend to increase as a function of $\Delta\lambda$ if the first decision (taken by the decision-making, first, network) is consistent with the evidence (i.e. correct), as shown at the top of Fig. 8.31a, and to decrease as a function of $\Delta\lambda$ if the first decision (taken by the decision-making, first, network) is inconsistent with the evidence (i.e. is an error), as also shown at the top of Fig. 8.31a.

The second type of neuron will be similar to that of the LC (lack of confidence in the prior decision) neurons shown in Fig. 8.31b in which the firing rate is high on individual trials on which the confidence decision is to abort the trial, and low if the confidence (second) decision is to stay with the first decision. (The firing rates of the LC population do not change much with $\Delta\lambda$ as shown by the lines in the thin boxes of Fig. 8.31b because the input from the saturating neurons has a fixed firing rate.) It is only when we categorize the neurons according to whether the first decision was correct or not that curves similar to those shown by thick lines in Fig. 8.31 and as reported by Kepecs et al. (2008) will be found, and such curves and analyses do not capture fully the properties of the confidence decision-related neurons, which are we propose as shown in the thin lines in Fig. 8.31 (Insabato, Pannunzi, Rolls & Deco 2010).

These two predicted effects have not been sought yet in neurophysiological investigations (Kepecs et al. 2008), as all the correct trials were averaged, and all the incorrect trials were averaged. We thus make the novel prediction that when an animal incorrectly judges its choice, acting with confidence or lack of confidence that is inappropriate, new types of neuronal firing activity from the confidence and lack of confidence neurons will be found (Insabato, Pannunzi, Rolls & Deco 2010).

8.8.3 Decisions about confidence estimates: neurophysiological evidence

The model we describe accounts for results obtained by Kepecs, Uchida, Zariwala & Mainen (2008) from a binary decision task. The rats had to perform a binary categorization task with a mixture of two pure odourants (A, caproic acid; B, 1-hexanol), by entering one of two ports to indicate that the mixture was more like odour A or odour B (see Fig. 8.32). Correct choices were rewarded after a delay of 0.3–2 s. Varying the relative concentration of the odourants allowed the difficulty of the trial to be altered.

Neural activity related to decision confidence should occur just after the decision is taken and before the trial outcome. Kepecs et al. (2008) therefore analysed recordings of neuronal activity during a delay period after a decision had been taken before a reward was given. The single neuron recordings were made in the rat orbitofrontal cortex. (Exactly what area in primates and humans corresponds to the area in which recordings were made is not yet clear.) The neurons were then divided into two groups based on whether they fired faster on correct or on error trials. Kepecs et al. (2008) found that the group of neurons ('negative outcome' neurons) with an increased firing rate on error trials had higher firing rates with easier stimuli. The same neurons fired at a substantially lower rate on correct trials, and on these trials the firing rates were lower when the decision was made easier (Fig. 8.32d). This produced the opposing V-shaped curves shown in Fig. 8.32d. These authors argued that this pattern of activity encoded decision confidence. The properties of these neurons, called 'negative outcome' neurons by Kepecs et al. (2008) (Fig. 8.32d), correspond to the Lack of Confidence (LC) neurons illustrated in Fig. 8.31b. We therefore interpret the 'negative outcome' neurons as being produced by a second network taking confidence decisions (about for example whether to abort a trial) based on the output of a first level decision-making network.

These 'negative outcome' neurons of Kepecs, Uchida, Zariwala & Mainen (2008) are very similar to the primate orbitofrontal cortex error neurons described by Thorpe, Rolls & Maddison (1983), which fire with a high rate which is prolonged for several seconds consistent

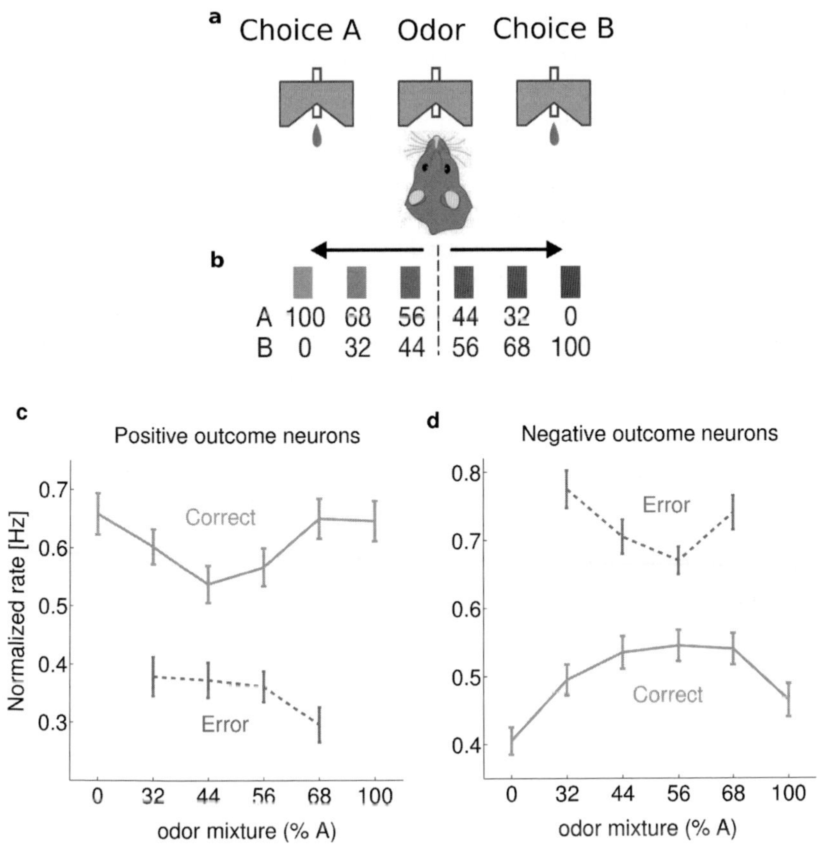

Fig. 8.32 (a) Odour mixture categorization task: when the rat enters the odour port, an odour mixture is delivered. Then the subject categorizes the mixture as A or B by moving left or right, according to the dominant odour. The stimulus is defined by the percentage of the two pure odourants A and B in the mixture as shown in (b). When odours are present in almost equal quantities, there is no bias to the decision process. Moving the stimulus towards pure odourants raises the bias towards one of the decisions and improves performance. (c) Mean normalized firing rate of the positive outcome selective neuronal population. These neurons fire faster on correct trials then on error trials, and increase their firing rate as the task becomes easier. On error trials, when the rat makes the wrong choice, these neurons fire more slowly, and decrease their firing rates more as the task becomes easier. If $\Delta\lambda$ is the discriminability of the stimuli, this is 0 for a 50% mixture of odours A and B, and $\Delta\lambda$ increases both to the left on the abscissa and to the right from 50% as the proportion of one of the odours in the mixture increases and the decision of which odour it is becomes easier. (d) Mean normalized firing rate of the negative outcome selective neuronal population in the orbitofrontal cortex as recorded by Kepecs et al. (2008). These neurons have sustained activity on error trials, increasing their firing rate further when the decision is made easier. On correct trials they fire slower, and decrease their firing rates as the decision becomes easier. (Reprinted by permission from Macmillan Publishers Ltd: *Nature*, 455 (7210), Adam Kepecs, Naoshige Uchida, Hatim A. Zariwala and Zachary F. Mainen, Neural correlates, computation and behavioural impact of decision confidence, pp. 227–231, copyright 2008, Nature Publishing Group.)

with attractor dynamics on error trials but not on correct trials of a visual discrimination task (see Fig. 4.38 and Section 4.5.5.5). In more detail, these neurons fire when an expected reward is not received, for example during extinction or reversal of a visual discrimination task. Particularly when these neurons fire in extinction (when an expected reward is not delivered), their firing reflects low confidence in a decision just taken, in a way rather analogous to that described by Kepecs et al. (2008). Although the mechanism just described can take decisions about confidence without an outcome (reward or punishment) being received, the underlying mechanisms for the computation of error may we suggest be rather similar for the error neurons of Thorpe, Rolls & Maddison (1983), which compute negative reward prediction error (Rolls & Grabenhorst 2008, Rolls 2009b). Because the reversal of the behaviour described by Thorpe, Rolls & Maddison (1983) takes place in one trial, the actual mechanism proposed is the reversal of a rule attractor by the prolonged firing of error neurons, with the rule attractor biasing conditional reward neurons found in the orbitofrontal cortex (Rolls 2008b, Deco & Rolls 2005a, Rolls 2009b).

The 'positive outcome' neurons of Kepecs et al. (2008) fired at a higher rate on correct than error trials, and increased their firing rates as the decisions became easier on correct trials (Fig. 8.32c). On incorrect trials, these 'positive outcome' neurons fired at lower and lower rates as the decision was made easier, that is as ΔI increased. These neurons thus had the same properties as the Confidence population of neurons in the Confidence Decision network, as illustrated in Fig. 8.31a. We thus interpret the 'positive outcome' neurons as being produced by the computational mechanism just described, in a second level attractor network that effectively 'monitors' a first level decision-making network, and takes decisions about decision confidence.

Kepecs et al. (2008) performed a second experiment to investigate if rats were able to make use of this information encoded by the orbitofrontal cortex neurons they described. The delay period was prolonged up to 8 s in order to allow the rat to reinitiate the trial. The subject could decide to leave the choice port and reinitiate the trial, or could wait for the reward to be delivered at the choice port. It was found that when the likelihood of a reward (i.e. the confidence) was low, due to the decision difficulty and the choice just made, the rat reinitiated the trial by leaving the choice port and returning to the odour port to sample a new mixture on a new trial. The probability that the rat would restart a trial as a function of stimulus difficulty and the choice just made was consistent with the responses of the neurons with activity described as encoding decision confidence: in our terminology, in taking decisions based on one's confidence in an earlier decision.

This finding strengthens the interpretation we place on the function of the Confidence and Lack of Confidence neurons. The mechanism we describe is however very different from that suggested by Kepecs et al. (2008). The mechanism we describe is consistent with the stochastic operations performed by attractor networks in the unifying and simple approach consistent with the underlying cortical architecture and function that is described in this book.

The model we described of decisions about confidence (Insabato, Pannunzi, Rolls & Deco 2010) thus is confirmed by and provides a computational account of the findings of Kepecs, Uchida, Zariwala & Mainen (2008). Moreover, the model makes predictions, not yet tested, about the firing rates of the different populations of neurons on trials on which the confidence decision network makes an error due to noise in the system.

8.8.4 Decisions about decisions: self-monitoring

In this section I consider the possible location of the networks that perform self-monitoring of decisions. The argument is as follows.

Sometimes it may be necessary to take a categorical decision based on the continuous value representation of confidence encoded as just described in the decision-making network. To make the decision based on confidence, we therefore need a second decision-making network, the confidence network shown in Fig. 8.26. In the case of Kepecs et al. (2008), the animal had to decide whether to stay and wait because confidence was high for a reward after the choice had been made, or whether to abort the trial and start a new trial because confidence in the decision just taken was low. It is for this type of choice that the second network is needed, and the way it operates is exactly in the same way as the first network in terms of how it takes the decision. The difference is primarily that the input to the second (confidence decision) network is the output of the decision-making network, the first network, the firing rates of which reflect and effectively encode the continuous-valued representation of confidence.

If the decision-making network and the confidence decision network are localized separately in the brain, one could predict some interesting dissociations neuropsychologically. For example, if the functions of the confidence decision network were impaired, one would predict good decision-making, but little ability to later decide whether one should have confidence in the decision just taken. Given that the decision network logically must come before the confidence decision network, and the hierarchical nature of cortical processing, one might predict that in humans the confidence network for decisions about the pleasantness of stimuli might be at the anterior end of the medial prefrontal cortex area 10 region implicated in choice decision-making (Rolls & Grabenhorst 2008, Grabenhorst, Rolls & Parris 2008b, Rolls, Grabenhorst & Parris 2010d, Shallice & Burgess 1991), or in another area connected to medial prefrontal cortex area 10.

8.8.5 Synthesis: decision confidence, noise, neuronal activity, the BOLD signal, and self-monitoring

8.8.5.1 Why there are larger BOLD signals for easy vs difficult decisions

The attractor neuronal network model of decision-making described in this chapter provides a firm foundation for understanding fMRI BOLD signals related to decision-making (Rolls, Grabenhorst & Deco 2010b). The model provides two reasons for the fMRI signal being larger on easy than on difficult trials during decision-making.

The first reason is that the neurons have somewhat higher firing rates on easy trials (e.g. those with a large ΔI) than on difficult trials, as shown in Fig. 8.15a. The reason for the faster response is that the difference in the inputs to the two attractors modifies the flow landscape so that the activity has a smaller barrier over which to jump towards one of the attractors (see Fig. 8.13c and Section 8.4). The fMRI BOLD signal thus starts sooner, even if by only a time in the order of 0.5 s, as shown in Fig. 8.15b.

The second reason is that the firing rates become higher in the winning attractor as ΔI increases, as shown in Fig. 8.15a, and this also contributes to a larger BOLD signal for easy vs difficult decisions. The firing rate of the winning attractor is higher with a large ΔI because the external input adds to the internal recurrent collateral synaptic effect (see Fig. 8.13a) to lead to a higher firing rate. This effect is increased because the external input to the D2 neurons is low, and so it competes less with the D1 attractor, also leading to higher rates in the D1 attractor with high ΔI.

Thus this approach from integrate-and-fire networks provides a foundation for understanding the shorter neuronal response times (Kim & Shadlen 1999, Shadlen & Newsome 2001) and the larger BOLD signals on easy than on difficult trials found in brain regions (Heekeren et al. 2004, Heekeren et al. 2008) that include for decisions about pleasantness the medial prefrontal cortex area 10 (Fig. 8.19). Very interestingly, the BOLD signal is linearly related to task easiness, as quantified by ΔI. This is predicted from the model (Figs. 8.17 and 8.18), and found experimentally (Fig. 8.20) (Rolls, Grabenhorst & Deco 2010b, Rolls, Grabenhorst & Deco 2010c).

8.8.5.2 Validation of BOLD signal magnitude related to the easiness of a decision as a signature of neural decision-making

The findings (Rolls, Grabenhorst & Deco 2010b) validate a larger BOLD signal on easy than on difficult trials as an fMRI signature of a region involved in decision-making, in that the areas that show this effect are areas implicated by other criteria in decision-making, including their larger activation on trials on which choice decisions must be made, rather than continuous ratings of affective value (Grabenhorst, Rolls & Parris 2008b, Rolls, Grabenhorst & Parris 2010d) (Fig. 8.19). The orbitofrontal and pregenual cortex, where continuous affective value but not choice is represented, do not show this easy vs difficult effect in the BOLD signal, as shown by the experimental fMRI results in Fig. 8.19.

8.8.5.3 Predictions of neuronal activity during decision-making

The model and its analysis described here also make predictions about the type of neuronal activity that will be found in brain areas involved in the choice part of decision-making, in which a categorical state must be reached. The predictions are that the neuronal activity will dynamically progress to a state in which there is a high firing of one population of neurons that occurs when one choice is made, with the other populations showing low activity, often below the spontaneous level, due to inhibition from the other attractor (especially when ΔI is high, as shown in Figs. 8.14 and 8.15a). This high vs low neuronal activity with almost a binary distribution of firing rates (as the decision is reached, either firing with a high firing rate, or a low firing rate, that predicts which decision is reached), is an important characteristic of a brain region performing the type of decision-making described here. However, although the firing rates are categorical in this sense, there is predicted to be some effect of ΔI on the firing rate when in the attractor, with as shown in Fig. 8.22a on correct trials an increase with ΔI of the winning population, with the additional prediction that on correct trials the firing rate of the losing populations will tend to become smaller as ΔI increases. Conversely, on error trials, as shown in Fig. 8.22a, there is predicted to be a decrease with ΔI of the winning population, with an increase of the (low) rate of the losing population as ΔI increases.

Another diagnostic property of the neuronal activity in this type of decision-making system is that the reaction times of the neurons (the time it takes to reach an attractor) will decrease as a function of ΔI, as shown in Fig. 8.15b.

Another fundamental property of this type of decision-making network is that it inherently shows statistical variation, with neuronal noise from the almost random, Poisson, spike times influencing the time when the system starts to fall into an attractor, and then a rapid change of firing rate, due to the supralinear positive feedback from the recurrent collateral synaptic connections (the recurrent collateral effect) starting to take off (see Section A.3 and Chapter 8). It is to indicate and quantify this trial by trial statistical variability that the figures of the simulations in this chapter show the standard deviation of the responses. This is a case where it is not the peristimulus time histogram (i.e. an average across trials of neuronal activity) that is a main important measure of the neuronal functionality, but just as important and interesting is what happens on a trial by trial basis, and especially its variability, as the statistical fluctuations unfold. Some examples of the noisy temporal evolution of the firing rate on individual trials are shown in Figs. 8.14 and 8.21.

8.8.5.4 Multiple types of decision are made, each in its own brain region

It has been argued that this decision-making categorization effect, where the attractor properties produced by for example the recurrent collateral effect make the decision on a given trial, is found in a number of different brain regions, each of which can be conceived of as making its own noise-influenced decision (Rolls 2008b, Rolls & Deco 2010) (see also

Section 8.11.1). For example, the lateral intraparietal area can be thought of as reaching a decision about the state of global motion in a noisy display (Shadlen & Newsome 1996, Gold & Shadlen 2002, Gold & Shadlen 2007, Churchland et al. 2008); the medial prefrontal cortex area 10 as making choices about pleasantness between rewarding (affective) thermal (Grabenhorst, Rolls & Parris 2008b) and olfactory (Rolls, Grabenhorst & Parris 2010d) stimuli; decisions about the intensity of odours as being related to larger activations in the dorsolateral prefrontal cortex and ventral premotor cortex (Rolls, Grabenhorst & Parris 2010d); and decisions about the frequency of vibrotactile stimuli to neuronal activity in the ventral premotor cortex (Romo & Salinas 2003, Deco, Rolls & Romo 2009b). Given that it is a property of a number of cortical regions that they can be involved in making choices between the inputs that are represented in those regions, we need not necessarily expect that at the neuronal level activity will always be related to the final behavioural choice of the subject, for there may be other decision-making processes in the final chain to behavioural output, including those involved in response selection (Rolls 2008b).

How then is neuronal activity different in brain systems not involved in choice decision-making? The difference it is suggested is that in other brain areas, neuronal activity will be required to represent the exact details about the sensory stimulus or affective state that is produced, and not to be driven into a noise-influenced categorical decision state. For example, when we have to make a decision between two stimuli of similar pleasantness, we can at the same time rate on a continuous scale exactly what the pleasantness of each stimulus is, yet, presumably with a different brain system, come on an individual trial to a categorical choice of one rather than the other stimulus (Rolls & Grabenhorst 2008, Grabenhorst, Rolls & Parris 2008b, Rolls, Grabenhorst & Parris 2010d). With respect to affect, representations correlated with continuous affective value (reward value) are found in brain regions such as the orbitofrontal cortex (O'Doherty et al. 2001a, Rolls 2005b, Rolls 2007c, Rolls 2008b, Rolls & Grabenhorst 2008), and here activations are much less influenced than in medial prefrontal cortex by which choice is made (Rolls & Grabenhorst 2008, Grabenhorst, Rolls & Parris 2008b, Rolls, Grabenhorst & Parris 2010d, Rolls, Grabenhorst & Deco 2010b).

It is suggested that the underlying computational basis for this is that in earlier cortical processing areas the recurrent collateral activity must not be allowed to be too strong, lest it produce a system that would fall into attractors where the internal recurrent collateral effect dominated the external input. This would distort the sensory signal, which should not occur in early sensory areas, where some approach to linearity can be useful so that undistorted signal is available for later processing. It is suggested that in contrast in later cortical processing areas where decisions are being taken or categorical states are being reached, the external inputs to the network must influence where the system reaches, but the recurrent collateral effects can be stronger so that an attractor state with categorical properties is reached. It could be a simple difference, genetically guided, between cortical areas that accounts for this difference, with the relative strength of the recurrent collateral synaptic connections being stronger in later cortical areas such as the prefrontal cortex, where this also serves the same purpose of enabling short-term memory to be maintained by the attractor even when no stimuli remain (Rolls 2008b). It could also be that transmitter effects, such as those produced by acetylcholine (Giocomo & Hasselmo 2007), could alter the relative balance between the external inputs to a network and the internal recurrent collateral effects, and thus alter dynamically how a network in the brain is being used for decision-making vs signal processing (Rolls 2008b).

8.8.5.5 The encoding of decision confidence in the brain

An interesting property of this network model of decision-making revealed by these analyses is that the degree of confidence in the decision is encoded in the firing rate of the attractor networks that take the decision, as shown in Fig. 8.15a (with the per cent correct, which is closely correlated with subjective confidence (Vickers & Packer 1982, Jonsson, Olsson & Olsson 2005), shown in Fig. 8.15c). (The higher firing rates when in the attractor on easy vs difficult trials are also clearly illustrated in Fig. 8.14.) In essence, the higher the firing rate of a particular attractor, the more confident or certain one is that the decision is correct. In fact, as shown in Fig. 8.15a, the difference of firing rates between the winning and losing populations also clearly reflects the confidence in the decision. In Section 8.7.8 we show how similar analyses follow through for confidence on correct vs error trials, and how these confidence estimates depend on ΔI. Thus confidence may not be a special property of a group of neurons (Kepecs, Uchida, Zariwala & Mainen 2008), but instead emerges as a property of the type of integrate-and-fire attractor network model of decision-making described here.

Consistent with this, activations in the medial prefrontal cortex, area 10, an area implicated by other criteria in decision-making, are correlated with the confidence in the decision, as indexed by increasing values of ΔI, as shown in Section 8.7.7 and Figs. 8.19 and 8.20.

Moreover, the theoretical approach described here is strongly supported by the evidence that neurons in the macaque parietal cortex involved in perceptual decision-making about motion stimuli have firing rates that are higher for decisions in which there is confidence (Kiani & Shadlen 2009).

The performance of the attractor network on error trials is also of interest in relation to the observation that when we make an incorrect choice, our confidence in our decision (or certainty) is likely to be low. As shown earlier, exactly this is represented in the firing rates of the neurons on incorrect trials, for as shown by the thin dotted curves in Fig. 8.22a, when an incorrect choice is made (and D2 wins the competition because of noise), the firing rate of the D2 attractor when winning decreases as ΔI increases (upper thin dotted line). The reason for this is that the external inputs, the evidence for the decision, are now working against the internal recurrent attractor dynamics, which have reached the wrong decision just because of the noise in the network. Thus on error trials, the confidence or certainty of a decision is also reflected in the firing rates of the attractors (Rolls, Grabenhorst & Deco 2010b).

I note that many further factors influence decision-making, including sensitivity to the non-reward that occurs on error trials, and impulsiveness (Rolls, Hornak, Wade & McGrath 1994a, Hornak, Bramham, Rolls, Morris, O'Doherty, Bullock & Polkey 2003, Hornak, O'Doherty, Bramham, Rolls, Morris, Bullock & Polkey 2004, Clark, Cools & Robbins 2004, Rolls & Grabenhorst 2008), both of which show important differences between individuals (Berlin, Rolls & Kischka 2004, Berlin & Rolls 2004, Berlin, Rolls & Iversen 2005), so that the inherent properties of the decision-making circuitry described here have an overlay that contributes to the final behaviour (see Chapter 10 in Rolls (2008b)).

Another interesting property of the decision-making framework described and analysed in this book, with quite clear neurophysiological and behavioural predictions, is that the percentage correct performance asymptotes to perfect at 100% with quite moderate levels of ΔI (Fig. 8.15c), whereas the neuronal responses continue to become higher as ΔI increases further (Fig. 8.15a), the BOLD signals become larger (Fig. 8.17b), and the reaction times decrease further (Fig. 8.15b).

Further, the inherent trial-by-trial variability in human choice reaction times, which has always been an enigma, can now be understood in terms of statistical fluctuations in decision-making networks in the brain. Further, a firm foundation for longer reaction times on error than on correct trials, and the relation to ΔI, has now been developed (see Fig. 8.22b).

What has been described in this chapter demonstrates that a major strength of the current approach is that the framework for decision-making incorporates effects from many levels, including the synaptic and biophysical levels, and the abstract level of statistical fluctuations in dynamical systems, and is able to make predictions all the way from synaptic currents, to neuronal activity, to fMRI signals, and to behavioural and subjective performance and confidence, and offers a quantitative and unifying approach to our understanding at all these levels (Rolls 2008b).

8.8.5.6 Self-monitoring: correction of previous decisions

The approach described in this section (8.8) indicates that an integrate-and-fire attractor neuronal decision-making network encodes confidence in its firing rates, and that adding a second attractor network allows decisions to be made about whether to change the decision made by the first network, and for example abort the trial or strategy (see Fig. 8.26). The second network, the confidence decision network, is in effect monitoring the decisions taken by the first network, and can cause a change of strategy or behaviour if the assessment of the decision taken by the first network does not seem a confident decision.

Now this is the type of description, and language used, to describe 'monitoring' functions, taken to be high level cognitive processes, possibly related to consciousness (Lycan 1997, Block 1995b). For example, in an experiment performed by Hampton (2001) (experiment 3), a monkey had to remember a picture over a delay. He was then given a choice of a 'test flag', in which case he would be allowed to choose from one of four pictures the one seen before the delay, and if correct earn a large reward (a peanut). If he was not sure that he remembered the first picture, he could choose an 'escape flag', to start another trial. With longer delays, when memory strength might be lower partly due to noise in the system, and confidence therefore in the memory on some trials might be lower, the monkey was more likely to choose the escape flag. The experiment is described as showing that the monkey is thinking about his own memory, that is, is a case of meta-memory, which may be related to consciousness (Heyes 2008). However, the decision about whether to escape from a trial can be taken just by adding a second decision network to the first decision network. Thus we can account for what seem like complex cognitive phenomena with a simple system of two attractor decision-making networks (Fig. 8.26). The design of Kepecs et al. (2008) was analogous, in that the rat could choose to abort a trial if decision confidence was low, and again this functionality can be implemented by two attractor decision-making networks, as described in Section 8.8.

The implication is that some types of 'self-monitoring' can be accounted for by simple, two-attractor network, computational processes. But what of more complex 'self-monitoring', such as is described as occurring in a commentary that might be based on reflection on previous events, and appears to be closely related to consciousness (Weiskrantz 1997). This approach has been developed into a higher-order syntactic theory (HOST) of consciousness (Rolls 1999a, Rolls 2004d, Rolls 2005b, Rolls 2007b, Rolls 2007g, Rolls 2008c), in which there is a credit assignment problem if a multi-step reasoned plan fails, and it may be unclear which step failed. Such plans are described as syntactic as there are symbols at each stage that must be linked together with the syntactic relationships between the symbols specified, but kept separate across stages of the plan. It is suggested that in this situation being able to have higher-order syntactic thoughts will enable one to think and reason about the first-order plan, and detect which steps are likely to be at fault. Now this type of 'self-monitoring' is much more complex, as it requires syntax. The thrust of the argument is that some types of 'self-monitoring' are computationally simple, for example in decisions made based on confidence in a first decision, and may have little to do with consciousness; whereas higher-order thought processes are very different in terms of the type of syntactic computation required, and may be more closely related to consciousness (Rolls 1999a, Rolls 2004d, Rolls 2005b, Rolls 2007b, Rolls 2007g, Rolls 2008c, Rolls 2011a) (see Chapter 10).

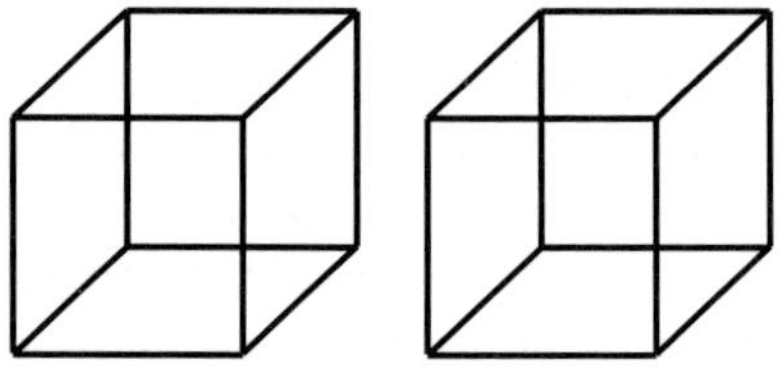

Fig. 8.33 Two Necker cubes. (It may be helpful to increase the viewing distance.)

8.9 Perceptual decisions

Many cortical areas can be conceived as performing a local type of decision-making using attractor dynamics of the type described (Rolls 2008b, Rolls & Deco 2010). Even memory recall is in effect the same local 'decision-making' process.

The somatosensory cortex and ventral premotor cortex are involved in decision-making when different vibrotactile frequencies must be compared (as described in this chapter).

The parietal cortex is involved in decision-making when the stimuli are for example optic flow patterns (Glimcher 2003, Gold & Shadlen 2007, Hedges, Gartshteyn, Kohn, Rust, Shadlen, Newsome & Movshon 2011, Kim & Shadlen 1999, Gold & Shadlen 2000, Schall 2001, Glimcher 2003, Glimcher 2004, Sugrue et al. 2005, Gold & Shadlen 2007, Churchland et al. 2010). For example, parietal cortex neurons with activity that precedes eye movements in area LIP show more activity if the expected utility is high, as described below (Glimcher 2003, Glimcher 2004, Platt & Glimcher 1999, McCoy & Platt 2005a, Platt & Padoa-Schioppa 2009). This modulation by expected utility, as influenced by both probability and reward value, of neurons studied in oculomotor tasks has been found in a number of areas with oculomotor-related activity, including the cingulate cortex and the superior colliculus (McCoy & Platt 2005a, Platt & Padoa-Schioppa 2009).

Another property of perception is that there may be categorically different interpretation of the perceptual input, and the decision-making process involved in taking decisions between the two (or more) possible interpretations may switch between the different categorizations of the sensory input to produce different perceptual states. Such perceptions can change 'spontaneously' from one to another interpretation of the world, even when the visual input is constant. A good example is the Necker cube, in which visual perception flips occasionally to make a different edge of the cube appear nearer to the observer (Fig. 8.33). It is hypothesized that the switching between these multistable states is due in part to the statistical fluctuations in the network due to the Poisson-like spike firing that is a form of noise in the system. This may or may not be supplemented by adaptation effects (of the synapses or neurons) in integrate-and-fire networks. It will be possible to test this hypothesis in integrate-and-fire simulations. [You may observe interesting effects in Fig. 8.33, in which when one cube flips which face appears closer, the other cube performs a similar flip, so that the two cubes remain for most of the time in the same configuration. This effect can be accounted for by short-range cortico-cortical excitatory connections between corresponding depth feature cue

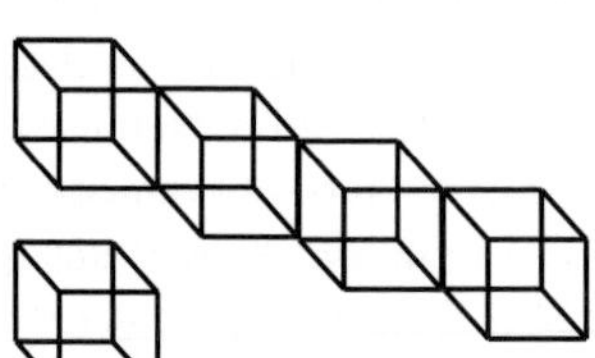

Fig. 8.34 Linked Necker cubes, and a companion.

combination neurons that normally help to produce a consistent interpretation of 3D objects. The underlying mechanism is that of attractor dynamics linking in this case corresponding features in different objects. When the noise in one of the attractors make the attractor flip, this in turn applies a bias to the other attractor, making it very likely that the attractor for the second cube will flip soon under the influence of its internal spiking-related noise. The whole configuration provides an interesting perceptual demonstration of the important role of noise in influencing attractor dynamics, and of the cross-linking between related attractors which helps the whole system to move towards energy minima, under the influence of noise. Another interesting example is shown in Fig. 8.34.]

The same approach provides a model of pattern and binocular rivalry, where one image is seen at a time even though two images are presented simultaneously, and indeed an attractor-based noise-driven model of perceptual alternations has been described (Moreno-Bote, Rinzel & Rubin 2007). When these are images of objects or faces, the system that is especially important in the selection is the inferior temporal visual cortex (Blake & Logothetis 2002, Maier, Logothetis & Leopold 2005), for it is here that representations of whole objects are present (Rolls 2008b, Rolls & Stringer 2006, Rolls 2009a, Rolls & Treves 2011, Rolls 2012e), and the global interpretation of one object can compete with the global interpretation of another object. These simulation models are highly feasible, in that the effects in integrate-and-fire simulations to influence switching between stable states not only of noise, but also of synaptic adaptation and neuronal adaptation which may contribute, have already been investigated (Deco & Rolls 2005a, Deco & Rolls 2005d, Moreno-Bote et al. 2007).

Further examples of analyses of perceptual decision-making are described in Appendix B.

The hippocampus is involved in (providing evidence for) decision-making when the allocentric places of stimuli must be associated with rewards or objects (Rolls & Kesner 2006, Rolls 2008b, Rolls 2010b, Rolls 2013c). There is evidence that the hippocampal memory recall process is also influenced by noise. It has been found that within each theta cycle, when tested in ambiguous places, hippocampal pyramidal neurons may stochastically represent one or other of the learned environments (Jezek, Henriksen, Treves, Moser & Moser 2011). This is an indication, predicted by Rolls & Treves (1998), that autoassociative memory recall can take place sufficiently rapidly to be complete within one theta cycle (120 ms), and that theta cycles could provide a mechanism for a fresh retrieval process to occur after a reset caused by the inhibitory part of each theta cycle, so that the memory can be updated rapidly to reflect a continuously changing environment, and not remain too long in an attractor state.

8.10 Comparison with other models of decision-making

In the attractor network model of decision-making described in this book and elsewhere (Wang 2002, Deco & Rolls 2006, Wang 2008, Rolls 2008b, Deco, Rolls & Romo 2009b, Rolls, Grabenhorst & Deco 2010b, Rolls, Grabenhorst & Deco 2010c, Rolls & Deco 2010), the decisions are taken probabilistically because of the finite size noise due to spiking activity in the integrate-and-fire dynamical network, with the probability that a particular decision is made depending on the biasing inputs provided by the input stimuli λ_1 and λ_2.

The model described here is different in a number of ways from accumulator or counter models which may include a noise term and which undergo a random walk in real time, which is a diffusion process (Ratcliff, Zandt & McKoon 1999, Carpenter & Williams 1995) (see further Appendix B, Wang (2002), Wang (2008), and Usher & McClelland (2001)). These accumulator / drift diffusion models accumulate evidence linearly from noisy inputs until a fixed threshold is reached, when a decision is deemed to have been taken, and are described in detail in Section B.1. They are phenomenological, mathematical, models which do not model the actual neuronal and synaptic mechanisms involved in the decision-making. Predictions from such phenomenological models (as contrasted with the mechanistic approach taken here, in which the neuronal and synaptic mechanisms are modelled in detail), about the implementation in the brain, and about how disorders of the mechanism can influence behaviour in for example dynamical neuropsychiatry (Section 8.11.12, Rolls & Deco (2010), Rolls (2012b)), are therefore much more limited.

First, in accumulator models, a mechanism for computing the difference between the stimuli is not described, whereas in the current model this is achieved, and scaled by λ, by the feedback inhibition included in the attractor network.

Second, in the current attractor network model the decision corresponds to high firing rates in one of the attractors, and there is no arbitrary threshold that must be reached.

Third, the noise in the current model is not arbitrary, but is accounted for by finite size noise effects of the spiking dynamics of the individual neurons with their Poisson-like spike trains in a system of limited size.

Fourth, because the attractor network has recurrent connections, the way in which it settles into a final attractor state (and thus the decision process) can naturally take place over quite a long time, as information gradually and stochastically builds up due to the positive feedback in the recurrent network, the weights in the network, and the biasing inputs, as shown in Figs. 8.6 and 8.7.

Fifth, the recurrent attractor network model produces longer response times in error trials than in correct trials (Wong & Wang 2006, Rolls et al. 2010c) (see Section 8.7), consistent with experimental findings (Roitman & Shadlen 2002). Longer reaction times in error trials can be realized in the diffusion model only with the additional assumption that the starting point varies stochastically from trial to trial (Ratcliff & Rouder 1998). Sixth, the diffusion model never reaches a steady state and predicts that performance can potentially improve indefinitely with a longer duration of stimulus processing, e.g. by raising the decision bound. In the recurrent attractor network model, ramping activity eventually stops as an attractor state is reached (Fig. 8.14). Consequently performance plateaus at sufficiently long stimulus-processing times (Wang 2002, Wang 2008).

Seventh, the attractor network model has been shown to be able to subtract negative signals as well as add positive evidence about choice alternatives, but the influence of newly arriving inputs diminishes over time, as the network converges non-linearly towards one of the attractor states representing the alternative choices (Wang 2002, Wang 2008). This is consistent with experimental evidence (Wong, Huk, Shadlen & Wang 2007). This violation of time-shift invariance cannot be accounted for by the inclusion of a leak in the linear accumulator model. In fact, in contrast to the recurrent attractor network model, the linear leaky competing accumulator model, which takes into account a leakage of integration and assumes competitive inhibition between accumulators selective for choice alternatives (Usher & McClelland 2001), actually predicts that later, not earlier, signals influence more the ultimate decision, because an earlier pulse is gradually 'forgotten' due to the leak and does not affect significantly the decision that occurs much later (Wong et al. 2007).

The approach described here offers therefore a new, alternative, approach to this type of linear diffusion model, in the sense that the integrate-and-fire attractor network model is nonlinear (due to the positive feedback in the attractor network), and is derived from and consistent with the underlying neurophysiological experimental data. The model thus differs from traditional linear diffusion models of decision-making used to account for example for human reaction time data (Luce 1986, Ratcliff & Rouder 1998, Ratcliff et al. 1999, Usher & McClelland 2001). The non-linear diffusion process that is a property of the attractor network model is analysed further in Section B.1.3.1.

The model of decision-making described here is also different to a model suggested by Sugrue, Corrado & Newsome (2005) in which it is suggested that the probabilistic relative value of each action directly dictates the instantaneous probability of choosing each action on the current trial. The present model shows how probabilistic decisions could be taken depending on the two biasing inputs (λ_1 and λ_2 in Fig. 8.1, which could be equal) to a biased competition attractor network subject to statistical fluctuations related to finite size noise in the dynamics of the integrate-and-fire network.

Reasons why the brain is inherently noisy are described by Faisal et al. (2008) and Rolls & Deco (2010), and include the quantal release of neurotransmitters at synapses, and the noise in ion channels opened by them. In addition, cortical neurons maintain their membrane potentials close to, the firing threshold and display a low spontaneous firing rate, so that small inputs can rapidly produce outputs without the need to charge up the neuronal membrane, and this make the neuronal spike times susceptible to statistical fluctuations, with a close to Poisson distribution of spike times (Softky & Koch 1993, Rolls 2008b, Battaglia & Treves 1998).

8.11 Applications and implications of this approach to decision-making

In this section I describe some applications and implications of this approach to decision-making, with further detail provided elsewhere (Rolls & Deco 2010, Rolls 2012d).

8.11.1 Multiple decision-making systems in the brain

Each cortical area can be conceived as performing a local type of decision-making using attractor dynamics of the type described (Rolls 2008b). Even memory recall is in effect the same local 'decision-making' process.

The orbitofrontal cortex for example is involved in providing evidence for decisions about which visual stimulus is currently associated with reward, in for example a visual discrimination reversal task. Its computations are about stimuli, primary reinforcers, and secondary reinforcers (Rolls 2005b). The orbitofrontal cortex appears to represent reward value on a continuous scale, with binary choice decisions being made in the immediately adjoining area anteriorly, the medial prefrontal cortex area 10, as described in Section 8.7 (Rolls & Grabenhorst 2008, Grabenhorst, Rolls & Parris 2008b, Rolls, Grabenhorst & Parris 2010d, Rolls, Grabenhorst & Deco 2010b, Rolls, Grabenhorst & Deco 2010c).

The dorsolateral prefrontal cortex takes an executive role in decision-making in a working memory task, in which information must be held available across intervening stimuli (Rolls 2008b). The dorsal and posterior part of the dorsolateral prefrontal cortex may be involved in short-term memory-related decisions about where to move the eyes (Rolls 2008b).

The parietal cortex is involved in decision-making when the stimuli are for example optic flow patterns (Glimcher 2003, Gold & Shadlen 2007, Hedges et al. 2011).

The hippocampus is involved in (providing evidence for) decision-making when the allocentric places of stimuli must be associated with rewards or objects (Rolls & Kesner 2006, Rolls 2008b, Rolls 2010b).

The somatosensory cortex and ventral premotor cortex are involved in decision-making when different vibrotactile frequencies must be compared (as described in this chapter).

The cingulate cortex may be involved when action–outcome decisions must be taken (Rushworth et al. 2004, Rolls 2005b, Rolls 2008b, Rolls 2009d, Grabenhorst & Rolls 2011) (Section 4.7).

In each of these cases, local cortical processing that is related to the type of decision being made takes place, and all cortical areas are not involved in any one decision. The style of the decision-making-related computation in each cortical area appears to be of the form described here, in which the local recurrent collateral connections enable the decision-making process to accumulate evidence across time, falling gradually into an attractor that represents the decision made in the network. Because there is an attractor state into which the network falls, this can be described statistically as a non-linear diffusion process, the noise for the diffusion being the stochastic spiking of the neurons, and the driving force being the biasing inputs.

If decision-making in the cortex is largely local and typically specialized, it leaves open the question of how one stream for behavioural output is selected. This type of 'global decision-making' may operate as follows (Rolls 2008b). The selection between all the different cortical processing streams might be taken in a structure that receives from all areas of the cortex. One such system is the basal ganglia. The hypothesis is that a second level of 'decision-making' takes place in for example the basal ganglia, which by competition between all the competing cortical inputs (including the explicit route described in Section 10.3.1) select one routing to behavioural output. The selection in this case appears to be by an evolutionarily old, primitive, and safe system that implements direct inhibition between the principal neurons of the network, which are GABA neurons in both the striatum and the globus pallidus, as described in Section 6.3 (page 287 ff.) and Fig. 6.14. It is assumed that these inhibitory connections are not associatively modifiable, so that these neurons do not form an attractor (or an anti-attractor)[29]. Without associatively modifiable connections between the principal neurons, the decision or selection process can be described as a linear diffusion, with the diffusion being driven by the biasing inputs, and the stochastic firing in the network implementing the diffusion. The basal ganglia would then according to this hypothesis select the strongest input to it from any cortical area (or combination of cortical areas, as described in Section 6.3).

The output of the basal ganglia could influence behaviour by two main methods, as described in Section 6.3. One is via connections to premotor or motor cortical areas or other motor systems (such as the nigro-collicular for eye movements). Forward associations of cortical inputs onto striatal neurons might allow for mapping into a motor response space as required for habit learning, for parts of the striatum do receive inputs from the motor cortex, and there are many movement-related neurons in the putamen and globus pallidus (see Section 6.3). The other main method would be by return connections to the neocortex via the thalamus, which could enable a processing stream selected in the basal ganglia to feed back to many cortical areas to influence their activity, and thus to contribute to the selection of a single output for behaviour. The single, or limited, output from the system as a whole is important, so that the motor system does not attempt to select many actions simultaneously. In this system, the threshold setting would be crucial, as with the threshold set too high there would be little behavioural output (which might correspond to Parkinson's disease), and if the threshold were too low, conflicting and inconsistent actions might be selected simultaneously. The dopamine pathways to the striatum, and the return feedback connections to the dopamine neurons from the striatum, may play a role in this threshold setting (Section 6.3).

It is thus suggested that decision-making is inherently a two-stage process. First, there is local computation in a specialized cortical area that performs processing on its specialized inputs which involves settling into an attractor, taking the different constraints or biases into

[29]A network with direct inhibitory connections between its principal neurons could form an attractor, which would be defined by a population with strong mutual inhibitory synaptic weights, and a low firing rate when in the attractor. The learning rule required would be: For low presynaptic firing and low postsynaptic firing, increase the synaptic weight; or equivalently: For high presynaptic firing and high postsynaptic firing, decrease the synaptic weight (i.e. associative LTD).

account to reach a local decision. This is inherently a non-linear diffusion process involving attractor dynamics. Of course this processing need not be restricted to only one cortical area, and forward and backward connections between connected areas may contribute to the attractor process, as described in this chapter. Indeed, when a decision is taken by a cortical area, the attractor into which it falls can be influenced by top-down biased competition from other areas, including for example a short-term memory system in for example the prefrontal cortex that holds active the current task or goal. Thus there is interaction between cortical areas in decision-making, perception, and memory recall, and this is part of the concept of the brain as a dynamical system described in this book. Second, there may be a more global competition to select one output stream for behaviour, and this may involve a linear diffusion process without inbuilt attractor short-term memory related dynamics, and may be implemented in a system such as the basal ganglia (Section 6.3.5.1 and Fig. 6.14).

8.11.2 Distributed decision-making

Although the model described here is effectively a single attractor network, we note that the network need not be localized to one brain region. Long-range connections between cortical areas enable networks in different brain areas to interact in the way needed to implement a single attractor network. The requirement is that the synapses between the neurons in any one pool be set up by Hebb-like associative synaptic modification, and this is likely to be a property of connectivity between areas (using forward and backprojections (Rolls 2008b)), as well as within areas (Rolls & Treves 1998, Rolls & Deco 2002). In this sense, the decision could be thought of as distributed across different brain areas. Consistent with this, Romo and colleagues have found neurons related to vibrotactile decisions not only in the ventral premotor cortex (VPC), but in a number of connected brain areas including the medial premotor cortex, as described in Section 8.5.

In order to achieve the desired probabilistic settling behaviour, the network we describe must not have very high inhibition, and, related to this, may sometimes not settle into one of its attractor states. In a forced choice task in which a decision must be reached on every trial, a possible solution is to have a second decision-making network, with parameters adjusted so that it will settle into one of its states (chosen at chance) even if a preceding network in the decision-making chain has not settled. This could be an additional reason for having a series of networks in different brain regions involved in the decision-making process.

In any case, we believe that there are decision-making networks, that is, networks that can reach a categorical state, in many cortical areas, each specializing in taking a decision about the information represented in that region (see Section 8.11.1). In this situation, a behavioural decision may reflect the operation of a number of partly separate, and partly sequential, decision-making processes.

8.11.3 Predicting a decision before the evidence is provided

There is a literature on how early one can predict from neural activity what decision will be taken (Hampton & O'Doherty 2007, Haynes & Rees 2005a, Haynes & Rees 2005b, Haynes & Rees 2006, Haynes, Sakai, Rees, Gilbert, Frith & Passingham 2007, Lau, Rogers & Passingham 2006, Pessoa & Padmala 2005, Rolls, Grabenhorst & Franco 2009). For example, when subjects held in mind in a delay period which of two tasks, addition or subtraction, they intended to perform, then it was possible to decode or predict with fMRI whether addition or subtraction would later be performed from medial prefrontal cortex activations with accuracies in the order of 70%, where chance was 50% (Haynes et al. 2007). A problem with such studies is that it is often not possible to know exactly when the decision was taken at the mental level,

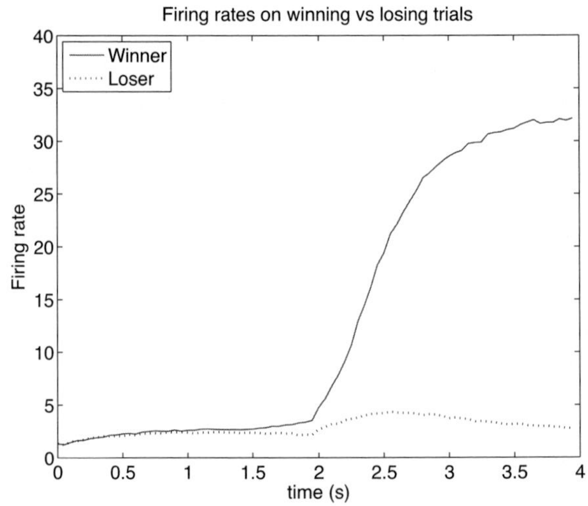

Fig. 8.35 Prediction of a decision before the evidence is applied. In this integrate-and-fire simulation of decision-making, the decision cues were turned on at t=2 s, with ΔI=0. The firing rate averaged over approximately 400 winning vs 400 losing trials for the attractor shows that the firing rate when the attractor will win is on average higher than that for when the attractor will lose at a time that starts in this case at approximately 1000 ms before the decision cues are applied. (At t=2 s with ΔI=0 the input firing rate on each of the 800 external input synapses onto every neuron of both of the selective attractor populations is increased from 3.00 to 3.04 Hz.) (Reproduced from Edmund T. Rolls and Gustavo Deco, Prediction of decisions from noise in the brain before the evidence is provided. *Frontiers in Neuroscience*, 5: (3) 33 ©2011, The Authors.)

or when preparation for the decision actually started, so it is difficult to know whether neural activity that precedes the decision itself in any way predicts the decision that will be taken (Rolls 2011a). In these circumstances, is there anything rigorous that our understanding of the neural mechanisms involved in the decision-making can provide? It turns out that there is (Rolls & Deco 2011b).

While investigating the speed of decision-making using a network of the type described in this chapter, Smerieri, Rolls & Feng (2010) studied the activity that preceded the onset of the decision cues. The results found in simulations in which the firing rate in the spontaneous firing period is measured before a particular attractor population won or lost the competition are illustrated in Fig. 8.35. The firing rate averaged over approximately 800 winning (correct) vs losing (error) trials for the attractor shows that the firing rate when the attractor will win is on average higher than that for when the attractor will lose at a time that starts in this case approximately 1000 ms before the decision cues are applied. Thus it is possible before the decision cues are applied to predict in this noisy decision-making attractor network something about what decision will be taken for periods in the order of 1 s before the decision cues are applied. (If longer time constants are used for some of the GABA inhibitory neurons in the network, the decision that will be taken can be predicted (probabilistically) for as much as 2 s before the decision cues are applied (Smerieri, Rolls & Feng 2010).)

What could be the mechanism? It appears to be as follows (Rolls & Deco 2011b). There will be noise (randomness, statistical fluctuations) in the neuronal firing that will lead, at different times in the period before the decision cues are applied, to low, but different, firing rates of the two selective populations of neurons that represent the different decisions. If the firing rate of say population D1 (representing decision 1) is higher than that of the D2 population at a time just as the decision-cues are being applied, this firing will add to the effect of the decision cues, and make it more likely that the D1 population will win. These fluctuations in the spontaneous firing rate will have a characteristic time course that will be influenced by the time constants of the synapses etc. in the system, so that if a population has somewhat higher firing at say 500 ms before the cues are applied, it will be a little more likely to also have higher firing some time later. This process is related to the integration that is being performed by the attractor network before the decision is taken, which is described more fully in Section B.1.3.1. By looking backwards in time one can see how long the effects of such statistical fluctuations can influence the decision that will be reached, and this is shown in Fig. 8.35 to be approximately 1000 ms in the network we have studied that is described in Section 8.7. I emphasize that this gradual increase of firing rate for the attractor that will win before the decision cues are applied is an effect found by averaging over very many trials, and that the fluctuations found on an individual trial (illustrated in Figs. 8.14 and 8.21) do not always reveal obvious changes of the type illustrated in Fig. 8.35 and Fig. B.6.

Thus we have a rigorous and definite answer and understanding of one way in which decisions that will be taken later are influenced by and can be probabilistically predicted from the prior state of the network. It is possible to make a probabilistic prediction of which decision will be taken from the prior activity of the system, before the decision cues are applied (Rolls & Deco 2011b). This conclusion emerges from a fundamental understanding of how noise in the brain produces statistical fluctuations that can influence neural processes (Rolls & Deco 2010). The non-deterministic operation of cortical attractor networks has implications for free will (Section 10.4).

8.11.4 The matching law

Another potential application of this model of decision-making is to probabilistic decision tasks. In such tasks, the proportion of choices reflects, and indeed may be proportional to, the expected value of the different choices. This pattern of choices is known as the matching law (Sugrue, Corrado & Newsome 2005). An example of a probabilistic decision task in which the choices of the human participants in the probabilistic decision task clearly reflected the expected value of the choices is described by Rolls, McCabe & Redoute (2008e) (Fig. 4.37).

A network of the type described here in which the biasing inputs λ_1 and λ_2 to the model are the expected values of the different choices alters the proportion of the decisions it makes as a function of the relative expected values in a way similar to that shown in Fig. 8.8, and provides a model of this type of probabilistic reward-based decision-making (Marti, Deco, Del Giudice & Mattia 2006). It was shown for example that the proportion of trials on which one stimulus was shown over the other was approximately proportional to the difference of the two values between which choices were being made. In setting the connection weights to the two attractors that represent the choices, the returns (the average reward per choice), rather than the incomes (the average reward per trial) of the two targets, are relevant (Soltani & Wang 2006).

This type of model also accounts for the observation that matching is not perfect, and the relative probability of choosing the more rewarding option is often slightly smaller than the relative reward rate ('undermatching'). If there were no neural variability, decision behaviour would tend to get stuck with the more rewarding alternative; stochastic spiking activity renders the network more exploratory and produces undermatching as a consequence (Soltani & Wang 2006).

8.11.5 Symmetry-breaking

It is of interest that the noise that contributes to the stochastic dynamics of the brain through the spiking fluctuations may be behaviourally adaptive, and that the noise should not be considered only as a problem in terms of how the brain works. This is the issue raised for example by the donkey in the medieval Duns Scotus paradox, in which a donkey situated between two equidistant food rewards might never make a decision and might starve.

The problem raised is that with a deterministic system, there is nothing to break the symmetry, and the system can become deadlocked. In this situation, the addition of noise can produce probabilistic choice, which is advantageous. We have shown here that stochastic neurodynamics caused for example by the relatively random spiking times of neurons in a finite sized cortical attractor network can lead to probabilistic decision-making, so that in this case the stochastic noise is a positive advantage.

8.11.6 The evolutionary utility of probabilistic choice

Probabilistic decision-making can be evolutionarily advantageous in another sense, in which sometimes taking a decision that is not optimal based on previous history may provide information that is useful, and which may contribute to learning. Consider for example a probabilistic decision task in which choice 1 provides rewards on 80% of the occasions, and choice 2 on 20% of the occasions. A deterministic system with knowledge of the previous reinforcement history would always make choice 1. But this is not how animals including humans behave. Instead (especially when the overall probabilities are low and the situation involves random probabilistic baiting, and there is a penalty for changing the choice), the proportion of choices made approximately matches the outcomes that are available, in what is called the matching law (Sugrue, Corrado & Newsome 2005, Corrado, Sugrue, Seung & Newsome 2005, Rolls, McCabe & Redoute 2008e) (Section 8.11.4). By making the less favoured choice sometimes, the organism can keep obtaining evidence on whether the environment is changing (for example on whether the probability of a reward for choice 2 has increased), and by doing this approximately according to the matching law minimizes the cost of the disadvantageous choices in obtaining information about the environment.

This probabilistic exploration of the environment is very important in trial-and-error learning, and indeed has been incorporated into a simple reinforcement algorithm in which noise is added to the system, and if this improves outcomes above the expected value, then changes are made to the synaptic weights in the correct direction (in the associative reward-penalty algorithm) (Sutton & Barto 1981, Barto 1985, Rolls 2008b) (Section A.5.1).

In perceptual learning, probabilistic exploratory behaviour may be part of the mechanism by which perceptual representations can be shaped to have appropriate selectivities for the behavioural categorization being performed (Sigala & Logothetis 2002, Szabo, Deco, Fusi, Del Giudice, Mattia & Stetter 2006).

Another example is in food foraging, which probabilistically may reflect the outcomes (Krebs & Davies 1991, Kacelnik & Brito e Abreu 1998), and is a way optimally in terms of costs and benefits to keep sampling and exploring the space of possible choices.

Another sense in which probabilistic decision-making may be evolutionarily advantageous is with respect to detecting signals that are close to threshold, in the process of *stochastic resonance* (Rolls & Deco 2010), as follows. If we had a deterministic neuron without noise and a fixed threshold above which spikes were emitted, then if the signal was below the threshold there would be no output, and if the signal was above threshold the neuron would emit a spike, and indeed continuous spike trains if the signal remained above threshold. In particular, if the signal was just below the threshold of the neuron, there would be no evidence that a signal close to threshold was present. However, if noise is present in the system (due for example to the afferent neurons having probabilistic spiking activity similar to that of a Poisson process), then occasionally with a signal close to threshold a spike would occur due to the summation of the signal and the noise. If the signal was a bit weaker, then the neuron might still occasionally spike, but at a lower average rate. If the signal was a bit closer to threshold, then the neuron would emit spikes at a higher average rate. Thus in this way some evidence about the presence of a subthreshold signal can be made evident in the spike trains emitted by a neuron if there is noise in the inputs to the neuron. The noise in this case is useful, and may have an adaptive function (cf. Faisal et al. (2008)). This process is known as stochastic resonance, and is a well known example of how noise can have beneficial effects in signal detection systems operating close to a threshold (Longtin 1993, Weisenfeld 1993, Stocks 2000, Riani & Simonotto 1994, Shang, Claridge-Chang, Sjulson, Pypaert & Miesenböck 2007, Faisal, Selen & Wolpert 2008, Goldbach, Loh, Deco & Garcia-Ojalvo 2008).

8.11.7 Unpredictable behaviour

An area where the spiking-related noise in the decision-making process may be evolutionarily advantageous is in the generation of unpredictable behaviour, which can be advantageous in a number of situations, for example when a prey is trying to escape from a predator, and perhaps in some social and economic situations in which organisms may not wish to reveal their intentions (Maynard Smith 1982, Maynard Smith 1984, Dawkins 1995). We note that such probabilistic decisions may have long-term consequences. For example, a probabilistic decision in a 'war of attrition' such as staring down a competitor e.g. in dominance hierarchy formation, may fix the relative status of the two individual animals involved, who then tend to maintain that relationship stably for a considerable period of weeks or more (Maynard Smith 1982, Maynard Smith 1984, Dawkins 1995).

Intrinsic indeterminacy may be essential for unpredictable behaviour (Glimcher 2005). For example, in interactive games like matching pennies or rock–paper–scissors, any trend that deviates from random choice by an agent could be exploited to his or her opponent's advantage.

8.11.8 Memory recall

The theory described here of decision-making is effectively a model of the stochastic dynamics of the recall of a memory in response to a recall cue. The memory might be a long-term memory, but the theory applies to the retrieval of any stored representation in the brain. The way in which the attractor is reached depends on the strength of the recall cue, and inherent noise in the attractor network performing the recall because of the spiking activity in a finite size system. The recall will take longer if the recall cue is weak. Spontaneous stochastic effects may suddenly lead to the memory being recalled, and this may be related to the sudden recovery of a memory which one tried to remember some time previously. These processes are considered further by Rolls (2008b).

The theory applies to a situation where the representation may be being 'recalled' by a single input, which is perceptual detection as described in Chapter 7 of Rolls & Deco (2010).

The theory also applies to a situation where the representation may be being 'recalled' by two or more competing inputs λ, which is decision-making as described in this chapter.

The theory also applies to short-term memory, in which the continuation of the recalled state as a persistent attractor is subject to stochastic noise effects, which may knock the system out of the short-term memory attractor, as described in Chapter 3 of Rolls & Deco (2010).

The theory also applies to attention, in which the continuation of the recalled state as a persistent attractor is subject to stochastic noise effects, which may knock the system out of the short-term memory attractor that is normally stable because of the non-linear positive feedback implemented in the attractor network by the recurrent collateral connections, as described by Rolls (2008b) and Rolls & Deco (2010).

8.11.9 Creative thought

Another way in which probabilistic decision-making may be evolutionarily advantageous is in creative thought, which is influenced in part by associations between one memory, representation, or thought, and another. If the system were deterministic, i.e. for the present purposes without noise, then the trajectory through a set of thoughts would be deterministic and would tend to follow the same furrow each time. However, if the recall of one memory or thought from another were influenced by the statistical noise due to the random spiking of neurons, then the trajectory through the state space would be different on different occasions, and we might be led in different directions on different occasions, facilitating creative thought (Rolls 2008b).

Of course, if the basins of attraction of each thought were too shallow, then the statistical noise might lead one to have very unstable thoughts that were too loosely and even bizarrely associated to each other, and to have a short-term memory and attentional system that is unstable and distractible, and indeed this is an account that we have proposed for some of the symptoms of schizophrenia (Rolls 2005b, Rolls 2008b, Loh, Rolls & Deco 2007a, Loh, Rolls & Deco 2007b, Rolls, Loh, Deco & Winterer 2008d, Rolls & Deco 2010, Rolls & Deco 2011a, Rolls 2012b) (see Section 8.11.12).

The stochastic noise caused by the probabilistic neuronal spiking plays an important role in these hypotheses, because it is the noise that destabilizes the attractors when the depth of the basins of attraction is reduced. If the basins of attraction were too deep, then the noise might be insufficient to destabilize attractors, and this leads to an approach to understanding obsessive-compulsive disorders (Rolls, Loh & Deco 2008c, Rolls 2012b) (see Section 8.11.12).

8.11.10 Decision-making with sequential inputs and with postponed responses

Extensions of the model of vibrotactile decision-making (Deco & Rolls 2006) described here, to account for sequential decision-making, and for decision-making in which the decision must be delayed, are provided in Sections B.2 and B.3.

8.11.11 Decision-making between the emotional and rational systems

Another application of this type of model is to taking decisions between the implicit and explicit systems in emotional decision-making (see Section 10.3.1 and Rolls (2005b)), where again the two different systems could provide the biasing inputs λ_1 and λ_2 to the model.

If decision-making in the cortex is largely local and typically specialized, it leaves open the question of how one stream for behavioural output is selected. This type of 'global decision-making' is considered in Sections 10.3.1 and 6.3.

8.11.12 Dynamical neuropsychiatry: schizophrenia

Schizophrenia is characterized by three main types of symptom: cognitive dysfunction, negative symptoms, and positive symptoms (Liddle 1987, Baxter & Liddle 1998, Mueser & McGurk 2004). I describe how the basic characteristics of these three categories might be produced by instability in the brain's dynamical systems in this section. First, it is useful to clarify how short-term memory attractor networks, which have the same architecture as a decision-making network, and in which the short-term memory attractor state can be thought of as a decision state resulting from the short-term memory initiating cue, requires two forms of stability to be controlled.

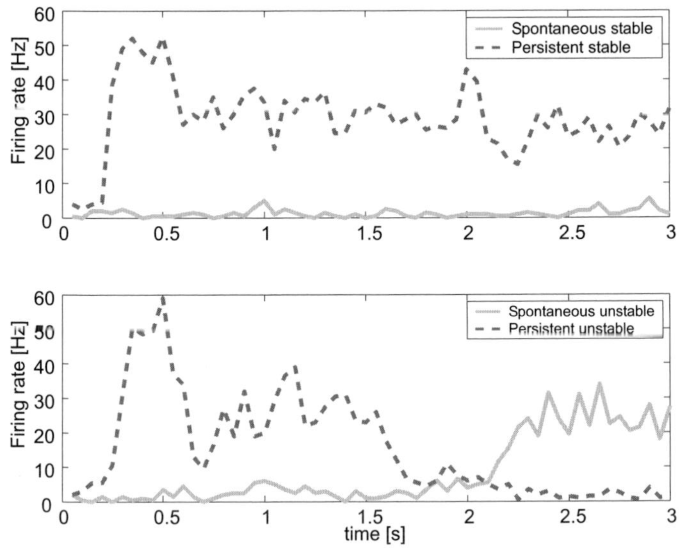

Fig. 8.36 Example trials of the integrate-and-fire attractor network simulations of short-term memory. The average firing rate of all the neurons in the S1 (short-term memory) pool is shown. Top. Normal operation. On a trial in which a recall stimulus was applied to S1 at 0–500 ms, firing continued normally until the end of the trial in the 'persistent' simulation condition. On a trial on which no recall stimulus was applied to S1, spontaneous firing continued until the end of the trial in the 'spontaneous' simulation condition. Bottom: Unstable operation. On this persistent condition trial, the firing decreased during the trial as the network fell out of the attractor because of the statistical fluctuations caused by the spiking dynamics. On the spontaneous condition trial, the firing increased during the trial because of the statistical fluctuations. In these simulations the network parameter was w_+=2.1. (Reproduced from Edmund T. Rolls, Marco Loh, and Gustavo Deco, An attractor hypothesis of obsessive-compulsive disorder, *European Journal of Neuroscience*, 28 (4) pp. 782–793, Copyright ©2008, The Authors, Journal Compilation ©Federation of European Neuroscience Societies and Blackwell Publishing Ltd.)

8.11.12.1 Short-term memory

An attractor or autoassociation network can provide a short-term memory (Rolls 2008b, Rolls & Deco 2010) (Section A.3). To illustrate this, and to clarify the concept of stability, Figure 8.36 shows examples of trials of integrate-and-fire attractor network simulations in which statistical fluctuations caused by the spiking-related noise have different impacts on the temporal dynamics (Rolls, Loh & Deco 2008c).

In the spontaneous state simulations, no cue was applied, and we are interested in whether the network remains stably in the spontaneous firing state, or whether it is unstable and on some trials due to statistical fluctuations enters one of the attractors, thus falsely retrieving a memory. Figure 8.36 (top) shows an example of a trial on which the network correctly stayed in the low spontaneous firing rate regime, and (bottom) another trial (labelled spontaneous unstable) in which statistical spiking-related fluctuations in the network caused it to enter incorrectly a high activity state, moving into one of the attractors even without a stimulus.

In the persistent state simulations (in which the short-term memory was implemented by the continuing neuronal firing), a strong excitatory input was given to the S1 neuronal population between 0 and 500 ms. Two such trials are shown in Fig. 8.36. In Fig. 8.36 (top), the S1 neurons (correctly) keep firing at approximately 30 Hz after the retrieval cue is removed at 500 ms. However, due to statistical fluctuations in the network related to the spiking activity, on the trial labelled persistent unstable the high firing rate in the attractor for S1 was not stable, and the firing decreased back towards the spontaneous level, in the example shown starting after 1.5 s (Fig. 8.36 bottom). This trial illustrates a failure to maintain a stable short-term memory state.

When an average was taken over many trials, for the persistent run simulations, in which the cue triggered the attractor into the high firing rate attractor state, the network was still in the high firing rate attractor state in the baseline condition on 88% of the runs. The noise had thus caused the network to fail to maintain the short-term memory on 12% of the runs.

The spontaneous state was unstable on approximately 10% of the trials, that is, on 10% of the trials the spiking noise in the network caused the network run in the condition without any initial retrieval cue to end up in a high firing rate attractor state. This is of course an error that is related to the spiking noise in the network.

I emphasize that the transitions to the incorrect activity states illustrated in Fig. 8.36 are caused by statistical fluctuations (noise) in the spiking activity of the integrate-and-fire neurons. Indeed, we used a mean-field approach with an equivalent network with the same parameters but without noise to establish parameter values where the spontaneous state and the high firing rate short-term memory ('persistent') state would be stable without the spiking noise, and then in integrate-and-fire simulations with the same parameter values examined the effects of the spiking noise (Loh, Rolls & Deco 2007a, Rolls, Loh & Deco 2008c).

8.11.12.2 Schizophrenia: cognitive symptoms

Dysfunction of working memory, the core of the cognitive symptoms of schizophrenia, may be related to instabilities of persistent attractor states (Durstewitz, Seamans & Sejnowski 2000, Wang 2001) which we have shown can be produced by reduced firing rates in attractor networks, in brain regions such as the prefrontal cortex (Rolls 2008b, Rolls & Deco 2010).

The *cognitive symptoms* of schizophrenia include distractibility, poor attention, and the dysexecutive syndrome in which behaviour is poorly organized in tasks with multiple components such as shopping for different items requiring visits to several shops (Liddle 1987, Green 1996, Mueser & McGurk 2004). The core of the cognitive symptoms is a working memory deficit in which there is a difficulty in maintaining items in short-term memory (Goldman-Rakic 1994, Goldman-Rakic 1999), which could directly or indirectly account for these cognitive symptoms (Rolls 2005b, Rolls 2008b). For example, with poor short-term memory systems in the prefrontal cortex, it becomes difficult to manipulate items in short-term memory which is a major property of what is termed working memory (Baddeley 1986), and which is important in planning (Chapter 10), an important part of executive function. A difficulty with short-term memory would also account for poor attention, in that a short-term memory in the prefrontal cortex holds the subject of attention in mind, e.g. an object or a place, and provides the source for a top-down influence on earlier stages of processing to affect how they operate by biassing the competition between incoming inputs (Rolls 2008b). A failure to maintain attention properly can be manifest by being very distractible.

We have sought an explanation for these cognitive symptoms by considering what computational processes might account for the dysfunctions of short-term memory and thus attention and executive function (Rolls 2005b, Loh et al. 2007a, Rolls et al. 2008d, Rolls & Deco 2011a, Rolls & Deco 2010, Rolls 2012b). I have suggested that if the short-term memory circuitry in the prefrontal cortex was too unstable because the firing in an attractor network became low, this would account for the cognitive symptoms (Rolls 2005b). The concept here is that an attractor network is stable if its firing rates are high, because then the positive feedback caused by the recurrent collateral connections between the neurons in the attractor and the inherent non-linearity of the system makes the system resistant to noise. The noise in the system corresponds to the random firing times of the neurons (for a given mean firing rate), or the firing produced by a distracting stimulus. An example of a trial in which the high firing rate implementing a short-term memory is correctly maintained is shown in Fig. 8.36 (top). Figure 8.36 (bottom) shows another trial in which the firing rate was not correctly maintained because of the noise, and the firing sank down into the spontaneous level of firing.

We tested this hypothesis with integrate-and-fire simulations, and showed that once a short-term memory state was started by a short input, the high firing rate state was less likely to be maintained, if a change that reduced the firing rate was present. The change we investigated was decreasing the efficacy of one class of the excitatory receptors on the neurons, NMDA receptors, which respond to the excitatory transmitter glutamate (Loh, Rolls & Deco 2007a, Rolls, Loh, Deco & Winterer 2008d). We chose this change to investigate because there is evidence that these excitatory receptors are less efficacious in patients with schizophrenia (Goff & Coyle 2001, Coyle, Tsai & Goff 2003, Coyle 2006, Coyle, Balu, Benneyworth, Basu & Roseman 2010, Bergeron & Coyle 2012), because spine density on cortical pyramidal cells is reduced in schizophrenia (Glausier & Lewis 2013) implying less excitatory input to the neurons, and because of other evidence consistent with this hypothesis of the cognitive symptoms of schizophrenia that is described in the next section.

For the cognitive symptoms, an aim of treatment might therefore be to increase the firing rates of neurons when in the high firing rate attractor state, to stabilize the attractor states required for short-term memory and attention. It is in this context very interesting that nicotine, self-administered by many patients with schizophrenia, acts in primates at nicotinic alpha7 cholinergic receptors (alpha7-nAChR) to facilitate the actions of NR2B glutamate receptors and thus to facilitate the maintenance of short-term memory in the dorsolateral prefrontal cortex (Yang, Paspalas, Jin, Picciotto, Arnsten & Wang 2013). Nicotine would in the same way be expected to ameliorate the negative symptoms of schizophrenia, by increasing the firing rates of neurons in the orbitofrontal and cingulate cortices where emotional and motivational states are represented, as described in the next subsection.

8.11.12.3 Negative symptoms

The *negative symptoms* of schizophrenia refer to the flattening of affect and a reduction in emotion. Behavioural indicators are blunted affect, emotional and passive withdrawal, poor rapport, lack of spontaneity, motor retardation, and disturbance of volition (Liddle 1987, Mueser & McGurk 2004). I proposed that these symptoms are related to decreases in firing rates in the orbitofrontal cortex and/or anterior cingulate cortex (Rolls 2005b), where neuronal firing rates and activations in fMRI investigations are correlated with reward value and pleasure, and which is involved in emotion (Rolls 2005b, Rolls 2006b, Rolls 2007c, Rolls & Grabenhorst 2008, Rolls 2008e, Grabenhorst & Rolls 2011) (Chapter 4). Consistent with this, imaging studies have identified a relationship between negative symptoms and prefrontal hypometabolism, i.e. a reduced activation of frontal areas (Wolkin, Sanfilipo, Wolf, Angrist, Brodie & Rotrosen 1992, Aleman & Kahn 2005).

We investigated this computational hypothesis in integrate-and-fire simulations, and showed that the same reduction in NMDA glutamate receptor function that could account for the instability of attractor networks also decreased the firing rates of the neurons in the networks (Loh, Rolls & Deco 2007a, Rolls, Loh, Deco & Winterer 2008d). We thus had a unifying account for the cognitive and negative functions of schizophrenia, in which the common cause was a reduction in NMDA glutamate receptor efficacy. When expressed in the dorsolateral prefrontal cortex, this can decrease the stability of attractor networks implementing short-term memory, by decreasing the firing rates of the neurons. When expressed in the orbitofrontal and cingulate cortex, the same change producing a decrease of firing rates can account for the negative symptoms, in that the amount of emotion, the effects of a reward or punisher, is related to the magnitude of the firing rate responses of orbitofrontal cortex neurons (Rolls 2005b, Rolls 2008b) (Section 4.5).

In this unifying approach, both the negative and cognitive symptoms thus could be caused by a reduction of the NMDA conductance (or other reduction in glutamate efficacy) in attractor networks. The proposed mechanism links the cognitive and negative symptoms of schizophrenia in an attractor framework and is consistent with a close relation between the cognitive and negative symptoms: blockade of NMDA receptors by dissociative anesthetics such as ketamine produces in normal subjects schizophrenic symptoms including both negative and cognitive impairments (Malhotra, Pinals, Weingartner, Sirocco, Missar, Pickar & Breier 1996, Newcomer, Farber, Jevtovic-Todorovic, Selke, Melson, Hershey, Craft & Olney 1999); agents that enhance NMDA receptor function reduce the negative symptoms and improve the cognitive abilities of schizophrenic patients (Goff & Coyle 2001); and the cognitive and negative symptoms occur early in the illness and precede the first episode of positive symptoms (Lieberman, Perkins, Belger, Chakos, Jarskog, Boteva & Gilmore 2001, Hafner, Maurer, Loffler, an der Heiden, Hambrecht & Schultze-Lutter 2003, Mueser & McGurk 2004). Consistent with this hypothesized role of a reduction in NMDA conductances being involved in schizophrenia, postmortem studies of schizophrenia have identified abnormalities in glutamate receptor density in regions such as the prefrontal cortex, thalamus, and the temporal lobe (Goff & Coyle 2001, Coyle et al. 2003, Coyle et al. 2010, Bergeron & Coyle 2012), brain areas that are active during the performance of cognitive tasks.

8.11.12.4 Positive symptoms

The *positive symptoms* of schizophrenia include bizarre (psychotic) trains of thoughts, hallucinations, and (paranoid) delusions (Liddle 1987, Mueser & McGurk 2004). We propose that these symptoms are related to shallow basins of attraction of both the spontaneous and persistent states in the temporal lobe semantic memory networks and to the statistical fluctuations caused by the probabilistic spiking of the neurons (Loh, Rolls & Deco 2007a, Rolls, Loh, Deco & Winterer 2008d, Rolls 2012b). The reduction in the stability of the high firing rate attractor states could result in thoughts moving too freely from one unstable thought to another loosely associated thought. The reduction in the stability of the spontaneous state, which is an attractor state in its own right, would mean that the system would suddenly jump from the spontaneous, quiet, state to a high firing rate attractor state even when no external stimulus is present, and resulting it is suggested in hallucinations, and in a feeling of a lack of control that is frequently present.

In the language of stochastic neurodynamics (Rolls & Deco 2010), these two different forms of instability could result in activations arising spontaneously, and thoughts moving too freely round the energy landscape, loosely from thought to weakly associated thought, leading to bizarre thoughts and associations, which may eventually over time be associated together in semantic memory to lead to false beliefs and delusions. Consistent with this, neuroimaging studies suggest higher activation especially in areas of the temporal lobe (Weiss & Heckers 1999, Shergill, Brammer, Williams, Murray & McGuire 2000, Scheuerecker, Ufer, Zipse, Frodl, Koutsouleris, Zetzsche, Wiesmann, Albrecht, Bruckmann, Schmitt, Moller & Meisenzahl 2008).

We suggest that the reduction in the stability of the high firing rate state is produced by a reduction in the NMDA receptor efficacy, which is present in schizophrenia (Goff & Coyle 2001, Coyle et al. 2003). We suggest that the reduction in the stability of the spontaneous (low) firing rate state is produced by a reduction in the inhibitory receptor GABA efficacy, which is present in schizophrenia (Wang, Tegner, Constantinidis & Goldman-Rakic 2004, Lewis, Hashimoto & Volk 2005, Volk & Lewis 2013), and which we suggest is especially related to the positive symptoms (Rolls 2005b, Loh et al. 2007a, Rolls et al. 2008d, Rolls & Deco 2011a, Rolls 2012b). Agents that act on cannabinoid receptors (such as cannabis) may decrease the firing of the GABA inhibitory neurons (Volk & Lewis 2013), and by reducing

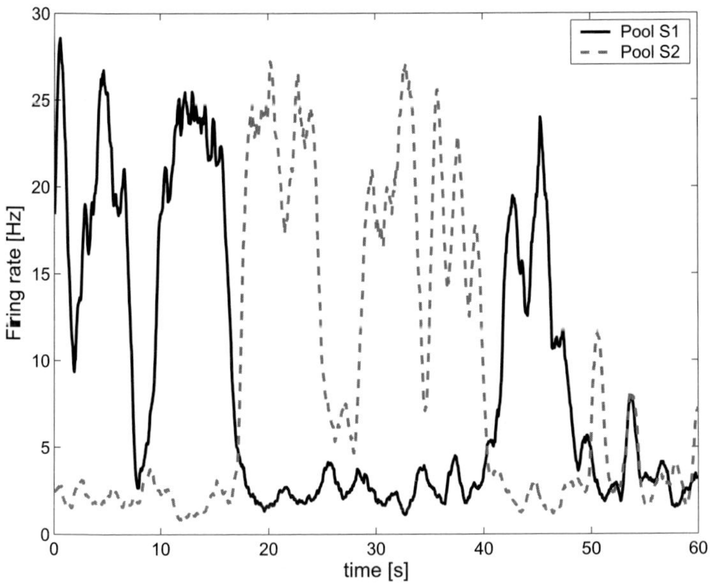

Fig. 8.37 Wandering between attractor states by virtue of statistical fluctuations caused by the randomness of the spiking activity. We simulated a single long trial (60 s) in the spontaneous test condition for the synaptic modification (−NMDA, −GABA). The two curves show the activity of the two selective pools over time smoothed with a 1 s sliding averaging window. The activity moves noisily between the attractor for the spontaneous (low firing) state and the two persistent (high firing) states S1 and S2. (Reproduced from Loh, M., Rolls, E. T. and Deco, G., A dynamical systems hypothesis of schizophrenia, *PLoS Computational Biology* 3, e228, figure 4 ©2007, The Authors.)

inhibition and therefore the stability of the spontaneous (low) firing state of excitatory neurons in attractor networks, may thereby tend to promote positive-like symptoms (Rolls 2012b).

When both NMDA and GABA are reduced one might think that these two counterbalancing effects (excitatory and inhibitory) would either cancel each other out or yield a tradeoff between the stability of the spontaneous and persistent state. However, this is not the case. The stability of both the spontaneous (i.e. low firing rate) state and the persistent (i.e. high firing rate) state is reduced. We relate this pattern to the positive symptoms of schizophrenia, in which both the spontaneous and attractor states are shallow, and the system merely jumps by the influence of statistical fluctuations between the different (spontaneous and high firing rate attractor) states.

To investigate more directly the wandering between spontaneous and several different persistent attractor states, we simulated the condition with decreased NMDA and GABA conductances over a long time period in which no cue stimulus input was given. Figure 8.37 shows the firing rates of the two selective short-term memory pools of neurons S1 and S2. The high activity switches between the two attractors due to the influence of fluctuations, which corresponds to spontaneous wandering in a shallow energy landscape, corresponding for example to sudden jumps between unrelated cognitive processes. These results are consistent with the mean-field flow analysis and demonstrate that the changes in the attractor landscape influence the behaviour at the stochastic level (Loh, Rolls & Deco 2007a, Rolls, Loh, Deco & Winterer 2008d, Rolls 2012b).

The positive symptoms (Fig. 8.38, right column) of schizophrenia include delusions, hallucinations, thought disorder, and bizarre behaviour. Examples of delusions are beliefs that others are trying to harm the person, impressions that others control the person's thoughts,

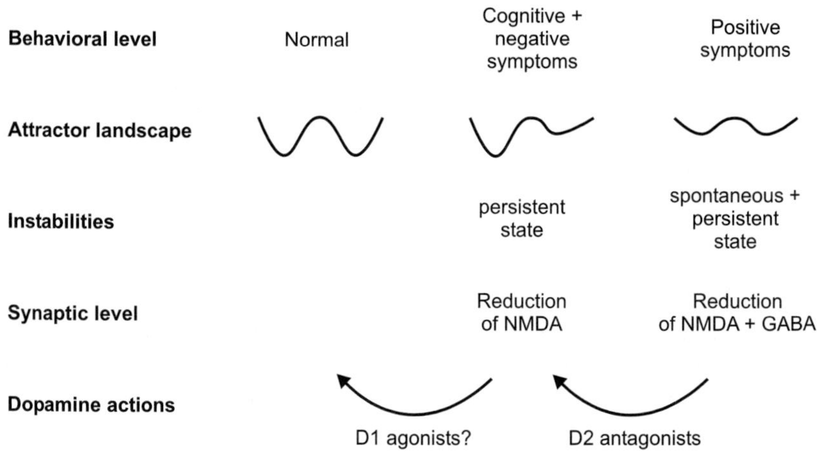

Fig. 8.38 Summary of the attractor hypothesis of schizophrenic symptoms and simulation results (see text). The first basin (from the left) in each energy landscape is the spontaneous state, and the second basin is the persistent attractor state. The vertical axis of each landscape is the energy potential. (Reproduced from Loh, M., Rolls, E. T. and Deco, G., A dynamical systems hypothesis of schizophrenia, *PLoS Computational Biology* 3, e228, figure 7 ©2007, The Authors.)

and delusions of grandeur. Hallucinations are perceptual experiences, which are not shared by others, and are frequently auditory but can affect any sensory modality. These symptoms may be related to activity in the temporal lobes (Liddle 1987, Epstein, Stern & Silbersweig 1999, Mueser & McGurk 2004). The attractor framework approach taken here hypothesizes that the basins of attraction of both spontaneous and persistent states are shallow (Fig. 8.38). Due to the shallowness of the spontaneous state, the system can jump spontaneously up to a high activity state causing hallucinations to arise and leading to bizarre thoughts and associations. This might be the cause for the higher activations in schizophrenics in temporal lobe areas which are identified in imaging experiments (Shergill et al. 2000, Scheuerecker et al. 2008).

Our general hypothesis regarding the attractor landscape is meant to describe the aberrant dynamics in cortical regions which could be caused by several pathways. A strength of this approach is that one can investigate in the simulations the effects of treatment with particular combinations of drugs designed to facilitate both glutamate transmission (including modulation with glycine or serine of the NMDA receptor, and nicotine) and GABA effects. Drug combinations identified in this way could be useful to explore, as combinations might work where treatment with a single drug on its own may not be effective, and possibilities can be systematically explored with the approach described here.

We thus have a new set of concepts related to the stability of brain states to bring to bear on the symptoms and causes of schizophrenia. We also have new ways of proposing new treatments based on the application of computational hypotheses that link synaptic receptor and neuronal effects of drugs to the effects that could be produced at the global level of the operation of cognitive systems involved in memory, attention, and the stability of memory and thus thought processes (Rolls 2012b, Rolls et al. 2008d, Rolls & Deco 2011a). For example, the antipsychotics such as the phenothiazines and the atypical neuroleptics may operate to control the positive symptoms by facilitating GABA transmission, in part by blocking dopamine D2 receptors, but do little to treat the cognitive and negative symptoms, for which other treatments (such as nicotine) are suggested (Rolls 2012b, Rolls, Loh, Deco & Winterer 2008d, Rolls & Deco 2011a, Pu, Guo, Liua, Yub, Xuea, Rolls, Feng & Liu 2013).

The points made about the stability of dynamical attractor systems in the brain clearly apply not only to short-term memory, but also to decision-making, top-down attention, and long-term memory, and their disorders including in aging (Rolls & Deco 2010), and in this sense we have a unifying computational neuroscience approach to many aspects of brain function (Rolls 2008b).

8.11.13 Dynamical neuropsychiatry: obsessive-compulsive disorder

8.11.13.1 The symptoms

Obsessive-compulsive disorder (OCD) is a chronically debilitating disorder with a lifetime prevalence of 2–3% (Robins, Helzer, Weissman, Orvaschel, Gruenberg, Burke & Regier 1984, Karno, Golding, Sorenson & Burnam 1988, Weissman, Bland, Canino, Greenwald, Hwu, Lee, Newman, Oakley-Browne, Rubio-Stipec, Wickramaratne et al. 1994). It is characterized by two sets of symptoms, obsessive and compulsive. Obsessions are unwanted, intrusive, recurrent thoughts or impulses that are often concerned with themes of contamination and 'germs', checking household items in case of fire or burglary, order and symmetry of objects, or fears of harming oneself or others. Compulsions are ritualistic, repetitive behaviours or mental acts carried out in relation to these obsessions e.g. washing, household safety checks, counting, rearrangement of objects in symmetrical array or constant checking of oneself and others to ensure no harm has occurred (Menzies, Chamberlain, Laird, Thelen, Sahakian & Bullmore 2008).

Patients with OCD experience the persistent intrusion of thoughts that they generally perceive as foreign and irrational but which cannot be dismissed. The anxiety associated with these unwanted and disturbing thoughts can be extremely intense; it is often described as a feeling that something is incomplete or wrong, or that terrible consequences will ensue if specific actions are not taken. Many patients engage in repetitive, compulsive behaviours that aim to discharge the anxieties associated with these obsessional thoughts. Severely affected patients can spend many hours each day in their obsessional thinking and resultant compulsive behaviours, leading to marked disability (Pittenger, Krystal & Coric 2006). While OCD patients exhibit a wide variety of obsessions and compulsions, the symptoms tend to fall into specific clusters. Common patterns include obsessions of contamination, with accompanying cleaning compulsions; obsessions with symmetry or order, with accompanying ordering behaviours; obsessions of saving, with accompanying hoarding; somatic obsessions; aggressive obsessions with checking compulsions; and sexual and religious obsessions (Pittenger, Krystal & Coric 2006).

8.11.13.2 A hypothesis about the increased stability of attractor networks and the symptoms of obsessive-compulsive disorder

I now describe an approach to how obsessive-compulsive disorders arise, and of the different symptoms, that has its foundations in a theoretical understanding of the stability of cortical systems in the brain (Rolls & Deco 2010). The aim is to show the way in which complex symptoms in psychiatric states, and their treatment, can be approached by an understanding of how the brain functions, and how neural dysfunctions could lead to psychiatric states. The description thus illustrates the neuro-approach to psychiatry, where the symptoms and their treatment can be approached by a theoretical understanding of cortical function from the level of ion channels through neuronal firing, to neuronal networks with their collective behaviour, to the global operation of the system.

The theory (Rolls, Loh & Deco 2008c, Rolls 2012b) is based on the top-down proposal that there is overstability of attractor neuronal networks in cortical and related areas in obsessive-compulsive disorders. The approach is top-down in that it starts with the set of symptoms and maps them onto the dynamical systems framework, and only after this considers detailed underlying biological mechanisms, of which there could be many, that might produce the effects. (In contrast, a complementary bottom-up approach starts from detailed neurobiological mechanisms, and aims to interpret their implications with a brain-like model for higher level phenomena.) We show by integrate-and-fire neuronal network simulations that the overstability could arise by for example overactivity in glutamatergic excitatory neurotransmitter synapses, which produces an increased depth of the basins of attraction, in the presence of which neuronal spiking-related and potentially other noise is insufficient to help the system move out of an attractor basin. I relate this top-down proposal, related to the stochastic dynamics of neuronal networks, to new evidence that there may be overactivity in glutamatergic systems in obsessive-compulsive disorders, and consider the implications for treatment (Rolls 2012b).

We hypothesize that cortical and related attractor networks become too stable in obsessive-compulsive disorder, so that once in an attractor state, the networks tend to remain there too long (Rolls, Loh & Deco 2008c, Rolls 2012b). The hypothesis is that the depths of the basins of attraction become deeper, and that this is what makes the attractor networks more stable. We further hypothesize that part of the mechanism for the increased depth of the basins of attraction is increased glutamatergic transmission, which increases the depth of the basins of attraction by increasing the firing rates of the neurons, and by increasing the effective value of the synaptic weights between the associatively modified synapses that define the attractor, as is made evident in Equation 8.1 on page 376. The synaptic strength is effectively increased if more glutamate is released per action potential at the synapse, or if in other ways the currents injected into the neurons through the NMDA (N-methyl-d-aspartate) and/or AMPA synapses are larger. In addition, if NMDA receptor function is increased, this could also increase the stability of the system because of the temporal smoothing effect of the long time constant of the NMDA receptors (Wang 1999). This increased stability of cortical and related attractor networks, and the associated higher neuronal firing rates, could occur in different brain regions, and thereby produce different symptoms, as follows.

If these effects occurred in high order motor areas, the symptoms could include inability to move out of one motor pattern, resulting for example in repeated movements or actions. In parts of the cingulate cortex and dorsal medial prefrontal cortex, this could result in difficulty in switching between actions or strategies (Rushworth, Behrens, Rudebeck & Walton 2007a, Rushworth et al. 2007b), as the system would be locked into one action or strategy. If an action was locked into a high order motor area due to increased stability of an attractor network, then lower order motor areas might thereby not be able to escape easily what they implement, such as a sequence of movements, so that the sequence would be repeated.

If occurring in the lateral prefrontal cortex (including the dorsolateral and ventrolateral parts), the increased stability of attractor networks could produce symptoms that include a difficulty in shifting attention, and in cognitive set shifting in which what is relevant to the task may shift from color to shape, etc. (Veale, Sahakian, Owen & Marks 1996, Watkins, Sahakian, Robertson, Veale, Rogers, Pickard, Aitken & Robbins 2005, Chamberlain, Fineberg, Blackwell, Robbins & Sahakian 2006, Chamberlain, Fineberg, Menzies, Blackwell, Bullmore, Robbins & Sahakian 2007). These are in fact important symptoms that can be found in obsessive-compulsive disorder (Menzies et al. 2008).

Planning may also be impaired in patients with OCD (Menzies et al. 2008), and this could arise because there is too much stability of attractor networks in the dorsolateral prefrontal cortex concerned with holding in mind the different short-term memory representations that encode the different steps of a plan (Rolls 2008b). Indeed, there is evidence for dorsolateral prefrontal cortex (DLPFC) dysfunction in patients with OCD, in conjunction with impairment on a version of the Tower of London task, a task often used to probe planning aspects of executive function (van den Heuvel, Veltman, Groenewegen, Cath, van Balkom, van Hartskamp, Barkhof & van Dyck 2005).

An increased firing rate of neurons in the orbitofrontal cortex, and anterior cingulate cortex, produced by hyperactivity of glutamatergic transmitter systems, would increase emotionality, which is frequently found in obsessive-compulsive disorder. Part of the increased anxiety found in obsessive-compulsive disorder could be related to an inability to complete tasks or actions in which one is locked. But part of our unifying proposal is that part of the increased emotionality in OCD may be directly related to increased firing produced by the increased glutamatergic activity in brain areas such as the orbitofrontal and anterior cingulate cortex (Rolls, Loh & Deco 2008c). The orbitofrontal cortex and anterior cingulate cortex are involved in emotion, in that they are activated by primary and secondary reinforcers that produce affective states (Rolls 2004c, Rolls 2005b, Rolls 2008b, Rolls & Grabenhorst 2008), and in that damage to these regions alters emotional behaviour and emotional experience (Rolls, Hornak, Wade & McGrath 1994a, Hornak, Rolls & Wade 1996, Hornak, Bramham, Rolls, Morris, O'Doherty, Bullock & Polkey 2003, Hornak, O'Doherty, Bramham, Rolls, Morris, Bullock & Polkey 2004, Berlin, Rolls & Kischka 2004, Berlin, Rolls & Iversen 2005). Indeed, negative emotions as well as positive emotions activate the orbitofrontal cortex, with the emotional states produced by negative events tending to be represented in the lateral orbitofrontal cortex and dorsal part of the anterior cingulate cortex (Kringelbach & Rolls 2004, Rolls 2005b, Rolls 2008b, Grabenhorst & Rolls 2011).

If the increased stability of attractor networks occurred in temporal lobe semantic memory networks, then this would result in a difficulty in moving from one thought to another, and possibly in stereotyped thoughts, which again may be a symptom of obsessive-compulsive disorder (Menzies et al. 2008). The obsessional states are thus proposed to arise because cortical areas concerned with cognitive functions have states that become too stable. The compulsive states are proposed to arise partly in response to the obsessional states, but also partly because cortical areas concerned with actions have states that become too stable.

The theory provides a unifying computational account of both the obsessional and compulsive symptoms, in that both arise due to increased stability of cortical attractor networks, with the different symptoms related to overstability in different cortical areas. The theory is also unifying in that a similar increase in glutamatergic activity in the orbitofrontal and anterior cingulate cortex could increase emotionality, as described earlier.

8.11.13.3 Glutamate and increased depth of the basins of attraction of attractor networks

We tested this approach in integrate-and-fire neuronal attractor network simulations, and showed that increased NMDA or AMPA excitatory receptor functionality (increased synaptic conductances) could produce overstability of noisy attractor networks, and could make them less distractible (Rolls, Loh & Deco 2008c).

We also showed that increasing the synaptic conductances activated by the GABA inhibitory neurons in the network could correct for the effect of increasing NMDA receptor activated synaptic currents on the persistent high firing rate type of test; and for the effect of increasing NMDA on the spontaneous state simulations when there was no initiating retrieval stimulus, and the network should remain in the low firing rate state until the end of the simulation run.

The implications for symptoms are that agents that increase GABA conductances might reduce and normalize the tendency to remain locked into an idea or concern or action; and would make it much less likely that the quiescent resting state would be left by jumping (because of the noisy spiking) towards a state representing a dominant idea or concern or action.

This simulation evidence, that an increase of glutamatergic synaptic efficacy can increase the stability of attractor networks and thus potentially provide an account for some of the symptoms of obsessive-compulsive disorder, is consistent with evidence that glutamatergic function may be increased in some brain systems in obsessive-compulsive disorder (Rosenberg, MacMaster, Keshavan, Fitzgerald, Stewart & Moore 2000, Rosenberg, MacMillan & Moore 2001, Rosenberg, Mirza, Russell, Tang, Smith, Banerjee, Bhandari, Rose, Ivey, Boyd & Moore 2004, Pittenger et al. 2006, Rolls 2012b, Pittenger, Bloch & Williams 2011) and that cerebro-spinal-fluid glutamate levels are elevated (Chakrabarty, Bhattacharyya, Christopher & Khanna 2005). Consistent with this, agents with antiglutamatergic activity such as riluzole, which can decrease glutamate transmitter release, may be efficacious in obsessive-compulsive disorder (Pittenger et al. 2006, Bhattacharyya & Chakraborty 2007, Pittenger et al. 2011).

Further evidence for a link between glutamate as a neurotransmitter and OCD comes from genetic studies. There is evidence for a significant association between the SLC1A1 glutamate transporter gene and OCD (Stewart, Fagerness, Platko, Smoller, Scharf, Illmann, Jenike, Chabane, Leboyer, Delorme, Jenike & Pauls 2007). This transporter is crucial in terminating the action of glutamate as an excitatory neurotransmitter and in maintaining extracellular glutamate concentrations within a normal range (Bhattacharyya & Chakraborty 2007). In addition, it has been postulated that N-methyl-d-aspartate (NMDA) receptors are involved in OCD, and specifically that polymorphisms in the $3'$ untranslated region of GRIN2B (glutamate receptor, ionotropic, N-methyl-d-aspartate 2B) were associated with OCD in affected families (Arnold, Rosenberg, Mundo, Tharmalingam, Kennedy & Richter 2004, Pittenger et al. 2011).

Thus we have seen how an increase in cortical excitability could increase the stability of cortical recurrent attractor networks, and that if expressed in different prefrontal systems, could produce some of the different types of symptoms found in different patients with obsessive-compulsive disorders (Rolls 2012b). Moreover, the approach links the low-level changes found in the increase in NMDA receptor efficacy in OCD to the systems-level effects such as overstability of cognitive and/or motor functioning. Implications for treatments are developed elsewhere (Rolls 2012b).

8.11.14 Decision-making, oscillations, and communication through coherence

Oscillations in the brain (Buzsáki 2006, Wang 2010) may influence decision-making. For example, theta oscillations (4–10 Hz) increased the speed of operation of a decision-making attractor network (Smerieri, Rolls & Feng 2010). The mechanisms involved may have included concentrating the spikes in the network close together to facilitate the speed of response of neurons, and increasing the firing rate above a threshold for part of the theta cycle in a mechanism like stochastic resonance (Smerieri et al. 2010, Rolls & Treves 2011). Gamma band (40–80 Hz) synchronization also has effects that could influence decision-making (Buehlmann & Deco 2010), though information transmission from one attractor decision-making network to another occurs at far lower values of the synaptic connection weights between the two networks than are required for gamma synchronization (Rolls, Webb & Deco 2012). This raises important questions (Rolls, Webb & Deco 2012, Rolls & Treves 2011) about the hypothesis of communication through coherence (Fries 2005, Fries 2009), that gamma band coherent oscillations between connected neural systems normally increase communication between the neural systems, at least in the context of connected decision-making attractor networks.

A mechanism by which oscillations may influence neuronal firing and decision-making is by resetting neuronal activity. For example, a process such as memory recall may occur within a single theta cycle, and then be quenched so that a new attempt at recall can be made in the next theta cycle. This has the potential advantage that in a changing, ambiguous, or uncertain situation, several attempts can be made at the memory recall, without previous attempts dominating the memory state for a period due to attractor dynamics in autoassociation networks (Rolls & Treves (1998) page 118). Effects consistent with this prediction have now been observed in the rat hippocampus (Jezek, Henriksen, Treves, Moser & Moser 2011): in response to an instantaneous transition between two familiar and similar spatial contexts, hippocampal neurons in one theta cycle indicated one place, and in another theta cycle another place. These findings indicate that, in hippocampal CA3, pattern-completion dynamics can occur within each individual theta cycle. Reset, with potentially different recall in different theta cycles, may facilitate rapid updating and correction of recall. Memory recall may be seen as the same neural network process as decision-making in an attractor network (Rolls 2008b).

9 Neuroeconomics and decision-making

9.1 Introduction

Reward magnitude value and punishment magnitude value are represented in the orbitofrontal cortex, as shown by investigations in which reward and punisher magnitudes have been parametrically varied (see Section 4.5). One type of evidence has been obtained with reward devaluation produced by sensory-specific satiety (Rolls, Sienkiewicz & Yaxley 1989b, Critchley & Rolls 1996c). Another has been with trial-by-trial variation of the monetary gain and loss, allowing correlation of activations of different parts of the orbitofrontal cortex with the magnitude of the gain or loss (O'Doherty, Kringelbach, Rolls, Hornak & Andrews 2001a). Another has been by correlation of subjective pleasantness ratings with activations in the orbitofrontal cortex (Rolls, Kringelbach & De Araujo 2003c, De Araujo, Rolls, Kringelbach, McGlone & Phillips 2003c, De Araujo, Rolls, Kringelbach, McGlone & Phillips 2003c, Kringelbach, O'Doherty, Rolls & Andrews 2003, Grabenhorst & Rolls 2008, Rolls, Grabenhorst & Parris 2008b, Rolls & Grabenhorst 2008, Grabenhorst, D'Souza, Parris, Rolls & Passingham 2010a, Grabenhorst & Rolls 2011). Another type of evidence comes from reward value reversal learning, in which it is found that single neurons in the primate orbitofrontal cortex reverse in one trial, a process that implies a rule reversal and may require the orbitofrontal cortex negative reward prediction error neurons (Thorpe, Rolls & Maddison 1983, Rolls, Critchley, Mason & Wakeman 1996a, Deco & Rolls 2005a) (Chapter 4).

As we have seen in Section 4.5, neurons in the orbitofrontal cortex represent value (or outcome, the value of the reward or punisher received); expected value; and negative reward prediction error. The representations of value and expected value include different representations by different neurons for different stimuli of positive and negative value ('reward value' and 'punisher value'), and of expected value ('expected reward value' and 'expected punisher value').

Moreover, different neurons in the orbitofrontal cortex convey information about which specific reward or punisher is being presented, using a sparse distributed representation (Rolls & Treves 2011, Rolls, Critchley, Verhagen & Kadohisa 2010a). Examples of the ways in which the coding specifies the detailed properties of each reward are provided in Fig. 5.15. This type of encoding provides a basis for sensory-specific satiety, and more generally for the devaluation of a specific reward without influencing other specific rewards. This type of value encoding provides also by stimulus-reinforcer association learning a representation that enables the expected value representation to be about a specific type of reward, or punisher. It is important that this is not a general reward signal, but that different neurons represent different types of reward. This provides the basis for different actions to be instrumentally learned to obtain different types of reward, or to avoid different types of punisher.

In the field of neuroeconomics, these concepts are developed and applied to decision-making when for example we must choose between different reward values available with different probabilities and at different times in the future, how we choose between different types of reward perhaps using a common scale, or when we consider the sensitivity of individuals to potential losses when taking decisions about which potential reward to choose. Decisions of this type are important in life, for example when individuals buy a house or car or simply shop for good value, or choose what type of insurance to buy, or decide what type of investment to make for their future, or take a gamble.

In Section 9.5 I consider some of the rapid advances being made in the neuroeconomics of decision-making. Extensive coverage of neuroeconomics is provided in the following sources: Glimcher (2011a), Padoa-Schioppa (2011), and Glimcher, Camerer, Fehr & Poldrack (2009). An issue that I aim to especially illuminate in this chapter is the biological basis for a 'common scale' vs a 'common currency' of value.

This research in neuroeconomics is linked to research in economics, and I start with a brief overview by way of background in Sections 9.2 and 9.3 of some different approaches that have been taken in classical and neoclassical microeconomics (Glimcher 2011a), the investigation of how choices are made by individuals. A more detailed treatment is provided by Glimcher (2011a). Some readers may wish to move at a first reading to Section 9.5.

In this chapter, following usage in economics, 'subjective' value usually refers to value to the individual of a commodity, taking the circumstances into account, and does not refer to conscious experience. Subjective value in economics implies just value to the individual . In other chapters, following usage in psychology and neuroscience, 'subjective' does refer to what is felt consciously, to phenomenal consciousness (see Chapter 10).

9.2 Classical economics

Blaise Pascal (1672) introduced the concept that when choosing between uncertain alternatives, the expected value (EV) for the choice could be calculated as the probability (p) of winning by the amount to be won (the value, V): $EV = p * V$. The choice should be made of the offer with the highest expected value.

Bernoulli (1738) considered whether a beggar with only one penny who finds a lottery ticket with a 50% probability of winning 20,000 florins (for which the EV is 10,000 florins) should accept an offer from a rich man of 7,000 florins for the lottery ticket. Pascal would have said 'yes'. But Bernoulli made the point that a better choice for the beggar (who currently had almost nothing) might just be a certain 7,000 florins than a possible value of 20,000 or 0 florins with a 50% chance. Bernoulli thus introduced the issue of *risk aversion*, and the concept of *utility* (U), a hidden variable that represents *subjective value* (the value to the individual): it might be more useful for the beggar to choose the certain 7,000 florins. The utility function was conceived as a function that increased with wealth, but increased less steeply as wealth increased (as a logarithmic function of wealth, Bernoulli thought). The expected utility (EU) of trading the lottery ticket was high for the beggar as his wealth was low and he was operating on the initial steeply rising part of the utility function, and of not trading it was low (taking into account the p of each possible outcome), so the beggar should trade the lottery ticket. More formally, $EU = p * U$, and the individual should make choices that would maximize EU. (However, the EU, as a hidden variable, and the exact shape of the utility function, is also measured by the choices, so there is some circularity, though once the function has been determined for an individual, further choices might become more predictable.)

This concept from classical economics is illustrated in Fig. 9.1. The Expected Utility (EU) is the product of an accurate representation of probability (in which the subjective weight for the effect of the probability is a linear function of the probability), multiplied by a utility function in which the utility U is a power function of the value V ($U = V^{\alpha}$). (A power α in the range $0 < \alpha < 1$ produces a utility function in which the utility increases less rapidly as the objective value of the good or offer increases.)

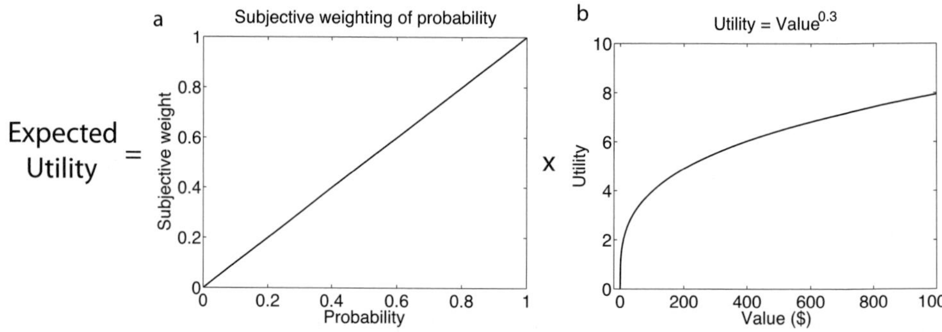

Fig. 9.1 In classical economics, expected utility EU is calculated by (a) a linear probability weighting of (b) Utility U which is a concave function of wealth (a measure of objective value V). In this example, $U = V^{0.3}$. (This material was originally published in *Foundations of Neuroeconomic Analysis* by Glimcher, P. and has been reproduced by permission of Oxford University Press http://ukcatalogue.oup.com/product/9780199744251.do#.Uf9ryqw2FLo.)

9.3 Neoclassical economics

9.3.1 Utility functions, WARP, and GARP

At the end of the 19th century, and in the 20th century, there were many attempts to understand better the **axioms** (rules) that govern economic choices, decisions.

Pareto (1906) realized that utility functions, as they are determined from choices, provide just a ranking (order or ordinal) measure, not a measure of the relative value of goods, i.e. not a ratio (cardinal) measure. He also aimed to simplify the assumptions that were being made about utility functions, and aimed to build an account based on as few assumptions as possible. One assertion he made (as a political economist, and now known as Pareto optimality), is that the resources of a society are not optimally allocated as long as it is possible to make at least one individual better off while keeping all others at least as well off as before.

Samuelson (1938) was also concerned that choices do not tell us about the utility function in a precise way. Samuelson defined what is now known as the Weak Axiom of Revealed Preferences (**WARP**): if a subject is observed to **choose A over B**, then we can assume that the subject cannot **prefer** B to A. If one adds the notion that 'more of a good thing is better than less of a good thing', then one can begin to make more specific statements about what choices tell us about utility, and therefore to make better predictions about future choices. WARP thus intended to show what still dominates economics, how a minimalist model with a few axioms (in Samuelson's case one main axiom) may be able to account for economic decision-making.

Houthakker (1950) developed a model in the style of WARP that could make stronger predictions about choice in a theorem now known as the Generalized Axiom of Revealed Preferences (**GARP**). GARP states as an assumption that choosers can never be satiated. GARP proposes that we can use observations like 'A is chosen over some set of alternatives B' to infer some of the choices subjects would make when asked to choose among a new set of alternatives. Houthakker proved that if a subject's observed behaviour obeys the assumptions of GARP then the subject has a monotonic utility function.

Subjects that have internally consistent preferences (i.e. that do not violate GARP or WARP) have behaviour that has been given the name *rationality* in economics, and the subject is described as a *rational actor*[30].

9.3.2 Expected Utility Theory

Expected Utility Theory, developed by von Neumann & Morgenstern (1944), provides a more detailed approach to the shape of the utility function. They introduced an object of choice called a *lottery* defined by a probability p and a value for each possible choice. The first axiom that they added was the *continuity axiom*. This states that there is some probability of winning prize C that is so small that adding it to either of the other prizes has no effect on the subject's choice between those other prizes. Essentially this specifies that probabilities have a continuous scale. The second axiom that they added was the *independence axiom*. This states that adding a common prize to each side of the choice relation, should not alter the subject's preferences. For example, if a subject prefers a 50% chance of winning \$100 over a 25% chance of winning \$200, the subject should also prefer a 50% chance of winning \$100 and a 5% chance of winning \$10 over a 25% chance of winning \$200 and a 5% chance of winning \$10.

von Neumann & Morgenstern (1944) proved that if we have a chooser who obeys GARP (i.e. has a monotonic utility function) and the continuity and independence axioms, then it is the same as saying that the chooser has some monotone utility function (as in GARP), and computes the desirability of any lottery by multiplying the probability of the gains or losses presented in the lottery by the utility of those gains and losses. That is, if a lottery has choices each with a probability p and a utility U, then the Expected Utility of each choice $EU = p*U$, and the subject should choose the option having the highest expected utility.

Expected utility theory, by introducing these two extra axioms, enables utilities to be measured relative to the utilities of other objects, and not just in terms of rank order. (This means that if A has a utility of 4 and B has a utility of 2, we can also say that A has a utility of 40 and B has a utility of 20. That is, ratios, relative utilities, are defined, but not the absolute utility values.)

9.3.3 Random Utility Models

The Expected Utility Theory of von Neumann & Morgenstern (1944) assumes that there is no noise, that is, no randomness, in the computations involved in the choices. It is a deterministic theory.

However, choices that are made take the general form illustrated in Fig. 8.8 on page 383, in which the percentage of the choice of A over B gradually increases as the difference between the value of A and B changes, which in models of decision-making we term $\Delta\lambda$. When $\Delta\lambda = 0$, the choice between the two options is 50%. It is noise in the system that makes the transition from choosing A to choosing B, gradual, with an approximately sigmoid shape to the curve. The more noise there is in the system, the shallower is this curve (Fig. 8.8). The whole treatment of decision-making processes in the brain formally incorporates this noise, as described in Chapter 8, in Appendix B, and in *The Noisy Brain* (Rolls & Deco 2010). Without noise in the system, the choices would jump from 0% to A to 100% to A just when A becomes larger than B. A deterministic system was considered in Expected Utility Theory (von Neumann & Morgenstern 1944).

In economics, noise has been introduced into the system to deal with this important issue that decision-making is probabilistic. Noise has been introduced in random utility models, in

[30]This definition holds only in this chapter. Elsewhere in this book it signifies reasoning.

which additional axioms (rules) assume that the utility inferred from the subject's choices can be treated as a stochastic (noisy, random) variable (McFadden 1974).

9.4 Behavioural economics

The traditional neoclassical models are inadequate to account for choice, as is shown in this section, which introduces new approaches now being used in the field of behavioural economics (Glimcher 2011a).

9.4.1 The Allais paradox

One inadequacy of neoclassical economics was demonstrated by Allais (1953), who showed that subjects do not obey the *independence axiom* of von Neumann & Morgenstern (1944).

Allais (1953) first asked 100 subjects to choose between two options:
(1A) a 100% chance of winning $1,000,000 (for which EV = $1,000,000), or
(1B) an 89% chance of winning $1,000,000, a 1% chance of winning $0, and a 10% chance of winning $5,000,000 (for which EV = $1,390,000).

The subjects mostly chose option 1A, that is, they is they showed a reasonable degree of risk aversion (i.e. to the 1% probability of winning $0).

Allais then asked the same subjects a second question, to choose between the following two options:
(2A) an 89% chance of winning $0, and an 11% chance of winning $1,000,000 (for which EV = $110,000), or
(2B) a 90% chance of winning $0, and an 10% chance of winning $5,000,000 (for which EV = $500,000)

Most of the subjects chose option 2B.

We can see that this is a disproof of the independence axiom as follows (Glimcher 2011a). Let us restate option 1A as follows:
(1A-restated) a 89% chance of winning $1,000,000 and an 11% chance of winning $1,000,000 (for which EV = $1,000,000).
Now imagine that we remove the 89% chance of winning $1,000,000 from both 1A-restated and 1B. What we get is an 11% chance of winning $1,000,000 versus a 10% chance of winning $5,000,000, which are exactly the gambles presented to Allais' subjects in question 2, so any subject who prefers option 1A and who obeys expected utility theory should also prefer option 2A, which is not what was found.

The root of Allais' concerns was his view that human subjects do not represent probabilities objectively, and his demonstration raised doubts about Expected Utility Theory in neoclassical economics.

9.4.2 Risk seeking over losses

Another effect that reveals some of the inadequacies of neoclassical economics is the 'risk seeking over losses' effect (Kahneman & Tversky 1979). They asked subjects whether they would prefer: (1A) a sure gain of $500 or (1B) a 50% chance to gain $1000. The EVs are the same, but most of the subjects (84%) chose 1A. Under this condition the subjects were risk averse.

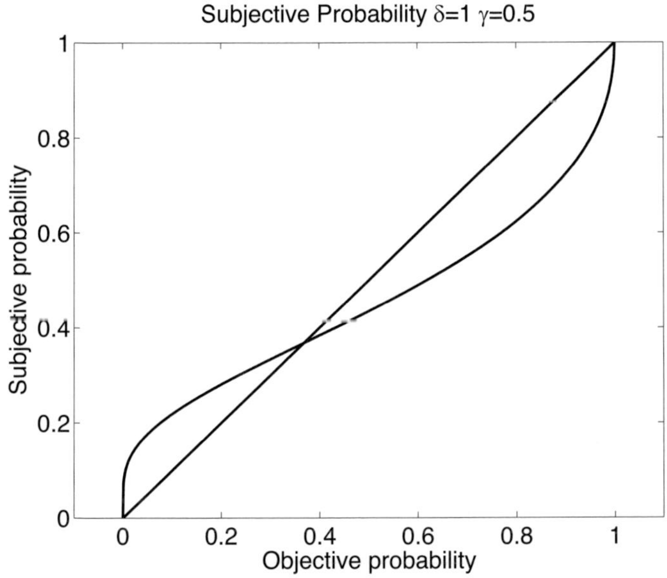

Fig. 9.2 Subjective probability π reflecting weighting of objective probability p by a probability weighting functions of the type used in prospect theory. $\delta = 1.0$ and $\gamma = 0.5$. (This material was originally published in *Foundations of Neuroeconomic Analysis* by Glimcher, P. and has been reproduced by permission of Oxford University Press http://ukcatalogue.oup.com/product/9780199744251.do#.Uf9ryqw2FLo.)

Next, Kahneman & Tversky (1979) asked the subjects a second question, (2A) whether they would choose a sure loss of $500, or (2B) a 50% chance of losing $1,000. 70% of the same subjects chose option 2B. Under this condition the subjects were risk seeking.

This result would not be predicted from the standard concave utility function (Fig. 9.1b) of neoclassical economics (see Glimcher (2011a) for more details).

Problems with neoclassical utility theory were thus raised by the Allais paradox, and risk seeking over losses. Problems were also raised by the Ellsberg (1961) paradox (in which subjects seemed to be thinking that there were both too many and too few items available in a lottery, indicating a difficulty in calculating probabilities rationally in the way assumed by expected utility theory); and by the endowment effect (Kahneman, Knetch & Thaler 1990) (in which 'gifts' seem to have a greater value than they would in a marketplace); and by other effects (Glimcher 2011a).

With this background of problems for neoclassical utility theory, developments emerged in the new field of Behavioral Economics, for example in the form of Prospect Theory.

9.4.3 Prospect Theory

Prospect theory (Kahneman & Tversky 1979, Tversky & Kahneman 1992) (reviewed by Glimcher (2011a) and Fox & Poldrack (2009)) introduces new ideas about how humans take account of probabilities, and how they appear to use a reference point, above which subjective value increases with a concave function, and below which it decreases, usually more rapidly, with a concave function. Kahneman and Tversky also accepted the idea that a number of different heuristics may influence choice depending on the context, with one example described below being the framing effect.

Prospect theory proposes that humans do not make choices based on actual probabilities, as von Neumann & Morgenstern (1944) proposed, but instead on a subjectivized form of

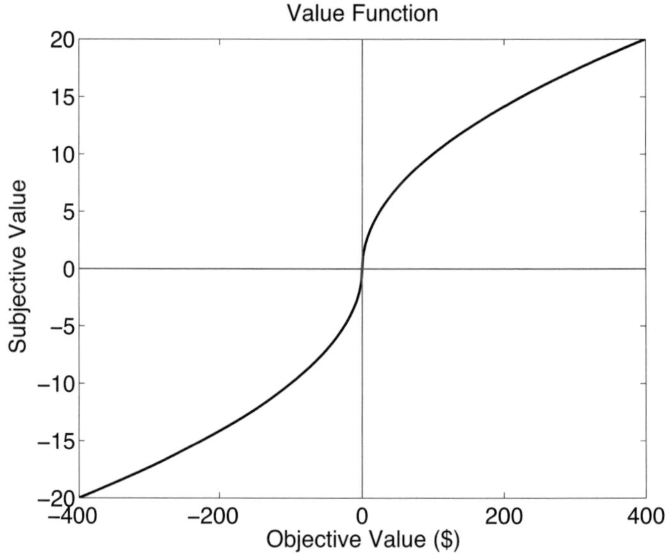

Fig. 9.3 Subjective value function used in prospect theory to relate subjective value to objective value. $\alpha = \beta = 0.5$. $\lambda = 1$. (This material was originally published in *Foundations of Neuroeconomic Analysis* by Glimcher, P. and has been reproduced by permission of Oxford University Press http://ukcatalogue.oup.com/product/9780199744251.do#.Uf9ryqw2FLo.)

probability (π), in which the objective probability p is weighted by a probability weighting function ($w(p)$). The overall effect of the probability weighting function is shown in Fig. 9.2. The effect is to reduce the subjective probability (π) of high probability events, and to increase the subjective probability of low probability events. (In summary, there is a tendency not to represent extreme values of objective probability accurately, but instead to have a subjective representation of probabilities that is moved towards a value at the crossover point with what would be produced by a linear weighting function. As a reminder, neoclassical utility theory assumed a linear probability weighting function, as illustrated in Fig. 9.1.)

A formulation of a probability weighting function $w(p)$ (Prelec 1998) is

$$w(p) = \exp[-\delta(\ln p)^\gamma] \tag{9.1}$$

where the free parameter γ controls the curvature, and δ controls where the function crosses the identity line, and $\delta, \gamma > 0$. In the example shown in Fig. 9.2, $\delta = 1.0$ and $\gamma = 0.5$. This type of probability function thus increases the subjective probability (π) of low objective probabilities (p); and decreases the subjective probability of high objective probabilities.

Prospect theory also moves away from assuming a monotonic utility function, and instead proposes that Subjective Value (SV the value to the subject) is related to Objective Value (V) around a reference point, above which Subjective Value increases with a concave function, and below which Subjective Value decreases with a (typically steeper) concave function, as illustrated in Fig. 9.3.

More formally, above the reference point

$$SV = V^\alpha \tag{9.2}$$

and below the reference point

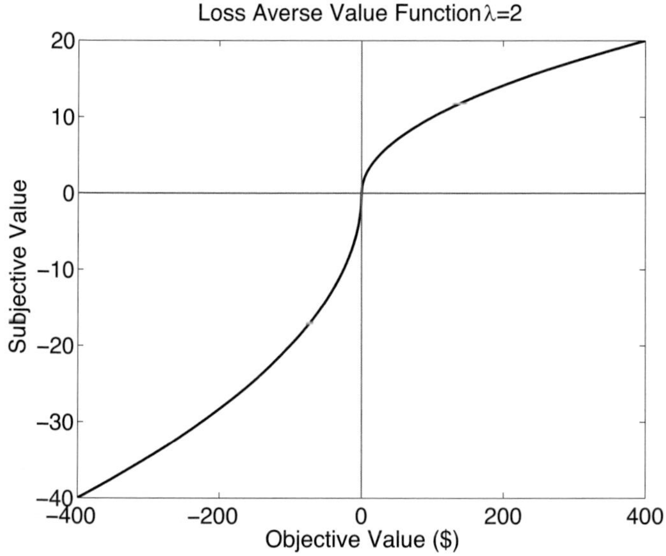

Fig. 9.4 Loss averse Subjective Value function with $\lambda > 1$ used in prospect theory to relate Subjective Value to Objective Value. $\alpha = \beta = 0.5$. $\lambda = 2$. (This material was originally published in *Foundations of Neuroeconomic Analysis* by Glimcher, P. and has been reproduced by permission of Oxford University Press http://ukcatalogue.oup.com/product/9780199744251.do#.Uf9ryqw2FLo.)

$$SV = -V^{\beta} \tag{9.3}$$

where α and β are < 1 and control the concavities of the functions.

The use of different functions above and below a reference point allows the data for a subject to reflect diminishing increases in subjective value or utility as objective value increases; and diminishing decreases in subjective loss value or utility as objective value decreases below the reference point.

To account for the fact that under many conditions humans are more sensitive to losses than to gains (loss aversiveness), Kahneman and Tversky proposed that the magnitude of the loss associated side of the subjective value function was steeper than the gains-associated side of the subjective value function. To achieve this, they weighted the loss side by an additional parameter λ

$$SV = -\lambda V^{\beta} \tag{9.4}$$

where λ, the loss aversion coefficient, captures the additional sensitivity of choosers to losses over gains. Thus a chooser who viewed a \$200 loss as equivalent to a \$100 gain would have λ=2. The parameter λ enables individual differences in loss sensitivity to be incorporated. An example of a loss aversive subjective value function with $\lambda > 1$ is shown in Fig. 9.4.

Overall, in prospect theory Expected Utility EU) would be calculated from the Subjective Value SV as

$$EU = \pi SV \tag{9.5}$$

by taking into account the subjectivized form of probability (π) described in Equation 9.1.

Prospect theory thus has five free parameters: δ and γ for the probability weighting function, and α, β and λ for the subjective value function. Although five free parameters is a large number, prospect theory can account for the Allais paradox, the endowment effect, and risk seeking in the domain of loss. To reduce the weakness of having this number of free parameters in full prospect theory, frequently α and β are assumed to be equal, and the probability weighting function is taken to cross the main diagonal of the graph at the value $1/e$ (Glimcher 2011a). Prospect theory also does not have much to say about how the reference point is set for the subjective value function.

The type of *framing effect* that could be accounted for by moving the reference point is as follows. Tversky & Kahneman (1981) read a group of subjects the following story: "Imagine that the U.S. is preparing for the outbreak of an usual Asian disease, which is expected to kill 600 people. Two alternative programs to combat the disease have been proposed". Then half of the subjects were asked to choose between the following first pair of options:
"(1) If program A is adopted, 200 people will be saved. If Program B is adopted, there is a 1/3 probability that 600 people will be saved." Under these conditions, 72% of the subjects picked A.
Then Tversky & Kahneman (1981) offered a second group of subjects two different options: "(2) If program C is adopted, 400 people will die. If Program D is adopted, there is a 1/3 probability that nobody will die, and a 2/3 probability that 600 people will die." Framed this way, 78% of their subjects now picked D, even though options A and C are numerically identical (as are B and D).

The objective values of options A and B are identical to the objective values of options C and D, yet these two sets of options present very different subjective experiences. In option A we consider the positive psychological experience of saving 200 people; in option C we confront the subjectively distasteful prospect of 400 deaths. Tversky & Kahneman (1981) argued that these differences affected the decisions that their subjects made in a way that could not be predicted from marginal utilities and a wealth level. Instead, some notion of subjective value was being used that was relative to the framework of the story being told to the subjects. This was one of the reasons why they introduced a moveable reference point for subjective value into prospect theory, which could then provide an account of framing effects.

Kahneman & Tversky (1979) had, in developing prospect theory, realized that a monotonic wealth-based marginal utility function is inadequate. Instead they introduced a reference-based utility function, a local reference point. The local reference point is important in assessing subjective value, and can be moved depending on the context, to account for example for framing effects in which different choices may be made if the contexts or frames of reference are different. Rather than computing marginal utilities against wealth as in the standard theory, utilities (not marginal utilities) could be computed directly as deviations from a baseline level of wealth, and then choices could be based on direct comparisons of these utilities (or strictly subjective value) rather than on comparisons of marginal utilities. One starts with a chooser's status quo, and then each gamble is represented as the chance of winning or losing utilities relative to the status-quo-like reference point. Moreover, prospect theory allows different loss vs gain functions for the computation of subjective value from objective value.

Prospect theory is a descriptive theory, and its parameters can be adjusted to fit the data. In contrast, classical and neoclassical economic theories attempted to set up a minimal number of axioms to predict choice.

Another limitation of prospect theory is that it is deterministic. This is a problem for predicting probabilistic choice even when the objective value V is fixed, as described in Section 9.3.3. This might be overcome by introducing noise, that is randomness or stochasticity, into for example the subjective value function defined in Equations 9.2 and 9.4. Alternatively (or probably additionally), stochasticity might be introduced into the choice mechanism that operates using the Expected Value or expected utility of Equation 9.5.

Overall, in classical economics and neoclassical economics, we have seen that models based on a minimal number of axioms or rules have not been able to account for choices that are made in a wide range of circumstances. Behavioural economics adopted a more descriptive approach, allowed heuristics to help account for different choice situations, but has not sufficiently clearly identified how parameters such as the location of the reference point are moved, or how probabilistic choices are made. Moreover, it has not provided an 'ultimate' explanation or account of what determines the value of a good to an individual subject, and how any common scale or currency might be set up. That might require for example an evolutionary explanation. Nor of course does economics have much to tell us about the underlying mechanisms for the valuation and choice, which is an important area with applications in medicine including neurology and psychiatry. We now turn to neuroeconomics to consider the rapid progress being made in this field about choice and decision-making by the brain.

9.5 Neuroeconomics

9.5.1 Overview of neuroeconomics

As we have seen in Section 4.5, neurons in the orbitofrontal cortex represent value (or outcome, the value of the reward or punisher received); expected value; and negative reward prediction error. The representations of value and expected value include different representations by different neurons of positive and negative value ('reward value' and 'punisher value', and of expected value ('expected reward value' and 'expected punisher value'). The representations are of reward value in that the neuronal responses to a reward such as the taste, sight or smell of food decrease when that particular food is devalued by feeding to satiety; and when the expected reward value of a visual stimulus is altered by its reversal during learning of the value of the (taste or flavor) outcome that is expected when the discriminative visual or olfactory stimulus is presented (Rolls 2005b, Rolls 2008b, Rolls & Grabenhorst 2008) (Section 4.5).

Thus the brain maintains representations of the values of different stimuli (including abstract reinforcers such as money (O'Doherty, Kringelbach, Rolls, Hornak & Andrews 2001a, Rolls, McCabe & Redoute 2008e)), and these representations are in the orbitofrontal cortex (Rolls 2005b, Rolls 2008b, Rolls & Grabenhorst 2008, Grabenhorst & Rolls 2011). We have argued and produced evidence that these reward value representations are on a common scale to facilitate the decision-making process (Grabenhorst, D'Souza, Parris, Rolls & Passingham 2010a, Grabenhorst & Rolls 2011) (see Section 9.5.2).

In slightly different terminology, value represents a common unit of measure to make a comparison between these reinforcing stimuli or 'goods' (Padoa-Schioppa 2011). In that terminology, a 'commodity' is a unitary amount of a specified good independently of the circumstances in which it is available (e.g. quantity, cost, delay, etc.). The value of each good is computed at the time of choice on the basis of multiple 'determinants', which include the specific commodity, its quantity, the current motivational state, the cost of obtaining it, the behavioural context of choice (i.e. the other choices that are currently available), etc. The collection of these determinants thus defines the value of the 'good'.

The hypothesis is that while choosing, individuals compute the values of different options independently of one another. It is argued that the 'net reward value', i.e. the value of each good minus the cost of obtaining it, must be computed and represented on a common scale of value as the input to the decision-making process, which makes the choice (Grabenhorst & Rolls 2011). The reason that the net value must be computed is that the decision-making process itself, performed it is suggested by an attractor decision-making network (Chapter 8), cannot by itself receive as inputs separate values and costs for each choice, for these variables related to a specific choice could not be related to each other in the decision-making attractor network.

A brain region that does appear to compute the actions needed to obtain a stimulus with the particular value, and which takes into account the costs of actions (which we have termed the extrinsic costs (Grabenhorst & Rolls 2011)), is the cingulate cortex (Rushworth et al. 2011, Grabenhorst & Rolls 2011), which receives value information about the goods in its anterior cingulate part from the orbitofrontal cortex (Rolls 2005b, Rolls 2009d, Grabenhorst & Rolls 2011). It is argued that the computation of net value in the orbitofrontal cortex does not depend on the sensori-motor contingencies of choice (the spatial configuration of the offers or the specific action that will implement the choice outcome), for the behavioural responses and actions are not represented in the orbitofrontal cortex, which represents the value of stimuli, and does not represent actions and responses (Thorpe, Rolls & Maddison 1983, Rolls 2005b, Padoa-Schioppa 2011). These action contingencies may, however, affect values in the form of action costs. In particular, the actions necessary to obtain different goods often bear different costs. It is still an interesting issue about whether these 'extrinsic costs' (the costs of the actions necessary to obtain a reward (Grabenhorst & Rolls 2011)) are represented in the orbitofrontal cortex.

The extrinsic costs that influence the value of a good and the value of a choice include
1. The action costs, including the difficulty of the actions needed to obtain the good, as just described;
2. the time delay (with future rewards being discounted as a function of the length of the delay, and differently discounted by different individuals);
3. the 'risk', i.e. the probability that the reward will be obtained;
4. the amount of the good obtained if it is chosen;
5. the quality of the good, e.g. one juice may be preferred over another;
6. ambiguity (i.e. poor knowledge about the probability that a reward if chosen will be obtained).

Intrinsic or internal costs and related factors that influence the value of stimuli include (Grabenhorst & Rolls 2011, Padoa-Schioppa 2011)
1. motivational state;
2. patience vs impatience or impulsiveness;
3. risk attitude, that is choice when the outcome is probabilistic, for example whether one is likely to gamble;
4. ambiguity attitude;
5. whether the stimulus which may have pleasant components has in addition unpleasant components.

Further factors important in understanding choices in the field of neuroeconomics, many described in more detail below, are:

The value of each good must be computed 'online' at the time of choice, for value is influenced by for example motivational state.

While choosing, individuals normally compute the values of different goods independently of one another. Such 'menu invariance' implies transitive preferences (Padoa-Schioppa 2011).

Absolute value is important for long-term choice and transitive preferences. This may be represented in the orbitofrontal cortex.

Relative value is useful for short-term choice, for example on a particular trial or a block

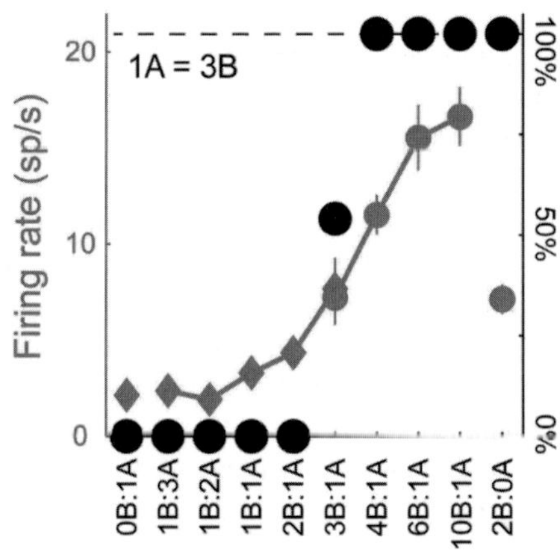

Fig. 9.5 Orbitofrontal cortex neuron encoding the offer value. On individual trials, the monkey was offered different numbers of drops of peppermint tea (juice B) versus 1 drop of grape juice (juice A). Black circles indicate the behavioural choice pattern (relative value in the upper left) and red symbols indicate the neuronal firing rate when the offer of different amounts of juice B was made vs 1 drop of juice A (1A). Red diamonds and circles refer, respectively, to trials in which the animal chose juice A and juice B. There is a sigmoid relationship between the firing rate of the neuron and the quantity of juice B offered to the monkey. (Reproduced from Padoa-Schioppa, C., Neurobiology of economic choice: a good-based model, *Annual Review of Neuroscience*, 34, pp. 333–359 ©2011, Annual Reviews.)

of trials, and may be separately represented in the orbitofrontal cortex.

In one neuroeconomics study that illustrates how the responses of orbitofrontal cortex neurons encode the value of a stimulus or choice, the value of the choice was manipulated by providing different numbers of drops of juice (quantity) of different quality (e.g. grape juice (A) and peppermint tea (B), which were termed commodities) to monkeys (Padoa-Schioppa & Assad 2006). The monkey preferred juice A. When offered one drop of juice A versus one drop of juice B (offer 1A:1B), the animals chose juice A. However, the animals were thirsty: they generally preferred larger amounts of juice to smaller amounts of juice. The amounts of the two juices offered against each other varied from trial to trial, which induced a commodity quantity trade-off in the choice pattern. For example in one session (Fig. 9.5), offer types (indicated by the number of small squares on a screen that were available for A and for B) included 0B:1A, 1B:2A, 1B:1A, 2B:1A, 3B:1A, 4B:1A, 6B:1A, 10B:1A and 3B:0A. The monkey generally chose 1A when 1B or 2B were available as the alternative, it was roughly indifferent between the two juices when offered 3B:1A, and it chose B when 4B, 6B or 10B were available (Fig. 9.5). In other words, the monkey assigned to 1A a value roughly equal to the value it assigned to 3B. A neuron recorded in the orbitofrontal cortex responded with a low rate (several spikes/s) when the offer was 2B or less, at an intermediate rate (approximately 10 spikes/s) when the offer was 3B or 4B, and at a high rate (approximately 17 spikes/s) when the offer was 6B or higher relative to 1A (Fig. 9.5). The neuron thus encoded the value of the offer, where the value assigned by the monkey reflected a commodity × quantity tradeoff.

The offer value neurons respond when the visual stimulus indicating the taste/flavor reward that will be obtained is shown (Padoa-Schioppa & Assad 2006, Padoa-Schioppa 2011). They thus correspond to the orbitofrontal cortex neurons described by Rolls and colleagues which respond to a visual stimulus, for example in a visual discrimination task, that indicates the value of the reward or punisher that will be obtained (Thorpe, Rolls & Maddison 1983, Rolls, Critchley, Mason & Wakeman 1996a, Critchley & Rolls 1996c). These visual neurons reflect reward value in that they respond to a particular visual stimulus when the value is high, and gradually respond less to the visual stimulus as gradually it becomes devalued by feeding to satiety (Critchley & Rolls 1996c) (Fig. 4.34). These visual neurons also respond to a visual stimulus when it signifies a high value, and do not respond when it is devalued by visual discrimination reversal learning so that it signifies after learning a low reward value (Rolls, Critchley, Mason & Wakeman 1996a) (Fig. 4.31). In addition, these studies show that other neurons reflect the punisher value of a visual stimulus, responding for example to a visual stimulus when it signifies the punisher of a taste of saline if the visual stimulus is selected (Fig. 4.32) (Thorpe, Rolls & Maddison 1983, Rolls, Critchley, Mason & Wakeman 1996a).

Padoa-Schioppa & Assad (2006) also described neurons that in the same task responded when the juice taste reward was delivered. Their taste neurons reflected value, in that they had for example (Padoa-Schioppa (2011) figure 2e) a large response when 4B or greater was delivered, an intermediate response when 3B was delivered, and no response when 2B or less was delivered. These neurons again correspond to the taste reward neurons of Rolls and colleagues analysed in the orbitofrontal cortex (Rolls, Yaxley & Sienkiewicz 1990, Rolls, Critchley, Verhagen & Kadohisa 2010a), which respond to a taste when it has a high value, and gradually respond less to that taste when it is gradually devalued by feeding to satiety (Rolls, Sienkiewicz & Yaxley (1989b), e.g. Fig. 4.22).

It is of interest that the visual reward and taste reward neurons in the orbitofrontal cortex described by Rolls and colleagues maintain their firing almost unchanged to other visual or taste stimuli when one visual or taste stimulus is devalued (Rolls, Sienkiewicz & Yaxley 1989b, Critchley & Rolls 1996c) (e.g. Fig. 4.22). These neurons thus reflect primarily *absolute reward value*, in that their firing rate to other rewards is little influenced when one of the visual or taste rewards on offer is devalued (see further Section 9.5.3). However, the small increase in firing rate sometimes found in sensory-specific satiety experiments to visual or taste food stimuli that have not been fed to satiety (Rolls, Sienkiewicz & Yaxley 1989b, Critchley & Rolls 1996c) (e.g. Fig. 4.34) may reflect a small proportion of *relative reward value* in the representations provided by these visual and taste orbitofrontal cortex neurons.

In the experiment illustrated in Fig. 9.5, offers varied on two dimensions: juice type (commodity), and juice amount (quantity). The same method can be applied when offers vary on other dimensions, such as probability, cost, delay, etc. For example, Kable & Glimcher (2007) conducted on human subjects an experiment on *temporal discounting*. People and animals often prefer smaller rewards delivered earlier to larger rewards delivered later – an important phenomenon with broad societal implications. In the study of Kable and Glimcher, subjects chose in each trial between a small amount of money delivered immediately and a larger amount of money delivered at a later time. For given delivery time t, the amount of money was varied, and the indifference point was identified: the amount of money delivered at time t such that the subject would be indifferent between the two options. This procedure was repeated for different delivery times t. Indifference points – fitted with a hyperbolic function – provided a measure of the subjective value choosers assigned to time-discounted money. The results of the fMRI experiment showed that the activation in the ventromedial prefrontal cortex (vmPFC) reflected the time-discounted values.

An interesting procedure to measure indifference points is to perform a 'second price auction'. For example in a study by Plassmann, O'Doherty & Rangel (2007), hungry human subjects were asked to declare the highest price they would be willing to pay for a given food (i.e., their indifference point, also called 'reservation price'). Normally, people would try to save money and declare a price lower than their true reservation price. However, second price auctions discourage them from doing so by randomly generating a second price after the subjects have declared their own price. If the second price is lower than the declared price, subjects get to buy the food and pay the second price; if the second price is higher than the declared price, subjects do not get to buy the food at all. In these conditions, the optimal strategy for subjects is to declare their true reservation price. This procedure thus measures for each subject the indifference point between food and money. Using this measure, Plassmann et al. (2007) confirmed that the BOLD signal in the orbitofrontal cortex reflects the subjective value assigned to different foods.

In summary, to measure the neural representation of subjective value, it is necessary to let the subject choose between alternative offers, infer values from the indifference point, and use that measure to interpret neural signals.

The findings are of course consistent with the reward value representations described previously in the orbitofrontal cortex based on neuronal recordings that show the encoding of value (Rolls, Sienkiewicz & Yaxley 1989b, Critchley & Rolls 1996c, Rolls, Critchley, Browning, Hernadi & Lenard 1999a, Rolls, Critchley, Verhagen & Kadohisa 2010a), and on BOLD signal activations in the human orbitofrontal cortex that are correlated with subjective pleasantness (Kringelbach, O'Doherty, Rolls & Andrews 2003, Grabenhorst, Rolls & Bilderbeck 2008a, Grabenhorst & Rolls 2008, Grabenhorst, Rolls, Parris & D'Souza 2010b).

A neuronal representation of value can be said to be 'abstract' (i.e., in the space of goods) if two conditions are met (Padoa-Schioppa 2011).

First, the encoding by neurons should be *independent of the sensori-motor contingencies* of choice, so that the neurons do not just encode movements. The relation of orbitofrontal cortex neuronal activity to the reward value of sensory stimuli including taste, olfactory, oral texture, and visual stimuli, and not to movements, for example of the mouth or arm, has been made clear since our earliest reports (Thorpe, Rolls & Maddison 1983, Rolls, Yaxley & Sienkiewicz 1990, Verhagen, Rolls & Kadohisa 2003, Rolls 2005b), and has been confirmed by Padoa-Schioppa & Assad (2006), who found that less than 5% of OFC neurons were significantly modulated by the spatial configuration of the offers on the monitor or by the direction of the eye movement. Similar independence of OFC representations of value from the details of actions has also been reported by others (Kennerley & Wallis 2009, Roesch & Olson 2005).

Second, the encoding should be *domain general*. In other words, the activity should represent the value of the good affected by all the relevant determinants (commodity, quantity, risk, cost, etc.). Current evidence for such an abstract representation is convincing for two brain areas, the orbitofrontal cortex (OFC) and the closely related ventromedial prefrontal cortex (vmPFC). Evidence that commodity and quantity affect value (subjective value, the value to the individual) and the representation in the OFC similarly has been described above (Padoa-Schioppa & Assad 2006, Padoa-Schioppa 2011) (see Fig. 9.5). The effects of risk, i.e. the probability of obtaining the good or reward, on subjective value have been shown to be reflected in the activations found in the human orbitofrontal cortex (Rolls, McCabe & Redoute 2008e, Peters & Buchel 2009). Under risk, the probabilities of different outcomes can be estimated, whereas under ambiguity, even these probabilities are not known. Choices of monetary offers under ambiguity vs risk (which are differently weighted in different subjects) also trade off as predicted by subjective value representations in the vmPFC (Levy, Snell, Nelson, Rustichini & Glimcher 2010). The delay of a reward decreases the value of the delayed reward and activations in the human vmPFC in a corresponding way (Kable & Glimcher 2007), and consistent results have been found at the single neuron level in monkeys (Roesch & Olson 2005). The cost in terms of the effort involved in obtaining a reward also decreases the neuronal responses in the OFC to a reward (Kennerley, Dahmubed, Lara & Wallis 2009), providing evidence that subjective value representations in the OFC do reflect the difficulty of the actions required to obtain the reward (though not the details of the actions themselves).This is an indication that what we have also termed the 'net value' of a reward, that is the value of the reward minus the cost/ effort required to obtain it, needs to be represented, for this 'net value' input is what is required to the decision-making network (Grabenhorst & Rolls 2011). This is needed because the attractor decision-making network cannot relate separate inputs for the rewards and for the costs of several alternatives, for which cost was to be bound to each reward could not be implemented in the decision-making network.

There is thus considerable evidence that the orbitofrontal cortex (OFC) and adjoining ventromedial prefrontal cortex (vmPFC) provide an abstract representation of value. Important properties of the representation are that the subjective value, the value to the individual, is represented and not the actions required to obtain the reward or 'good'; and that the representation is domain general, that is reflects the value when it is altered in a number of ways including the magnitude of the good, risk, delay, and the cost/effort required to obtain the good. The single neuron data, including much that we have obtained, indicates that the representation at the neuronal level is specific for each different type of reward or good, with a common scale of value, but no conversion into a common currency, as described further in Section 9.5.2. The view that there is a representation of value in the orbitofrontal cortex and vmPFC, which may be the source of value effects in other brain regions, has now been accepted by Levy & Glimcher (2012). However, as the data that they review is from fMRI studies, they are not able to make the distinction as clear about no conversion into a common currency, for the fMRI activations reflect the responses of very many different single neurons, and do not provided clear evidence that different types of reward are represented by separate neurons in a sparse distributed representation (Rolls 2005b, Rolls 2008b, Rolls & Treves 2011, Rolls, Critchley, Verhagen & Kadohisa 2010a) (see also Chapters 4 and 5).

The effect of the value representations in the orbitofrontal cortex on other brain areas is indeed a point of great interest. As described in Chapter 4, there are projections from the orbitofrontal cortex to the anterior cingulate cortex, with many rewards represented in the human pregenual cingulate cortex, and many punishers in the anterodorsal cingulate cortex (Rolls 2005b, Rolls & Grabenhorst 2008, Grabenhorst & Rolls 2011) (Fig. 4.47). Indeed, we (Rolls 2005b, Rolls & Grabenhorst 2008, Rolls 2009d, Grabenhorst & Rolls 2011) have argued that the function of the value representation in the anterior cingulate cortex is to provide the representation of (reward) outcome necessary for action–outcome learning implemented in the cingulate cortex, as described in Chapter 4. In this context, it is of interest that single neurons in the monkey anterior cingulate cortex encoded post-decision variables such as chosen value and chosen juice taste value, but not pre-decision variables such as offer value (e.g. the sight of the food or of a symbol that indicated what was available for choice) (Cai & Padoa-Schioppa 2012). This is in contrast to the orbitofrontal cortex, in which the offer value is also encoded. This evidence is thus consistent with the hypothesis that the OFC represents subjective value in a way that can be an input to a choice decision-making system (in for example medial prefrontal cortex area 10) because the OFC represents the expected value of the outcome (e.g. the sight of food, or an offer value (Thorpe, Rolls & Maddison 1983, Rolls, Critchley, Mason & Wakeman 1996a, Rolls, McCabe & Redoute 2008e, Padoa-Schioppa & Assad 2006, Padoa-Schioppa 2011)), whereas the cingulate cortex is involved in learning associations between actions and outcomes such as whether a juice or monetary reward was obtained (Chapter 4).

It is of interest that insofar as a representation of value exists in rodents (Schoenbaum, Roesch, Stalnaker & Takahashi 2009), it does not appear to meet the conditions for abstraction described above (Padoa-Schioppa 2011). For example, neurons in the rodent OFC may be spatially selective and thus represent responses (Feierstein, Quirk, Uchida, Sosulski & Mainen 2006, Roesch, Taylor & Schoenbaum 2006). Further, experiments that manipulated two determinants of value found that different neuronal populations in the rat OFC represent reward magnitude and time delay – a striking difference with primates (Roesch & Olson 2005, Roesch, Taylor & Schoenbaum 2006). Differences in the anatomy and connections of the rat from the primate orbitofrontal cortex are apparent (e.g. with the rat having only agranular regions (Wise 2008), see Fig. 1.1 and Section 1.3), and it is possible that an abstract representation of value may have emerged later in evolution in parallel with the expansion of the frontal lobe.

9.5.2 A common scale of value for different goods in the orbitofrontal cortex, but no conversion to a common currency

9.5.2.1 Reward-specific / value-specific representations

Single neurons in the orbitofrontal cortex encode different specific rewards (Chapters 4 and 5) (Rolls 2005b, Rolls & Grabenhorst 2008, Grabenhorst & Rolls 2011). They do this by responding to different combinations of taste, olfactory, somatosensory, visual, and auditory stimuli including socially relevant stimuli such as face expression (Rolls 2005b, Rolls, Critchley, Browning & Inoue 2006a, Rolls & Grabenhorst 2008). Part of the adaptive utility of this reward-specific representation is that it provides for sensory-specific satiety as implemented by a decrease in the responsiveness of reward-specific neurons (Rolls 2005b, Rolls & Grabenhorst 2008). This is a fundamental property of every reward system that helps to ensure that a variety of different rewards is selected over time. Representations of both reward outcome and expected value are specific for the particular reward: not only do different neurons respond to different primary reinforcers, but different neurons also encode the conditioned stimuli for different outcomes, with different neurons responding for example to the sight or odour of stimuli based on the outcome that is expected (Thorpe, Rolls & Maddison 1983, Rolls, Critchley, Mason & Wakeman 1996a) (Chapters 4 and 5).

9.5.2.2 Topology of reward and punishment systems

Different types of reward tend to be represented in the human medial OFC and pregenual ACC, and different types of punisher tend to be represented in the lateral OFC and dorsal part of ACC (Fig. 4.47). The punishers include negative reward prediction error encoded by neurons that fire only when an expected reward is not received (Thorpe, Rolls & Maddison 1983). To compute this OFC signal, inputs are required from neurons that respond to the expected value of a stimulus (exemplified in the OFC by neurons with responses to the sight of food), and from other neurons that respond to the magnitude of the reward outcome (exemplified in the OFC by neurons that respond to the taste of food) (Chapters 4 and 5 (Rolls 2005b, Rolls 2009b)). All these signals are reflected in activations found for expected monetary value and for monetary reward outcome in the human medial OFC (O'Doherty, Kringelbach, Rolls, Hornak & Andrews 2001a, Rolls, McCabe & Redoute 2008e), and for monetary loss and negative reward prediction error for social reinforcers in the human lateral OFC (O'Doherty, Kringelbach, Rolls, Hornak & Andrews 2001a, Kringelbach & Rolls 2003). This topological organization with different types of specific reward represented close together in the OFC may allow for comparison between different rewards implemented by lateral inhibition as part of a process of scaling different specific rewards to the same range (Rolls 2005b, Rolls & Grabenhorst 2008, Grabenhorst & Rolls 2011).

9.5.2.3 A common scale for different specific rewards

A classical view of economic decision theory (Bernoulli 1738) implies that decision-makers convert the value of different goods into a common scale of utility. Ecological (McFarland & Sibly 1975), psychological (Cabanac 1992), and some neuroeconomic (Montague & Berns 2002) approaches similarly suggest that the values of different kinds of rewards are converted

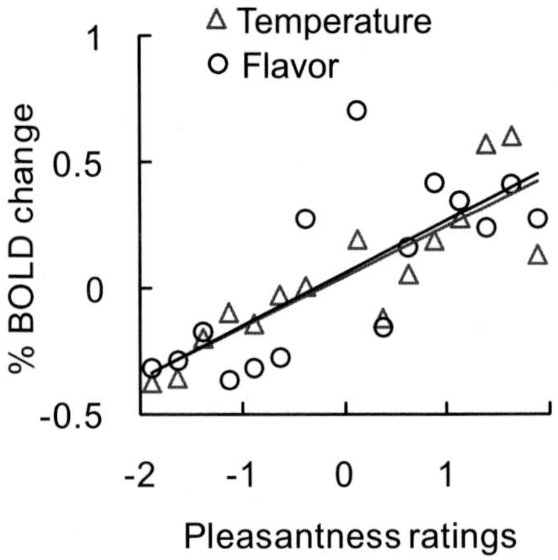

Fig. 9.6 A common scale for the subjective pleasure for different primary rewards: Neural activations in the orbitofrontal cortex correlate with the subjective pleasantness ratings for flavor stimuli in the mouth and somatosensory temperature stimuli delivered to the hand. The regression lines describing the relationship between neural activity (% BOLD signal change) and subjective pleasantness ratings were indistinguishable for both types of reward. (Reprinted from *NeuroImage*, 51 (3), Fabian Grabenhorst, Arun A. D'Souza, Benjamin A. Parris, Edmund T. Rolls, and Richard E. Passingham, A common neural scale for the subjective pleasantness of different primary rewards, pp. 1265–74, Copyright (2010), with permission from Elsevier.)

into a common currency. We have argued that different specific rewards must be represented on the same scale, but not converted into a common currency, as the specific goal selected (i.e. the particular reward selected) must be the output of the decision process so that the appropriate action for that particular goal can then be chosen (Rolls 2005b, Rolls 2008b, Rolls & Grabenhorst 2008, Grabenhorst & Rolls 2011). The key difference between the two concepts of common currency and common scaling lies in the specificity with which rewards are represented at the level of single neurons. While a common currency view implies convergence of different types of rewards onto the same neurons (a process in which information about reward identity is lost), a common scaling view implies that different rewards are represented by different neurons (thereby retaining reward identity in information processing), with the activity of the different neurons scaled to be in the same value range.

To investigate the possibility of common scaling, we performed an fMRI study in which we were able to show that even fundamentally different primary rewards, taste in the mouth and warmth on the hand, produced activations in the human OFC that were scaled to the same range as evaluated by reports made during the neuroimaging of the subjective pleasantness of the set of stimuli (Grabenhorst, D'Souza, Parris, Rolls & Passingham 2010a) (Fig. 9.6). In this case, value was measured by human subjective ratings on the same scale of pleasantness.

A different study found that the decision value for different categories of goods (food, non-food consumables, and monetary gambles) during purchasing decisions correlated with activations in the adjacent vmPFC (Chib, Rangel, Shimojo & O'Doherty 2009). Further fMRI studies with similar indications are reviewed by Levy & Glimcher (2012).

Importantly, because of the limited spatial resolution of fMRI, these studies do not answer whether it is the same or different neurons in these areas that encode the value of different rewards. However, as shown most clearly by single neuron recording studies, the representations in the OFC provide evidence about the exact nature of each reward (Chapters 4 and 5 (Rolls 2005b, Rolls & Grabenhorst 2008, Grabenhorst & Rolls 2011). Moreover, as described in Section 9.5.1, in economic decision-making, neurons in the macaque OFC encode the economic value of the specific choice options on offer, for example different juice rewards (Padoa-Schioppa & Assad 2006). For many of these 'offer value' neurons, the relationship between neuronal firing rate and value was invariant with respect to the different types of juice that were available (Padoa-Schioppa & Assad 2008), suggesting that different types of juice are evaluated on a common value scale.

With our current computational understanding of how decisions are made in attractor neural networks (Chapter 8 and Appendix B (Deco & Rolls 2006, Wang 2008, Rolls 2008b, Rolls & Deco 2010, Deco, Rolls, Albantakis & Romo 2013)), it is important that different rewards are expressed on a similar scale for decision-making networks to operate correctly but retain information about the identity of the specific reward. The computational reason is that one type of reward (e.g. food reward) should not dominate all other types of reward and always win in the competition, as this would be maladaptive. Making different rewards approximately equally rewarding makes it likely that a range of different rewards will be selected over time (and depending on factors such as motivational state), which is adaptive and essential for survival (Rolls 2005b). The exact scaling into a decision-making attractor network will be set by the number of inputs from each source, their firing rates, and the strengths of the synapses that introduce the different inputs into the decision-making network. Importantly, common scaling need not imply conversion into a new representation that is of a common currency of general reward (Rolls & Grabenhorst 2008, Grabenhorst & Rolls 2011). In the decision process itself it is important to know which reward has won, and the mechanism is likely to involve competition between different rewards represented close together in the cerebral cortex, with one of the types of reward winning the competition, rather than convergence of different rewards onto the same neuron (Rolls 2005b, Rolls 2008b, Rolls & Deco 2010). A great advantage is that whichever attractor in the decision-making network wins, has the additional property that it represents and maintains active in an attractor short-term memory the specific reward that has won, and this allows behaviour to be directed to perform actions to obtain that reward. The continuing firing of the specific reward decision attractor maintains active the goal for the action to direct the action until the action is completed. If the representation was in a common currency, the action system would have no evidence about the goal (e.g. food reward, monetary reward) that actions should be performed to acquire. Actions are typically different for different goals.

This brain organization, with specific value systems scaled on a common scale by neuronal representations in the orbitofrontal cortex but with no conversion to a common currency is an elegant aspect of brain design. One of the features of this book is that it describes this organization.

This organization may be compared with that proposed by Glimcher (2011a), where he proposes (page 407) that fairly direct inputs from sensory transduction systems to the dopamine neurons carry 'experienced subjective value', and points to evidence that the serotonergic neurons of the midbrain raphe also encode 'experienced SV' for primary rewards. This is completely different to the organization described in this book, in which representations through Tier 1 of cortical areas build invariant representations of stimuli and objects in the world that do not reflect reward value. Then in Tier 2, mainly the orbitofrontal cortex, reward value representations are built, that are specific to different types of reward (Fig. 4.2). It is these specific reward systems that I argue provide the inputs to reward-related decision-making systems (in Tier 3). Moreover, inputs to the dopamine neurons, insofar as they reflect reward prediction error, would be likely to receive their inputs from the orbitofrontal cortex, perhaps via the ventral striatum, as described in Chapter 6. However, for Glimcher (2011a), the dopamine neurons seem to carry the reward signal to other parts of the brain. That is not what the evidence described in this book shows, for, apart from other considerations, the dopamine neurons would be poor (see Section 6.2.4) at carrying any specific reward signal of the type that is needed as the input to a decision mechanism for choosing between different rewards, and that are represented in the orbitofrontal cortex.

9.5.2.4 An 'ultimate' evolutionary approach to reward value scaling

My approach instead is to produce a theory in which different specific rewards are encoded by different neurons in the orbitofrontal cortex, with the different rewards represented on the same scale of value. What is the 'ultimate' explanation for how the scale is set to be appropriate for different rewards?

My hypothesis is that the scaling of each type of primary reward is defined by the fitness provided to the genes that specify in the process of evolution each type of primary reward (Chapter 3). If genes made one type of reward value too high, that would decrease the fitness of those genes, as an animal might for example always find eating, but not reproducing, most rewarding. So there are processes in evolution to ensure that the magnitude of each type of gene-specified reward is set to a value that, in combination with other rewards, maximizes reproductive success. The concept is that genes are in competition with each other, and must make compromises with each other, to optimize their reproductive success.

Of course, due to the variation that is part of the process of evolution by natural selection, different individuals will have a different profile of values for each gene-specified reward, leading to individual differences in behaviour and leading to a basis for understanding personality (Section 2.7).

In addition to this genetic specification of rewards and of the value of each on a common scale, there are many heuristics that also contribute to the successful operation of this system, which is at the heart of emotion and emotion-related decision-making. These heuristics include sensory-specific satiety, to ensure that different types of reward are sampled, which of course is adaptive; and incentive motivation, the increase in the value of a reward after its initial presentation, which helps animals to lock efficiently onto one reward for more than too brief periods of time for efficiency (see Section 3.3). Another useful adaptation relevant to this 'ultimate' account of value scaling is relearning of the value of genetically programmed rewards, for example *taste aversion learning*, in which an innately rewarding taste can be reconfigured to be treated as aversive if the taste is paired with sickness (Scott 2011). In an analogous way, *conditioned appetite and conditioned satiety* allow gene-specified flavour rewards to be recalibrated in terms of the amount of energy with which the rewarding stimulus is associated (Booth 1985).

Of course gene-specified 'primary' rewards may provide a foundation, and many other stimuli can become rewarding by virtue of associations with these primary rewards. Examples include stimuli associated with wealth, power, and status, which themselves may be genetically specified to be rewarding because of their value (to the relevant genes) for promoting reproductive success (of those genes) (see Chapters 3 and 7).

The different gene-specified rewards can themselves be regarded as heuristics to optimize the reproductive success of the genes. For example, the steeper loss than gain subjective value function in prospect theory illustrated in Fig. 9.4 can be understood as a biological adaptation to the situation in which a single loss to an individual such as an injury or loss of reputation might spell disaster in terms of reproductive success, whereas each gain in value may be of benefit to but not crucial to reproductive success, as there will remain other opportunities for gains to be made. The gene-specified value system can be seen to be quite different to one that a rational agent might use when dealing with economic gains and losses, where rational calculations might lead to a strategy where sensitivity to losses and gains is much more equal, as this might optimize long-term economic success. This really highlights a major difference between classical economic approaches that assume a rational agent performing calculations about economic benefit, and the much more biologically realistic interpretation of much economic decision-making as frequently (unless explicit rational calculations are relied upon) involving choices influenced by the gene-specified heuristic value in evolution of different types of economic choice. In the biologically plausible case, there may be many types of value and potential costs associated with a stimulus, and these influences on value both combine and compete with each other to influence whether that stimulus, or another stimulus, is chosen. Thus in the biologically realistic economic choice situation, many factors may influence the value of a stimulus, and it may be a simplification to think of a single parameter, such as economic gain, being optimized.

This approach, with a specification of many different specific and competing rewards specified by different competing ('selfish') genes, provides a rich basis for understanding both emotion, decision-making, and the specification of value for both emotion and for decision-making including economic decision-making.

9.5.3 Absolute value and relative value are both represented in the orbitofrontal cortex

For economic decision-making it is useful to have separate representations of absolute and relative valuation signals, as described next.

9.5.3.1 A representation of absolute reward value: menu invariance

A representation of the *absolute value* of rewards is important for stable long-term preferences and consistent economic choices (Padoa-Schioppa & Assad 2008, Padoa-Schioppa 2011, Glimcher, Camerer, Fehr & Poldrack 2009). Such a representation should not be influenced by the value of other available rewards. There is evidence for absolute value coding in the orbitofrontal cortex. For example, in sensory-specific satiety experiments, the responses of neurons to the food eaten to satiety decrease to zero, while the responses of the neurons to other stimuli changes rather little, even though their relative value has changed (see e.g. Fig. 4.22 (Rolls, Sienkiewicz & Yaxley 1989b)). Indeed, as satiety progresses, the neuronal responses to the food gradually decrease, and so does whether and how vigorously the animal will select that food for ingestion, so that the neuronal firing encodes exactly how rewarding the stimulus is, not its relative value relative for example to no reward (see e.g. Fig. 4.22). In another type of experiment, it was found that the responses of some orbitofrontal cortex neurons that encoded the value of a specific stimulus did not depend on what other stimuli were available at the same time (Padoa-Schioppa & Assad 2008). This has been referred to as *menu invariance*. In the experiment, juices of three types A, B, and C could be offered as a choice between any two on a given trial, viz A:B, B:C, and C:A. The firing rate to for example juice C was not affected by whether the choice was between C and A or B.

This absolute value representation in the orbitofrontal cortex may provide a neurobiological foundation for *transitivity*, a fundamental trait of economic choice (Padoa-Schioppa & Assad 2008). Transitivity of choice refers to a situation in which if A is preferred to B (A>B), and B is preferred to C, then A should be preferred to C. Further, preference transitivity is a hallmark of rational choice behaviour and one of the most fundamental assumptions of economic theory (Kreps 1990).

9.5.3.2 A representation of relative reward value

In contrast, to select the option with the highest subjective value in a specific choice situation, it may be useful to represent the *relative value* of each option. For example, in the parietal cortex, neurons encode the relative value of the options associated with specific eye movements (Kable & Glimcher 2009). The apparent difference in value coding between the orbitofrontal cortex and parietal cortex has led to the suggestion that absolute value signals encoded in

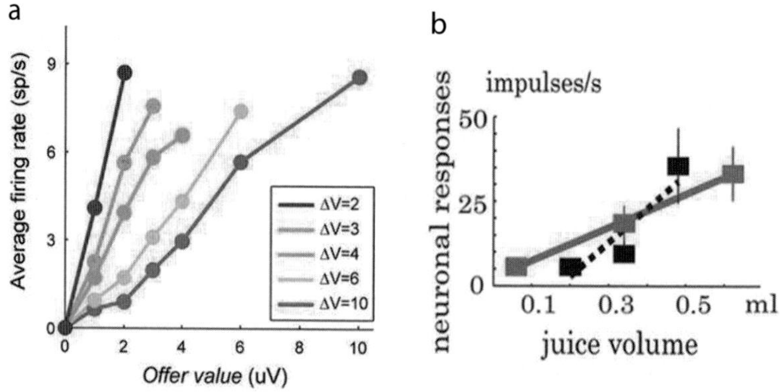

Fig. 9.7 Scaling of value: a representation of relative reward value. (a) Padoa-Schioppa (2009) found that some neurons in the orbitofrontal cortex that encode the offer value of different types of juice adapt their sensitivity to the value range of juice rewards available in a given session, while keeping their neuronal activity range constant. Each line shows the average neuronal response for a given value range. (b) Kobayashi et al. (2010) found that neurons in the orbitofrontal cortex adapt their sensitivity of value coding to the statistical distribution of reward values, in that the reward sensitivity slope adapted to the standard deviation of the probability distribution of juice volumes available in different groups of trials (solid vs dashed line). These findings indicate that the range of the value scale in the orbitofrontal cortex can be adjusted to reflect the range of rewards that are available at a given time. Reproduced with permission. (See colour plates section.) ((a) Reproduced from Padoa-Schioppa, C., Range-adapting representation of economic value in the orbitofrontal cortex. *Journal of Neuroscience* 29 (44) pp. 14004–14014, ©2009, The Society for Neuroscience. (b) Reproduced from Kobayashi, S., Pinto de Carvalho, O. and Schultz, W., Adaptation of reward sensitivity in orbitofrontal neurons, *Journal of Neuroscience* 30 (2) pp. 534–544, ©2010, The Society for Neuroscience.)

the orbitofrontal cortex are subsequently rescaled in the parietal cortex to encode relative value in order to maximize the difference between the choice options for action selection (Kable & Glimcher 2009). However, there is also evidence for relative encoding of value in the orbitofrontal cortex, in that neuronal responses to a food reward can depend on the value of the other reward that is available in a block of trials (Tremblay & Schultz 1999, Padoa-Schioppa 2009, Kobayashi, Pinto de Carvalho & Schultz 2010), as described next.

Some neurons in the orbitofrontal cortex show an adaptive *scaling of reward value*. These neurons adapt the sensitivity with which reward value is encoded to the range of values that is available at a given time (Padoa-Schioppa 2009, Kobayashi et al. 2010). The basic result is illustrated in Fig. 9.7a, which depicts the activity of 937 offer value neurons from the orbitofrontal cortex (Padoa-Schioppa 2009). Different neurons were recorded in different sessions and the range of values offered to the monkey varied from session to session. What was found was that the distribution of firing rate responses measured for the population across sessions did not depend on the range of values offered to the monkey within a session. In other words, orbitofrontal cortex neurons adapted their gain (i.e., the slope of the relation between the firing rate and the reward value) in such a way that a given range of firing rates described different ranges of values in different behavioural conditions. Kobayashi et al. (2010) showed that this adaptation to the range of rewards available at any one time (Fig. 9.7b) can take place within 15 trials. Thus relative reward value is represented by some neurons in the orbitofrontal cortex.

This scaling of value may be useful when values computed in different behavioural conditions can vary substantially. For example the same individual might choose sometimes between goods worth a few dollars and at other times between goods worth many thousands of dollars (e.g. when choosing between different houses for sale). However, any representation of value is ultimately limited to a finite range of neuronal firing rates, typically in the region of 0–50 spikes/s in the orbitofrontal cortex. The scaling of reward value by orbitofrontal cortex neurons may, for a given range of possible values, produce an optimal (i.e. maximally sensitive) representation of value at any one time that would fully exploit the range of possible firing rates. This is a similar hypothesis to that of the regression of emotional, that is reward-produced, states towards an average level that may occur in order to allow an individual, whatever the environment, to be maximally sensitive to a change of reward value, so that a local reward gradient can be climbed efficiently (Rolls (2005b) and Section 2.4).

This adaptive *scaling of reward value* is also evident in positive and negative contrast effects, which also make the system optimally sensitive to the local reward gradient, by dynamically altering the sensitivity of the reward system so that small changes can be detected (Section 2.4).

9.5.3.3 Both relative and absolute reward are represented in the orbitofrontal cortex

As a comment on the relative and absolute value representations described in Sections 9.5.3.1 and 9.5.3.2, it should be noted that the 'absolute value' representation described in Section 9.5.3.1 was found in an experiment where the different values were being offered close together in time, whereas the 'relative reward' value representation described was found after a number of trials, approximately 15 (Padoa-Schioppa 2009, Kobayashi et al. 2010), had been allowed for rescaling. The two findings are therefore not necessarily inconsistent, and might just show that the value system in the orbitofrontal cortex can rescale given a number of trials where the values available in the task are found to be within a given range.

Given that representations of both absolute value and relative value are needed for economic decision-making, Grabenhorst & Rolls (2009) tested explicitly whether both types of representation are present *simultaneously* in the human orbitofrontal cortex. In a task in which two odours were successively delivered on each trial, we found that BOLD activations to the second odour in the antero-lateral orbitofrontal cortex tracked the relative subjective pleasantness (i.e. the pleasantness of the second odour relative to the pleasantness of the first odour on that trial) (Fig. 9.8). In contrast, in the medial and mid-orbitofrontal cortex, activations tracked the absolute pleasantness of the odour, which was obtained across the whole experiment and very probably reflected the long-term pleasantness / value of the odour (Fig. 9.8). Thus, both relative and absolute subjective value signals, both of which provide important inputs to decision-making processes, are separately and simultaneously represented in the human orbitofrontal cortex, and both representations are of the type important in economic decision-making (Grabenhorst & Rolls 2009).

In sensory-specific satiety experiments, it is found that neuronal responses to the taste or flavour eaten to satiety decrease to zero. However, it is of interest that there is often a small increase in the firing rates of the neurons to the other stimuli not eaten to satiety (see example in Fig. 4.34). This may reflect a small degree of relative value encoding in these neurons. The same small effect is sometimes evident in human subjective pleasantness ratings during sensory-specific satiety experiments (e.g. Rolls, Rolls, Rowe & Sweeney (1981a)).

Thus separate representations are found of absolute, long-term, value, and of relative value as it depends on the behavioural context of the current choice.

My assessment, based on evidence from the thousands of neurons that I have recorded in the orbitofrontal cortex, is that absolute value is the more dominant representation. For example, the neuron illustrated in Fig. 4.22 (Rolls et al. 1989b) showed almost no alteration in its firing to fruit juice (blackcurrant juice, BJ) when the other item on the 'menu', glucose solution, was devalued by feeding glucose to satiety. This is thus 'menu invariance', and reflects a representation of absolute value. Any increase in firing of such a neuron to the foods

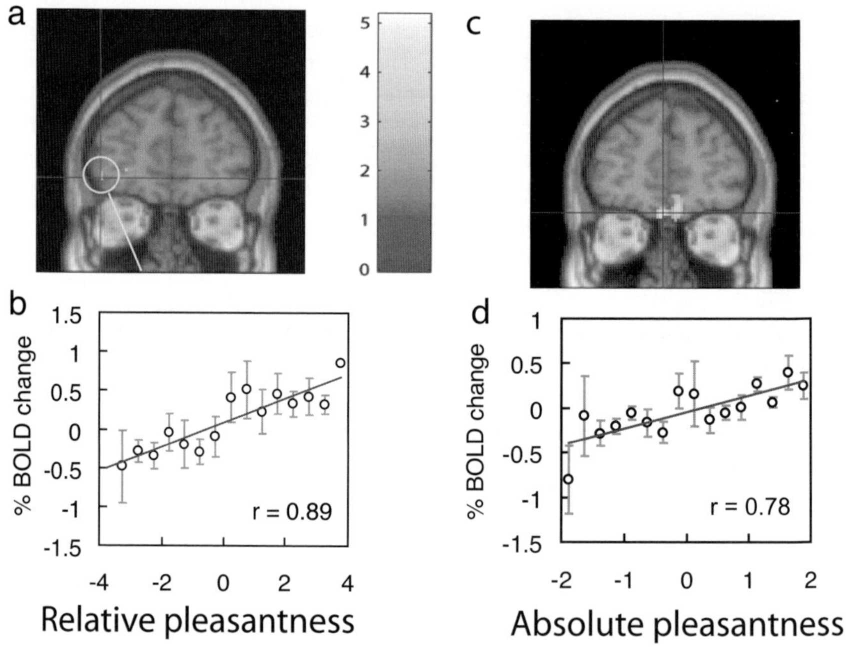

Fig. 9.8 Absolute and relative value representations in the human orbitofrontal cortex. On each trial, the subjects rated the pleasantness (value) of the second odour of a pair of 4 odours used in the experiment. a-b. Relative pleasantness: positive correlation between the BOLD signal and the difference in pleasantness of the second odor compared to the first odor. a. A significant correlation was found in the anterior lateral orbitofrontal cortex at [-44 48 -8]. b. There was a positive correlation between the BOLD signal in this brain region measured at the time of the second odor and the difference in the pleasantness of the second odor compared to the first (i.e. positive values on the abscissa are when the second odor is more pleasant) (r=0.89). c-d. Absolute pleasantness: positive correlation between the BOLD signal and the absolute value of the pleasantness ratings given to the (second) odor in (c) the medial orbitofrontal cortex [-2 50 -20]. d. The correlation between the BOLD signal in the medial orbitofrontal cortex and the pleasantness ratings (r=0.78). (See colour plates section.) (Reprinted from *NeuroImage*, 48 (1), Fabian Grabenhorst and Edmund T. Rolls, Different representations of relative and absolute subjective value in the human brain, pp. 258–68, Copyright 2009, with permission from Elsevier.)

not fed to satiety (which might reflect relative value) is typically small. Similarly, when a fat stimulus (cream) was fed to satiety and an orbitofrontal cortex neuron stopped responding to the cream, the same neuron changed its response very little to the taste of glucose, which remained rewarding (Fig. 5.17 after Rolls, Critchley, Browning, Hernadi & Lenard (1999a)). The same type of absolute value representation is found in neurons in a region that receives from the orbitofrontal cortex, the lateral hypothalamus (Figs. 5.3 and 5.10, Rolls, Murzi, Yaxley, Thorpe & Simpson (1986)).

Correspondingly, from a computational neuroscience perspective, an absolute value representation is much more important than a relative value representation, for absolute value is needed for transitivity of choice and choices between rewards available in the long term; and a choice decision-making network can make choices based on absolute value, and has no need for a partial solution to the decision problem to be performed by a relative value representation, as described in Chapter 8.

9.5.4 The representation of expected reward value

Decision under uncertainty refers to choice when the probabilities and magnitudes of the expected rewards and punishers available for each choice are not made known explicitly to the subject, but must be discovered by sampling the choices. Examples of such decision tasks include the probabilistic monetary reward and loss tasks by which the representation of monetary reward value and monetary loss value in the orbitofrontal cortex was discovered (O'Doherty, Kringelbach, Rolls, Hornak & Andrews (2001a), see Sections 4.5.5.4 and 4.5.5.4), which was also used to investigate the sensitivity of patients with orbitofrontal cortex damage to changes in the probability of the reward and loss outcomes of particular choices (Hornak, O'Doherty, Bramham, Rolls, Morris, Bullock & Polkey (2004), see Section 4.5.6), the Iowa Gambling task (Bechara et al. 1994, Bechara et al. 1996, Bechara et al. 1997, Damasio 1994, Bechara et al. 2005) (see Section 2.6.1), probabilistic tasks used to compare brain areas sensitive to reward outcome, expected value, and errors between these (Rolls, McCabe & Redoute 2008e), and all decision tasks in non-human animals in which explicit instructions about the probabilities and possible outcomes cannot be provided. Further examples include investing in the stock market, and betting on the outcome in a sport. This is also known as decision under ambiguity.

Decision under risk refers to choice when the probability distributions and magnitudes of the expected rewards and punishers available for each choice are made known explicitly by instruction to the subject. Examples include betting on the flip of a coin, or entering a lottery with a known number of tickets.

We have seen that in microeconomics, **expected value** (and possibly **expected utility**), can be thought of as the probability of obtaining the reward multiplied by the reward value (Glimcher 2003, Glimcher 2004, Kahneman & Tversky 1984). If the probability of obtaining a reward is low, then we are less likely to choose it than when the probability is high.

Some dopamine neurons show increasing responses to conditioned stimuli predicting reward with increasing probability (Fiorillo, Tobler & Schultz 2003), and decrease their firing to predicted reward omission (Tobler et al. 2003). Their responses may thus reflect expected value. However, it also appears that at least some dopamine neurons have activity that is high when reward uncertainty is high (which occurs when reward probability is 0.5) (Fiorillo et al. 2003). As noted in Section 6.2.4, this dual coding (of positive reward prediction error, and of reward uncertainty) raises problems in how receiving neurons might use this multiplexed information.

Parietal cortex neurons with activity that precedes eye movements in for example area LIP show more activity if the expected utility is high (Glimcher 2003, Glimcher 2004, Platt & Glimcher 1999, McCoy & Platt 2005a). This modulation or responsiveness by expected utility, as influenced by both probability and reward value, of neurons studied in oculomotor tasks has been found in a number of areas with oculomotor-related activity, including the cingulate cortex and the superior colliculus (McCoy & Platt 2005a, Platt & Padoa-Schioppa 2009).

For both the dopamine and the parietal cortex neurons, it seems unlikely that the actual computation of probability multiplied by reward value is performed in those areas, as reward stimuli are not known to be encoded there. It is likely, as we have seen, that expected value, reflecting reward magnitude and probability, is reflected in the activity of neurons in the orbitofrontal cortex.

9.5.5 Delay of reward, emotional choice, and rational choice

Another factor that can influence decisions for rewards is the delay before the reward is obtained. If the reward will not be available for a long time, then we discount the reward value, and this is termed *temporal discounting*. Most models assume an exponential decrease in the reward value as a function of the delay until the reward is obtained, as rational choice entails treating each moment of delay equally (Frederick, Loewenstein & O'Donoghue 2002, McClure, Laibson, Loewenstein & Cohen 2004). Impulsive preference changes may reflect a disproportionate valuation of rewards available in the immediate future (Ainslie 1992, Benabou & Pycia 2002, Rachlin 2000, Montague & Berns 2002, Metcalfe & Mischel 1999). It is possible that there are two systems that influence decisions in these circumstances.

One is a rational, logic-based, system requiring syntactic manipulation of symbols (see Chapter 10 and Fig. 10.4) that can treat each moment of delay equally, and calculate choice based on an exponential decrease of reward value with increasing delay. This rational decision system might involve language or mathematical systems in the brain, and the ability to hold several items in a working memory while the trade-offs of different long-term courses of action are compared.

A different more emotion-based system that can operate implicitly might operate according to heuristics that have become built into the system during evolution which might value disproportionately immediate rewards compared to delayed rewards. This emotion-based system might involve the orbitofrontal cortex, which as we have seen (Section 4.5) represents different types of reward and punisher (e.g. monetary gain and loss), and lesions of which in humans lead to impairments in changing behaviour when rewards are received less often for particular choices (Hornak, O'Doherty, Bramham, Rolls, Morris, Bullock & Polkey 2004, Berlin, Rolls & Kischka 2004), to impulsive choices (Berlin, Rolls & Iversen 2005), and to impairments in gambling tasks (Bechara et al. 1994, Bechara et al. 1998). This suggested dissociation of decision systems is the same concept as that encompassed by the hypothesis of dual routes to action considered in Section 10.3.1 and by Rolls (1999a) (see Fig. 10.4).

Consistent with the point being made about evolutionarily old emotion-based decision systems vs a recent rational system present in humans is that humans trade off immediate costs/benefits against cost/benefits that are delayed by as much as decades, whereas non-human primates have not been observed to engage in unpreprogrammed delay of gratification involving more than a few minutes (Rachlin 1989, Kagel, Battalio & Green 1995)[31].

Moreover, individual differences in sensitivity to rewards and punishers could lead to personality differences with respect to impulsive behaviour (see Section 2.7), and indeed patients with Borderline Personality Disorder behave similarly with respect to their impulsive behaviour to patients with orbitofrontal cortex lesions (Berlin, Rolls & Kischka 2004, Berlin & Rolls 2004, Berlin, Rolls & Iversen 2005).

Consistent with dual emotional and rational bases for decisions in humans, a 'quasi-hyperbolic' time discounting function that splices together two discounting functions – an emotional one that distinguishes sharply between present and future, and a rational one that discounts exponentially and more shallowly – provides a good fit to experimental data including retirement saving, credit-card borrowing, and procrastination (Laibson 1997, Angeletos, Laibson, Repetto, Tobacman & Weinberg 2001, O'Donoghue & Rabin 1999). This dual mechanism process can be modelled formally by

$$r(t) = \beta \gamma^t r(0) \tag{9.6}$$

where $r(t)$ is the time discounted reward value at time t, and $r(0)$ is the reward value if received immediately at time $t = 0$ (McClure, Laibson, Loewenstein & Cohen 2004). β $(0 < \beta \leq 1)$ (or in fact its inverse) represents the uniform downweighting of future compared to immediate rewards, and is the parameter that encompasses the effects of emotion on decision-making in this formulation. β is 1 at time zero, and is set to a value that scales a reward at any future time

[31] Seasonal food storage is not an exception, in that it appears to be stereotyped and instinctive, and hence is unlike the generalizable nature of human planning (McClure, Laibson, Loewenstein & Cohen 2004).

relative to the value at time 0. If $\beta = 0.8$, this indicates that relative to a reward of value r at time zero, the reward at any future time would have a value of 0.8. In this sense, it models the role of emotion in decision making as down-valuing a reward at any future time compared to immediately by a uniform discounting factor β. The γ ($\gamma \leq 1$) parameter is the discount rate in the standard exponential formula that treats a given delay equivalently independently of when it occurs (i.e. in any time interval, the value decreases by a fixed proportion of the value it has already reached), and encompasses the rational route to decision-making. In the model, it produces exponential decay of the value of a reward according to how long it is delayed. It is used in the model to capture the effects of long-term economic planning for the future.

McClure, Laibson, Loewenstein & Cohen (2004) performed an fMRI investigation in which smaller immediate rewards (today) could be chosen vs larger delayed rewards (given after delays of up to six weeks). (The monetary rewards were in the range \$5–\$40.) Brain areas that showed more activation for immediate vs delayed rewards (and reflected the β emotional parameter) included the medial orbitofrontal cortex, the medial prefrontal cortex/pregenual cingulate cortex, and the ventral striatum. Brain areas where activations reflected the decisions being made and the decision difficulty but which were not preferentially activated in relation to the immediate reward parameter β included the lateral prefrontal cortex (a brain region implicated in higher level cognitive functions including working memory and executive functions (Miller & Cohen 2001, Deco & Rolls 2003, Passingham & Wise 2012)), and a part of the parietal cortex implicated in numerical processing (Dehaene, Dehaene-Lambertz & Cohen 1998). (Activations in these prefrontal and parietal areas reflect the effects of the γ^t variable in Equation 9.6.) Thus emotional decisions that emphasize the importance of immediate rewards may preferentially activate reward-related areas ('β areas') such as the medial orbitofrontal cortex, pregenual cingulate cortex, and the ventral striatum, whereas difficult decisions requiring cost–benefit analysis about the value of long-term rewards preferentially activate a more cognitive system ('γ areas') that may be involved in rational thought and multistep calculation.

9.5.6 The representation of negative reward prediction error

To trigger behaviour, including economic behaviour, when an expected value is not obtained, it appears to be useful to have a neuronal system that detects a mismatch between expected reward value (e.g. the sight of food) and the reward outcome (e.g. the taste of food). Evidence that exactly this representation is provided by a small proportion of neurons in the orbitofrontal cortex (Thorpe, Rolls & Maddison 1983, Kringelbach & Rolls 2003) is described in Section 4.5.5.5. It is likely that this representation is computed in the orbitofrontal cortex, for the representations needed for this computation, the expected value, and the reward outcome, are both present in the orbitofrontal cortex (Thorpe, Rolls & Maddison 1983, Rolls, Sienkiewicz & Yaxley 1989b, Rolls, Critchley, Mason & Wakeman 1996a, Critchley & Rolls 1996c, O'Doherty, Kringelbach, Rolls, Hornak & Andrews 2001a, Rolls, McCabe & Redoute 2008e). It is of interest that the negative reward prediction error neurons appear to be context specific, so that it may be possible to learn that in one context a stimulus is no longer associated with reward, but to not necessarily generalize this to other contexts (Thorpe, Rolls & Maddison 1983) (see Section 4.5.5.5).

9.5.7 The representation of positive reward prediction error

As described in Chapter 6, some dopamine neurons may respond when there is a positive reward prediction error, that is when the reward outcome (e.g. the taste reward) is higher than the expected reward outcome. These neuronal responses have been interpreted as part of a reinforcement learning system to shape habit, stimulus-response, learning, in brain regions such as the basal ganglia (Schultz 1998, Schultz et al. 1997, Waelti et al. 2001, Schultz 2004, Schultz 2006, Schultz 2013). Questions that arise, and are discussed in Chapter 6, include the source of the inputs to these neurons, which is hardly addressed in descriptions of their properties and possible functions (Schultz 1998, Schultz, Dayan & Montague 1997, Waelti, Dickinson & Schultz 2001, Schultz 2004, Schultz 2006, Schultz 2013).

9.5.8 Reward prediction error, temporal difference error, and choice

The expected utility may alter from time to time, for example during a trial. For example, there is a negative reward prediction error when a reward is predicted but not obtained. Similarly, there is a positive reward prediction error when a reward is not expected but is obtained. The reward prediction error may be defined as the difference between the reward obtained and the reward predicted (see Section A.5.2). The firing of some dopamine neurons may reflect these reward prediction errors (Schultz 1998, Schultz et al. 1997, Waelti et al. 2001, Schultz 2004, Glimcher 2011b, Schultz 2013) (but see Section 6.2.4).

O'Doherty et al. (2004) related reward prediction error correlated activations of the ventral striatum to a 'critic' that learns to predict a future reward because these activations occurred even when no action was required in a Pavlovian conditioning task, and reward prediction error correlated activations of the dorsal striatum to an 'actor' because it showed stronger activation during instrumental learning than Pavlovian association[32].

The hypothesis that dopamine neuron firing provides a reward prediction error signal (Schultz 1998, Schultz et al. 1997, Waelti et al. 2001, Schultz 2004, Schultz 2013) appears to be inconsistent with the evidence that dopamine neuron firing and activations of parts of the striatum are also produced by aversive, novel, or intense/salient stimuli (Zink et al. 2003, Zink et al. 2004, Bromberg-Martin et al. 2010a) (see Section 6.2.4). Indeed, Zink et al. (2004) argue, from an fMRI investigation in which caudate and nucleus accumbens activations were greater when responses were made to obtain money than when money was given passively, that the activity in these regions is not related to reward value or predictions, but instead to *saliency*, that is to an arousing event to which attentional and/or behavioural resources are redirected (see further Section 6.1).

Reward prediction error encoding is in contrast to that of many neurons in the head of the caudate nucleus, which fire in relation to predicted rewards (Rolls, Thorpe & Maddison 1983c). They do this in that they start firing as soon as a cue such as a tone, or a light that precedes the tone, is given to indicate that a trial is starting, and continue to respond if a visual stimulus is shown indicating that a juice reward will be obtained, and stop responding if a different visual stimulus is shown indicating that aversive saline will be obtained (see Section 6.3.3.4).

The reward prediction error approach to changes in expected utility can be developed into a temporal difference learning approach, in which the temporal difference error depends on the difference in the reward value prediction at two successive time steps (see Appendix 1, Section A.5.3 and Equation A.29). This temporal difference error is useful in some temporal difference reinforcement learning algorithms for producing learning that optimizes predictions, and thus how to learn optimal actions as events unfold in time, for example during a trial (see Appendix 1, Section A.5.3). Temporal difference models have been applied to model the activity of dopamine neurons (Suri & Schultz 2001), and of fMRI activations related to the anticipation of reward (O'Doherty et al. 2003a).

Seymour et al. (2004) took the temporal difference approach in an fMRI analysis of a more complicated, second-order, pain conditioning task, with two successive visual cues to

[32]See Section A.5.3 for a description of the functions of a 'critic' and an 'actor' in reward prediction learning.

predict either low or high pain. The second cue was fully predictive of the strength of the subsequently experienced pain. The first cue only allowed a probabilistic prediction. Thus in a low proportion (18%) of the trials, the expectation evoked by the first cue was reversed by the second cue. The punisher value (pain) prediction thus alters on some trials after the second cue is delivered, generating a temporal difference prediction error. After many conditioning trials, the punisher prediction value becomes good on the 82% of trials where the first cue does predict the second cue, and during the learning the temporal difference error at the time the second cue is shown becomes low. However, on the 18% of trials where the first cue makes the incorrect prediction of the second cue, temporal difference prediction errors remain when the second cue is presented. The temporal difference error was correlated with activations in the ventral putamen (a part of the ventral striatum), the right insular cortex (probably providing a somatosensory representation of the left hand to which the pain was delivered), the right head of the caudate nucleus, and the substantia nigra (a region where dopamine neurons are located), suggesting that these areas are involved in learning expectations of pain. It should be noted that this was a conditioning procedure, and that although pain expectations were being learned, decisions and actions were not being made by the subjects.

The temporal difference approach was taken in an fMRI study of a decision task by Rolls, McCabe & Redoute (2008e) described in Section 6.3.3.1. They showed in a probabilistic decision task in which the expected utility was systematically varied that temporal difference (reward prediction) errors were reflected in activity in the ventral striatum (see Fig. 6.9 on page 296). However, the findings showed that care is needed in interpreting fMRI signals as related to temporal difference (reward prediction) errors, for the correlation with TD error was related to the fact that in the ventral striatum, the activations were related to the reward actually obtained on each trial, and changed at the point in each trial at which this information was made available to the participant (see Section 6.3.3.1). Thus the ventral striatal activation was related to decision-making in so far as its activation reflected the reward actually provided on a given trial.

9.5.9 Conclusions

We have seen how neuroeconomics is bringing new approaches to economics, and can be linked now to the mechanisms involved in decision-making and in emotion. It is shown in this book that values can be thought of as reflecting many different gene specified rewards and punishers, goals for action, that can influence reproductive success. Thus value representations can be of many of the different types of reward summarized in Table 2.1 and many more, including food and water rewards; rewards associated with courtship and reproduction including wealth, power, success and conspicuous consumption; kin and reciprocal altruism and related rewards including empathy, trust, forgiveness, and giving. In this context, many of the value representations that influence choice including economic choice can be seen as heuristics designed in the course of evolution to increase reproductive success. Clearly humans can perform rational, that is reasoned, thought, and can perform calculations about expected value, and expected utility to the individual taking into account the costs involved of each choice. However, rational evaluation and choice, which has hitherto held sway in economics, thus is clearly not the only route that humans use for economic decision-making, which instead I suggest should now be considered as reflecting the operation of many heuristics, that is the operation of many routes, many of them short-cuts, to obtaining different 'values', often in competition with each other, and all designed for reproductive success (see further Section 9.5.2.4). Of course, one of these routes is the 'rational', reasoning, route, but the point is that it is not the only route by which economic decisions are taken. The influences of some of these further factors, including empathy, trust, regret, inequity and other social factors are described further in some of the chapters in Glimcher, Camerer, Fehr & Poldrack (2009).

For reasons discussed in this chapter, classical microeconomics with its approach of a few axioms and a rational actor can no longer be considered as what really may account for the behaviour of humans and other animals. Instead, classical (micro)economics may be replaced by an understanding in neuroeconomics of how heuristics guided by evolution make different rewards and costs become differently scaled in different individuals, and further how choices are sometimes selected by a decision-making process based on in-built and probabilistic heuristics rather than by correctly computed calculations in a rational, reasoning, decision-making actor.

In addition, I make the point that value, and how and why it is computed, provide close links between emotion (which is elicited by rewarding and punishing stimuli, that is by stimuli with value), neuroeconomics (which considers how value is represented to help understand decisions), and decision-making mechanisms themselves, which utilize representations of reward and punisher value, and the costs of obtaining or avoiding the stimuli, and may be taken by a more emotional or reasoning route, as considered in the next chapter (especially in Section 10.3.1).

Because emotion, value as investigated in neuroeconomics, and decision-making are closely related, our overall understanding can be enhanced by considering all of them together, which is an important aim of this book.

10 Emotional feelings and consciousness: a theory of consciousness

10.1 Introduction

It might be possible to build a computer that would perform the functions of emotions described in Chapter 3, and yet we might not want to ascribe emotional feelings to the computer. We might even build the computer with some of the main processing stages present in the brain, and implemented using neural networks that simulate the operation of the real neural networks in the brain (see Chapter 4, Rolls & Treves (1998), Rolls (2008b), and Appendices A and B), yet we might not still wish to ascribe emotional feelings to this computer. This point often arises in discussions with undergraduates, who may say that they follow the types of point made about emotion in Chapter 4, yet believe that almost the most important aspect of emotions, the feelings, have not been accounted for, nor their neural basis described. In a sense, the functions of reward and punishment in emotional behaviour are described in Chapters 2 and 3, but what about the subjective aspects of emotion, what about the pleasure?

A similar point arises in Chapter 5, where parts of the taste, olfactory, and visual systems in which the reward value of the taste, smell, and sight of food is represented are described. Although the neuronal representation in the orbitofrontal cortex is clearly related to the reward value of food, and in humans the activations found with functional neuroimaging are directly (indeed linearly) correlated with the reported subjective pleasantness of the stimuli (see Chapters 4 and 5), is this where the pleasantness (the subjective hedonic aspect) of the taste, smell, and sight of food is represented and produced? Again, we could (in principle at least) build a computer with neural networks to simulate each of the processing stages for the taste, smell, and sight of food which are described in Chapter 5, and yet would probably not wish to ascribe feelings of pleasantness to the system we have simulated on the computer.

What is it about neural processing that makes it feel like something when some types of information processing are taking place? It is clearly not a general property of processing in neural networks, for there is much processing, for example that in the autonomic nervous system concerned with the control of our blood pressure and heart rate, of which we are not aware. Is it then that awareness arises when a certain type of information processing is being performed? If so, what type of information processing? And how do emotional feelings, and sensory events, come to feel like anything? These 'feels' are called qualia. These are great mysteries that have puzzled philosophers for centuries. They are at the heart of the problem of consciousness, for why it should feel like something at all is the great mystery.

Other aspects of consciousness may be easier to analyse, such as the fact that often when we 'pay attention' to events in the world, we can process those events in some better way. These are referred to as 'process' or 'access' aspects of consciousness, as opposed to the 'phenomenal' or 'feeling' aspects of consciousness referred to in the preceding paragraph (Block 1995b, Chalmers 1996, Allport 1988, Koch 2004, Block 1995a).

The puzzle of qualia, that is of the phenomenal aspect of consciousness, seems to be rather different from normal investigations in science, in that there is no agreement on criteria by which to assess whether we have made progress. So, although the aim of this chapter is to address the issue of consciousness, especially of qualia, what is written cannot be regarded as being as firmly scientific as the other chapters in this book. For most of the work in those, there is good evidence for most of the points made, and there would be no hesitation or difficulty in adjusting the view of how things work as new evidence is obtained. However, in the work on qualia, the criteria are much less clear. Nevertheless, the reader may well find these issues interesting, because although not easily solvable, they are very important issues to consider if we wish to really say that we understand some of the very complex and interesting issues about brain function, and ourselves.

With these caveats in mind, I consider in this chapter the general issue of consciousness and its functions, and how feelings, and pleasure, come to occur as a result of the operation of our brains. A view on consciousness, influenced by contemporary cognitive neuroscience, is outlined next. I outline a theory of what the processing is that is involved in consciousness, of its adaptive value in an evolutionary perspective, and of how processing in our visual and other sensory systems can result in subjective or phenomenal states, the 'raw feels' of conscious awareness. However, this view on consciousness that I describe is only preliminary, and theories of consciousness are likely to develop considerably. Partly for these reasons, this theory of consciousness, at least, should not be taken to have practical implications.

10.2 A Higher-Order Syntactic Thought (HOST) theory of consciousness

10.2.1 Multiple routes to action

A starting point is that many actions can be performed relatively automatically, without apparent conscious intervention. An example sometimes given is driving a car. Another example is the identification of a visual stimulus that can occur without conscious awareness as described in Section 10.8.3. Another example is much of the sensory processing and actions that involve the dorsal stream of visual processing to the parietal cortex, such as posting a letter through a box at the correct orientation even when one may not be aware of what the object is (Milner & Goodale 1995, Goodale 2004, Milner 2008). Another example is blindsight, in which humans with damage to the visual cortex may be able to point to objects even when they are not aware of seeing an object (Weiskrantz 1997, Weiskrantz 1998, Weiskrantz 2009). Similar evidence applies to emotions, some of the processing for which can occur without conscious awareness (De Gelder et al. 1999, Phelps & LeDoux 2005, LeDoux 2008). Consistent with the hypothesis of multiple routes to action, only some of which involve conscious awareness, is the evidence that split-brain patients may not be aware of actions being performed by the 'non-dominant' hemisphere (Gazzaniga & LeDoux 1978, Gazzaniga 1988, Gazzaniga 1995). Also consistent with multiple, including non-verbal, routes to action, patients with focal brain damage, for example to the prefrontal cortex, may emit actions, yet comment verbally that they should not be performing those actions (Rolls, Hornak, Wade & McGrath 1994a, Hornak, Bramham, Rolls, Morris, O'Doherty, Bullock & Polkey 2003). In both these types of patient, confabulation may occur, in that a verbal account of why the action was performed may be given, and this may not be related at all to the environmental event that actually triggered the action (Gazzaniga & LeDoux 1978, Gazzaniga 1988, Gazzaniga 1995).

Such implicit (not phenomenally conscious) actions could involve control of behaviour by brain systems that are old in evolutionary terms such as the basal ganglia. It is of interest that the basal ganglia (and cerebellum) do not have backprojection systems to most of the parts of the cerebral cortex from which they receive inputs (see Section 6.3 and Rolls & Treves (1998)). In contrast, parts of the brain such as the hippocampus and amygdala, involved

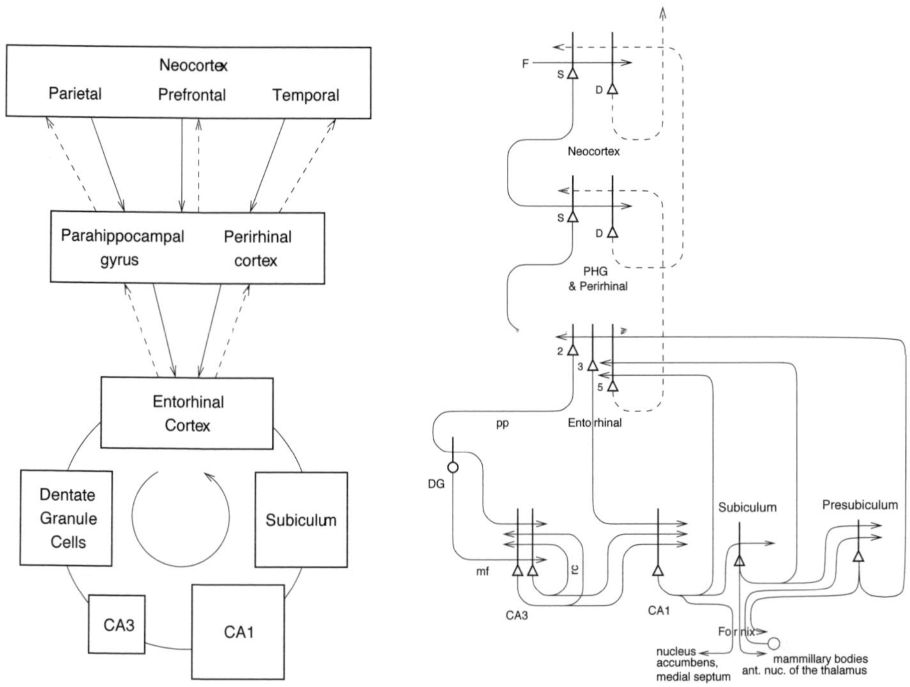

Fig. 10.1 Forward connections (solid lines) from areas of cerebral association neocortex via the parahippocampal gyrus and perirhinal cortex, and entorhinal cortex, to the hippocampus; and backprojections (dashed lines) via the hippocampal CA1 pyramidal cells, subiculum, and parahippocampal gyrus back to the neocortex. There is great convergence in the forward connections down to the single network implemented in the CA3 pyramidal cells; and great divergence again in the backprojections. Left: block diagram. Right: more detailed representation of some of the principal excitatory neurons in the pathways. Abbreviations: D, Deep pyramidal cells; DG, dentate granule cells; F, forward inputs to areas of the association cortex from preceding cortical areas in the hierarchy. mf: mossy fibres; PHG, parahippocampal gyrus and perirhinal cortex; pp, perforant path; rc, recurrent collaterals of the CA3 hippocampal pyramidal cells; S, superficial pyramidal cells; 2, pyramidal cells in layer 2 of the entorhinal cortex; 3, pyramidal cells in layer 3 of the entorhinal cortex; 5, 6, pyramidal cells in the deep layers of the entorhinal cortex. The thick lines above the cell bodies represent the dendrites.

in functions such as episodic memory and emotion respectively, about which we can make (verbal) declarations (hence declarative memory, Squire (1992)) do have major backprojection systems to the high parts of the cerebral cortex from which they receive forward projections (see Figs. 10.1, 4.72 and 4.74) (Rolls 2008b). It may be that evolutionarily newer parts of the brain, such as the language areas and parts of the prefrontal cortex, are involved in an alternative type of control of behaviour, in which actions can be planned with the use of a (language) system that allows relatively arbitrary (syntactic) manipulation of semantic entities (symbols).

The general view that there are many routes to behavioural output is supported by the evidence that there are many input systems to the basal ganglia (from almost all areas of the cerebral cortex), and that neuronal activity in each part of the striatum reflects the activity in the overlying cortical area (see Section 6.3). The evidence is consistent with the possibility that different cortical areas, each specialized for a different type of computation, have their outputs directed to the basal ganglia, which then select the strongest input, and map this into action (via outputs directed, for example, to the premotor cortex). The view is also supported

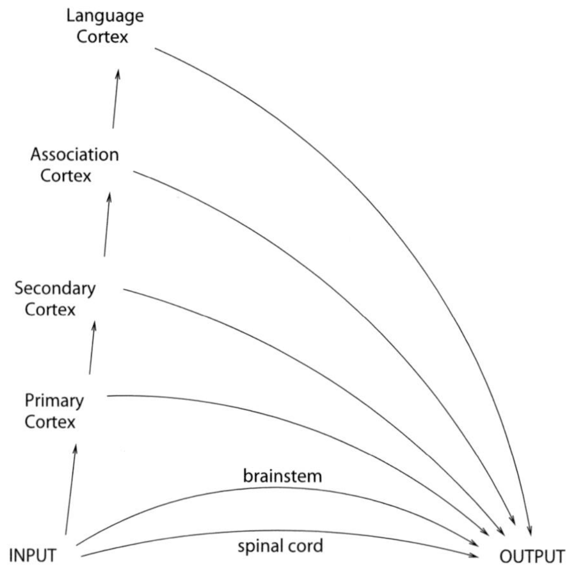

Fig. 10.2 Schematic illustration indicating many possible routes from input systems to action (output) systems. Cortical information-processing systems are organized hierarchically, and there are routes to output systems from most levels of the hierarchy.

by the evidence that the cingulate cortex is involved in actions performed for goals (Section 4.7). Within this scheme, the language areas would offer one of many routes to action, but a route particularly suited to planning actions, because of the syntactic manipulation of semantic entities which may make long-term planning possible. A schematic diagram of this suggestion is provided in Fig. 10.2.

It is accordingly possible that sometimes in normal humans when actions are initiated as a result of processing in a specialized brain region such as those involved in some types of rewarded behaviour, the language system may subsequently elaborate a coherent account of why that action was performed (i.e. confabulate). This would be consistent with a general view of brain evolution in which, as areas of the cortex evolve, they are laid on top of existing circuitry connecting inputs to outputs, and in which each level in this hierarchy of separate input–output pathways may control behaviour according to the specialized function it can perform (see schematic in Fig. 10.2). (It is of interest that mathematicians may get a hunch that something is correct, yet not be able to verbalize why. They may then resort to formal, more serial and language-like, theorems to prove the case, and these seem to require conscious processing. This is a further indication of a close association between linguistic processing, and consciousness. The linguistic processing need not, as in reading, involve an inner articulatory loop.)

We may next examine some of the advantages and behavioural functions that language, present as the most recently added layer to the above system, would confer.

One major advantage would be the ability to plan actions through many potential stages and to evaluate the consequences of those actions without having to perform the actions. For this, the ability to form propositional statements, and to perform syntactic operations on the semantic representations of states in the world, would be important.

Also important in this system would be the ability to have second-order thoughts about the type of thought that I have just described (e.g. I think that he thinks that ..., involving 'theory of mind'), as this would allow much better modelling and prediction of others' behaviour, and therefore of planning, particularly planning when it involves others[33]. This capability for higher-order thoughts would also enable reflection on past events, which would also be useful in planning. In contrast, non-linguistic behaviour would be driven by learned reinforcement associations, learned rules etc., but not by flexible planning for many steps ahead involving a model of the world including others' behaviour. (For an earlier view that is close to this part of the argument see Humphrey (1980).) [The examples of behaviour from non-humans that may reflect planning may reflect much more limited and inflexible planning. For example, the dance of the honey-bee to signal to other bees the location of food may be said to reflect planning, but the symbol manipulation is not arbitrary. There are likely to be interesting examples of non-human primate behaviour that reflect the evolution of an arbitrary symbol manipulation system that could be useful for flexible planning, cf. Cheney & Seyfarth (1990), Byrne & Whiten (1988), and Whiten & Byrne (1997).]

It is important to state that the language ability referred to here is not necessarily human verbal language (though this would be an example). What it is suggested is important to planning is the syntactic manipulation of symbols, and it is this syntactic manipulation of symbols that is the sense in which language is defined and used here. The type of syntactic processing need not be at the natural language level (which implies a universal grammar), but could be at the level of mentalese (Rolls 2005b, Rolls 2004d, Fodor 1994).

I understand **reasoning, and rationality**, to involve syntactic manipulations of symbols in the way just described. Reasoning thus typically may involve multiple steps of 'if .. then' conditional statements, all executed as a one-off or one-time process (see below), and is very different from associatively learned conditional rules typically learned over many trials, such as 'if yellow, a left choice is associated with reward'.

10.2.2 A computational hypothesis of consciousness

It is next suggested that this arbitrary symbol-manipulation using important aspects of language processing and used for planning but not in initiating all types of behaviour is close to what consciousness is about. In particular, consciousness may *be* the state that arises in a system that can think about (or reflect on) its own (or other peoples') thoughts, that is in a system capable of second- or higher-order thoughts (Rosenthal 1986, Rosenthal 1990, Rosenthal 1993, Dennett 1991, Rolls 1995a, Carruthers 1996, Rolls 1997a, Rolls 1997b, Rolls 1999a, Gennaro 2004, Rolls 2004d, Rosenthal 2004, Rolls 2005b, Rosenthal 2005, Rolls 2007b, Rolls 2008c, Rolls 2007g, Rolls 2011a, Lau & Rosenthal 2011, Rosenthal 2012, Rolls 2013b). On this account, a mental state is non-introspectively (i.e. non-reflectively) conscious if one has a roughly simultaneous thought that one is in that mental state. Following from this, introspective consciousness (or reflexive consciousness, or self consciousness) is the attentive, deliberately focused consciousness of one's mental states. It is noted that not all of the higher-order thoughts need themselves be conscious (many mental states are not). However, according to the analysis, having a higher-order thought about a lower-order thought is necessary for the lower-order thought to be conscious.

A slightly weaker position than Rosenthal's (and mine) on this is that a conscious state corresponds to a first-order thought that has the capacity to cause a second-order thought

[33] Second-order thoughts are thoughts about thoughts. Higher-order thoughts refer to second-order, third-order, etc., thoughts about thoughts... (A thought may be defined briefly as an intentional mental state, that is a mental state that is about something. Thoughts include beliefs, and are usually described as being propositional (Rosenthal 2005). An example of a thought is "It is raining". A more detailed definition is as follows. A thought may be defined as an occurrent mental state (or event) that is intentional – that is a mental state that is about something – and also propositional, so that it is evaluable as true or false. Thoughts include occurrent beliefs or judgements. An example of a thought would be an occurrent belief that the earth moves around the sun / that Maurice's boat goes faster with two sails / that it never rains in southern California.)

or judgement about it (Carruthers 1996). Another position that is close in some respects to that of Carruthers and the present position is that of Chalmers (1996), that awareness is something that has direct availability for behavioural control, which amounts effectively for him in humans to saying that consciousness is what we can report (verbally) about[34]. This analysis is consistent with the points made above that the brain systems that are required for consciousness and language are similar. In particular, a system that can have second- or higher-order thoughts about its own operation, including its planning and linguistic operation, must itself be a language processor, in that it must be able to bind correctly to the symbols and syntax in the first-order system. According to this explanation, the feeling of anything is the state that is present when linguistic processing that involves second- or higher-order thoughts is being performed.

It might be objected that this hypothesis captures some of the process aspects of consciousness, that is, what is useful in an information processing system, but does not capture the phenomenal aspect of consciousness. (Chalmers, following points made in his 1996 book, might make this point.) I agree that there is an element of 'mystery' that is invoked at this step of the argument, when I say that it feels like something for a machine with higher-order thoughts to be thinking about its own first- or lower-order thoughts. But the return point is the following: if a human with second-order thoughts is thinking about its own first-order thoughts, surely it is very difficult for us to conceive that this would not feel like something? (Perhaps the higher-order thoughts in thinking about the first-order thoughts would need to have in doing this some sense of continuity or self, so that the first-order thoughts would be related to the same system that had thought of something else a few minutes ago. But even this continuity aspect may not be a requirement for consciousness. Humans with anterograde amnesia cannot remember what they felt a few minutes ago, yet their current state does feel like something.)

As a point of clarification, I note that according to this theory, a language processing system (let alone a working memory (LeDoux 2008)) is not sufficient for consciousness. What defines a conscious system according to this analysis is the ability to have higher-order thoughts, and a first order language processor (that might be perfectly competent at language) would not be conscious, in that it could not think about its own or others' thoughts. One can perfectly well conceive of a system that obeyed the rules of language (which is the aim of some connectionist modelling), and implemented a first-order linguistic system, that would not be conscious. [Possible examples of language processing that might be performed non-consciously include computer programs implementing aspects of language, or ritualized human conversations, e.g., about the weather. These might require syntax and correctly grounded semantics, and

[34]Chalmers (1996) is not entirely consistent about this. Later in the same book he advocates a view that experiences are associated with information-processing systems, e.g. experiences are associated with a thermostat (p. 297). He does not believe that the brain has experiences, but that he has experiences. This leads him to suggest that experiences are associated with information processing systems such as the thermostat in the same way as they are associated with him. "If there is experience associated with thermostats, there is probably experience everywhere: wherever there is a causal interaction, there is information, and wherever there is information, there is experience." (p. 297). He goes on to exclude rocks from having experiences, in that "a rock, unlike a thermostat, is not picked out as an information-processing system". My response to this is that of course there is mutual information between the physical world (e.g. the world of tastants, the chemical stimuli that can produce tastes) and the conscious world (e.g. of taste) – if there were not, the information represented in the conscious processing system would not be useful for any thoughts or operations on or about the world. And according to the view I present here, the conscious processing system is good at some specialized types of processing (e.g. planning ahead using syntactic processing with semantics grounded in the real world, and reflecting on and correcting such plans), for which it would need reliable information about the world. Clearly Chalmers' view on consciousness is very much weaker than mine, in that he allows thermostats to be associated with consciousness, and in contrast to the theory presented here, does not suggest any special criteria for the types of information processing to be performed in order for the system to be aware of its thoughts, and of what it is doing.

yet be performed non-consciously. A more complex example, illustrating that syntax could be used, might be "If A does X, then B will probably do Y, and then C would be able to do Z." A first order language system could process this statement. Moreover, the first order language system could apply the rule usefully in the world, provided that the symbols in the language system (A, B, X, Y etc.) are grounded (have meaning) in the world.]

A second clarification is that the plan would have to be a unique string of steps, in much the same way as a sentence can be a unique and one-off (or one-time) string of words. The point here is that it is helpful to be able to think about particular one-off plans, and to correct them; and that this type of operation is very different from the slow learning of fixed rules by trial and error, or the application of fixed rules by a supervisory part of a computer program.

10.2.3 Adaptive value of processing in the system that is related to consciousness

It is suggested that part of the evolutionary *adaptive significance* of this type of higher-order thought is that it enables correction of errors made in first-order linguistic or in non-linguistic processing. Indeed, the ability to reflect on previous events is extremely important for learning from them, including setting up new long-term semantic structures. It was shown above that the hippocampus may be a system for such 'declarative' recall of recent memories (see also Squire, Stark & Clark (2004)). Its close relation to 'conscious' processing in humans (Squire has classified it as a declarative memory system) may be simply that it enables the recall of recent memories, which can then be reflected upon in conscious, higher-order, processing. Another part of the adaptive value of a higher-order thought system may be that by thinking about its own thoughts in a given situation, it may be able to understand better the thoughts of another individual in a similar situation, and therefore predict that individual's behaviour better (Humphrey 1980, Humphrey 1986) (cf. Barlow (1997)).

As a point of clarification, I note that according to this theory, a language processing system is not sufficient for consciousness. What defines a conscious system according to this analysis is the ability to have higher-order thoughts, and a first-order language processor (which might be perfectly competent at language) would not be conscious, in that it could not think about its own or others' thoughts. One can perfectly well conceive of a system that obeyed the rules of language (which is the aim of much connectionist modelling), and implemented a first-order linguistic system, that would not be conscious. [Possible examples of language processing that might be performed non-consciously include computer programs implementing aspects of language, or ritualized human conversations, e.g. about the weather. These might require syntax and correctly grounded semantics, and yet be performed non-consciously. A more complex example, illustrating that syntax could be used, might be 'If A does X, then B will probably do Y, and then C would be able to do Z.' A first-order language system could process this statement. Moreover, the first-order language system could apply the rule usefully in the world, provided that the symbols in the language system (A, B, X, Y etc.) are grounded (have meaning) in the world.]

In line with the argument on the adaptive value of higher-order thoughts and thus consciousness given above, that they are useful for correcting lower-order thoughts, I now suggest that correction using higher-order thoughts of lower-order thoughts would have adaptive value primarily if the lower-order thoughts are sufficiently complex to benefit from correction in this way. The nature of the complexity is specific – that it should involve syntactic manipulation of symbols, probably with several steps in the chain, and that the chain of steps should be a one-off (or in American usage, 'one-time', meaning used once) set of steps, as in a sentence or in a particular plan used just once, rather than a set of well learned rules. The first or lower-order thoughts might involve a linked chain of 'if ... then' statements that would be involved in planning, an example of which has been given above, and this type of cognitive processing is thought to be a primary basis for human skilled performance (Anderson 1996). It is partly because complex lower-order thoughts such as these that involve syntax and language would benefit from correction by higher-order thoughts that I suggest that there is a close link between this reflective consciousness and language.

The *computational hypothesis* is that by thinking about lower-order thoughts, the higher-order thoughts can discover what may be weak links in the chain of reasoning at the lower-order level, and having detected the weak link, might alter the plan, to see if this gives better success. In our example above, if it transpired that C could not do Z, how might the plan have failed? Instead of having to go through endless random changes to the plan to see if by trial and error some combination does happen to produce results, what I am suggesting is that by thinking about the previous plan, one might, for example, using knowledge of the situation and the probabilities that operate in it, guess that the step where the plan failed was that B did not in fact do Y. So by thinking about the plan (the first- or lower-order thought), one might correct the original plan in such a way that the weak link in that chain, that 'B will probably do Y', is circumvented.

To draw a parallel with neural networks: there is a **'credit assignment'** problem in such multistep syntactic plans, in that if the whole plan fails, how does the system assign credit or blame to particular steps of the plan? [In multilayer neural networks, the credit assignment problem is that if errors are being specified at the output layer, the problem arises about how to propagate back the error to earlier, hidden, layers of the network to assign credit or blame to individual synaptic connection; see Rumelhart, Hinton & Williams (1986) and Rolls (2008b).] **My suggestion is that this solution to the credit assignment problem for a one-off syntactic plan is the function of higher-order thoughts, and is why systems with higher-order thoughts evolved. The suggestion I then make is that if a system were doing this type of processing (thinking about its own thoughts), it would then be very plausible that it should feel like something to be doing this.** I even suggest to the reader that it is not plausible to suggest that it would not feel like anything to a system if it were doing this.

I emphasize that the plan would have to be a unique string of steps, in much the same way as a sentence can be a unique and one-off string of words. The point here is that it is helpful to be able to think about particular one-off plans, and to correct them; and that this type of operation is very different from the slow learning of fixed rules by trial and error, or the application of fixed rules by a supervisory part of a computer program.

10.2.4 Symbol grounding

A further point in the argument should be emphasized for clarity. The system that is having syntactic thoughts about its own syntactic thoughts (higher-order syntactic thoughts or HOSTs) would have to have its symbols grounded in the real world for it to feel like something to be having higher-order thoughts. The intention of this clarification is to exclude systems such as a computer running a program when there is in addition some sort of control or even overseeing program checking the operation of the first program. We would want to say that in such a situation it would feel like something to be running the higher level control program only if the first-order program was symbolically performing operations on the world and receiving input about the results of those operations, and if the higher-order system understood what the first order system was trying to do in the world.

The symbols (or symbolic representations) are symbols in the sense that they can take part in syntactic processing. The symbolic representations are grounded in the world in that they refer to events in the world. The symbolic representations must have a great deal of information about what is referred to in the world, including the quality and intensity of sensory events, emotional states, etc. The need for this is that the reasoning in the symbolic system must be about stimuli, events, and states, and remembered stimuli, events and states, and for the reasoning to be correct, all the information that can affect the reasoning must be represented in the symbolic system, including for example just how light or strong the touch was, etc. Indeed, it is pointed out (Rolls 2005b) that it is no accident that the shape of the multidimensional phenomenal (sensory etc.) space does map so clearly onto the space defined by neuronal activity in sensory systems, for if this were not the case, reasoning about the state of affairs in the world would not map onto the world, and would not be useful. Good examples of this close correspondence are found in the taste system, in which subjective space maps simply onto the multidimensional space represented by neuronal firing in primate cortical taste areas. In particular, if a two-dimensional space reflecting the distances between the representations of different tastes provided by macaque neurons in the cortical taste areas is constructed, then the distances between the subjective ratings by humans of different tastes is very similar (see Section 5.4.6.3, Figs. 5.19 and 5.20, Kadohisa, Rolls & Verhagen (2005b) and Smith-Swintosky, Plata-Salaman & Scott (1991)). Similarly, the changes in human subjective ratings of the pleasantness of the taste, smell and sight of food parallel very closely the responses of neurons in the macaque orbitofrontal cortex (Chapters 4 and 5).

The representations in the first-order linguistic processor that the HOSTs process include beliefs (for example "Food is available", or at least representations of this), and the HOST system would then have available to it the concept of a thought (so that it could represent "I believe [or there is a belief] that food is available"). However, as argued by Rolls (1999a, 2005b), representations of sensory processes and emotional states must be processed by the first-order linguistic system, and HOSTs may be about these representations of sensory processes and emotional states capable of taking part in the syntactic operations of the first-order linguistic processor. Such sensory and emotional information may reach the first-order linguistic system from many parts of the brain, including those such as the orbitofrontal cortex and amygdala implicated in emotional states. When the sensory information is about the identity of the taste, the inputs to the first-order linguistic system must come from the primary taste cortex, in that the identity and intensity of taste, independently of its pleasantness (in that the representation is independent of hunger) must come from the primary taste cortex (Fig. 4.45). In contrast, when the information that reaches the first-order linguistic system is about the pleasantness of taste, it must come from the secondary taste (orbitofrontal) cortex, in that there the representation of taste depends on hunger and is linearly related to pleasantness (Rolls & Grabenhorst 2008) (Fig. 4.44).

The issue of symbol grounding is considered further in Section 10.6. A related view has been developed by the philosopher Ruth Millikan (1984).

10.2.5 Qualia

This analysis does not yet give an account for sensory qualia ('raw sensory feels', for example why 'red' feels red), for emotional qualia (e.g. why a rewarding touch produces an emotional feeling of pleasure), or for motivational qualia (e.g. why food deprivation makes us feel hungry). The view I suggest on such **qualia** is as follows. Information processing in and from our sensory systems (e.g. the sight of the colour red) may be relevant to planning actions using language and the conscious processing thereby implied. Given that these inputs must be represented in the system that plans, we may ask whether it is more likely that we would be conscious of them or that we would not. I suggest that it would be a very special-purpose system that would allow such sensory inputs, and emotional and motivational states, to be part of (linguistically based) planning, and yet remain unconscious (given that the processing being performed by this system is inherently conscious, as suggested above). It seems to be much more parsimonious to hold that we would be conscious of such sensory, emotional, and motivational qualia because they would be being used (or are available to be used) in this type of (linguistically based) higher-order thought processing system, and this is what I propose.

The explanation of emotional and motivational subjective feelings or qualia that this discussion has led towards is thus that they should be felt as conscious because they enter into a specialized linguistic symbol-manipulation system, which is part of a higher-order thought system that is capable of reflecting on and correcting its lower-order thoughts involved for example in the flexible planning of actions. It would require a very special machine to enable this higher-order linguistically-based thought processing, which is conscious by its nature, to occur without the sensory, emotional and motivational states (which must be taken into account by the higher-order thought system) becoming felt qualia. The sensory, emotional, and motivational qualia are thus accounted for by the evolution of a linguistic (i.e. syntactic) system that can reflect on and correct its own lower-order processes, and thus has adaptive value.

This account implies that it may be especially animals with a higher-order belief and thought system and with linguistic (i.e. syntactic, not necessarily verbal) symbol manipulation that have qualia. It may be that much non-human animal behaviour, provided that it does not require flexible linguistic planning and correction by reflection, could take place according to reinforcement-guidance (using, e.g., stimulus–reinforcer association learning in the amygdala and orbitofrontal cortex as described in Chapter 4, and rule-following [implemented, e.g., using habit or stimulus–response learning in the basal ganglia, see Section 6.3]). Such behaviours might appear very similar to human behaviour performed in similar circumstances, but need not imply qualia. It would be primarily by virtue of a system for reflecting on flexible, linguistic, planning behaviour that humans (and animals close to humans, with demonstrable syntactic manipulation of symbols, and the ability to think about these linguistic processes) would be different from other animals, and would have evolved qualia.

It is of interest to comment on how the evolution of a system for flexible planning might affect emotions. Consider grief which may occur when a reward is terminated and no immediate action is possible. It may be adaptive by leading to a cessation of the formerly rewarded behaviour and thus facilitating the possible identification of other positive reinforcers in the environment. In humans, grief may be particularly potent because it becomes represented in a system which can plan ahead, and understand the enduring implications of the loss. Thus *depression* in humans may be much more severe than in animals without a reasoning system, because the explicit, reasoning, system can see how bad the non-reward or punisher really is, can foresee the consequences for the future using reasoning, and using re-entrant processing between the explicit and implicit systems may produce positive feedback as a result of rumination. In this situation, thinking about or verbally discussing emotional states may help, because this can lead towards the identification of new or alternative reinforcers, and of the realization that for example negative consequences may not be as bad as feared.

10.2.6 Pathways

In order for processing in a part of our brain to be able to reach consciousness, appropriate pathways must be present. Certain constraints arise here. For example, in the sensory pathways, the nature of the representation may change as it passes through a hierarchy of processing levels, and in order to be conscious of the information in the form in which it is represented in early processing stages, the early processing stages must have access to the part of the brain necessary for consciousness. An example is provided by processing in the taste system. In the primate primary taste cortex, neurons respond to taste independently of hunger, yet in the secondary taste cortex, food-related taste neurons (e.g. responding to sweet taste) only respond to food if hunger is present, and gradually stop responding to that taste during feeding to satiety (see Chapter 5) (Rolls 1989a, Rolls 1997c, Rolls & Scott 2003, Rolls 2012c). Now the quality of the tastant (sweet, salt, etc.) and its intensity are not affected by hunger, but the pleasantness of its taste is reduced to zero (neutral) (or even becomes unpleasant) after we have eaten it to satiety. The implication of this is that for quality and intensity information about taste, we must be conscious of what is represented in the primary taste cortex (or perhaps in another area connected to it that bypasses the secondary taste cortex), and not of what is represented in the secondary taste cortex (Fig. 4.45). In contrast, for the pleasantness of a taste, consciousness of this could not reflect what is represented in the primary taste cortex, but instead what is represented in the secondary taste cortex (or in an area beyond it) (Fig. 4.44).

The same argument applies for reward in general, and therefore for emotion, which in primates is not represented early on in processing in the sensory pathways (nor in or before the inferior temporal cortex for vision), but in the areas to which these object analysis systems project, such as the orbitofrontal cortex, where the reward value of visual stimuli is reflected in the responses of neurons to visual stimuli (see Chapter 4).

It is also of interest that reward signals (e.g., the taste of food when we are hungry) are associated with subjective feelings of pleasure (Chapters 4 and 5). I suggest that this correspondence arises because pleasure is the subjective state that represents in the conscious system a signal that is positively reinforcing (rewarding), and that inconsistent behaviour would result if the representations did not correspond to a signal for positive reinforcement in both the conscious and the non-conscious processing systems.

Do these arguments mean that the conscious sensation of, e.g., taste quality (i.e. identity and intensity) is represented or occurs in the primary taste cortex, and of the pleasantness of taste in the secondary taste cortex, and that activity in these areas is sufficient for conscious sensations (qualia) to occur? I do not suggest this at all. Instead the arguments I have put forward above suggest that we are only conscious of representations when we have high-order thoughts about them. The implication then is that pathways must connect from each of the brain areas in which information is represented about which we can be conscious, to the system that has the higher-order thoughts, which as I have argued above, requires language (understood as syntactic manipulation of symbols). Thus, in the example given, there must be connections to the language areas from the primary taste cortex, which need not be direct, but which must bypass the secondary taste cortex, in which the information is represented differently (Rolls 2005b, Rolls 1989a). There must also be pathways from the secondary taste cortex, not necessarily direct, to the language areas so that we can have higher-order thoughts about the pleasantness of the representation in the secondary taste cortex. There would also need to be pathways from the hippocampus, implicated in the recall of declarative memories, back to the language areas of the cerebral cortex (at least via the cortical areas that receive backprojections from the hippocampus, see Fig. 10.1, which would in turn need connections to the language areas). A schematic diagram incorporating this anatomical prediction about human cortical neural connectivity in relation to consciousness is shown in Fig. 10.3.

10.2.7 Consciousness and causality

One question that has been discussed is whether there is a causal role for consciousness (e.g. Armstrong & Malcolm (1984)). The position to which the above arguments lead is that indeed conscious processing does have a causal role in the elicitation of behaviour, but only under the set of circumstances when higher-order thoughts play a role in correcting or influencing lower-order thoughts. The sense in which the consciousness is causal is then, it is suggested, that the higher-order thought is causally involved in correcting the lower-order thought; and

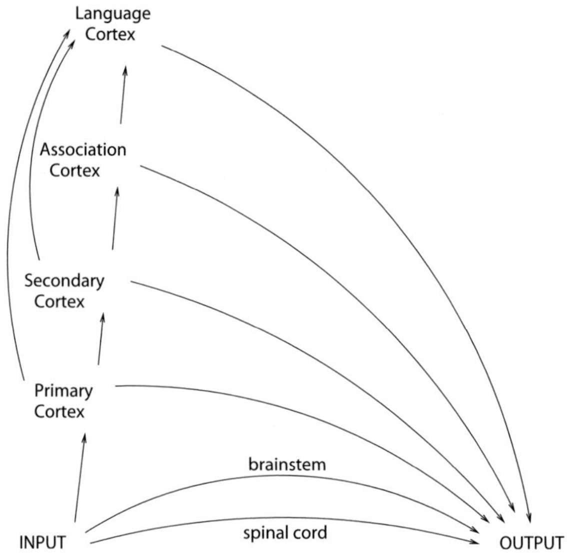

Fig. 10.3 Schematic illustration indicating that early cortical stages in information processing may need access to language areas that bypass subsequent levels in the hierarchy, so that consciousness of what is represented in early cortical stages, and which may not be represented in later cortical stages, can occur. Higher-order linguistic thoughts (HOLTs) could be implemented in the language cortex itself, and would not need a separate cortical area. Backprojections, a notable feature of cortical connectivity, with many probable functions including recall (Rolls and Treves 1998, Rolls 2008d, Treves and Rolls 1994), probably reciprocate all the connections shown.

that it is a property of the higher-order thought system that it feels like something when it is operating. As we have seen, some behavioural responses can be elicited when there is not this type of reflective control of lower-order processing, nor indeed any contribution of language. There are many brain-processing routes to output regions, and only one of these involves conscious, verbally represented processing that can later be recalled (see Fig. 10.2 and Section 10.3.1).

I suggest that these concepts may help us to understand what is happening in experiments of the type described by Libet and many others (Libet 2002) in which consciousness appears to follow with a measurable latency the time when a decision was taken. This is what I predict, if the decision is being made by an implicit perhaps reward/emotion or habit-related process, for then the conscious processor confabulates an account of or commentary on the decision, so that inevitably the conscious account follows the decision. On the other hand, I predict that if the rational (multistep, reasoning) route is involved in taking the decision, as it might be during planning, or a multistep task such as mental arithmetic, then the conscious report of when the decision was taken, and behavioural or other objective evidence on when the decision was taken, would correspond much more. Under those circumstances, the brain processing taking the decision would be closely related to consciousness, and it would not be a case of just confabulating or reporting on a decision taken by an implicit processor. It would be of interest to test this hypothesis in a version of Libet's task (Libet 2002) in which reasoning was required. The concept that the rational, conscious, processor is only in some tasks involved in taking decisions is extended further in the section on dual routes to action below.

10.2.8 Consciousness, a computational system for higher-order syntactic manipulation of symbols, and a commentary or reporting functionality

I now consider some clarifications of the present proposal, and how it deals with some issues that arise when considering theories of the phenomenal aspects of consciousness.

First, the present proposal has as its foundation the type of computation that is being performed, and suggests that it is a property of a higher-order syntactic thought (HOST) system used for correcting multistep plans with its representations grounded in the world that it would feel like something for a system to be doing this type of processing. To do this type of processing, the system would have to be able to recall previous multistep plans, and would require syntax to keep the symbols in each step of the plan separate. In a sense, the system would have to be able to recall and take into consideration its earlier multistep plans, and in this sense *report* to itself, on those earlier plans. Some approaches to consciousness take the ability to report on or make a *commentary* on events as being an important marker for consciousness (Weiskrantz 1997), and the computational approach I propose suggests why there should be a close relation between consciousness and the ability to report or provide a commentary, for the ability to report is involved in using higher-order syntactic thoughts to correct a multistep plan.

Second, the implication of the present approach is that the type of linguistic processing or reporting need not be verbal, using natural language, for what is required to correct the plan is the ability to manipulate symbols syntactically, and this could be implemented in a much simpler type of mentalese or syntactic system (Fodor 1994, Jackendoff 2002, Rolls 2004d) than verbal language or natural language which implies a universal grammar.

Third, this approach to consciousness suggests that the information must be being processed in a system capable of implementing HOSTs for the information to be conscious, and in this sense is more specific than global workspace hypotheses (Baars 1988, Dehaene & Naccache 2001, Dehaene, Changeux, Naccache, Sackur & Sergent 2006). Indeed, the present approach suggests that a workspace could be sufficiently global to enable even the complex processing involved in driving a car to be performed, and yet the processing might be performed unconsciously, unless HOST (supervisory, monitory, correcting) processing was involved.

Fourth, the present approach suggests that it just is a property of HOST computational processing with the representations grounded in the world that it feels like something. There is to some extent an element of mystery about why it feels like something, why it is phenomenal, but the explanatory gap does not seem so large when one holds that the system is recalling, reporting on, reflecting on, and reorganizing information about itself in the world in order to prepare new or revised plans. In terms of the physicalist debate (see for a review Davies (2008)), an important aspect of my proposal is that it is a necessary property of this type of (HOST) computational processing that it feels like something (the philosophical description is that this is an absolute metaphysical necessity), and given this view, then it is up to one to decide whether this view is consistent with one's particular view of physicalism or not (Rolls 2008c). Similarly, the possibility of a zombie is inconsistent with the present hypothesis, which proposes that it is by virtue of performing processing in a specialized system that can perform higher-order syntactic processing with the representations grounded in the world that phenomenal consciousness is necessarily present.

An implication of these points is that my theory of consciousness is a computational theory. It argues that it is a property of a certain type of computational processing that it feels like something. In this sense, although the theory spans many levels from the neuronal to the computational, it is unlikely that any particular neuronal phenomena such as oscillations are necessary for consciousness, unless such computational processes happen to rely on some particular neuronal properties not involved in other neural computations but necessary for higher-order syntactic computations. It is these computations and the system that implements them that this computational theory argues are necessary for consciousness.

These are my initial thoughts on why we have consciousness, and are conscious of sensory, emotional and motivational qualia, as well as qualia associated with first-order linguistic thoughts. However, as stated above, one does not feel that there are straightforward criteria in this philosophical field of enquiry for knowing whether the suggested theory is correct; so it is likely that theories of consciousness will continue to undergo rapid development; and current theories should not be taken to have practical implications.

10.3 Selection between conscious vs unconscious decision-making, and free will

10.3.1 Dual major routes to action: implicit and explicit

According to the present formulation, there are two major types of route to action performed in relation to reward or punishment in humans. Examples of such actions include those associated with emotional and motivational behaviour.

The first ('implicit') route is via the brain systems that have been present in non-human primates such as monkeys, and to some extent in other mammals, for millions of years. These systems include the amygdala and, particularly well-developed in primates, the orbitofrontal cortex. These systems control behaviour in relation to previous associations of stimuli with reinforcement. The computation which controls the action thus involves assessment of the reinforcement-related value of a stimulus. This assessment may be based on a number of different factors:

One is the previous reinforcement history, which involves stimulus–reinforcer association learning using the amygdala, and its rapid updating especially in primates using the orbitofrontal cortex. This stimulus–reinforcer association learning may involve quite specific information about a stimulus, for example of the energy associated with each type of food, by the process of conditioned appetite and satiety (Booth 1985).

A second is the current motivational state, for example whether hunger is present, whether other needs are satisfied, etc.

A third factor that affects the computed reward value of the stimulus is whether that reward has been received recently. If it has been received recently but in small quantity, this may increase the reward value of the stimulus. This is known as incentive motivation or the 'salted nut' phenomenon. The adaptive value of such a process is that this positive feedback of reward value in the early stages of working for a particular reward tends to lock the organism on to behaviour being performed for that reward. This means that animals that are for example almost equally hungry and thirsty will show hysteresis in their choice of action, rather than continually switching from eating to drinking and back with each mouthful of water or food. This introduction of hysteresis into the reward evaluation system makes action selection a much more efficient process in a natural environment, for constantly switching between different types of behaviour would be very costly if all the different rewards were not available in the same place at the same time. (For example, walking half a mile between a site where water was available and a site where food was available after every mouthful would be very inefficient.) The amygdala is one structure that may be involved in this increase in the reward value of stimuli early on in a series of presentations, in that lesions of the amygdala (in rats) abolish the expression of this reward-incrementing process which is

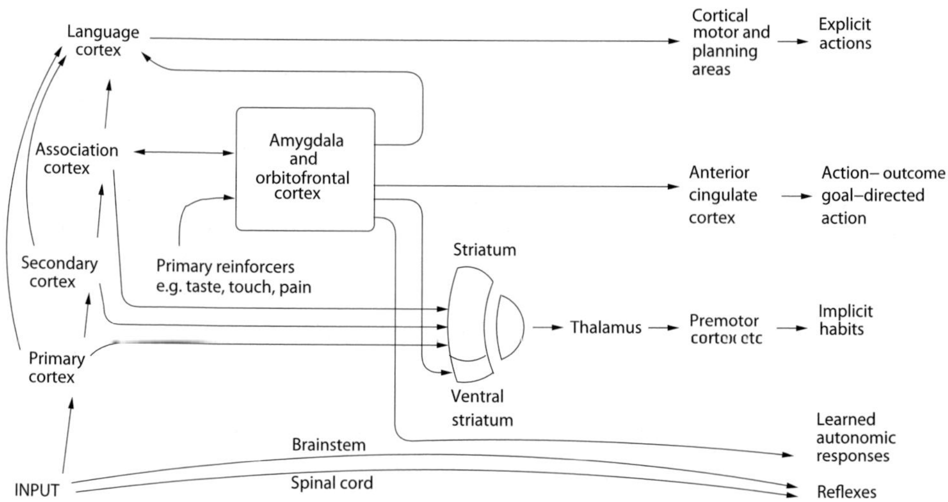

Fig. 10.4 Dual routes to the initiation of actions in response to rewarding and punishing stimuli. The inputs from different sensory systems to brain structures such as the orbitofrontal cortex and amygdala allow these brain structures to evaluate the reward- or punishment-related value of incoming stimuli, or of remembered stimuli. One type of route is via the language systems of the brain, which allow explicit (verbalizable) decisions involving multistep syntactic planning to be implemented. The other type of route may be implicit, and includes the anterior cingulate cortex for action–outcome, goal-dependent, learning; and the striatum and rest of the basal ganglia for stimulus–response habits. Outputs for autonomic responses can also be produced using outputs from the orbitofrontal cortex and anterior cingulate cortex (some of which are routed via the anterior insular cortex) and amygdala.

normally evident in the increasing rate of working for a food reward early on in a meal (Rolls & Rolls 1973b, Rolls 2005b).

A fourth factor is the computed absolute value of the reward or punishment expected or being obtained from a stimulus, e.g. the sweetness of the stimulus (set by evolution so that sweet stimuli will tend to be rewarding, because they are generally associated with energy sources), or the pleasantness of touch (set by evolution to be pleasant according to the extent to which it brings animals of the opposite sex together, and depending on the investment in time that the partner is willing to put into making the touch pleasurable, a sign that indicates the commitment and value for the partner of the relationship, as in social grooming).

After the reward value of the stimulus has been assessed in these ways, behaviour is then initiated based on approach towards or withdrawal from the stimulus. A critical aspect of the behaviour produced by this type of 'implicit' system is that it is aimed directly towards obtaining a sensed or expected reward, by virtue of connections to brain systems such as the basal ganglia which are concerned with the initiation of actions (see Fig. 10.4). The expectation may of course involve behaviour to obtain stimuli associated with reward, which might even be present in a fixed chain or sequence.

Now part of the way in which the behaviour is controlled with this first ('implicit') route is according to the reward value of the outcome. At the same time, the animal may only work for the reward if the cost is not too high. Indeed, in the field of behavioural ecology animals are often thought of as performing optimally on some cost–benefit curve (see, e.g., Krebs & Kacelnik (1991)). This does not at all mean that the animal thinks about the long-term rewards, and performs a cost–benefit analysis using a lot of thoughts about the costs, other rewards (short and long term) available and their costs, etc. (see Section 9.5.5). Instead, it should be taken to mean that in evolution the system has evolved in such a way that the way in which the reward varies with the different energy densities or amounts of food and the delay before it is received can be used as part of the input to a mechanism that has also been built to track the costs of obtaining the food (e.g. energy loss in obtaining it, risk of predation, etc.), and to then select given many such types of reward and the associated cost, the current behaviour that provides the most 'net reward'. Part of the value of having the computation expressed in this reward-minus-cost form is that there is then a suitable 'currency', or net reward value, to enable the animal to select the behaviour with currently the most net reward gain (or minimal aversive outcome).

Part of the evidence that this implicit route often controls emotional behaviour in humans is that humans with orbitofrontal cortex damage have impairments in selecting the correct action during visual discrimination reversal, yet can state explicitly what the correct action should be (Rolls, Hornak, Wade & McGrath 1994a, Rolls 1999c). The implication is that the intact orbitofrontal cortex is normally involved in making rapid emotion-related decisions, and that this emotion-related decision system is a separate system from the explicit system, which by serial reasoning can provide an alternative route to action. The explicit system may simply comment on the success or failure of actions that are initiated by the implicit system, and the explicit system may then be able to switch in to control mode to correct failures of the implicit system. Consistent evidence that an implicit system can control human behaviour is that in psychophysical and neurophysiological studies, it has been found that face stimuli presented for 16 ms and followed immediately by a mask are not consciously perceived, yet produce above chance identification (Rolls & Tovee 1994, Rolls, Tovee, Purcell, Stewart & Azzopardi 1994b, Rolls, Tovee & Panzeri 1999b, Rolls 2003, Rolls 2006a). In a similar backward masking paradigm, it was found that happy vs angry face expressions could influence how much beverage was wanted and consumed even when the faces were not consciously perceived (Winkielman & Berridge 2005, Winkielman & Berridge 2003). Thus unconscious emotion-related stimuli (in this case face expressions) can influence actions, and there is no need for processing to be conscious for actions to be initiated. Further, in blindsight, humans with damage to the primary visual cortex may not be subjectively aware of stimuli, yet may be able to guess what the stimulus was, or to perform reaching movements towards it (Weiskrantz 1998, Weiskrantz 2009). Further, humans with striate cortex lesions may be influenced by emotional stimuli which are not perceived consciously (De Gelder, Vroomen, Pourtois & Weiskrantz 1999). Thus actions and emotions can be initiated without the necessity for the conscious route to be in control, and we should not infer that all actions require conscious processing.

The second ('explicit') route in (at least) humans involves a computation with many 'if ... then' statements, to implement a plan to obtain a reward. In this case, the reward may actually be deferred as part of the plan, which might involve working first to obtain one reward, and only then to work for a second more highly valued reward, if this was thought to be overall an optimal strategy in terms of resource usage (e.g. time). In this case, syntax is required, because the many symbols (e.g. names of people) that are part of the plan must be correctly linked or bound. Such linking might be of the form: 'if A does this, then B is likely to do this, and this will cause C to do this ...'. The requirement of syntax for this type of planning implies that an output to language systems in the brain is required for this type of planning (see Fig. 10.4). **Thus the explicit language system in humans may allow working for deferred rewards by enabling use of a one-off, individual, plan appropriate for each situation.** This explicit system may allow immediate rewards to be deferred, as part of a long-term plan. This ability to defer immediate rewards and plan syntactically in this way for the long term may be an important way in which the explicit system extends the capabilities of the implicit emotion systems that respond more directly to rewards and punishers, or to rewards and punishers with fixed expectancies such as can be learned by reinforcement learning (see Appendix 1, Section A.5).

Consistent with the point being made about evolutionarily old emotion-based decision systems vs a recent rational system present in humans (and perhaps other animals with syntactic processing) is that humans trade off immediate costs/benefits against cost/benefits that are delayed by as much as decades, whereas non-human primates have not been observed to engage in unpreprogrammed delay of gratification involving more than a few minutes (Rachlin 1989, Kagel, Battalio & Green 1995, McClure, Laibson, Loewenstein & Cohen 2004) (though this is a potentially interesting area for further investigation, see Section 9.5.5).

Another building block for such planning operations in the brain may be the type of short-term memory in which the prefrontal cortex is involved. This short-term memory may be, for example in non-human primates, of where in space a response has just been made. A development of this type of short-term response memory system in humans to enable multiple short-term memories to be held in place correctly, preferably with the temporal order of the different items in the short-term memory coded correctly, may be another building block for the multiple step 'if .... then' type of computation in order to form a multiple step plan. Such short-term memories are implemented in the (dorsolateral and inferior convexity) prefrontal cortex of non-human primates and humans (Goldman-Rakic 1996, Petrides 1996, Rolls & Deco 2002, Deco & Rolls 2003, Rolls 2008b), and may be part of the reason why prefrontal cortex damage impairs planning and executive function (Shallice & Burgess 1996, Burgess 2000).

Of these two routes (see Fig. 10.4), it is the second that I have suggested above is related to consciousness. The hypothesis is that consciousness is the state that arises by virtue of having the ability to think about one's own thoughts, which has the adaptive value of enabling one to correct long multistep syntactic plans. This latter system is thus the one in which explicit, declarative, processing occurs. Processing in this system is frequently associated with reason and rationality, in that many of the consequences of possible actions can be taken into account. The actual computation of how rewarding a particular stimulus or situation is, or will be, probably still depends on activity in the orbitofrontal cortex and amygdala, as the reward value of stimuli is computed and represented in these regions, and in that it is found that verbalized expressions of the reward (or punishment) value of stimuli are dampened by damage to these systems. (For example, damage to the orbitofrontal cortex renders painful input still identifiable as pain, but without the strong affective, 'unpleasant', reaction to it.)

This language system that enables long-term planning may be contrasted with the first system in which behaviour is directed at obtaining the stimulus (including the remembered stimulus) which is currently most rewarding, as computed by brain structures that include the orbitofrontal cortex and amygdala. There are outputs from this system, perhaps those directed at the basal ganglia and cingulate cortex, which do not pass through the language system, and behaviour produced in this way is described as implicit, and verbal declarations cannot be made directly about the reasons for the choice made. When verbal declarations are made about decisions made in this first ('implicit') system, those verbal declarations may be confabulations, reasonable explanations or fabrications, of reasons why the choice was made. These reasonable explanations would be generated to be consistent with the sense of continuity and self that is a characteristic of reasoning in the language system.

The question then arises of how decisions are made in animals such as humans that have both the implicit, direct reward-based, and the explicit, rational, planning systems (see Fig. 10.4). One particular situation in which the first, implicit, system may be especially important is when rapid reactions to stimuli with reward or punishment value must be made, for then the direct connections from structures such as the orbitofrontal cortex to the basal ganglia may allow rapid actions. Another is when there may be too many factors to be taken into account easily by the explicit, rational, planning, system, then the implicit system may be used to guide action.

In contrast, when the implicit system continually makes errors, it would then be beneficial for the organism to switch from automatic, direct, action based on obtaining what the orbitofrontal cortex system decodes as being the most positively reinforcing choice currently available, to the explicit conscious control system which can evaluate with its long-term planning algorithms what action should be performed next. Indeed, it would be adaptive for the explicit system to be regularly assessing performance by the more automatic system, and to switch itself in to control behaviour quite frequently, as otherwise the adaptive value of having the explicit system would be less than optimal.

Another factor that may influence the balance between control by the implicit and explicit systems is the presence of pharmacological agents such as alcohol, which may alter the balance towards control by the implicit system, may allow the implicit system to influence more the explanations made by the explicit system, and may within the explicit system alter the relative value it places on caution and restraint vs commitment to a risky action or plan.

There may also be a flow of influence from the explicit, verbal system to the implicit system, in that the explicit system may decide on a plan of action or strategy, and exert an influence on the implicit system that will alter the reinforcement evaluations made by and the signals produced by the implicit system. An example of this might be that if a pregnant woman feels that she would like to escape a cruel mate, but is aware that she may not survive in the jungle, then it would be adaptive if the explicit system could suppress some aspects of her implicit behaviour towards her mate, so that she does not give signals that she is displeased with her situation[35]. Another example might be that the explicit system might, because of its long-term plans, influence the implicit system to increase its response to for example a positive reinforcer. One way in which the explicit system might influence the implicit system is by setting up the conditions in which, for example, when a given stimulus (e.g. person) is present, positive reinforcers are given, to facilitate stimulus–reinforcement association learning by the implicit system of the person receiving the positive reinforcers. Conversely, the implicit system may influence the explicit system, for example by highlighting certain stimuli in the environment that are currently associated with reward, to guide the attention of the explicit system to such stimuli.

However, it may be expected that there is often a conflict between these systems, in that the first, implicit, system is able to guide behaviour particularly to obtain the greatest immediate reinforcement, whereas the explicit system can potentially enable immediate rewards to be deferred, and longer-term, multistep, plans to be formed. This type of conflict will occur in animals with a syntactic planning ability, that is in humans and any other animals that have the ability to process a series of 'if ... then' stages of planning. This is a property of the human language system, and the extent to which it is a property of non-human primates is not yet fully clear. In any case, such conflict may be an important aspect of the operation of at least the human mind, because it is so essential for humans to decide correctly, at every moment, whether to invest in a relationship or a group that may offer long-term benefits, or whether to pursue immediate benefits directly (Nesse & Lloyd 1992)[36].

[35] In the literature on self-deception, it has been suggested that unconscious desires may not be made explicit in consciousness (or actually repressed), so as not to compromise the explicit system in what it produces; see, e.g., Alexander (1975), Alexander (1979), Trivers (1976), Trivers (1985); and the review by Nesse & Lloyd (1992).

[36] As Nesse & Lloyd (1992) describe, some psychoanalysts ascribe to a somewhat similar position, for they hold that intrapsychic conflicts usually seem to have two sides, with impulses on one side and inhibitions on the other. Analysts describe the source of the impulses as the id, and the modules that inhibit the expression of impulses, because of external and internal constraints, the ego and superego respectively (Leak & Christopher 1982, Trivers 1985, Nesse & Lloyd 1992). The superego can be thought of as the conscience, while the ego is the locus of executive functions

Some investigations on deception in non-human primates have been interpreted as showing that animals can plan to deceive others (see, e.g., Griffin (1992), Byrne & Whiten (1988), and Whiten & Byrne (1997)), that is to utilize 'Machiavellian intelligence'. For example, a baboon might 'deliberately' mislead another animal in order to obtain a resource such as food (e.g. by screaming to summon assistance in order to have a competing animal chased from a food patch) or sex (e.g. a female baboon who very gradually moved into a position from which the dominant male could not see her grooming a subadult baboon) (see Dawkins (1993)). The attraction of the Machiavellian argument is that the behaviour for which it accounts seems to imply that there is a concept of another animal's mind, and that one animal is trying occasionally to mislead another, which implies some planning. However, such observations tend by their nature to be field-based, and may have an anecdotal character, in that the previous experience of the animals in this type of behaviour, and the reinforcements obtained, are not known (Dawkins 1993). It is possible, for example, that some behavioural responses that appear to be Machiavellian may have been the result of previous instrumental learning in which reinforcement was obtained for particular types of response, or of observational learning, with again learning from the outcome observed. However, in any case, most examples of Machiavellian intelligence in non-human primates do not involve multiple stages of 'if ... then' planning requiring syntax to keep the symbols apart (but may involve associative learning which might lead to a description of the type 'if the dominant male sees me grooming a subadult male, I will be punished') (see Dawkins (1993)). Nevertheless, the possible advantage of such Machiavellian planning could be one of the adaptive guiding factors in evolution that provided advantage to a multistep, syntactic system that enables long-term planning, the best example of such a system being human language.

Another, not necessarily exclusive, advantage of the evolution of a linguistic multi-step planning system could well be not Machiavellian planning, but planning for social co-operation and advantage. Perhaps in general an 'if ... then' multistep syntactic planning ability is useful primarily in evolution in social situations of the type: 'if X does this, then Y does that; then I would/should do that, and the outcome would be ... '. It is not yet at all clear whether such planning is required in order to explain the social behaviour of social animals such as hunting dogs, or socializing monkeys (Dawkins 1993).

However, in humans, members of 'primitive' hunting tribes spend hours recounting tales of recent events (perhaps who did what, when; who then did what, etc.), perhaps to help learn from experience about good strategies, necessary for example when physically weak men take on large animals (see Pinker & Bloom (1992)).

Thus, social co-operation may be as powerful a driving force in the evolution of syntactical planning systems as Machiavellian intelligence. What is common to both is that they involve social situations. However, such a syntactic planning system would have advantages not only in social systems, for such planning may be useful in obtaining resources purely in a physical (non-social) world. An example might be planning how to cross terrain given current environmental constraints in order to reach a particular place[37].

that balance satisfaction of impulses with anticipated internal and external costs. A difference of the present position is that it is based on identification of dual routes to action implemented by different systems in the brain, each with its own selective advantage.

[37]Tests of whether such multistep planning might be possible in even non-human primates are quite difficult to devise. One example might be to design a multistep maze. On a first part of the trial, the animal might be allowed to choose for itself, given constraints set on that trial to ensure trial unique performance, a set of choices through a maze. On the second part of that trial, the animal would be required to run through the maze again, remembering and repeating every choice just made in the first part of that trial. This part of the design is intended to allow recall of a multistep plan. To test on probe occasions whether the plan is being recalled, and whether the plan can be corrected by a higher-order thought process, the animal might be shown after the first part of a trial, that one of its previous free choices was not now available. The test would be to determine whether the animal can make a set of choices

The thrust of this argument thus is that much complex animal, including human, behaviour can take place using the implicit, non-conscious, route to action. We should be very careful not to postulate intentional states (i.e. states with intentions, beliefs, and desires) unless the evidence for them is strong, and it seems to me that a flexible, one-off, linguistic processing system that can handle propositions is needed for intentional states. What the explicit, linguistic, system does allow is exactly this flexible, one-off, multistep planning-ahead type of computation, which allows us to defer immediate rewards based on such a plan.

Emotions as actions, and emotions as affects, are sometimes contrasted. My view on this is that sometimes emotions can lead to actions implicitly, without the need for conscious processing. However, when emotions involve longer term planning, then representation and processing in the explicit system is required, and affective feelings will then be inextricably linked to the processing.

This discussion of dual routes to action has been with respect to the behaviour produced. There is of course in addition a third output of brain regions such as the orbitofrontal cortex and amygdala involved in emotion, which is directed to producing autonomic and endocrine responses. Although it has been argued in Chapter 2 that the autonomic system is not normally in a circuit through which behavioural responses are produced (i.e. against the James–Lange and related theories), there may be some influence from effects produced through the endocrine system (and possibly the autonomic system, through which some endocrine responses are controlled) on behaviour, or on the dual systems just discussed that control behaviour. For example, during female orgasm the hormone oxytocin may be released, and this may influence the implicit system to help develop positive reinforcement associations and thus attachment to her lover.

10.3.2 The Selfish Gene vs The Selfish Phenotype

I have provided evidence in Section 10.3.1 that there are two main routes to decision-making and action. The first route selects actions by gene-defined goals for action, and is closely associated with emotion. The second route involves multistep planning and reasoning which requires syntactic processing to keep the symbols involved at each step separate from the symbols in different steps. (This second route is used by humans and perhaps by closely related animals.) Now the 'interests' of the first and second routes to decision-making and action are different. As argued very convincingly by Richard Dawkins in *The Selfish Gene* (Dawkins 1976, Dawkins 1989), and by others (Hamilton 1964, Ridley 1993a, Hamilton 1996), many behaviours occur in the interests of the survival of the genes, not of the individual (nor of the group), and much behaviour can be understood in this way. I have extended this approach by arguing that an important role for some genes in evolution is to define the goals for actions that will lead to better survival of those genes; that emotions are the states associated with these gene-defined goals; and that the defining of goals for actions rather that actions themselves is an efficient way for genes to operate, as it leaves flexibility of choice of action open until the animal is alive (Rolls 2005b). This provides great simplification of the genotype as action details do not need to be specified, just rewarding and punishing stimuli, and also flexibility of action in the face of changing environments faced by the genes. Thus the interests that are implied when the first route to action is chosen are those of the 'selfish genes', not those of the individual.

However, the second route to action allows, by reasoning, decisions to be taken that might not be in the interests of the genes, might be longer term decisions, and might be

that indicate corrections to the multistep plan, in which the trajectory has to be altered before the now unavailable choice point is reached.

in the interests of the individual. An example might be a choice not to have children, but instead to devote oneself to science, medicine, music, or literature. The reasoning, rational, system presumably evolved because taking longer-term decisions involving planning rather than choosing a gene-defined goal might be advantageous at least sometimes for genes. But an unforeseen consequence of the evolution of the rational system might be that the decisions would, sometimes, not be to the advantage of any genes in the organism. After all, evolution by natural selection operates utilizing genetic variation like a Blind Watchmaker (Dawkins 1986a). In this sense, the interests when the second route to decision-making is used are at least sometimes those of the 'selfish phenotype'. (Indeed, we might euphonically say that the interests are those of the '*selfish phene*' (where the etymology is Gk φαινω (phaino), 'appear', referring to appearance, hence the thing that one observes, the individual). Hence the decision-making referred to in Section 10.3.1 is between a first system where the goals are gene-defined, and a second rational system in which the decisions may be made in the interests of the genes, or in the interests of the phenotype and not in the interests of the genes. Thus we may speak of the choice as sometimes being between the 'Selfish Genes' and the 'Selfish Phenes'.

Now what keeps the decision-making between the 'Selfish Genes' and the 'Selfish Phenes' more or less under control and in balance? If the second, rational, system chose too often for the interests of the 'Selfish Phene', the genes in that phenotype would not survive over generations. Having these two systems in the same individual will only be stable if their potency is approximately equal, so that sometimes decisions are made with the first route, and sometimes with the second route. If the two types of decision-making, then, compete with approximately equal potency, and sometimes one is chosen, and sometimes the other, then this is exactly the scenario in which stochastic processes in the decision-making mechanism are likely to play an important role in the decision that is taken. The same decision, even with the same evidence, may not be taken each time a decision is made, because of noise in the system.

The system itself may have some properties that help to keep the system operating well. One is that if the second, rational, system tends to dominate the decision-making too much, the first, gene-based emotional system might fight back over generations of selection, and enhance the magnitude of the reward value specified by the genes, so that emotions might actually become stronger as a consequence of them having to compete in the interests of the selfish genes with the rational decision-making process.

Another property of the system may be that sometimes the rational system cannot gain all the evidence that would be needed to make a rational choice. Under these circumstances the rational system might fail to make a clear decision, and under these circumstances, basing a decision on the gene-specified emotions is an alternative. Indeed, Damasio (1994) argued that under circumstances such as this, emotions might take an important role in decision-making. In this respect, I agree with him, basing my reasons on the arguments above. He called the emotional feelings gut feelings, and, in contrast to me, hypothesized that actual feedback from the gut was involved. His argument seemed to be that if the decision was too complicated for the rational system, then send outputs to the viscera, and whatever is sensed by what they send back could be used in the decision-making, and would account for the conscious feelings of the emotional states. My reading of the evidence is that the feedback from the periphery is not necessary for the emotional decision-making, or for the feelings, nor would it be computationally efficient to put the viscera in the loop given that the information starts from the brain (Section 2.6.1).

Another property of the system is that the interests of the second, rational, system, although involving a different form of computation, should not be too far from those of the gene-defined emotional system, for the arrangement to be stable in evolution by natural selection. One way that this could be facilitated would be if the gene-based goals felt pleasant or unpleasant in the rational system, and in this way contributed to the operation of the second, rational, system. This is something that I propose is the case.

10.3.3 Decision-making between the implicit and explicit systems

Decision-making as implemented in neural networks in the brain is now becoming understood, and is described in Chapter 8. As shown there, two attractor states, each one corresponding to a decision, compete in an attractor single network with the evidence for each of the decisions acting as biases to each of the attractor states. The non-linear dynamics, and the way in which noise due to the random spiking of neurons makes the decision-making probabilistic, makes this a biologically plausible model of decision-making consistent with much neurophysiological and fMRI data (Wang 2002, Rolls & Deco 2010, Deco, Rolls, Albantakis & Romo 2013).

I propose (Rolls 2005b, Rolls 2008b) that this model applies to taking decisions between the implicit (unconscious) and explicit (conscious) systems in emotional decision-making, where the two different systems could provide the biasing inputs λ_1 and λ_2 to the model. An implication is that noise will influence with probabilistic outcomes which system takes a decision.

When decisions are taken, sometimes confabulation may occur, in that a verbal account of why the action was performed may be given, and this may not be related at all to the environmental event that actually triggered the action (Gazzaniga & LeDoux 1978, Gazzaniga 1988, Gazzaniga 1995, Rolls 2005b, LeDoux 2008, Rolls 2012d). It is accordingly possible that sometimes in normal humans when actions are initiated as a result of processing in a specialized brain region such as those involved in some types of rewarded behaviour, the language system may subsequently elaborate a coherent account of why that action was performed (i.e. confabulate). This would be consistent with a general view of brain evolution in which, as areas of the cortex evolve, they are laid on top of existing circuitry connecting inputs to outputs, and in which each level in this hierarchy of separate input–output pathways may control behaviour according to the specialized function it can perform. This hierarchical overlaying is an important concept advanced in this book as being important for understanding emotion, the different brain systems involved in different aspects of emotion and decision-making, and the relation between the implicit and explicit systems. When a new layer is added, previous layers may lose some of their importance, as appears to occur in the taste system in which in primates the subcortical processing from the brainstem nucleus of the solitary tract is lost; when the granular orbitofrontal cortex of primates becomes relatively more important than the amygdala; and when language areas are added on top of existing circuitry (Fig. 10.4).

10.4 Determinism

These thoughts raise the issue of free will in decision-making, and of determinism (Rolls 2012g).

There are a number of senses in which our behaviour might be deterministic. One sense might be genetic determinism, and we have already seen that there are far too few genes to determine the structure and function of our brains, and thus to determine our behaviour (Rolls & Stringer 2000, Rolls 2012f). Moreover, development, and the environment with the opportunities it provides for brain self-organization and learning, play a large part in brain structure and function, and thus in our behaviour.

Another sense might be that if there were random factors that influence the operation of the brain, then our behaviour might be thought not to be completely predictable and deterministic. It is this that I consider here, a topic developed in *The Noisy Brain: Stochastic Dynamics as a Principle of Brain Function* (Rolls & Deco 2010), in which we show that there is noise or randomness in the brain, and argue that this can be advantageous[38].

Neurons emit action potentials, voltage spikes, which transmit information along axons to other neurons. These all-or-none spikes are a safe way to transmit information along axons, for they do not lose amplitude and degrade along a long axon. In most brain systems, an increase in the firing rate of the spikes carries the information. For example, taste neurons in the taste cortex fire faster if the particular taste to which they respond is present, and neurons in the inferior temporal visual cortex fire faster if for example one of the faces to which they are tuned is seen (Rolls 2005b, Rolls 2008b). However, for a given mean firing rate (e.g. 50 spikes/s), the exact timing of each spike is quite random, and indeed is close to a Poisson distribution which is what is expected for a random process in which the timing of each spike is independent of the other spikes. Part of the neuronal basis of this randomness of the spike firing times is that each cortical neuron is held close to its threshold for firing and even produces occasional spontaneous firing, so that when an input is received, some at least of the cortical neurons will be so close to threshold that they emit a spike very rapidly, allowing information processing to be rapid (Rolls 2008b, Rolls & Deco 2010).

This randomness in the firing time of individual neurons results in probabilistic behaviour of the brain (Chapter 8). For example, in decision-making, if the population of neurons that represents decision 1 has by chance more randomly occurring spikes in a short time, that population may win the competition (implemented through inhibitory interneurons) with a different population of neurons that represents decision 2. Decision-making is by this mechanism probabilistic. For example, if the odds are equal for decision 1 and decision 2, each decision will be taken probabilistically on 50% of the occasions or trials. This is highly adaptive, and is much better than getting stuck between two equally attractive rewards and unable to make a decision, as in the medieval tale of Duns Scotus about the donkey who starved because it could not choose between two equally attractive foods (Rolls & Deco 2010).

However, given that the brain operates with some degree of randomness due to the statistical fluctuations produced by the random spiking times of neurons, brain function is to some extent non-deterministic, as defined in terms of these statistical fluctuations. That is, the behaviour of the system, and of the individual, can vary from trial to trial based on these statistical fluctuations, in ways that are described in Chapter 8 and by Rolls & Deco (2010). Indeed, given that each neuron has this randomness, and that there are sufficiently small numbers of synapses on the neurons in each network (between a few thousand and 20,000) that these statistical fluctuations are not smoothed out, and that there are a number of different networks involved in typical thoughts and actions each one of which may behave probabilistically, and with 10^{11} neurons in the brain each with this number of synapses, the system has so many degrees of freedom that it operates effectively as a non-deterministic system. (Philosophers may wish to argue about different senses of the term deterministic, but it is being used here in a precise, scientific, and quantitative way, which has been clearly defined.)

[38]This randomness is not a property of chaotic systems, which although complex, are not random in the sense that the same trajectory is followed from a given starting position (Peitgen, Jürgens & Saupe 2004).

10.5 Free will

Do we have free will when we make a choice? Given the distinction made between the implicit system that seeks for gene-specified rewards, and the explicit system that can use reasoning to defer an immediate goal and plan many steps ahead for longer-term goals, do we have free will when both the implicit and the explicit systems have made the choice?

Free will would in Rolls' view (Rolls 2005b, Rolls 2008c, Rolls 2008b, Rolls 2010a, Rolls 2011a, Rolls 2012g, Rolls 2012d) involve the use of language to check many moves ahead on a number of possible series of actions and their outcomes, and then with this information to make a choice from the likely outcomes of different possible series of actions. (If, in contrast, choices were made only on the basis of the reinforcement value of immediately available stimuli, without the arbitrary syntactic symbol manipulation made possible by language, then the choice strategy would be much more limited, and we might not want to use the term free will, as all the consequences of those actions would not have been computed.) It is suggested that when this type of reflective, conscious, information processing is occurring and leading to action, the system performing this processing and producing the action would have to believe that it could cause the action, for otherwise inconsistencies would arise, and the system might no longer try to initiate action. This belief held by the system may partly underlie the feeling of free will. At other times, when other brain modules are initiating actions (in the implicit systems), the conscious processor (the explicit system) may confabulate and believe that it caused the action, or at least give an account (possibly wrong) of why the action was initiated. The fact that the conscious processor may have the belief even in these circumstances that it initiated the action may arise as a property of it being inconsistent for a system that can take overall control using conscious verbal processing to believe that it was overridden by another system. This may be the underlying computational reason why confabulation occurs (Section 10.3.1).

The interesting view we are led to is thus that when probabilistic choices influenced by stochastic dynamics (Rolls & Deco 2010) are made between the implicit and explicit systems, we may not be aware of which system made the choice. Further, when the stochastic noise has made us choose with the implicit system, we may confabulate and say that we made the choice of our own free will, and provide a guess at why the decision was taken. In this scenario, the stochastic dynamics of the brain plays a role even in how we understand free will (Rolls 2010a, Rolls 2012d, Rolls 2012g).

The implication of this argument is that a good use of the term free will is when the term refers to the operation of the rational, planning, explicit (conscious) system that can think many moves ahead, and choose from a number of such computations the multistep strategy that best optimizes the goals of the explicit system with long-term goals. When on the other hand our implicit system has taken a decision, and we confabulate a spurious account with our explicit system, and pronounce that we took the decision for such and such a (confabulated) reason of our own "free will", then my view is that the feeling of free will was an illusion (Rolls 2005b, Rolls 2010a, Rolls 2012d, Rolls 2012g).

Before leaving these thoughts, it may be worth commenting on the feeling of continuing self-identity that is characteristic of humans. Why might this arise? One suggestion is that if one is an organism that can think about its own long-term multistep plans, then for those plans to be consistently and thus adaptively executed, the goals of the plans would need to remain stable, as would memories of how far one had proceeded along the execution path of each plan. If one felt each time one came to execute, perhaps on another day, the next step of a plan, that the goals were different, or if one did not remember which steps had already been taken in a multistep plan, the plan would never be usefully executed. So, given that it does feel like something to be doing this type of planning using higher-order thoughts, it would have to feel as if one were the same agent, acting towards the same goals, from day to day, for which autobiographical memory would be important.

Thus it is suggested that the feeling of continuing self-identity falls out of a situation in which there is an actor with consistent long-term goals, and long-term recall. If it feels like anything to be the actor, according to the suggestions of the higher-order thought theory, then it should feel like the same thing from occasion to occasion to be the actor, and no special further construct is needed to account for self-identity. Humans without such a feeling of being the same person from day to day might be expected to have, for example, inconsistent goals from day to day, or a poor recall memory. It may be noted that the ability to recall previous steps in a plan, and bring them into the conscious, higher-order thought system, is an important prerequisite for long-term planning which involves checking each step in a multistep process.

Conscious feelings of self will be likely to be of value to the individual. Indeed, it would be maladaptive if feelings of self-identity, and continuation of the self, were not wanted by the individual, for that would lead to the brain's capacity for feelings about self-identity to leave the gene pool, due for example to suicide. This wish for feelings and thoughts about the self to continue may lead to the wish and hope that this will occur after death, and this may be important as a foundation for religions (Rolls 2012d).

10.6 Content and meaning in representations: How are representations grounded in the world?

In Section 10.2 I suggested that representations need to be grounded in the world for a system with higher-order thoughts to be conscious. I therefore now develop somewhat what I understand by representations being grounded in the world.

It is possible to analyse how the firing of populations of neurons encodes information about stimuli in the world (Rolls & Treves 1998, Rolls 2008b, Rolls & Treves 2011). For example, from the firing rates of small numbers of neurons in the primate inferior temporal visual cortex, it is possible to know which of 20 faces has been shown to the monkey (Abbott, Rolls & Tovee 1996, Rolls, Treves & Tovee 1997d, Rolls & Treves 2011). Similarly, a population of neurons in the anterior part of the macaque temporal lobe visual cortex has been discovered that has a view-invariant representation of objects (Booth & Rolls 1998, Rolls 2012e). From the firing of a small ensemble of neurons in the olfactory part of the orbitofrontal cortex, it is possible to know which of eight odours was presented (Rolls, Critchley & Treves 1996b, Rolls, Critchley, Verhagen & Kadohisa 2010a). From the firing of small ensembles of neurons in the hippocampus, it is possible to know where in allocentric space a monkey is looking (Rolls, Treves, Robertson, Georges-François & Panzeri 1998b). In each of these cases, the number of stimuli that is encoded increases exponentially with the number of neurons in the ensemble, so this is a very powerful representation (Abbott, Rolls & Tovee 1996, Rolls, Treves & Tovee 1997d, Rolls & Treves 1998, Rolls & Deco 2002, Rolls, Aggelopoulos, Franco & Treves 2004, Franco, Rolls, Aggelopoulos & Treves 2004, Aggelopoulos, Franco & Rolls 2005, Rolls 2008b, Rolls & Treves 2011). What is being measured in each example is the mutual information between the firing of an ensemble of neurons and which stimuli are present in the world. In this sense, one can read off the code that is being used at the end of each of these sensory systems.

However, what sense does the representation make to the animal? What does the firing of each ensemble of neurons 'mean'? What is the content of the representation? In the visual system, for example, it is suggested that the representation is built by a series of appropriately connected competitive networks, operating with a modified Hebb-learning rule (Rolls 1992b, Rolls 1994b, Wallis & Rolls 1997, Rolls 2000c, Rolls & Milward 2000, Stringer & Rolls 2000, Rolls & Stringer 2001a, Rolls & Deco 2002, Elliffe, Rolls & Stringer 2002, Stringer & Rolls 2002, Deco & Rolls 2004, Rolls 2008b, Rolls 2012e). Now competitive networks categorize their inputs without the use of a teacher (Kohonen 1989, Hertz et al. 1991, Rolls 2008b). So which particular neurons fire as a result of the self-organization to represent a particular object or stimulus is arbitrary. What meaning, therefore, does the particular ensemble that fires to an object have? How is the representation grounded in the real world? The fact that there is mutual information between the firing of the ensemble of cells in the brain and a stimulus or event in the world (Rolls & Treves 1998, Rolls 2008b, Rolls & Treves 2011) does not fully answer this question.

One answer to this question is that there may be meaning in the case of objects and faces that it is an object or face, and not just a particular view. This is the case in that the representation may be activated by any view of the object or face. This is a step, suggested to be made possible by a short-term memory in the learning rule that enables different views of objects to be associated together (Wallis & Rolls 1997, Rolls & Treves 1998, Rolls & Milward 2000, Rolls 2008b, Rolls 2012e). But it still does not provide the representation with any meaning in terms of the real world. What actions might one make, or what emotions might one feel, if that arbitrary set of temporal cortex visual cells was activated?

This leads to one of the answers I propose. I suggest that one type of meaning of representations in the brain is provided by their reward (or punishment) value: activation of these representations is the goal for actions. In the case of primary reinforcers such as the taste of food or pain, the activation of these representations would have meaning in the sense that the animal would work to obtain the activation of the taste of food neurons when hungry, and to escape from stimuli that cause the neurons representing pain to be activated. Evolution has built the brain so that genes specify these primary reinforcing stimuli, and so that their representations in the brain should be the targets for actions (see Chapter 3). In the case of other ensembles of neurons in, for example, the visual cortex that respond to objects with the colour and shape of a banana, and which 'represent' the sight of a banana in that their activation is always and uniquely produced by the sight of a banana, such representations come to have meaning only by association with a primary reinforcer, involving the process of stimulus–reinforcer association learning.

The second sense in which a representation may be said to have meaning is by virtue of sensory–motor correspondences in the world. For example, the touch of a solid object such as a table might become associated with evidence from the motor system that attempts to walk through the table result in cessation of movement. The representation of the table in the inferior temporal visual cortex might have 'meaning' only in the sense that there is mutual information between the representation and the sight of the table until the table is seen just before and while it is touched, when sensory–sensory association between inputs from different sensory modalities will be set up that will enable the visual representation to become associated with its correspondences in the touch and movement worlds. In this second sense, meaning will be conferred on the visual sensory representation because of its associations in the sensory–motor world. Related views have been developed by the philosopher Ruth Millikan (1984). Thus it is suggested that there are two ways by which sensory representations can be said to be grounded, that is to have meaning, in the real world.

It is suggested that the symbols used in language become grounded in the real world by the same two processes.

In the first, a symbol such as the word 'banana' has meaning because it is associated with primary reinforcers such as the flavour of the banana, and with secondary reinforcers such as the sight of the banana. These reinforcers have 'meaning' to the animal in that evolution has built animals as machines designed to do everything that they can to obtain these reinforcers, so that they can eventually reproduce successfully and pass their genes onto the next generation[39]. In this sense, obtaining reinforcers may have life-threatening 'meaning' for animals, though of course the use of the word 'meaning' here does not imply any subjective state, just that the animal is built as a survival for reproduction machine[40].

In the second process, the word 'table' may have meaning because it is associated with sensory stimuli produced by tables such as their touch, shape, and sight, as well as other functional properties, such as, for example, being load-bearing, and obstructing movement if they are in the way (see Section 10.2).

This section (10.6) thus adds to Section 10.2 on a higher-order syntactic thought (HOST) theory of consciousness, by addressing the sense in which the thoughts may need to be grounded in the world. The HOST theory holds that the thoughts 'mean' something to the individual, in the sense that they may be about the survival of the individual (the phenotype, Section 10.3.2) in the world, which the rational, thought, system aims to maximize (Rolls 2012d).

10.7 The causal role of consciousness: a theory of the relation between the mind and the brain

Does consciousness cause our behaviour? Before discussing the causal role of consciousness, I summarize my view on the *relation between the mind and the brain*.

What is the causal relation between mental events and neurophysiological events, part of the mind–body problem? My view is that the relationship between mental events and neurophysiological events is similar (apart from the problem of consciousness) to the relationship between the program running in a computer (the software) and the hardware on the computer. We can consider that the software and hardware in terms of causality are at different levels of explanation. The program moving from one step to the next is one level of explanation, and the hardware implementation by the transistor-transistor logic (TTL) is another. A crucial point is that the processes described at the different levels take place at the same point in time, so that we should not think of one as causing the other. Completion of one step of the program may cause the next step to be performed, and causality operates here, with a time delay. Similarly, the hardware operations involved in performing one step of the program can be thought of as causing the next step of hardware operations to be performed, so again causality operates here, with a time delay. But on this analysis, for a given step of the program, causality would not operate between the software and the hardware, and these would just be different levels of explanation. The implication of this account for understanding the relation between the mind and the brain is that the mind and the operations performed by the brain are different levels of explanation, and that the mind should not be thought of as causing brain changes, and vice versa, for they would be happening at the same point in time. This analysis is consistent with the requirement for causality '*post hoc, ergo propter hoc*' ('after this, therefore because of this', a necessary but not sufficient condition for causality). I now favour this account of the relation between the mind and the brain (having considered other possibilities before (Rolls 2012d, Rolls 2013b)), because it is consistent with the condition of *post hoc, ergo propter hoc*.

[39]The fact that some stimuli are reinforcers but may not be adaptive as goals for action is no objection. Genes are limited in number, and can not allow for every eventuality, such as the availability to humans of (non-nutritive) saccharin as a sweetener. The genes can just build reinforcement systems the activation of which is generally likely to increase the fitness of the genes specifying the reinforcer (or may have increased their fitness in the recent past).

[40]This is a novel, Darwinian, approach to the issue of symbol grounding.

Some philosophers taking an intentional stance think of one mental event as causing another mental event, and that this is a convenient level of explanation for at least providing an account to the behaviour of others (Dennett 1987). That is consistent with what I have summarized in the preceding paragraph, provided that we realize that it is neuronal operations that implement syntactic thought and hence reasoning. That is, the neuronal networks in the brain have evolved to the stage where they can implement a language of thought. With my approach, there is nothing 'extra' that remains unexplained at the mental level, and that somehow operates in a different way to that just described. To elaborate further, the style of computation implemented by the brain is based on the (dot or inner product) similarity between input firing rate vectors and synaptic weight vectors, and is very poor at logical operations (see Rolls (2012d) Sections 2.14–2.16 for my thoughts on the differences between computations in the brain and in digital computers). Nevertheless, as a result of training, our neuronal networks have evolved to have the capability to learn to follow syntactic rules that enable us to perform logical operations such as AND, XOR, and odd or even parity determination, in a serial manner characteristic of language. As a result of this, we can think of humans as intentional systems, with beliefs etc. represented in a language of thought, but all implemented by neuronal networks that implement syntax (Rolls 2012d).

The view that I currently hold about the causal role of consciousness is that the information processing that is related to consciousness (activity in a linguistic system capable of higher-order thoughts, and used for planning and correcting the operation of lower-order linguistic systems) can play a causal role in producing our behaviour (see Fig. 10.4). It is, I postulate, a property of processing in this system (capable of higher-order thoughts) that it feels like something to be performing that type of processing. It is in this sense that I suggest that consciousness can act causally to influence our behaviour – consciousness is the property that occurs when a linguistic system is thinking about its lower-order thoughts, which may be useful in correcting plans.

The hypothesis that it does feel like something when this processing is taking place is at least to some extent testable: humans performing this type of higher-order linguistic processing, for example recalling episodic memories and comparing them with current circumstances, who denied being conscious, would prima facie constitute evidence against the theory. Most humans would find it very implausible though to posit that they could be thinking about their own thoughts, and reflecting on their own thoughts, without being conscious. This type of processing does appear, for most humans, to be necessarily conscious.

In this context, I provide a short specification of what might have to be implemented in a neural network to implement conscious processing. First, a linguistic system, not necessarily verbal, but implementing syntax between symbols implemented in the environment would be needed. This system would be necessary for a multi-step one-off planning system. Then a higher-order thought system also implementing syntax and able to think about the representations in the first-order linguistic system, and able to correct the reasoning in the first-order linguistic system in a flexible manner, would be needed. The system would also need to have its representations grounded in the world, as discussed in Section 10.6. So my view is that consciousness can be implemented in neural networks (and that this is a topic worth discussing), but that the neural networks would have to implement the type of higher-order linguistic processing described in this chapter, and also would need to be grounded in the world.

10.8 Comparison with other theories of consciousness

10.8.1 Higher-order thought theories

Some ways in which the current theory may be different from other higher-order thought theories (Rosenthal 2004, Rosenthal 2005, Rosenthal 2012, Gennaro 2004, Carruthers 2000) is that it provides an account of the evolutionary, adaptive, value of a higher-order thought system in helping to solve a credit assignment problem that arises in a multistep syntactic plan, links this type of processing to consciousness, and therefore emphasizes a role for syntactic processing in consciousness. The type of syntactic processing need not be at the natural language level (which implies a universal grammar), but could be at the level of mentalese or simpler, as it involves primarily the syntactic manipulation of symbols (Fodor 1994, Rolls 2005b).

The current theory holds that it is higher-order linguistic thoughts (HOLTs) (or higher-order syntactic thoughts, HOSTs (Rolls 2004d, Rolls 2007b, Rolls 2011a, Rolls 2012d)) that are closely associated with consciousness, and this might differ from Rosenthal's higher-order thoughts (HOTs) theory (Rosenthal 1986, Rosenthal 1990, Rosenthal 1993, Rosenthal 2004, Rosenthal 2005, Rosenthal 2012) in the emphasis in the current theory on language. Language in the current theory is defined by syntactic manipulation of symbols, and does not necessarily imply verbal (or natural) language.

The reason that strong emphasis is placed on language is that it is as a result of having a multistep, flexible, 'one-off', reasoning procedure that errors can be corrected by using 'thoughts about thoughts'. This enables correction of errors that cannot be easily corrected by reward or punishment received at the end of the reasoning, due to the credit assignment problem. That is, there is a need for some type of supervisory and monitoring process, to detect where errors in the reasoning have occurred. It is having such a HOST brain system, and it becoming engaged (even if only a little), that according to the HOST theory is associated with phenomenal consciousness.

This suggestion on the adaptive value in evolution of such a higher-order linguistic thought process for multistep planning ahead, and correcting such plans, may also be different from earlier work. Put another way, this point is that *credit assignment* when reward or punishment is received is straightforward in a one-layer network (in which the reinforcement can be used directly to correct nodes in error, or responses), but is very difficult in a multistep linguistic process executed once. Very complex mappings in a multilayer network can be learned if hundreds of learning trials are provided. But once these complex mappings are learned, their success or failure in a new situation on a given trial cannot be evaluated and corrected by the network. Indeed, the complex mappings achieved by such networks (e.g. networks trained by backpropagation of errors or by reinforcement learning) mean that after training they operate according to fixed rules, and are often quite impenetrable and inflexible (Rumelhart, Hinton & Williams 1986, Rolls 2008b). In contrast, to correct a multistep, single occasion, linguistically based plan or procedure, recall of the steps just made in the reasoning or planning, and perhaps related episodic material, needs to occur, so that the link in the chain that is most likely to be in error can be identified. This may be part of the reason why there is a close relationship between declarative memory systems, which can explicitly recall memories, and consciousness.

Some computer programs may have supervisory processes. Should these count as higher-order linguistic thought processes? My current response to this is that they should not, to the extent that they operate with fixed rules to correct the operation of a system that does not itself involve linguistic thoughts about symbols grounded semantically in the external world. If on the other hand it were possible to implement on a computer such a high-order linguistic thought–supervisory correction process to correct first-order one-off linguistic thoughts with symbols grounded in the real world (as described at the end of Section 10.6), then prima facie this process would be conscious. If it were possible in a thought experiment to reproduce the neural connectivity and operation of a human brain on a computer, then prima facie it would also have the attributes of consciousness[41]. It might continue to have those attributes for as long as power was applied to the system.

Another possible difference from earlier theories is that raw sensory feels are suggested to arise as a consequence of having a system that can think about its own thoughts. Raw sensory feels, and subjective states associated with emotional and motivational states, may not necessarily arise first in evolution.

A property often attributed to consciousness is that it is *unitary*. The current theory would account for this by the limited syntactic capability of neuronal networks in the brain, which render it difficult to implement more than a few syntactic bindings of symbols simultaneously (Rolls & Treves 1998, McLeod, Plunkett & Rolls 1998, Rolls 2008b). This limitation makes it difficult to run several 'streams of consciousness' simultaneously. In addition, given that a linguistic system can control behavioural output, several parallel streams might produce maladaptive behaviour (apparent as, e.g. indecision), and might be selected against. The close relationship between, and the limited capacity of, both the stream of consciousness, and auditory–verbal short-term working memory, may be that both implement the capacity for syntax in neural networks.

The hypothesis that syntactic binding is necessary for consciousness is one of the postulates of the theory I am describing (for the system I describe must be capable of correcting its own syntactic thoughts). The fact that the binding must be implemented in neuronal networks may well place limitations on consciousness that lead to some of its properties, such as its unitary nature.

The theory (Rolls 1997b, Rolls 2004d, Rolls 2006a, Rolls 2007b, Rolls 2007g, Rolls 2008c, Rolls 2010a, Rolls 2011a, Rolls 2012d) holds that consciousness arises by virtue of a system that can think linguistically about its own linguistic thoughts. The advantages for a system of being able to do this have been described, and this has been suggested as the reason why consciousness evolved. The evidence that consciousness arises by virtue of having a system that can perform higher-order linguistic processing is however, and I think might remain, circumstantial. [Why must it feel like something when we are performing a certain type of information processing? The evidence described here suggests that it does feel like something when we are performing a certain type of information processing, but does not produce a strong reason for why it has to feel like something. It just does, when we are using this linguistic processing system capable of higher-order thoughts.] The evidence, summarized above, includes the points that we think of ourselves as conscious when, for example, we recall earlier events, compare them with current events, and plan many steps ahead. Evidence also comes from neurological cases, from, for example, split-brain patients (who may confabulate conscious stories about what is happening in their other, non-language, hemisphere); and from cases such as frontal lobe patients who can tell one consciously what they should be doing, but nevertheless may be doing the opposite. (The force of this type of case is that much of our behaviour may normally be produced by routes about which we cannot verbalize, and are not conscious about.)

This raises discussion of the *causal role of consciousness*. Does consciousness cause our behaviour? The view that I currently hold is that the information processing that is related to consciousness (activity in a linguistic system capable of higher-order thoughts, and used for

[41] This is a functionalist position. Apparently Damasio (2003) does not subscribe to this view, for he suggests that there is something in the 'stuff' (the 'natural medium') that the brain is made of that is also important. It is difficult for a person with this view to make telling points about consciousness from neuroscience, for it may always be the 'stuff' that is actually important.

planning and correcting the operation of lower-order linguistic systems) can play a causal role in producing our behaviour (see Fig. 10.4), but as part of a 'levels of explanation' account of the relation between mental events and brain events (Section 10.7). It is, I postulate, a property of processing in this system (capable of higher-order thoughts) that it feels like something to be performing that type of processing. It is in this sense that I suggest that consciousness can act causally to influence our behaviour – consciousness is the property that occurs when a linguistic system is thinking about its lower-order thoughts, which may be useful in correcting plans.

The hypothesis that it does feel like something when this processing is taking place is at least to some extent testable (cf. Lau & Rosenthal (2011)): humans performing this type of higher-order linguistic processing, for example recalling episodic memories and comparing them with current circumstances, who denied being conscious, would prima facie constitute evidence against the theory. Most humans would find it very implausible though to posit that they could be thinking about their own thoughts, and reflecting on their own thoughts, without being conscious. This type of processing does appear, for most humans, to be necessarily conscious.

It is suggested that qualia, raw sensory, and emotional, 'feels', arise secondarily to having evolved such a higher-order thought system, and that sensory and emotional processing feels like something because once this emotional processing has entered the planning, higher-order thought, system, it would be unparsimonious for it not to feel like something, given that all the other processing in this system I suggest does feel like something.

The adaptive value of having sensory and emotional feelings, or qualia, is thus suggested to be that such inputs are important to the long-term planning, explicit, processing system. Raw sensory feels, and subjective states associated with emotional and motivational states, may not necessarily arise first in evolution.

Reasons why the ventral visual system is more closely related to explicit than implicit processing include the fact that representations of objects and individuals need to enter the planning, hence conscious, system, and are considered in more detail by Rolls (2003) and by Rolls (2008b).

10.8.2 Oscillations and temporal binding

The postulate of Crick & Koch (1990) that oscillations and synchronization are necessary bases of consciousness might possibly be related to the present theory if it turns out that oscillations or neuronal synchronization are the way the brain implements syntactic binding. However, the fact that oscillations and neuronal synchronization are especially evident in anaesthetized cats does not impress as strong evidence that oscillations and synchronization are critical features of consciousness, for most people would hold that anaesthetized cats are not conscious. The fact that oscillations and stimulus-dependent neuronal synchronization are much more difficult to demonstrate in the temporal cortical visual areas of awake behaving monkeys (Tovee & Rolls 1992, Franco, Rolls, Aggelopoulos & Treves 2004, Aggelopoulos, Franco & Rolls 2005, Rolls 2008b, Rolls & Treves 2011) might just mean that during the evolution of primates the cortex has become better able to avoid parasitic oscillations, as a result of developing better feedforward and feedback inhibitory circuits (Rolls 2008b).

The suggestion that syntax in real neuronal networks is implemented by temporal binding (Malsburg 1990, Singer 1999) seems unlikely (Rolls 2008b, Rolls & Treves 2011). For example, the code about which visual stimulus has been shown can be read off from the end of the visual system without taking the temporal aspects of the neuronal firing into account; much of the information about which stimulus is shown is available in short times of 30–50 ms, and cortical neurons need fire for only this long during the identification of objects

(Tovee, Rolls, Treves & Bellis 1993, Rolls & Tovee 1994, Tovee & Rolls 1995, Rolls & Treves 1998, Rolls 2003, Rolls 2006a, Rolls 2008b, Rolls & Treves 2011) (these are rather short time-windows for the expression of multiple separate populations of synchronized neurons); and stimulus-dependent synchronization of firing between neurons is not a quantitatively important way of encoding information in the primate temporal cortical visual areas involved in the representation of objects and faces (Tovee & Rolls 1992, Rolls & Treves 1998, Rolls & Deco 2002, Rolls, Franco, Aggelopoulos & Reece 2003b, Rolls, Aggelopoulos, Franco & Treves 2004, Franco, Rolls, Aggelopoulos & Treves 2004, Aggelopoulos, Franco & Rolls 2005, Rolls 2008b, Rolls & Treves 2011, Rolls 2012e) – see Section A.1.6.

Further, even the hypothesis that information transmission is facilitated by coherent (phase locked) oscillations (communication through coherence (Fries 2005, Fries 2009)) has considerable difficulties (Rolls, Webb & Deco 2012), in that although there is much emphasis on finding coherence in the brain, there is much less causal evidence that coherence affects the transmission of information. In a test of this, it was found in an integrate-and-fire model of two connected networks in which causal effects of gamma oscillations (approximately 50 Hz) could be analysed, that information transmission between coupled networks occurs at very much lower strengths of the connecting synapses than are required to make the oscillations coherent (Rolls, Webb & Deco 2012). The finding was thus that information transmission does not require, and is little influenced by, gamma oscillations. The implication is that great care is needed to test whether coherence in the brain has causal effects in influencing information transmission, at least in the gamma band (Rolls, Webb & Deco 2012, Rolls & Treves 2011).

10.8.3 A high neural threshold for information to reach consciousness

Part in fact of Rolls' theory of consciousness is that it provides a computational reason why the threshold for information to reach consciousness is higher than the threshold for information to influence behaviour in what is referred to as subliminal processing (Dehaene, Changeux, Naccache, Sackur & Sergent 2006).

Evidence that explicit, conscious, processing may have a higher threshold in sensory processing than implicit processing is considered by Rolls (2003, 2006a, 2011a) based on neurophysiological and psychophysical investigations of backward masking (Rolls & Tovee 1994, Rolls, Tovee, Purcell, Stewart & Azzopardi 1994b, Rolls, Tovee & Panzeri 1999b, Rolls 2003, Rolls 2006a, Rolls 2008b, Rolls 2012e). It is suggested there that part of the adaptive value of this is that if linguistic processing is inherently serial and slow, it may be maladaptive to interrupt it unless there is a high probability that the interrupting signal does not arise from noise in the system. In the psychophysical and neurophysiological studies, it was found that face stimuli presented for 16 ms and followed immediately by a masking stimulus were not consciously perceived by humans, yet produced above chance identification, and firing of inferior temporal cortex neurons in macaques for approximately 30 ms. If the mask was delayed for 20 ms, the neurons fired for approximately 50 ms, and the test face stimuli were more likely to be perceived consciously. In a similar backward masking paradigm, it was found that happy vs angry face expressions could influence how much beverage was wanted and consumed even when the faces were not consciously perceived (Winkielman & Berridge 2005, Winkielman & Berridge 2003). This is further evidence that unconscious emotional stimuli can influence behaviour.

10.8.4 James–Lange theory and Damasio's somatic marker hypothesis about feelings

The theory described here is also different from other theories of consciousness and affect. James and Lange (James 1884, Lange 1885) held that emotional feelings arise when feedback from the periphery (about for example heart rate) reach the brain, but had no theory of why some stimuli and not others produced the peripheral changes, and thus of why some but not other events produce emotional feelings.

Moreover, the evidence that feedback from peripheral autonomic and proprioceptive systems is essential for emotions is very weak, in that for example blocking peripheral feedback does not eliminate emotions, and producing peripheral, e.g. autonomic, changes does not elicit emotion (Reisenzein 1983, Schachter & Singer 1962, Rolls 1999a) (see Section 2.6.1).

Damasio's theory of emotion (Damasio 1994, Damasio 2003) is a similar theory to the James–Lange theory (and is therefore subject to some of the same objections), but holds that the peripheral feedback is used in decision-making rather than in consciousness. He does not formally define emotions, but holds that body maps and representations are the basis of emotions. When considering consciousness, he assumes that all consciousness is self-consciousness (Damasio 2003) (p. 184), and that the foundational images in the stream of the mind are images of some kind of body event, whether the event happens in the depth of the body or in some specialized sensory device near its periphery (Damasio 2003) (p. 197). His theory does not appear to be a fully testable theory, in that he suspects that "the ultimate quality of feelings, a part of why feelings feel the way they feel, is conferred by the neural medium" (Damasio 2003) (p. 131). Thus presumably if the processes he discusses (Damasio 1994, Damasio 2003) were implemented in a computer, then the computer would not have all the same properties with respect to consciousness as the real brain. In this sense he appears to be arguing for a non-functionalist position, and something crucial about consciousness being related to the particular biological machinery from which the system is made. In this respect the theory seems somewhat intangible.

10.8.5 LeDoux's approach to emotion and consciousness

LeDoux's approach to emotion (LeDoux 1992, LeDoux 1995, LeDoux 1996, LeDoux 2008, LeDoux 2011) is largely (to quote him) one of automaticity, with emphasis on brain mechanisms involved in the rapid, subcortical, mechanisms involved in fear. LeDoux (1996), in line with Johnson-Laird (1988) and Baars (1988), emphasizes the role of working memory in consciousness, where he views working memory as a limited-capacity serial processor that creates and manipulates symbolic representations (p. 280). He thus holds that much emotional processing is unconscious, and that when it becomes conscious it is because emotional information is entered into a working memory system. However, LeDoux (1996) concedes that consciousness, especially its phenomenal or subjective nature, is not completely explained by the computational processes that underlie working memory (p. 281).

10.8.6 Panksepp's approach to emotion and consciousness

Panksepp's (1998) approach to emotion and consciousness has its origins in neuroethological investigations of brainstem systems that when activated lead to behaviours like fixed action patterns, including escape, flight and fear behaviour. A flavour of his views about consciousness includes his postulate that "feelings may emerge when endogenous sensory and emotional systems within the brain that receive direct inputs from the outside world as well as the neurodynamics of the SELF (a Simple Ego-type Life Form) begin to reverberate with each other's changing neuronal firing rhythms" (Panksepp 1998) (p. 309).

10.8.7 Global workspace theories of consciousness

Rolls' approach to consciousness suggests that the information must be being processed in a system capable of implementing HOSTs for the information to be conscious, and in this sense is more specific than global workspace hypotheses (Baars 1988, Dehaene & Naccache 2001, Dehaene et al. 2006). Indeed, the present approach suggests that a workspace could be sufficiently global to enable even the complex processing involved in driving a car to be performed, and yet the processing might be performed unconsciously, unless HOST (supervisory, monitory, correcting) processing was involved.

10.8.8 Monitoring and consciousness

An attractor network in the brain with positive feedback implemented by excitatory recurrent collateral connections between the neurons can implement decision-making (Wang 2002, Deco & Rolls 2006, Wang 2008, Rolls & Deco 2010) (see Chapter 8). As explained in detail elsewhere (Rolls & Deco 2010), if the external evidence for the decision is consistent with the decision taken (which has been influenced by the noisy neuronal firing times), then the firing rates in the winning attractor are supported by the external evidence, and become especially high. If the external evidence is contrary to the noise-influenced decision, then the firing rates of the neurons in the winning attractor are not supported by the external evidence, and are lower than expected (Fig. 8.15). In this way the confidence in a decision is reflected in, and encoded by, the firing rates of the neurons in the winning attractor population of neurons (Section 8.7) (Rolls & Deco 2010).

If we now add a second attractor network to read the firing rates from the first decision-making network, the second attractor network can take a decision based on the confidence expressed in the firing rates in the first network (Insabato, Pannunzi, Rolls & Deco 2010). The second attractor network allows decisions to be made about whether to change the decision made by the first network, and for example abort the trial or strategy (see Fig. 8.26). The second network, the confidence decision network, is in effect monitoring the decisions taken by the first network, and can cause a change of strategy or behaviour if the assessment of the decision taken by the first network does not seem a confident decision. This is described in detail elsewhere (Insabato, Pannunzi, Rolls & Deco 2010, Rolls & Deco 2010), but Fig. 8.26 shows the simple system of two attractor networks that enables confidence-based (second-level) decisions to be made, by monitoring the output of the first, decision-making, network.

Now this is the type of description, and language used, to describe 'monitoring' functions, taken to be a high-level cognitive process, possibly related to consciousness (Block 1995b, Lycan 1997). For example, in an experiment performed by Hampton (2001) (experiment 3), a monkey had to remember a picture over a delay. He was then given a choice of a 'test flag', in which case he would be allowed to choose from one of four pictures the one seen before the delay, and if correct earn a large reward (a peanut). If he was not sure that he remembered the first picture, he could choose an 'escape flag', to start another trial. With longer delays, when memory strength might be lower partly due to noise in the system, and confidence therefore in the memory on some trials might be lower, the monkey was more likely to choose the escape flag. The experiment is described as showing that the monkey is thinking about his own memory, that is, is a case of meta-memory, which may be related to consciousness (Heyes 2008). However, the decision about whether to escape from a trial can be taken just by adding a second decision network to the first decision network. Thus we can account for what seem like complex cognitive phenomena with a simple system of two attractor decision-making networks (Fig. 8.26) (Rolls & Deco 2010, Rolls 2012d).

The implication is that some types of 'self-monitoring' can be accounted for by simple, two-attractor network, computational processes. But what of more complex 'self-monitoring', such as is described as occurring in a commentary that might be based on reflection on previous events, and appears to be closely related to consciousness (Weiskrantz 1997). This approach has been developed into my higher-order syntactic theory (HOST) of consciousness (Section 10.2 (Rolls 1997b, Rolls 2004d, Rolls 2005b, Rolls 2007b, Rolls 2008c, Rolls 2007g, Rolls 2010a, Rolls 2011a, Rolls 2012d)), in which there is a credit assignment problem if a multi-step reasoned plan fails, and it may be unclear which step failed. Such plans are described as syntactic as there are symbols at each stage that must be linked together with the syntactic relationships between the symbols specified, but kept separate across stages of the plan. It is suggested that in this situation being able to have higher-order syntactic thoughts will enable one to think and reason about the first-order plan, and detect which steps are likely to be at fault.

Now this type of 'self-monitoring' is much more complex, as it requires syntax. The thrust of the argument is that some types of 'self-monitoring' are computationally simple, for example in decisions made based on confidence in a first decision (Rolls & Deco 2010), and may have little to do with consciousness; whereas higher-order thought processes are very different in terms of the type of syntactic computation required, and may be more closely related to consciousness (Rolls 1997b, Rolls 2003, Rolls 2004d, Rolls 2005b, Rolls 2007b, Rolls 2008c, Rolls 2007g, Rolls 2010a, Rolls 2011a, Rolls 2012d).

Thus the theory of consciousness described in this chapter is different from some other theories of consciousness.

11 Conclusions, and broader issues

11.1 Conclusions

Let us evaluate where we have reached in this book, before we consider some broader issues, including the background that this biological approach to emotion provides for understanding some issues that arise in aesthetics, ethics, and economics, which are developed further in *Neuroculture: On the Implications of Brain Science* (Rolls 2012d).

1. We have a scientific approach to emotion, its nature, and its functions (Chapters 2 and 3). It has been shown that this approach can help with classifying different emotions (Chapter 2), and in understanding what information processing systems in the brain are involved in emotion, and how they are involved (Chapters 4–6).

2. We have reached a quite specific view about how brains are designed around reward and punishment value systems, because this is the way that genes can build a complex system that will produce appropriate but flexible behaviour to increase their fitness, as described in Chapter 3. The way that evolution by natural selection does this is to build us with reward and punishment systems that will direct our behaviour towards goals in such a way that survival and in particular reproductive fitness are achieved. By specifying goals, rather than particular responses, genes leave much more open the possible behavioural strategies that might be required to increase their fitness. Specifying particular responses would be inefficient in terms of behavioural flexibility as environments change during evolution, and also would be more genetically costly to specify (in terms of the information to be encoded and the possibility of error). This view of the evolutionarily adaptive value for genes to build organisms using reward- and punishment-decoding and action systems in the brain places one squarely in line as a scientist from Darwin, and is a key part of my theory of emotion that will I envisage stand the test of time.

The theory helps us to understand much of sensory information processing in the brain, followed by reward and punishment value encoding, followed by action selection to obtain the goals identified by the sensory/reinforcer decoding systems. Value coding systems must be separate from purely sensory or motor systems, and while a goal is being sought, or if a goal is not obtained, the value-related representation must remain to direct further goal-directed behaviour, and it is these continuing goal-related states to which emotion is related.

3. The importance of reward and punishment systems in brain design helps us to understand not only the significance and importance of emotion, but also of motivational behaviour, which frequently involves working to obtain goals that are specified by the current state of internal signals to achieve homeostasis (see Chapter 5 on hunger and Rolls (2005b) on thirst) or are influenced by internal hormonal signals (Chapter 7 on sexual behaviour). Indeed, motivation may be seen as a state in which one is working for a goal, and emotion as a state that occurs when the goal, a reinforcer, is obtained or is not obtained, and that may persist afterwards. The concept of gene-defined reinforcers providing the goals for action helps to understand the relation between motivational states (or desires) and emotion, as the organism must be built to be motivated to obtain the goals, and to be placed in a different state (emotion) when the goal is or is not achieved by the action. Emotional states may be motivating, as in frustrative non-reward. The close but clear relation between motivation and emotion is that both involve what humans describe as affective states (e.g. feeling hungry, liking the taste of a food, feeling happy because of a social reinforcer), and both are about goals.

4. We have outlined in Chapters 4–6 what may be the fundamental architectural and design principles of the brain for sensory, reward value, and punishment value information processing in primates *including humans*. These architectural principles include the following:

(a) For potential secondary reinforcers, analysis is to the stage of invariant object identification before reward and punisher associations are learned. The reason for this is to enable correct generalization to other instances of the same or similar objects, even when a reward or punisher has been associated with one instance previously.

(b) The representation of the object is (appropriately) in a form that is ideal as an input to pattern associators that allow the reinforcement associations to be learned. The representations are appropriately encoded in that they can be decoded by dot product decoding of the type that is very neuronally plausible; are distributed so allowing excellent generalization and graceful degradation; have relatively independent information conveyed by different neurons in the ensemble thus allowing very high capacity; and allow much of the information to be read off very quickly, in periods of 20–50 ms (see Chapter 4, Appendix A, and Rolls (2008b) and Rolls & Treves (2011)).

(c) An aim of processing in the ventral visual system (which projects to the inferior temporal visual cortex) is to help select the goals, or objects with reward or punisher associations, for actions. Action is concerned with the identification and selection of goals, for action, in the environment. The ventral visual system is crucially involved in this. I thus disagree with Milner & Goodale (1995) that the dorsal visual system is for the control of action, and the ventral visual system for 'perception', e.g. perceptual and cognitive representations. The ventral visual system is concerned with selecting the goals for action. It does this by providing invariant representations of objects, with a representation that is appropriate for interfacing to systems [such as the amygdala and orbitofrontal cortex, see Chapter 4, and Figs. 4.2 and 4.3, and 10.4 in which association cortex would correspond in vision to the inferior temporal visual cortex] which determine using pattern association the reward or punishment value of the object, as part of the process of selecting which goal is appropriate for action. Some of the evidence for this described in Chapter 4 is that large lesions of the temporal lobes (which damage the ventral visual system and some of its outputs such as the amygdala) produce the Kluver-Bucy syndrome, in which monkeys select objects indiscriminately, independently of their reward value, and place them in their mouths. The dorsal visual system helps with executing those actions, for example with shaping the hand appropriately to pick up a selected object. (Often this type of sensori-motor operation is performed implicitly, i.e. without conscious awareness.) In so far as explicit planning about future goals and actions requires knowledge of objects and their reward or punisher associations, it is the ventral visual system that provides the appropriate input for planning future actions. Further, for the same reason, I propose that when explicit, or conscious, planning is required, activity in the ventral visual system will be closely related to consciousness, because it is to objects, represented in the ventral visual system, that we normally apply multi-step planning processes.

(d) For primary reinforcers, the reward decoding may occur after several stages of processing, as in the primate taste system in which reward is decoded only after the primary taste cortex. The architectural principle here is that in primates there is one main taste information-processing stream in the brain, via the thalamus to the primary taste cortex, and the information about the identity of the taste is not biased by modulation of how good the taste is before this, so that the taste representation in the primary cortex can be used for purposes that are not reward-dependent. One example might be learning where a particular taste can be found in the environment, even when the primate is not hungry and therefore the taste is not currently rewarding. In the case of other sensory systems, the reinforcement value may be made explicit early on in sensory processing. This occurs, for example, in the pain system. The architectural basis of this is that there are different channels (nerve fibres) for pain and touch, so that the affective value and the identity of a tactile stimulus can be carried by separate parallel information channels, allowing separate representation and processing of each.

(e) In non-primates including, for example, rodents, the design principles may involve less sophisticated design features, partly because the stimuli being processed are simpler. For example, view-invariant object recognition is probably much less developed in non-primates, with the recognition that is possible being based more on physical similarity in terms of texture, colour, simple features, etc. (Rolls & Deco 2002, Rolls 2008b). It may be because there is less sophisticated cortical processing of visual stimuli in this way that other sensory systems are also organized more simply in rodents, with, for example, some (but not total, only perhaps 30%) modulation of taste processing by hunger early in sensory processing in rodents (Scott, Yan & Rolls 1995, Rolls & Scott 2003) (Section 1.3). Further, while it is appropriate usually to have emotional responses to well-processed objects (e.g. the sight of a particular person), there are instances, such as a loud noise or a pure tone associated with punishment, where it may be possible to tap off a sensory representation early in sensory information processing that can be used to produce emotional responses, and this may occur, for example, in rodents, where the subcortical auditory system provides afferents to the amygdala (see Chapter 4).

(f) Another design principle is that the outputs of the reward and punishment value systems must be treated by the action system as being the goals for action. The action systems must be built to try to maximize the activation of the representations produced by rewarding events, and to minimize the activation of the representations produced by punishers or stimuli associated with punishers. Drug addiction produced by the psychomotor stimulants such as amphetamine and cocaine can be seen as activating the brain at the stage where the outputs of the amygdala and orbitofrontal cortex, which provide representations of whether stimuli are associated with rewards or punishers, are fed into the ventral striatum to influence approach behaviour. The fact that addiction is persistent may be related to the fact that because the outputs of the amygdala and orbitofrontal cortex are after the stage of stimulus–reinforcer learning, and after sensory-specific satiety as been computed, the action system has to be built to interpret the representations they provide as meaning reward value, and a goal for action.

5. Especially in primates, the visual processing in emotional and social behaviour requires sophisticated representation of individuals, and for this there are many neurons devoted to face processing (Rolls 2011c). In addition, there is a separate system that encodes face gesture, movement, and view, as all are important in social behaviour, for interpreting whether a particular individual, with his or her own reinforcement associations, is producing threats or appeasements (Rolls 2011c, Rolls 2012e).

6. After mainly unimodal processing to the object level, sensory systems then project into convergence zones. Those especially important for reward and punishment, emotion and motivation, are the orbitofrontal cortex and amygdala, where primary reinforcers are represented to encode **outcome value**. These parts of the brain appear to be especially important in emotion and motivation not only because they are the parts of the brain where in primates the primary (unlearned) reinforcing value of stimuli is represented, but also because they are the parts of the brain that perform pattern-association learning between potential secondary reinforcers and primary reinforcers to compute **expected value**. They are thus the parts of the brain involved in learning the emotional and motivational **reward value** of stimuli.

The orbitofrontal cortex is involved in the rapid, one-trial, reversal of emotional behaviour when the reinforcement contingencies change, and this may be implemented by switching a rule, as described in Section 4.5.7. These orbitofrontal cortex neurons may be described as *expected value* neurons. This rapid, rule-based, reversal and re-valuation of stimuli to encode their current reward value in one trial and using rules may be a computation made possible by the development of the granular orbitofrontal cortex and connected areas that are not present in rodents (Section 1.3).

7. The different reward valuation systems are specified to have values scaled appropriately by genes to lead to their selection in such a way that reproductive success is maximized. In addition, the reward systems are specific, encode the value of specific rewards and punishers, and have tendencies to self-regulate, so that they operate on a common value scale that leads to the selection of different rewards with appropriately balanced probabilities, and often depending on modulation by internal motivational signals. The presence of many different reward value systems operating with a **common scale of value** helps each reward to be selected to maximize reproductive success. There is no conversion to a common currency, as this would no longer encode the specific reward to which the action system should direct action. The value of a reward or punisher specified by genes may be rescaled by learning, as in taste aversion learning (Scott 2011) and conditioned appetite and satiety (Booth 1985).

8. A principle that assists the selection of different behaviours is sensory-specific satiety, which builds up when a reward is repeated for a number of minutes. A principle that helps behaviour to lock on to one goal for at least a useful period is incentive motivation, the process by which early on in the presentation of a reward there is reward potentiation. There are probably simple neurophysiological bases for these time-dependent processes in the reward (as opposed to the early sensory) systems that involve synaptic habituation and (non-associative) facilitation respectively.

9. With the advances made in the last 30 years in understanding the brain mechanisms involved in reward and punishment, and emotion and motivation, the basis for addiction to drugs is becoming clearer, with dopamine playing an important role, particularly in the conditioned reinforcing effects of stimuli associated with drug usage, which influence 'wanting' for the addictive substance. Further, now that we are starting to understand how different brain systems contribute to emotion, this provides a better foundation for developing pharmacological treatments for depression and anxiety that may target particular brain areas (Chapter 6).

10. The representation in the orbitofrontal cortex appears indeed to represent economic value, in that neuronal responses and neural activations appear to be related closely to what is chosen, and also to the conscious subjective value or pleasantness rating placed on a 'good'. The orbitofrontal cortex activity reflects by these measures of **economic value** the effects of risk (the probability that a reward will be available), of ambiguity (whether the outcome probability is known), of temporal discounting, and of the tradeoff between the amount of the good that is available and the value of the good. Value is represented on a continuous scale in the orbitofrontal cortex, and indeed orbitofrontal cortex activations are linearly related to the subjective pleasantness (medially) or unpleasantness (laterally) of stimuli or events.

11. The reward value placed on different rewards and the punishment value placed on different non-rewards or punishers will be different between different individuals, as a result of genetic variation for natural selection. Also, most humans cannot perform economic calculations of the expected value of different choices, as the human brain operates primarily by similarity comparisons and not by logical calculations of the type implemented in computers (Rolls 2008b, Rolls 2012d). For these reasons, classical microeconomics with its approach of a few axioms and a rational actor can no longer be considered as what really may account for the behaviour of humans and other animals. Instead, classical (micro)economics may be replaced by an understanding in neuroeconomics of how heuristics guided by evolution make different rewards and costs become differently scaled in different individuals, and further how choices may be selected by a decision-making process based on in-built and probabilistic heuristics rather than by correctly computed calculations in a rational, reasoning, decision-making actor.

12. The orbitofrontal cortex represents the value of stimuli. Its neurons respond to stimulus value, and not to behavioural responses. The orbitofrontal cortex provides outputs to:

(a) the anterior cingulate cortex for goal-directed actions taking into account the costs of the actions (Sections 4.6.1.2 and 4.7), and for which positive value is represented in the pregenual anterior cingulate cortex and negative value more dorsally, for interfacing to motor / action representations in the mid-cingulate cortex;

(b) the basal ganglia for stimulus-response habits (Sections 4.6.1.2, 6.3 and 6.8);

(c) with the amygdala implements Pavlovian learning processes which enable stimuli to elicit approach or withdrawal as well as affective states which may become the goals for instrumental actions;

(d) with the amygdala implements Pavlovian learning processes which enable autonomic and endocrine responses to be elicited by conditioned stimuli (Section 4.6.1.1).

13. Decision-making is now understood as a non-linear competition between different attractor states in an attractor neuronal network that results in a single winner. The decision variables bias the neurons in the different possible attractor states. The mechanism is understood at the level of integrate-and-fire neurons with biophysically realistic parameters. The decision-making is probabilistic because of statistical fluctuations introduced by the approximately Poisson nature of the timing of the spikes of the neurons for a given mean firing rate.

This understanding is replacing the artificial drift-diffusion mathematical models of decision-making with fitted parameters, not only because the attractor model is more realistic, but also because it allows the exploration of how biological parameters such as ion channel conductances and the effects of different transmitters expressed through different ion channels influence the operation and stability of the decision-making system. This is enabling medically relevant implications to be investigated, for example to neuropsychiatric disorders including schizophrenia and obsessive-compulsive disorder (Sections 8.11.12 and 8.11.13).

14. The attractor approach to decision-making is a unifying approach, for the same mechanism applies not only to decision-making, but also to the operation of short-term memory systems, to the recall of information from long-term memory systems, and to top-down attention (Rolls 2008b). Part of the basis for this is that attractor states are a natural property of cortical systems, which are characterized by excitatory local recurrent collaterals which implement positive feedback; associative synaptic plasticity of these connections; and inhibition between the neurons implemented by GABA neurons (Rolls 2008b).

15. The probabilistic operation of the decision-making process caused by the spiking-related statistical fluctuations in finite-sized neuronal networks has many advantages, including different decisions and memory recall on different occasions even with similar inputs, giving rise to non-deterministic behaviour of the system. This probabilistic behaviour has a useful impact in many situations, including sometimes choosing less favourable options to update knowledge, predator avoidance, social interactions, and creativity (Rolls & Deco 2010). The probabilistic behaviour of the mechanism also makes the brain non-deterministic, and there are implications for free-will.

16. These non-linear decision-making attractor networks that result not only in 'decisions' but also in categorization are found in many parts of the cortex, typically after earlier stages of more linear processing performing analysis of the stimulus. There is not therefore just one decision-maker in the brain, but multiple decision processes for different types of decision. One type of decision for example is the direction of global optic flow made in the dorsal visual system (Rolls 2008b, Rolls & Deco 2010). In the context of value and hence emotion systems, there is evidence that the more anterior, ventromedial parts of the prefrontal cortex (vmPFC), including medial prefrontal cortex area 10, are involved in the decision-making between stimuli of different value, and follow in the hierarchy the more linear representation of reward value in the orbitofrontal cortex.

17. With respect to the dopamine system, it appears that the activity of the dopamine neurons does not represent reward, and is not correlated with hedonic or emotional states (see Chapter 6). Part of the evidence for this is that the dopamine neurons may fire in relation to a reward prediction error, rather than in relation to reward itself, and that damage to the dopaminergic system does not impair hedonic responses or 'liking'. Dopamine pathways do influence systems involved in Pavlovian (classically conditioned) incentive salience effects mediated by the ventral striatum, and may thereby influence 'wanting'. However, there are inconsistencies with the dopamine reward prediction error hypothesis, with respect for example to whether the dopamine system is implicated in salience (as many dopamine neurons respond to aversive, novel, and alerting stimuli) vs reward error prediction, and whether a reward prediction error signal could facilitate the learning of stimuli associated with punishment (see Chapter 6 and Section 6.3.7).

18. In addition to the implicit system for action selection, in humans and perhaps related animals there is also an explicit system that can use language to compute actions to obtain deferred rewards using a one-off plan. The language system enables one-off multistep plans that require the syntactic organization of symbols to be formulated in order to obtain rewards and avoid punishers. There are thus two separate systems for producing actions to rewarding and punishing stimuli in humans and potentially in related animals. These systems may weight different courses of action differently, and produce conflict in decision-making, in that each can produce behaviour for different goals (immediate vs long-term goals involving multiple step planning). Understanding our evolutionary history is useful in enabling us to understand our emotional decision-making processes, and the conflicts that may be inherent in how they operate.

19. It is argued that the decisions taken by the emotional system are in the interests of selfish genes, in which the value systems have their foundations. The reasoning, rational, system enables longer-term decisions to be taken by planning ahead, and for the decisions to be in the interests of the individual, the phenotype, instead of the genes. This is another important sense (additional to the sense that genes and environment usually make joint contributions) in which the behaviour of humans and other animals with reasoning systems can be said to be not determined by our genes.

This rational, reasoning, 'explicit' decision-making system provides a basis for the operation of societies in which social contracts underpinned by reasoned understanding provide a basis for stability, and for gene-specified emotional value systems not to provide the only goal (Rolls 2012d). Understanding the emotional system is very important, for it has major influences on behaviour, and helps us to understand not only individual differences and personality, but also influences on behaviour that may have their origins partly in the different interests of males and females (Chapter 7). Understanding the emotional and the rational systems, and their very different types of computation, has many implications for understanding processes as far ranging as aesthetics, economics, politics, and religion (Rolls 2012d).

20. Pleasure is a subjective state reported in humans that is associated with a reward. Just as reward is specific, with many different types of reward, so is pleasure. It is possible that emotional feelings (including pleasure), part of the much larger problem of consciousness, arise as part of a process that involves thoughts about thoughts, which have the adaptive value of helping to correct one-off multistep plans. This is the approach described in Chapter 10, but there seems to be no clear way to choose which theory of consciousness is moving in the right direction, and caution must be exercised here, and current theories should not be taken to have implications.

21. Functional neuroimaging and neuropsychological data in humans (see Chapters 4 and 6) are consistent with many of the conclusions based on primate data including neurophysiology which provide the fundamental evidence needed to make computational models of how the brain functions as an information processing system exchanging information between its computing elements, the neurons (see Appendices A and B and Rolls (2008b)). In addition, the human findings provide interesting new evidence on how top-down cognitive and attentional effects can influence emotions in areas such as the orbitofrontal and anterior cingulate cortex (Section 4.5.5.7). The mechanisms by which cognitive states have top-down effects on emotion are probably similar to the biased competition mechanisms that subserve top-down attentional effects (Rolls & Deco 2002, Deco & Rolls 2003, Deco & Rolls 2005c, Rolls 2008b), though whole linked processing streams of cortical processing may be influenced in a top-down biased activation process (Rolls 2013a) (see also Section 4.12).

22. In relation to animal welfare, the suggestion arises that in addition to being guided by health, it may be useful to be guided by how the animals set their priorities for different rewards and punishers. This follows from the hypothesis that the brain is designed round reward/punisher evaluation systems, and behaviour optimizes obtaining the goals defined by the genes. The degree to which different genes make different reinforcers important, and how they depend on for example motivational state, then directly influence the value the animal places on a provision. The value or choice of the reinforcer thus provides a useful measure of its 'importance to the animal'. When making these measures of the value of different instrumental reinforcers, it is important to be aware of the many factors that can influence the selection of a reinforcer. Examples are the fact that the choice of a reinforcer is very sensitive to incentive motivational effects, priming, delay of reinforcement, and shows rapid extinction if the reinforcer is of low value, as shown by the behaviour when tested under zero drive conditions (Rolls 2005b). We may also note that the reinforcer value systems in the brain are generally different to the systems involved in autonomic and endocrine responses (see Chapter 4). The implication is that the systems (for reinforcer value vs autonomic/endocrine responses) have evolved separately, and that the autonomic/endocrine responses elicited in emotion-provoking situations may not necessarily be a good guide to the instrumental reinforcing value (as measured by choice) or 'importance' of the resource to the animal.

23. The processes and systems involved in emotion have evolved considerably. Some of the principles described in this book include the following:
1. There may be no cortical area in rodents that is homologous to most of the primate including human orbitofrontal cortex (Wise 2008).
2. The primate including human orbitofrontal cortex (OFC) implements reward value, as shown by devaluation experiments such as feeding to satiety.
3. Value is not represented at earlier stages of processing in primates including humans. Invariant visual object recognition is used for many functions including memory formation, so perception is kept separate from emotion.
4. In contrast, in rodents, value is represented even in the first taste relay in the brain, the nucleus of the solitary tract: there is no clear separation between perception and emotion. In rodents, even the taste pathways are connected differently, with subcortical connections bypassing the cortex (including orbitofrontal cortex) and making connections via a pontine taste area directly to the hypothalamus and amygdala.
5. In primates and humans, the orbitofrontal cortex implements one-trial rule-based reversal learning, and this is important in rapidly updating social behaviour. This is rapid updating of value-based representations. Maintaining the current rule in short-term memory and using this to bias neurons in the orbitofrontal cortex (Deco & Rolls 2005a) may be one computation that granular prefrontal cortex facilitates. Rodents may not be able to perform this.
6. The value representation in the primate and human orbitofrontal cortex is domain general, in that the amount and value of goods, and temporal discounting, operate transitively (as shown by trade-offs), providing a basis for economic decision-making. There is evidence that this is not the case in rodents.
7. Goal value-directed choice is usual in primates and humans, whereas fixed action patterns such as pecking in birds are more common elsewhere.
8. Goal-directed choice may be the best measure of value and emotion, for there are many partly separate neural circuits for different emotion-related responses, e.g. autonomic output, freezing, fixed action patterns, and unconditioned approach or withdrawal.
9. In humans, and perhaps some primates, syntactic reasoning and thereby planning allows selfish gene-specified (emotion-related) rewards to be rejected in favour of the long-term interests of the individual, the phenotype.

11.2 Decision-making

We have shown how rewards and punishers provide a basis for understanding emotion. Rewards and punishers, and emotion, are important in decision-making. I integrate some of the themes of this book by showing how there are different types of choice or decision that are made about rewards and punishers (see also Cardinal et al. (2002), Berridge & Robinson (2003) and Rolls (2008b)), and how emotion is related to these different types of decision (see Fig. 10.4).

11.2.1 Selection of mainly autonomic responses, and their classical conditioning

Responses produced by primary rewards and punishers, such as salivation, a change of heart rate, or arousal, can become classically conditioned (see Section 4.6.1.1 on page 160), and this is a form of stimulus–response (CS–UCS) learning. These responses are important for fitness, and are being selected, but hardly merit the term 'decision'. Brain regions such as the amygdala, orbitofrontal cortex, and anterior cingulate cortex are involved in these responses.

11.2.2 Selection of approach or withdrawal, and their classical conditioning; fixed action patterns

Rewards and punishers also lead to approach or withdrawal, and these effects can be classically conditioned (see Section 4.6.1.1). This is an important way in which genes can influence the behaviour that is selected, and this might be thought of as a very simple, automated, 'decision'. However, there is little flexibility in the response that is selected, in that the behaviour is either approach (e.g. to a sweet taste), or withdrawal/rejection (e.g. to a bitter taste), and in this sense behaviour is being selected by the reinforcer, but the 'decision' is essentially an automated type of behaviour. This type of approach behaviour to rewards can be classically conditioned, resulting in conditioned 'incentive salience' or 'wanting' effects (Berridge & Robinson 1998, Berridge & Robinson 2003), and this learning is implemented via the amygdala and ventral striatum, is under control of dopamine (Cardinal et al. 2002), and contributes to addiction (Robinson & Berridge 2003). Fixed action patterns, such as pecking for grain in birds, or pecking by chicks at a releasing stimulus such as a red spot on the herring gulls' beak to obtain food (Tinbergen 1951, Tinbergen 1963, Panksepp 1998) do not require intervening emotional states of the type required for action–outcome goal-directed instrumental learning.

11.2.3 Selection of fixed stimulus–response habits

Stimulus–response connections can be reinforced by rewards or punishers to produce fixed habits (see Section 4.6.1.2 on page 162). Habits typically arise when behavioural responses are overlearned, and it is suggested that action–outcome learning sets up the correct stimulus–response conditions for a habit learning system to implement fixed responses to stimuli (Section 4.6.1.2). Once a habit has been learned, we may think of the behavioural selection as being a rather fixed type of 'decision'. The basal ganglia may be especially involved in habit learning (see Sections 6.3 and 6.3.7), though it does receive inputs that may be important in this process from the amygdala and orbitofrontal cortex. Reinforcement learning (see Section A.5) using reward prediction errors implemented in dopamine neuron firing may or not be important in this habit learning (see Sections 6.3 and 6.3.7).

11.2.4 Selection of arbitrary behaviours to obtain goals, action–outcome learning, and emotional learning

The real power of emotion, and rewards and punishers, occurs when goals for actions are specified by genes, and arbitrary actions can then be performed (instrumentally) to achieve the goals (see Chapters 2 and 3). The type of learning is action–outcome learning (see Sections 4.6.1.2, 4.7 and 6.8). Motivated behaviour is made to obtain, terminate or avoid the goal, and when the reward or punisher is or is not obtained, terminated, or avoided, emotional states occur that may be further motivating. Although in evolution Darwinian processes lead to gene-defined goals, it is also the case that in humans goals may be generated by other processes, including cultural processes.

The orbitofrontal cortex is important in representing the rewards and punishers, and in performing rapid stimulus–reinforcer association learning and reversal. This is the fundamental type of learning involved in producing learned emotional or affective states, and is stimulus–stimulus learning.

The orbitofrontal cortex is thus very important in emotion and affective states. The orbitofrontal cortex is not itself involved in action–outcome association learning, in that actions appear not to be represented in the orbitofrontal cortex (see Section 4.5). It is important for action–outcome learning though, in that it represents the affective outcomes. Brain regions such as the cingulate cortex may be involved in action–outcome association learning (see Section 4.7.5), and receive inputs about the outcomes, and predicted outcomes, from the orbitofrontal cortex.

11.2.5 The roles of the prefrontal cortex in the selection of action, in decision-making, and in attention

First we consider the functions of the dorsolateral prefrontal cortex in short-term memory. Then we consider how this functionality enables the dorsolateral prefrontal cortex to participate in certain types of decision-making, selection of action, and top-down attention that require a short-term or working memory.

A common way that the brain implements a short-term memory is to maintain the firing of neurons during a short memory period after the end of a stimulus (Fuster 2000, Fuster 2008, Goldman-Rakic 1995, Rolls 2008b) (Section A.3). In the inferior temporal cortex this firing may be maintained for a few hundred ms even when the monkey is not performing a memory task (Rolls & Tovee 1994, Rolls, Tovee, Purcell, Stewart & Azzopardi 1994b, Rolls, Tovee & Panzeri 1999b, Desimone 1996). In more ventral temporal cortical areas such as the entorhinal cortex the firing may be maintained for longer periods in delayed match to sample tasks (Suzuki, Miller & Desimone 1997), and in the prefrontal cortex for even tens of seconds (Fuster 2000, Fuster 2008). In the dorsolateral (area 46) and inferior convexity (area 12/47) prefrontal cortex (for diagram see Fig. 4.1 on page 68) the firing of the neurons may be related to the memory of spatial responses or objects (Goldman-Rakic 1996, Wilson, O'Sclaidhe & Goldman-Rakic 1993) or both (Rao, Rainer & Miller 1997), and in the principal sulcus / arcuate sulcus region to the memory of places for eye movements (Funahashi, Bruce & Goldman-Rakic 1989). The firing may be maintained by the operation of associatively modified recurrent collateral connections between nearby pyramidal cells producing attractor states in autoassociative networks (see Section A.3).

For the short-term memory to be maintained during periods in which new stimuli are to be perceived, there must be separate networks for the perceptual and short-term memory functions, and indeed two coupled networks (with one in the inferior temporal visual cortex for perceptual functions, and another in the prefrontal cortex for maintaining the short-term memory during intervening stimuli) provide a precise model of the interaction of perceptual and short-term memory systems (Renart, Parga & Rolls 2000, Renart, Moreno, Rocha, Parga & Rolls 2001, Rolls 2008b) (see Fig. 11.1). In particular, this model shows how a prefrontal cortex attractor (autoassociation) network could be triggered by a sample visual stimulus represented in the inferior temporal visual cortex in a delayed match to sample task, and could keep this attractor active during a memory interval in which intervening stimuli are shown. Then when the sample stimulus reappears in the task as a match stimulus, the inferior temporal cortex module shows a large response to the match stimulus, because it is activated both by the visual incoming match stimulus, and by the consistent backprojected memory of the sample stimulus still being represented in the prefrontal cortex memory module (see Fig. 11.1).

This computational model makes it clear that in order for ongoing perception to occur unhindered in posterior cortex (parietal and temporal lobe) networks, there must be a separate set of modules that is capable of maintaining a representation over intervening stimuli. This is

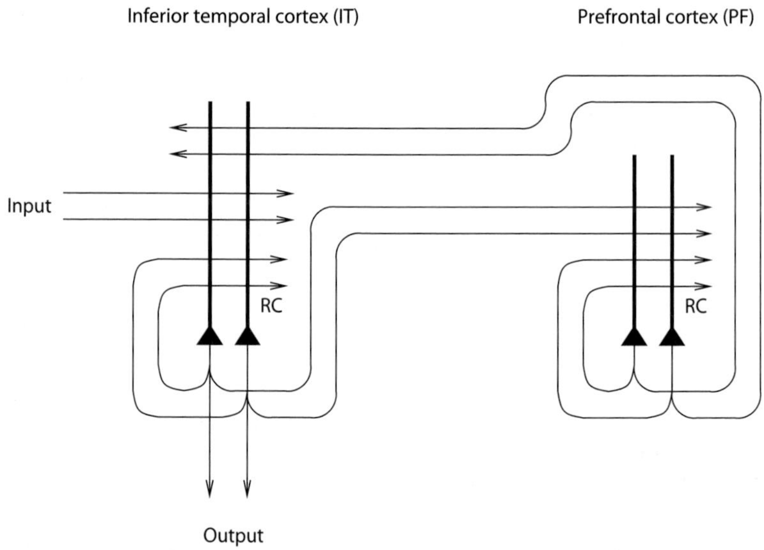

Fig. 11.1 A short-term memory autoassociation network in the prefrontal cortex could hold active a working memory representation by maintaining its firing in an attractor state. The prefrontal module would be loaded with the to-be-remembered stimulus by the posterior module (in the temporal or parietal cortex) in which the incoming stimuli are represented. Backprojections from the prefrontal short-term memory module to the posterior module would enable the working memory to be unloaded, to for example influence on-going perception (see text). RC – recurrent collateral connections.

the fundamental understanding offered for the evolution and functions of the dorsolateral prefrontal cortex, and it is this ability to provide multiple separate short-term attractor memories that provides I suggest the basis for its functions in planning (Rolls 2008b).

Renart, Parga & Rolls (2000) and Renart, Moreno, Rocha, Parga & Rolls (2001) performed analyses and simulations which showed that for working memory to be implemented in this way, the connections between the perceptual and the short-term memory modules (see Fig. 11.1) must be relatively weak. As a starting point, they used the neurophysiological data showing that in delayed match to sample tasks with intervening stimuli, the neuronal activity in the inferior temporal visual cortex (IT) is driven by each new incoming visual stimulus (Miller, Li & Desimone 1993, Miller & Desimone 1994), whereas in the prefrontal cortex, neurons start to fire when the sample stimulus is shown, and continue the firing that represents the sample stimulus even when the potential match stimuli are being shown (Miller, Erickson & Desimone 1996). The architecture studied by Renart, Parga & Rolls (2000) was as shown in Fig. 11.1, with both the intramodular (recurrent collateral) and the intermodular (forward IT to PF, and backward PF to IT) connections trained on the set of patterns with an associative synaptic modification rule. A crucial parameter is the strength of the intermodular connections, g, which indicates the relative strength of the intermodular to the intramodular connections. (This parameter measures effectively the relative strengths of the currents injected into the neurons by the inter-modular relative to the intra-modular connections, and the importance of setting this parameter to relatively weak values for useful interactions between coupled attractor networks was highlighted by Renart, Parga & Rolls (1999a) and Renart, Parga & Rolls (1999b), as shown in Section A.4.) The patterns themselves were sets of random numbers, and the simulation utilized a dynamical approach with neurons with continuous (hyperbolic tangent) activation functions (see (Shiino & Fukai 1990, Kuhn 1990, Kuhn, Bos & van Hemmen 1991, Amit & Tsodyks 1991)). The external current injected into IT by the incoming

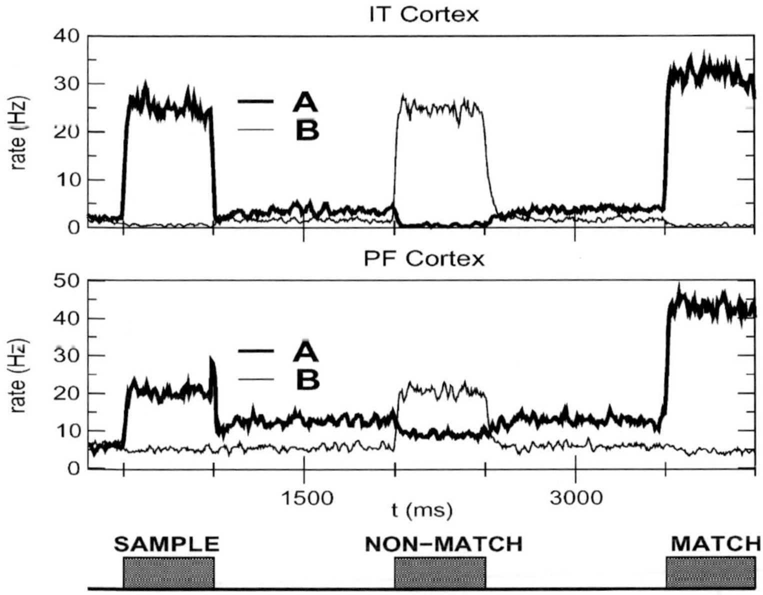

Fig. 11.2 Interaction between the prefrontal cortex (PF) and the inferior temporal cortex (IT) in a delayed match to sample task with intervening stimuli with the architecture illustrated in Fig. 11.1. Above: activity in the IT attractor module. Below: activity in the PF attractor module. The thick lines show the firing rates of the set of neurons with activity selective for the Sample stimulus (which is also shown as the Match stimulus, and is labelled **A**), and the thin lines the activity of the neurons with activity selective for the Non-Match stimulus, which is shown as an intervening stimulus between the Sample and Match stimulus and is labelled **B**. A trial is illustrated in which **A** is the Sample (and Match) stimulus. The prefrontal cortex module is pushed into an attractor state for the sample stimulus by the IT activity induced by the sample stimulus. Because of the weak coupling to the PF module from the IT module, the PF module remains in this Sample-related attractor state during the delay periods, and even while the IT module is responding to the non-match stimulus. The PF module remains in its Sample-related state even during the Non-Match stimulus because once a module is in an attractor state, it is relatively stable. When the Sample stimulus reappears as the Match stimulus, the PF module shows higher Sample stimulus-related firing, because the incoming input from IT is now adding to the activity in the PF attractor network. This in turn also produces a match enhancement effect in the IT neurons with Sample stimulus-related selectivity, because the backprojected activity from the PF module matches the incoming activity to the IT module. (Reprinted from *Neurocomputing*, 38-40, Alfonso Renart, Ruben Moreno, Jaime de la Rocha, Nestor Parga, and Edmund T Rolls, A model of the IT–PF network in object working memory which includes balanced persistent activity and tuned inhibition, pp. 1525–31, Copyright (2001), with permission from Elsevier.)

visual stimuli was sufficiently strong to trigger the IT module into a state representing the incoming stimulus. When the sample was shown, the initially silent PF module was triggered into activity by the weak ($g > 0.002$) intermodular connections. The PF module remained firing to the sample stimulus even when IT was responding to potential match stimuli later in the trial, provided that g was less than 0.024, because then the intramodular recurrent connections could dominate the firing (see Fig. 11.2). If g was higher than this, then the PF module was pushed out of the attractor state produced by the sample stimulus. The IT module responded to each incoming potentially matching stimulus provided that g was not greater than approximately 0.024. Moreover, this value of g was sufficiently large that a larger response of the IT module was found when the stimulus matched the sample stimulus (the match enhancement effect found neurophysiologically, and a mechanism by which the matching stimulus can be identified). This simple model thus shows that the operation of the prefrontal cortex in short-term memory tasks such as delayed match to sample with intervening stimuli, and its relation to posterior perceptual networks, can be understood by the interaction of two weakly coupled attractor networks, as shown in Figs. 11.1 and 11.2.

This approach emphasizes that in order to provide a good brain lesion test of prefrontal cortex short-term memory functions, the task set should require a short-term memory for stimuli over an interval in which other stimuli are being processed, because otherwise the posterior cortex perceptual modules could implement the short-term memory function by their own recurrent collateral connections. This approach also emphasizes that there are many at least partially independent modules for short-term memory functions in the prefrontal cortex (e.g. several modules for delayed saccades; one or more for delayed spatial (body) responses in the dorsolateral prefrontal cortex; one or more for remembering visual stimuli in the more ventral prefrontal cortex; and at least one in the left prefrontal cortex used for remembering the words produced in a verbal fluency task – see Section 10.3 of Rolls & Treves (1998)).

This computational approach thus provides a clear understanding of why a separate (prefrontal) mechanism is needed for working memory functions. This understanding then provides a basis for understanding the contributions of the dorsolateral prefrontal cortex to attention and decision-making (Rolls & Deco 2002, Deco & Rolls 2003, Deco & Rolls 2005b, Deco & Rolls 2005c), as summarized next.

Attention can control or influence decision-making. One way in which it does this is by a top-down influence of information held in a short-term memory in the prefrontal cortex on earlier perceptual modules in the temporal and parietal lobes, or on reward-related representations in the orbitofrontal and anterior cingulate cortex. The general architecture is that illustrated in Fig. 11.1 and shown in more detail in Fig. 11.3. The information to which attention must be paid, for example spatial position in a scene, is loaded into the dorsolateral prefrontal cortex short-term memory, and this then biases competition between different representations in the parietal or temporal cortex (Desimone & Duncan 1995, Rolls & Deco 2002, Deco & Rolls 2004, Deco & Rolls 2005b). This *biased competition* is understood at the detailed level of an integrate-and-fire neuronal network model in which the top-down bias can have highly non-linear effects on the competition between competing perceptual representations (Deco & Rolls 2005c, Deco & Rolls 2006). Top-down attention can also bias whole cortical processing streams towards emotion-related vs perceptual processing (Grabenhorst & Rolls 2008, Rolls, Grabenhorst, Margot, da Silva & Velazco 2008a, Grabenhorst & Rolls 2010, Ge, Feng, Grabenhorst & Rolls 2012, Luo, Ge, Grabenhorst, Feng & Rolls 2013), and the processes involved are now being understood with a biased activation theory of top-down attention (Rolls 2013a) (Section 4.5.5.8, Fig. 4.46).

Another way in which attention can influence decision-making is by influencing the mapping from stimuli to responses. This is needed for example in tasks in which the rule is sometimes that one aspect of a stimulus, for example its spatial position, must be mapped to a particular spatial response, yet at other times the rule is that a different aspect of the stimulus, for example which object is being shown, must be mapped to a particular response. The prefrontal cortex contributes to this type of decision-making in two ways. First it provides a short-term memory which holds active the current rule. Second, if there is a delay between the stimulus and the response, short-term memory networks in the prefrontal cortex can bridge the delay. This type of rule-based mapping task has been studied using single neuron recording by Asaad, Rainer & Miller (1998) and Asaad, Rainer & Miller (2000), and neurons have been described that encode and hold active in the delay period the object and spatial properties of the stimuli, combinations of each of these stimulus properties with the response required, and the responses. Deco & Rolls (2003) have developed a model of this type of decision-making

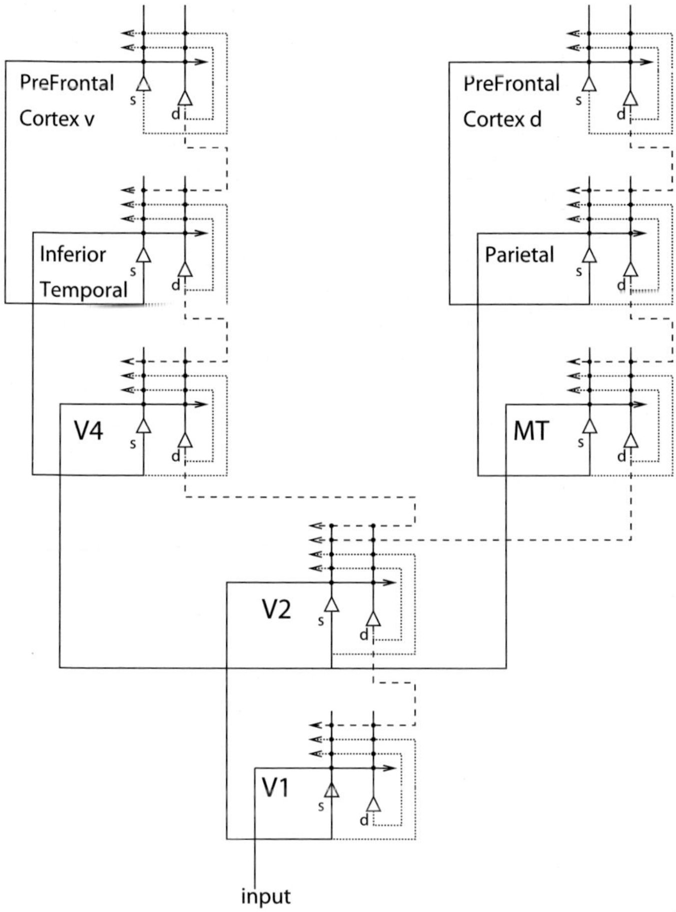

Fig. 11.3 The overall architecture of the model of object and spatial processing and attention, including the prefrontal cortical areas that provide the short-term memory required to hold the object or spatial target of attention active. Forward projections between areas are shown as solid lines, and backprojections as dashed lines. The triangles represent pyramidal cell bodies, with the thick vertical line above them the dendritic trees. The cortical layers in which the cells are concentrated are indicated by s (superficial, layers 2 and 3) and d (deep, layers 5 and 6). The prefrontal cortical areas most strongly reciprocally connected to the inferior temporal cortex 'what' processing stream are labelled v to indicate that they are in the more ventral part of the lateral prefrontal cortex, area 46, close to the inferior convexity in macaques. The prefrontal cortical areas most strongly reciprocally connected to the parietal visual cortical 'where' processing stream are labelled d to indicate that they are in the more dorsal part of the lateral prefrontal cortex, area 46, in and close to the banks of the principal sulcus in macaques (see text). V1 is the primary visual cortex, and V2, V4 and MT are other visual cortical areas (see Rolls and Deco 2002 *Computational Neuroscience of Vision* for further details).

in which rule-encoding neurons in a short-term attractor network keep the current rule active, and this operates as in attentional networks to bias the competition at the level of the stimulus-response combination neurons. The formal architecture of the model is similar to that of the model shown in Fig. 4.52, though the types of neuron are different. This biased competition operates in such a way that when the correct combination neurons are biased, the mapping automatically occurs from the correct aspect of the stimulus (its spatial position or object identity) to the correct response after the delay period. One interesting aspect of this model of how the prefrontal cortex implements this type of decision-making is that the network maps from stimuli to responses by having separate attractors for the stimuli, for the combinations of stimuli and responses, and for the responses. These attractor networks are hierarchically coupled by using asymmetrical feedforward vs feedback connections from stimulus neurons, through stimulus-response combination neurons, to response neurons, to perform the desired stimulus-to-motor response transform (Deco & Rolls 2003). Another interesting aspect of this model of decision-making is that it can perform reversal, which it does by altering the rule module output to bias instead a different set of stimulus-response combination neurons that implement the reverse mapping (Deco & Rolls 2005a). Another interesting aspect of the model is that it implements the short-term memory functions required because it consists of a set of attractor networks (described in Section A.3). The model is also very interesting for it shows how at the start of the delay period neurons can have firing that is part of a network that holds the stimulus representation active, but later in the delay period can have firing that reflects the behavioural response that will be made (Deco, Ledberg, Almeida & Fuster 2005) (see also Takeda & Funahashi (2002)). The network model of decision-making shows that individual neurons can change their activity from stimulus-related to response-related at different times in the delay period, and that this is an interesting property of hierarchically connected attractor networks. The model itself is described in detail by Deco & Rolls (2003) (see also Deco & Rolls (2005b)). The model also provides a basis for understanding how, as the rewarded rules change in the Wisconsin card sorting task, the mapping can change from one stimulus dimension (e.g. the colour of the items on the cards) to another (e.g. the number of items on the cards), which is an example of an extradimensional shift which depends on the dorsolateral prefrontal cortex (Dias, Robbins & Roberts 1996).

If a prefrontal cortex module is to control behaviour in a working memory task, then it must be capable of assuming some type of executive control. There may be no need to have a single central executive that is additional to the control that must be capable of being exerted by short-term memory modules. This is in contrast to what has traditionally been assumed for the prefrontal cortex (Shallice & Burgess 1996). The concept of executive function in the prefrontal cortex may thus be implicit in its capability to function as a short-term memory that can control behaviour. Further, the role of the prefrontal cortex in executive function may be limited to situations in which a short-term or working memory functionality is required. For example, the execution of 'free-will' tasks in which subjects make decisions about which finger to raise is impaired by damage to the prefrontal cortex, and causes activation of the prefrontal cortex (Frith, Friston, Liddle & Frackowiak 1991, Jahanshahi, Jenkins, Brown, Marsden, Passingham & Brooks 1995, Jahanshahi, Dinberger, Fuller & Frith 2000), yet is a task which places demands on a working memory for previous responses, as the subjects try to make different responses from trial to trial to demonstrate their 'free will'. The impairment in verbal fluency tasks (in which a large number of different words must be produced with a given first letter) produced by left prefrontal cortex lesions (Baldo, Shimamura, Delis, Kramer & Kaplan 2001) may similarly be related to a difficulty in utilizing short-term memory to remember which words have already been produced, so that further words can be different. It has also been argued that the prefrontal cortex may be especially involved in working memory in which items must be manipulated, for example in planning an optimal route or shopping expedition (Shallice 1982, Shallice & Burgess 1996, Petrides 1996). The rearrangement of items is essentially a syntactic function in which symbols must be flexibly related or linked to each other in particular ways (see Section 10.2), and this manipulation of syntactic relations may not itself be a function of the dorsolateral prefrontal cortex, damage to which does not impair syntactic and linguistic operations in general, which may depend more on specialized brain regions such as Broca's area (Kolb & Whishaw 2008, Caplan 1996). Thus the dorsolateral prefrontal cortex may provide the short-term memory capability which is required when several items must be held in short-term memory for manipulation by another processing region. Overall, the implication of these concepts is that the off-line short-term memory functionality provided by the prefrontal cortex is fundamental to what it provides for brain computation, and that this functionality is useful in a number of tasks which are predicated on short-term memory such as attention, executive function (when short-term memory is required), planning, free-will, verbal fluency, and manipulation of items (which must be held in a short-term memory in order to be manipulated). All of these functions use the short-term memory functionality provided by the dorsolateral prefrontal cortex, but other parts of the computation depend on other brain regions. It may be noted that when decisions require not delay-related processing but instead reward and punishment evaluation, then it is the other part of the prefrontal cortex, the orbitofrontal cortex, that is involved (see Section 11.2.4).

This model (Deco & Rolls 2003) of decision-making with delays also has interesting implications for understanding disorders of attention and decision-making that follow frontal lobe damage or interference with dopamine systems. For example, Deco & Rolls (2003) simulated the effect of blockade of dopamine receptors, one effect of which is to limit the maximum current that can flow through NMDA receptor activated ion channels (Chen, Greengard & Yan 2004, Seamans & Yang 2004). The effect of this in the model of decision-making is to limit the rate of firing of the population of neurons that are in the current attractor, and this makes the attractor basin shallow (Deco & Rolls 2003, Rolls & Deco 2010, Rolls, Loh, Deco & Winterer 2008d). The implication of this is that attention can too easily be shifted if dopamine is low, so that the current attentional rule can not be stably maintained, and so that the biasing effect of the attentional rule does not produce such strong biasing, leading also to incorrect mappings between stimuli and responses. This is consistent with previous work showing that in simpler, single attractor, networks, D1 agonists, which can increase NMDA and GABA receptor mediated currents can increase the depth and width of basins of attraction (Durstewitz & Seamans 2002), which could affect working memory. The approach was extended to produce a theory of the cognitive impairments in schizophrenia (Rolls 2005b, Loh, Rolls & Deco 2007a, Rolls, Loh, Deco & Winterer 2008d, Rolls & Deco 2010, Rolls 2012b) (Section 8.11.12) and in normal aging (Rolls & Deco 2010).

11.2.6 Selection of optimal actions by explicit rational thought

In Section 10.3.1 the hypothesis was developed that an explicit rational planning system allows immediate rewards encoded by an implicit emotional reward evaluation to be deferred. In this sense there are dual routes to action, one emotional, and the second rational and syntactic (see Fig. 10.4). Further evidence for these two types of decision-making was described in Section 9.5.5 in which the influence of immediate vs delayed rewards was considered. In delayed reward decisions, a rational, logic-based, system requiring syntactic manipulation of symbols that can treat each moment of delay equally, and calculate choice based on an exponential decrease of reward value with increasing delay, is involved. This rational decision system might involve language or mathematical systems in the brain, and the ability to hold several items in a working memory while the trade-offs of different long-term courses of action are compared.

A different more emotion-based system might operate according to heuristics that have become built into the system during evolution that might disproportionately value immediate rewards compared to delayed rewards.

Consistent with the point being made about evolutionarily old emotion-based decision systems vs a recent rational system present in humans is that humans trade off immediate costs/benefits against cost/benefits that are delayed by as much as decades, whereas non-human primates have not been observed to engage in unpreprogrammed delay of gratification involving more than a few minutes (Rachlin 1989, Kagel et al. 1995). Moreover, as described in Section 9.5.5, there appear to be different systems involved in these types of decision, with the orbitofrontal and pregenual cingulate cortices implicated in immediate emotion-related reward-based decision-making, and the lateral prefrontal cortex and parietal cortex implicated in long-term cost–benefit planning-related decision-making.

We have seen, especially in Chapters 3 and 7, that goals specified by genes contribute to much animal behaviour. What are some of the implications when this is coupled with a rational, reasoning, system, as for example in humans? Some of the following thoughts are prompted by the characters portrayed by Richard Wagner in Rheingold. One biologically influenced goal for a woman (e.g. Fricka) might be resources, such as a castle, which might be useful to bring up and defend her children, and to keep her husband (Wotan) at home, not roving the world looking for variety and potentially squandering her resources. A biologically influenced goal for a man might be competition (including fighting) for resources, land, wealth (gold) etc. to make himself attractive to women, and to increase the chances that his offspring will survive sufficiently long to have a reasonable chance of reproducing themselves. (The latter would of course be facilitated by inheritance of wealth, resources, territory, a home, etc.) Another goal for a man might be roving the world in search of variety (Wotan), which could promote further reproductive success by pairing with other genes. Now, and this is where we move forwards, what happens if the basic biological goals common to many animals are coupled with rational thinking? The rational planning ahead can now be put to the use of the biologically specified goals, resulting in great plans to obtain resources (gold in Rheingold) which will give the man power, again something that may be biologically attractive to women as it brings wealth, resources, and protection. These great plans lead to alliances and language-supported agreements, promoted by reciprocal altruism, which, to ensure that they are not broken, lead to legal agreements. These agreements should not be broken to maintain the man's reputation, but the man may be tempted to break the agreements if it is to the man's advantage, and the man calculates using reasoning that breaking the agreement is likely to succeed and to maintain resources without having long-term implications for difficulties ahead. This brings agreements and treaties into conflict with biological goals. The result therefore of combining a reasoning system with the biologically, gene-influenced, goals is that whole complex social systems of bartering, agreements, broken agreements, treachery, agreements kept to maintain reputation, attraction to members of the opposite sex for what they can provide in terms of (gene) reproductive success, and the whole underlying biology, become amplified by utilizing the resources of reasoning. The reasoning system may even choose to do things for the individual that are not in the interests of reproductive success (e.g. Alberich forswearing love, for wealth and the comforts that it brings). Thus adding reasoning can make the whole biological scenario with its goals into a complex web of planned behaviour that is often in the interests of the genes, and may go beyond this in the interests of the individual.

Wagner, and for that matter Shakespeare, were able to portray in drama many of the complex behaviours that can arise from these processes in humans. But they did not have an understanding of the underlying factors that cause these emotion and reasoning-related behaviours to arise, and nor do most individuals today in society. However, with the concepts described in this book, we do now have a grasp of how by working together, these emotional, gene-specified value or goal systems, and reasoning systems, can produce the rich web of human behaviour, and an understanding of the underlying forces that influence it. However, these emotional systems only influence our behaviour, and the goal-defining gene-related effects are coupled with effects of the environment, and of development, including epigenetics. Beyond this, not only is our behaviour not 'determined' in this sense by our genes, but our reasoning system can allow us to go beyond these gene-influenced goals, and to choose a behaviour that is not in the interests of genes, but could be in the interests of for example making a social contract with others to live by rules and laws that are in the interests of individuals in the society. (This theme is developed much more by Rolls (2012d) in *Neuroculture*.) The rational system can thus mean that the rather unpleasant individuals portrayed in Rheingold need not be where society is forced to go in an eternal Ring or cycle, but instead that we can choose with our rational systems to make choices that enable peacefulness and adequate provision to be set up in society, now that we have a grasp of some of the forces that are acting within humans to influence their pleasures and desires. In this sense, as scientists we can see even better that our behaviour is not 'determined' by our genes, for the rational system can make choices that are not subject to the goals that our genes promote.

This scientific understanding of behaviour should lead to societies that, with this understanding, can support the goals, desires, and pleasures that are influenced by genes and by the reasoning system, without producing harm to others. I emphasize that rationality, reasoning, enables humans to go beyond gene-specified or gene-influenced goals. These and related concepts have many implications, including for ethics, religion, aesthetics, politics, and economics (see further *Neuroculture: On the Implications of Brain Science* (Rolls 2012d)).

11.3 Emotion and ethics

I have argued in this book that much of the foundation of our emotional behaviour arises from specification by genes of primary reinforcers that provide goals for our actions. We have emotional reactions in certain circumstances, such as when we see that we are about to suffer pain, when we fall in love, or if someone does not return a favour in a reciprocal interaction. What is the relation between our emotions, and what we think is right, that is our ethical principles? If we think something is right, such as returning something that has been on loan, is this a fundamental and absolute ethical principle, or might it have arisen from deep-seated biologically-based systems shaped to be adaptive by natural selection operating in evolution to select genes that tend to promote the survival of those genes?

Many principles that we regard as ethical principles *might* arise in this biological way (see Rolls (2012d)). For example, as noted in Chapter 2, guilt might arise when there is a conflict between an available reward and a rule or law of society. Jealousy is an emotion that might be aroused in a male if the faithfulness of his partner seems to be threatened by her liaison (e.g. flirting) with another male. In this case the reinforcement contingency that is operating is produced by a punisher, and it may be that males are specified genetically to find this punishing because it indicates a potential threat to their paternity and parental investment, as described in Chapters 7 and 3. Similarly, a female may become jealous if her partner has a liaison with another female, because the resources available to the 'wife' useful to bring up her children are threatened. Again, the punisher here may be gene-specified, as described in Chapter 3. Such emotional responses might influence what we build into some of the ethical principles that surround marriage and partnerships for raising children.

Many other similar examples can be surmised from the area of evolutionary psychology (see e.g. Ridley (1993a, 1996) and Buss (2012)). For example, there may be a set of reinforcers that are genetically specified to help promote social cooperation and even reciprocal altruism, and that might thus influence what we regard as ethical, or at least what we are willing to accept as ethical principles. Such genes might specify that emotion should be elicited, and behavioural changes should occur, if a cooperating partner defects or 'cheats' (Cosmides &

Tooby 1999). Moreover, the genes may build brains with genetically specified rules that are useful heuristics for social cooperation, such as acting with a strategy of 'generous tit-for tat', which can be more adaptive than strict 'tit-for-tat', in that being generous occasionally is a good strategy to help promote further cooperation that has failed when both partners defect in a strict 'tit-for-tat' scenario (Ridley 1996). Genes that specify good heuristics to promote social cooperation may thus underlie such complex emotional states as feeling forgiving.

It is suggested that many apparently complex emotional states have their origins in designing animals to perform well in such sociobiological and socioeconomic situations (Ridley 1996, Glimcher 2003, Glimcher 2004). In this way, many principles that humans accept as ethical may be closely related to strategies that are useful heuristics for promoting social cooperation, and emotional feelings associated with ethical behaviour may be at least partly related to the adaptive value of such gene-specified strategies.

The situation is clarified by the ideas I have advanced in Chapter 10 and in this chapter about a rational syntactically based reasoning system and how this interacts with an evolutionarily older emotional system with gene-specified rewards. The rational system enables us for example to defer immediate gene-specified rewards, and make longer-term plans for actions that in the long term may have more useful outcomes. This rational system enables us to make reasoned choices, and to reason about what is right. Indeed, it is because of the linguistic system that the naturalistic fallacy becomes an issue. In particular, we should not believe that what is right is what is natural (*the naturalistic fallacy*), because we have a rational system that can go beyond simpler gene-specified rewards and punishers that may influence our actions through brain systems that operate at least partly implicitly, i.e. unconsciously. I now consider further the relation between the biological underpinnings to emotion, and ethics, morals, and morality.

There are many reasons why people have particular moral beliefs, and believe that it is good to act in particular ways. It is possible that biology can help to explain why certain types of behaviour are adopted perhaps implicitly by humans, and become incorporated for consistency into explicit rules for conduct. This approach does not, of course, replace other approaches to what is moral, but it may help in implementing moral beliefs held for other reasons to have some insight into some of the directions that the biological underpinnings of human behaviour might lead. Humans may be better able to decide explicitly what to do when they have knowledge and insight into the biological underpinnings. It is in this framework that the following points are made, with no attempt made to lead towards any suggestions about what is 'right' or 'wrong'. The arguments that follow are based on the hypothesis that there are biological underpinnings based on the types of reward and punishment systems that have been built into our genes during evolution for at least some of the types of behaviour held to be moral.

One type of such biological underpinning is kin selection. This would tend to produce supportive behaviour towards individuals likely to be related, especially towards children, grandchildren, siblings etc., depending on how closely they are genetically related. This does tend to occur in human societies, and is part of what is regarded as 'right', and indeed it is a valued 'right' to be able to pass on goods, possessions, wealth, etc., to children. The underlying basis here would be genes for kin altruism[42].

Another such underpinning might be the fact that many animals, and especially primates, co-operate with others in order to achieve ends which turn out to be on average to their

[42]Kin selection genes spread because of kin altruism. Such genes direct their bodies to aid relatives because those relatives have a high chance of having the same relative-helping gene. This is a specific mechanism, and it happens to be incorrect to think that genes direct their bodies to aid relatives because those bodies 'share genes' in general (see Hamilton (1964); and the chapter on inclusive fitness in Dawkins (1995)).

advantage, including genetic advantage. One example includes the coalitions formed by groups of males in order to obtain a female for one of the groups, followed by reciprocation of the good turn later (see Ridley (1996)). This is an example of altruism, in this case by groups of primates, which is to the advantage of both groups or individuals provided that neither individual or group cheats, in which case the rules for social interaction must change to keep the strategy stable. Another such underpinning, in this case for property 'rights', might be the territory guarding behaviour that is so common from fish to primates. Another such underpinning might be the jealousy and guarding of a partner shown by males who invest parental care in their partner's offspring. This occurs in many species of birds, and also in humans, with both exemplars showing male parental investment because of the immaturity of the children. This might be a biological underpinning to the 'right' to fidelity in a female partner.

The suggestion I make is that in all these cases, and in many others, there are biological underpinnings that determine what we find rewarding or punishing, designed into genes by evolution to lead to appropriate behaviour that helps to increase the fitness of the genes. When these implicit systems for rewards and punishers start to be expressed explicitly (in language) in humans, the explicit rules, rights, and laws that are formalized are those that set out in language what the biological underpinnings 'want' to occur[43]. Clearly in formulating the explicit rights and laws, some compromise is necessary in order to keep the society stable. When the rights and laws are formulated in small societies, it is likely that individuals in that society will have many of the same genes, and rules such as 'help your neighbour' (but 'make war with "foreigners" ') will probably be to the advantage of one's genes. However, when the society increases in size beyond a small village (in the order of 1000), then the explicitly formalized rules, rights, and laws may no longer produce behaviour that turns out to be to the advantage of an individual's genes. In addition, it may no longer be possible to keep track of individuals in order to maintain the stability of 'tit-for-tat' co-operative social strategies (Dunbar 1996, Ridley 1996)[44]. In such cases, other factors doubtless come into play to additionally influence what groups hold to be right. For example, a group of subjects in a society might demand the 'right' to free speech because it is to their economic advantage.

Thus overall it is suggested that many aspects of what a society holds as right and moral, and of what becomes enshrined in explicit 'rights' and laws, are related to biological underpinnings, which have usually evolved because of the advantage to the individual's genes, but that as societies develop other factors also start to influence what is believed to be 'right' by groups of individuals, related to socioeconomic factors. In both cases, the laws and rules of the society develop so that these 'rights' are protected, but often involve compromise in such a way that a large proportion of the society will agree to, or can be made subject to, what is held as right.

To conclude this discussion, we note that what is natural does not necessarily imply what is 'right' (the naturalistic fallacy, pointed out by G. E. Moore) (see, e.g., Singer (1981)). However, our notions of what we think of as right may be related to biological underpinnings, and the point of this discussion is that it can only give helpful insight into human behaviour to realize this. Other ways in which a biological approach, based on what our brains have evolved to treat as rewarding or punishing, can illuminate moral issues, and rights, follow.

[43] Before the rules are explicitly formalized, conventions may be developed and spread using language, for example in the form of verbal traditions handed down from generation to generation that may provide possible models for behaviour, such as Homer's *Odyssey*.

[44] A limit on the size of the group for reciprocal altruism might be set by the ability both to have direct evidence for and remember person–reinforcer associations for large numbers of different individual people. In this situation, reputation passed on verbally from others who have the direct experience of whether an individual can be trusted to reciprocate might be a factor in the adaptive value of language and gossip (Dunbar 1996, Dunbar 1993).

'Pain is a worse state than no pain'. This is a statement held as true by some moral philosophers, and is said to hold with no reference to biological underpinnings. It is a self-evident truth, and certain implications for behaviour may follow from the proposition. A biological approach to pain is that the elicitation of pain has to be punishing (in the sense that animals will work to escape or avoid it), as pain is the state elicited by stimuli signalling a dimension of environmental conditions that reduces survival and therefore gene fitness.

'Incest is morally wrong. One should not marry a brother or sister. One should not have intercourse with any close relation.' The biological underpinning is that children of close relations have an increased chance of having double-recessive genes, which are sometimes harmful to the individual and reduce fitness. In addition, breeding out may produce hybrid vigour. It is presumably for this reason that many animals as well as humans have behavioural strategies (influenced by the properties of reward systems) that reduce inbreeding (e.g. philopatry, that is only one sex remaining in the natal unit at the time of puberty; and mate selection influenced by the olfactory receptor/major histocompatibility genes as described in Section 7.9). At the same time, it may be adaptive (for genes) to pair with another animal that has many of the same genes, for this may help complex gene sequences to be passed intact into the next generation. This may underlie the fact that quails have mechanisms that enable them to recognize their cousins, and make them appear attractive, an example of kin selection (Bateson 1983). In humans, if one were part of a strong society (in which one's genes would have a good chance not to be eliminated by other societies), then it could be advantageous (whether male or female) to invest resources with someone else who would provide maximum genetic and resource potential for one's children, which on average across a society of relatively small size and not too mobile would be a person with relatively similar genes and resources (wealth, status etc.) to oneself. In an exception to this, in certain societies there has been a tradition of marrying close relations (e.g. the Pharaohs of Egypt), and part of the reason for this could be maintaining financial and other resources within the (genetic) family.

There may be several reasons why particular behavioural conduct may be selected. A first is that the conduct may be good for the individual and for the genes of the individual, at least on average. An example might be a prohibition on killing others in the same society (while at the same time defending that kin group in times of war). The advantage here could be for one's own genes, which would be less at risk in a society without large numbers of killings. A second reason is that particular codes of conduct might effectively help one's genes by making society stable. An example here might be a prohibition on theft, which would serve to protect property. A third reason is that the code of conduct might actually be to other, powerful, individuals' advantage, and might have been made for that reason into a rule that others in society are persuaded to follow. A general rule in society might be that honesty is a virtue, but the rule might be given a special interpretation or ignored by members of society too powerful to challenge. As discussed in Chapter 7, different aspects of behaviour could have different importance for males and females (Goetz & Shackelford 2009). This could lead men and women to put different stress on different rules of society, because they have different importance for men and women. One example might be being unfaithful. Because this could be advantageous to men's genes, this may be treated by men as a less serious error of conduct than by women. However, within men there could be differential condemnation, with men predisposed to being faithful being more concerned about infidelity in other men, because it is a potential threat to them. In the same way, powerful men who can afford to have liaisons with many women may be less concerned about infidelity than less powerful men, whose main genetic investment may be with one woman.

Society may set down certain propositions of what is 'right'. One reason for this is that it may be too difficult on every occasion, and for everyone, to work out explicitly what all the payoffs of each rule of conduct are. A second reason is that what is promulgated as 'right' could actually be to someone else's advantage, and it would not be wise to expose this fully. One way to convince members of society not to do what is apparently in their immediate interest is to promise a reward later. Such deferred rewards are often offered by religions (Rolls 2012d). The ability to work for a deferred reward using a one-off plan in this way becomes possible, it was suggested earlier in this chapter, with the evolution of the explicit, propositional, system.

The overall view that one is led to is that some of our moral beliefs may be explicit, verbal, formulations of what may reflect factors built genetically by kin selection into behaviour, namely a tendency to favour kin, because they are likely to share some of an individual's genes. In a small society this explicit formulation may be 'appropriate' (from the point of view of the genes), in that many members of that society will be related to that individual. When the society becomes larger, the relatedness may decrease, yet the explicit formulation of the rules or laws of society may not change. In such a situation, it is presumably appropriate for society to make it clear to its members that its rules for what is acceptable and 'right' behaviour are set in place so that individuals can live in safety, and with some expectation of help from society in general.

Other factors that can influence what is held to be right might reflect socioeconomic advantage to groups or alliances of individuals. It would be then in a sense up to individuals to decide whether they wished to accept the rules, with the costs and benefits provided by the rules of that society, in a form of Social Contract. Individuals who did not agree to the social contract might wish to transfer to another society with a different place on the continuum of costs and potential benefits to the individuals, or to influence the laws and policies of their own society. Individuals who attempt to cheat the system would be expected to pay a cost in terms of punishment meted out by the society in accordance with its rules. This approach is developed further in *Neuroculture* (Rolls 2012d).

11.4 Emotion and aesthetics

Those interested in literature are sometimes puzzled by the following situation, which can perhaps be clarified by the theory of emotion developed here. The puzzle is that emotions often seem very intense in humans, indeed sometimes so intense that they produce behaviour that does not seem to be adaptive, such as fainting instead of producing an active escape response, or freezing instead of avoiding, or vacillating endlessly about emotional situations and decisions, or falling hopelessly in love even when it can be predicted to be without hope or to bring ruin. The puzzle is not only that the emotion is so intense, but also that even with our rational, reasoning, capacities, humans still find themselves in these situations, and may find it difficult to produce reasonable and effective decisions and behaviour for resolving the situation. The reasons for this include, I suggest, the following.

In humans, the reward and punishment systems may operate implicitly in comparable ways to those in other animals. But in addition to this, humans have the explicit system, which enables us consciously to look and predict many steps ahead (using language and syntax) the consequences of environmental events, and also to reflect on previous events (see Chapter 10). The consequence of this explicit processing is that we can see the full impact of rewarding and punishing events, both looking ahead to see how this will impact us, and reflecting back to previous situations that we can see may never be repeated. For example, in humans grief occurs with the loss of a loved one, and this may be much more intense than might occur simply because of failure to receive a positively reinforcing stimulus, because we can look ahead to see that the person will never be present again, can process all the possible consequences of that, and can remember all the previous occasions with that person. In another example, someone may faint at the sight of blood, and this is more likely to occur in humans because we appreciate the full consequences of major loss of blood, which we all know is life-threatening.

Thus what happens is that reinforcing events can have a very much greater reinforcing value in humans than in other animals, because we have so much cognitive, especially linguistic, processing that leads us to evaluate and appreciate many reinforcing events far more fully than can other animals. Thus humans may decode reinforcers to have supernormal intensity relative to what is usual in other animals, and the supernormal appreciated intensity of the decoded reinforcers leads to super-strong emotions. The emotional states can then be so strong that they are not necessarily adaptive, and indeed language has brought humans out of the environmental conditions under which our emotional systems evolved. For example, the autonomic responses to the sight of blood may be so strong, given that we know the consequences of loss of blood, that we faint rather than helping. Another example is that panic and anxiety states can be exacerbated by feeling the heart pounding, because we are able to use our explicit processing system to think and worry about all the possible causes. One can think of countless other examples from life, and indeed make up other examples, which of course is part of what novelists do.

A second reason for such strong emotions in humans is that the stimuli that produce emotions may be much stronger than those in which our emotional systems evolved. For example, with man-made artefacts (such as cars and guns which may injure many people simultaneously, or a large bus speeding towards one, both of which produce super-normal stimuli), the sights and related stimuli that can be produced in terms of damage to humans are much more intense that those present when our emotional systems evolved. In this way, the things we see can in some cases produce super-strong emotions. Indeed, the strength and sometimes maladaptive consequences of human emotions have preoccupied literature and literary theorists for the last 2,400 years, since Aristotle.

A third reason for the intensely mobilizing, and sometimes immobilizing, effects of emotions in humans is that we can evaluate linguistically, with reasoning, the possible courses of action open to us in emotional situations. Because we can evaluate the possible effects of reinforcers many steps ahead in our plans, and because language enables us to produce flexible one-off plans for actions, and enables us to work for deferred rewards based on one-off plans (see Chapter 10), the ways in which reinforcers are used in decision-making becomes much more complex than in those animals that cannot produce similar one-off plans using language. The consequence of this is that decision-making can become very difficult, with so many potential but uncertain reinforcement outcomes, that humans may vacillate. They are trying to compute by this explicit method the most favourable outcome of each plan in terms of the net reinforcements received, rather than using reinforcement implicitly to select the highest currently available reinforcer.

A fourth reason for complexity in the human emotional system is that there are, it is suggested, two routes to action for emotions in humans, an implicit (unconscious) and an explicit route (see Chapter 10). These systems may not always agree. The implicit system may tend to produce one type of behaviour, typically for immediately available rewards. The explicit system may tend to produce another planned course of action to produce better deferred rewards. Conflict between these systems can lead to many difficult situations, will involve conscience (what is right as conceived by the explicit system) and the requirement to abide by laws (which assume a rational explicit system responsible for our actions). It appears that the implicit system does often control our behaviour, as shown by the effects of frontal lobe damage in humans, which may produce deficits in reward-reversal tasks, even when the human can explicitly state the correct behaviour in the situation (see Chapters 4 and 10). The conflicts that arise between these implicit and explicit systems are again some of the very stuff on which literature often capitalizes.

A fifth reason for complexity in the human emotional system is that we, as social animals, with major investments in our children who benefit from long-term parental co-operation, and with advantages to be gained from social alliances if the partners can be trusted, may be built to try to estimate the goals and reliability of those we know. For example, it may matter to a woman with children whether her partner has been attracted by / is in love with / a different woman, as this could indicate a reduction of help and provision. Humans may thus be very interested in the emotional lives of each other, as this may impact on their own lives. Indeed, humans will, for this sort of reason, be very interested in who is co-operating with whom, and gossip about this may even have acted as a selective pressure for the evolution of language (Dunbar 1996, Dunbar 1993). In these circumstances, fascination with unravelling the thoughts and emotions of others (using the capacity described as theory of mind (Frith & Frith 2003, Gallagher & Frith 2003)), and empathy which may facilitate this (Singer, Seymour, O'Doherty, Kaube, Dolan & Frith 2004), would have adaptive value, though it is difficult computationally to model the minds and interactions of groups of other people, and to keep track of who knows what about whom, as this requires many levels of nested syntactical reference. Our resulting fascination with this, and perhaps the value of experience of as wide a range of situations as possible, may then be another reason why human emotions, and guessing others' emotions in complex social situations, may also be part of the stuff of novelists, playwrights, and poets. Indeed, it may be important for us to find it attractive to engage in this type of processing because of its potential adaptive value, and this may be part of the reason why we find drama, novels, and poetry so fascinating.

A sixth reason for complexity in the human emotional system is that high level cognitive processing can reach down in to the emotional systems and influence how they respond. This was demonstrated in the experiment by DeAraujo, Rolls et al. (2005) in which it was shown that processing at the linguistic level, in the form of a word label, can influence processing as far down in sensory processing as the secondary olfactory cortex in the orbitofrontal cortex, the first stage in cortical processing at which the reward- or punishment-related (hence affective) significance of stimuli is made explicit in the neuronal representations of stimuli (see Fig. 4.42). An implication of this is that cognitive factors such as the current cultural, cognitive, interpretation of literature or music may influence how the literature or music is perceived emotionally (Reddy 2001). Correspondingly, when in the 18th and 19th centuries sentiment developed as a cultural aspect of emotion in literature, the great cognitive emphasis on sentiment can be predicted to have influenced how people responded emotionally to novels written at that time. Thus the current cognitive and cultural context may have an effect not just on the high-level cognitive processing involved in emotion, but may also reach down into the systems (such as the orbitofrontal cortex) where emotion is first made explicit in brain processing, and influence at that level the emotional feelings that occur.

When at the performance of a drama or when reading a novel, the emotional feelings that occur may be partly related to the empathetic states that are being elicited as part of the way in which we are built to try to understand the feelings of others, so as better to predict their behaviour. Of course at the drama or when reading a novel, we know with our explicit system that these are not real events that have direct consequences for us, and top-down cognitive attentional processes (see Section 4.5.5.7) may influence to what extent we allow the incoming events to elicit emotional responses in us, using probably a biased competition attentional mechanism (Rolls & Deco 2002, Deco & Rolls 2003, Deco & Rolls 2005c, Rolls 2013a).

This approach is developed further, and applied to aesthetics more widely, in *Neuroculture* (Rolls 2012d) and elsewhere (Rolls 2011d, Rolls 2014b, Rolls 2014c).

11.5 Close

This book started by raising the following questions. What are emotions? Why do we have emotions? What is their adaptive value? What are the brain mechanisms of emotion, and how can disorders of emotion be understood? Why does it feel like something to have an emotion? Why do emotions sometimes feel so intense? How do we take decisions? When we know what emotions are, why we have them, how they are produced by our brains, and why it feels like something to have an emotion, and how decisions are taken, we will have a broad-ranging explanation of emotion and decision-making. It is in this sense that the title of this book is *Emotion and Decision-Making Explained*. How close have we come to this?

This book provides answers to these questions. The 'why' question is answered by a Darwinian, evolutionary, theory of the adaptive value of emotion in terms of the design of animals and the brain, for the book shows that if genes specify a range of rewards and punishers (primary reinforcers) as the goals for action, then this is an efficient way for genes to influence adaptively the behaviour of the organism to promote fitness (of the genes). Part of the adaptive value, simplicity, and efficiency of this design is that the behaviour itself is not determined or specified by the genes, which need to specify just the goals for actions. This means that during the lifetime of the organism, appropriate actions to obtain the goals can be learned, allowing great flexibility of the behaviour. Another part of the adaptive value of the design is that arbitrary, previously neutral, stimuli can become associated with a primary reinforcer by stimulus–reinforcer association learning, so that there is great flexibility in learning in the lifetime of the organism about which stimuli are associated with primary reinforcers, and should also act as emotional stimuli, and lead towards attainment of the goals specified by the primary reinforcers. This is I believe a fundamental approach to understanding why we have emotions.

This Darwinian account of the 'why' question fits naturally with the operational definition of emotions as states (with particular functions) elicited by instrumental reinforcers (Chapter 2), for the reinforcers define the goals for action, that is rewards and punishers, and it is the rewards and punishers that are operationally related to emotional states. The definition thus should not be thought of as a behaviourist definition of emotion, but as a definition linked to the deep biological adaptive value of designing animals around reward and punishment systems. In addition, the definition is not behaviourist in the sense that cognitive states can elicit emotions, and that emotions can influence cognitive states (see for example Sections 2.8 and 4.12). Further, the definition is not limited to an account of a narrow range of emotions, but can encompass a very wide range of emotions, as outlined in Chapter 2. An advantage of the approach is that it clearly specifies what emotions are, and what their adaptive value is.

The 'how' question about the implementation of emotion in the brain is addressed not only by a wealth of data from neuroscience, but also by a set of principles of the brain organization for emotion set out at the start of this chapter. An advantage of the approach to emotion described here is that it leads to well formulated questions about how to investigate the brain mechanisms that underlie emotion, for the approach indicates that it is important to understand where primary reinforcers are decoded and represented in the brain, how and where stimulus–reinforcer association learning occurs in the brain, how action–outcome (i.e. action–reinforcer) learning occurs, and the ways in which rewards and punishers influence decision-making as outlined in Section 11.2.

In relation to decision-making, it is shown that there are multiple routes via which rewards and punishers, that is emotion-provoking stimuli and the states they elicit, can influence behaviour (see Section 11.2). An important division is into the implicit ways in which rewards directly influence choice via processes such as Pavlovian approach and action–outcome learning, and an explicit route via which immediate rewards can be deferred using a long-term one-off explicit plan which may enable alternative rewards to be obtained in the long term. This is the 'dual routes to action' account developed in Chapter 10 and Section 11.2.

In relation to emotional feelings, it is emphasized that this is part of the much larger problem of consciousness. My own approach to this is described in Chapter 10, but it is pointed out that this is just one approach, that there do not seem to be clear criteria by which any particular theory can be confirmed, and that in the circumstances such theories should not be taken to have practical implications. Nevertheless, these are interesting issues.

It is also shown how a scientific approach to emotion can illuminate some of the biological underpinnings on top of which ethical and moral principles are developed (Section 11.3). A scientific approach to emotion also provides comments about the role of emotion in literature and aesthetics (Section 11.4 and Rolls (2012d)).

This approach to emotion also fits well with the development of a precise and quantitative understanding of how emotion and decision-making are implemented, using the computational approaches illustrated in Appendices 1 and 2, Chapters 4, 8 and 9, and by Rolls (2008b) and Rolls & Deco (2010).

In this book, I show how it is now possible to follow processing in the brain from the sensory representation and perception of objects including visual and taste objects that are independent of reward value; to brain regions where reward value (both outcome value and expected value) are represented, which are crucial components of decision-making; to brain mechanisms that actually implement the choice part of the decision-making, with a mechanism that is common to categorization and decision-making in other brain systems and cortical areas. I believe that this represents a major advance in neuroscience that we are able to understand at the level of mechanisms all of these processes, and to see how they are linked together in the brain to implement much of our behaviour. Moreover, all of this neural understanding is linked to an understanding of the adaptive value of this organization of behaviour, how emotion is a key component, and even how the subjective feeling of pleasure may arise and be related to these processes.

Thus we may suggest that we are getting closer to a scientific understanding and explanation of emotion and of decision-making; and that we have some useful principles and guidelines for investigations that will further enhance our understanding[45].

[45]The front cover, 'Adam and Eve' painted in c. 1528 by Lucas Cranach the Elder (Uffizi Gallery, Florence), provides an early interpretation of early human emotions, and emotion-related decision-making. This book provides a more recent, scientific, approach to emotions, and to decision-making.

Appendix 1 Neural networks and emotion-related learning

A.1 Neurons in the brain, the representation of information, and neuronal learning mechanisms

A.1.1 Introduction

In Chapters 3 and 4, the type of learning that is important in learned emotional responses was characterized as stimulus–reinforcer association learning. This is a particular case of pattern-association learning, in which the to-be-associated or conditioned stimulus is the potential secondary reinforcer, and the unconditioned stimulus is the primary reinforcer (see Fig. 4.5). In Chapter 4, it was indicated that many of the properties required of emotional learning (e.g. generalization and graceful degradation) arise in pattern associators if the correct type of distributed representation is present (Section 4.4). In this Appendix the relevant properties of biologically plausible pattern-association memories (such as may be present in the orbitofrontal cortex and amygdala and used for stimulus–reinforcer association learning) are presented more formally, to provide a foundation for research into the neural basis of emotional learning. In Section A.3 an introduction to autoassociation or attractor networks is given, as this type of network is involved in decision-making, memory, attention, and in maintaining mood states. In Section A.4 an introduction to how attractor networks can interact is given, as this may be relevant to understanding how mood states influence cognitive processing, and vice versa. A fuller analysis of these neural networks, and of other neural networks that, for example, by competitive learning build representations of sensory stimuli, is provided by Rolls & Treves (1998) in *Neural Networks and Brain Function*, by Rolls & Deco (2002) in *Computational Neuroscience of Vision*, and by Rolls (2008b) in *Memory, Attention, and Decision-Making*.

Before starting the description of pattern-association neuronal networks, a brief review of the evidence on synaptic plasticity, and the rules by which synaptic strength is modified, much based on studies with long-term potentiation, is provided.

After describing pattern-association and autoassociation neural networks, an overview of another learning algorithm, called reinforcement learning, which might be relevant to learning in systems that receive rewards and punishers and which has been supposed to be implemented using the dopamine pathways (Barto 1995, Schultz et al. 1995b, Houk et al. 1995, Schultz 2013), is provided in Section A.5.

A.1.2 Neurons in the brain, and their representation in neuronal networks

Neurons in the vertebrate brain typically have, extending from the cell body, large dendrites which receive inputs from other neurons through connections called synapses. The synapses operate by chemical transmission. When a synaptic terminal receives an all-or-nothing action potential from the neuron of which it is a terminal, it releases a transmitter that crosses the synaptic cleft and produces either depolarization or hyperpolarization in the postsynaptic

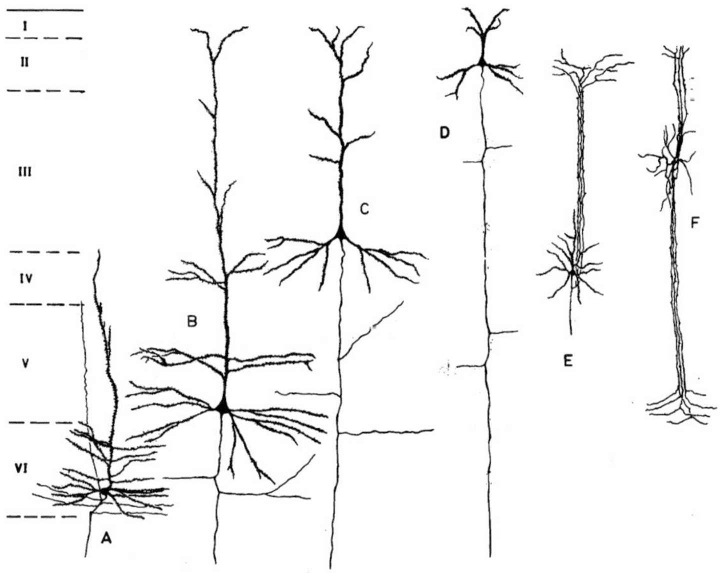

Fig. A.1 Examples of neurons found in the brain. Cell types in the cerebral neocortex are shown. The different laminae of the cortex are designated I–VI, with I at the surface. Cells A–E are pyramidal cells in the different layers. Cell E is a spiny stellate cell, and F is a double bouquet cell. (Reproduced from Edward G. Jones and Alan Peters, *Cerebral Cortex: Functional Properties of Cortical Cells* (vol 2), figure 7 ©1984, Springer Science and Business Media with kind permission.)

neuron, by opening particular ionic channels. (A textbook such as Kandel, Schwartz, Jessell, Siegelbaum & Hudspeth (2012) gives further information on this process.) Summation of a number of such depolarizations or excitatory inputs within the time constant of the receiving neuron, which is typically 15–25 ms, produces sufficient depolarization that the neuron fires an action potential. There are often 5,000–20,000 inputs per neuron. Examples of cortical neurons are shown in Fig. A.1, and further examples are shown elsewhere (Rolls 2008b, Shepherd 2004, Shepherd & Grillner 2010).

Once firing is initiated in the cell body (or axon initial segment of the cell body), the action potential is conducted in an all-or-nothing way to reach the synaptic terminals of the neuron, whence it may affect other neurons. Any inputs the neuron receives that cause it to become hyperpolarized make it less likely to fire (because the membrane potential is moved away from the critical threshold at which an action potential is initiated), and are described as inhibitory. The neuron can thus be thought of in a simple way as a computational element that sums its inputs within its time constant and, whenever this sum, minus any inhibitory effects, exceeds a threshold, produces an action potential that propagates to all of its outputs. This simple idea is incorporated in many neuronal network models using a formalism of a type described in the next Section.

A.1.3 A formalism for approaching the operation of single neurons in a network

Let us consider a neuron i as shown in Fig. A.2, which receives inputs from axons that we label j through synapses of strength w_{ij}. The first subscript (i) refers to the receiving neuron, and the second subscript (j) to the particular input. j counts from 1 to C, where C is the number of synapses or connections received by the neuron. The firing rate of the ith neuron

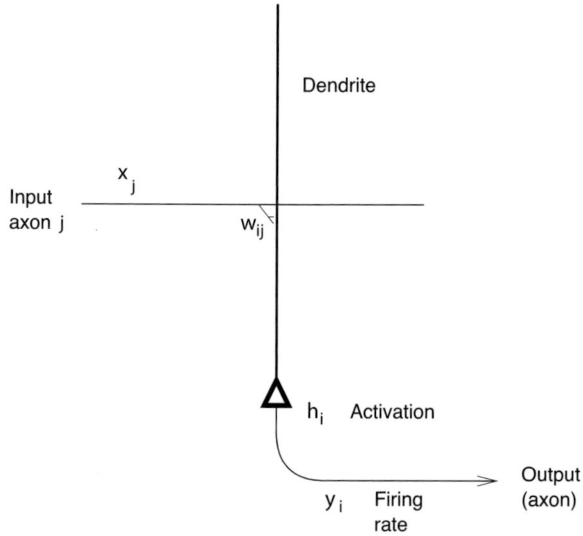

Fig. A.2 Notation used to describe an individual neuron in a network model. By convention, we generally represent the dendrite as thick, and vertically oriented (as this is the normal way that neuroscientists view cortical pyramidal cells under the microscope); and the axon as thin. The cell body or soma is indicated between them. The firing rate we also call the activity of the neuron.

is denoted as y_i, and that of the jth input to the neuron as x_j. To express the idea that the neuron makes a simple linear summation of the inputs it receives, we can write the activation of neuron i, denoted h_i, as

$$h_i = \sum_j^C x_j w_{ij} \tag{A.1}$$

where $\sum_j^C$ indicates that the sum is over the C input axons (or synaptic connections) indexed by j to each neuron. The multiplicative form here indicates that activation should be produced by an axon only if it is firing, and depending on the strength of the synapse w_{ij} from input axon j onto the dendrite of the receiving neuron i. Equation A.1 indicates that the strength of the activation reflects how fast each axon j is firing (that is x_j), and how strong its synapse w_{ij} is. The sum of all such activations expresses the idea that summation (of synaptic currents in real neurons) occurs along the length of the dendrite, to produce activation at the cell body, where the activation h_i is converted into firing y_i. This conversion can be expressed as

$$y_i = \mathrm{f}(h_i) \tag{A.2}$$

which indicates that the firing rate is a function (f) of the activation. The function is called the activation function in this case. (The activation is equivalent to the depolarization of the neuron measured electrophysiologically.) The function at its simplest could be linear, so that the firing rate would be proportional to the activation (see Fig. A.3). Real neurons have thresholds, with firing occurring only if the activation is above the threshold. A threshold linear activation function is shown in Fig. A.3b. This has been useful in formal analysis of the properties of neural networks. Neurons also have firing rates that become saturated at a maximum rate, and we could express this as the sigmoid activation function shown in Fig. A.3c. Another simple activation function, used in some models of neural networks, is the binary threshold function (Fig. A.3d), which indicates that if the activation is below threshold, there is no firing, and that if the activation is above threshold, the neuron fires maximally.

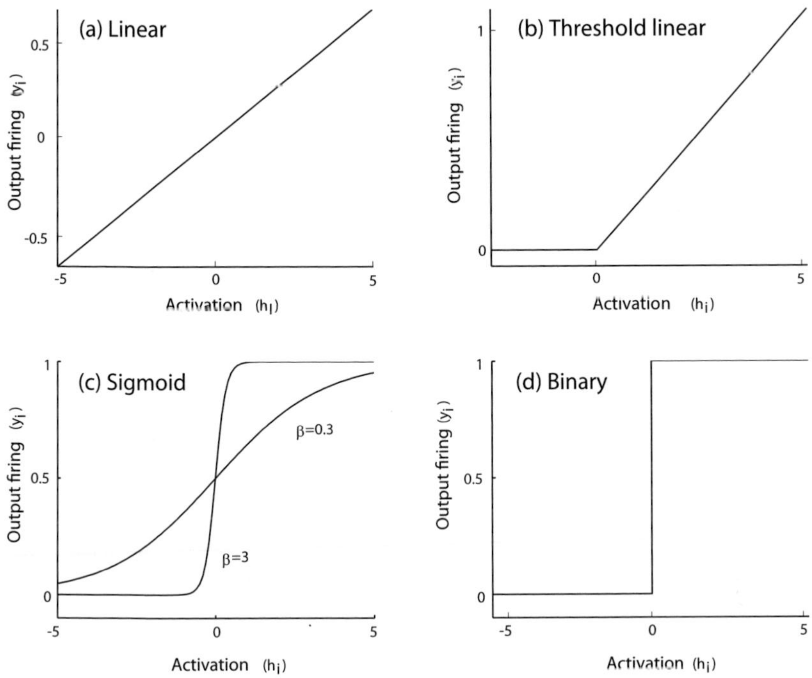

Fig. A.3 Different types of activation function. The activation function relates the output activity (or firing rate), y_i, of the neuron (i) to its activation, h_i. (a) Linear. (b) Threshold linear. (c) Sigmoid. (One mathematical exemplar of this class of activation function is $y_i = 1/(1 + \exp(-2\beta h_i))$.) The output of this function, also sometimes known as the logistic function, is 0 for an input of $-\infty$, 0.5 for 0, and 1 for $+\infty$. The function incorporates a threshold at the lower end, followed by a linear portion, and then an asymptotic approach to the maximum value at the top end of the function. The parameter β controls the steepness of the almost linear part of the function round $h_i = 0$. If β is small, the output goes smoothly and slowly from 0 to 1 as h_i goes from $-\infty$ to $+\infty$. If β is large, the curve is very steep, and approximates a binary threshold activation function.) (d) Binary threshold.

Some non-linearity in the activation function is an advantage, for it enables many useful computations to be performed in neuronal networks, including removing interfering effects of similar memories, and enabling neurons to perform logical operations, such as firing only if several inputs are present simultaneously.

A property implied by Equation A.1 is that the postsynaptic membrane is electrically short, and so summates its inputs irrespective of where on the dendrite the input is received. In real neurons, the transduction of current into firing frequency (the analogue of the transfer function of Equation A.2) is generally studied not with synaptic inputs but by applying a steady current through an electrode into the soma. Examples of the resulting curves, which illustrate the additional phenomenon of firing rate adaptation, are reproduced in Fig. A.4.

A.1.4 Synaptic modification

For a neuronal network to perform useful computation, that is to produce a given output when it receives a particular input, the synaptic weights must be set up appropriately. This is often performed by synaptic modification occurring during learning.

A simple learning rule that was originally presaged by Donald Hebb (1949) proposes that

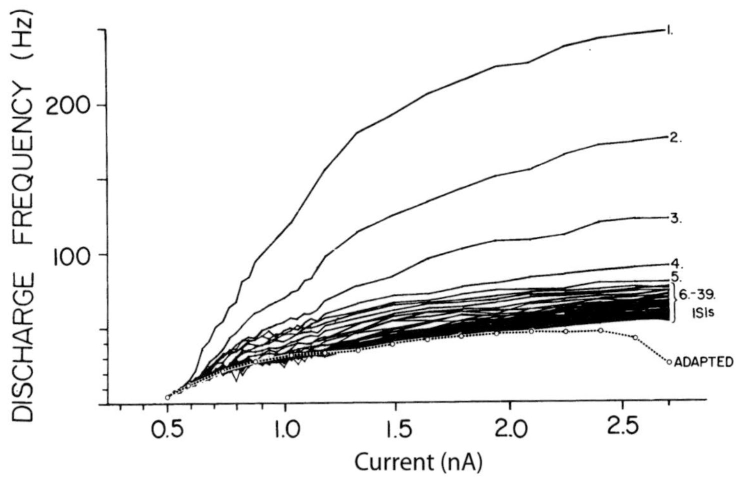

Fig. A.4 Frequency current plot (the closest experimental analogue of the activation function) for a CA1 pyramidal cell. The firing frequency (in Hz) in response to the injection of 1.5 s long, rectangular depolarizing current pulses has been plotted against the strength of the current pulses (in nA) (abscissa). The first 39 interspike intervals (ISIs) are plotted as instantaneous frequency (1/ISI, where ISI is the inter-stimulus interval), together with the average frequency of the adapted firing during the last part of the current injection (circles and broken line). The plot indicates a current threshold at approximately 0.5 nA, a linear range with a tendency to saturate, for the initial instantaneous rate, above approximately 200 Hz, and the phenomenon of adaptation, which is not reproduced in simple non-dynamical models (see further Appendix A5 of Rolls and Treves 1998). (Reproduced from *Experimental Brain Research*, 53 (2), pp. 431–443, Current-to-frequency transduction in CA1 hippocampal pyramidal cells: slow prepotentials dominate the primary range firing, Lanthorn, T., Storm, J. and Andersen, P. (c) 1984, Springer Science and Business Media, with kind permission.)

synapses increase in strength when there is conjunctive presynaptic and postsynaptic activity. The Hebb rule can be expressed more formally as follows:

$$\delta w_{ij} = \alpha y_i x_j. \tag{A.3}$$

where δw_{ij} is the change of the synaptic weight w_{ij} that results from the simultaneous (or conjunctive) presence of presynaptic firing x_j and postsynaptic firing y_i (or strong depolarization), and α is a learning rate constant that specifies how much the synapses alter on any one pairing. The presynaptic and postsynaptic activity must be present approximately simultaneously (to within perhaps 100–500 ms in the real brain).

The Hebb rule is expressed in this multiplicative form to reflect the idea that both presynaptic and postsynaptic activity must be present for the synapses to increase in strength. The multiplicative form also reflects the idea that strong pre- and postsynaptic firing will produce a larger change of synaptic weight than smaller firing rates. The Hebb rule thus captures what is typically found in studies of associative Long-Term Potentiation (LTP) in the brain, described in Section A.1.5.

One useful property of large neurons in the brain, such as cortical pyramidal cells, is that with their short electrical length, the postsynaptic term, y_i, is available on much of the dendrite of a cell. The implication of this is that once sufficient postsynaptic activation has been produced, any active presynaptic terminal on the neuron will show synaptic strengthening. This enables associations between coactive inputs, or correlated activity in input axons, to be learned by neurons using this simple associative learning rule.

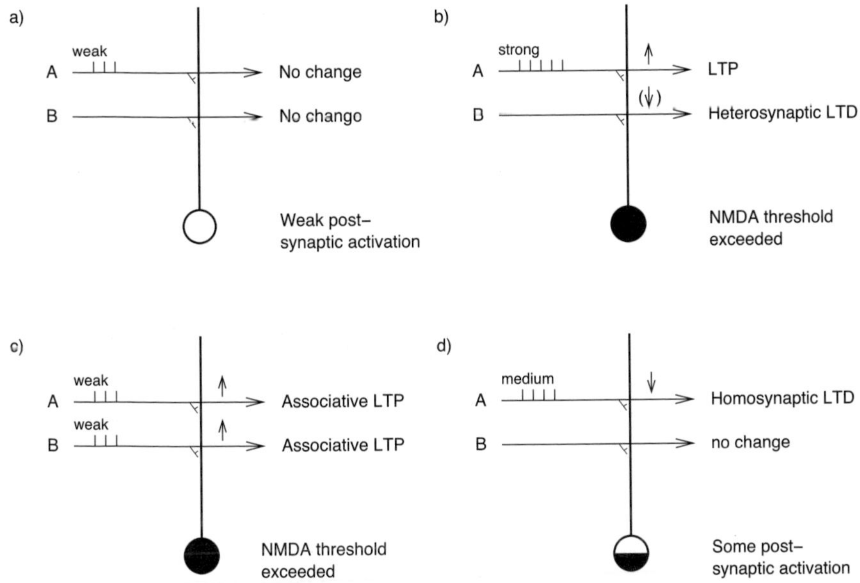

Fig. A.5 Schematic illustration of synaptic modification rules as revealed by Long-Term Potentiation (LTP) and Long-Term Depression (LTD). The activation of the postsynaptic neuron is indicated by the extent to which its soma is black. There are two sets of inputs to the neuron: A and B. (a) A weak input (indicated by 3 spikes) on the set A of input axons produces little postsynaptic activation, and there is no change in synaptic strength. (b) A strong input (indicated by 5 spikes) on the set A of input axons produces strong postsynaptic activation, and the active synapses increase in strength. This is LTP. It is homosynaptic in that the synapses that increase in strength are the same as those through which the neuron is activated. LTP is synapse-specific, in that the inactive axons, B, do not show LTP. They either do not change in strength, or they may weaken. The weakening is called heterosynaptic LTD, because the synapses that weaken are other than those through which the neuron is activated (hetero- is Greek for other). (c) Two weak inputs present simultaneously on A and B summate to produce strong postsynaptic activation, and both sets of active synapses show LTP. (d) Intermediate strength firing on A produces some activation, but not strong activation, of the postsynaptic neuron. The active synapses become weaker. This is homosynaptic LTD, in that the synapses that weaken are the same as those through which the neuron is activated (homo- is Greek for same).

A.1.5 Long-Term Potentiation and Long-Term Depression as models of synaptic modification

Long-Term Potentiation (LTP) and Long-Term Depression (LTD) provide useful models of some of the synaptic modifications that occur in the brain (Feldman 2009). The synaptic changes found appear to be synapse–specific, and to depend on information available locally at the synapse. LTP and LTD may thus provide a good model of the biological synaptic modifications involved in real neuronal network operations in the brain. We next therefore describe some of the properties of LTP and LTD, and evidence that implicates them in learning in at least some brain systems. Even if they turn out not to be the basis for the synaptic modifications that occur during learning, they have many of the properties that would be needed by some of the synaptic modification systems used by the brain.

Long-term potentiation (LTP) is a use-dependent and sustained increase in synaptic strength that can be induced by brief periods of synaptic stimulation. It is usually measured as a sustained increase in the amplitude of electrically evoked responses in specific neural pathways following brief trains of high-frequency stimulation (see Fig. A.5b). For example, high frequency stimulation of the Schaffer collateral inputs to the hippocampal CA1 cells results in a larger response recorded from the CA1 cells to single test pulse stimulation of the pathway. LTP is long-lasting, in that its effect can be measured for hours in hippocampal slices, and in chronic in vivo experiments in some cases it may last for months. LTP becomes evident rapidly, typically in less than 1 minute. LTP is in some brain systems associative. This is illustrated in Fig. A.5c, in which a weak input to a group of cells (e.g. the commissural input to CA1) does not show LTP unless it is given at the same time as (i.e. associatively with) another input (which could be weak or strong) to the cells. The associativity arises because it is only when sufficient activation of the postsynaptic neuron to exceed the threshold of NMDA receptors (see below) is produced that any learning can occur. The two weak inputs summate to produce sufficient depolarization to exceed the threshold. This associative property is shown very clearly in experiments in which LTP of an input to a single cell only occurs if the cell membrane is depolarized by passing current through it at the same time as the input arrives at the cell. The depolarization alone or the input alone is not sufficient to produce the LTP, and the LTP is thus associative. Moreover, in that the presynaptic input and the postsynaptic depolarization must occur at about the same time (within approximately 500 ms), the LTP requires temporal contiguity. LTP is also synapse-specific, in that for example an inactive input to a cell does not show LTP even if the cell is strongly activated by other inputs (Fig. A.5b, input B).

These spatiotemporal properties of LTP can be understood in terms of actions of the inputs on the postsynaptic cell, which in the hippocampus has two classes of receptor, NMDA (N-methyl-D-aspartate) and K–Q (kainate–quisqualate), both activated by the glutamate released by the presynaptic terminals. The NMDA receptor channels are normally blocked by Mg^{2+}, but when the cell is strongly depolarized by strong tetanic stimulation of the type necessary to induce LTP, the Mg^{2+} block is removed, and Ca^{2+} entering via the NMDA receptor channels triggers events that lead to the potentiated synaptic transmission (see Fig. A.6). Part of the evidence for this is that NMDA antagonists such as AP5 (D-2-amino-5-phosphonopentanoate) block LTP. Further, if the postsynaptic membrane is voltage clamped to prevent depolarization by a strong input, then LTP does not occur. The voltage-dependence of the NMDA receptor channels introduces a threshold and thus a non-linearity that contributes to a number of the phenomena of some types of LTP, such as cooperativity (many small inputs together produce sufficient depolarization to allow the NMDA receptors to operate), associativity (a weak input alone will not produce sufficient depolarization of the postsynaptic cell to enable the NMDA receptors to be activated, but the depolarization will be sufficient if there is also a strong input), and temporal contiguity between the different inputs that show LTP (in that if inputs occur non-conjunctively, the depolarization shows insufficient summation to reach the required level, or some of the inputs may arrive when the depolarization has decayed). Once the LTP has become established (which can be within one minute of the strong input to the cell), the LTP is expressed through the K–Q receptors, in that AP5 blocks only the establishment of LTP, and not its subsequent expression (Bliss & Collingridge 1993, Nicoll & Malenka 1995, Fazeli & Collingridge 1996, Feldman 2009).

There are a number of possibilities about what change is triggered by the entry of Ca^{2+} to the postsynaptic cell to mediate LTP. One possibility is that somehow a messenger reaches the presynaptic terminals from the postsynaptic membrane and, if the terminals are active, causes them to release more transmitter in future whenever they are activated by an action potential. Consistent with this possibility is the observation that, after LTP has been induced, more transmitter appears to be released from the presynaptic endings. Another possibility is that the postsynaptic membrane changes just where Ca^{2+} has entered, so that K–Q receptors become more responsive to glutamate released in future. Consistent with this possibility is the observation that after LTP, the postsynaptic cell may respond more to locally applied

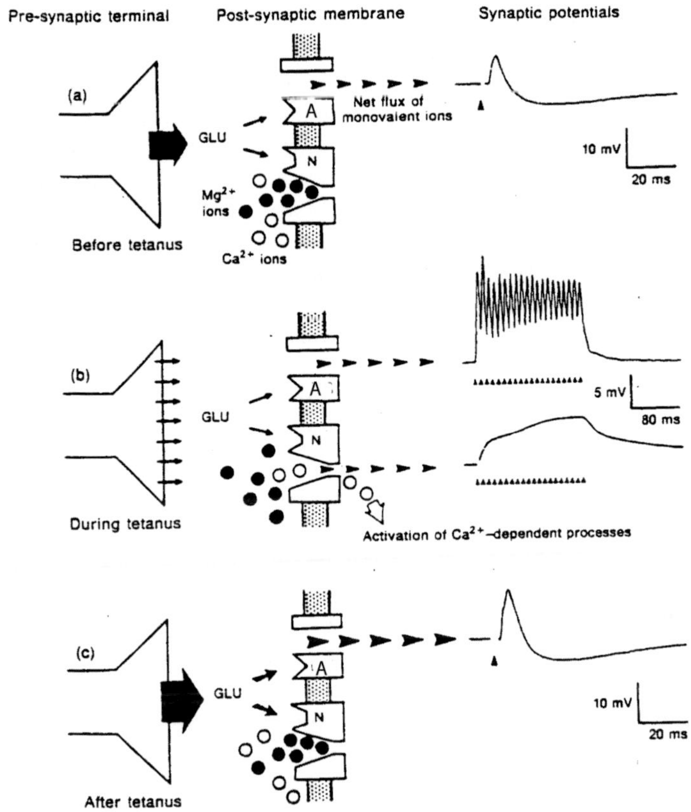

Fig. A.6 The mechanism of induction of LTP in the CA1 region of the hippocampus. (a) Neurotransmitter (e.g. L-glutamate) is released and acts upon both K–Q (kainate–quisqualate) and NMDA (N) receptors. The NMDA receptors are blocked by magnesium and the excitatory synaptic response (EPSP) is therefore mediated primarily by ion flow through the channels associated with K–Q receptors. (b) During high-frequency activation, the magnesium block of the ion channels associated with NMDA receptors is released by depolarization. Activation of the NMDA receptor by transmitter now results in ions moving through the channel. In this way, calcium enters the postsynaptic region to trigger various intracellular mechanisms that eventually result in an alteration of synaptic efficacy. (c) Subsequent low-frequency stimulation results in a greater EPSP. See text for further details. (Reprinted from *Trends in Neurosciences*, 10 (7), G.L. Collingridge and T.V.P. Bliss, NMDA receptors – their role in long-term potentiation, pp. 288–93, Copyright (1987), with permission from Elsevier.)

glutamate (using a microiontophoretic technique).

The rule that underlies associative LTP is thus that synapses connecting two neurons become stronger if there is conjunctive presynaptic and (strong) postsynaptic activity. This learning rule for synaptic modification is sometimes called the Hebb rule, after Donald Hebb of McGill University who drew attention to this possibility, and its potential importance in learning (Hebb 1949).

In that LTP is long-lasting, develops rapidly, is synapse-specific, and is in some cases associative, it is of interest as a potential synaptic mechanism underlying some forms of memory. Evidence linking it directly to some forms of learning comes from experiments in which it has been shown that the drug AP5, infused so that it reaches the hippocampus to block NMDA receptors, blocks spatial learning mediated by the hippocampus (see Morris (1989),

Martin, Grimwood & Morris (2000)). The task learned by the rats was to find the location relative to cues in a room of a platform submerged in an opaque liquid (milk). Interestingly, if the rats had already learned where the platform was, then the NMDA infusion did not block performance of the task. This is a close parallel to LTP, in that the learning, but not the subsequent expression of what had been learned, was blocked by the NMDA antagonist AP5. Although there is still some uncertainty about the experimental evidence that links LTP to learning (see for example Martin, Grimwood & Morris (2000)), there is a need for a synapse-specific modifiability of synaptic strengths on neurons if neuronal networks are to learn (see Section A.2). If LTP is not always an exact model of the synaptic modification that occurs during learning, then something with many of the properties of LTP is nevertheless needed, and is likely to be present in the brain given the functions known to be implemented in many brain regions (see Rolls & Treves (1998)).

In another model of the role of LTP in memory, Davis (2000) has studied the role of the amygdala in learning associations to fear-inducing stimuli. He has shown that blockade of NMDA synapses in the amygdala interferes with this type of learning, consistent with the idea that LTP also provides a useful model of this type of learning (see further Chapter 4).

Long-Term Depression (LTD) can also occur (Feldman 2009). It can in principle be associative or non-associative. In associative LTD, the alteration of synaptic strength depends on the pre- and post-synaptic activities. There are two types. Heterosynaptic LTD occurs when the postsynaptic neuron is strongly activated, and there is low presynaptic activity (see Fig. A.5b input B, and Table A.1). Heterosynaptic LTD is so-called because the synapse that weakens is other than (hetero-) the one through which the postsynaptic neuron is activated. Heterosynaptic LTD is important in associative neuronal networks, and in competitive neuronal networks (see Chapter 7 of Rolls & Deco (2002)). In competitive neural networks it would be helpful if the degree of heterosynaptic LTD depended on the existing strength of the synapse, and there is some evidence that this may be the case (see Chapter 7 of Rolls & Deco (2002)). Homosynaptic LTD occurs when the presynaptic neuron is strongly active, and the postsynaptic neuron has some, but low, activity (see Fig. A.5d and Table A.1). Homosynaptic LTD is so-called because the synapse that weakens is the same as (homo-) the one that is active. Heterosynaptic and homosynaptic LTD are found in the neocortex (Artola & Singer 1993, Singer 1995, Frégnac 1996) and hippocampus (Christie 1996), and in many cases are dependent on activation of NMDA receptors (see also Fazeli & Collingridge (1996)). LTD in the cerebellum is evident as weakening of active parallel fibre to Purkinje cell synapses when the climbing fibre connecting to a Purkinje cell is active (Ito 1984, Ito 1989, Ito 1993a, Ito 1993b).

An interesting time-dependence of LTP and LTD has been observed, with LTP occurring especially when the presynaptic spikes precede by a few ms the postsynaptic activation, and LTD occurring when the presynaptic spikes follow the postsynaptic activation by a few ms (Markram, Lübke, Frotscher & Sakmann 1997, Bi & Poo 1998, Feldman 2012). This type of temporally asymmetric Hebbian learning rule, demonstrated in the neocortex and the hippocampus, can induce associations over time, and not just between simultaneous events. Networks of neurons with such synapses can learn sequences (Minai & Levy 1993), enabling them to predict the future state of the postsynaptic neuron based on past experience (Abbott & Blum 1996) (see further Koch (1999), Markram, Pikus, Gupta & Tsodyks (1998) and Abbott & Nelson (2000)). This mechanism, because of its apparent time-specificity for periods in the range of tens of ms, could also encourage neurons to learn to respond to temporally synchronous presynaptic firing (Gerstner, Kreiter, Markram & Herz 1997), and indeed to decrease the synaptic strengths from neurons that fire at random times with respect to the synchronized group. This mechanism might also play a role in the normalization of the strength of synaptic connection strengths onto a neuron. Under the somewhat steady state conditions of the firing of neurons in the higher parts of the ventral visual system on the 10 ms timescale that are observed not only when single stimuli are presented for 500 ms (see Fig. 4.11), but also when macaques have found a search target and are looking at it (in the experiments described in Section 4.4.4.3), the average of the presynaptic and postsynaptic rates are likely to be the important determinants of synaptic modification. Part of the reason for this is that correlations between the firing of simultaneously recorded inferior temporal cortex neurons are not common, and if present are not very strong or typically restricted to a short time window in the order of 10 ms (Rolls & Treves 2011, Franco et al. 2004, Aggelopoulos et al. 2005). This point is also made in the context that each neuron has thousands of inputs, several tens of which are normally likely to be active when a cell is firing above its spontaneous firing rate and is strongly depolarized. This may make it unlikely statistically that there will be a strong correlation between a particular presynaptic spike and postsynaptic firing, and thus that this is likely to be a main determinant of synaptic strength under these natural conditions. Further points are that cortical neurons often fire to effective stimuli with firing rates of 50 or more spikes/s (Rolls 2008b, Rolls & Treves 2011); that usually LTP and not LTD is observed with high firing rates; and that with these high firing rates, the issue arises of whether one neuron is firing before or after another neuron.

A.1.6 Distributed representations

When considering the operation of many neuronal networks in the brain, it is found that many useful properties arise if each input to the network (arriving on the axons as a firing rate vector $\mathbf{x}$) is encoded in the activity of an ensemble or population of the axons or input lines (distributed encoding), and is not signalled by the activity of a single input, which is called local encoding. We start with some definitions, and then highlight some of the differences, and summarize some evidence that shows the type of encoding used in some brain regions. Then in Section A.2.8 (e.g. Table A.2), we show how many of the useful properties of the neuronal networks described depend on distributed encoding. Rolls (2008b) and Rolls & Treves (2011) review evidence on the encoding actually found in cortical areas.

A.1.6.1 Definitions

A *local representation* is one in which all the information that a particular stimulus or event occurred is provided by the activity of one of the neurons. In a famous example, a single neuron might be active only if one's grandmother was being seen. An implication is that most neurons in the brain regions where objects or events are represented would fire only very rarely. A problem with this type of encoding is that a new neuron would be needed for every object or event that has to be represented. There are many other disadvantages of this type of encoding, many of which are made apparent in this book. Moreover, there is evidence that objects are represented in the brain by a different type of encoding.

A *fully distributed representation* is one in which all the information that a particular stimulus or event occurred is provided by the activity of the full set of neurons. If the neurons are binary (e.g. either active or not), the most distributed encoding is when half the neurons are active for any one stimulus or event.

A *sparse distributed representation* is a distributed representation in which a small proportion of the population of neurons is active at any one time. In a sparse representation with binary neurons, less than half of the neurons are active for any one stimulus or event. For binary neurons, we can use as a measure of the sparseness the proportion of neurons in the active state. For neurons with real, continuously variable, values of firing rates, the sparseness a of the representation can be measured, by extending the binary notion of the proportion of neurons that are firing, as

$$a = \frac{(\sum_{i=1}^{N} y_i/N)^2}{\sum_{i=1}^{N} y_i^2/N} \tag{A.4}$$

where y_i is the firing rate of the ith neuron in the set of N neurons (Treves & Rolls 1991, Rolls & Treves 2011, Franco, Rolls, Aggelopoulos & Jerez 2007).

Coarse coding utilizes overlaps of receptive fields, and can compute positions in the input space using differences between the firing levels of coactive cells (e.g. colour-tuned cones in the retina). The representation implied is very distributed. Fine coding (in which for example a neuron may be 'tuned' to the exact orientation and position of a stimulus) implies more local coding.

A.1.6.2 Advantages of different types of coding

One advantage of distributed encoding is that the similarity between two representations can be reflected by the correlation between the two patterns of activity that represent the different stimuli. We have already introduced the idea that the input to a neuron is represented by the activity of its set of input axons x_j, where j indexes the axons, numbered from $j = 1, C$ (see Fig. A.2 and Equation A.1). Now the set of activities of the input axons is a vector (a vector is an ordered set of numbers; Appendix 1 of Rolls & Treves (1998) and of Rolls (2008b) provides a summary of some of the concepts involved). We can denote as $\mathbf{x}_1$ the vector of axonal activity that represents stimulus 1, and $\mathbf{x}_2$ the vector that represents stimulus 2. Then the similarity between the two vectors, and thus the two stimuli, is reflected by the correlation between the two vectors. The correlation will be high if the activity of each axon in the two representations is similar; and will become more and more different as the activity of more and more of the axons differs in the two representations. Thus the similarity of two inputs can be represented in a graded or continuous way if (this type of) distributed encoding is used. This enables generalization to similar stimuli, or to incomplete versions of a stimulus (if it is for example partly seen or partly remembered), to occur. With a local representation, either one stimulus or another is represented, and similarities between different stimuli are not encoded.

Another advantage of distributed encoding is that the number of different stimuli that can be represented by a set of C components (e.g. the activity of C axons) can be very large. A simple example is provided by the binary encoding of an 8-element vector. One component can code for which of two stimuli has been seen, 2 components (or bits in a computer byte) for 4 stimuli, 3 components for 8 stimuli, 8 components for 256 stimuli, etc. That is, the number of stimuli increases exponentially with the number of components (or in this case, axons) in the representation. (In this simple binary illustrative case, the number of stimuli that can be encoded is 2^C.) Put the other way round, even if a neuron has only a limited number of inputs (e.g. a few thousand), it can nevertheless receive a great deal of information about which stimulus was present. This ability of a neuron with a limited number of inputs to receive information about which of potentially very many input events is present is probably one factor that makes computation by the brain possible. With local encoding, the number of stimuli that can be encoded increases only linearly with the number C of axons or components (because a different component is needed to represent each new stimulus). (In our example, only 8 stimuli could be represented by 8 axons.)

In the real brain, there is now good evidence that in a number of brain systems, including the high-order visual and olfactory cortices, and the hippocampus, distributed encoding with the above two properties, of representing similarity, and of exponentially increasing encoding capacity as the number of neurons in the representation increases, is found (Rolls & Tovee 1995, Abbott, Rolls & Tovee 1996, Rolls, Treves & Tovee 1997d, Rolls,

Treves, Robertson, Georges-François & Panzeri 1998b, Rolls, Aggelopoulos, Franco & Treves 2004, Franco, Rolls, Aggelopoulos & Jerez 2007, Rolls 2008b, Rolls, Critchley, Verhagen & Kadohisa 2010a, Rolls & Treves 2011). For example, in the primate inferior temporal visual cortex, the number of faces or objects that can be represented increases approximately exponentially with the number of neurons in the population (see Chapter 4). If we consider instead the information about which stimulus is seen, we see that this rises approximately linearly with the number of neurons in the representation (see Chapter 4). This corresponds to an exponential rise in the number of stimuli encoded, because information is a log measure (see Rolls & Treves (2011)). A similar result has been found for the encoding of position in space by the primate hippocampus (Rolls, Treves, Robertson, Georges-François & Panzeri 1998b). Similar results have been found for the encoding of information about taste and olfactory stimuli in the orbitofrontal cortex (Rolls, Critchley, Verhagen & Kadohisa 2010a, Rolls & Treves 2011). It is particularly important that the information can be read from the ensemble of neurons using a simple measure of the similarity of vectors, the correlation (or dot product) between two vectors. The importance of this is that it is essentially vector similarity operations that characterize the operation of many neuronal networks (see Section A.2). The neurophysiological results show that both the ability to reflect similarity by vector correlation, and the utilization of exponential coding capacity, are properties of real neuronal networks found in the brain.

To emphasize one of the points being made here, although the binary encoding used in the 8-bit vector described above has optimal capacity for binary encoding, it is not optimal for vector similarity operations. For example, the two very similar numbers 127 and 128 are represented by 01111111 and 10000000 with binary encoding, yet the correlation or bit overlap of these vectors is 0. The brain in contrast uses a code that has the attractive property of exponentially increasing capacity with the number of neurons in the representation, though it is different from the simple binary encoding of numbers used in computers; and at the same time the brain codes stimuli in such a way that the code can be read off with simple dot product or correlation-related decoding, which is what is specified for the elementary neuronal network operation shown in Equation A.1 (see Rolls (2008b)).

A.2 Pattern association memory

A fundamental operation of most nervous systems is to learn to associate a first stimulus with a second that occurs at about the same time, and to retrieve the second stimulus when the first is presented. The first stimulus might be the sight of food, and the second stimulus the taste of food. After the association has been learned, the sight of food would enable its taste to be retrieved. In classical conditioning, the taste of food might elicit an unconditioned response of salivation, and if the sight of the food is paired with its taste, then the sight of that food would by learning come to produce salivation. Pattern associators are thus used where the outputs of the visual system interface to learning systems in the orbitofrontal cortex and amygdala that learn associations between the sight of objects and their taste or touch in stimulus–reinforcer association learning (see Chapter 4). Pattern association is also used throughout the visual processing cortical areas, as it is the architecture that describes the backprojection connections from one cortical area to the preceding cortical area (Rolls & Deco 2002, Rolls 2008b). Pattern association thus contributes to implementing top-down influences in vision, including the effects of attention from higher to lower cortical areas, and thus between the object and spatial processing streams (Rolls & Deco 2002); the effects of mood on memory and visual information processing (see Section 4.12); the recall of visual memories; and the operation of visual short-term memory (Rolls 2008b).

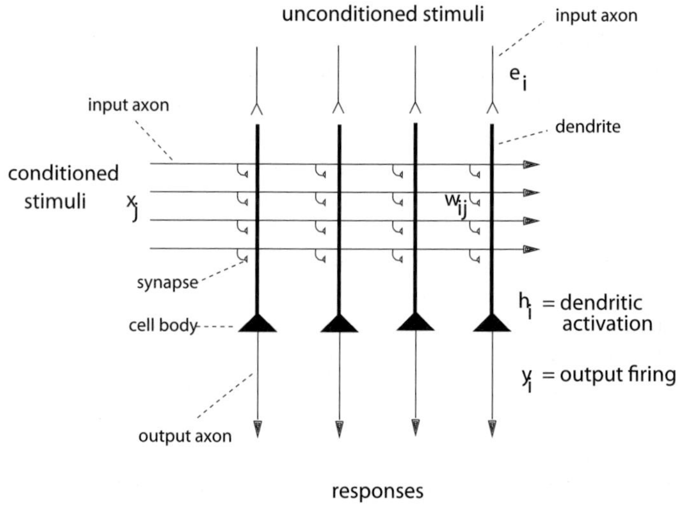

Fig. A.7 A pattern association memory. An unconditioned stimulus has activity or firing rate e_i for the ith neuron, and produces firing y_i of the ith neuron. An unconditioned stimulus may be treated as a vector, across the set of neurons indexed by i, of activity $\mathbf{e}$. The firing rate response can also be thought of as a vector of firing $\mathbf{y}$. The conditioned stimuli have activity or firing rate x_j for the jth axon, which can also be treated as a vector $\mathbf{x}$.

A.2.1 Architecture and operation

The essential elements necessary for pattern association, forming what could be called a prototypical pattern associator network, are shown in Fig. A.7. What we have called the second or unconditioned stimulus pattern is applied through unmodifiable synapses generating an input to each neuron, which, being external with respect to the synaptic matrix we focus on, we can call the external input e_i for the ith neuron. (We can also treat this as a vector, $\mathbf{e}$, as indicated in the legend to Fig. A.7. Vectors and simple operations performed with them are summarized in Appendix A of Rolls (2008b).) This unconditioned stimulus is dominant in producing or forcing the firing of the output neurons (y_i for the ith neuron, or the vector $\mathbf{y}$). At the same time, the first or conditioned stimulus pattern consisting of the set of firings on the horizontally running input axons in Fig. A.7 (x_j for the jth axon) (or equivalently the vector $\mathbf{x}$) is applied through modifiable synapses w_{ij} to the dendrites of the output neurons. The synapses are modifiable in such a way that if there is presynaptic firing on an input axon x_j paired during learning with postsynaptic activity on neuron i, then the strength or weight w_{ij} between that axon and the dendrite increases. This simple learning rule is often called the Hebb rule, after Donald Hebb who in 1949 formulated the hypothesis that if the firing of one neuron was regularly associated with another, then the strength of the synapse or synapses between the neurons should increase[46]. After learning, presenting the pattern $\mathbf{x}$ on the input axons will activate the dendrite through the strengthened synapses. If the cue or conditioned stimulus pattern is the same as that learned, the postsynaptic neurons will be activated, even in the absence of the external or unconditioned input, as each of the firing axons produces

[46] In fact, the terms in which Hebb put the hypothesis were a little different from an association memory, in that he stated that if one neuron regularly comes to elicit firing in another, then the strength of the synapses should increase. He had in mind the building of what he called cell assemblies. In a pattern associator, the conditioned stimulus need not produce before learning any significant activation of the output neurons. The connections must simply increase if there is associated pre- and postsynaptic firing when, in pattern association, most of the postsynaptic firing is being produced by a different input.

through a strengthened synapse some activation of the postsynaptic element, the dendrite. The total activation h_i of each postsynaptic neuron i is then the sum of such individual activations. In this way, the 'correct' output neurons, that is those activated during learning, can end up being the ones most strongly activated, and the second or unconditioned stimulus can be effectively recalled. The recall is best when only strong activation of the postsynaptic neuron produces firing, that is if there is a threshold for firing, just like real neurons. The advantages of this are evident when many associations are stored in the memory, as will soon be shown.

Next we introduce a more precise description of the above by writing down explicit mathematical rules for the operation of the simple network model of Fig. A.7, which will help us to understand how pattern association memories in general operate. (In this description we introduce simple vector operations, and, for those who are not familiar with these, refer the reader to for example Appendix 1 of Rolls (2008b).) We have denoted above a conditioned stimulus input pattern as $\mathbf{x}$. Each of the axons has a firing rate, and if we count or index through the axons using the subscript j, the firing rate of the first axon is x_1, of the second x_2, of the jth x_j, etc. The whole set of axons forms a vector, which is just an ordered (1, 2, 3, etc.) set of elements. The firing rate of each axon x_j is one element of the firing rate vector $\mathbf{x}$. Similarly, using i as the index, we can denote the firing rate of any output neuron as y_i, and the firing rate output vector as $\mathbf{y}$. With this terminology, we can then identify any synapse onto neuron i from neuron j as w_{ij} (see Fig. A.7). In this book, the first index, i, always refers to the receiving neuron (and thus signifies a dendrite), while the second index, j, refers to the sending neuron (and thus signifies a conditioned stimulus input axon in Fig. A.7). We can now specify the learning and retrieval operations as follows:

A.2.1.1 Learning

The firing rate of every output neuron is forced to a value determined by the unconditioned (or external or forcing stimulus) input. In our simple model this means that for any one neuron i,

$$y_i = \mathrm{f}(e_i) \tag{A.5}$$

which indicates that the firing rate is a function of the dendritic activation, taken in this case to reduce essentially to that resulting from the external forcing input (see Fig. A.7). The function f is called the activation function (see Fig. A.3), and its precise form is irrelevant, at least during this learning phase. For example, the function at its simplest could be taken to be linear, so that the firing rate would be just proportional to the activation.

The Hebb rule can then be written as follows:

$$\delta w_{ij} = \alpha y_i x_j \tag{A.6}$$

where δw_{ij} is the change of the synaptic weight w_{ij} that results from the simultaneous (or conjunctive) presence of presynaptic firing x_j and postsynaptic firing or activation y_i, and α is a learning rate constant that specifies how much the synapses alter on any one pairing.

The Hebb rule is expressed in this multiplicative form to reflect the idea that both presynaptic and postsynaptic activity must be present for the synapses to increase in strength. The multiplicative form also reflects the idea that strong pre- and postsynaptic firing will produce a larger change of synaptic weight than smaller firing rates. It is also assumed for now that before any learning takes place, the synaptic strengths are small in relation to the changes that can be produced during Hebbian learning. We will see that this assumption can be relaxed later when a modified Hebb rule is introduced that can lead to a reduction in synaptic strength under some conditions.

A.2.1.2 Recall

When the conditioned stimulus is present on the input axons, the total activation h_i of a neuron i is the sum of all the activations produced through each strengthened synapse w_{ij} by each active neuron x_j. We can express this as

$$h_i = \sum_{j=1}^{C} x_j w_{ij} \tag{A.7}$$

where $\sum_{j=1}^{C}$ indicates that the sum is over the C input axons (or connections) indexed by j to each neuron.

The multiplicative form here indicates that activation should be produced by an axon only if it is firing, and only if it is connected to the dendrite by a strengthened synapse. It also indicates that the strength of the activation reflects how fast the axon x_j is firing, and how strong the synapse w_{ij} is. The sum of all such activations expresses the idea that summation (of synaptic currents in real neurons) occurs along the length of the dendrite, to produce activation at the cell body, where the activation h_i is converted into firing y_i. This conversion can be expressed as

$$y_i = \mathrm{f}(h_i) \tag{A.8}$$

where the function f is again the activation function. The form of the function now becomes more important. Real neurons have thresholds, with firing occurring only if the activation is above the threshold. A threshold linear activation function is shown in Fig. A.3b. This has been useful in formal analysis of the properties of neural networks. Neurons also have firing rates that become saturated at a maximum rate, and we could express this as the sigmoid activation function shown in Fig. A.3c. Yet another simple activation function, used in some models of neural networks, is the binary threshold function (Fig. A.3d), which indicates that if the activation is below threshold, there is no firing, and that if the activation is above threshold, the neuron fires maximally. Whatever the exact shape of the activation function, some non-linearity is an advantage, for it enables small activations produced by interfering memories to be minimized, and it can enable neurons to perform logical operations, such as to fire or respond only if two or more sets of inputs are present simultaneously.

A.2.2 A simple model

An example of these learning and recall operations is provided in a simple form as follows. The neurons will have simple firing rates, which can be 0 to represent no activity, and 1 to indicate high firing. They are thus binary neurons, which can assume one of two firing rates. If we have a pattern associator with six input axons and four output neurons, we could represent the network before learning, with the same layout as in Fig. A.7, as shown in Fig. A.8:

	UCS			
	1	1	0	0
	↓	↓	↓	↓
CS				
1 →	0	0	0	0
0 →	0	0	0	0
1 →	0	0	0	0
0 →	0	0	0	0
1 →	0	0	0	0
0 →	0	0	0	0

Fig. A.8 Pattern association: before synaptic modification. The unconditioned stimulus (UCS) firing rates are shown as 1 if high and 0 if low as a row vector being applied to force firing of the four output neurons. The six conditioned stimulus (CS) firing rates are shown as a column vector being applied to the vertical dendrites of the output neurons which have initial synaptic weights of 0.

where $\mathbf{x}$ or the conditioned stimulus (CS) is 101010, and $\mathbf{y}$ or the firing produced by the unconditioned stimulus (UCS) is 1100. (The arrows indicate the flow of signals.) The synaptic weights are initially all 0.

After pairing the CS with the UCS during one learning trial, some of the synaptic weights will be incremented according to Equation A.6, so that after learning this pair the synaptic weights will become as shown in Fig. A.9:

	UCS			
	1	1	0	0
	↓	↓	↓	↓
CS				
1 →	1	1	0	0
0 →	0	0	0	0
1 →	1	1	0	0
0 →	0	0	0	0
1 →	1	1	0	0
0 →	0	0	0	0

Fig. A.9 Pattern association: after synaptic modification. The synapses where there is conjunctive pre- and post-synaptic activity have been strengthened to value 1.

We can represent what happens during recall, when, for example, we present the CS that has been learned, as shown in Fig. A.10:

CS					
1 →	1	1	0	0	
0 →	0	0	0	0	
1 →	1	1	0	0	
0 →	0	0	0	0	
1 →	1	1	0	0	
0 →	0	0	0	0	
	↓	↓	↓	↓	
	3	3	0	0	Activation h_i
	1	1	0	0	Firing y_i

Fig. A.10 Pattern association: recall. The activation h_i of each neuron i is converted with a threshold of 2 to the binary firing rate y_i (1 for high, and 0 for low).

The activation of the four output neurons is 3300, and if we set the threshold of each output neuron to 2, then the output firing is 1100 (where the binary firing rate is 0 if below threshold, and 1 if above). The pattern associator has thus achieved recall of the pattern 1100, which is correct.

We can now illustrate how a number of different associations can be stored in such a pattern associator, and retrieved correctly. Let us associate a new CS pattern 110001 with the UCS 0101 in the same pattern associator. The weights will become as shown next in Fig. A.11 after learning:

	U	C	S	
	0	1	0	1
	↓	↓	↓	↓
CS				
1 →	1	2	0	1
1 →	0	1	0	1
0 →	1	1	0	0
0 →	0	0	0	0
0 →	1	1	0	0
1 →	0	1	0	1

Fig. A.11 Pattern association: synaptic weights after learning a second pattern association.

If we now present the second CS, the retrieval is as shown in Fig. A.12:

CS					
1 →	1	2	0	1	
1 →	0	1	0	1	
0 →	1	1	0	0	
0 →	0	0	0	0	
0 →	1	1	0	0	
1 →	0	1	0	1	
	↓	↓	↓	↓	
	1	4	0	3	Activation h_i
	0	1	0	1	Firing y_i

Fig. A.12 Pattern association: recall with the second CS.

The binary output firings were again produced with the threshold set to 2. Recall is perfect.

This illustration shows the value of some threshold non-linearity in the activation function of the neurons. In this case, the activations did reflect some small cross-talk or interference from the previous pattern association of CS1 with UCS1, but this was removed by the threshold operation, to clean up the recall firing. The example also shows that when further associations are learned by a pattern associator trained with the Hebb rule, Equation A.6, some synapses will reflect increments above a synaptic strength of 1. It is left as an exercise to the reader to verify that recall is still perfect to CS1, the vector 101010. (The activation vector $\mathbf{h}$ is 3401, and the output firing vector $\mathbf{y}$ with the same threshold of 2 is 1100, which is perfect recall.)

A.2.3 The vector interpretation

The way in which recall is produced, Equation A.7, consists for each output neuron i of multiplying each input firing rate x_j by the corresponding synaptic weight w_{ij} and summing the products to obtain the activation h_i. Now we can consider the firing rates x_j where j varies from 1 to N', the number of axons, to be a vector. (A vector is simply an ordered set of numbers – see Appendix 1 of Rolls (2008b).) Let us call this vector $\mathbf{x}$. Similarly, on a neuron i, the synaptic weights can be treated as a vector, $\mathbf{w}_i$. (The subscript i here indicates that this is the weight vector on the ith neuron.) The operation we have just described to obtain the activation of an output neuron can now be seen to be a simple multiplication operation of two vectors to produce a single output value (called a scalar output). This is the inner product or dot product of two vectors, and can be written

$$h_i = \mathbf{x} \cdot \mathbf{w}_i. \tag{A.9}$$

The inner product of two vectors indicates how similar they are. If two vectors have corresponding elements the same, then the dot product will be maximal. If the two vectors are similar but not identical, then the dot product will be high. If the two vectors are completely different, the dot product will be 0, and the vectors are described as orthogonal. (The term orthogonal means at right angles, and arises from the geometric interpretation of vectors, which is summarized in Appendix 1 of Rolls (2008b).) Thus the dot product provides a direct measure of how similar two vectors are.

It can now be seen that a fundamental operation many neurons perform is effectively to compute how similar an input pattern vector $\mathbf{x}$ is to their stored weight vector $\mathbf{w}_i$. The similarity measure they compute, the dot product, is a very good measure of similarity, and indeed, the standard (Pearson product-moment) correlation coefficient used in statistics is the same as a normalized dot product with the mean subtracted from each vector, as shown in Appendix 1 of Rolls (2008b). (The normalization used in the correlation coefficient results in the coefficient varying always between $+1$ and -1, whereas the actual scalar value of a dot product clearly depends on the length of the vectors from which it is calculated.)

With these concepts, we can now see that during learning, a pattern associator adds to its weight vector a vector $\delta\mathbf{w}_i$ that has the same pattern as the input pattern $\mathbf{x}$, if the postsynaptic neuron i is strongly activated. Indeed, we can express Equation A.6 in vector form as

$$\delta\mathbf{w}_i = \alpha y_i \mathbf{x}. \tag{A.10}$$

We can now see that what is recalled by the neuron depends on the similarity of the recall cue vector $\mathbf{x}_r$ to the originally learned vector $\mathbf{x}$. The fact that during recall the output of each neuron reflects the similarity (as measured by the dot product) of the input pattern $\mathbf{x}_r$ to each of the patterns used originally as $\mathbf{x}$ inputs (conditioned stimuli in Fig. A.7) provides a simple way to appreciate many of the interesting and biologically useful properties of pattern associators, as described next.

A.2.4 Properties

A.2.4.1 Generalization

During recall, pattern associators generalize, and produce appropriate outputs if a recall cue vector $\mathbf{x}_r$ is similar to a vector that has been learned already. This occurs because the recall operation involves computing the dot (inner) product of the input pattern vector $\mathbf{x}_r$ with the synaptic weight vector $\mathbf{w}_i$, so that the firing produced, y_i, reflects the similarity of the current input to the previously learned input pattern $\mathbf{x}$. (Generalization will occur to input cue or conditioned stimulus patterns $\mathbf{x}_r$ that are incomplete versions of an original conditioned stimulus $\mathbf{x}$, although the term completion is usually applied to the autoassociation networks described in Section A.3.)

This is an important property of pattern associators, for input stimuli during recall will rarely be absolutely identical to what has been learned previously, and automatic generalization to similar stimuli is extremely useful, and has great adaptive value in biological systems.

Generalization can be illustrated with the simple binary pattern associator considered above. (Those who have appreciated the vector description just given might wish to skip this illustration.) Instead of the second CS, pattern vector 110001, we will use the similar recall cue 110100, as shown in Fig. A.13:

CS					
1 →	1	2	0	1	
1 →	0	1	0	1	
0 →	1	1	0	0	
1 →	0	0	0	0	
0 →	1	1	0	0	
0 →	0	1	0	1	
	↓	↓	↓	↓	
	1	3	0	2	Activation h_i
	0	1	0	1	Firing y_i

Fig. A.13 Pattern association: generalization using an input vector similar to the second CS.

It is seen that the output firing rate vector, 0101, is exactly what should be recalled to CS2 (and not to CS1), so correct generalization has occurred. Although this is a small network trained with few examples, the same properties hold for large networks with large numbers of stored patterns, as described more quantitatively in the section on capacity below and in Appendix A3 of Rolls & Treves (1998).

A.2.4.2 Graceful degradation or fault tolerance

If the synaptic weight vector $\mathbf{w}_i$ (or the weight matrix, which we can call $\mathbf{W}$) has synapses missing (e.g. during development), or loses synapses, then the activation h_i or $\mathbf{h}$ is still reasonable, because h_i is the dot product (correlation) of $\mathbf{x}$ with $\mathbf{w}_i$. The result, especially after passing through the activation function, can frequently be perfect recall. The same property arises if for example one or some of the conditioned stimulus (CS) input axons are lost or damaged. This is a very important property of associative memories, and is not a property of conventional computer memories, which produce incorrect data if even only 1 storage location (for 1 bit or binary digit of data) of their memory is damaged or cannot be accessed. This property of graceful degradation is of great adaptive value for biological systems.

We can illustrate this with a simple example. If we damage two of the synapses in Fig. A.12 to produce the synaptic matrix shown in Fig. A.14 (where x indicates a damaged synapse which has no effect, but was previously 1), and now present the second CS, the retrieval is as follows:

CS					
1 →	1	2	0	1	
1 →	0	1	0	x	
0 →	1	1	0	0	
0 →	0	0	0	0	
0 →	1	x	0	0	
1 →	0	1	0	1	
	↓	↓	↓	↓	
	1	4	0	2	Activation h_i
	0	1	0	1	Firing y_i

Fig. A.14 Pattern association: graceful degradation when some synapses are damaged (x).

The binary output firings were again produced with the threshold set to 2. The recalled vector, 0101, is perfect. This illustration again shows the value of some threshold non-linearity in the activation function of the neurons. It is left as an exercise to the reader to verify that recall is still perfect to CS1, the vector 101010. (The output activation vector **h** is 3301, and the output firing vector **y** with the same threshold of 2 is 1100, which is perfect recall.)

A.2.4.3 The importance of distributed representations for pattern associators

A distributed representation is one in which the firing or activity of all the elements in the vector is used to encode a particular stimulus. For example, in a conditioned stimulus vector CS1 that has the value 101010, we need to know the state of all the elements to know which stimulus is being represented. Another stimulus, CS2, is represented by the vector 110001. We can represent many different events or stimuli with such overlapping sets of elements, and because in general any one element cannot be used to identify the stimulus, but instead the information about which stimulus is present is distributed over the population of elements or neurons, this is called a distributed representation (see Section A.1.6). If, for binary neurons, half the neurons are in one state (e.g. 0), and the other half are in the other state (e.g. 1), then the representation is described as fully distributed. The CS representations above are thus fully distributed. If only a smaller proportion of the neurons is active to represent a stimulus, as in the vector 100001, then this is a sparse representation. For binary representations, we can quantify the sparseness by the proportion of neurons in the active (1) state.

In contrast, a local representation is one in which all the information that a particular stimulus or event has occurred is provided by the activity of one of the neurons, or elements in the vector. One stimulus might be represented by the vector 100000, another stimulus by the vector 010000, and a third stimulus by the vector 001000. The activity of neuron or element 1 would indicate that stimulus 1 was present, and of neuron 2, that stimulus 2 was present. The representation is local in that if a particular neuron is active, we know that the stimulus represented by that neuron is present. In neurophysiology, if such cells were present, they might be called 'grandmother cells' (cf. Barlow (1972, 1995, 2008b)), in that one neuron might represent a stimulus in the environment as complex and specific as one's grandmother. Where the activity of a number of cells must be taken into account in order to represent a stimulus (such as an individual taste), then the representation is sometimes described as using ensemble encoding.

The properties just described for associative memories, generalization, and graceful degradation are only implemented if the representation of the CS or $\mathbf{x}$ vector is distributed. This occurs because the recall operation involves computing the dot (inner) product of the input pattern vector $\mathbf{x}_r$ with the synaptic weight vector $\mathbf{w}_i$. This allows the activation h_i to reflect the similarity of the current input pattern to a previously learned input pattern $\mathbf{x}$ only if several or many elements of the $\mathbf{x}$ and $\mathbf{x}_r$ vectors are in the active state to represent a pattern. If local encoding were used, e.g. 100000, then if the first element of the vector (which might be the firing of axon 1, i.e. x_1, or the strength of synapse $i1$, w_{i1}) is lost, the resulting vector is not similar to any other CS vector, and the activation is 0. In the case of local encoding, the important properties of associative memories, generalization and graceful degradation do not thus emerge. Graceful degradation and generalization are dependent on distributed representations, for then the dot product can reflect similarity even when some elements of the vectors involved are altered. If we think of the correlation between Y and X in a graph, then this correlation is affected only a little if a few X, Y pairs of data are lost (see Appendix 1 of Rolls (2008b)).

A.2.5 Prototype extraction, extraction of central tendency, and noise reduction

If a set of similar conditioned stimulus vectors $\mathbf{x}$ are paired with the same unconditioned stimulus e_i, the weight vector $\mathbf{w}_i$ becomes (or points towards) the sum (or with scaling, the average) of the set of similar vectors $\mathbf{x}$. This follows from the operation of the Hebb rule in Equation A.6. When tested at recall, the output of the memory is then best to the average input pattern vector denoted $< \mathbf{x} >$. If the average is thought of as a prototype, then even though the prototype vector $< \mathbf{x} >$ itself may never have been seen, the best output of the neuron or network is to the prototype. This produces 'extraction of the prototype' or 'central tendency'. The same phenomenon is a feature of human memory performance (see McClelland & Rumelhart (1986) Chapter 17), and this simple process with distributed representations in a neural network accounts for the psychological phenomenon.

If the different exemplars of the vector $\mathbf{x}$ are thought of as noisy versions of the true input pattern vector $< \mathbf{x} >$ (with incorrect values for some of the elements), then the pattern associator has performed 'noise reduction', in that the output produced by any one of these vectors will represent the output produced by the true, noiseless, average vector $< \mathbf{x} >$.

A.2.6 Speed

Recall is very fast in a real neuronal network, because the conditioned stimulus input firings x_j ($j = 1, C$ axons) can be applied simultaneously to the synapses w_{ij}, and the activation h_i can be accumulated in one or two time constants of the dendrite (e.g. 10–20 ms). Whenever the threshold of the cell is exceeded, it fires. Thus, in effectively one step, which takes the brain no more than 10–20 ms, all the output neurons of the pattern associator can be firing with rates that reflect the input firing of every axon. This is very different from a conventional digital computer, in which computing h_i in Equation A.7 would involve C multiplication and addition operations occurring one after another, or $2C$ time steps.

The brain performs parallel computation in at least two senses in even a pattern associator. One is that for a single neuron, the separate contributions of the firing rate x_j of each axon j multiplied by the synaptic weight w_{ij} are computed in parallel and added in the same time step. The second is that this can be performed in parallel for all neurons $i = 1, N$ in the network, where there are N output neurons in the network. It is these types of parallel processing that enable these classes of neuronal network in the brain to operate so fast, in effectively so few steps.

Learning is also fast ('one-shot') in pattern associators, in that a single pairing of the conditioned stimulus $\mathbf{x}$ and the unconditioned stimulus (UCS) $\mathbf{e}$ which produces the unconditioned output firing $\mathbf{y}$ enables the association to be learned. There is no need to repeat the pairing in order to discover over many trials the appropriate mapping. This is extremely important for biological systems, in which a single co-occurrence of two events may lead to learning that could have life-saving consequences. (For example, the pairing of a visual stimulus with a potentially life-threatening aversive event may enable that event to be avoided in future.) Although repeated pairing with small variations of the vectors is used to obtain the useful properties of prototype extraction, extraction of central tendency, and noise reduction, the essential properties of generalization and graceful degradation are obtained with just one pairing. The actual time scales of the learning in the brain are indicated by studies of associative synaptic modification using long-term potentiation paradigms (LTP, see Section A.1.5). Co-occurrence or near simultaneity of the CS and UCS is required for periods of as little as 100 ms, with expression of the synaptic modification being present within typically a few seconds.

A.2.7 Local learning rule

The simplest learning rule used in pattern association neural networks, a version of the Hebb rule, is, as shown in Equation A.6 above,

$$\delta w_{ij} = \alpha y_i x_j.$$

This is a local learning rule in that the information required to specify the change in synaptic weight is available locally at the synapse, as it is dependent only on the presynaptic firing rate x_j available at the synaptic terminal, and the postsynaptic activation or firing y_i available on the dendrite of the neuron receiving the synapse (see Fig. A.15b). This makes the learning rule biologically plausible, in that the information about how to change the synaptic weight does not have to be carried from a distant source, where it is computed, to every synapse. Such a non-local learning rule would not be biologically plausible, in that there are no appropriate connections known in most parts of the brain to bring in the synaptic training or teacher signal to every synapse.

Evidence that a learning rule with the general form of Equation A.6 is implemented in at least some parts of the brain comes from studies of long-term potentiation, described in Section A.1.5. Long-term potentiation (LTP) has the synaptic specificity defined by Equation A.6, in that only synapses from active afferents, not those from inactive afferents, become strengthened. Synaptic specificity is important for a pattern associator, and most other types of neuronal network, to operate correctly. The number of independently modifiable synapses on each neuron is a primary factor in determining how many different memory patterns can be stored in associative memories (see Sections A.2.7.1 and A.3.3.6).

Another useful property of real neurons in relation to Equation A.6 is that the postsynaptic term, y_i, is available on much of the dendrite of a cell, because the electrotonic length of the dendrite is short. In addition, active propagation of spiking activity from the cell body along the dendrite may help to provide a uniform postsynaptic term for the learning. Thus if a neuron is strongly activated with a high value for y_i, then any active synapse onto the cell will be capable of being modified. This enables the cell to learn an association between the pattern of activity on all its axons and its postsynaptic activation, which is stored as an addition to its weight vector $\mathbf{w}_i$. Then later on, at recall, the output can be produced as a vector dot product

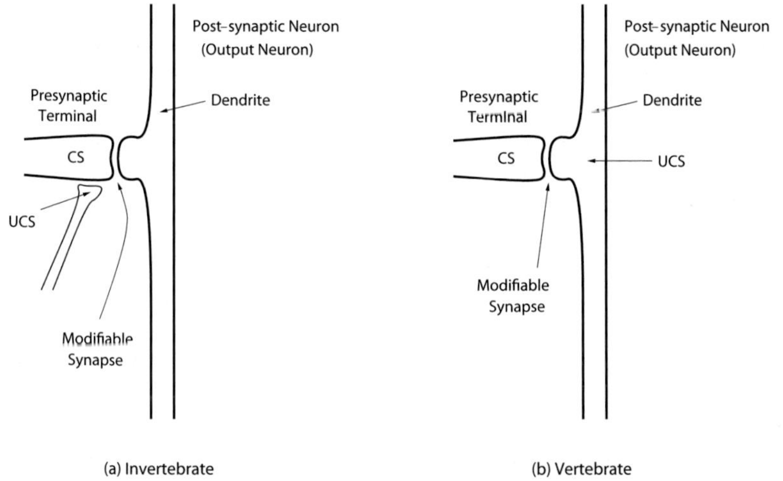

Fig. A.15 (b) In vertebrate pattern association learning, the unconditioned stimulus (UCS) may be made available at all the conditioned stimulus (CS) terminals onto the output neuron because the dendrite of the postsynaptic neuron is electrically short, so that the effect of the UCS spreads for long distances along the dendrite. (a) In contrast, in at least some invertebrate association learning systems, the unconditioned stimulus or teaching input makes a synapse onto the presynaptic terminal carrying the conditioned stimulus.

operation between the input pattern vector $\mathbf{x}$ and the weight vector $\mathbf{w}_i$, so that the output of the cell can reflect the correlation between the current input vector and what has previously been learned by the cell.

It is interesting that at least many invertebrate neuronal systems may operate very differently from those described here, as described by Rolls & Treves (1998) (see Fig. A.15a).

A.2.7.1 Capacity

The question of the storage capacity of a pattern associator is considered in detail in Appendix A3 of Rolls & Treves (1998). It is pointed out there that, for this type of associative network, the number of memories that it can hold simultaneously in storage has to be analysed together with the retrieval quality of each output representation, and then only for a given quality of the representation provided in the input. This is in contrast to autoassociative nets (Section A.3), in which a critical number of stored memories exists (as a function of various parameters of the network), beyond which attempting to store additional memories results in it becoming impossible to retrieve essentially anything. With a pattern associator, instead, one will always retrieve something, but this something will be very small (in information or correlation terms) if too many associations are simultaneously in storage and/or if too little is provided as input.

The conjoint quality-capacity input analysis can be carried out, for any specific instance of a pattern associator, by using formal mathematical models and established analytical procedures (see e.g. Treves (1995)). This, however, has to be done case by case. It is anyway useful to develop some intuition for how a pattern associator operates, by considering what its capacity would be in certain well-defined simplified cases.

Linear associative neuronal networks These networks are made up of units with a linear activation function, which appears to make them unsuitable to represent real neurons with their positive-only firing rates. However, even purely linear units have been considered as provisionally relevant models of real neurons, by assuming that the latter operate sometimes in the linear regime of their transfer function. (This implies a high level of spontaneous activity, and may be closer to conditions observed early on in sensory systems rather than in areas more specifically involved in memory.) As usual, the connections are trained by a Hebb (or similar) associative learning rule. The capacity of these networks can be defined as the total number of associations that can be learned independently of each other, given that the linear nature of these systems prevents anything more than a linear transform of the inputs. This implies that if input pattern C can be written as the weighted sum of input patterns A and B, the output to C will be just the same weighted sum of the outputs to A and B. If there are N' input axons, then there can be only at most N' mutually independent input patterns (i.e. none able to be written as a weighted sum of the others), and therefore the capacity of linear networks, defined above, is just N', or equal to the number of inputs to each neuron. In general, a random set of less than N' vectors (the CS input pattern vectors) will tend to be mutually independent but not mutually orthogonal (at 90 deg to each other) (see Appendix 1 of Rolls (2008b)). If they are not orthogonal (the normal situation), then the dot product of them is not 0, and the output pattern activated by one of the input vectors will be partially activated by other input pattern vectors, in accordance with how similar they are (see Equations A.9 and A.10). This amounts to interference, which is therefore the more serious the less orthogonal, on the whole, is the set of input vectors.

Since input patterns are made of elements with positive values, if a simple Hebbian learning rule like the one of Equation A.6 is used (in which the input pattern enters directly with no subtraction term), the output resulting from the application of a stored input vector will be the sum of contributions from all other input vectors that have a non-zero dot product with it (see Appendix 1 of Rolls (2008b)), and interference will be disastrous. The only situation in which this would not occur is when different input patterns activate completely different input lines, but this is clearly an uninteresting circumstance for networks operating with distributed representations. A solution to this issue is to use a modified learning rule of the following form:

$$\delta w_{ij} = \alpha y_i (x_j - x) \tag{A.11}$$

where x is a constant, approximately equal to the average value of x_j. This learning rule includes (in proportion to y_i) increasing the synaptic weight if $(x_j - x) > 0$ (long-term potentiation), and decreasing the synaptic weight if $(x_j - x) < 0$ (heterosynaptic long-term depression). It is useful for x to be roughly the average activity of an input axon x_j across patterns, because then the dot product between the various patterns stored on the weights and the input vector will tend to cancel out with the subtractive term, except for the pattern equal to (or correlated with) the input vector itself. Then up to N' input vectors can still be learned by the network, with only minor interference (provided of course that they are mutually independent, as they will in general tend to be).

This modified learning rule can also be described in terms of a contingency table (Table A.1) showing the synaptic strength modifications produced by different types of learning rule, where LTP indicates an increase in synaptic strength (called Long-Term Potentiation in neurophysiology), and LTD indicates a decrease in synaptic strength (called Long-Term Depression in neurophysiology). Heterosynaptic long-term depression is so-called because it is the decrease in synaptic strength that occurs to a synapse that is other than that through which the postsynaptic cell is being activated. This heterosynaptic long-term depression is the type of change of synaptic strength that is required (in addition to LTP) for effective subtraction of the average presynaptic firing rate, in order, as it were, to make the CS vectors appear more orthogonal to the pattern associator. The rule is sometimes called the Singer–Stent rule, after work by Singer (1987) and Stent (1973), and was discovered in the brain by Levy (Levy (1985); Levy & Desmond (1985); see Brown, Kairiss & Keenan (1990)). Homosynaptic long-

Table A.1 Effects of pre- and post-synaptic activity on synaptic modification

		Post-synaptic activation	
		0	high
Presynaptic firing	0	No change	Heterosynaptic LTD
	high	Homosynaptic LTD	LTP

term depression is so-called because it is the decrease in synaptic strength that occurs to a synapse which is (the same as that which is) active. For it to occur, the postsynaptic neuron must simultaneously be inactive, or have only low activity. (This rule is sometimes called the BCM rule after the paper of Bienenstock, Cooper and Munro (1982); see Rolls & Deco (2002), Chapter 7).

Associative neuronal networks with non-linear neurons With non-linear neurons, that is with at least a threshold in the activation function so that the output firing y_i is 0 when the activation h_i is below the threshold, the capacity can be measured in terms of the number of different clusters of output pattern vectors that the network produces. This is because the non-linearities now present (one per output neuron) result in some clustering of the outputs produced by all possible (conditioned stimulus) input patterns $\mathbf{x}$. Input patterns that are similar to a stored input vector can produce, due to the non-linearities, output patterns even closer to the stored output; and vice versa sufficiently dissimilar inputs can be assigned to different output clusters thereby increasing their mutual dissimilarity. As with the linear counterpart, in order to remove the correlation that would otherwise occur between the patterns because the elements can take only positive values, it is useful to use a modified Hebb rule of the form shown in Equation A.11.

With fully distributed output patterns, the number p of associations that leads to different clusters is of order C, the number of input lines (axons) per output neuron (that is, of order N' for a fully connected network), as shown in Appendix A3 of Rolls & Treves (1998). If sparse patterns are used in the output, or alternatively if the learning rule includes a non-linear postsynaptic factor that is effectively equivalent to using sparse output patterns, the coefficient of proportionality between p and C can be much higher than one, that is, many more patterns can be stored than inputs onto each output neuron (see Appendix A3 of Rolls & Treves (1998)). Indeed, the number of different patterns or prototypes p that can be stored can be derived for example in the case of binary units (Gardner 1988) to be

$$p \approx C/[a_o log(1/a_o)] \tag{A.12}$$

where a_o is the sparseness of the output firing pattern $\mathbf{y}$ produced by the unconditioned stimulus. p can in this situation be much larger than C (see Rolls & Treves (1990), and Appendix A3 of Rolls & Treves (1998)). This is an important result for encoding in pattern associators, for it means that provided that the activation functions are non-linear (which is the case with real neurons), there is a very great advantage to using sparse encoding, for then many more than C pattern associations can be stored. Sparse representations may well be present in brain regions involved in associative memory (see Chapter 12 of Rolls & Treves (1998)) for this reason.

Input A	1	0	1
Input B	0	1	1
Required Output	1	1	0

Fig. A.16 A non-linearly separable mapping.

The non-linearity inherent in the NMDA receptor-based Hebbian plasticity present in the brain may help to make the stored patterns more sparse than the input patterns, and this may be especially beneficial in increasing the storage capacity of associative networks in the brain by allowing participation in the storage of especially those relatively few neurons with high firing rates in the exponential firing rate distributions typical of neurons in sensory systems (see Rolls (2008b)).

A.2.7.2 Interference

Interference occurs in linear pattern associators if two vectors are not orthogonal, and is simply dependent on the angle between the originally learned vector and the recall cue or CS vector (see Appendix 1 of Rolls (2008b)), for the activation of the output neuron depends simply on the dot product of the recall vector and the synaptic weight vector (Equation A.9). Also in non-linear pattern associators (the interesting case for all practical purposes), interference may occur if two CS patterns are not orthogonal, though the effect can be controlled with sparse encoding of the UCS patterns, effectively by setting high thresholds for the firing of output units. In other words, the CS vectors need not be strictly orthogonal, but if they are too similar, some interference will still be likely to occur.

The fact that interference is a property of neural network pattern associator memories is of interest, for interference is a major property of human memory. Indeed, the fact that interference is a property of human memory and of neural network association memories is entirely consistent with the hypothesis that human memory is stored in associative memories of the type described here, or at least that network associative memories of the type described represent a useful exemplar of the class of parallel distributed storage network used in human memory.

It may also be suggested that one reason that interference is tolerated in biological memory is that it is associated with the ability to generalize between stimuli, which is an invaluable feature of biological network associative memories, in that it allows the memory to cope with stimuli that will almost never be identical on different occasions, and in that it allows useful analogies that have survival value to be made.

A.2.7.3 Expansion recoding and pattern separation

If patterns are too similar to be stored in associative memories, then one solution that the brain seems to use repeatedly is to expand the encoding to a form in which the different stimulus patterns are less correlated, that is, more orthogonal, before they are presented as CS stimuli to a pattern associator. The problem can be highlighted by a non-linearly separable mapping (which captures part of the eXclusive OR (XOR) problem), in which the mapping that is desired is as shown in Fig. A.16. The neuron has two inputs, A and B.

This is a mapping of patterns that is impossible for a one-layer network, because the patterns are not linearly separable[47]. A solution is to remap the two input lines A and B to three input lines 1–3, that is to use expansion recoding, as shown in Fig. A.17. This can be

[47] See Appendix 1 of Rolls (2008b). There is no set of synaptic weights in a one-layer net that could solve the problem shown in Fig. A.16. Two classes of patterns are not linearly separable if no hyperplane can be positioned

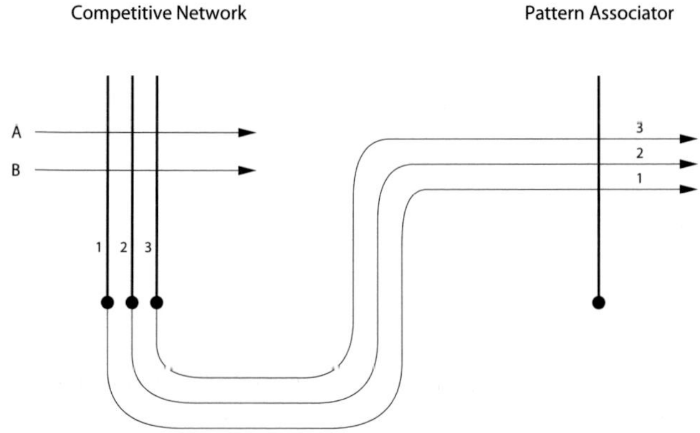

Fig. A.17 Expansion recoding. A competitive network followed by a pattern associator that can enable patterns that are not linearly separable to be learned correctly.

	Synaptic weight
Input 1 (A=1, B=0)	1
Input 2 (A=0, B=1)	1
Input 3 (A=1, B=1)	0

Fig. A.18 Synaptic weights on the dendrite of the output neuron in Fig. A.17.

performed by a competitive network (see Rolls (2008b)). The synaptic weights on the dendrite of the output neuron could then learn the following values using a simple Hebb rule, Equation A.6, and the problem could be solved as in Fig. A.18. The whole network would look like that shown in Fig. A.17.

Rolls & Treves (1998) show that competitive networks could help with this type of recoding, and could provide very useful preprocessing for a pattern associator in the brain. It is possible that the lateral nucleus of the amygdala performs this function, for it receives inputs from the temporal cortical visual areas, and may preprocess them before they become the inputs to associative networks at the next stage of amygdala processing (see Fig. 4.56). Pattern separation is a major function of the dentate gyrus/mossy fibre connections in the hippocampal system (Rolls 2008b, Rolls 2010b).

A.2.8 Implications of different types of coding for storage in pattern associators

Throughout this Section, we have made statements about how the properties of pattern associators – such as the number of patterns that can be stored, and whether generalization and graceful degradation occur – depend on the type of encoding of the patterns to be associated. (The types of encoding considered, local, sparse distributed, and fully distributed, are described above.) We draw together these points in Table A.2.

The amount of information that can be stored in each pattern in a pattern associator is considered in Appendix A3 of Rolls & Treves (1998).

in their N-dimensional space so as to separate them (see Appendix 1 of Rolls (2008b)). The XOR problem has the additional constraint that $A = 0, B = 0$ must be mapped to Output = 0.

Table A.2 Coding in associative memories*

	Local	**Sparse distributed**	**Fully distributed**
Generalization, Completion, Graceful degradation	No	Yes	Yes
Number of patterns that can be stored	N (large)	of order $C/[a_o \log(1/a_o)]$ (can be larger)	of order C (usually smaller than N)
Amount of information in each pattern (values if binary)	Minimal ($\log(N)$ bits)	Intermediate ($Na_o \log(1/a_o)$ bits)	Large (N bits)

* N refers here to the number of output units, and C to the average number of inputs to each output unit. a_o is the sparseness of output patterns, or roughly the proportion of output units activated by a UCS pattern. Note: logs are to the base 2.

In conclusion, the architecture and properties of pattern association networks make them very appropriate for stimulus–reinforcer association learning. Their high capacity enables them to learn the correct reinforcement associations for very large numbers of different stimuli.

A.3 Autoassociation memory: attractor networks

In this section an introduction to autoassociation or attractor networks is given, as this type of network may be relevant to understanding how mood states are maintained.

Autoassociative memories, or attractor neural networks, store memories, each one of which is represented by a different set of the neurons firing. The memories are stored in the recurrent synaptic connections between the neurons of the network, for example in the recurrent collateral connections between cortical pyramidal cells. Autoassociative networks can then recall the appropriate memory from the network when provided with a fragment of one of the memories. This is called completion. Many different memories can be stored in the network and retrieved correctly. A feature of this type of memory is that it is content addressable: that is, the information in the memory can be accessed if just the contents of the memory (or a part of the contents of the memory) are used. This is in contrast to a conventional computer, in which the address of what is to be accessed must be supplied, and used to access the contents of the memory. Content addressability is an important simplifying feature of this type of memory, which makes it suitable for use in biological systems. The issue of content addressability will be amplified below.

An autoassociation memory can be used as a short-term memory, in which iterative processing round the recurrent collateral connections between the principal neurons in the network keeps a representation active by continuing, persistent, neuronal firing. Used in this way, attractor networks provide the basis for the implementation of short-term memory in the dorsolateral prefrontal cortex. In this cortical area, the short-term memory provides the basis for keeping a memory active even while perceptual areas such as the inferior temporal visual cortex must respond to each incoming visual stimulus in order for it to be processed, to produce behavioural responses, and for it to be perceived (Renart, Moreno, Rocha, Parga & Rolls 2001). The implementation of short-term memory in the prefrontal cortex which can maintain neuronal firing even across intervening stimuli provides an important foundation for attention, in which an item or items must be held in mind for a period and during this time bias other brain areas by top-down processing using cortico-cortical backprojections (Rolls 2008b, Deco & Rolls 2004, Deco & Rolls 2005c), or determine how stimuli are

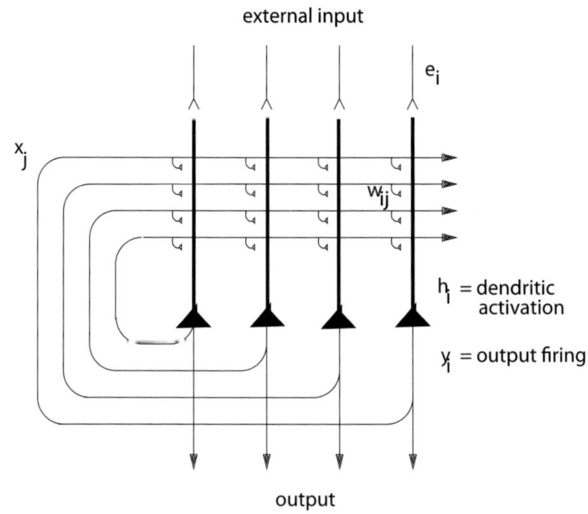

Fig. A.19 The architecture of an autoassociative neural network.

mapped to responses (Deco & Rolls 2003) or to rewards (see Deco & Rolls (2005a)) with rapid, one-trial, task switching and decision-making. This dorsolateral prefrontal cortex short-term memory system also provides a computational foundation for executive function, in which several items must be held in a working memory so that they can be performed with the correct priority and order (Rolls 2008b). In brain areas involved in emotion, attractor networks may play a role in maintaining a mood state, at least in the short term after for example frustrative non-reward (see Chapters 2 and 3), and possibly in the longer term. Other functions for autoassociation networks including perceptual short-term memory which may be used in the learning of invariant representations, constraint satisfaction, and episodic memory are described by Rolls & Treves (1998) and Rolls (2008b).

A.3.1 Architecture and operation

The prototypical architecture of an autoassociation memory is shown in Fig. A.19. The external input e_i is applied to each neuron i by unmodifiable synapses. This produces firing y_i of each neuron, or a vector of firing on the output neurons $\mathbf{y}$. Each output neuron i is connected by a recurrent collateral connection to the other neurons in the network, via modifiable connection weights w_{ij}. This architecture effectively enables the output firing vector $\mathbf{y}$ to be associated during learning with itself. Later on, during recall, presentation of part of the external input will force some of the output neurons to fire, but through the recurrent collateral axons and the modified synapses, other neurons in $\mathbf{y}$ can be brought into activity. This process can be repeated a number of times, and recall of a complete pattern may be perfect. Effectively, a pattern can be recalled or recognized because of associations formed between its parts. This of course requires distributed representations.

Next we introduce a more precise and detailed description of the above, and describe the properties of these networks. Ways to analyse formally the operation of these networks are introduced in Appendix A4 of Rolls & Treves (1998) and by Amit (1989).

A.3.1.1 Learning

The firing of every output neuron i is forced to a value y_i determined by the external input e_i. Then a Hebb-like associative local learning rule is applied to the recurrent synapses in the network:

$$\delta w_{ij} = \alpha y_i y_j. \tag{A.13}$$

(The term y_j in this Equation is the presynaptic term shown as x_j in Fig. A.19, and this is due to the fact that the recurrent collateral connections connect the outputs of the network back as inputs.) It is notable that in a fully connected network, this will result in a symmetric matrix of synaptic weights, that is the strength of the connection from neuron 1 to neuron 2 will be the same as the strength of the connection from neuron 2 to neuron 1 (both implemented via recurrent collateral synapses).

It is a factor that is sometimes overlooked that there must be a mechanism for ensuring that during learning y_i does approximate e_i, and must not be influenced much by activity in the recurrent collateral connections, otherwise the new external pattern $\mathbf{e}$ will not be stored in the network, but instead something will be stored that is influenced by the previously stored memories. Mechanisms that may facilitate this are described by Rolls & Treves (1998) and Rolls (2008b).

A.3.1.2 Recall

During recall, the external input e_i is applied, and produces output firing, operating through the non-linear activation function described below. The firing is fed back by the recurrent collateral axons shown in Fig. A.19 to produce activation of each output neuron through the modified synapses on each output neuron. The activation h_i produced by the recurrent collateral effect on the ith neuron is, in the standard way, the sum of the activations produced in proportion to the firing rate of each axon y_j operating through each modified synapse w_{ij}, that is,

$$h_i = \sum_j y_j w_{ij} \tag{A.14}$$

where $\sum_j$ indicates that the sum is over the C input synapses each from a separate axon to each neuron, indexed by j.

The output firing y_i is a function of the activation h_i produced by the recurrent collateral effect (internal recall) and by the external input (e_i):

$$y_i = \mathrm{f}(h_i + e_i) \tag{A.15}$$

The activation function should be nonlinear, and may be for example binary threshold, linear threshold, sigmoid, etc. (see Fig. A.3). The threshold at which the activation function operates is set in part by the effect of the inhibitory neurons in the network (not shown in Fig. A.19). The connectivity is that the pyramidal cells have collateral axons that excite the inhibitory interneurons, which in turn connect back to the population of pyramidal cells to inhibit them by a mixture of shunting (divisive) and subtractive inhibition using GABA (gamma-amino-butyric acid) synaptic terminals, as described by Rolls (2008b).

There are many fewer inhibitory neurons than excitatory neurons [in the order of 5–10%, and of connections to and from inhibitory neurons, and partly for this reason the inhibitory neurons are considered to perform generic functions such as threshold setting, rather than to store patterns by modifying their synapses (see Rolls (2008b))]. The non-linear activation function can minimize interference between the pattern being recalled and other patterns stored in the network, and can also be used to ensure that what is a positive feedback system remains stable. The network can be allowed to repeat this recurrent collateral loop a number of times. Each time the loop operates, the output firing becomes more like the originally stored pattern, and this progressive recall is usually complete within 5–15 iterations.

A.3.2 Introduction to the analysis of the operation of autoassociation networks

With complete connectivity in the synaptic matrix, and the use of a Hebb rule, the matrix of synaptic weights formed during learning is symmetric. The learning algorithm is fast, 'one-shot', in that a single presentation of an input pattern is all that is needed to store that pattern.

During recall, a part of one of the originally learned stimuli can be presented as an external input. The resulting firing is allowed to iterate repeatedly round the recurrent collateral system, gradually on each iteration recalling more and more of the originally learned pattern. Completion thus occurs. If a pattern is presented during recall that is similar but not identical to any of the previously learned patterns, then the network settles into a stable recall state in which the firing corresponds to that of the most similar previously learned pattern. The network can thus generalize in its recall to the most similar previously learned pattern. The activation function of the neurons should be non-linear, since a purely linear system would not produce any categorization of the input patterns it receives, and therefore would not be able to effect anything more than a trivial (i.e. linear) form of completion and generalization.

Recall can be thought of in the following way, relating it to what occurs in pattern associators. The external input $\mathbf{e}$ is applied, produces firing $\mathbf{y}$, which is applied as a recall cue on the recurrent collaterals as $\mathbf{y}^{\mathrm{T}}$. (The notation $\mathbf{y}^{\mathrm{T}}$ signifies the transpose of $\mathbf{y}$, which is implemented by the application of the firing of the neurons $\mathbf{y}$ back via the recurrent collateral axons as the next set of inputs to the neurons.) The activity on the recurrent collaterals is then multiplied with the synaptic weight vector stored during learning on each neuron to produce the new activation h_i which reflects the similarity between $\mathbf{y}^{\mathrm{T}}$ and one of the stored patterns. Partial recall has thus occurred as a result of the recurrent collateral effect. The activations h_i after thresholding (which helps to remove interference from other memories stored in the network, or noise in the recall cue) result in firing y_i, or a vector of all neurons $\mathbf{y}$, which is already more like one of the stored patterns than, at the first iteration, the firing resulting from the recall cue alone, $\mathbf{y} = \mathrm{f}(\mathbf{e})$. This process is repeated a number of times to produce progressive recall of one of the stored patterns.

Autoassociation networks operate by effectively storing associations between the elements of a pattern. Each element of the pattern vector to be stored is simply the firing of a neuron. What is stored in an autoassociation memory is a set of pattern vectors. The network operates to recall one of the patterns from a fragment of it. Thus, although this network implements recall or recognition of a pattern, it does so by an association learning mechanism, in which associations between the different parts of each pattern are learned. These memories have sometimes been called autocorrelation memories (Kohonen 1977), because they learn correlations between the activity of neurons in the network, in the sense that each pattern learned is defined by a set of simultaneously active neurons. Effectively each pattern is associated by learning with itself. This learning is implemented by an associative (Hebb-like) learning rule.

Formal approaches to the operation of these networks have been described by Hopfield (1982), Amit (1989), Hertz, Krogh & Palmer (1991), and Rolls & Treves (1998).

A.3.3 Properties

The internal recall in autoassociation networks involves multiplication of the firing vector of neuronal activity by the vector of synaptic weights on each neuron. This inner product vector multiplication allows the similarity of the firing vector to previously stored firing vectors to be provided by the output (as effectively a correlation), if the patterns learned are distributed. As a result of this type of 'correlation computation' performed if the patterns are distributed, many important properties of these networks arise, including pattern completion (because part of a pattern is correlated with the whole pattern), and graceful degradation (because a damaged synaptic weight vector is still correlated with the original synaptic weight vector). Some of these properties are described next.

A.3.3.1 Completion

One important and useful property of these memories is that they complete an incomplete input vector, allowing recall of a whole memory from a small fraction of it. The memory recalled in response to a fragment is that stored in the memory that is closest in pattern similarity (as measured by the dot product, or correlation). Because the recall is iterative and progressive, the recall can be perfect.

A.3.3.2 Generalization

The network generalizes in that an input vector similar to one of the stored vectors will lead to recall of the originally stored vector, provided that distributed encoding is used. The principle by which this occurs is similar to that described for a pattern associator.

A.3.3.3 Graceful degradation or fault tolerance

If the synaptic weight vector $\mathbf{w}_i$ on each neuron (or the weight matrix) has synapses missing (e.g. during development), or loses synapses (e.g. with brain damage or aging), then the activation h_i (or vector of activations $\mathbf{h}$) is still reasonable, because h_i is the dot product (correlation) of $\mathbf{y}^{\mathrm{T}}$ with $\mathbf{w}_i$. The same argument applies if whole input axons are lost. If an output neuron is lost, then the network cannot itself compensate for this, but the next network in the brain is likely to be able to generalize or complete if its input vector has some elements missing, as would be the case if some output neurons of the autoassociation network were damaged.

A.3.3.4 Speed

The recall operation is fast on each neuron on a single iteration, because the pattern $\mathbf{y}^{\mathrm{T}}$ on the axons can be applied simultaneously to the synapses $\mathbf{w}_i$, and the activation h_i can be accumulated in one or two time constants of the dendrite (e.g. 10–20 ms). If a simple implementation of an autoassociation net such as that described by Hopfield (1982) is simulated on a computer, then 5–15 iterations are typically necessary for completion of an incomplete input cue $\mathbf{e}$. This might be taken to correspond to 50–200 ms in the brain, rather too slow for any one local network in the brain to function. However, it transpires (see Rolls (2008b), Treves (1993), Battaglia & Treves (1998), Appendix A5 of Rolls & Treves (1998), and Panzeri, Rolls, Battaglia & Lavis (2001)) that if the neurons are treated not as McCulloch–Pitts neurons which are simply 'updated' at each iteration, or cycle of time steps (and assume the active state if the threshold is exceeded), but instead are analysed and modelled as 'integrate-and-fire' neurons in real continuous time, then the network can effectively 'relax' into its recall state very rapidly, in one or two time constants of the synapses[48] This corresponds to perhaps 20 ms in the brain. One factor in this rapid dynamics of autoassociative networks with brain-like 'integrate-and-fire' membrane and synaptic properties is that with some spontaneous activity, some of the neurons in the network are close to threshold already before the recall cue is applied, and hence some of the neurons are very quickly pushed by the recall cue into firing, so that information starts to be exchanged very rapidly (within 1–2 ms of brain time) through the modified synapses by the neurons in the network. The progressive exchange of information starting early on within what would otherwise be thought of as an iteration period

[48]Integrate-and-fire neurons are described in Appendix B.

(of perhaps 20 ms, corresponding to a neuronal firing rate of 50 spikes/s), is the mechanism accounting for rapid recall in an autoassociative neuronal network made biologically realistic in this way. Further analysis of the fast dynamics of these networks if they are implemented in a biologically plausible way with 'integrate-and-fire' neurons is provided in Appendix A5 of Rolls & Treves (1998), by Rolls (2008b), and by Treves (1993).

Learning is fast, 'one-shot', in that a single presentation of an input pattern $\mathbf{e}$ (producing $\mathbf{y}$) enables the association between the activation of the dendrites (the postsynaptic term h_i) and the firing of the recurrent collateral axons $\mathbf{y}^{\mathrm{T}}$, to be learned. Repeated presentation with small variations of a pattern vector is used to obtain the properties of prototype extraction, extraction of central tendency, and noise reduction, because these arise from the averaging process produced by storing very similar patterns in the network.

A.3.3.5 Local learning rule

The simplest learning used in autoassociation neural networks, a version of the Hebb rule, is (as in Equation A.13)

$$\delta w_{ij} = \alpha y_i y_j.$$

The rule is a local learning rule in that the information required to specify the change in synaptic weight is available locally at the synapse, as it is dependent only on the presynaptic firing rate y_j available at the synaptic terminal, and the postsynaptic activation or firing y_i available on the dendrite of the neuron receiving the synapse. This makes the learning rule biologically plausible, in that the information about how to change the synaptic weight does not have to be carried to every synapse from a distant source where it is computed. As with pattern associators, since firing rates are positive quantities, a potentially interfering correlation is induced between different pattern vectors. This can be removed by subtracting the mean of the presynaptic activity from each presynaptic term, using a type of long-term depression. This can be specified as

$$\delta w_{ij} = \alpha y_i (y_j - z) \tag{A.16}$$

where α is a learning rate constant. This learning rule includes (in proportion to y_i) increasing the synaptic weight if $(y_j - z) > 0$ (long-term potentiation), and decreasing the synaptic weight if $(y_j - z) < 0$ (heterosynaptic long-term depression). This procedure works optimally if z is the average activity $< y_j >$ of an axon across patterns.

Evidence that a learning rule with the general form of Equation A.13 is implemented in at least some parts of the brain comes from studies of long-term potentiation, described in Section A.1.5. One of the important potential functions of heterosynaptic long-term depression is its ability to allow in effect the average of the presynaptic activity to be subtracted from the presynaptic firing rate (see Appendix A3 of Rolls & Treves (1998) and Rolls & Treves (1990)).

A.3.3.6 Capacity

One measure of storage capacity is to consider how many orthogonal (i.e. uncorrelated) patterns could be stored, as with pattern associators. If the patterns are orthogonal, there will be no interference between them, and the maximum number p of patterns that can be stored will be the same as the number N of output neurons in a fully connected network.

With non-linear neurons used in the network, the capacity can be measured in terms of the number of input patterns $\mathbf{y}$ (produced by the external input $\mathbf{e}$, see Fig. A.19) that can be stored in the network and recalled later whenever the network settles within each stored pattern's basin of attraction. The first quantitative analysis of storage capacity (Amit, Gutfreund & Sompolinsky 1987) considered a fully connected Hopfield (1982) autoassociator model, in which units are binary elements with an equal probability of being 'on' or 'off' in each pattern, and the number C of inputs per unit is the same as the number N of output units. (Actually it is equal to $N-1$, since a unit is taken not to connect to itself.) Learning is taken to occur by clamping the desired patterns on the network and using a modified Hebb rule, in which the mean of the presynaptic and postsynaptic firings is subtracted from the firing on any one learning trial (this amounts to a covariance learning rule, and is described more fully in Appendix A4 of Rolls & Treves (1998)). With such fully distributed random patterns, the number of patterns that can be learned is (for C large) $p \approx 0.14C = 0.14N$.

Treves & Rolls (1991) have extended this analysis to autoassociation networks that are much more biologically relevant in the following ways. First, some or many connections between the recurrent collaterals and the dendrites are missing (this is referred to as diluted connectivity, and results in a non-symmetric synaptic connection matrix in which w_{ij} does not equal w_{ji}, one of the original assumptions made in order to introduce the energy formalism in the Hopfield model). Second, the neurons need not be restricted to binary threshold neurons, but can have a threshold linear activation function (see Fig. A.3). This enables the neurons to assume real continuously variable firing rates, which are what is found in the brain (Rolls & Tovee 1995, Treves, Panzeri, Rolls, Booth & Wakeman 1999). Third, the representation need not be fully distributed (with half the neurons 'on', and half 'off'), but instead can have a small proportion of the neurons firing above the spontaneous rate, which is what is found in parts of the brain such as the hippocampus that are involved in memory (see (Treves & Rolls 1994, Rolls & Treves 1998, Rolls 2008b, Rolls & Treves 2011). Such a representation is defined as being sparse, and the population sparseness a of the representation can be measured, by extending the binary notion of the proportion of neurons that are firing, as

$$a = \frac{(\sum_{i=1}^{N} y_i/N)^2}{\sum_{i=1}^{N} y_i^2/N} \tag{A.17}$$

where y_i is the firing rate of the ith neuron in the set of N neurons. (It should be noted that this is the sparseness of the representation provided by the population of neurons to a single stimulus, though the value is similar to that of the single neuron sparseness which defines the tuning of a single neuron to a set of stimuli, consistent with the low correlations between the tuning of different neurons (Franco, Rolls, Aggelopoulos & Jerez 2007, Rolls 2008b, Rolls & Treves 2011). Treves & Rolls (1991) have shown that such a network does operate efficiently as an autoassociative network, and can store (and recall correctly) a number of different patterns p as follows:

$$p \approx \frac{C^{\mathrm{RC}}}{a \ln(\frac{1}{a})} k \tag{A.18}$$

where C^{RC} is the number of synapses on the dendrites of each neuron devoted to the recurrent collaterals from other neurons in the network, and k is a factor that depends weakly on the detailed structure of the rate distribution, on the connectivity pattern, etc., but is roughly in the order of 0.2–0.3.

The main factors that determine the maximum number of memories that can be stored in an autoassociative network are thus the number of connections on each neuron devoted to the recurrent collaterals, and the sparseness of the representation. For example, for C^{RC} = 12,000 and $a = 0.02$, p is calculated to be approximately 36,000. This storage capacity can be realized, with little interference between patterns, if the learning rule includes some form of heterosynaptic Long-Term Depression that counterbalances the effects of associative

Long-Term Potentiation (Treves & Rolls (1991); see Appendix A4 of Rolls & Treves (1998)). It should be noted that the number of neurons N (which is greater than C^{RC}, the number of recurrent collateral inputs received by any neuron in the network from the other neurons in the network) is not a parameter that influences the number of different memories that can be stored in the network. The implication of this is that increasing the number of neurons (without increasing the number of connections per neuron) does not increase the number of different patterns that can be stored (see Rolls & Treves (1998) Appendix A4), although it may enable simpler encoding of the firing patterns, for example more orthogonal encoding, to be used, and simpler connectivity rules by reducing the probability of more than one connection between any pair of neurons which decreases the storage capacity (Rolls 2012f). These latter points may account in part for why there are generally in the brain more neurons in a recurrent network than there are connections per neuron. Another advantage of having many neurons in the network may be related to the fact that within any integration time period of 20 ms not all neurons will have fired a spike if the average firing rate is less than 50 Hz. Having large numbers of neurons may enable the vector of neuronal firing to contribute to recall efficiently even though not every neuron can contribute in a short time period.

The non-linearity inherent in the NMDA receptor-based Hebbian plasticity present in the brain may help to make the stored patterns more sparse than the input patterns, and this may be especially beneficial in increasing the storage capacity of associative networks in the brain by allowing participation in the storage of especially those relatively few neurons with high firing rates in the exponential firing rate distributions typical of neurons in sensory systems (see Rolls & Treves (1998) and Rolls (2008b)).

A.3.3.7 Context

The environmental context in which learning occurs can be a very important factor that affects retrieval in humans and other animals. Placing the subject back into the same context in which the original learning occurred can greatly facilitate retrieval.

Context effects arise naturally in association networks if some of the activity in the network reflects the context in which the learning occurs. Retrieval is then better when that context is present, for the activity contributed by the context becomes part of the retrieval cue for the memory, increasing the correlation of the current state with what was stored. (A strategy for retrieval arises simply from this property. The strategy is to keep trying to recall as many fragments of the original memory situation, including the context, as possible, as this will provide a better cue for complete retrieval of the memory than just a single fragment.)

The effects that mood has on memory including visual memory retrieval may be accounted for by backprojections from brain regions such as the amygdala in which the current mood, providing a context, is represented, to brain regions involved in memory such as the perirhinal cortex, and in visual representations such as the inferior temporal visual cortex (see Rolls & Stringer (2001b) and Section 4.12). The very well-known effects of context in the human memory literature could arise in the simple way just described. An implication of the explanation is that context effects will be especially important at late stages of memory or information processing systems in the brain, for there information from a wide range of modalities will be mixed, and some of that information could reflect the context in which the learning takes place. One part of the brain where such effects may be strong is the hippocampus, which is implicated in the memory of recent episodes, and which receives inputs derived from most of the cortical information processing streams, including those involved in spatial representations (see Chapter 6 of Rolls & Treves (1998), Rolls (1996a), and Rolls (1999b)).

It is now known that reward-related information is associated with place-related information in the primate hippocampus, and this provides a particular neural system in which mood context can influence memory retrieval (Rolls & Xiang 2005).

A.3.3.8 Memory for sequences

One of the first extensions of the standard autoassociator paradigm that has been explored in the literature is the capability to store and retrieve not just individual patterns, but whole sequences of patterns. Hopfield (1982) suggested that this could be achieved by adding to the standard connection weights, which associate a pattern with itself, a new, asymmetric component, that associates a pattern with the next one in the sequence. In practice this scheme does not work very well, unless the new component is made to operate on a slower time scale than the purely autoassociative component (Kleinfeld 1986, Sompolinsky & Kanter 1986). With two different time scales, the autoassociative component can stabilize a pattern for a while, before the heteroassociative component moves the network, as it were, into the next pattern. The heteroassociative retrieval cue for the next pattern in the sequence is just the previous pattern in the sequence. A particular type of 'slower' operation occurs if the asymmetric component acts after a delay τ. In this case, the network sweeps through the sequence, staying for a time of order τ in each pattern.

If implemented with integrate-and-fire neurons with biologically plausible dynamics, this type of sequence memory will either step through its remembered sequence with uncontrollable speed, or not step through the sequence. A proposal that attractor networks with adapting synapses could be used to retain memory sequences is an interesting alternative (Deco & Rolls 2005d).

A.4 Coupled attractor networks

In this Section A.4 an introduction to how attractor networks can interact is given, as this may be relevant to understanding how mood states influence cognitive processing, and vice versa.

It is prototypical of the cerebral neocortical areas that there are recurrent collateral connections between the neurons within an area or module, and forward connections to the next cortical area in the hierarchy, which in turn sends backprojections (see Rolls (2008b)). This architecture, made explicit in Fig. 4.75 on page 217, immediately suggests, given that the recurrent connections within a module, and the forward and backward connections, are likely to be associatively modifiable, that the operation incorporates at least to some extent interactions between coupled attractor (autoassociation) networks. For these reasons, it is important to analyse the rules that govern the interactions between coupled attractor networks. This has been done using the formal type of model described by Rolls (2008b) introduced here (see also Renart, Parga & Rolls (1999a), Renart, Parga & Rolls (1999b), Renart, Parga & Rolls (2000), Renart, Moreno, Rocha, Parga & Rolls (2001), and Deco & Rolls (2003)).

One boundary condition is when the coupling between the networks is so weak that there is effectively no interaction. This holds when the coupling parameter g between the networks is less than approximately 0.002, where the coupling parameter indicates the relative strength of the intermodular to the intramodular connections, and measures effectively the relative strengths of the currents injected into the neurons by the inter-modular relative to the intramodular (recurrent collateral) connections (Renart, Parga & Rolls 1999a). At the other extreme, if the coupling parameter is strong, all the networks will operate as a single attractor network, together able to represent only one state (Renart, Parga & Rolls 1999a). This critical value of the coupling parameter (at least for reciprocally connected networks with symmetric synaptic strengths) is relatively low, in the region of 0.024 (Renart, Parga & Rolls 1999a). This is one reason why cortico-cortical backprojections are predicted to be quantitatively relatively weak, and for this reason it is suggested end on the apical parts of the dendrites of cortical pyramidal cells (see Rolls (2008b)). In the strongly coupled regime when the system of networks operates as a single attractor, the total storage capacity (the number of patterns that can be stored and correctly retrieved) of all the networks will be set just by the number of synaptic connections received from other neurons in the network, a number in the order of a few thousand. This is one reason why connected cortical networks are thought not to act in the strongly coupled regime, because the total number of memories that could be represented in the whole of the cerebral cortex would be so small, in the order of a few thousand, depending on the sparseness of the patterns (see Equation A.18) (O'Kane & Treves 1992).

Between these boundary conditions, that is in the region where the inter-modular coupling parameter g is in the range 0.002–0.024, it has been shown that interesting interactions can occur (Renart, Parga & Rolls 1999a, Renart, Parga & Rolls 1999b). In a bimodular architecture, with forward and backward connections between the modules, the capacity of one module can be increased, and an attractor is more likely to be found under noisy conditions, if there is a consistent pattern in the coupled attractor. By consistent we mean a pattern that during training was linked associatively by the forward and backward connections, with the pattern being retrieved in the first module. This provides a quantitative model for understanding some of the effects that backprojections can produce by supporting particular states in earlier cortical areas (Renart, Parga & Rolls 1999a). The total storage capacity of the two networks is however in line with O'Kane & Treves (1992), not a great deal greater than the storage capacity of one of the modules alone. Thus the help provided by the attractors in falling into a mutually compatible global retrieval state (in e.g. the scenario of a hierarchical system) is where the utility of such coupled attractor networks must lie. Another interesting application of such weakly coupled attractor networks is in coupled perceptual and short-term memory systems in the brain, described by Rolls (2008b). Thus the most interesting scenario for coupled attractor networks is when they are weakly coupled, for then interactions occur whereby how well one module responds to its own inputs can be influenced by the states of the other modules, but it can retain partly independent representations. This emphasizes the importance of weak interactions between coupled modules in the brain (Renart, Parga & Rolls 1999a, Renart, Parga & Rolls 1999b, Renart, Parga & Rolls 2000).

If a multimodular architecture is trained with each of many patterns (which might be visual stimuli) in one module associated with one of a few patterns (which might be mood states) in a connected module, then interesting effects due to this asymmetry are found, as described in Section 4.12 and by Rolls & Stringer (2001b).

An interesting issue that arises is how rapidly a system of interacting attractor networks such as that illustrated in Fig. 4.75 settles into a stable state. Is it sufficiently rapid for the interacting attractor effects described to contribute to cortical information processing? It is likely that the settling of the whole system is quite rapid, if it is implemented (as it is in the brain) with synapses and neurons that operate with continuous dynamics, where the time constant of the synapses dominates the retrieval speed, and is in the order of 15 ms for each module, as described by Rolls (2008b) and by Panzeri, Rolls, Battaglia & Lavis (2001). It is shown there that a multimodular attractor network architecture can process information in approximately 15 ms per module (assuming an inactivation time constant for the synapses of 10 ms).

Attractor networks can be coupled together with stronger forward than backward connections. This provides a model of how the prefrontal cortex could map sensory inputs (in one attractor), through intermediate attractors that respond to combinations of sensory inputs and the behavioural responses being made, to further attractors that encode the response to be made (Deco & Rolls 2003). Having attractors at each stage enables the prefrontal cortex to bridge delays between parts of a task. The hierarchical organization of the attractors achieved by the stronger forward than backward connections enables the mapping to be from sensory input to motor output. The presence of intermediate attractors with neurons that respond to combinations of the stimuli and the behavioural responses to be made allows a top-down attentional input to bias the competition implemented by the intermediate level attractors to enable the behaviour to be switched from one cognitive mapping to another (Deco & Rolls 2003). The whole architecture has been modelled at the integrate-and-fire neuronal level, and simulates the activity of the different populations of neurons just described which are types of neuron recorded in the prefrontal cortex when monkeys are performing this decision task (see Deco & Rolls (2003)).

The cortico-cortical backprojection connectivity described can be interpreted as a system that allows the forward-projecting neurons in one cortical area to be linked autoassociatively with the backprojecting neurons in the next cortical area (see Fig. 4.75 and Rolls (2008b)). It is interesting to note that if the forward and backprojection synapses were associatively modifiable, but there were no recurrent connections in each of the modules, then the whole system could still operate (with the right parameters) as an attractor network.

A.5 Reinforcement learning

In supervised networks, an error signal is provided for each output neuron in the network, and whenever an input to the network is provided, the error signals specify the magnitude and direction of the error in the output produced by each neuron. These error signals are then used to correct the synaptic weights in the network in such a way that the output errors for each input pattern to be learned gradually diminish over trials (see Rolls (2008b)). These networks have an architecture that might be similar to that of the pattern associator shown in Fig. A.7, except that instead of an unconditioned stimulus, there is an error correction signal provided for each output neuron. Such a network trained by an error-correcting (or delta) rule is known as a one-layer perceptron. The architecture is not very plausible for most brain regions, in that it is not clear how an individual error signal could be computed for each of thousands of neurons in a network, and fed into each neuron as its error signal and then used in a delta rule synaptic correction (see Rolls & Treves (1998) and Rolls (2008b)).

The architecture can be generalized to a multilayer feedforward architecture with many layers between the input and output (Rumelhart, Hinton & Williams 1986), but the learning is very non-local and rather biologically implausible (see Rolls & Treves (1998) and Rolls (2008b)), in that an error term (magnitude and direction) for each neuron in the network must be computed from the errors and synaptic weights of all subsequent neurons in the network that any neuron influences, usually on a trial-by-trial basis, by a process known as error backpropagation. Thus although computationally powerful, an issue with perceptrons and multilayer perceptrons that makes them generally biologically implausible for many brain regions is that a separate error signal must be supplied for each output neuron, and that with multilayer perceptrons, computed error backpropagation must occur.

When operating in an environment, usually a simple binary or scalar signal representing success or failure of the whole network or organism is received. This is usually action-dependent feedback that provides a single evaluative measure of the success or failure. Evaluative feedback tells the learner whether or not, and possibly by how much, its behaviour has improved; or it provides a measure of the 'goodness' of the behaviour. Evaluative feedback does not directly tell the learner what it should have done, and although it may provide an index of the degree (i.e. magnitude) of success, it does not include directional information telling the learner how to change its behaviour towards a target, as does error-correction learning (see Barto (1995)). Partly for this reason, there has been some interest in networks that can be taught with such a single reinforcement signal. In this Section, approaches to such networks are described. It is noted that such networks are classified as reinforcement networks in which there is a single teacher, and that these networks attempt to perform an

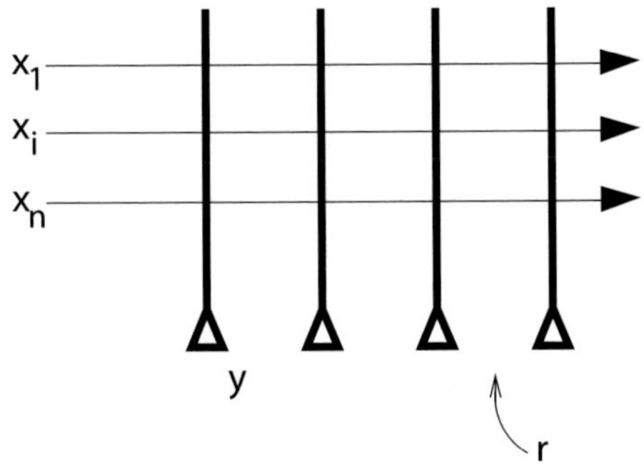

Fig. A.20 A network trained by a single reinforcement input r. The inputs to each neuron are $x_j, j = 1, C$; and y is the output of one of the output neurons.

optimal mapping between an input vector and an output neuron or set of neurons. They thus solve the same class of problems as single layer and multilayer perceptrons. They should be distinguished from pattern-association networks in the brain, which might learn associations between previously neutral stimuli and primary reinforcers such as taste (signals which might be interpreted appropriately by a subsequent part of the brain), but do not attempt to produce arbitrary mappings between an input and an output, using a single reinforcement signal.

A class of problems to which such reinforcement networks might be applied are motor-control problems. It was to such a problem that Barto and Sutton (Barto 1985, Sutton & Barto 1981) applied a reinforcement learning algorithm, the associative reward–penalty algorithm described next. The algorithm can in principle be applied to multilayer networks, and the learning is relatively slow. The algorithm is summarized by Rolls & Treves (1998) and Hertz, Krogh & Palmer (1991). More recent developments in reinforcement learning are described by Sutton & Barto (1998) and reviewed by Dayan & Abbott (2001), and some of these developments are described in Section A.5.3.

A.5.1 Associative reward–penalty algorithm of Barto and Sutton

The terminology of Barto and Sutton is followed here (see Barto (1985)).

A.5.1.1 Architecture

The architecture, shown in Fig. A.20, uses a single reinforcement signal, r, = +1 for reward, and –1 for penalty. The inputs x_i take real (continuous) values. The output of a neuron, y, is binary, +1 or –1. The weights on the output neuron are designated w_i.

A.5.1.2 Operation

1. An input vector is applied to the network, and produces activation, h, in the normal way as follows:

$$h = \sum_{j=1}^{C} x_j w_j \tag{A.19}$$

where $\sum_{j=1}^{C}$ indicates that the sum is over the C input axons (or connections) indexed by j to each neuron.

2. The output y is calculated from the activation with a noise term η included. The principle of the network is that if the added noise on a particular trial helps performance, then whatever

change it leads to should be incorporated into the synaptic weights, in such a way that the next time that input occurs, the performance is improved.

$$y = \begin{cases} +1 & \text{if } h + \eta \geq 0, \\ -1 & \text{else.} \end{cases} \tag{A.20}$$

where η = the noise added on each trial.

3. Learning rule. The weights are changed as follows:

$$\delta w_j = \begin{cases} \rho(y - \mathrm{E}[y|h])x_j & \text{if } r = +1, \\ \rho\lambda(-y - \mathrm{E}[y|h])x_j & \text{if } r = -1. \end{cases} \tag{A.21}$$

ρ and λ are learning-rate constants. (They are set so that the learning rate is higher when positive reinforcement is received than when negative reinforcement is received.) $\mathrm{E}[y|h]$ is the expectation of y given h (usually a sigmoidal function of h with the range ± 1). $\mathrm{E}[y|h]$ is a (continuously varying) indication of how the neuron usually responds to the current input pattern, i.e. if the actual output y is larger than normally expected, by computing $h = \sum w_j x_j$, because of the noise term, and the reinforcement is +1, increase the weight from x_j; and vice versa. The expectation could be the prediction generated before the noise term is incorporated.

This network combines an associative capacity with its properties of generalization and graceful degradation, with a single 'critic' or error signal for the whole network (Barto 1985). [The term $y - \mathrm{E}[y|h]$ in Equation A.21 can be thought of as an error for the output of the neuron: it is the difference between what occurred, and what was expected to occur. The synaptic weight is adjusted according to the sign and magnitude of the error of the postsynaptic firing, multiplied by the presynaptic firing, and depending on the reinforcement r received. The rule is similar to a Hebb synaptic modification rule (Equation A.6), except that the postsynaptic term is an error instead of the postsynaptic firing rate, and the learning is modulated by the reinforcement.] The network can solve difficult problems (such as balancing a pole by moving a trolley that supports the pole from side to side, as the pole starts to topple). Although described for single-layer networks, the algorithm can be applied to multilayer networks. The learning rate is very slow, for there is a single reinforcement signal on each trial for the whole network, not a separate error signal for each neuron in the network as is the case in a perceptron trained with an error rule (see Rolls (2008b) and Rolls & Treves (1998)).

This associative reward–penalty reinforcement-learning algorithm is certainly a move towards biological relevance, in that learning with a single reinforcer can be achieved. That single reinforcer might be broadcast throughout the system by a general projection system. It is not clear yet how a biological system might store the expected output $\mathrm{E}[y|h]$ for comparison with the actual output when noise has been added, and might take into account the sign and magnitude of this difference. Nevertheless, this is an interesting algorithm, which is related to the temporal difference reinforcement learning algorithm described in Section A.5.3.

A.5.2 Error correction or delta rule learning, and classical conditioning

In classical or Pavlovian associative learning, a number of different types of association may be learned (see Section 4.6.1.1). This type of associative learning may be performed by networks with the general architecture and properties of pattern associators (see Section A.2 and Fig. A.7). However, the time course of the acquisition and extinction of these associations can be expressed concisely by a modified type of learning rule in which an error correction term is used (introduced in Section A.5.1), rather than the postsynaptic firing y itself as in

Equation A.6. Use of this modified, error correction, type of learning also enables some of the properties of classical conditioning to be explained (see Dayan & Abbott (2001) for review), and this type of learning is therefore described briefly here. The rule is known in learning theory as the Rescorla–Wagner rule, after Rescorla & Wagner (1972).

The Rescorla–Wagner rule is a version of error correction or delta-rule learning, and is based on a simple linear prediction of the expected reward value, denoted by v, associated with a stimulus representation x ($x = 1$ if the stimulus is present, and $x = 0$ if the stimulus is absent). The expected reward value v is expressed as the input stimulus variable x multiplied by a weight w

$$v = wx. \tag{A.22}$$

The error in the reward prediction is the difference between the expected reward v and the actual reward obtained r, i.e.

$$\Delta = r - v \tag{A.23}$$

where Δ is the reward prediction error. The value of the weight w is learned by a rule designed to minimize the expected squared error $< (r - v)^2 >$ between the actual reward r and the predicted reward v. The angle brackets indicate an average over the presentations of the stimulus and reward. The delta rule will perform the required type of learning:

$$\delta w = k(r - v)x \tag{A.24}$$

where δw is the change of synaptic weight, k is a constant that determines the learning rate, and the term $(r - v)$ is the error Δ in the output (equivalent to the error in the postsynaptic firing, rather than the postsynaptic firing y itself as in Equation A.6). Application of this rule during conditioning with the stimulus x presented on every trial results in the weight w approaching the asymptotic limit $w = r$ exponentially over trials as the error Δ becomes zero. In extinction, when $r = 0$, the weight (and thus the output of the system) exponentially decays to $w = 0$. This rule thus helps to capture the time course over trials of the acquisition and extinction of conditioning. The rule also helps to account for a number of properties of classical conditioning, including blocking, inhibitory conditioning, and overshadowing (see Dayan & Abbott (2001)).

How this functionality is implemented in the brain is not yet clear. We consider one suggestion (Schultz et al. 1995b, Schultz 2004, Schultz 2013) after we introduce a further sophistication of reinforcement learning which allows the time course of events within a trial to be taken into account.

A.5.3 Temporal Difference (TD) learning

An important advance in the area of reinforcement learning was the introduction of algorithms that allow for learning to occur when the reinforcement is delayed or received over a number of time steps, and which allow effects within a trial to be taken into account (Sutton & Barto 1998, Sutton & Barto 1990). A solution to these problems is the addition of an adaptive critic that learns through a time difference (TD) algorithm how to predict the future value of the reinforcer. The time difference algorithm takes into account not only the current reinforcement just received, but also a temporally weighted average of errors in predicting future reinforcements. The temporal difference error is the error by which any two temporally adjacent error predictions are inconsistent (see Barto (1995)). The output of the critic is used as an effective reinforcer instead of the instantaneous reinforcement being received (see Sutton & Barto (1998), Sutton & Barto (1990) and Barto (1995)). This is a solution to the temporal credit assignment problem, and enables future rewards to be predicted. Summaries are provided by Doya (1999), Schultz et al. (1997) and Dayan & Abbott (2001).

In reinforcement learning, a learning agent takes an *action* $\mathbf{u}(t)$ in response to the *state* $\mathbf{x}(t)$ of the environment, which results in the change of the state

$$\mathbf{x}(t+1) = \mathrm{F}(\mathbf{x}(t), \mathbf{u}(t)), \tag{A.25}$$

and the delivery of the reinforcement signal, or *reward*

$$r(t+1) = \mathrm{R}(\mathbf{x}(t), \mathbf{u}(t)). \tag{A.26}$$

In the above equations, $\mathbf{x}$ is a vector representation of inputs x_j, and Equation A.25 indicates that the next state $\mathbf{x}(t+1)$ at time $(t+1)$ is a function F of the state at the previous time step of the inputs and actions at that time step in a closed system. In Equation A.26 the reward at the next time step is determined by a reward function R which uses the current sensory inputs and action taken. The time t may refer to time within a trial.

The goal is to find a *policy* function G which maps sensory inputs $\mathbf{x}$ to actions

$$\mathbf{u}(t) = \mathrm{G}(\mathbf{x}(t)) \tag{A.27}$$

which maximizes the cumulative sum of the rewards based on the sensory inputs.

The current action $\mathbf{u}(t)$ affects all future states and accordingly all future rewards. The maximization is realized by the use of the *value function* V of the states to predict, given the sensory inputs $\mathbf{x}$, the cumulative sum (possibly discounted as a function of time) of all future rewards $\mathrm{V}(\mathbf{x})$ (possibly within a learning trial) as follows:

$$\mathrm{V}(\mathbf{x}) = E[r(t+1) + \gamma r(t+2) + \gamma^2 r(t+3) + ...] \tag{A.28}$$

where $r(t)$ is the reward at time t, and $E[\cdot]$ denotes the expected value of the sum of future rewards up to the end of the trial. $0 \leq \gamma \leq 1$ is a discount factor that makes rewards that arrive sooner more important than rewards that arrive later, according to an exponential decay function. (If $\gamma = 1$ there is no discounting.) It is assumed that the presentation of future cues and rewards depends only on the current sensory cues and not the past sensory cues. The right hand side of Equation A.28 is evaluated for the dynamics in Equations A.25–A.27 with the initial condition $\mathbf{x}(t) = \mathbf{x}$. The two basic ingredients in reinforcement learning are the estimation (which we term $\hat{\mathrm{V}}$) of the value function V, and then the improvement of the policy or action $\mathbf{u}$ using the value function (Sutton & Barto 1998).

The basic algorithm for learning the value function is to minimize the *temporal difference* (TD) *error* $\Delta(t)$ for time t within a trial, and this is computed by a 'critic' for the estimated value predictions $\hat{\mathrm{V}}(\mathbf{x}(t))$ at successive time steps as

$$\Delta(t) = [r(t) + \gamma\hat{\mathrm{V}}(\mathbf{x}(t))] - \hat{\mathrm{V}}(\mathbf{x}(t-1)) \tag{A.29}$$

where $\hat{\mathrm{V}}(\mathbf{x}(t)) - \hat{\mathrm{V}}(\mathbf{x}(t-1))$ is the difference in the reward value prediction at two successive time steps, giving rise to the terminology temporal difference learning. If we introduce the term $\hat{v}$ as the estimate of the cumulated reward by the end of the trial, we can define it as a function $\hat{\mathrm{V}}$ of the current sensory input $\mathbf{x}(t)$, i.e. $\hat{v} = \hat{\mathrm{V}}(\mathbf{x})$, and we can also write Equation A.29 as

$$\Delta(t) = r(t) + \gamma\hat{v}(t) - \hat{v}(t-1) \tag{A.30}$$

which draws out the fact that it is differences at successive timesteps in the reward value predictions $\hat{v}$ that are used to calculate Δ.

$\Delta(t)$ is used to improve the estimates $\hat{v}(t)$ by the 'critic', and can also be used (by an 'actor') to choose appropriate actions.

For example, when the value function is represented (in the critic) as

$$\hat{\mathrm{V}}(\mathbf{x}(t)) = \sum_{j=1}^{n} w_j^{\mathrm{C}} x_j(t) \qquad \text{(A.31)}$$

the learning algorithm for the (value) weight w_j^{C} in the critic is given by

$$\delta w_j^{\mathrm{C}} = k_c \Delta(t) x_j(t-1) \qquad \text{(A.32)}$$

where δw_j^{C} is the change of synaptic weight, k_c is a constant that determines the learning rate for the sensory input x_j, and $\Delta(t)$ is the Temporal Difference error at time t. Under certain conditions this learning rule will cause the estimate $\hat{v}$ to converge to the true value (Dayan & Sejnowski 1994).

A simple way of improving the policy of the actor is to take a stochastic action

$$u_i(t) = \mathrm{g}(\sum_{j=1}^{n} w_{ij}^{\mathrm{A}} x_j(t) + \mu_i(t)), \qquad \text{(A.33)}$$

where g() is a scalar version of the policy function G, w_{ij}^{A} is a weight in the actor, and $\mu_i(t)$ is a noise term. The TD error $\Delta(t)$ as defined in Equation A.29 then signals the unexpected delivery of the reward $r(t)$ or the increase in the state value $\hat{\mathrm{V}}(\mathbf{x}(t))$ above expectation, possibly due to the previous choice of action $u_i(t-1)$. The learning algorithm for the action weight w_{ij}^{A} in the actor is given by

$$\delta w_{ij}^{\mathrm{A}} = k_a \Delta(t)(u_i(t-1) - < u_i >) x_j(t-1), \qquad \text{(A.34)}$$

where $< u_i >$ is the average level of the action output, and k_a is a learning rate constant in the actor.

Thus, the TD error $\Delta(t)$, which signals the error in the reward prediction at time t, works as the main teaching signal in both learning the value function (implemented in the critic), and the selection of actions (implemented in the actor). The usefulness of a separate critic is that it enables the TD error to be calculated based on the difference in reward value predictions at two successive time steps as shown in Equation A.29.

The algorithm has been applied to modelling the time course of classical conditioning (Sutton & Barto 1990). The algorithm effectively allows the future reinforcement predicted from past history to influence the responses made, and in this sense allows behaviour to be guided not just by immediate reinforcement, but also by 'anticipated' reinforcements. Different types of temporal difference learning are described by Sutton & Barto (1998). An application is to the analysis of decisions when future rewards are discounted with respect to immediate rewards (Dayan & Abbott 2001, Tanaka, Doya, Okada, Ueda, Okamoto & Yamawaki 2004). Another application is to the learning of sequences of actions to take within a trial (Suri & Schultz 1998).

The possibility that dopamine neuron firing may provide an error signal useful in training neuronal systems to predict reward has been discussed in Section 6.2.4. It has been proposed that the firing of the dopamine neurons can be thought of as an error signal about reward prediction, in that the firing occurs in a task when a reward is given, but then moves forward in time within a trial to the time when a stimulus is presented that can be used to predict when the taste reward will be obtained (Schultz et al. 1995b) (see Fig. 6.4). The argument is that there is no prediction error when the taste reward is obtained if it has been signalled by a preceding conditioned stimulus, and that is why the dopamine midbrain neurons do not respond at the time of taste reward delivery, but instead, at least during training, to the onset of the conditioned stimulus (Waelti, Dickinson & Schultz 2001). If a different conditioned stimulus is shown that normally predicts that no taste reward will be given, there is no firing of the dopamine neurons to the onset of that conditioned stimulus.

This hypothesis has been built into models of learning in which the error signal is used to train synaptic connections in dopamine pathway recipient regions (such as presumably the striatum and orbitofrontal cortex) (Houk et al. 1995, Schultz 2004, Schultz et al. 1997, Waelti et al. 2001, Dayan & Abbott 2001, Schultz 2013). Some difficulties with the hypothesis are discussed in Section 6.2.4. The difficulties include the fact that dopamine is released in large quantities by aversive stimuli (see Section 6.2.4); that error computations for differences between the expected reward and the actual reward received on a trial are computed in the primate orbitofrontal cortex, where expected reward, actual reward, and error neurons are all found, and lesions of which impair the ability to use changes in reward contingencies to reverse behaviour (see Section 4.5.5.5); that the tonic, sustained, firing of the dopamine neurons in the delay period of a task with probabilistic rewards reflects reward uncertainty, and not the expected reward, nor the magnitude of the prediction error (see Section 6.2.4 and Shizgal & Arvanitogiannis (2003)); and that reinforcement learning is suited to setting up connections that might be required in fixed tasks such as motor habit or sequence learning, for reinforcement learning algorithms seek to set weights correctly in an 'actor', but are not suited to tasks where rules must be altered flexibly, as in rapid one trial reversal, for which a very different type of mechanism is described in Section 4.5.7.

Overall, reinforcement learning algorithms are certainly a move towards biological relevance, in that learning with a single reinforcer can be achieved in systems that might learn motor habits or fixed sequences. Whether a single prediction error is broadcast throughout a neural system by a general projection system, such as the dopamine pathways in the brain, which distribute to large parts of the striatum and the prefrontal cortex, remains to be clearly established.

Appendix 2 Decision-making models

In this Appendix, a wide range of approaches to decision-making is reviewed, and then the implementation of the biologically plausible model of decision-making described in Chapter 8 is described.

B.1 Overview of different models of decision-making

In the following, the most common models of two-alternative forced choice (2AFC) decision-making and their theoretical origins (Deco, Rolls, Albantakis & Romo 2013) are reviewed. I start with basic, linear, conceptual and not biologically realistic models, which successfully capture aspects of decision-behaviour, followed by attempts to implement these models in a physiologically plausible way. Then I turn to the implementation of nonlinear attractor models and describe in Sections B.1.3.1–B.6 the biophysically-inspired implementation of an attractor model with spiking neurons that is described in Chapters 8 and 8.7. The objective is to provide an intuitive overview. Consequently, the formal presentation is restricted to the basic equations and characteristics of the models, and citations are provided to the original publications for detailed theoretical analyses.

B.1.1 Sequential-sampling models: sequential probability ratio test, drift-diffusion, and race models

Present conceptual models of decision behaviour considering noisy evidence build on signal detection theory (SDT), developed to describe categorical choices under uncertainty (Green & Swets 1966, Tanner & Swets 1954). SDT typically assumes fixed, short stimulus times that are out of the subject's control. The class of models summarized as 'sequential sampling models' forms the logical extension of SDT to temporally stretched streams of (noisy) data (Stone 1960, Wald 1947). In addition to the probability of correct responses, these models give predictions on subjects' reaction times in two-alternative forced choice (2AFC) paradigms. To form a decision, evidence for each of the two alternatives is integrated over time. Whether an independent integration for each alternative (e.g. a race model), or an integration of the difference in evidence (e.g. a drift-diffusion model) gives a better account of experimental two-alternative forced choice data, is, however, still open to debate, although the latter seems to fit a wider set of experimental observations (Bogacz, Brown, Moehlis, Holmes & Cohen 2006, Ratcliff, Cherian & Segraves 2003, Ratcliff & Smith 2004).

B.1.1.1 Signal detection theory and the sequential probability ratio test (SPRT)

In simple perceptual two-alternative forced choice tasks, subjects are often faced with problems such as: 'Has a dim light been flashed or not?' or: 'Which of two similar images has been presented?' Signal detection theory (SDT) provides a prescription for these kinds of decisions, where one of two hypotheses has to be chosen on the basis of a single observation in the presence of uncertainty, or noise (Gold & Shadlen 2007). If the sensory observation

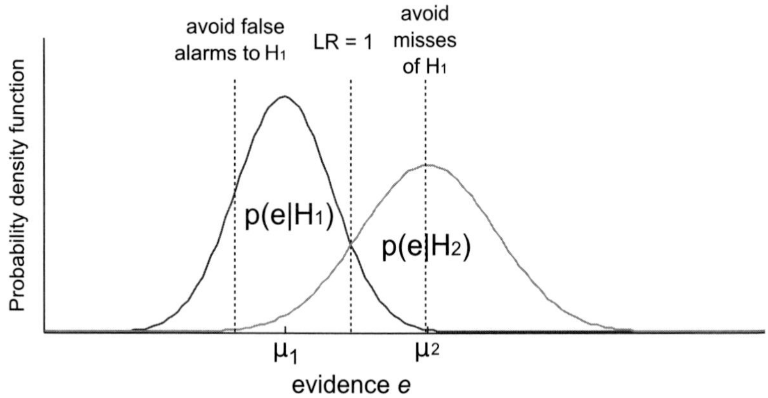

Fig. B.1 Signal detection theory in two-alternative forced choice tasks. Because of uncertainty the probability density functions (PDFs) of the two alternative hypotheses overlap. A choice is made depending on the desired level of accuracy for one of the alternatives. Comparing the likelihood ratio (LR) to 1 minimizes the total number of errors.

is informative about the hypotheses, it provides 'evidence' favoring one alternative. We will generally refer to information that is indicative of a choice as evidence e. The two hypotheses H_1 and H_2 stand for the two choice-alternatives. The conditional probability $\mathrm{P}(e|H_1)$ denotes the probability of observing evidence e if H_1 is true.

Depending on the signal-to-noise ratio μ/σ and the similarity of the hypotheses $\mu_1 - \mu_2$, the probability density functions (PDFs) of the two alternatives overlap to some degree (Fig. B.1).

The smaller the signal-to-noise ratio, the higher the overlap of the PDF. Likewise, the more distinguishable the stimuli, the smaller the overlap. In the case of sensory stimuli the PDFs are often assumed to be normally distributed with means $\mu_1 \neq \mu_2$ and standard deviations $\sigma_1 = \sigma_2$.

The *a posteriori* probability $P(H_1|e)$ that hypothesis H_1 is true given the evidence e can be determined according to Bayes' theorem from the conditional probability $P(e|H_1)$, the prior, or *a priori* probability of the hypothesis $P(H_1)$, and the total probability of the evidence $P(e)$:

$$\mathrm{P}(H_1|e) = \frac{\mathrm{P}(e|H_1)\mathrm{P}(H_1)}{\mathrm{P}(e)}, \tag{B.1}$$

The prior $P(H_1)$ thereby denotes the probability that H_1 is true before any evidence has been obtained. If equal priors are assumed for both alternatives, H_1 is more likely to be correct than H_2 if the 'likelihood ratio' $\mathrm{LR}(e) = \mathrm{P}(e|H_1)/\mathrm{P}(e|H_2)$ is larger than 1.

Choosing H_1 if $\mathrm{LR} > 1$ is the optimal strategy, in the sense that it provides the lowest overall error rate. In the case of equal rewards or costs, it also indicates the optimal choice in terms of the highest reward. For some decisions, however, the consequences of a false alarm, for example, are negligible compared to missing a signal. Because of the noise, mistakes are inevitable. Still, the kind of errors, i.e. false alarms or misses, can be adjusted by the decision criterion (Fig. B.1). Generally, the desired level of accuracy for one of the alternatives determines the decision threshold, or bound, B. For unequal prior probabilities, but identical rewards, H_1 should be chosen if $LR(e) > B = \mathrm{P}(H_2)/\mathrm{P}(H_1)$ (Green & Swets 1966). In sensorimotor tasks, unequal priors arise for instance if one stimulus is presented more often than the other.

If not just one, but multiple pieces of evidence e_1 .... e_N are available over time, as for instance in the random-dot motion (RDM) task, the likelihood ratio has to be updated with each new sample of evidence. With the simplifying assumption that all evidence samples e_1 ... e_N are independent, the likelihood ratio becomes

$$\mathrm{LR}(e) = \frac{\mathrm{P}(H_1|e_1...e_N)}{\mathrm{P}(H_2|e_1...e_N)} = \prod_{n-1}^{N} \frac{\mathrm{P}e_n|H_1}{\mathrm{P}e_n|H_2}. \tag{B.2}$$

A decision bound $B = 1$ again minimizes the error rate, as it determines the most likely hypothesis (Neyman & Pearson 1933). From the perspective of two-alternative forced choice problems, Equation B.2 applies to the 'interrogation' paradigm, where the decision is based on a fixed sample of evidence.

In the 'free response' paradigm, where the decision-maker is allowed to control the decision time autonomously, she or he is faced with the additional problem of when to end the evidence accumulation. Accordingly, optimality in free response tasks is often assessed as the strategy that yields the shortest expected reaction time (RT) for a given error rate.

The sequential probability ratio test (SPRT) provides a solution to this specific optimality problem (Wald 1947). Here, the momentary likelihood ratio LR(e) is again calculated as in Equation B.2, but instead of one, there are now two decision bounds B_1 and B_2 and the sampling process continues as long as

$$B_2 < \mathrm{LR}(e) < B_1, \mathrm{with} B_2 < B_1. \tag{B.3}$$

In other words, if B_1 is crossed, alternative 1 is selected, if B_2 is crossed, alternative 2 is selected, and while the evidence for both alternatives is insufficient, meaning below a certain level of significance, the decision process continues. Interestingly, a decision rule equivalent to Equation B.3 can be obtained using any quantity that is monotonically related to the likelihood ratio LR if B is scaled appropriately (Green & Swets 1966). Hence, by taking the logarithm of Equations B.2 and B.3, the decision process can be written as a simple addition:

$$\log(B_2) < \log(\mathrm{LR}(e)) = \Sigma_{n-1}^{N} \log \frac{\mathrm{P}(e_n|H_1)}{\mathrm{P}(e_n|H_2)} < \log(B_1). \tag{B.4}$$

Moreover, the temporal evolution of the log-likelihood ratio (logLR) can be described as a discrete decision variable V, starting at $V_0 = 0$, which is subsequently updated at each time step, according to

$$V^n = V^{n-1} + \log \frac{\mathrm{P}(e_n|H_1)}{\mathrm{P}(e_n|H_2)}. \tag{B.5}$$

Using the log-likelihood ratio to express the sequential probability ratio test has the further advantage that evidence in favor of H_1 intuitively adds to V with a positive value, while evidence supporting H_2 contributes negatively. In that sense, the trajectory of the decision variable $V(t)$ for noisy evidence is analogous to a one-dimensional 'random walk' bounded by a positive and negative threshold.

In the limit of infinitesimally small time steps, equivalent to continuous sampling, the discrete sequential probability ratio test / random walk model converges to the drift-diffusion model (DDM) described in the next section. A more detailed theoretical description of optimality, including the case of unequal priors, and the continuum limit of the sequential probability ratio test, is provided elsewhere (Bogacz et al. 2006).

Before we turn to the drift-diffusion model, we briefly discuss how the theory presented above might relate to real neural computations during decision-making and the random-dot motion task in particular. According to Shadlen and colleagues (Churchland, Kiani & Shadlen 2008, Gold & Shadlen 2001, Gold & Shadlen 2002, Gold & Shadlen 2007, Roitman &

Shadlen 2002, Shadlen & Newsome 2001), decision-related neural activity in area LIP (lateral intraparietal cortex) is consistent with the notion of an 'accumulation-to-bound' process, while area MT (middle temporal cortical visual area) encodes the absolute amount of visual motion present in the random dot motion stimulus and might consequently provide decision evidence to LIP (Britten, Shadlen, Newsome & Movshon 1992, Britten, Shadlen, Newsome & Movshon 1993). Could LIP activity actually correspond to a neural decision variable in the mathematical sense of the sequential probability ratio test?

As the brain is unlikely to store the complete distribution of possible neural responses to every encountered stimulus, it probably has no access to the PDFs of the neural populations, which would be necessary to infer the likelihood ratio LR (Gold & Shadlen 2001) (but see Ma, Beck, Latham & Pouget (2006)).

However, motivated by the apparent analogy between the trajectory of V and visual cortical area LIP firing rates, Gold and Shadlen (2001, 2002, 2007) argued that a quantity approximating the logLR could indeed be computed in the brain. More precisely, knowledge about the probability density functions would not be explicitly necessary to implement a decision rule approximating the optimal sequential probability ratio test, if the output firing rates of two antagonistic sensory neurons or neural populations were used as evidence. One example would be the responses I_1 and I_2 of two populations of visual cortical area MT neurons, one selective for rightward, the other for leftward motion, which respond to their preferred and null direction with mean firing rates $\mu_1 > \mu_2$, and roughly equal variance σ. In that case, the optimal logLR decision rule will depend only on the firing rate difference $I_1 - I_2$, apart from a scaling factor.

This largely holds true for a variety of possible probability density functions (PDFs) (Gold & Shadlen 2001). In particular:

$$\log \mathrm{LR}_{\text{left,right}} = \frac{\mu_1 - \mu_2}{\sigma^2}(I_1 - I_2) \tag{B.6}$$

if I_1 and I_2 are sampled from normal distributions, which is a plausible assumption for the average firing rate of a neural population. However, the responses of single neurons might better be described by a Poisson distribution. In that case

$$\log \mathrm{LR}_{\text{left,right}} = \log(\frac{\mu_1}{\mu_2})(I_1 - I_2). \tag{B.7}$$

Knowing the sign of the difference $I_1 - I_2$ in MT activity would hence be sufficient for downstream areas like cortical area LIP to elicit a left or right saccade according to a sequential probability ratio test optimal rule.

Furthermore, a study by Platt & Glimcher (1999) revealed that both the prior probability of getting a reward, and the expected magnitude of the reward, could modulate LIP activity, consistent with the suggestion that LIP activity might be a neural correlate of the decision-variable V (Equation B.5).

As a final note on the sequential probability ratio test (SPRT), the argument of Gold and Shadlen (2001, 2002, 2007) can also be extended to multiple alternatives, or neural populations, which results in a comparison between the neural population with the highest rate and the average rate of the other populations ('the max-vs-average test') (Ditterich 2010). However, contrary to the 2-alternative case, the resulting statistical test is not optimal. Interestingly, the optimal algorithm for decisions between more than two alternatives is still unknown (McMillen & Holmes 2006). The multihypothesis SPRT was shown to approximate optimality for small error rates (Dragalin, Tartakovsky & Veeravalli 1999). For moderate error rates, the physiologically plausible max-vs-average test performs almost as well as the multihypothesis SPRT (Ditterich 2010).

B.1.1.2 The drift-diffusion model (DDM)

The continuum limit of the sequential probability ratio test represents the most basic form of the drift-diffusion model. A continuous decision variable $\nu(t)$ is accumulating the evidence difference between the two choice-alternatives, or hypotheses (Laming 1968, Ratcliff 1978, Stone 1960). In the unbiased case with equal prior probabilities, $\nu(t)$ is integrated over time according to

$$d\nu(t) = \mu dt + \sigma dW, \qquad \nu(0) = 0, \tag{B.8}$$

with symmetric decision bounds $b_1 = -b_2$, and the accumulation time interval dt (assumed to be very small). Equation B.8 is the continuous extension of Equation B.5. The right side of Equation B.8 denotes the new noisy evidence obtained during dt. It is composed of a constant drift μdt, with drift rate μ, and the diffusion term σdW, which represents white noise drawn from a Gaussian distribution with mean 0 and variance $\sigma^2 dt$. (dW is proportional to $N(0,1) \cdot \sqrt{dt}$, as the variance of uncorrelated stochastic random variables is additive with successive time-steps, which leads to a square-root behaviour for the standard deviation (Usher & McClelland 2001).) The correct alternative is determined by μ, which, in the case of the random dot motion task, can be interpreted as the amount of coherent motion. Using the terminology of the sequential probability ratio test, if $\mu > 0$, H_1 is correct; if $\mu < 0$, H_2 is correct. Which alternative is eventually chosen by the drift-diffusion model, however, is also subject to noise, depending on σ, and the height of the decision bounds b_1 and b_2. Still, the drift-diffusion model, as a continuous implementation of the sequential probability ratio test, solves two-alternative forced choice problems optimally: it will on average return a decision in the shortest possible time for a specified level of accuracy (Bogacz et al. 2006).

Solutions of Equation B.8 are normally distributed with probability density $p(\nu, t) = N(\mu t, \sigma\sqrt{t})$, if the decision bounds are ignored (Gardiner 1985). Consequently, the variance across trials of the temporal evolution of ν increases linearly with t. This can be appreciated in Fig. B.2, where several example trials of ν and their variance are displayed.

Due to the threshold nonlinearity of the decision bounds, the reaction time distributions of correct and error trials are typically left-skewed, with equal means (Fig. B.2b). Treated as a so called 'first-passage time problem', error rates (ER) and mean reaction times (meanRT) of the basic drift-diffusion model can be expressed as

$$\text{ER} = \frac{1}{1 + e^{2\mu b/\sigma^2}} \tag{B.9}$$

$$\text{meanRT} = \frac{b}{\mu} \tanh\left(\frac{\mu b}{\sigma^2}\right) + t_{\text{ND}} \tag{B.10}$$

where t_{ND} denotes the 'non-decision' time (e.g. the time related to sensory and motor processes which add to the reaction time RT).

Contrary to the theoretical predictions of the basic drift-diffusion model, error responses in 2-alternative forced choice tasks can have significantly different mean RTs than correct responses, depending on experimental specifications, e.g. stressing accuracy or speed, or the difficulty of a condition (Luce 1986, Pleskac & Busemeyer 2010, Ratcliff & Smith 2004). A more general, extended version of the drift-diffusion model includes trial-to-trial variability in the drift rate and the starting point (Ratcliff & McKoon 2008, Ratcliff & Rouder 1998). A normally distributed drift rate with mean μ and standard deviation s_μ leads to longer RTs on error trials, as errors will occur more often in trials where μ is small. Drawing the starting point $\nu(0)$ from a uniform distribution ranging from $-s_\nu$ to s_ν produces on average shorter error RTs, because errors are more likely for a bias towards bound b_2 and hence reach the threshold faster. Physiologically, this variability can be explained by trial-to-trial differences in attention, premature sampling, or other variable perceptual biases.

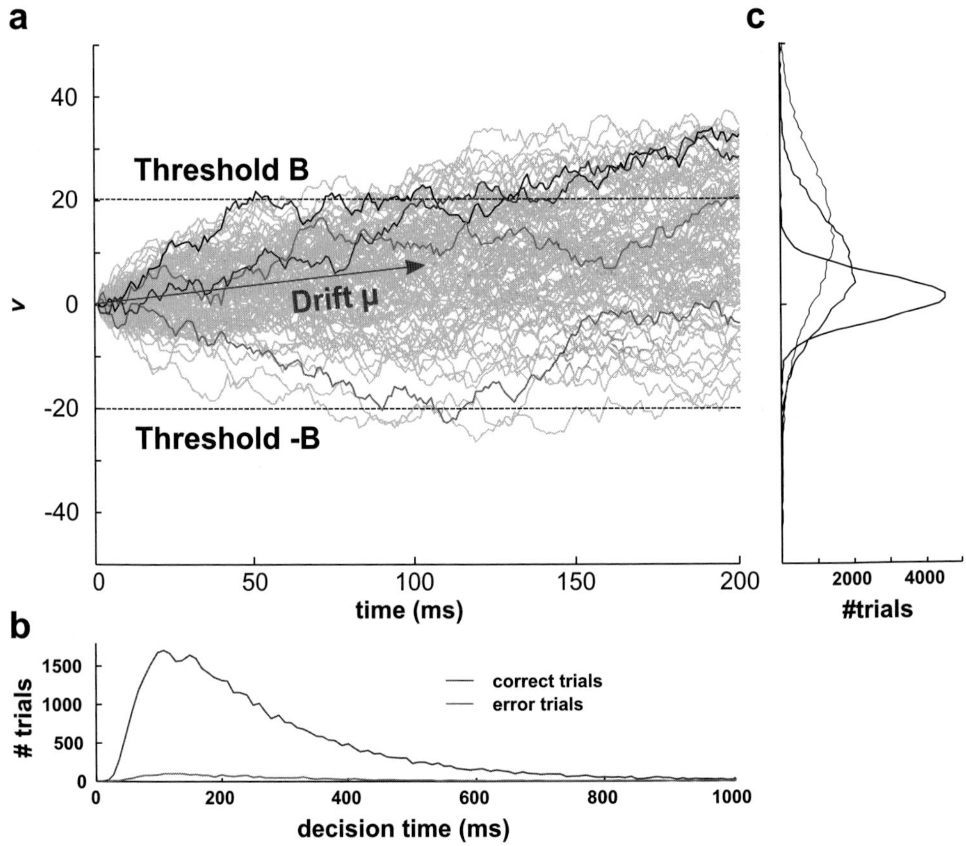

Fig. B.2 Basic drift-diffusion model. (a) 100 example traces of the time evolution of $v(t)$. Three correct trials are labelled in blue, one error trial in orange. (b) Left-skewed RT Histograms of correct and error choices from 50,000 trials. (c) The variance of ν increases with time. The distribution of ν for 50,000 trials is given for t = 20 ms, 100 ms and 200 ms (bold to narrow lines). Model parameters: μ = 0.07, σ = 1, dt = 1 ms, B = 20. (See colour plates section.) (Reprinted from *Progress in Neurobiology* 103, G. Deco, E. T. Rolls, L. Albantakis and R. Romo. Brain mechanisms for perceptual and reward-related decision-making, pp. 194–213, Copyright 2013, with permission from Elsevier.)

The extended drift-diffusion model version is hardly tractable analytically. RT distributions and ERs can only be obtained numerically. Typically, the drift-diffusion model is fitted to a particular set of behavioural data by minimizing the deviation between a simulated data set and the experimental data set (Vandekerckhove & Tuerlinckx 2007).

A simplified deterministic version of the DDM has also been proposed by Reddi and Carpenter (2000). Their 'LATER' model produces variability in reaction times by varying the drift rate across trials, without any within-trial noise. For the random dot motion task, where the stimulus itself is explicitly stochastic, this might not seem a plausible model. However, trial-to-trial variability alone can be sufficient to fit the behavioural data of certain two-alternative forced choice tasks (Brown & Heathcote 2008).

Nevertheless, the drift-diffusion model has the advantage that reaction times and accuracy are directly related above the decision threshold. In experiments, more pressure for speed typically leads to faster RTs and lower accuracy. This negative correlation is known as the 'speed-accuracy tradeoff' (SAT). By adjusting the decision bounds, the DDM can reproduce the negative speed-accuracy tradeoff correlation (Palmer, Huk & Shadlen 2005). In the absence of noise, as for the LATER model, the threshold influences reaction times, but has no effect on accuracy.

The reverse conclusion of the speed-accuracy tradeoff is that perfect accuracy could be achieved with unlimited processing time. Accordingly, the drift-diffusion model implements perfect integration of the evidence difference in the sense that no information is 'forgotten' or overly emphasized. Nonetheless, participants' accuracy as a function of RT often reaches an asymptote, especially in difficult tasks, and the assumption of perfect integration may not hold true for neural systems. These discrepancies can be solved by introducing a 'leakage' term $\lambda\nu$ to the drift rate in Equation B.8. Information loss over time is modeled according to:

$$d\nu(t) = (\lambda\nu + \mu)dt + \sigma dW, \qquad \nu(0) = 0, \tag{B.11}$$

with $\lambda < 0$, corresponding to a stable Ornstein-Uhlenbeck (O-U) process (Busemeyer & Townsend 1993). This can be pictured by a diffusion of ν in a curved instead of a flat landscape, where ν approaches a stable fixed point $\nu^* = -\mu/\lambda$, where $d\nu = 0$. In the opposite case of $\lambda > 0$ both the mean and variance of ν grow exponentially, as ν is repelled from the now unstable fixed point (an unstable O-U process).

B.1.1.3 The race model

In the drift-diffusion model a single integrator accumulates the evidence difference between two alternatives, whereas in the race model (Vickers 1970, Vickers 1979) separate integrators ν_1, and ν_2 are used for each alternative:

$$d\nu_1 = I_1 dt + \sigma dW_1 \tag{B.12}$$

$$d\nu_2 = I_2 dt + \sigma dW_2 \tag{B.13}$$

with $\nu_1(0) = \nu_2(0) = 0$, where I_1 and I_2 denote the average incoming evidence, respectively. As for the drift-diffusion model, white noise is sampled from a normal distribution, $N(0, \sigma^2 dt)$. In the free-response mode, a decision is made as soon as one of the two integrators exceeds a threshold B. (We again assume equal prior probabilities. Therefore both integrators have the same decision bound B.) The two integrators thus perform a 'race to threshold' against each other.

Except for the case of perfectly anticorrelated noise in the two accumulators, the race model is not equivalent to the drift-diffusion model and thus is not optimal (Bogacz et al. 2006). Nevertheless, in contrast to the drift-diffusion model, the race model can easily be extended to multiple-choice decisions, simply by adding more integrators.

Moreover, in the race model, ν can be interpreted as the population activity of two neural populations, receiving inputs from distinct populations of up-stream sensory neurons. For the drift-diffusion model, however, it remains unclear how the difference in evidence might be computed physiologically.

This problem has been addressed in subsequent 'connectionist' models of two-alternative forced choice decision-making (Fig. B.3). These abstract neural network models implement the diffusion process with inhibition between two integrators and will be reviewed in the following section.

B.1.2 Biologically motivated rate models

As we have seen, the drift-diffusion model (DDM) is an intuitively appealing model of two-alternative forced choice decision-making and, moreover, achieves optimality according to the sequential probability ratio test (SPRT). But, is there a way to implement this drift-diffusion concept in a physiologically plausible manner? Several models have been proposed, which

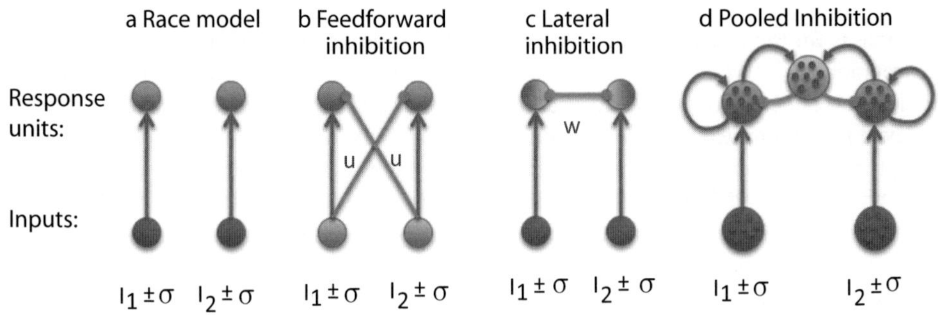

Fig. B.3 Two-alternative forced choice (2AFC) decision models with two integrators. The connections that terminate with arrows denote excitatory connections, and those that terminate with circles denote inhibitory connections. The two inputs to each of the four models are $I_1 \pm \sigma$ and $I_2 \pm \sigma$. (See colour plates section.) (Adapted from Bogacz, R., Brown, E., Moehlis, J., Holmes, P. and Cohen, J. D., The physics of optimal decision making: a formal analysis of models of performance in two-alternative forced choice tasks, *Psychological Review* 113 (4), pp. 700–765 ©2006, The American Psychological Association.)

effectively compute evidence subtraction with different inhibitory mechanisms (Fig. B.3). Although these models all have two separate integrators just like the race model, dynamically they are more closely related to the drift-diffusion model (Bogacz et al. 2006).

B.1.2.1 Feedforward inhibition (FFI)

Mazurek, Roitman, Ditterich & Shadlen (2003) proposed a feedforward inhibition (FFI) model directly motivated by neuronal activity from MT and LIP during the random dot motion task (Britten et al. 1993, Shadlen & Newsome 2001). The model instantiates the hypothesis that two populations of movement-sensitive MT neurons provide evidence in favor or against the opposed motion directions, which is then integrated in area LIP (Fig. B.3b). A decision is made when the pooled activity reaches a threshold. The two LIP populations thus correspond to the response units, which receive excitatory inputs from one population of MT neurons, and inhibitory inputs from the other, according to:

$$d\nu_1 = I_1 dt + \sigma dW_1 - u(I_2 dt + \sigma dW_2) \quad \text{(B.14)}$$

$$d\nu_2 = I_2 dt + \sigma dW_2 - u(I_1 dt + \sigma dW_1) \quad \text{(B.15)}$$

with $\nu_1(0) = \nu_2(0) = 0$, and where u denotes the inhibitory feedforward (FF) connection weight. In this simple version of the feedforward inhibition model, integration is perfect without leakage.

Just as with the basic drift-diffusion model, the feedforward inhibition model cannot account for the slower error reaction times (RTs) found experimentally in the random dot motion task without further extensions. Ditterich (2006a) and Ditterich (2006b) subsequently suggested that a time-variant version of the feedforward inhibition, including for example a within-trial increase of the input gain, could account quite well quantitatively for both the behavioural and neural data of Roitman and Shadlen (2002). An additional leak term further improved the fit to the neural data.

In addition, Niwa & Ditterich (2008) successfully applied a 3-alternative version of the feedforward inhibition model to their random dot motion experiment with three possible directions of motion. Theoretically, the FFI model can be extended to any number of choice-alternatives, if the inhibitory weights are adapted accordingly. This assumption might be plausible in an experiment where trials with different numbers of alternatives are present in separate blocks of trials. By contrast, if the different trials are randomly interleaved, as in Churchland et al. (2008), sufficient neural plasticity to adapt the connection weights is hardly practical in the short time between trials.

B.1.2.2 Lateral inhibition and the leaky competing accumulator (LCA) model

Apart from feedforward inhibition, lateral inhibition between the two integrators, here the two LIP populations, could effectively support a diffusion process through competition within LIP (Fig. B.3c). This picture is consistent with the established assessment that long range cortical connections are mostly excitatory, and inhibition thus acts locally within a cortical column (Lund, Angelucci & Bressloff 2003, Rolls 2008b). Usher & McClelland (2001) proposed a model called the 'leaky competing accumulator' (LCA) model, which in its simplest form can be written as:

$$d\nu_1 = (-k\nu_1 - w\nu_2 + I_1)dt + \sigma dW_1 \tag{B.16}$$

$$d\nu_2 = (-k\nu_2 - w\nu_1 + I_2)dt + \sigma dW_2 \tag{B.17}$$

with $\nu_1(0) = \nu_2(0) = 0$. Here, $k > 0$ is the decay rate, or leak, equivalent to $\lambda < 0$ in the Ohrnstein-Uhlenbeck model (Equation B.11), and w denotes the inhibitory connection strength between the integrator units. Usher & McClelland (2001) further incorporated non-linearity in their model in the form of a threshold-linear activation function, which prevents the firing rates from dropping below zero. The leaky competing accumulator model accounts for correct and error RT distributions without the need for trial-to-trial, or within-trial, variability.

Interestingly, the authors also addressed multi-choice decision-making with the leaky competing accumulator model and found that the model captures the positive log-linear relation between reaction time and the number of alternatives, known as Hick's law (Hick 1952). (Hick's law is that the reaction time increases linearly as a function of the log of the number of alternatives between which a choice is being made.)

To summarize, Bogacz et al. (2006) demonstrated that for a particular parameter range, namely large and balanced leakage and inhibition, the dynamics of the leaky competing accumulator and the feedforward inhibition model approximate a one-dimensional linear diffusion process equivalent to the drift-diffusion model with perfect integration. Moreover, the leaky competing accumulator and consequently also the basic drift-diffusion model are approximated by a more physiologically-plausible connectionist model with pooled inhibition and recurrent excitation, if self-excitation balances the decay and the inhibition is strong (Fig. B.3d). However, whether the brain actually works in a parameter regime of perfect linear integration has been called into question by a random dot motion study with time-varying evidence (Huk & Shadlen 2005, Wong & Huk 2008). For an accurate description of real neural dynamics, nonlinear attractor states that arise from strong recurrent connections between the neurons is a very plausible approach, which is described in Chapter 8. The details of how these attractor network models with integrate-and-fire neurons are implemented, and further evidence about how they operate, are provided in Section B.1.3.

B.1.3 Attractor models

Neural networks with interconnected neurons, such as the pooled inhibition model displayed in Fig. B.3d, form nonlinear dynamical systems, whose long-term behaviour is determined by 'fixed points', or 'steady states'. These fixed points can be attractive, or repellent, and their existence depends on different parameters of the system, in this case for example the recurrent connection weights, or the inputs to the neural network. A useful analogy of the

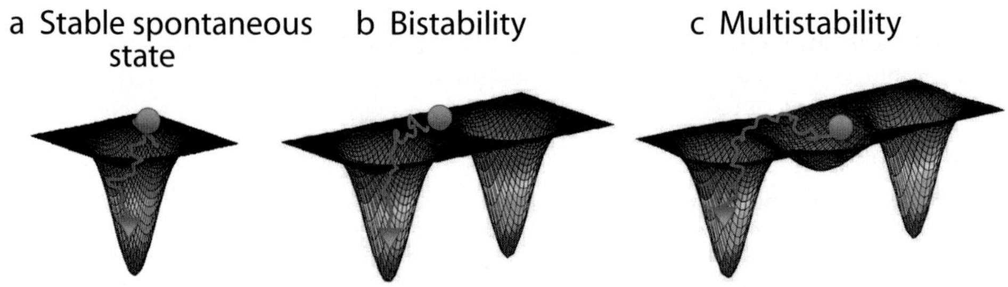

Fig. B.4 Schematic presentation of possible attractor configurations in the attractor network of binary decision-making. Stable fixed points, or attractors, are illustrated as valleys in the 'energy landscape', and the hills correspond to unstable, repellent fixed points. Depending on the network parameters and inputs, (a) one, (b) two, or (c) three attractors can be simultaneously stable. (b) In the bistable case, the two decision attractors, but not the spontaneous state, are stable. The system (blue dot) will eventually move from the unstable spontaneous state into one of the two decision states. (c) In the multistable case, the spontaneous state as well as the two decision attractors are stable states. Transitions from the spontaneous state to a decision-attractor can happen due to noise fluctuations that are large enough to drive the system from the spontaneous state across the 'hill', or unstable fixed point, into the 'basin of attraction' of one of the decision-attractors. (See colour plates section.)

system's trajectory through state space is a particle that moves on an energy landscape with valleys, corresponding to attractors or stable fixed points, and hills, corresponding to unstable, repellent fixed points (Fig. B.4). Decision-making can be implemented in an attractor network with at least two stable fixed points ('bistability'), representing the two choice alternatives. The decision process is then regarded as the transition from an initial starting point towards one of the two attractors. Once such a decision-attractor is reached, this state will persist except where it is destabilized by high levels of noise or perturbations, and can thus be produce persistent neural activity. This is an advantage, for the decision state can be maintained in the attractor short-term memory that may provide the goal for an action while the action is being produced (Rolls 2008b).

In the pooled inhibition model, decision-attractors emerge through strong recurrent connections, which form positive feedback loops of activity in the excitatory neural populations. Runaway activity is averted through negative feedback from the inhibitory neural population.

The biophysically-realistic attractor model that forms the basis of our theoretical work is a spiking-neuron implementation of the pooled inhibition model (Wang 2002). Many of the properties of this model of decision-making have been described in Chapter 8. One of the biologically realistic features of the model is that due to the nonlinear response properties of the spiking neurons, and background Poisson activity representing inputs from other cortical areas, the model can maintain a low spontaneous firing rate (Amit & Brunel 1997). Therefore, depending on the magnitude of the (e.g. sensory) inputs and the strength of the recurrent connections, the model can work in three different dynamical regimes: (1) only the spontaneous state of low firing is stable, (2) a bistable regime of categorical decision-making, and (3) a 'multistable regime', where the spontaneous and the decision attractors are all stable states while the decision inputs are being applied (Fig. B.4). In the multistable regime, transitions from the spontaneous state to a decision-attractor can happen due to noise fluctuations (i.e. randomness in the firing times of the neurons in the system and its inputs) that are large enough to drive the system across the 'hill', or unstable fixed point, into the 'basin of attraction' of one of the decision-attractors.

B.1.3.1 Biophysically-realistic attractor model with spiking neurons

Although the connectionist models discussed above schematically describe neural processes in area MT and LIP, they still lack a direct connection between model variables and real neuronal parameters. In contrast, neurons are modelled in the biophysically detailed implementation of the pooled inhibition model (Wang (2002), Rolls & Deco (2010), and Chapter 8), where single neurons are modeled as leaky integrate-and-fire (LIF) neurons (Tuckwell 1988) with conductance-based synaptic responses, described by realistic synaptic kinetics. The model was initially developed to account for (persistent) neural activity of prefrontal cortex neurons during working memory tasks (Brunel & Wang 2001). Its application to decision-making was inspired by the experimental observation that neurons, which exhibit ramping activity, characteristically show persistent neural firing in delayed memory or decision tasks (Gnadt & Andersen 1988, Shadlen & Newsome 2001). Wang (2002) successfully applied the spiking-neuron attractor model to behavioural and neurophysiological decision-making data measured from primates performing a binary random dot motion discrimination task (Roitman & Shadlen 2002). In this context, the attractor network can again be viewed as the representation of a local microcircuit in area LIP, or in many other cortical areas (Rolls 2008b, Rolls & Deco 2010).

Physiological neuronal firing rates are obtained by averaging over the simulated action potentials, or output 'spikes', of distinct neural populations or 'pools' of leaky integrate-and-fire neurons in the network. Each leaky integrate-and-fire neuron is characterized by its subthreshold membrane potential V

$$C_{\mathrm{m}}\frac{dV(t)}{dt} = -g_{\mathrm{m}}(V(t) - V_{\mathrm{L}}) - I_{\mathrm{syn}}(t), \qquad \text{(B.18)}$$

where C_{m} is the membrane capacitance taken to be 0.5 nF for excitatory neurons and 0.2 nF for inhibitory neurons; g_{m} is the membrane leak conductance taken to be 25 nS for excitatory neurons and 20 nS for inhibitory neurons; V_{L} is the resting potential of –70 mV, and I_{syn} is the total synaptic current. When the membrane potential V of a leaky integrate-and-fire neuron reaches the firing threshold V_{th}, it is reset to V_{reset} and a spike is emitted to all connected neurons with a subsequent absolute refractory period of τ_{ref}. Thus LIF neurons do not explicitly model action potentials, but give a realistic account of the subthreshold membrane potential. The total synaptic current is given by a sum of glutamatergic, AMPA ($I_{\mathrm{AMPA,rec}}$) and NMDA ($I_{\mathrm{NMDA,rec}}$) mediated, currents from the excitatory recurrent collateral connections, one AMPA ($I_{\mathrm{AMPA,ext}}$) mediated external excitatory current, and one inhibitory GABAergic current (I_{GABA}):

$$I_{\mathrm{syn}}(t) = I_{\mathrm{AMPA,ext}}(t) + I_{\mathrm{AMPA,rec}}(t) + I_{\mathrm{NMDA,rec}}(t) + I_{\mathrm{GABA}}(t). \qquad \text{(B.19)}$$

The attractor network is organized into separate populations of LIF neurons, termed 'pools', which share common inputs and connectivities (Fig. B.5a, after Masquelier, Albantakis & Deco (2011)). As in the connectionist version, the spiking neuron model contains one homogenous pool of inhibitory neurons, globally connected to all neurons in the network. The two 'integrator units' of the connectionist version are implemented by two 'selective pools' of excitatory neurons (S1, S2 in Fig. B.5a), which respond selectively to one of the two possible decisions, for example directions of coherent motion and, hence, reflect the possible choice-alternatives in for example the random dot motion task. Moreover, a third excitatory pool of 'nonselective' neurons represents the activity of surrounding neurons that are not selective to either input (e.g. direction of motion). More generally, there is one specific (or decision) pool for each possible decision alternative.

All neurons in the network receive an external background input simulated by uncorrelated, stochastic Poisson spike trains applied independently to the individual neurons. This

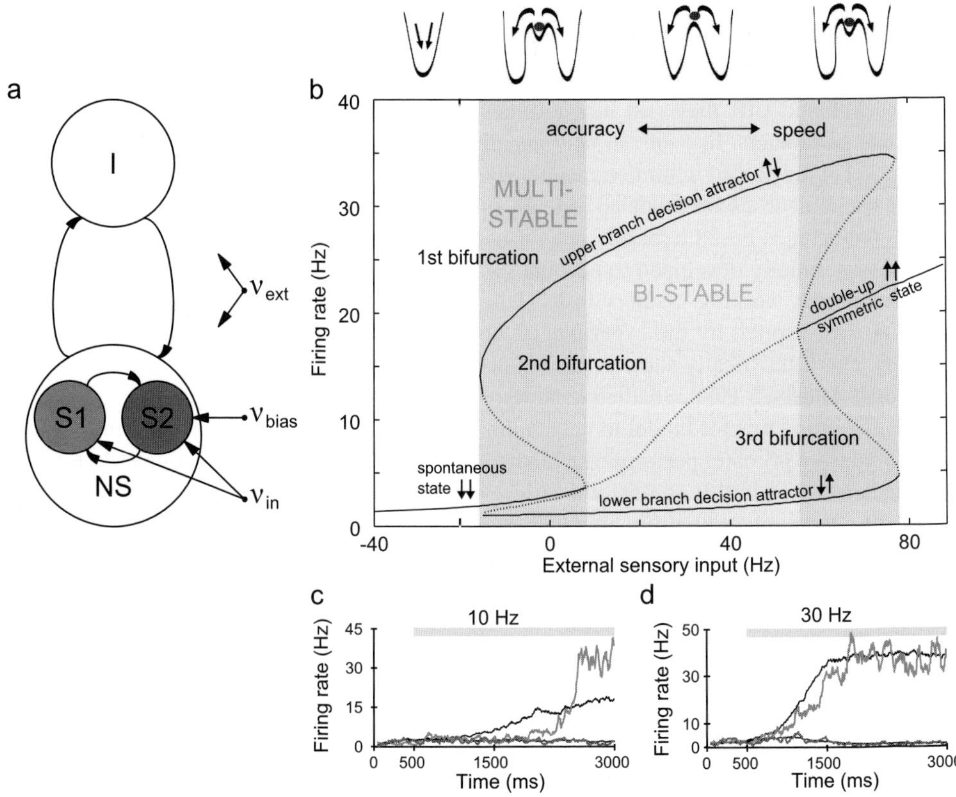

Fig. B.5 Biophysically-realistic attractor network of decision-making. (a) Schematic representation of the network. The excitatory neurons are organized into three pools: the nonselective neurons (NS) and the two selective, decision-making, pools (S1, S2) that receive the inputs encoding each stimulus (with rate ν_{in} in the terminology of this Appendix). An additional bias (ν_{bias}) can be applied to one of the two selective pools. All neurons also receive an input (ν_{ext}) that simulates the spontaneous activity in the surrounding cerebral cortex. (b) Stable (solid lines) and unstable (dotted lines) fixed points depend on the external sensory input. They were calculated with the mean-field approximation of the network (Brunel and Wang, 2001). (c,d) Single trial (colored traces) and mean (black, averaged over 20 trials) temporal evolution of the firing rate of the selective pools for different inputs, denoted by the grey bars (ν_{bias} = 0). (c) Noise-induced transition from the spontaneous state to the decision state (with low inputs, in the multistable regime). (d) Input-driven transition (in the bistable regime). Simulations were performed with a synaptic strength of w_+ = 1.68 within selective populations; all other parameters were taken from Wang (2002). (See colour plates section.) (Adapted from Masquelier, T., Albantakis, L. and Deco, G., The timing of vision – how neural processing links to different temporal dynamics, *Frontiers in Psychology* 2, 151 ©The Authors.)

background activity determines the spontaneous firing rate of all network neurons and is the main source of noise in the network together with finite-size effects due to the limited number of neurons (Rolls & Deco 2010). Here, the term 'finite-size noise' describes the variance in the recurrent inputs caused by their Poisson-like spike firing times, which tend to zero when the size of the network is increased. In addition to the background input, the selective pools receive time-dependent external inputs through the same input connections that correspond to the decision evidence λ, such as, for instance, the decision sensory stimuli in the random dot motion experiment. (ν_{in} refers to the total input to each decision pool, and consists of the background activity which is held constant, plus the evidence about the decision λ. In this case $\lambda_1 = \lambda_2 = \lambda_{\text{in}}$.)

As explained above for the general case, decision-attractors emerge in the network due to the strong recurrent connectivity w_+ of neurons within one selective pool, while the connections between the two selective pools are weaker than average $w_- < 1$. (This is consistent with an associative, Hebbian, synaptic learning rule, as it is assumed that the activity of neurons that are selective for the same feature has been correlated in the past, while neurons encoding opposite directions instead fired in an anticorrelated manner (Rolls 2008b, Rolls & Deco 2010).)

Fig. B.5b shows an example of a typical attractor landscape for strong w_+ as a function of increasing external inputs ν_{in} applied equally to both selective pools. Without any external sensory inputs to the selective pools (0 Hz), the system will naturally rest in its spontaneous state with similarly low firing rates in all excitatory neural pools.

If a sensory stimulus is applied to the model, which increases the external inputs to the selective pools sufficiently (> 10 Hz), the spontaneous state becomes unstable in a 'subcritical pitchfork bifurcation' leading to bistability between the decision attractors (the gray area in Fig. B.5b). The network then operates in a region of categorical decision-making, where one selective pool will settle at the upper decision branch with high firing rate ('winner'), while the other will decay to the lower branch ('loser'). In this case, the transition from the spontaneous state to the decision state is 'input-driven' and can be gradual, in the order of several hundred milliseconds, even on single trials (Fig. B.5d). These gradual transitions between attractor states, corresponding to the decision process, are a distinguishing feature of the biophysically-realistic attractor model, and rely on the slow kinetics of the NMDA receptors ($\tau_{\text{NMDA,decay}} = 100$ ms). Consequently, the network's behaviour is not just dominated by its steady states, but also exhibits prolonged responses to momentary sensory inputs, with a characteristic time constant of up to a second, during which the model effectively integrates the incoming inputs (Wang 2008).

As depicted schematically in Fig. B.4c, in the multistable regimes decision-making is also possible. There, the transition from the spontaneous or symmetric state to a decision state is induced by noise fluctuations, and can be rather sharp in a single trial (Fig. B.5c). Nevertheless, the trial-averaged activity appears to build up slowly, as observed experimentally in decision-related neurons. This ramping activity is, however, obtained in a conceptually different way compared to the bistable regime: in the multistable regime, the gradual build-up is an artifact of averaging across trials each with abrupt transitions at random times (Marti, Deco, Mattia, Gigante & Del Giudice 2008).

For sufficiently strong connection weights w_+, as in the example of Fig. B.5, the network can exhibit persistent activity, meaning that the high firing rates of the 'winner' population can be sustained even after all the external sensory inputs that provided the evidence for the decision are switched off. This is because at 0 Hz, with only background activity, the system is already in the multistable regime, where the decision states are stable in addition to the spontaneous state. Under these conditions, the decision states would only destabilize if negative inputs were applied to the selective populations, or if synaptic or neuronal adaptation occurred in the winning population related to its high firing rate, or if a strong input was applied to the losing population which would then lead to a new competition implemented through the inhibitory neurons. Persistent activity is a characteristic feature of all biophysically-realistic attractor models that we will describe, unless otherwise stated. Therefore, the bifurcation between the multistable regime at low inputs and the bistable regime is the first bifurcation with relevance to the decision-making process ('second bifurcation' in Fig. B.5).

In the vicinity of this 'second bifurcation', slow integration is enhanced above the intrinsically slow kinetics mediated by the NMDA receptors, as the effective time constant of the system increases even beyond that related to the NMDA receptors close to the third bifurcation (Roxin & Ledberg 2008, Wong & Wang 2006). Therefore, in this dynamical region

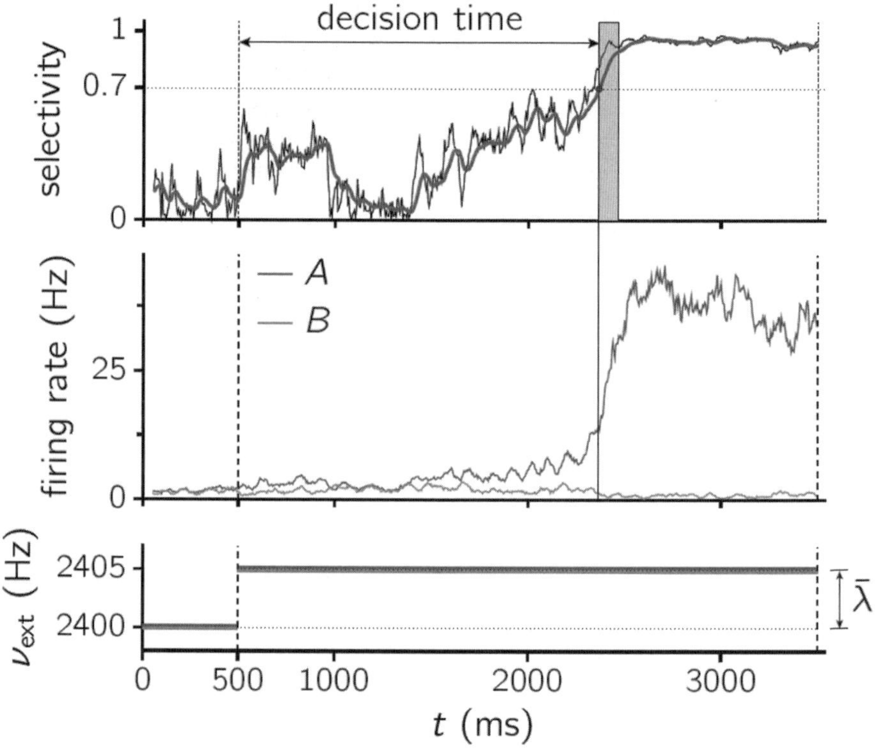

Fig. B.6 Development of the selectivity index (top), the average activity of populations A and B (middle), and the stimulation applied (bottom), for a single decision-making trial with a stable spontaneous state (the 'multistable regime'). The green line in the top panel is the low-pass filtered selectivity. (The selectivity index was $\mid \nu_1 - \nu_2 \mid / (\nu_1 + \nu_2)$.) From 0 to 500 ms no stimulation was applied (λ =0). From 500 ms to the end of the trial, λ was set to a constant value different from zero ($\nu_{\text{ext}} = \nu_0 + \lambda$ for the selective cells). The decision time, DT, was the time between stimulus onset and the time at which the low-pass filtered selectivity index crossed the threshold of 0.7 and stayed above it for at least 100 ms. The shaded area shows the time window within which the signal (green line) was required to be greater than the threshold. N = 2000, w_+ = 1.75, λ = 5 Hz. (See colour plates section.) (Reproduced from Marti, D., Deco, G., Mattia, M., Gigante, G. and Del Giudice, P., A fluctuation-driven mechanism for slow decision processes in reverberant networks, *PLoS ONE* 3: e2534, figure 4 ©2008, The Authors.)

performance is high and reaction times are rather long, because of long stimulus-integration times. For this reason, previous analyses of the binary attractor model particularly concentrated on the dynamics in the proximity of the second bifurcation, where the spontaneous state destabilizes (Marti, Deco, Mattia, Gigante & Del Giudice 2008, Wang 2002, Wong & Wang 2006).

The decision process being described for the 'multistable regime' can be visualized with Fig. B.6. We use the term 'multistable regime' to refer to the scenario in which the spontaneous state is stable even when the decision cues are being applied. It is stable in the system without noise, that is in an infinite size network in which the noise disappears, and to which the mean field analysis applies. Of course in a smaller system, with several thousand synapses per neuron, the noise from the close to Poisson neuronal spiking times becomes significant and causes statistical fluctuations, and this can make the system eventually jump out of the spontaneous state. Fig. B.6 shows the operation of a decision-making network in which the

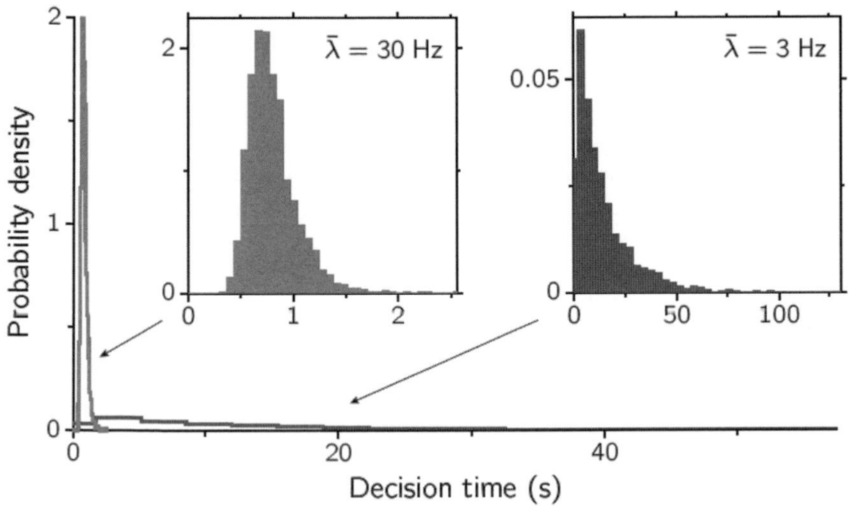

Fig. B.7 Distributions of decision times for a regime with a spontaneous stable state (blue, right, λ = 3 Hz) and without a spontaneous stable state (red, left, λ = 30 Hz), from a sample of 4000 trials each. The two insets show the distributions separately (note the different scales). N = 4500, w_+ = 1.75. (See colour plates section.) (Reproduced from Marti, D., Deco, G., Mattia, M., Gigante, G. and Del Giudice, P., A fluctuation-driven mechanism for slow decision processes in reverberant networks, *PLoS ONE* 3: e2534, figure 4 ©2008, The Authors.)

spontaneous state is stable (without noise, as just described, and established with a mean field analysis) (Marti, Deco, Mattia, Gigante & Del Giudice 2008). After 500 ms, the decision cues are applied, with $\lambda_1 = \lambda_2$ and ν_{ext} increased in each of the two decision pools to 2405 Hz across the 800 synapses for external inputs to each neuron. It can be seen that over the time period from 500 to approximately 2300 ms the firing rates in the two decision pools fluctuate at just above the spontaneous rate of 3 spikes/s. This is the period in which we can describe the system as 'accumulating or integrating evidence', even though it is in this case just related to the statistical fluctuations. In the time period from approximately 1500–2300 ms the statistical fluctuations cause the firing rates of the neurons by chance in pool A to gradually increase above those in pool B. Finally, when pool A reaches a firing rate of approximately 5 spikes/s, the attractor dynamics in pool A become so strong that the pool suddenly increases its firing rate to reach the high firing rate attractor state in less that 40 ms. The decisions in this multistable regime are thus dependent on the statistical fluctuations which cause one of the decision pools to jump out of the low firing rate state that is close to the spontaneous state.

In this regime, the reaction or decision times can be very variable and long, because it is primarily a matter of waiting for the statistical fluctuations to produce sufficiently large effects that one of the pools reaches the critical level of firing at which the decision has been taken and that pool moves rapidly to a high and stable firing rate state in a decision attractor state. These long and variable decision times in the 'multistable regime' are illustrated in Fig. B.7 (right, blue).

The same 'multistable regime' can still apply, with a stable spontaneous state even when the decision cues are applied, when λ_1 does not equal λ_2. In this case the reaction time is still dominated by the statistical fluctuations, but the system is also being driven slowly on average towards one of the pools having a slightly higher firing rate in the decision period, until suddenly again at about 5 spikes/s in this system (the bifurcation point) one of the pools wins and rapidly then enters the high firing rate attractor state. In this case, the decision-making is still probabilistic, and is influenced by the noise, but gradually the percentage correct increases and the decision time decreases as $\Delta\lambda$ increases. This is illustrated in Fig. 8.15 (in which ΔI corresponds to $\Delta\lambda$). This regime applies in general when the external decision cues λ are similar to each other, and when the λs are small. The decision will in this case be difficult, less than 100% correct. The 'multistable' regime may not apply if the mean value of λ is high, even for a difficult decision where $\lambda_1 = \lambda_2$, for the high mean value of λ may force the system out of the state where the spontaneous state is stable when the decision cues are being applied.

The 'bistable' regime (with two decision pools) applies when the spontaneous state (in the infinite size limit when the mean field analysis applies) is not stable. In this case, the system starts moving immediately towards one of the decision states, and although the noise can influence the decision, the system cannot wait in the spontaneous state for long just for a statistical fluctuation to cause a decision. In this regime, the decision times will be faster, and much less variable, as illustrated in Fig. B.7 (left, red).

The variability of decision times around the mean can be measured with the coefficient of variation, CV = $\sigma / < RT >$ (the standard deviation of the reaction times divided by the mean reaction time). The CV of the reaction times tends for sufficiently large N, the number of neurons in the network (i.e. with low noise), to the value 1 as the mean value of λ is decreased below the bifurcation value, the critical level of the inputs λ at which the system crosses into a high firing rate attractor state. This asymptotic value, together with the histogram in Fig. B.7 (right, blue), suggest that in this 'multistable' regime and in the limit of vanishing noise, decisions are essentially Poisson processes, with exponentially distributed decision times. This Poissonian character is gradually lost as the mean value of the external inputs λ increases and the deterministic component of the dynamics takes over from the stochastic one, leading to more peaked, gamma-like reaction time distributions such as those shown in Fig. B.7 (left, red) and hence to lower CV values (Marti, Deco, Mattia, Gigante & Del Giudice 2008). [In more detail, it is found that for mean values of λ (i.e. $\overline{\lambda}$) < $\overline{\lambda_c}$ (the critical value of $\overline{\lambda}$ at which the spontaneous firing rates are no longer stable), the value of the CV of the decision times is essentially insensitive to the amount of noise (while the mean value of the decision times strongly depends on N in the same region), consistent with the picture of an approximate Poisson statistics for the noise-driven decision process in the 'multistable' regime. For $\overline{\lambda} > \overline{\lambda_c}$ the converse is observed, the strong dependence of the CV on $\overline{\lambda}$ being due to the fact that for increasing noise (decreasing N) the representative point in the (ν_A, ν_B) plane drops off the symmetric ridge down from the unstable spontaneous state at more widely distributed times (Marti et al. 2008).]

Overall, we can describe the operation of the decision-making attractor network system as being fluctuation-driven in the regime when the spontaneous state is stable with the decision cues applied, and as being in a relaxation regime when the spontaneous state is not stable with the decision cues applied. The transition from the fluctuation-driven to the relaxation regime as the mean value of λ is increased is more abrupt the lower is the presence of noise in the system, that is the larger the system is in terms of the number of neurons N (Marti et al. 2008).

The operation of the system in the multistable regime with a stable spontaneous state as well as stable decision states provides a way to account for the wide range of decision times and their variability with distributions exhibiting long tails that are frequently found experimentally (Roitman & Shadlen 2002, Luce 1986, Hanes & Schall 1996, Burbeck & Luce 1982). This approach has been explored in the context of perceptual alternations in a paper by Moreno-Bote, Rinzel & Rubin (2007), which considers a broad class of attractor-based models that are consistent with the properties of perceptual rivalry. Among these, the model accounts for the observed narrow distribution of dominance durations as well as for the associated mean value of the order of seconds, substantially higher than the intrinsic synaptic and neuronal time scales. As described in Chapter 8, the principle of noise-driven transitions is also important in explaining the neurophysiological and behavioural signatures of Weber's law, in the context of a two-forced choice vibrotactile task (Deco & Rolls 2006).

Exploring the network dynamics at the other end of the bistable regime when the mean value of λ is high is also of interest. For sufficiently high external sensory inputs, the network enters a different type of multistable regime. Crossing the 'third bifurcation', a symmetric 'double-up' state can become stable, where both selective pools fire with intermediate, elevated rates. This double-up symmetric state has recently been deployed to explain LIP responses to static visual stimuli, as for example the response targets in the random dot motion paradigm (Albantakis & Deco 2009, Furman & Wang 2008, Wong et al. 2007). Assuming high selective inputs with R-target onset, the high firing rates of LIP neurons prior to the motion stimulus (Churchland, Kiani & Shadlen 2008, Huk & Shadlen 2005, Kiani & Shadlen 2009, Roitman & Shadlen 2002) can be reproduced with the attractor model in the double-up state. Changes of mind, and thus the possibility to reevaluate a first choice, also emerge naturally in the attractor network close to the 'third bifurcation' (Albantakis & Deco 2011).

The integrate-and-fire attractor model of decision-making that we have been exploring provides we believe also a foundation for the implementation of short-term memory in the brain (Rolls 2008b). The item to be remembered is provided as an input to the attractor network, and, perhaps in competition with other inputs and certainly of background noise present in the inputs, the attractor enters a high firing rate state. The high firing rate state continues as it is stable when the input from the item to be remembered is removed. The 'double-up' states just referred to correspond to having two items simultaneously active in the same short-term memory attractor network. If the global inhibition is reduced, it has been shown that it is possible to increase the number of items that can be maintained simultaneously active (Rolls, Dempere-Marco & Deco 2013). If the inhibition is reduced too far, the spontaneous state becomes unstable (i.e. the system jumps into a high firing state even without any input applied). In practice, with a sparseness of 0.1 (which measures the proportion of the excitatory neurons in each decision pool), and non-overlapping representations (which have generally been used in these investigations), it has been possible to maintain 4–5 populations of neurons simultaneously active. Interestingly, if synaptic facilitation is introduced, this enables more short-term memories to be maintained active simultaneously (Rolls, Dempere-Marco & Deco 2013). In the case described, 9 of the 10 possible short-term memories can be maintained active simultaneously with synaptic facilitation.

Across the bistable regime, in between the two bifurcations (2nd and 3rd), higher external inputs to both selective populations lead to faster reaction times and less accuracy, congruent with a speed-accuracy tradeoff (Roxin & Ledberg 2008, Wong & Wang 2006). This dependency of decision-behaviour on the amount of unbiased external sensory inputs to both selective populations explicitly arises from the nonlinearity of the attractor model. In linear models, such as the drift-diffusion model, changes in the common sensory evidence to both decision alternatives would not affect decision behaviour. This is clear in the case of the drift-diffusion model, as the drift-diffusion model characteristically accumulates only the difference between the evidence for the two alternatives. Indeed, input-dependent decision behaviour might provide a means to distinguish between linear and nonlinear modeling approaches.

Further, although the integrate-and-fire attractor model of decision-making would automatically provide an upper bound for the neuronal activity of the winning selective population, the model's decision is typically determined by a fixed firing rate threshold independent of the applied amount of sensory inputs, in line with neurophysiological evidence from LIP neurons. How this decision threshold is read out or adjusted by down-stream areas is not explicitly included in the attractor model. Nevertheless, possible extensions have been suggested, which implement the decision threshold involving cortico-collicular and cortico-basal ganglia circuits (Bogacz & Gurney 2007, Lo & Wang 2006).

Taken together, the characteristic features of the biophysically realistic integrate-and-fire spiking neuron attractor model are:

1. strong recurrent connections within the selective neural populations, which generate attractor states,
2. global feedback inhibition enabling winner-take-all competition,
3. stochasticity because of finite-size effects and random Poisson inputs to the network,
4. a long synaptic time-constant (NMDA) facilitating the integration of incoming neural activity.

B.1.3.2 Mean-field approximation

Simulating populations of individual and realistic neurons as described above is necessary to simulate realistic neuronal dynamics, physiological responses and behaviour. Nevertheless, to gain an analytical understanding of the population dynamics, a reduced, mathematically tractable description can yield deeper insights into the essential, collective model behaviour (Rolls & Deco 2010). Several such approaches are reviewed in this and the next subsections.

Taking a mean-field approach, Brunel & Wang (2001) considerably reduced the state variables of the network by replacing the different populations of spiking neurons with an approximation of their average population activity. Because of the recurrent connections in the network, the population firing rates have to be determined self-consistently based on the input currents to the neural pools, which in turn depend on the firing rates. Equalizing the pre- and postsynaptic activity, the possible fixed points or steady states of the population firing rates can be obtained.

Several approximations have to be assumed in order to arrive at a closed system of one nonlinear equation for each population in the network. First, postulating that individual neurons fire spikes independently, according to a stationary Poisson process, the net input is treated as a Gaussian random process. This assumption generally holds in the limit of infinitely large networks, where each neuron receives a large number of presynaptic currents, which each deflect the membrane potential only minimally compared to the voltage distance between the resting and threshold potential. Second, only fast AMPA-mediated external inputs are assumed to contribute to the fluctuations in the synaptic current. Fluctuations in the NMDA and GABA currents are neglected as they are considered to filter out, due to the longer synaptic time constants.

Finding a self-consistent solution for the population rates is further complicated by the nonlinear properties of the NMDA receptors. NMDA saturation is approximated by calculating the average NMDA gating variable as a nonlinear function of the presynaptic rate. In addition, the voltage dependence of the NMDA conductance is linearized around the average neural potential.

For the detailed mathematical derivation we refer to the original publication (Brunel & Wang 2001), to Section B.5, to Renart, Brunel and Wang (2003), to Deco and Rolls (2006), and to Rolls and Deco (2010). Solving the mean-field equations is computationally much less intense than running simulations with the full spiking network. The mean-field analysis thus allows calculation of the steady state firing rates of the attractor model for a wide range of parameters. This makes it feasible to scan the parameter space in order to find a parameter set matching experimental findings.

In sum, by solving the mean-field equations for a set of initial conditions (here the initial firing rates of each neural population) one obtains the approximate average firing rate of each pool when the system has settled into a stationary state after the period of dynamical transients. The mean-field reduction, however, does not provide an accurate description of the temporal dynamics.

B.1.3.3 Two-dimensional reduction

Based on the mean-field approach, Wong & Wang (2006) further reduced the biophysically-realistic spiking-neuron model to a two-variable system. In particular, they fitted a simplified input–output function to the complex first-passage time formula used in the mean-field to describe the output firing rates as a function of the mean synaptic inputs. With the assumption that the network dynamics are dominated by the slow NMDA receptors, they further set the firing rate of the nonselective pool to a constant mean firing rate (2 Hz) and linearized the input-output relation of the inhibitory neurons. In this way, inhibition could be incorporated as mutual negative inputs between the selective pools. The nonselective and interneurons could thus be eliminated, leaving two neural units with self-excitation and effective mutual inhibition.

The two-dimensional reduction is particularly useful to perform phase-plane analyses in order to elucidate the different dynamical regimes of the network. To simulate the noisy temporal evolution of the spiking neural network, Wong & Wang (2006) explicitly added a noise term to the external inputs, described by an Ohrnstein-Uhlenbeck process (white noise filtered by a short, AMPA receptor synaptic time constant). The two-dimensional reduction can thus be viewed as a closely related connectionist version of the full spiking model. In this way, it can also account for decision-related behaviour and neural activity, albeit without explicit analogy to real neural parameters (Wong et al. 2007).

B.1.3.4 Nonlinear diffusion

Instead of a two-component system of rate equations as in Wong & Wang (2006), Roxin & Ledberg (2008) derived a one-dimensional nonlinear diffusion equation to describe the asymptotic behaviour of winner-take-all models in the proximity of the bifurcation to bistability, where the spontaneous state destabilizes. Their reduction is universally valid for all winner-take-all models, but also makes it possible to relate the variables of the nonlinear diffusion process to those of the full spiking-neuron model, and thus to neurobiologically meaningful quantities. A particularly relevant prediction based on this one-dimensional reduction is that the speed-accuracy tradeoff can be implemented by changes in the common inputs to both selective neural populations, instead of, or in addition to, an alteration of the decision-threshold.

A novel *top-down* methodology has been introduced that allows an effective reduction of a high-dimensional spiking neurodynamical system in a data-driven fashion (Deco, Marti, Ledberg, Reig & Sanchez Vives 2009a, Rolls & Deco 2010). The idea is to depart from the high-dimensional data first by reducing the dimensionality with techniques such as principal component analysis or principal curves. After this reduction, one fits the underlying dynamics by a system of mean-field-like reduced Langevin equations. In particular, a system of Langevin equations is used that describes the stochastic dynamics by assuming an underlying potential (or energy function). The advantage of using this type of potential-based stochastic system is that for this system, the associated Fokker–Planck equation, which expresses the evolution of the probabilistic distribution of the variable, can be solved analytically at least for stationary conditions, so that we have a closed form for the asymptotic probabilistic distribution of the reduced data. In this schema, the underlying fluctuations can be explicitly extracted (Deco et al. 2009a, Rolls & Deco 2010). The resulting system can be interpreted as a nonlinear diffusion system, which can be used for linking the underlying cortical dynamics with behaviour. In fact, it is usual in psychophysics to describe the behavioural data by (linear) diffusion models, as described earlier in this Appendix. The top-down approach described offers therefore an extension of this type of model, in the sense that the new diffusion models described used for fitting behaviour are nonlinear (due to the positive feedback in the attractor network), and are derived from the underlying neurophysiological experimental data. The model thus differs from traditional linear diffusion models of decision-making used to account for example for human reaction time data (Luce 1986, Ratcliff & Rouder 1998, Ratcliff, Zandt & McKoon 1999, Usher & McClelland 2001).

B.1.4 Distinguishing model approaches

As we have seen, models on the accumulation of noisy evidence, as for instance in the random-dot motion paradigm, come with a huge variety. Although they differ in fundamental features, such as network structure and connectivity, in practice, it may be very difficult to distinguish between them on the basis of just behavioural data or mean firing rates (Bogacz et al. 2006, Ditterich 2010).

Ratcliff & Smith (2004) evaluated four types of sequential sampling models and the leaky competing accumulator (LCA) model against three sets of psychophysical two-alternative forced-choice experiments. In particular they compared the three models described above, the drift-diffusion model (DDM), the Ornstein-Uhlenbeck model (Equation B.11), and the race model, and a so-called ‘Poisson counter’ model (Townsend & Ashby 1983), all with trial-to-trial variability in drift, starting point, and non-decision time. (The Poisson counter model resembles the race model, with the difference that evidence is counted in discrete units, delivered at random times, with exponentially distributed intervals. Therefore, it can be interpreted as an independent accumulation of two spike trains.)

Of all models considered, only the Poisson counter model failed to match the empirical data, and faster mean decision times on error trials presented problems for the race model. The Poisson counter model also proved inferior to the drift-diffusion model when compared to the neural activity of superior colliculus build-up neurons from macaque monkeys performing a two-alternative forced-choice task (Ratcliff et al. 2003). The activity pattern predicted by the drift-diffusion model, however, resembled the observed neuronal firing rates, suggesting that build-up cells in the superior colliculus might participate in a diffusion-like decision process.

Because of the mutual similarity between the models (Bogacz et al. 2006, Ratcliff & Smith 2004), finding new analytical methods and well designed experiments to distinguish the different approaches is a major challenge in the field of perceptual decision-making.

One approach along that line was conducted by Huk & Shadlen (2005). By adding brief motion pulses to a standard random dot motion stimulus, they first of all provided strong physiological support for a temporal integration in area LIP. However, their findings revealed a departure from perfect integration, as the effect of the motion pulse decreased with its onset time. Later motion pulses thus influenced behaviour and neural activity less than earlier motion pulses. Neither a perfect drift-diffusion model, nor leaky integrators, could reproduce this experimental finding, while the time-varying dynamics of the attractor model explained both the behavioural and the neuronal data (Wong & Huk 2008, Wong, Huk, Shadlen & Wang 2007). Still, time-varying effects such as decreasing decision bounds, or an ‘urgency’ signal, might produce decreased sensitivity to later perturbations also in the drift-diffusion model and leaky competing accumulator model.

Recently, multiple-choice decision tasks have received increasing attention in the context of distinctions between models (Churchland et al. 2011, Ditterich 2010, Leite & Ratcliff 2010, Purcell, Heitz, Cohen, Schall, Logan & Palmeri 2010). Analysing higher-order statistical properties of neurophysiological data from their 2- and 4-alternative random dot motion task, Churchland et al. (2011, 2008) were able to distinguish between models categorized by their different sources of variability. Models with just one source of variability, such as the LATER model (Section B.1.1.2) and a model by Cisek, Puskas & El-Murr (2009) with fixed slope, but a random distribution of firing rates at each time-step, failed to account for the higher-order measures, although they agreed with behaviour and mean firing rates. On the other hand, all different model implementations of a stochastic accumulation-to-threshold tested in Churchland et al.'s (2011) study could account for variance and within-trial correlations, in addition to the behavioural data and first-order firing rates. In particular, the tested models included the drift-diffusion model (Ratcliff & Rouder 1998), a model based on probabilistic population codes (Beck et al. 2008), and the reduced version of the attractor model by Wong, Huk, Shadlen & Wang (2007).

Based on human behavioural data from a random dot motion task with three alternatives and three motion components, Ditterich (2010) aimed to distinguish more detailed aspects of conceptual accumulation-to-bound models with regard to their goodness of fit and their neurophysiological predictions. Perfect integrators were compared to leaky, saturating integrators, with either feedback or feedforward inhibition. As we have seen, in the case of two alternatives, most of the discussed models proved equivalent to the drift-diffusion model for certain parameter ranges (Bogacz et al. 2006). Therefore, it might not be too surprising that none of the models could be excluded based only on the fits to behavioural data of a 3-alternative random dot motion task (Niwa & Ditterich 2008). Yet, the models differ substantially in their neurophysiological predictions on how the integrator states should evolve over time (see Table 2 in Ditterich (2010)). Neuronal recordings from monkeys performing the same task will hopefully soon provide clarification. Moreover, feedforward and feedback inhibition respectively suggest either negative or positive correlation between the integrator units, which might be tested with multi-electrode recordings. Finally, in the case of an equal amount of motion coherence in all three directions, Niwa & Ditterich (2008) measured faster mean reaction times for higher coherence levels. While models with feedforward inhibition require a scaling of the variance of the sensory signals in order to account for this effect, conceptual models with feedback inhibition could explain the result just with a change of the mean input (Ditterich 2010).

Considering the evidence presented in this section, so far two types of decision-making models have proven particularly successful: on the one hand, the extended drift-diffusion model and its connectionist implementations account for a wide range of behavioural data. They also conceptually represent neural activity during the decision-making period. On the other hand, the physiologically-detailed attractor model (Rolls & Deco 2010, Wang 2002, Deco & Rolls 2006, Wang 2008) and its reductions (Wong & Wang 2006), which mimic real neuronal dynamics, accurately simulate behavioural data and area LIP activity during the random dot motion task, and in other decision-making tasks including vibrotactile decision-making in areas such as the ventral premotor cortex (Deco & Rolls 2006), value-based decision-making in the medial prefrontal cortex, and many other types of decision-making (Rolls 2008b, Rolls, Grabenhorst & Deco 2010b, Rolls, Grabenhorst & Deco 2010c, Rolls & Deco 2010, Grabenhorst & Rolls 2011) (see Chapter 8), and also memory and attention (Rolls 2008b). Moreover, they account for persistent activity, and the nonlinear, time-dependent, effects of events that interrupt the decision-making process (Wong & Huk 2008, Wong et al. 2007).

With respect to the biologically plausible attractor decision-making networks, the dynamics relevant to the decision-making depend on the stability of the spontaneous firing activity state (i.e., the low firing rate state in which no decision has yet been made). If, once the second stimulus is presented, the spontaneous state destabilizes, then the dynamics rapidly evolves toward one of the two decision states (Wong & Wang 2006). This corresponds to a so called 'ballistic scenario' consistent with a linear diffusion model. On the other hand, if the spontaneous state does not lose stability but is instead bistable with the decision states, hence leading to multistability between three possible fixed points (with a multistable region between the first and second bifurcation), then, only a sufficiently strong perturbation would drive the system from the stable spontaneous state to one of the two decision states (Deco & Rolls 2006, Rolls & Deco 2010). This differs from the earlier ballistic scenario, in which the system will evolve towards one of the two choices even in the absence of fluctuations (Wong & Wang 2006). Thus, in the multistable regime, fluctuations, perhaps noise-driven, are essential for decision-making. Computational analysis of this scenario showed that behaviour consistent with Weber's law for decision-making (that the difference between the decision cues $\Delta\lambda$ / the intensity of the decision cues λ is a constant) is more consistent with a fluctuation-driven scenario in a multistable regime (Deco & Rolls 2006, Deco et al. 2007). In particular, experimental behavioural evidence showing behaviour that conforms to Weber's law for the decision-making involved in the discrimination of two vibrotactile stimuli in humans suggests that the neurodynamical mechanisms and computational principle underlying this process are consistent with a fluctuation-driven scenario in a multistable regime (Deco & Rolls 2006, Deco et al. 2007) (Chapter 8).

B.2 Synaptic facilitation and sequential decision-making

Most models of decision-making deal with simultaneous presentation of the stimuli to be discriminated, λ_1 and λ_2. But in some tasks, such as the vibrotactile discrimination task, the stimuli are presented sequentially, and the decision is then about whether the second stimulus applied to the finger is higher or lower in vibrotactile frequency than the first stimulus (Romo, Hernandez & Zainos 2004). One way in which this has been modeled is to assume that there is a short-term memory of the first stimulus, and then to analyse the decision-making between the remembered first stimulus and the second stimulus, both applied simultaneously to the attractor decision-making network as λ_1 and λ_2 (Deco & Rolls 2006). This approach also assumes that λ_1 and λ_2 are represented by different neurons, that is, that a place code (Rolls & Treves 2011) is used.

By introducing synaptic facilitation into the attractor model, we have been able to develop a model of decision-making that can account for the memory of the first stimulus as well as the temporal evolution of how the stimuli are encoded in the neuronal firing rates. This means that the model for example captures when and how the vibrotactile flutter frequencies of both the first and the second stimulus are reflected in the neural firing rates (Deco, Rolls & Romo 2010).

The model accounts for the presence and usefulness of partial differential neurons of the type illustrated in Fig. B.8 in the ventral premotor cortex, which is implicated in vibrotactile decision-making (Romo et al. 2004). In the ventral premotor cortex (VPC) some neurons reflect the decision-making itself, responding for example if the first vibrotactile stimulus (f_1) applied to the hand is higher in flutter frequency than the second (f_2), while other neurons respond to the decision $f_1 > f_2$ (see Fig. 2GHI of Romo et al. (2004) with an example shown in Fig. 8.5). In addition to these neurons, the so called 'partial differential' neurons reflect the memory of f_1. Partial differential neurons respond to f_1 during the presentation of f_1, do not respond in the first part of the delay period, then gradually ramp up towards the end of the delay period to a firing frequency that reflects f_1, and then during the decision period when

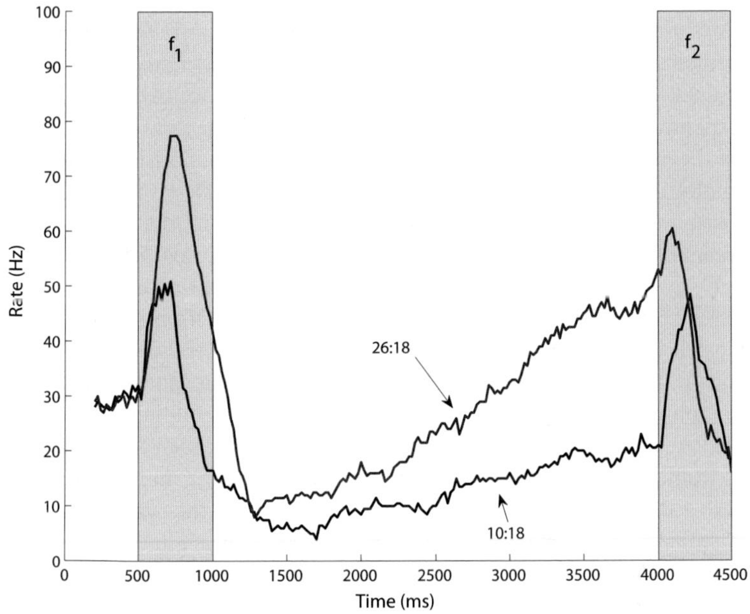

Fig. B.8 Activity of a single neuron of the 'partially differential' type recorded in the ventral premotor cortex (VPC) during the vibrotactile decision-making task, after Romo et al. (2004), as illustrated in Fig. 2JLK of that paper. The f_1 period was from 500-1000 ms, there was then a delay period, and the f_2 period when f_2 was applied and the decision was made was from 4000–4500 ms. f_2 was in both cases 18 Hz. When f_1 was 26 Hz (red plot), the firing rate during f_1, and at the end of the delay period, and during the comparison period when f_2 was being applied was higher than when f_1 was 10 Hz (black plot). Thus the firing of this type of neuron during f_2 helps in the decision that $f_1 > f_2$ when f_1 is 26 Hz, and that $f_1 < f_2$ when f_1 is 10 Hz. Approximately 30 trials were used to generate these peristimulus time histograms for each pair for this single neuron. (See colour plates section.) (Reproduced from Deco, G., Rolls, E. T. and Romo, R., Synaptic dynamics and decision-making, *Proceedings of the National Academy of Sciences* 107 (16), pp. 7545–7549, figure 1 ©2010, National Academy of Sciences.)

f_2 is presented are influenced by f_2 (Romo et al. 2004). The responses of partial differential neurons may be related to the decision-making (Romo et al. 2004), for as shown in Fig. B.8, if $f_1 > f_2$ the firing during f_2 is higher than when $f_1 < f_2$, for a given f_2.

To simulate the neuronal activity during the delay period the model utilizes synaptic facilitation, a process implemented using a phenomenological model of calcium-mediated transmission (Mongillo, Barak & Tsodyks 2008). Synaptic facilitation is caused by the increased accumulation of residual calcium at the presynaptic terminals, which increases the probability of neurotransmitter release (Zucker & Regehr 2002). This type of synaptic facilitation is common in higher cortical areas such as the prefrontal cortex (Hempel, Hartman, Wang, Turrigiano & Nelson 2000, Wang, Markram, Goodman, Berger, Ma & Goldman-Rakic 2006, Zucker & Regehr 2002). The synaptic efficacy of the recurrent connections between excitatory neurons is modulated by the utilization parameter u (the fraction of resources used) reflecting the calcium level. When a spike reaches the presynaptic terminal, calcium influx in the presynaptic terminal causes an increase of u which increases the release probability of transmitter and thus the strength of that synapse. The decay time constant of the synaptic facilitation is regulated by a parameter τ_F which has been determined experimentally to be around 1–2 s (Wang et al. 2006), i.e. large enough to be able to sustain memory and allow comparison for short delays (3 s in our case).

Another difference between the attractor network with synaptic facilitation modeling the partial differential neurons and the basic attractor model is that here the recurrent connections are not sufficient to maintain the attractor state without external sensory inputs. Consequently, the model responds to the first stimulus f_1, but then the firing decreases when f_1 is removed. Subsequently the firing gradually increases again due to a non-specific increase in excitation that is externally applied during the delay period after f_1 (Deco et al. 2010). This non-specific increase in excitation, in conjunction with the synaptic facilitation, which remains in the recurrent collateral connections of the network neurons that recently fired due to the application of f_1, is sufficient to reinstate these neurons into firing. This principle usefully models the delay-related firing shown in Fig. B.8 (Deco, Rolls & Romo 2010). Then when f_2 is presented, the firing rate of the partial differential neurons reflects the vibrotactile frequencies of both f_1 and f_2 (Deco, Rolls & Romo 2010). Other neurons respond to f_2 and not to f_1. If both these neuron types (the partial differential and the f_2 responding neurons) form the λ_1 and λ_2 inputs to a separate attractor decision-making network, then the correct decision can be computed from λ_1 which reflects a combination of f_1 and f_2, and λ_2 which reflects only f_2. Provided that the inputs from these two types of neuron to the attractor decision-making network are scaled appropriately by synaptic strengths that are trained during a learning period, one population in the attractor decision-making network will respond when $f_1 > f_2$, and the other when $f_1 < f_2$. This is possible because the firing of the partial differential neurons reflects f_2 as well as f_1. The decision-making attractor network then compares the firing of the partial differential neurons with the firing of the f_2 neurons. The decision taken will be in one direction if f_1 is high in frequency relative to f_2, and in the other direction if f_1 is low in frequency relative to f_2. In effect, the partial differential neurons allow the value of f_2 to be taken into account in making the decision, so that the attractor network can subtract the exact value of f_2 from the decision reached, and reflect just the difference between f_1 and f_2 (Deco, Rolls & Romo 2010).

We argue that it is inevitable given the rate encoding with broad tuning of the neurons in VPC to the vibrotactile stimuli, that f_1 will be contaminated by f_2, and that a solution of the type we propose is needed. Indeed, we argue that the partial differential neurons of the type illustrated in Fig. B.8 are fundamental to the solution of the decision-making problem by this brain region (Deco, Rolls & Romo 2010).

B.3 Synaptic facilitation, graded firing rates, and postponed decisions

In the preceding section we showed that a synaptic facilitation mechanism allows the attractor network to maintain the memory of f_1 during the delay between the stimuli f_1 and f_2 in a sequential decision-making task (Deco, Rolls & Romo 2010).

In addition to being necessary to perform sequential decision-making tasks, memory also plays a role in tasks where the decision is postponed for a period after the evidence has been provided (Lemus, Hernandez, Luna, Zainos, Nacher & Romo 2007). Using an information theoretic approach to single-cell neurophysiological data recorded during a sequential tactile discrimination task with postponed decisions (Lemus et al. 2007), we were able to analyse at what time during the trial information about the forthcoming action becomes available. In particular, we found that information about the forthcoming action becomes available from the activity of neurons recorded in the medial premotor cortex in a sequential decision-making task after the second stimulus is applied that provides the information for a decision about whether the first or second stimulus was higher in vibrotactile frequency (Martinez-Garcia,

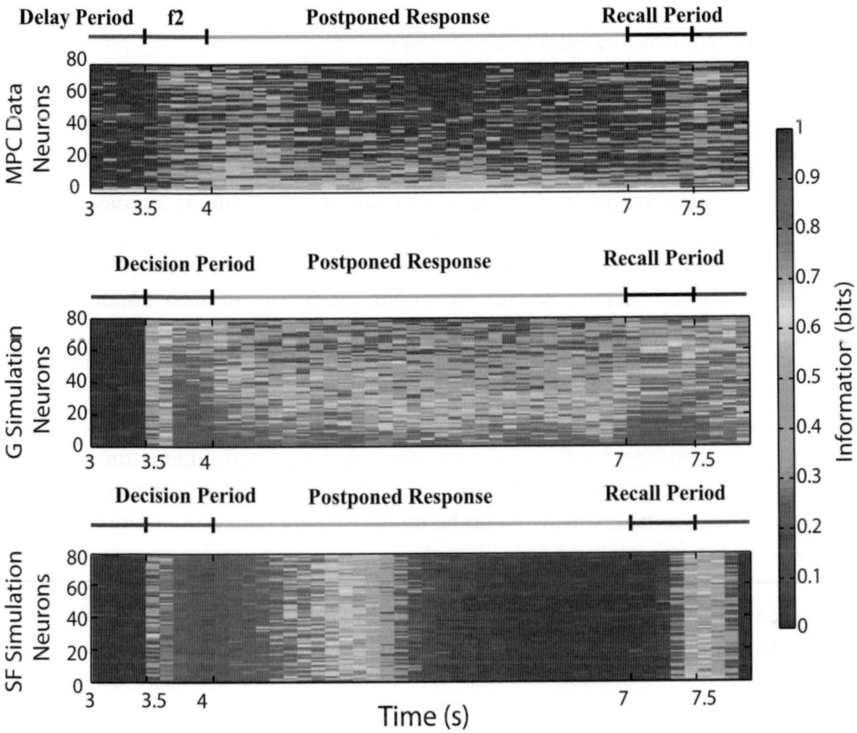

Fig. B.9 Mutual information analyses as a function of time. (Top) Eighty neurons from the medial premotor cortex. Each row corresponds to a different neuron. In the experiment the f_2 stimuli have been applied from 3.5–4.0 s. The postponed response delay period is 4.0–7.0 s. The behavioural response can be started with a response signal given at 7.0 s. The mutual information shown was calculated between firing rate windows of 200 ms (sliding every 100 ms) and the response made by the monkey. (Middle) Eighty neurons from decision pool 1 of the graded firing rate simulation. Each row is a single neuron. The rows are sorted by the amount of information during the decision period, 3.5–4.0 s, which corresponds to the f_2 period for the medial premotor cortex neurons. The postponed response period is 4–7 s. The non-selective external input is applied at t = 7.0–7.5 s, labelled recall period. The mutual information of the simulated firing rates was calculated between the firing rate in a 200 ms sliding window and the firing in the decision period. (Bottom) Synaptic Facilitation simulation (conventions as in Middle). (See colour plates section.) (Reproduced from Martinez-Garcia, M., Rolls, E. T., Deco, G. and Romo, R., Neural and computational mechanisms of postponed decisions, *Proceedings of the National Academy of Sciences* 108 (28), pp. 11626–11631, figure 2 ©2011, National Academy of Sciences.)

Rolls, Deco & Romo 2011). After this 'decision period' the information then decays in a 3 s delay period in which the decision is postponed and the neuronal activity declines before the behavioural response can be made. The information then increases again when the behavioural response is required in the 'recall period' (top panel Fig. B.9).

We were able to model the observed neuronal activity using an attractor decision-making network in which information reflecting the decision is maintained at a low level during the postponed response delay period, and is then selectively restored by a non-specific input when the response is required (Martinez-Garcia, Rolls, Deco & Romo 2011).

One mechanism for the short-term memory is synaptic facilitation which can implement a mechanism for postponed decisions that can be correct even when there is little neuronal firing during the delay period before the postponed decision, as illustrated in Fig. B.9 (bottom panel).

A second mechanism to model the experimental data is graded firing rates by different neurons in the delay period (Fig. B.9, middle panel). Importantly, also in this scenario, the information about the decision can be restored by the application of the non-specific input during the recall period. This is because the higher firing rate neurons of the 'winner' population continue firing during the postponed response period, and help to activate the whole population and thus retrieve the decision information when the non-specific input is applied.

To conclude, either mechanism, synaptic facilitation or graded firing rates, can account for the experimentally observed activity of medial premotor cortex neurons and the time course of the information about the decision during the decision-making and delay period before the response is made (Martinez-Garcia, Rolls, Deco & Romo 2011), though the graded firing rate model does seem closer to the actual neurophysiological data in that some of the neurons do maintain some firing in the delay period in the real neurophysiological data (Fig. B.9 top panel). The two mechanisms have in common the property that a non-specific input can restore the firing specifically in the correct attractor population of neurons. The relative contribution of the two mechanisms could be tested experimentally by increasing the delay between the decision formation and recall, as the synaptic memory decays away within a few seconds, and this would predict that delays of more than a few seconds without much firing before the delayed response could occur would not be possible.

B.4 The integrate-and-fire formulation used in the model of decision-making

Deco & Rolls (2006) used the mathematical formulation of integrate-and-fire (IF) neurons and synaptic currents described by Brunel & Wang (2001), but extended for example to multiple interacting networks, and typically run with the spontaneous state as a stable state even when the decision cues are applied (see Section B.1.3.1). A brief summary of the framework follows as used in many of our investigations of decision-making, short-term memory, attention, and dynamical neuropsychiatry (Deco & Rolls 2003, Deco, Rolls & Horwitz 2004, Deco & Rolls 2005a, Deco & Rolls 2005d, Deco & Rolls 2005c, Rolls & Deco 2006, Loh, Rolls & Deco 2007a, Loh, Rolls & Deco 2007b, Rolls, Loh, Deco & Winterer 2008d, Rolls, Loh & Deco 2008c, Rolls, Grabenhorst & Deco 2010b, Rolls, Grabenhorst & Deco 2010c, Insabato, Pannunzi, Rolls & Deco 2010, Deco, Rolls & Romo 2010, Smerieri, Rolls & Feng 2010, Rolls & Deco 2011a, Rolls & Deco 2011b, Webb, Rolls, Deco & Feng 2011, Martinez-Garcia, Rolls, Deco & Romo 2011, Rolls 2012b, Rolls & Webb 2012, Rolls, Webb & Deco 2012, Deco, Rolls, Albantakis & Romo 2013, Rolls, Dempere-Marco & Deco 2013).

The dynamics of the sub-threshold membrane potential V of a neuron are given by the equation:

$$C_{\rm m}\frac{dV(t)}{dt} = -g_{\rm m}(V(t) - V_{\rm L}) - I_{\rm syn}(t), \tag{B.20}$$

where $C_{\rm m}$ is the membrane capacitance taken to be 0.5 nF for excitatory neurons and 0.2 nF for inhibitory neurons; $g_{\rm m}$ is the membrane leak conductance taken to be 25 nS for excitatory neurons and 20 nS for inhibitory neurons; $V_{\rm L}$ is the resting potential of –70 mV, and $I_{\rm syn}$ is the synaptic current. The firing threshold is taken to be $V_{\rm thr} = -50$ mV, and the reset potential $V_{\rm reset} = -55$ mV (see McCormick, Connors, Lighthall & Prince (1985)).

The synaptic current is given by a sum of glutamatergic, AMPA ($I_{\rm AMPA,rec}$) and NMDA ($I_{\rm NMDA,rec}$) mediated, currents from the excitatory recurrent collateral connection, one AMPA

($I_{\text{AMPA,ext}}$) mediated external excitatory current, and one inhibitory GABAergic current (I_{GABA}):

$$I_{\text{syn}}(t) = I_{\text{AMPA,ext}}(t) + I_{\text{AMPA,rec}}(t) + I_{\text{NMDA,rec}}(t) + I_{\text{GABA}}(t). \tag{B.21}$$

The synaptic currents are defined by:

$$I_{\text{AMPA,ext}}(t) = g_{\text{AMPA,ext}}(V(t) - V_{\text{E}}) \sum_{j=1}^{N_{\text{ext}}} s_j^{\text{AMPA,ext}}(t) \tag{B.22}$$

$$I_{\text{AMPA,rec}}(t) = g_{\text{AMPA,rec}}(V(t) - V_{\text{E}}) \sum_{j=1}^{N_{\text{E}}} w_j s_j^{\text{AMPA,rec}}(t) \tag{B.23}$$

$$I_{\text{NMDA,rec}}(t) = \frac{g_{\text{NMDA}}(V(t) - V_{\text{E}})}{1 + [\text{Mg}^{++}] \exp(-0.062V(t))/3.57} \times \sum_{j=1}^{N_{\text{E}}} w_j s_j^{\text{NMDA}}(t) \tag{B.24}$$

$$I_{\text{GABA}}(t) = g_{\text{GABA}}(V(t) - V_{\text{I}}) \sum_{j=1}^{N_{\text{I}}} s_j^{\text{GABA}}(t) \tag{B.25}$$

where $V_{\text{E}} = 0$ mV, $V_{\text{I}} = -70$ mV, w_j are the synaptic weights, each receptor has its own fraction s_j of open channels, and its own synaptic conductance g. The NMDA synaptic current is dependent on the potential and controlled by the extracellular concentration of magnesium ($[\text{Mg}^{++}] = 1$ mM) (Jahr & Stevens 1990). The values for the synaptic conductances for excitatory neurons are $g_{\text{AMPA,ext}} = 2.08$ nS, $g_{\text{AMPA,rec}} = 0.104$ nS, $g_{\text{NMDA}} = 0.327$ nS and $g_{\text{GABA}} = 1.287$ nS; and for inhibitory neurons $g_{\text{AMPA,ext}} = 1.62$ nS, $g_{\text{AMPA,rec}} = 0.081$ nS, $g_{\text{NMDA}} = 0.258$ nS and $g_{\text{GABA}} = 1.002$ nS. These values are obtained from the ones used by Brunel & Wang (2001) by multiplication by a factor which corrects for the difference in the number of neurons used in our model and Brunel and Wang's model. In their work the conductances were calculated so that in an unstructured network the excitatory neurons have a spontaneous spiking rate of 3 Hz and the inhibitory neurons a spontaneous rate of 9 Hz.

The fractions of open channels are described by:

$$\frac{ds_j^{\text{AMPA,ext}}(t)}{dt} = -\frac{s_j^{\text{AMPA,ext}}(t)}{\tau_{\text{AMPA}}} + \sum_k \delta(t - t_j^k) \tag{B.26}$$

$$\frac{ds_j^{\text{AMPA,rec}}(t)}{dt} = -\frac{s_j^{\text{AMPA,rec}}(t)}{\tau_{\text{AMPA}}} + \sum_k \delta(t - t_j^k) \tag{B.27}$$

$$\frac{ds_j^{\text{NMDA}}(t)}{dt} = -\frac{s_j^{\text{NMDA}}(t)}{\tau_{\text{NMDA,decay}}} + \alpha x_j(t)(1 - s_j^{\text{NMDA}}(t)) \tag{B.28}$$

$$\frac{dx_j(t)}{dt} = -\frac{x_j(t)}{\tau_{\text{NMDA,rise}}} + \sum_k \delta(t - t_j^k) \tag{B.29}$$

$$\frac{ds_j^{\text{GABA}}(t)}{dt} = -\frac{s_j^{\text{GABA}}(t)}{\tau_{\text{GABA}}} + \sum_k \delta(t - t_j^k), \tag{B.30}$$

where the rise time constant for NMDA synapses is $\tau_{\text{NMDA,rise}} = 2$ ms (Spruston, Jonas & Sakmann 1995, Hestrin, Sah & Nicoll 1990), the rise time constants for AMPA and GABA are neglected because they are smaller than 1 ms, and $\alpha = 0.5$ ms^{-1}. All synapses have a delay of 0.5 ms. The decay time constant for the AMPA synapses is $\tau_{\text{AMPA}} = 2$ ms

(Spruston et al. 1995, Hestrin et al. 1990), for NMDA synapses is $\tau_{\text{NMDA,decay}} = 100$ ms (Spruston et al. 1995, Hestrin et al. 1990), and for GABA synapses $\tau_{\text{GABA}} = 10$ ms (Salin & Prince 1996, Xiang, Huguenard & Prince 1998). The sums over k represent a sum over spikes formulated as δ-peaks ($\delta(t)$) emitted by presynaptic neuron j at time t_j^k.

B.5 The mean-field approach used in the model of decision-making

The mean-field approximation used by Deco & Rolls (2006) and in their other papers referred to in Section B.4 was derived by Brunel & Wang (2001), assuming that the network of integrate-and-fire neurons is in a stationary state. In this formulation the potential of a neuron is calculated as:

$$\tau_x \frac{dV(t)}{dt} = -V(t) + \mu_x + \sigma_x \sqrt{\tau_x}\eta(t) \tag{B.31}$$

where $V(t)$ is the membrane potential, x labels the populations, τ_x is the effective membrane time constant, μ_x is the mean value the membrane potential would have in the absence of spiking and fluctuations, σ_x measures the magnitude of the fluctuations, and η is a Gaussian process with absolute exponentially decaying correlation function with time constant τ_{AMPA}. The quantities μ_x and σ_x^2 are given by:

$$\mu_x = \frac{(T_{\text{ext}}\nu_{\text{ext}} + T_{\text{AMPA}} n_x^{\text{AMPA}} + \rho_1 n_x^{\text{NMDA}})V_{\text{E}} + \rho_2 n_x^{\text{NMDA}} \langle V \rangle + T_{\text{I}} n_x^{\text{GABA}} V_{\text{I}} + V_{\text{L}}}{S_x} \tag{B.32}$$

$$\sigma_x^2 = \frac{g_{\text{AMPA,ext}}^2 (\langle V \rangle - V_{\text{E}})^2 N_{\text{ext}} \nu_{\text{ext}} \tau_{\text{AMPA}}^2 \tau_x}{g_{\text{m}}^2 \tau_{\text{m}}^2}. \tag{B.33}$$

where ν_{ext} Hz is the external incoming spiking rate, ν_{I} is the spiking rate of the inhibitory population, $\tau_{\text{m}} = C_{\text{m}}/g_{\text{m}}$ with the values for the excitatory or inhibitory neurons depending on the population considered, and the other quantities are given by:

$$S_x = 1 + T_{\text{ext}}\nu_{\text{ext}} + T_{\text{AMPA}} n_x^{\text{AMPA}} + (\rho_1 + \rho_2) n_x^{\text{NMDA}} + T_{\text{I}} n_x^{\text{GABA}} \tag{B.34}$$

$$\tau_x = \frac{C_{\text{m}}}{g_{\text{m}} S_x} \tag{B.35}$$

$$n_x^{\text{AMPA}} = \sum_{j=1}^{p} r_j w_{jx}^{\text{AMPA}} \nu_j \tag{B.36}$$

$$n_x^{\text{NMDA}} = \sum_{j=1}^{p} r_j w_{jx}^{\text{NMDA}} \psi(\nu_j) \tag{B.37}$$

$$n_x^{\text{GABA}} = \sum_{j=1}^{p} r_j w_{jx}^{\text{GABA}} \nu_j \tag{B.38}$$

$$\psi(\nu) = \frac{\nu\tau_{\text{NMDA}}}{1 + \nu\tau_{\text{NMDA}}} \left(1 + \frac{1}{1 + \nu\tau_{\text{NMDA}}} \sum_{n=1}^{\infty} \frac{(-\alpha\tau_{\text{NMDA,rise}})^n T_n(\nu)}{(n+1)!} \right) \tag{B.39}$$

$$T_n(\nu) = \sum_{k=0}^{n} (-1)^k \binom{n}{k} \frac{\tau_{\text{NMDA,rise}}(1 + \nu\tau_{\text{NMDA}})}{\tau_{\text{NMDA,rise}}(1 + \nu\tau_{\text{NMDA}}) + k\tau_{\text{NMDA,decay}}} \tag{B.40}$$

$$\tau_{\text{NMDA}} = \alpha\tau_{\text{NMDA,rise}}\tau_{\text{NMDA,decay}} \tag{B.41}$$

$$T_{\text{ext}} = \frac{g_{\text{AMPA,ext}}\tau_{\text{AMPA}}}{g_{\text{m}}} \tag{B.42}$$

$$T_{\text{AMPA}} = \frac{g_{\text{AMPA,rec}} N_{\text{E}} \tau_{\text{AMPA}}}{g_{\text{m}}} \tag{B.43}$$

$$\rho_1 = \frac{g_{\text{NMDA}} N_{\text{E}}}{g_{\text{m}} J} \tag{B.44}$$

$$\rho_2 = \beta \frac{g_{\text{NMDA}} N_{\text{E}}(\langle V_x \rangle - V_{\text{E}})(J - 1)}{g_{\text{m}} J^2} \tag{B.45}$$

$$J = 1 + \gamma \exp(-\beta \langle V_x \rangle) \tag{B.46}$$

$$T_{\text{I}} = \frac{g_{\text{GABA}} N_{\text{I}} \tau_{\text{GABA}}}{g_{\text{m}}} \tag{B.47}$$

$$\langle V_x \rangle = \mu_x - (V_{\text{thr}} - V_{\text{reset}})\nu_x \tau_x, \tag{B.48}$$

where p is the number of excitatory populations, r_x is the fraction of neurons in the excitatory x population, $w_{j,x}$ the weight of the connections from population x to population j, ν_x is the spiking rate of the x excitatory population, $\gamma = [\text{Mg}^{++}]/3.57$, $\beta = 0.062$ and the average membrane potential $\langle V_x \rangle$ has a value between -55 mV and -50 mV.

The spiking rate of a population as a function of the defined quantities is then given by:

$$\nu_x = \phi(\mu_x, \sigma_x), \tag{B.49}$$

where

$$\phi(\mu_x, \sigma_x) = \left(\tau_{\text{rp}} + \tau_x \int_{\beta(\mu_x,\sigma_x)}^{\alpha(\mu_x,\sigma_x)} du \sqrt{\pi} \exp(u^2)[1 + \text{erf}(u)] \right)^{-1} \tag{B.50}$$

$$\alpha(\mu_x, \sigma_x) = \frac{(V_{\text{thr}} - \mu_x)}{\sigma_x} \left(1 + 0.5 \frac{\tau_{\text{AMPA}}}{\tau_x} \right) + 1.03 \sqrt{\frac{\tau_{\text{AMPA}}}{\tau_x}} - 0.5 \frac{\tau_{\text{AMPA}}}{\tau_x} \tag{B.51}$$

$$\beta(\mu_x, \sigma_x) = \frac{(V_{\text{reset}} - \mu_x)}{\sigma_x} \tag{B.52}$$

with erf(u) the error function and τ_{rp} the refractory period which is considered to be 2 ms for excitatory neurons and 1 ms for inhibitory neurons. To solve the equations defined by (B.49) for all xs we integrate numerically (B.48) and the differential equation below, which has fixed point solutions corresponding to Equation B.49:

$$\tau_x \frac{d\nu_x}{dt} = -\nu_x + \phi(\mu_x, \sigma_x). \tag{B.53}$$

B.6 The model parameters used in the simulations of decision-making

The fixed parameters of the model are shown in Table B.1, and not only provide information about the values of the parameters used in the simulations, but also enable them to be compared to experimentally measured values.

Table B.1 Parameters used in the integrate-and-fire simulations

N_{E}	800
N_{I}	200
r	0.1
w_+	2.2
w_{I}	1.015
N_{ext}	800
ν_{ext}	2.4 kHz
C_{m} (excitatory)	0.5 nF
C_{m} (inhibitory)	0.2 nF
g_{m} (excitatory)	25 nS
g_{m} (inhibitory)	20 nS
V_{L}	–70 mV
V_{thr}	–50 mV
V_{reset}	–55 mV
V_{E}	0 mV
V_{I}	–70 mV
$g_{\mathrm{AMPA,ext}}$ (excitatory)	2.08 nS
$g_{\mathrm{AMPA,rec}}$ (excitatory)	0.104 nS
g_{NMDA} (excitatory)	0.327 nS
g_{GABA} (excitatory)	1.25 nS
$g_{\mathrm{AMPA,ext}}$ (inhibitory)	1.62 nS
$g_{\mathrm{AMPA,rec}}$ (inhibitory)	0.081 nS
g_{NMDA} (inhibitory)	0.258 nS
g_{GABA} (inhibitory)	0.973 nS
$\tau_{\mathrm{NMDA,decay}}$	100 ms
$\tau_{\mathrm{NMDA,rise}}$	2 ms
τ_{AMPA}	2 ms
τ_{GABA}	10 ms
α	0.5 ms^{-1}

Appendix 3 Glossary

Instrumental reinforcers are stimuli that, if their occurrence, termination, or omission is made contingent upon the making of an action, alter the probability of the future emission of that action (Gray 1975, Mackintosh 1983, Dickinson 1980, Lieberman 2000, Mazur 2012). Rewards and punishers are instrumental reinforcing stimuli. The notion of an action here is that an arbitrary action, e.g. turning right vs turning left, will be performed in order to obtain the reward or avoid the punisher, so that there is no pre-wired connection between the response and the reinforcer. Some stimuli are **primary (unlearned) reinforcers** (e.g., the taste of food if the animal is hungry, or pain); while others may become reinforcing by learning, because of their association with such primary reinforcers, thereby becoming '**secondary reinforcers**'. This type of learning may thus be called '**stimulus–reinforcer association learning**', and occurs via a stimulus–stimulus associative learning process.

A **positive reinforcer** (such as food) increases the probability of emission of an action on which it is contingent, the process is termed **positive reinforcement**, and the outcome is a **reward** (such as food).

A **negative reinforcer** (such as a painful stimulus) increases the probability of emission of an actione that causes the negative reinforcer to be omitted (as in **active avoidance**) or terminated (as in **escape**), and the procedure is termed **negative reinforcement**.

Punishment refers to procedures in which the probability of an action is decreased. Punishment thus describes procedures in which an action decreases in probability if it is followed by a painful stimulus, as in **passive avoidance**. Punishment can also be used to refer to a procedure involving the omission or termination of a reward ('**extinction**' and '**time out**' respectively), both of which decrease the probability of responses (Gray 1975, Mackintosh 1983, Dickinson 1980, Lieberman 2000, Mazur 2012).

A **punisher** when delivered acts instrumentally to decrease the probability of actions on which it is contingent, or when not delivered (escaped from or avoided) acts as a negative reinforcer in that it then increases the probability of the action on which its non-delivery is contingent. Note that my definition of a punisher, which is similar to that of an aversive stimulus, is of a stimulus or event that can either decrease the probability of actions on which it is contingent, or increase the probability of actions on which its non-delivery is contingent. The term **punishment** is restricted to situations where the probability of an action is being decreased.

Emotions are states elicited by instrumental reinforcers, where the states have the set of functions described in Chapter 3. My argument is that an affectively positive or 'appetitive' stimulus (which produces a state of pleasure) acts operationally as a **reward**, which when delivered acts instrumentally as a positive reinforcer, or when not delivered (omitted or terminated) acts to decrease the probability of responses on which it is contingent. Conversely

I argue that an affectively negative or aversive stimulus (which produces an unpleasant state) acts operationally as a **punisher**, which when delivered acts instrumentally to decrease the probability of actions on which it is contingent, or when not delivered (escaped from or avoided) acts as a negative reinforcer in that it then increases the probability of the action on which its non-delivery is contingent[49].

Classical conditioning or **Pavlovian conditioning**. When a **conditioned stimulus (CS)** (such as a tone) is paired with a primary reinforcer or **unconditioned stimulus (US)** (such as a painful stimulus), then there are opportunities for a number of types of association to be formed. Some of these involve 'classical conditioning' or 'Pavlovian conditioning', in which no action is performed that affects the contingency between the conditioned stimulus and the unconditioned stimulus. Typically an **unconditioned response (UR)**, for example an alteration of heart rate, is produced by the US, and will come to be elicited by the CS as a **conditioned response (CR)**. These responses are typically autonomic (such as the heart beating faster), or endocrine (for example the release of adrenaline (epinephrine in American usage) by the adrenal gland). In addition, the organism may learn to perform an instrumental response with the skeletal muscles in order to alter the probability that the primary reinforcer will be obtained. In our example, the experimenter might alter the contingencies so that when the tone sounded, if the organism performed a response such as pressing a lever, then the painful stimulus could be avoided. In the instrumental learning situation there are still opportunities for many classically conditioned responses, including emotional states such as fear, to occur. The associative processes involved in classical conditioning, and the influences that these processes may have on instrumental performance, are described in Section 4.6.1.

Motivated behaviour occurs when an animal will perform an instrumental (i.e. arbitrary operant) response to obtain a reward or to escape from or avoid a punisher. If this criterion of an arbitrary operant response is not met, and only a fixed response can be performed, then the term **drive** can be used to describe the state of the animal when it will work to obtain or escape from the stimulus.

Fitness is the reproductive potential of genes. Through the process of natural selection and reproduction, fit genes are selected for the next generation.

Long-term potentiation (LTP) is the increase in synaptic strength that can occur during learning. It is typically associative, depending on conjunctive presynaptic activity and postsynaptic depolarization.

Long-term depression (LTP) is the decrease in synaptic strength that can occur during learning. It is typically associative, occurring when the presynaptic activity is low and the postsynaptic depolarization is high (heterosynaptic long-term depression), or when the presynaptic activity is high, and the postsynaptic activity is only moderate (homosynaptic long-term depression) (see Fig. A.5).

[49]Note that my definition of a punisher, which is similar to that of an aversive stimulus, is of a stimulus or event that can either decrease the probability of actions on which it is contingent, or increase the probability of actions on which its non-delivery is contingent. The term punishment is restricted to situations where the probability of an action is being decreased.

References

Abbott LF & Blum KI (1996). Functional significance of long-term potentiation for sequence learning and prediction. *Cerebral Cortex* 6: 406–416.

Abbott LF & Nelson SB (2000). Synaptic plasticity: taming the beast. *Nature Neuroscience* 3: 1178–1183.

Abbott LF, Rolls ET, & Tovee MJ (1996). Representational capacity of face coding in monkeys. *Cerebral Cortex* 6: 498–505.

Abbott LF, Varela JA, Sen K, & Nelson SB (1997). Synaptic depression and cortical gain control. *Science* 275: 220–224.

Abeles M (1991). *Corticonics: Neural Circuits of the Cerebral Cortex*. Cambridge University Press, Cambridge.

Abercrombie ED, Keefe KA, DiFrischia DS, & Zigmond MJ (1989). Differential effect of stress on in vivo dopamine release in striatum, nucleus accumbens, and medial frontal cortex. *Journal of Neurochemistry* 52: 1655–1658.

Ackley DH (1987). *A Connectionist Machine for Genetic Hill-Climbing*. Kluwer Academic Publishers, Dordrecht.

Adams CD (1982). Variations in the sensitivity of instrumental responding to reinforcer devaluation. *Quarterly Journal of Experimental Psychology B* 34: 77–98.

Adams CD & Dickinson A (1981). Instrumental responding following reinforcer devaluation. *Quarterly Journal of Experimental Psychology B* 33: 109–121.

Adams JE (1976). Naloxone reversal of analgesia produced by brain stimulation in the human. *Pain* 2: 161–166.

Adelmann PK & Zajonc RB (1989). Facial efference and the experience of emotion. *Annual Review of Psychology* 40: 249–280.

Adolphs R (2003). Cognitive neuroscience of human social behavior. *Nature Reviews Neuroscience* 4: 165–178.

Adolphs R, Tranel D, Damasio H, & Damasio AR (1994). Impaired recognition of emotion in facial expressions following bilateral damage to the human amygdala. *Nature* 372: 669–672.

Adolphs R, Tranel D, Damasio H, & Damasio AR (1995). Fear and the human amygdala. *Journal of Neuroscience* 15: 5879–5891.

Adolphs R, Tranel D, Hamann S, Young AW, Calder AJ, Phelps EA, Anderson A, Lee GP, & Damasio AR (1999). Recognition of facial emotion in nine individuals with bilateral amygdala damage. *Neuropsychologia* 37: 1111–1117.

Adolphs R, Damasio H, Tranel D, Cooper G, & Damasio AR (2000a). A role for somatosensory cortices in the visual recognition of emotion as revealed by three-dimensional lesion mapping. *The Journal of Neuroscience* 20: 2683–2690.

Adolphs R, Tranel D, & Denburg N (2000b). Impaired emotional declarative memory following unilateral amygdala damage. *Learning and Memory* 7: 180–186.

Adolphs R, Tranel D, & Baron-Cohen S (2002). Amygdala damage impairs recognition of social emotions from facial expressions. *Journal of Cognitive Neuroscience* 14: 1–11.

Adolphs R, Gosselin F, Buchanan TW, Tranel D, Schyns P, & Damasio AR (2005). A mechanism for impaired fear recognition after amygdala damage. *Nature* 433: 68–72.

Aggelopoulos NC & Rolls ET (2005). Natural scene perception: inferior temporal cortex neurons encode the positions of different objects in the scene. *European Journal of Neuroscience* 22: 2903–2916.

Aggelopoulos NC, Franco L, & Rolls ET (2005). Object perception in natural scenes: encoding by inferior temporal cortex simultaneously recorded neurons. *Journal of Neurophysiology* 93: 1342–1357.

Aggleton JP (1992). The functional effects of amygdala lesions in humans, a comparison with findings from monkeys. In Aggleton JP, editor, *The Amygdala*, chap. 19, 485–503. Wiley-Liss, New York.

Aggleton JP, editor (2000). *The Amygdala, A Functional Analysis*. Oxford University Press, Oxford, 2nd edn.

Aggleton JP & Passingham RE (1981). Syndrome produced by lesions of the amygdala in monkeys (Macaca mulatta). *Journal of Comparative and Physiological Psychology* 95: 961–977.

Aggleton JP & Passingham RE (1982). An assessment of the reinforcing properties of foods after amygdaloid lesions in rhesus monkeys. *Journal of Comparative and Physiological Psychology* 96: 71–77.

Aggleton JP, Burton MJ, & Passingham RE (1980). Cortical and subcortical afferents to the amygdala in the rhesus monkey (Macaca mulatta). *Brain Research* 190: 347–368.

Aiello LC & Wheeler P (1995). The expensive-tissue hypothesis: the brain and the digestive system in human and primate evolution. *Current Anthropology* 36: 199–221.

Aigner TG, Mitchell SJ, Aggleton JP, DeLong MR, Struble RG, Price DL, Wenk GL, Pettigrew KD, & Mishkin M (1991). Transient impairment of recognition memory following ibotenic acid lesions of the basal forebrain in macaques. *Experimental Brain Research* 86: 18–26.

Ainslie G (1992). *Picoeconomics*. Cambridge University Press, Cambridge.

Akert K, Gruesen RA, Woolsey CN, & Meyer DR (1961). Kluver-Bucy syndrome in monkeys with neocortical ablations of temporal lobe. *Brain* 84: 480–498.

Akil H, Mayer DJ, & Liebeskind JC (1976). Antagonism of stimulation-produced analgesia by naloxone, a narcotic antagonist. *Science* 191: 961–962.

Albantakis L & Deco G (2009). The encoding of alternatives in multiple-choice decision making. *Proceedings of the National Academy of Sciences USA* 106: 10308–10313.

Albantakis L & Deco G (2011). Changes of mind in an attractor model of decision-making. *PLoS Computational Biology* 7: e1002086.

Aleman A & Kahn RS (2005). Strange feelings: do amygdala abnormalities dysregulate the emotional brain in schizophrenia? *Progress in Neurobiology* 77: 283–298.

Alexander GE, Crutcher MD, & DeLong MR (1990). Basal ganglia thalamo-cortical circuits: parallel substrates for motor, oculomotor, 'prefrontal' and 'limbic' functions. *Progress in Brain Research* 85: 119–146.

Alexander RD (1975). The search for a general theory of behavior. *Behavioral Sciences* 20: 77–100.

Alexander RD (1979). *Darwinism and Human Affairs*. University of Washington Press, Seattle.

Allais M (1953). Le comportement do l'homme rational devant le risque. critique des postulats et axiomes de l'ecole americaine. *Econometrica* 21: 503–546.

Allport A (1988). What concept of consciousness? In Marcel AJ & Bisiach E, editors, *Consciousness in Contemporary Science*, 159–182. Oxford University Press, Oxford.

Amaral DG (2003). The amygdala, social behavior, and danger detection. *Annals of the New York Academy of Sciences* 1000: 337–347.

Amaral DG & Price JL (1984). Amygdalo-cortical projections in the monkey (Macaca fascicularis). *Journal of Comparative Neurology* 230: 465–496.

Amaral DG, Price JL, Pitkanen A, & Carmichael ST (1992). Anatomical organization of the primate amygdaloid complex. In Aggleton JP, editor, *The Amygdala*, chap. 1, 1–66. Wiley-Liss, New York.

Amaral DG, Bauman MD, Capitanio JP, Lavenex P, Mason WA, Mauldin-Jourdain ML, & Mendoza SP (2003). The amygdala: is it an essential component of the neural network for social cognition? *Neuropsychologia* 41: 517–522.

Amit DJ (1989). *Modelling Brain Function*. Cambridge University Press, New York.

Amit DJ & Brunel N (1997). Model of global spontaneous activity and local structured activity during delay periods in the cerebral cortex. *Cerebral Cortex* 7: 237–252.

Amit DJ & Tsodyks MV (1991). Quantitative study of attractor neural network retrieving at low spike rates. I. Substrate – spikes, rates and neuronal gain. *Network* 2: 259–273.

Amit DJ, Gutfreund H, & Sompolinsky H (1987). Statistical mechanics of neural networks near saturation. *Annals of Physics (New York)* 173: 30–67.

Amsel A (1958). The role of frustrative non-reward in non-continuous reward situations. *Psychological Bulletin* 55: 102–119.

Amsel A (1962). Frustrative non-reward in partial reinforcement and discrimination learning: some recent history and a theoretical extension. *Psychological Review* 69: 306–328.

Anand BK & Brobeck JR (1951). Localization of a feeding center in the hypothalamus of the rat. *Proceedings of the Society for Experimental Biology and Medicine* 77: 323–324.

Anderson AK & Phelps EA (2001). Lesions of the human amygdala impair enhanced perception of emotionally salient events. *Nature* 17: 305–309.

Anderson AK, Christoff K, Stappen I, Panitz D, Ghahremani DG, Glover G, Gabrieli JD, & Sobel N (2003). Dissociated neural representations of intensity and valence in human olfaction. *Nature Neuroscience* 6: 196–202.

Anderson JR (1996). ACT: a simple theory of complex cognition. *American Psychologist* 51: 355–365.

Anderson ME (1978). Discharge patterns of basal ganglia neurons during active maintenance of postural stability and adjustment to chair tilt. *Brain Research* 143: 325–338.

Anderson SW, Bechara A, Damasio H, Tranel D, & Damasio AR (1999). Impairment of social and moral behaviour related to early damage in human prefrontal cortex. *Nature Neuroscience* 2: 1032–1037.

Andrew RJ (1963). Evolution of facial expression. *Science* 142: 1034–1041.

Angeletos GM, Laibson D, Repetto A, Tobacman J, & Weinberg S (2001). The hyperbolic buffer stock model: calibration, simulation, and empirical evaluation. *Journal of Economic Perspectives* 15: 47–68.

Aou S, Oomura Y, Lenard L, Nishino H, Inokuchi A, Minami T, & Misaki H (1984). Behavioral significance of monkey hypothalamic glucose-sensitive neurons. *Brain Research* 302: 69–74.

Apanius V, Penn D, Slev PR, Ruff LR, & Potts WK (1997). The nature of selection on the major histocompatibility complex. *Critical Reviews in Immunology* 17: 179–224.

Argiolas A & Melis MR (2013). Neuropeptides and central control of sexual behavior from the past to the present: A review. *Progress in Neurobiology* doi: 10.1016/j.pneurobio.2013.06.006.

Armstrong DM & Malcolm M (1984). *Consciousness and Causality*. Blackwell, Oxford.

Arnold PD, Rosenberg DR, Mundo E, Tharmalingam S, Kennedy JL, & Richter MA (2004). Association of a glutamate (NMDA) subunit receptor gene (GRIN2B) with obsessive-compulsive disorder: a preliminary

study. *Psychopharmacology (Berl)* 174: 530–538.
Aron AR, Fletcher PC, Bullmore ET, Sahakian BJ, & Robbins TW (2003). Stop-signal inhibition disrupted by damage to inferior frontal gyrus in humans. *Nature Neuroscience* 6: 115–116.
Artola A & Singer W (1993). Long term depression: related mechanisms in cerebellum, neocortex and hippocampus. In Baudry M, Thompson RF, & Davis JL, editors, *Synaptic Plasticity: Molecular, Cellular and Functional Aspects*, chap. 7, 129–146. MIT Press, Cambridge, MA.
Asaad WF, Rainer G, & Miller EK (1998). Neural activity in the primate prefrontal cortex during associative learning. *Neuron* 21: 1399–1407.
Asaad WF, Rainer G, & Miller EK (2000). Task-specific neural activity in the primate prefrontal cortex. *Journal of Neurophysiology* 84: 451–459.
Avena NM & Hoebel BG (2003a). Amphetamine-sensitised rats show sugar-induced hyperactivity (cross-sensitization) and sugar hyperphagia. *Pharmacology, Biochemistry and Behaviour* 74: 635–639.
Avena NM & Hoebel BG (2003b). A diet promoting sugar dependency causes behavioural cross-sensitisation to a low dose of amphetamine. *Neuroscience* 122: 17–20.
Baars BJ (1988). *A Cognitive Theory of Consciousness*. Cambridge University Press, New York.
Baddeley A (1986). *Working Memory*. Oxford University Press, New York.
Baddeley RJ, Abbott LF, Booth MJA, Sengpiel F, Freeman T, Wakeman EA, & Rolls ET (1997). Responses of neurons in primary and inferior temporal visual cortices to natural scenes. *Proceedings of the Royal Society B* 264: 1775–1783.
Baker RR (1996). *Sperm Wars*. Fourth Estate, London.
Baker RR & Bellis MA (1993). Human sperm competition: ejaculate manipulation by females and a function for the female orgasm. *Animal Behaviour* 46: 887–909.
Baker RR & Bellis MA (1995). *Human Sperm Competition: Copulation, Competition and Infidelity*. Chapman and Hall, London.
Baldo JV, Shimamura AP, Delis DC, Kramer J, & Kaplan E (2001). Verbal and design fluency in patients with frontal lobe lesions. *Journal of the International Neuropsychological Society* 7: 586–596.
Balleine BW (1992). Instrumental performance following a shift in primary motivation depends upon incentive learning. *Journal of Experimental Psychology* 18: 236–250.
Balleine BW (1994). Asymmetrical interactions between thirst and hunger in Pavlovian–instrumental transfer. *Quarterly Journal of Experimental Psychology B* 47: 211–231.
Balleine BW & Dickinson A (1991). Instrumental performance following reinforcer devaluation depends upon incentive learning. *Quarterly Journal of Experimental Psychology B* 43: 279–296.
Balleine BW & Dickinson A (1998). The role of incentive learning in instrumental outcome revaluation by sensory-specific satiety. *Animal Learning and Behavior* 26: 46–59.
Balleine BW & O'Doherty JP (2010). Human and rodent homologies in action control: corticostriatal determinants of goal-directed and habitual action. *Neuropsychopharmacology* 35: 48–69.
Balleine BW, Liljeholm M, & Ostlund SB (2009). The integrative function of the basal ganglia in instrumental conditioning. *Behavioral Brain Research* 199: 43–52.
Bar-On R (1997). *The Emotional Intelligence Inventory (EQ-i): Technical Manual*. MultiHealth Systems, Toronto.
Barbas H (1988). Anatomic organization of basoventral and mediodorsal visual recipient prefrontal regions in the rhesus monkey. *Journal of Comparative Neurology* 276: 313–342.
Barbas H (1993). Organization of cortical afferent input to the orbitofrontal area in the rhesus monkey. *Neuroscience* 56: 841–864.
Barbas H (1995). Anatomic basis of cognitive–emotional interactions in the primate prefrontal cortex. *Neuroscience and Biobehavioral Reviews* 19: 499–510.
Barbas H (2007). Specialized elements of orbitofrontal cortex in primates. *Annals of the New York Academy of Sciences* 1121: 10–32.
Barbas H & Pandya DN (1989). Architecture and intrinsic connections of the prefrontal cortex in the rhesus monkey. *Journal of Comparative Neurology* 286: 353–375.
Barbas H, Zikopoulos B, & Timbie C (2011). Sensory pathways and emotional context for action in primate prefrontal cortex. *Biological Psychiatry* 69: 1133–1139.
Barlow H (1995). The neuron doctrine in perception. In Gazzaniga MS, editor, *The Cognitive Neurosciences*, chap. 26, 415–435. MIT Press, Cambridge, MA.
Barlow H (1997). Single neurons, communal goals, and consciousness. In Ito M, Miyashita Y, & Rolls ET, editors, *Cognition, Computation, and Consciousness*, chap. 7, 121–136. Oxford University Press, Oxford.
Barlow HB (1972). Single units and sensation: a neuron doctrine for perceptual psychology. *Perception* 1: 371–394.
Baron-Cohen S, Wheelwright S, & Joliffe T (1997). Is there a 'language of the eyes'? Evidence from normal adults, and adults with autism or Asperger syndrome. *Visual Cognition* 4: 311–331.
Baron-Cohen S, Ring HA, Bullmore ET, Wheelwright S, Ashwin C, & Williams SCR (2000). The amygdala theory of autism. *Neuroscience and Biobehavioral Reviews* 24: 355–364.
Barrett L, Dunbar R, & Lycett J (2002). *Human Evolutionary Psychology*. Palgrave, Basingstoke.
Barsh GS & Schwartz MW (2002). Genetic approaches to studying energy balence: perception and integration.

Nature Reviews Genetics 3: 589–600.
Barsh GS, Farooqi IS, & O'Rahilly S (2000). Genetics of body weight regulation. *Nature* 404: 644–651.
Barson JR, Karatayev O, Chang GQ, Johnson DF, Bocarsly ME, Hoebel BG, & Leibowitz SF (2009). Positive relationship between dietary fat, ethanol intake, triglycerides, and hypothalamic peptides: counteraction by lipid-lowering drugs. *Alcohol* 43: 433–441.
Barto AG (1985). Learning by statistical cooperation of self-interested neuron-like computing elements. *Human Neurobiology* 4: 229–256.
Barto AG (1995). Adaptive critics and the basal ganglia. In Houk JC, Davis JL, & Beiser DG, editors, *Models of Information Processing in the Basal Ganglia*, chap. 11, 215–232. MIT Press, Cambridge, MA.
Barton RA & Aggleton JP (2000). Primate evolution and the amygdala. In Aggleton JP, editor, *The Amygdala: A Functional Analysis*, 479–508. Oxford University Press, Oxford, 2nd edn.
Basbaum AI & Jessell TM (2013). Pain. In Kandel E, Schwartz JH, Jessell TM, Siegelbaum SA, & Hudspeth AJ, editors, *Principles of Neural Science*, chap. 24, 530–576. McGraw-Hill, New York, 5th edn.
Bateson P (1983). *Mate Choice*. Cambridge University Press, Cambridge.
Battaglia F & Treves A (1998). Stable and rapid recurrent processing in realistic autoassociative memories. *Neural Computation* 10: 431–450.
Baum MJ, Everitt BJ, Herbert J, & Keverne EB (1977). Hormonal basis of proceptivity and receptivity in female primates. *Archives of Sexual Behavior* 6: 173–192.
Bauman MD, Lavenex P, Mason WA, Capitanio JP, & Amaral DG (2004). The development of social behaviour following neonatal amygdala lesions in rhesus monkeys. *Journal of Cognitive Neuroscience* 16: 1388–1411.
Baxter MG & Murray EA (2000). Reinterpreting the behavioural effects of amygdala lesions in non-human primates. In Aggleton JP, editor, *The Amygdala: A Functional Analysis*, chap. 16, 545–568. Oxford University Press, Oxford, 2nd edn.
Baxter MG & Murray EA (2002). The amygdala and reward. *Nature Reviews Neuroscience* 3: 563–573.
Baxter RD & Liddle PF (1998). Neuropsychological deficits associated with schizophrenic syndromes. *Schizophrenia Research* 30: 239–249.
Baylis GC & Rolls ET (1987). Responses of neurons in the inferior temporal cortex in short term and serial recognition memory tasks. *Experimental Brain Research* 65: 614–622.
Baylis GC, Rolls ET, & Leonard CM (1985). Selectivity between faces in the responses of a population of neurons in the cortex in the superior temporal sulcus of the monkey. *Brain Research* 342: 91–102.
Baylis GC, Rolls ET, & Leonard CM (1987). Functional subdivisions of temporal lobe neocortex. *Journal of Neuroscience* 7: 330–342.
Baylis LL & Gaffan D (1991). Amygdalectomy and ventromedial prefrontal ablation produce similar deficits in food choice and in simple object discrimination learning for an unseen reward. *Experimental Brain Research* 86: 617–622.
Baylis LL & Rolls ET (1991). Responses of neurons in the primate taste cortex to glutamate. *Physiology and Behavior* 49: 973–979.
Baylis LL, Rolls ET, & Baylis GC (1994). Afferent connections of the orbitofrontal cortex taste area of the primate. *Neuroscience* 64: 801–812.
Bear MF & Singer W (1986). Modulation of visual cortical plasticity by acetylcholine and noradrenaline. *Nature* 320: 172–176.
Beauchamp GK & Yamazaki K (2003). Chemical signalling in mice. *Biochemical Society Transactions* 31: 147–151.
Beaver JD, Lawrence AD, Ditzhuijzen Jv, Davis MH, Woods A, & Calder AJ (2006). Individual differences in reward drive predict neural responses to images of food. *Journal of Neuroscience* 26: 5160–5166.
Bechara A, Damasio AR, Damasio H, & Anderson SW (1994). Insensitivity to future consequences following damage to human prefrontal cortex. *Cognition* 50: 7–15.
Bechara A, Tranel D, Damasio H, & Damasio AR (1996). Failure to respond autonomically to anticipated future outcomes following damage to prefrontal cortex. *Cerebral Cortex* 6: 215–225.
Bechara A, Damasio H, Tranel D, & Damasio AR (1997). Deciding advantageously before knowing the advantageous strategy. *Science* 275: 1293–1295.
Bechara A, Damasio H, Tranel D, & Anderson SW (1998). Dissociation of working memory from decision making within the human prefrontal cortex. *Journal of Neuroscience* 18: 428–437.
Bechara A, Damasio H, Damasio AR, & Lee GP (1999). Different contributions of the human amygdala and ventromedial prefrontal cortex to decision making. *Journal of Neurosience* 19: 5473–5481.
Bechara A, Damasio H, & Damasio AR (2000). Emotion, decision making and the orbitofrontal cortex. *Cerebral Cortex* 10: 295–307.
Bechara A, Damasio H, Tranel D, & Damasio AR (2005). The Iowa Gambling Task and the somatic marker hypothesis: some questions and answers. *Trends in Cognitive Sciences* 9: 159–162.
Beck JM, Ma WJ, Kiani R, Hanks T, Churchland AK, Roitman J, Shadlen MN, Latham PE, & Pouget A (2008). Probabilistic population codes for Bayesian decision making. *Neuron* 60: 1142–1152.
Beckstead RM & Norgren R (1979). An autoradiographic examination of the central distribution of the trigeminal, facial, glossopharyngeal, and vagal nerves in the monkey. *Journal of Comparative Neurology* 184: 455–472.

Beckstead RM, Morse JR, & Norgren R (1980). The nucleus of the solitary tract in the monkey: projections to the thalamus and brainstem nuclei. *Journal of Comparative Neurology* 190: 259–282.
Begg DP & Woods SC (2013a). Interactions between the central nervous system and pancreatic islet secretions: a historical perspective. *Advances in Physiology Education* 37: 53–60.
Begg DP & Woods SC (2013b). The endocrinology of food intake. *Nature Reviews Endocrinology* doi: 10.1038/nrendo.2013.136.
Beluzzi JD, Grant N, Garsky V, Sarantakis D, Wise CD, & Stein L (1976). Analgesia induced in vivo by central administration of enkephalin in rat. *Nature* 260: 625–626.
Ben-Ari ET (2000). Choosy females. *BioScience* 50: 7–12.
Ben-Ze'ev A (2000). *The Subtlety of Emotions*. MIT Press, Cambridge, MA.
Benabou R & Pycia M (2002). Dynamic inconsistency and self-control: a planner–doer interpretation. *Economics Letters* 77: 419–424.
Bergeron R & Coyle JT (2012). NAAG, NMDA receptor and psychosis. *Current Medicinal Chemistry* 19: 1360–1364.
Berglund A & Rosenqvist G (2001). Male pipefish prefer ornamented females. *Animal Behaviour* 61: 345–350.
Berlin H & Rolls ET (2004). Time perception, impulsivity, emotionality, and personality in self-harming borderline personality disorder patients. *Journal of Personality Disorders* 18: 358–378.
Berlin H, Rolls ET, & Kischka U (2004). Impulsivity, time perception, emotion, and reinforcement sensitivity in patients with orbitofrontal cortex lesions. *Brain* 127: 1108–1126.
Berlin H, Rolls ET, & Iversen SD (2005). Borderline Personality Disorder, impulsivity, and the orbitofrontal cortex. *American Journal of Psychiatry* 58: 234–245.
Berliner DL, Monti-Bloch L, Jennings-White C, & Diaz-Sanchez V (1996). The functionality of the human vomeronasal organ (VNO): evidence for steroid receptors. *Journal of Steroid Biochemistry and Molecular Biology* 58: 259–265.
Bermond B, Fasotti L, Niewenhuyse B, & Schuerman J (1991). Spinal cord lesions, peripheral feedback and intensities of emotional feelings. *Cognition and Emotion* 5: 201–220.
Berner LA, Bocarsly ME, Hoebel BG, & Avena NM (2011). Pharmacological interventions for binge eating: lessons from animal models, current treatments, and future directions. *Current Pharmaceutical Design* 17: 1180–1187.
Bernoulli D (1738). Learning the value of information in an uncertain world. *Econometrica (1954)* 22: 22–36.
Berntson GG, Norman GJ, Bechara A, Bruss J, Tranel D, & Cacioppo JT (2011). The insula and evaluative processes. *Psychological Science* 22: 80–66.
Berridge KC (1996). Food reward: brain substrates of wanting and liking. *Neuroscience and Biobehavioral Reviews* 20: 1–25.
Berridge KC & Robinson TE (1998). What is the role of dopamine in reward: hedonic impact, reward learning, or incentive salience? *Brain Research Reviews* 28: 309–369.
Berridge KC & Robinson TE (2003). Parsing reward. *Trends in Neurosciences* 26: 507–513.
Berridge KC, Flynn FW, Schulkin J, & Grill HJ (1984). Sodium depletion enhances salt palatability in rats. *Behavioral Neuroscience* 98: 652–660.
Berridge KC, Robinson TE, & Aldridge JW (2009). Dissecting components of reward: 'liking', 'wanting', and learning. *Current Opinion in Pharmacology* 9: 65–73.
Bertino M, Beauchamp GK, & Engelman K (1991). Naltrexone, an opioid blocker, alters taste perception and nutrient intake in humans. *American Journal of Physiology* 261: 59–63.
Bertram BCR (1975). Social factors influencing reproduction in wild lions. *Journal of Zoology* 177: 463–482.
Betzig LL (1986). *Despotism and Differential Reproduction*. Aldine, New York.
Betzig LL, editor (1997). *Human Nature: a Critical Reader*. Oxford University Press, New York.
Bhattacharyya S & Chakraborty K (2007). Glutamatergic dysfunction–newer targets for anti-obsessional drugs. *Recent Patents CNS Drug Discovery* 2: 47–55.
Bi GQ & Poo MM (1998). Activity-induced synaptic modifications in hippocampal culture, dependence on spike timing, synaptic strength and cell type. *Journal of Neuroscience* 18: 10464–10472.
Bienenstock EL, Cooper LN, & Munro PW (1982). Theory for the development of neuron selectivity: orientation specificity and binocular interaction in visual cortex. *Journal of Neuroscience* 2: 32–48.
Birkhead T (2000). *Promiscuity*. Faber and Faber, London.
Birkhead TR & Moller AP (1992). *Sperm Competition in Birds*. Academic Press, London.
Birkhead TR & Pizzari T (2002). Postcopulatory sexual selection. *Nature Reviews Genetics* 3: 262–273.
Birkhead TR, Chaline N, Biggins JD, Burke T, & Pizzari T (2004). Nontransivity of paternity in a bird. *Evolution* 58: 416–420.
Bjorklund A & Lindvall O (1986). Catecholaminergic brainstem regulatory systems. In Mountcastle VB, Bloom FE, & Geiger SR, editors, *Handbook of Physiology: The Nervous System*, vol. 4, Intrinsic systems of the Brain, 155–236. American Psychological Society, Bethesda.
Blair HT, Schafe GE, Bauer EP, Rodrigues SM, & LeDoux JE (2001). Synaptic plasticity in the lateral amygdala: a cellular hypothesis of fear conditioning. *Learning and Memory* 8: 229–242.
Blair HT, Tinkelman A, Moita MAP, & LeDoux JE (2003). Associative plasticity in neurons of the lateral amygdala

during auditory fear conditioning. *Annals of the New York Academy of Sciences* 985: 485–487.
Blair RJ, Morris JS, Frith CD, Perrett DI, & Dolan RJ (1999). Dissociable neural responses to facial expressions of sadness and anger. *Brain* 122: 883–893.
Blair RJR (2003). Facial expressions, their communicatory functions and neuro-cognitive substrates. *Philosophical Transactions of the Royal Society of London B* 358: 561–572.
Blake R & Logothetis NK (2002). Visual competition. *Nature Reviews Neuroscience* 3: 13–21.
Blaney PH (1986). Affect and memory: a review. *Psychological Bulletin* 99: 229–246.
Blaustein JD & Erskine MS (2002). Feminine sexual behavior. In Pfaff DW, Arnold AP, Etgen AM, Fahrbach SE, & Rubin RT, editors, *Hormones, Brain and Behavior*, vol. 1, chap. 2, 139–214. Academic Press, San Diego, CA.
Bliss TVP & Collingridge GL (1993). A synaptic model of memory: long-term potentiation in the hippocampus. *Nature* 361: 31–39.
Block N (1995a). Two neural correlates of consciousness. *Trends in Cognitive Sciences* 9: 46–52.
Block N (1995b). On a confusion about a function of consciousness. *Behavioral and Brain Sciences* 18: 22–47.
Blood AJ & Zatorre RJ (2001). Intensely pleasureable responses to music correlate with activity of brain regions implicated in reward and emotion. *Proceedings of the National Academy of Sciences USA* 98: 11818–11823.
Blood AJ, Zatorre RJ, Bermudez P, & Evans AC (1999). Emotional responses to pleasant and unpleasant music correlate with activity in paralimbic brain regions. *Nature Neuroscience* 2: 382–387.
Blumberg J & Kreiman G (2010). How cortical neurons help us see: visual recognition in the human brain. *The Journal of Clinical Investigation* 120: 3054–3063.
Boden MA, editor (1996). *The Philosophy of Artificial Life*. Oxford University Press, Oxford.
Bogacz R & Gurney K (2007). The basal ganglia and cortex implement optimal decision making between alternative actions. *Neural Computation* 19: 442–477.
Bogacz R, Brown E, Moehlis J, Holmes P, & Cohen JD (2006). The physics of optimal decision making: a formal analysis of models of performance in two-alternative forced-choice tasks. *Psychological Review* 113: 700–765.
Boorman ED, Behrens TE, Woolrich MW, & Rushworth MF (2009). How green is the grass on the other side? Frontopolar cortex and the evidence in favor of alternative courses of action. *Neuron* 62: 733–743.
Booth DA (1985). Food-conditioned eating preferences and aversions with interoceptive elements: learned appetites and satieties. *Annals of the New York Academy of Sciences* 443: 22–37.
Booth MCA & Rolls ET (1998). View-invariant representations of familiar objects by neurons in the inferior temporal visual cortex. *Cerebral Cortex* 8: 510–523.
Borsini F & Rolls ET (1984). Role of noradrenaline and serotonin in the basolateral region of the amygdala in food preferences and learned taste aversions in the rat. *Physiology and Behavior* 33: 37–43.
Boussaoud D, Desimone R, & Ungerleider LG (1991). Visual topography of area TEO in the macaque. *Journal of Computational Neurology* 306: 554–575.
Bowlby J (1969). *Attachment and Loss: Volume 1 Attachment*. Hogarth Press, London.
Bowlby J (1973). *Attachment and Loss: Volume 2 Separation*. Hogarth Press, London.
Bowlby J (1980). *Attachment and Loss: Volume 3 Loss*. Hogarth Press, London.
Bowles S & Gintis H (2005). Prosocial emotions. In Blume LE & Durlauf SN, editors, *The Economy as an Evolving Complex System III*. Santa Fe Institute, Santa Fe, NM.
Boyd R, Gintis H, Bowles S, & Richerson PJ (2003). The evolution of altruistic punishment. *Proceedings of the National Academy of Sciences USA* 100: 3531–3535.
Bray GA, Inoue S, & Nishizawa Y (1981). Hypothalamic obesity: the autonomic hypothesis and the lateral hypothalamus. *Diabetologia* 20 (Suppl.): 366–378.
Brebner K, Childress AR, & Roberts DC (2002). A potential role for GABA (B) agonists in the treatment of psychostimulant addiction. *Alcohol and Alcoholism* 37: 478–484.
Bressler SL, Tang W, Sylvester CM, Shulman GL, & Corbetta M (2008). Top-down control of human visual cortex by frontal and parietal cortex in anticipatory visual spatial attention. *Journal of Neuroscience* 28: 10056–10061.
Brevers D, Cleeremans A, Verbruggen F, Bechara A, Kornreich C, Verbanck P, & Noel X (2012). Impulsive action but not impulsive choice determines problem gambling severity. *PLoS ONE* 7: e50647.
Britten KH, Shadlen MN, Newsome WT, & Movshon JA (1992). The analysis of visual motion: a comparison of neuronal and psychophysical performance. *Journal of Neuroscience* 12: 4745–4765.
Britten KH, Shadlen MN, Newsome WT, & Movshon JA (1993). Responses of neurons in macaque mt to stochastic motion signals. *Visual Neuroscience* 10: 1157–1169.
Brodersen KH, Wiech K, Lomakina EI, Lin CS, Buhmann JM, Bingel U, Ploner M, Stephan KE, & Tracey I (2012). Decoding the perception of pain from fmri using multivariate pattern analysis. *Neuroimage* 63: 1162–1170.
Brody C, Hernandez A, Zainos A, & Romo R (2003). Timing and neural encoding of somatosensory parametric working memory in macaque prefrontal cortex. *Cerebral Cortex* 13: 1196–1207.
Bromberg-Martin ES, Matsumoto M, & Hikosaka O (2010a). Dopamine in motivational control: rewarding, aversive, and alerting. *Neuron* 68: 815–834.
Bromberg-Martin ES, Matsumoto M, Hong S, & Hikosaka O (2010b). A pallidus-habenula-dopamine pathway

signals inferred stimulus values. *Journal of Neurophysiology* 104: 1068–1076.
Brothers L & Ring B (1993). Mesial temporal neurons in the macaque monkey with responses selective for aspects of social stimuli. *Behavioural Brain Research* 57: 53–61.
Brown SD & Heathcote A (2008). The simplest complete model of choice response time: linear ballistic accumulation. *Cognitive Psychology* 57: 153–178.
Brown TH, Kairiss EW, & Keenan CL (1990). Hebbian synapses: biophysical mechanisms and algorithms. *Annual Review of Neuroscience* 13: 475–511.
Brown VJ, Desimone R, & Mishkin M (1995). Responses of cells in the tail of the caudate nucleus during visual discrimination learning. *Journal of Neurophysiology* 74: 1083–1094.
Brunel N & Wang XJ (2001). Effects of neuromodulation in a cortical network model of object working memory dominated by recurrent inhibition. *Journal of Computational Neuroscience* 11: 63–85.
Brunel N & Wang XJ (2003). What determines the frequency of fast network oscillations with irregular neural discharges? I. Synaptic dynamics and excitation-inhibition balance. *Journal of Neurophysiology* 90: 415–430.
Brunello N, Mendlewicz J, Kasper S, Leonard B, Montgomery S, Craig Nelson J, Paykel E, Versiani M, & Racagni G (2002). The role of noradrenaline and selective noradrenaline reuptake inhibition in depression. *European Neuropsychopharmacology* 12: 461–475.
Buck L & Axel R (1991). A novel multigene family may encode odorant receptors: a molecular basis for odor recognition. *Cell* 65: 175–187.
Buck L & Bargmann CI (2013). Smell and taste: the chemical senses. In Kandel E, Schwartz JH, Jessell TH, Siegelbaum SA, & Hudspeth AJ, editors, *Principles of Neural Science*, chap. 32, 712–742. McGraw-Hill, New York, 5th edn.
Buckholtz JW, Treadway MT, Cowan RL, Woodward ND, Benning SD, Li R, Ansari MS, Baldwin RM, Schwartzman AN, Shelby ES, Smith CE, Cole D, Kessler RM, & Zald DH (2010). Mesolimbic dopamine reward system hypersensitivity in individuals with psychopathic traits. *Nature Neuroscience* 13: 419–421.
Buehlmann A & Deco G (2010). Optimal information transfer in the cortex through synchronization. *PLoS Computational Biology* 6: e1000934.
Buot A & Yelnik J (2012). Functional anatomy of the basal ganglia: limbic aspects. *Revue Neurologique (Paris)* 168: 569–575.
Burbeck S & Luce R (1982). Evidence from auditory simple reaction times for both change and level detectors. *Perception and Psychophysics* 32: 117–133.
Burgess PW (2000). Strategy application disorder: the role of the frontal lobes in human multitasking. *Psychological Research* 63: 279–288.
Burton MJ, Rolls ET, & Mora F (1976). Effects of hunger on the responses of neurones in the lateral hypothalamus to the sight and taste of food. *Experimental Neurology* 51: 668–677.
Busemeyer JR & Townsend JT (1993). Decision field theory: a dynamic-cognitive approach to decision making in an uncertain environment. *Psychological Review* 100: 432–459.
Bush G, Luu P, & Posner MI (2000). Cognitive and emotional influences in anterior cingulate cortex. *Trends in Cognitive Sciences* 4: 215–222.
Bush G, Vogt BA, Holmes J, Dales AM, Greve D, Jenike MA, & Rosen BR (2002). Dorsal anterior cingulate cortex: a role in reward-based decision making. *Proceedings of the National Academy of Sciences USA* 99: 523–528.
Buss DM (1989). Sex differences in human mate preferences: evolutionary hypotheses tested in 37 cultures. *Behavioural and Brain Sciences* 12: 1–14.
Buss DM (1994). *The Evolution of Desire: Strategies of Human Mating*. Basic Books, New York.
Buss DM (2003). *Evolution of Desire. Strategies of Human Mating*. Basic Books, New York, NY, 2nd edn.
Buss DM (2012). *Evolutionary Psychology: The New Science of the Mind*. Allyn and Bacon, Boston, MA, 4th edn.
Buss DM & Schmitt DP (1993). Sexual strategies theory: an evolutionary perspective on human mating. *Psychological Review* 100: 204–232.
Buss DM, Abbott M, Angeleitner A, Asherian A, Biaggio A, Blancovillasenor A, Bruchonschweitzer M, Chu H, Czapinski J, DeRaad B, Ekehammar B, Ellohamy N, Fioravanti M, Georgas J, Gjerde P, Guttman R, Hazan F, Iwawaki S, Janakiramaiah N, Khosroshani F, Kreitler S, Lachenicht L, Lee M, Liik K, Little B, Mika S, Moadelshahid M, Moane G, Montero M, Mundycastle AC, Niit T, Nsenduluka E, Pienkowski R, Pirttila-Backman AM, Deleon JP, Rousseau J, Runco MA, Safir MP, Samuels C, Sanitioso R, Serpell R, Smid N, Spencer C, Tadinac M, Todorova EN, Troland K, Vandenbrande L, Van Heck G, Vanlangenhove L, & Yang KS (1990). International preferences in selecting mates: a study of 37 cultures. *Journal of Cross-Cultural Psychology* 21: 5–47.
Bussey TJ & Everitt BJ (1997). Dissociable effects of cingulate and medial frontal cortex lesions on stimulus–reward learning using a novel Pavlovian autoshaping procedure for the rat: implications for the neurobiology of emotion. *Behavioral Neuroscience* 111: 908–919.
Butter CM (1969). Perseveration in extinction and in discrimination reversal tasks following selective prefrontal ablations in Macaca mulatta. *Physiology and Behavior* 4: 163–171.
Butter CM & Snyder DR (1972). Alterations in aversive and aggressive behaviors following orbitofrontal lesions in

rhesus monkeys. *Acta Neurobiologica Experimentalis* 32: 525–565.
Butter CM, McDonald JA, & Snyder DR (1969). Orality, preference behavior, and reinforcement value of non-food objects in monkeys with orbital frontal lesions. *Science* 164: 1306–1307.
Butter CM, Snyder DR, & McDonald JA (1970). Effects of orbitofrontal lesions on aversive and aggressive behaviors in rhesus monkeys. *Journal of Comparative Physiology and Psychology* 72: 132–144.
Buxton RB & Frank LR (1997). A model for the coupling between cerebral blood flow and oxygen metabolism during neural stimulation. *Journal of Cerebral Blood Flow and Metabolism* 17: 64–72.
Buxton RB, Wong EC, & Frank LR (1998). Dynamics of blood flow and oxygenation changes during brain activation: the balloon model. *Magnetic Resonance in Medicine* 39: 855–864.
Buzsáki G (2006). *Rhythms of the Brain.* Oxford University Press, Oxford.
Byrne RW & Whiten A (1988). *Machiavellian Intelligence: Social Expertise and the Evolution of Intellect in Monkeys, Apes and Humans.* Clarendon Press, Oxford.
Caan W, Perrett DI, & Rolls ET (1984). Responses of striatal neurons in the behaving monkey. 2. Visual processing in the caudal neostriatum. *Brain Research* 290: 53–65.
Cabanac M (1971). Physiological role of pleasure. *Science* 173: 1103–1107.
Cabanac M (1992). Pleasure: the common currency. *Journal of Theoretical Biology* 155: 173–200.
Cabanac M & Duclaux R (1970). Specificity of internal signals in producing satiety for taste stimuli. *Nature* 227: 966–967.
Cabanac M & Fantino M (1977). Origin of olfacto-gustatory alliesthesia: Intestinal sensitivity to carbohydrate concentration? *Physiology and Behavior* 10: 1039–1045.
Cacioppo JT, Klein DJ, Berntson GC, & Hatfield E (1993). The psychophysiology of emotion. In Lewis M & Hatfield JM, editors, *Handbook of Emotions*, 119–145. Guildford, New York.
Cador M, Robbins TW, & Everitt BJ (1989). Involvement of the amygdala in stimulus–reward associations: interaction with the ventral striatum. *Neuroscience* 30: 77–86.
Caggiula AR (1970). Analysis of the copulation-reward properties of posterior hypothalamic stimulation in male rats. *Journal of Comparative and Physiological Psychology* 70: 399–412.
Cahusac PMB, Rolls ET, Miyashita Y, & Niki H (1993). Modification of the responses of hippocampal neurons in the monkey during the learning of a conditional spatial response task. *Hippocampus* 3: 29–42.
Cai X & Padoa-Schioppa C (2012). Neuronal encoding of subjective value in dorsal and ventral anterior cingulate cortex. *Journal of Neuroscience* 32: 3791–3808.
Calabresi P, Maj R, Pisani A, Mercuri NB, & Bernardi G (1992). Long-term synaptic depression in the striatum: physiological and pharmacological characterization. *Journal of Neuroscience* 12: 4224–4233.
Calder AJ, Young AW, Rowland D, Perrett DI, Hodges JR, & Etcoff NL (1996). Facial emotion recognition after bilateral amygdala damage: differentially severe impairment of fear. *Cognitive Neuropsycology* 13: 699–745.
Calder AJ, Keane J, Manes F, Antoun N, & Young AW (2000). Impaired recognition and experience of disgust following brain injury. *Nature Neuroscience* 3: 1077–1078.
Calder AJ, Keane J, Lawrence AD, & Manes F (2004). Impaired recognition of anger following damage to the ventral striatum. *Brain* 127: 1958–1969.
Camille N, Tsuchida A, & Fellows LK (2011). Double dissociation of stimulus-value and action-value learning in humans with orbitofrontal or anterior cingulate cortex damage. *Journal of Neuroscience* 31: 15048–15052.
Campfield LA, Smith FJ, Guisez Y, Devos R, & Burn P (1995). Recombinant mouse ob protein: evidence for a peripheral signal linking adiposity and central neural networks. *Science* 269: 546–549.
Canli T, Zhao Z, Desmond JE, Kang E, Gross J, & Gabrieli JD (2001). An fMRI study of personality influences on brain reactivity to emotional stimuli. *Behavioral Neuroscience* 115: 33–42.
Canli T, Sivers H, Whitfield SL, Gotlib IH, & Gabrieli JD (2002). Amygdala response to happy faces as a function of extraversion. *Science* 296: 2191.
Cannistraro PA & Rauch SL (2003). Neural circuitry of anxiety: evidence from structural and functional neuroimaging studies. *Psychopharmacology Bulletin* 37: 8–25.
Cannon WB (1927). The James–Lange theory of emotion: a critical examination and an alternative theory. *American Journal of Psychology* 39: 106–124.
Cannon WB (1929). *Bodily Changes in Pain, Hunger, Fear and Rage.* Appleton, New York, 2nd edn.
Cannon WB (1931). Again the James–Lange theory of emotion: a critical examination and an alternative theory. *Psychological Review* 38: 281–295.
Caplan D (1996). *Language: Structure, Processing and Disorders.* MIT Press, Cambridge, MA.
Cardinal N & Everitt BJ (2004). Neural and psychological mechanisms underlying appetitive learning: links to drug addiction. *Current Opinion in Neurobiology* 14: 156–162.
Cardinal RN, Pennicott DR, Sugathapala CL, Robbins TW, & Everitt BJ (2001). Impulsive choice induced in rats by lesions of the nucleus accumbens core. *Science* 292: 2499–2501.
Cardinal RN, Parkinson JA, Hall J, & Everitt BJ (2002). Emotion and motivation: the role of the amygdala, ventral striatum, and prefrontal cortex. *Neuroscience and Biobehavioral Reviews* 26: 321–352.
Carlson NR (2012). *Physiology of Behavior.* Pearson, Boston, 11th edn.
Carmichael ST & Price JL (1994). Architectonic subdivision of the orbital and medial prefrontal cortex in the

macaque monkey. *Journal of Comparative Neurology* 346: 366–402.

Carmichael ST & Price JL (1995a). Limbic connections of the orbital and medial prefrontal cortex in macaque monkeys. *Journal of Comparative Neurology* 363: 615–641.

Carmichael ST & Price JL (1995b). Sensory and premotor connections of the orbital and medial prefrontal cortex of macaque monkeys. *Journal of Comparative Neurology* 363: 642–664.

Carmichael ST, Clugnet MC, & Price JL (1994). Central olfactory connections in the macaque monkey. *Journal of Comparative Neurology* 346: 403–434.

Carpenter RHS & Williams M (1995). Neural computation of log likelihood in control of saccadic eye movements. *Nature* 377: 59–62.

Carruthers P (1996). *Language, Thought and Consciousness*. Cambridge University Press, Cambridge.

Carruthers P (2000). *Phenomenal Consciousness*. Cambridge University Press, Cambridge.

Carter SC (1998). Neuroendocrine perpectives on social attachment and love. *Psychoneuroendocrinology* 23: 779–818.

Cavanna AE & Trimble MR (2006). The precuneus: a review of its functional anatomy and behavioural correlates. *Brain* 129: 564–583.

Celada P, Puig MV, Armagos-Bosch M, Adell A, & Artigas F (2004). The therapeutic role of 5-HT_{1A} and 5-HT_{2A} receptors in depression. *Journal of Psychiatry and Neuroscience* 29: 252–265.

Chakrabarty K, Bhattacharyya S, Christopher R, & Khanna S (2005). Glutamatergic dysfunction in OCD. *Neuropsychopharmacology* 30: 1735–1740.

Chalmers DJ (1996). *The Conscious Mind*. Oxford University Press, Oxford.

Chamberlain SR, Fineberg NA, Blackwell AD, Robbins TW, & Sahakian BJ (2006). Motor inhibition and cognitive flexibility in obsessive-compulsive disorder and trichotillomania. *American Journal of Psychiatry* 163: 1282–1284.

Chamberlain SR, Fineberg NA, Menzies LA, Blackwell AD, Bullmore ET, Robbins TW, & Sahakian BJ (2007). Impaired cognitive flexibility and motor inhibition in unaffected first-degree relatives of patients with obsessive-compulsive disorder. *American Journal of Psychiatry* 164: 335–338.

Chandrashekar J, Hoon MA, Ryba NJ, & Zuker CS (2006). The receptors and cells for mammalian taste. *Nature* 444: 288–294.

Chaudhari N & Roper SD (2010). The cell biology of taste. *Journal of Cell Biology* 190: 285–296.

Chaudhari N, Landin AM, & Roper S (2000). A metabolic glutamate receptor variant functions as a taste receptor. *Nature Neuroscience* 3: 113–119.

Chen G, Greengard P, & Yan Z (2004). Potentiation of NMDA receptor currents by dopamine D1 receptors in prefrontal cortex. *Proceedings of the National Academy of Sciences USA* 101: 2596–2600.

Cheney DL & Seyfarth RM (1990). *How Monkeys See the World*. University of Chicago Press, Chicago.

Chevalier-Skolnikoff S (1973). Facial expression of emotion in non-human primates. In Ekman P, editor, *Darwin and Facial Expression*, 11–89. Academic Press, New York.

Chiavaras MM & Petrides M (2001). Three-dimensional probabilistic atlas of the human orbitofrontal sulci in standardised stereotaxic space. *Neuroimage* 13: 479–496.

Chib VS, Rangel A, Shimojo S, & O'Doherty JP (2009). Evidence for a common representation of decision values for dissimilar goods in human ventromedial prefrontal cortex. *Journal of Neuroscience* 29: 12315–12320.

Childress AR, Mozley PD, McElgin W, Fitzgerald J, Reivich M, & O'Brien CP (1999). Limbic activation during cue-induced cocaine craving. *American Journal of Psychiatry* 156: 11–18.

Cho YK, Li CS, & Smith DV (2002). Gustatory projections from the nucleus of the solitary tract to the parabrachial nuclei in the hamster. *Chemical Senses* 27: 81–90.

Christie BR (1996). Long-term depression in the hippocampus. *Hippocampus* 6: 1–2.

Churchland AK, Kiani R, & Shadlen MN (2008). Decision-making with multiple alternatives. *Nature Neuroscience* 11: 693–702.

Churchland AK, Kiani R, Chaudhuri R, Wang XJ, Pouget A, & Shadlen MN (2011). Variance as a signature of neural computations during decision making. *Neuron* 69: 818–831.

Churchland MM, Yu BM, Cunningham JP, Sugrue LP, Cohen LR, Corrado GS, Newsome WT, Clark AM, Hosseini P, Scott BB, Bradley DC, Smith MA, Kohn A, Movshon A, Armstrong KM, Moore T, Chang SW, Snyder LH, Lisberger SG, Priebe NJ, Finn IM, Ferster D, Ryu SI, Santhanam G, Sahani M, & Shenoy KV (2010). Stimulus onset quenches neural variability: a widespread cortical phenomenon. *Nature Neuroscience* 13: 369–378.

Churchland PS & Winkielman P (2012). Modulating social behavior with oxytocin: how does it work? What does it mean? *Hormones and Behavior* 61: 392–399.

Cisek P, Puskas GA, & El-Murr S (2009). Decisions in changing conditions: the urgency-gating model. *Journal of Neuroscience* 29: 11560–=11571.

Clark DA & Beck AT (2010). Cognitive theory and therapy of anxiety and depression: convergence with neurobiological findings. *Trends in Cognitive Science* 14: 418–424.

Clark JM, Clark AJM, Bartle A, & Winn P (1991). The regulation of feeding and drinking in rats with lesions of the lateral hypothalamus made by N-methyl-D-aspartate. *Neuroscience* 45: 631–640.

Clark L, Cools R, & Robbins TW (2004). The neuropsychology of ventral prefrontal cortex: decision-making and reversal learning. *Brain and Cognition* 55: 41–53.

Coghill RC, Talbot JD, Evans AC, Meyer E, Gjedde A, Bushnell MC, & Duncan GH (1994). Distributed processing of pain and vibration in the human brain. *Journal of Neuroscience* 14: 4095–4108.

Colantuoni C, Rada P, McCarthy J, Patten C, Avena NM, Chadeayne A, & Hoebel BG (2002). Evidence that intermittent, excessive sugar intake causes endogenous opioid dependence. *Obesity Research* 10: 478–488.

Collingridge GL & Bliss TVP (1987). NMDA receptors: their role in long-term potentiation. *Trends in Neurosciences* 10: 288–293.

Colwill RM & Rescorla RA (1985). Postconditioning devaluation of a reinforcer affects instrumental responding. *Journal of Experimental Psychology* 11: 120–132.

Colwill RM & Rescorla RA (1988). Associations between the discriminative stimulus and the reinforcer in instrumental learning. *Journal of Experimental Psychology* 14: 155–164.

Colwill RM & Rescorla RA (1990). Evidence for the hierarchical structure of instrumental learning. *Animal Learning and Behaviour* 18: 71–82.

Cone RD (2005). Anatomy and regulation of the central melanocortin system. *Nature Neuroscience* 8: 571–578.

Cooper JR, Bloom FE, & Roth RH (2003). *The Biochemical Basis of Neuropharmacology*. Oxford University Press, Oxford, 8th edn.

Corbetta M & Shulman GL (2002). Control of goal-directed and stimulus-driven attention in the brain. *Nature Reviews Neuroscience* 3: 201–215.

Cornell CE, Rodin J, & Weingarten H (1989). Stimulus-induced eating when satiated. *Physiology and Behavior* 45: 695–704.

Corr PJ & McNaughton N (2012). Neuroscience and approach/avoidance personality traits: a two stage (valuation-motivation) approach. *Neuroscience and Biobehavioural Reviews* 36: 2339–2254.

Corrado GS, Sugrue LP, Seung HS, & Newsome WT (2005). Linear-nonlinear-Poisson models of primate choice dynamics. *Journal of the Experimental Analysis of Behavior* 84: 581–617.

Corwin RL & Buda-Levin A (2004). Behavioral models of binge-type eating. *Physiology and Behavior* 82: 123–130.

Cosmides I & Tooby J (1999). Evolutionary psychology. In Wilson R & Keil F, editors, *MIT Encyclopedia of the Cognitive Sciences*, 295–298. MIT Press, Cambridge, MA.

Cowley JJ & Brooksbank BWL (1991). Human exposure to putative pheromones and changes in aspects of social behaviour. *Journal of Steroid Biochemistry and Molecular Biology* 39: 647–659.

Coyle JT (2006). Glutamate and schizophrenia: beyond the dopamine hypothesis. *Cellular and Molecular Neurobiology* 26: 365–384.

Coyle JT, Tsai G, & Goff D (2003). Converging evidence of NMDA receptor hypofunction in the pathophysiology of schizophrenia. *Annals of the New York Academy of Sciences* 1003: 318–327.

Coyle JT, Balu D, Benneyworth M, Basu A, & Roseman A (2010). Beyond the dopamine receptor: novel therapeutic targets for treating schizophrenia. *Dialogues in Clinical Neuroscience* 12: 359–382.

Craig AD (2009). How do you feel–now? The anterior insula and human awareness. *Nature Reviews Neuroscience* 10: 59–70.

Craig AD (2011). Significance of the insula for the evolution of human awareness of feelings from the body. *Annals of the New York Academy of Sciences* 1225: 72–82.

Craig AD, Chen K, Bandy D, & Reiman EM (2000). Thermosensory activation of insular cortex. *Nature Neuroscience* 3: 184–190.

Crews FT & Boettiger CA (2009). Impulsivity, frontal lobes and risk for addiction. *Pharmacology Biochemistry and Behavior* 93: 237–247.

Crick FHC & Koch C (1990). Towards a neurobiological theory of consciousness. *Seminars in the Neurosciences* 2: 263–275.

Critchley HD (2005). Neural mechanisms of autonomic, affective, and cognitive integration. *Journal of Comparative Neurology* 493: 154–166.

Critchley HD & Harrison NA (2013). Visceral influences on brain and behavior. *Neuron* 77: 624–638.

Critchley HD & Rolls ET (1996a). Responses of primate taste cortex neurons to the astringent tastant tannic acid. *Chemical Senses* 21: 135–145.

Critchley HD & Rolls ET (1996b). Olfactory neuronal responses in the primate orbitofrontal cortex: analysis in an olfactory discrimination task. *Journal of Neurophysiology* 75: 1659–1672.

Critchley HD & Rolls ET (1996c). Hunger and satiety modify the responses of olfactory and visual neurons in the primate orbitofrontal cortex. *Journal of Neurophysiology* 75: 1673–1686.

Cromwell HC & Schultz W (2003). Effects of expectations for different reward magntitudes on neuronal activity in primate striatum. *Journal of Neurophysiology* 89: 2823–2838.

Croxson PL, Walton ME, O'Reilly JX, Behrens TE, & Rushworth MF (2009). Effort-based cost-benefit valuation and the human brain. *Journal of Neuroscience* 29: 4531–4541.

Crutcher MD & DeLong MR (1984a). Single cell studies of the primate putamen. I. Functional organisation. *Experimental Brain Research* 53: 233–243.

Crutcher MD & DeLong MR (1984b). Single cell studies of the primate putamen. II. Relations to direction of

movements and pattern of muscular activity. *Experimental Brain Research* 53: 244–258.
Cullen E (1957). Adaptations in the kittiwake to cliff-nesting. *Ibis* 99: 275–302.
Cummings DE & Schwartz MW (2003). Genetics and pathophysiology of human obesity. *Annual Reviews of Medicine* 54: 453–471.
Cummings DE, Frayo RS, Marmonier C, Aubert R, & Chapolet D (2004). Plasma ghrelin levels and hunger scores in humans initiating meals voluntarily without time- and food-related cues. *American Journal of Physiology - Endocrinology and Metabolism* 287: 297–304.
Cunningham MR, Roberts AR, Barbee AP, & Druen PB (1995). Their ideas of beauty are, on the whole, the same as ours: consistency and variability in the cross-cultural perception of female physical attractiveness. *Journal of Personality and Social Psychology* 68: 261–279.
Dahlström A & Fuxe K (1965). Evidence for the existence of monoamine-containing neurons in the central nervous system: demonstration of monoamines in the cell bodies of brain stem neurons. *Acta Physiologia Scandinavica* 62: 1–55.
Daly M & Wilson M (1988). *Homicide*. Aldine De Gruyter, New York.
Damasio A, Damasio H, & Tranel D (2013). Persistence of feelings and sentience after bilateral damage of the insula. *Cerebral Cortex* 23: 833–846.
Damasio AR (1994). *Descartes' Error: Emotion, Reason, and the Human Brain*. Grosset/Putnam, New York.
Damasio AR (1996). The somatic marker hypothesis and the possible functions of the prefrontal cortex [and discussion]. *Philosophical Transactions of the Royal Society of London. Series B: Biological Sciences* 351: 1413–1420.
Damasio AR (2003). *Looking for Spinoza*. Heinemann, London.
Damasio AR, Grabowski TJ, Bechara A, Damasio H, Ponto LLB, Parvizi J, & Hichwa RD (2000). Subcortical and cortical brain activity during the feeling of self-generated emotions. *Nature Neuroscience* 3: 1049–1056.
Damasio H, Grabowski T, Frank R, Galaburda AM, & Damasio AR (1994). The return of Phineas Gage: clues about the brain from the skull of a famous patient. *Science* 264: 1102–1105.
Darwin C (1859). *The Origin of Species*. John Murray [reprinted (1982) by Penguin Books Ltd], London.
Darwin C (1871). *The Descent of Man, and Selection in Relation to Sex*. John Murray [reprinted (1981) by Princeton University Press], London.
Darwin C (1872). *The Expression of the Emotions in Man and Animals*. University of Chicago Press. [reprinted (1998) (3rd edn) ed. P. Ekman. Harper Collins], Glasgow.
Davidson RJ (1992). Anterior cerebral asymmetry and the nature of emotion. *Brain and Cognition* 6: 245–268.
Davidson RJ (2003). Affective neuroscience and psychophysiology: toward a synthesis. *Psychophysiology* 40: 655–665.
Davidson RJ, Ekman P, Saron C, Senulis J, & Friesen WV (1990). Approach/withdrawal and cerebral asymmetry. *Journal of Personality and Social Research* 58: 330–341.
Davies M (2008). Consciousness and explanation. In Weiskrantz L & Davies M, editors, *Frontiers of Consciousness*, chap. 1, 1–54. Oxford University Press, Oxford.
Davis M (1992). The role of the amygdala in conditioned fear. In Aggleton JP, editor, *The Amygdala*, chap. 9, 255–306. Wiley-Liss, New York.
Davis M (1994). The role of the amygdala in emotional learning. *International Review of Neurobiology* 36: 225–266.
Davis M (2000). The role of the amygdala in conditioned and unconditioned fear and anxiety. In Aggleton JP, editor, *The Amygdala: a Functional Analysis*, chap. 6, 213–287. Oxford University Press, Oxford, 2nd edn.
Davis M (2011). NMDA receptors and fear extinction: implications for cognitive behavioral therapy. *Dialogues in Clinical Neuroscience* 13: 463–474.
Davis M, Campeau S, Kim M, & Falls WA (1995). Neural systems and emotion: the amygdala's role in fear and anxiety. In McGaugh JL, Weinberger NM, & Lynch G, editors, *Brain and Memory: Modulation and Mediation of Neuroplasticity*, 3–40. Oxford University Press, New York.
Davis M, Antoniadis EA, Amaral DG, & Winslow JT (2008). Acoustic startle reflex in rhesus monkeys: a review. *Reviews in Neuroscience* 19: 171–185.
Dawkins MS (1986a). *Unravelling Animal Behaviour*. Longman, Harlow, 1st edn.
Dawkins MS (1993). *Through Our Eyes Only? The Search for Animal Consciousness*. Freeman, Oxford.
Dawkins MS (1995). *Unravelling Animal Behaviour*. Longman, Harlow, 2nd edn.
Dawkins R (1976). *The Selfish Gene*. Oxford University Press, Oxford.
Dawkins R (1982). *The Extended Phenotype*. Freeman, Oxford.
Dawkins R (1986b). *The Blind Watchmaker*. Longman, Harlow.
Dawkins R (1989). *The Selfish Gene*. Oxford University Press, Oxford, 2nd edn.
Dayan P & Abbott LF (2001). *Theoretical Neuroscience*. MIT Press, Cambridge, MA.
Dayan P & Sejnowski TJ (1994). TD(λ) converges with probability 1. *Machine Learning* 14: 295–301.
De Araujo IET & Rolls ET (2004). Representation in the human brain of food texture and oral fat. *Journal of Neuroscience* 24: 3086–3093.
De Araujo IET, Rolls ET, & Stringer SM (2001). A view model which accounts for the response properties of hippocampal primate spatial view cells and rat place cells. *Hippocampus* 11: 699–706.

De Araujo IET, Kringelbach ML, Rolls ET, & Hobden P (2003a). Representation of umami taste in the human brain. *Journal of Neurophysiology* 90: 313–319.

De Araujo IET, Kringelbach ML, Rolls ET, & McGlone F (2003b). Human cortical responses to water in the mouth, and the effects of thirst. *Journal of Neurophysiology* 90: 1865–1876.

De Araujo IET, Rolls ET, Kringelbach ML, McGlone F, & Phillips N (2003c). Taste-olfactory convergence, and the representation of the pleasantness of flavour in the human brain. *European Journal of Neuroscience* 18: 2059–2068.

De Araujo IET, Rolls ET, Velazco MI, Margot C, & Cayeux I (2005). Cognitive modulation of olfactory processing. *Neuron* 46: 671–679.

De Gelder B, Vroomen J, Pourtois G, & Weiskrantz L (1999). Non-conscious recognition of affect in the absence of striate cortex. *NeuroReport* 10: 3759–3763.

de Lafuente V & Romo R (2005). Neuronal correlates of subjective sensory experience. *Nature Neuroscience* 8: 1698–1703.

Deadwyler S, Hayashizaki S, Cheer J, & Hampson RE (2004). Reward, memory and substance abuse: functional neuronal circuits in the nucleus accumbens. *Neuroscience and Biobehavioral Reviews* 27: 703–711.

Debiec J, LeDoux JE, & Nader K (2002). Cellular and systems reconsolidation in the hippocampus. *Neuron* 36: 527–538.

Debiec J, Doyere V, Nader K, & LeDoux JE (2006). Directly reactivated, but not indirectly reactivated, memories undergo reconsolidation in the amygdala. *Proceedings of the National Academy of Sciences USA* 103: 3428–3433.

Deco G & Marti D (2007). Deterministic analysis of stochastic bifurcations in multi-stable neurodynamical systems. *Biological Cybernetics* 96: 487–496.

Deco G & Rolls ET (2002). Object-based visual neglect: a computational hypothesis. *European Journal of Neuroscience* 16: 1994–2000.

Deco G & Rolls ET (2003). Attention and working memory: a dynamical model of neuronal activity in the prefrontal cortex. *European Journal of Neuroscience* 18: 2374–2390.

Deco G & Rolls ET (2004). A neurodynamical cortical model of visual attention and invariant object recognition. *Vision Research* 44: 621–644.

Deco G & Rolls ET (2005a). Synaptic and spiking dynamics underlying reward reversal in the orbitofrontal cortex. *Cerebral Cortex* 15: 15–30.

Deco G & Rolls ET (2005b). Attention, short term memory, and action selection: a unifying theory. *Progress in Neurobiology* 76: 236–256.

Deco G & Rolls ET (2005c). Neurodynamics of biased competition and cooperation for attention: a model with spiking neurons. *Journal of Neurophysiology* 94: 295–313.

Deco G & Rolls ET (2005d). Sequential memory: a putative neural and synaptic dynamical mechanism. *Journal of Cognitive Neuroscience* 17: 294–307.

Deco G & Rolls ET (2006). A neurophysiological model of decision-making and Weber's law. *European Journal of Neuroscience* 24: 901–916.

Deco G & Thiele A (2011). Cholinergic control of cortical network interactions enables feedback-mediated attentional modulation. *European Journal of Neuroscience* 34: 146–157.

Deco G, Rolls ET, & Horwitz B (2004). 'What' and 'where' in visual working memory: a computational neurodynamical perspective for integrating fMRI and single-neuron data. *Journal of Cognitive Neuroscience* 16: 683–701.

Deco G, Ledberg A, Almeida R, & Fuster J (2005). Neural dynamics of cross-modal and cross-temporal associations. *Experimental Brain Research* 166: 325–336.

Deco G, Scarano L, & Soto-Faraco S (2007). Weber's law in decision making: integrating behavioral data in humans with a neurophysiological model. *Journal of Neuroscience* 27: 11192–11200.

Deco G, Marti D, Ledberg A, Reig R, & Sanchez Vives MS (2009a). Effective reduced diffusion-models: a data driven approach to the analysis of neuronal dynamics. *PLoS Computational Biology* 5: e1000587.

Deco G, Rolls ET, & Romo R (2009b). Stochastic dynamics as a principle of brain function. *Progress in Neurobiology* 88: 1–16.

Deco G, Rolls ET, & Romo R (2010). Synaptic dynamics and decision-making. *Proceedings of the National Academy of Sciences* 107: 7545–7549.

Deco G, Rolls ET, Albantakis L, & Romo R (2013). Brain mechanisms for perceptual and reward-related decision-making. *Progress in Neurobiology* 103: 194–213.

Dehaene S & Naccache L (2001). Towards a cognitive neuroscience of consciousness: basic evidence and a workspace framework. *Cognition* 79: 1–37.

Dehaene S, Dehaene-Lambertz G, & Cohen L (1998). Abstract representations of numbers in the animal and human brain. *Trends in Neurosciences* 21: 355–361.

Dehaene S, Changeux JP, Naccache L, Sackur J, & Sergent C (2006). Conscious, preconscious, and subliminal processing: a testable taxonomy. *Trends in Cognitive Sciences* 10: 204–211.

Delgado MR, Nystrom LE, Fissell C, Noll DC, & Fiez JA (2000). Tracking the human hemodynamic responses to

reward and punishment in the striatum. *Journal of Neurophysiology* 84: 3072–3077.
Delgado MR, Jou RL, & Phelps EA (2011). Neural systems underlying aversive conditioning in humans with primary and secondary reinforcers. *Frontiers in Neuroscience* 5: 71.
DeLong M & Wichmann T (2010). Changing views of basal ganglia circuits and circuit disorders. *Clinical EEG and Neuroscience* 41: 61–67.
DeLong MR, Georgopoulos AP, Crutcher MD, Mitchell SJ, Richardson RT, & Alexander GE (1984). Functional organization of the basal ganglia: Contributions of single-cell recording studies. In *Functions of the Basal Ganglia. CIBA Foundation Symposium*, 64–78. Pitman, London.
Dennett DC (1987). *The Intentional Stance*. MIT Press, Cambridge, MA.
Dennett DC (1991). *Consciousness Explained*. Penguin, London.
Derbyshire SWG, Vogt BA, & Jones AKP (1998). Pain and Stroop interference tasks activate separate processing modules in anterior cingulate cortex. *Experimental Brain Research* 118: 52–60.
Desimone R (1996). Neural mechanisms for visual memory and their role in attention. *Proceedings of the National Academy of Sciences USA* 93: 13494–13499.
Desimone R & Duncan J (1995). Neural mechanisms of selective visual attention. *Annual Review of Neuroscience* 18: 193–222.
DeVries AC, DeVries MB, Taymans SE, & Carter CS (1996). The effects of stress on social preferences are sexually dimorphic in prairie voles. *Proceedings of the National Academy of Science USA* 93: 11980–11984.
Di Lorenzo PM (1990). Corticofugal influence on taste responses in the parabrachial pons of the rat. *Brain Research* 530: 73–84.
Di Marzo V & Matias I (2005). Endocannabinoid control of food intake and energy balance. *Nature Neuroscience* 8: 585–590.
Diamond J (1997). *Why is Sex Fun?* Weidenfeld and Nicholson, London.
Dias R, Robbins TW, & Roberts AC (1996). Dissociation in prefrontal cortex of affective and attentional shifts. *Nature* 380: 69–72.
DiChiara G, Acquas E, & Carboni E (1992). Drug motivation and abuse: a neurobiological perspective. *Annals of the New York Academy of Sciences* 654: 207–219.
Dickinson A (1980). *Contemporary Animal Learning Theory*. Cambridge University Press, Cambridge.
Dickinson A (1985). Actions and habits – the development of behavioural autonomy. *Philosophical Transactions of the Royal Society of London B* 308: 67–78.
Dickinson A (1986). Re-examination of the role of the instrumental contingency in the sodium-appetitive irrelevant incentive effect. *Quarterly Journal of Experimental Psychology B* 38: 161–172.
Dickinson A (1994). Instrumental conditioning. In Mackintosh NJ, editor, *Animal Learning and Cognition*, 45–80. Academic Press, San Diego.
Dickinson A & Balleine B (1994). Motivational control of goal-directed action. *Animal Learning and Behaviour* 22: 1–18.
Dickinson A & Dawson GR (1987a). Pavlovian processes in the motivational control of instrumental performance. *Quarterly Journal of Experimental Psychology B* 39: 201–213.
Dickinson A & Dawson GR (1987b). The role of the instrumental contigency in the motivational control of performance. *Quarterly Journal of Experimental Psychology B* 39: 77–93.
Dickinson A & Dearing MF (1979). Appetitive-aversive interactions and inhibitory processes. In Dickinson A & Boakes RA, editors, *Mechanisms of Learning and Motivation*, 203–231. Erlbaums, Hillsdale, NJ.
Dickinson A, Nicholas DJ, & Adams CD (1983). The effects of the instrumental training contingency on susceptibility to reinforcer devaluation. *Quarterly Journal of Experimental Psychology B* 35: 35–51.
Dickinson A, Balleine B, Watt A, Gonzalez F, & Boakes RA (1995). Motivational control after extended instrumental training. *Animal Learning and Behaviour* 23: 197–206.
Ditterich J (2006a). Evidence for time-variant decision making. *European Journal of Neuroscience* 24: 3628–3241.
Ditterich J (2006b). Stochastic models of decisions about motion direction: Behavior and physiology. *Neural Networks* 19: 981–1012.
Ditterich J (2010). A comparison between mechanisms of multi-alternative perceptual decision making: ability to explain human behavior, predictions for neurophysiology, and relationship with decision theory. *Frontiers in Neuroscience* 4: 184.
Divac I (1975). Magnocellular nuclei of the basal forebrain project to neocortex, brain stem, and olfactory bulb. Review of some functional correlates. *Brain Research* 93: 385–398.
Divac I & Oberg RGE (1979). Current conceptions of neostriatal functions. In Divac I & Oberg RGE, editors, *The Neostriatum*, 215–230. Pergamon, New York.
Divac I, Rosvold HE, & Szwarcbart MK (1967). Behavioral effects of selective ablation of the caudate nucleus. *Journal of Comparative and Physiological Psychology* 63: 184–190.
Dixson AF (1998). Sexual behaviour and evolution of the seminal vesicles in primates. *Folia Primatologica* 69: 300–306.
Dolan RJ, Fletcher P, Morris J, Kapur N, Deakin JFW, & Frith CD (1996). Neural activation during covert processing of positive emotional facial expressions. *Neuroimage* 4: 194–200.

Dolan RJ, Fink GR, Rolls ET, Booth M, Holmes A, Frackowiak RSJ, & Friston KJ (1997). How the brain learns to see objects and faces in an impoverished context. *Nature* 389: 596–599.

Douglas RJ, Markram H, & Martin KAC (2004). Neocortex. In Shepherd GM, editor, *The Synaptic Organization of the Brain*, chap. 12, 499–558. Oxford University Press, Oxford, 5th edn.

Doya K (1999). What are the computations of the cerebellum, the basal ganglia and the cerebral cortex? *Neural Networks* 12: 961–974.

Doyere V, Debiec J, Monfils MH, Schafe GE, & LeDoux JE (2007). Synapse-specific reconsolidation of distinct fear memories in the lateral amygdala. *Nature Neuroscience* 10: 414–416.

Dragalin VP, Tartakovsky AG, & Veeravalli VV (1999). Multihypothesis sequential probability ratio tests - Part I: Asymptotic optimality. *IEEE Transactions on Information Theory* 45: 2448–2461.

Drevets WC (2007). Orbitofrontal cortex function and structure in depression. *Annals of the New York Academy of Sciences* 1121: 499–527.

Drevets WC & Raichle ME (1992). Neuroanatomical circuits in depression: implications for treatment mechanisms. *Psychopharmacology Bulletin* 28: 261–274.

Dulac C & Kimchi T (2007). Neural mechanisms underlying sex-specific behaviors in vertebrates. *Current Opinion in Neurobiology* 17: 675–683.

Dulac C & Torello AT (2003). Molecular detection of pheromone signals in mammals: from genes to behaviour. *Nature Reviews Neuroscience* 4: 551–562.

Duman RS & Aghajanian GK (2012). Synaptic dysfunction in depression: potential therapeutic targets. *Science* 338: 68–72.

Dunbar R (1993). Co-evolution of neocortex size, group size and language in humans. *Behavioural and Brain Sciences* 16: 681–735.

Dunbar R (1996). *Grooming, Gossip, and the Evolution of Language*. Faber and Faber, London.

Dunn LT & Everitt BJ (1988). Double dissociations of the effects of amygdala and insular cortex lesions on conditioned taste aversion, passive avoidance, and neophobia in the rat using the excitotoxin ibotenic acid. *Behavioral Neuroscience* 102: 3–23.

Dunnett SB & Iversen SD (1982a). Sensorimotor impairments following localised kainic acid and 6-hydroxydopamine lesions of the neostriatum. *Brain Research* 248: 121–127.

Dunnett SB & Iversen SD (1982b). Neurotoxic lesions of ventrolateral but not anteromedial neostriatum impair differential reinforcement of low rates (DRL) performance. *Behavioural Brain Research* 6: 213–226.

Dunnett SB, Lane DM, & Winn P (1985). Ibotenic acid lesions of the lateral hypothalamus: comparison with 6-hydroxydopamine-induced sensorimotor deficits. *Neuroscience* 14: 509–518.

Durstewitz D & Seamans JK (2002). The computational role of dopamine D1 receptors in working memory. *Neural Networks* 15: 561–572.

Durstewitz D, Seamans JK, & Sejnowski TJ (2000). Neurocomputational models of working memory. *Nature Neuroscience* 3 Suppl: 1184–1191.

Easton A & Gaffan D (2000). Amygdala and the memory of reward: the importance of fibres of passage from the basal forebrain. In Aggleton JP, editor, *The Amygdala: a Functional Analysis*, chap. 17, 569–586. Oxford University Press, Oxford, 2nd edn.

Easton A, Ridley RM, Baker HF, & Gaffan D (2002). Unilateral lesions of the cholinergic basal forebrain and fornix in one hemisphere and inferior temporal cortex in the opposite hemisphere produce severe learning impairments in rhesus monkeys. *Cerebral Cortex* 12: 729–736.

Eggert F, Holler C, Luszyk D, Muller-Ruchholtz W, & Ferstl R (1996). MHC-associated and MHC-independent urinary chemosignals in mice. *Physiology and Behavior* 59: 57–62.

Eisenberger NI & Lieberman MD (2004). Why rejection hurts: a common neural alarm system for physical and social pain. *Trends in Cognitive Neuroscience* 8: 294–300.

Ekman P (1982). *Emotion in the Human Face*. Cambridge University Press, Cambridge, 2nd edn.

Ekman P (1992). An argument for basic emotions. *Cognition and Emotion* 6: 169–200.

Ekman P (1993). Facial expression and emotion. *American Psychologist* 48: 384–392.

Ekman P (1998). Introduction. In *C.Darwin: The Expression of the Emotions in Man and Animals, 1872, 3rd Edition 1998*, xxi–xxxvi. Harper Collins, Glasgow.

Ekman P (2003). *Emotions Revealed: Understanding Faces and Feelings*. Weidenfeld and Nicolson, London.

Ekman P, Friesen WV, & Ellsworth PC (1972). *Emotion in the Human Face: Guidelines for Research and Integration of Findings*. Pergamon Press, Oxford.

Ekman P, Levenson RW, & Friesen WV (1983). Autonomic nervous system activity distinguishes between the emotions. *Science* 221: 1208–1210.

Elithorn A, Piercy MF, & Crosskey MA (1955). Prefrontal leucotomy and the anticipation of pain. *Journal of Neurology, Neurosurgery and Psychiatry* 18: 34–43.

Elliffe MCM, Rolls ET, & Stringer SM (2002). Invariant recognition of feature combinations in the visual system. *Biological Cybernetics* 86: 59–71.

Ellis BJ & Symons D (1990). Sex differences in sexual fantasy: an evolutionary psychological approach. *Journal of Sex Research* 27: 527–555.

Ellsberg D (1961). Risk, ambiguity, and the Savage axioms. *Economics* 75: 643–669.

Elmquist JK, Elias CF, & Saper CB (1999). From lesions to leptin: hypothalamic control of food intake and body weight. *Neuron* 22: 221–232.

Engelhardt A, Pfeifer JB, Heistermann M, Niemitz C, Van Hoof JARAM, & Jodges JK (2004). Assessment of females' reproductive status by male longtailed macques, Macaca fascicularis, under natural conditions. *Animal Behaviour* 67: 915–924.

Enomoto K, Matsumoto N, Nakai S, Satoh T, Sato TK, Ueda Y, Inokawa H, Haruno M, & Kimura M (2011). Dopamine neurons learn to encode the long-term value of multiple future rewards. *Proceedings of the National Academy of Sciences U S A* 108: 15462–15467.

Epstein J, Stern E, & Silbersweig D (1999). Mesolimbic activity associated with psychosis in schizophrenia. Symptom-specific PET studies. *Annals of the New York Academy of Sciences* 877: 562–574.

Eslinger P & Damasio A (1985). Severe disturbance of higher cognition after bilateral frontal lobe ablation: patient EVR. *Neurology* 35: 1731–1741.

Estes WK (1948). Discriminative conditioning II Effects of Pavlovian conditioned stimulus upon a subsequently established operant response. *Journal of Experimental Psychology* 38: 173–177.

Etcoff NL (1989). Asymmetries in recognition of emotion. In Boller F & Grafman F, editors, *Handbook of Psychology*, vol. 3, 363–382. Elsevier, Amsterdam.

Evarts EV & Wise SP (1984). Basal ganglia outputs and motor control. In *Functions of the Basal Ganglia. CIBA Foundation Symposium*, vol. 107, 83–96. Pitman, London.

Everitt B (1997). Craving cocaine cues: cognitive neuroscience meets drug addiction research. *Trends in Cognitive Sciences* 1: 1–2.

Everitt BJ (1990). Sexual motivation: a neural and behavioural analysis of the mechanisms underlying appetitive and copulatory responses of male rats. *Neuroscience and Biobehavioral Reviews* 14: 217–232.

Everitt BJ & Robbins TW (1992). Amygdala-ventral striatal interactions and reward-related processes. In Aggleton JP, editor, *The Amygdala*, chap. 15, 401–429. Wiley, Chichester.

Everitt BJ & Robbins TW (2013). From the ventral to the dorsal striatum: Devolving views of their roles in drug addiction. *Neuroscience and Biobehavioural Reviews* doi: 10.1016/j.neubiorev.2013.02.010.

Everitt BJ, Cador M, & Robbins TW (1989). Interactions between the amygdala and ventral striatum in stimulus–reward association: studies using a second order schedule of sexual reinforcement. *Neuroscience* 30: 63–75.

Everitt BJ, Morris KA, O'Brien A, & Robbins TW (1991). The basolateral amygdala-ventral striatal system and conditioned place preference: further evidence of limbic-striatal interactions underlying reward-related processes. *Neuroscience* 42: 1–18

Everitt BJ, Cardinal RN, Hall J, Parkinson JA, & Robbins TW (2000). Differential involvement of amygdala subsystems in appetitive conditioning and drug addiction. In Aggleton JP, editor, *The Amygdala: a Functional Analysis*, chap. 10, 353–390. Oxford University Press, Oxford, 2nd edn.

Everitt BJ, Cardinal RN, Parkinson JA, & Robbins TW (2003). Appetitive behaviour: impact of amygdala-dependent mechanisms of emotional learning. *Annals of the New York Academy of Sciences* 985: 233–250.

Everitt BJ, Belin D, Economidou D, Pelloux Y, Dalley JW, & Robbins TW (2008). Review. neural mechanisms underlying the vulnerability to develop compulsive drug-seeking habits and addiction. *Philosopjical Transactions of the Royal Society London B Biological Sciences* 363: 3125–3135.

Ewart W (1993). Hepatic and other parenteral visceral afferents affecting ingestive behaviour. In Booth DA, editor, *The Neurophysiology of Ingestion*. Manchester University Press, Manchester.

Eysenck HJ & Eysenck SBG (1968). *Personality Structure and Measurement*. R. R. Knapp, San Diego.

Eysenck HJ & Eysenck SBG (1985). *Personality and Individual Differences: a Natural Science Approach*. Plenum, New York.

Faisal A, Selen L, & Wolpert D (2008). Noise in the nervous system. *Nature Reviews Neuroscience* 9: 292–303.

Farooqi IS & O'Rahilly S (2009). Leptin: a pivotal regulator of human energy homeostasis. *American Journal of Clinical Nutrition* 89: 980S–984S.

Farooqi IS, Keogh JM, Kamath S, Jones S, Gibson WT, Trussell R, Jebb SA, Lip GYH, & O'Rahilly S (2001). Partial leptin deficiency and human adiposity. *Nature* 414: 34–35.

Farrow TF, Zheng Y, Wilkinson ID, Spence SA, Deakin JF, Tarrier N, Griffiths PD, & Woodruff PW (2001). Investigating the functional anatomy of empathy and forgiveness. *NeuroReport* 12: 2433–2438.

Fazeli MS & Collingridge GL, editors (1996). *Cortical Plasticity: LTP and LTD*. Bios, Oxford.

Feierstein CE, Quirk MC, Uchida N, Sosulski DL, & Mainen ZF (2006). Representation of spatial goals in rat orbitofrontal cortex. *Neuron* 51: 495–507.

Feinstein JS, Adolphs R, Damasio A, & Tranel D (2011). The human amygdala and the induction and experience of fear. *Current Biology* 21: 34–38.

Feldman DE (2009). Synaptic mechanisms for plasticity in neocortex. *Annual Reviews of Neuroscience* 32: 33–55.

Feldman DE (2012). The spike-timing dependence of plasticity. *Neuron* 75: 556–571.

Fellows LK (2007). The role of orbitofrontal cortex in decision making: a component process account. *Annalls of the New York Academy of Sciences* 1121: 421–430.

Fellows LK (2011). Orbitofrontal contributions to value-based decision making: evidence from humans with frontal

lobe damage. *Annals of the New York Academy of Sciences* 1239: 51–58.
Fellows LK & Farah MJ (2003). Ventromedial frontal cortex mediates affective shifting in humans: evidence from a reversal learning paradigm. *Brain* 126: 1830–1837.
Fellows LK & Farah MJ (2005). Different underlying impairments in decision-making after ventromedial and dorsolateral frontal lobe damage in humans. *Cerebral Cortex* 15: 58–63.
Ferguson JN, Aldag JM, Insel TR, & Young LJ (2001). Oxytocin in the medial amygdala is essential for social recognition in the mouse. *Journal of Neuroscience* 21: 8278–8285.
File SE (1987). The contribution of behavioural studies to the neuropharmacology of anxiety. *Neuropharmacology* 26: 877–886.
Fiorillo CD, Tobler PN, & Schultz W (2003). Discrete coding of reward probability and uncertainty by dopamine neurons. *Science* 299: 1898–1902.
Fiorino DF, Coury A, & Phillips AG (1997). Dynamic changes in nucleus accumbens dopamine efflux during the Coolidge effect in male rats. *Journal of Neuroscience* 17: 4849–4855.
Fisher RA (1930). *The Genetical Theory of Natural Selection*. Clarendon Press, Oxford.
Fisher RA (1958). *The Genetical Theory of Natural Selection*. Dover, New York, 2nd edn.
Fodor JA (1994). *The Elm and the Expert: Mentalese and its Semantics*. MIT Press, Cambridge, MA.
Fox CR & Poldrack RA (2009). Prospect theory and the brain. In Glimcher PW, Camerer CF, Fehr E, & Poldrack RA, editors, *Neuroeconomics. Decision Making and the Brain*, chap. 11, 145–173. Academic Press, London.
Francis S, Rolls ET, Bowtell R, McGlone F, O'Doherty J, Browning A, Clare S, & Smith E (1999). The representation of pleasant touch in the brain and its relationship with taste and olfactory areas. *NeuroReport* 10: 453–459.
Franco L, Rolls ET, Aggelopoulos NC, & Treves A (2004). The use of decoding to analyze the contribution to the information of the correlations between the firing of simultaneously recorded neurons. *Experimental Brain Research* 155: 370–384.
Franco L, Rolls ET, Aggelopoulos NC, & Jerez JM (2007). Neuronal selectivity, population sparseness, and ergodicity in the inferior temporal visual cortex. *Biological Cybernetics* 96: 547–560.
Frederick S, Loewenstein T, & O'Donoghue (2002). Time discounting and time preference: a critical review. *Journal of Economic Literature* 40: 351–401.
Freeman WJ & Watts JW (1950). *Psychosurgery in the Treatment of Mental Disorders and Intractable Pain*. Thomas, Springfield, IL, 2nd edn.
Freese JL & Amaral DG (2009). Neuroanatomy of the primate amygdala. In Whalen PJ & Phelps EA, editors, *The Human Amygdala*, chap. 1, 3–42. Guilford, New York.
Frégnac Y (1996). Dynamics of cortical connectivity in visual cortical networks: an overview. *Journal of Physiology, Paris* 90: 113–139.
Frey S & Petrides M (2002). Orbitofrontal cortex and memory formation. *Neuron* 36: 171–176.
Frey S, Kostopoulos P, & Petrides M (2000). Orbitofrontal involvement in the processing of unpleasant auditory information. *European Journal of Neuroscience* 12: 3709–3712.
Friedman DP, Murray EA, O'Neill JB, & Mishkin M (1986). Cortical connections of the somatosensory fields of the lateral sulcus of macaques: evidence for a corticolimbic pathway for touch. *Journal of Comparative Neurology* 252: 323–347.
Fries P (2005). A mechanism for cognitive dynamics: neuronal communication through neuronal coherence. *Trends in Cognitive Sciences* 9: 474–480.
Fries P (2009). Neuronal gamma-band synchronization as a fundamental process in cortical computation. *Annual Reviews of Neuroscience* 32: 209–224.
Frijda NH (1986). *The Emotions*. Cambridge University Press, Cambridge.
Friston KJ, Buechel C, Fink GR, Morris J, Rolls ET, & Dolan RJ (1997). Psychophysiological and modulatory interactions in neuroimaging. *Neuroimage* 6: 218–229.
Frith CD, Friston K, Liddle PF, & Frackowiak RS (1991). Willed action and the prefrontal cortex in man: a study with PET. *Proceedings of the Royal Society of London B* 244: 241–246.
Frith U (2001). Mind blindness and the brain in autism. *Neuron* 32: 969–979.
Frith U & Frith CD (2003). Development and neurophysiology of mentalizing. *Philosophical Transactions of the Royal Society London B* 358: 459–473.
Fujisawa TX & Cook ND (2011). The perception of harmonic triads: an fMRI study. *Brain Imaging Behav* 5: 109–125.
Fulton JF (1951). *Frontal Lobotomy and Affective Behavior. A Neurophysiological Analysis*. W. W. Norton, New York.
Funahashi S, Bruce C, & Goldman-Rakic P (1989). Mnemonic coding of visual space in monkey dorsolateral prefrontal cortex. *Journal of Neurophysiology* 61: 331–349.
Furl N, Hadj-Bouziane F, Liu N, Averbeck BB, & Ungerleider LG (2012). Dynamic and static facial expressions decoded from motion-sensitive areas in the macaque monkey. *Journal of Neuroscience* 32: 15952–15962.
Furman M & Wang XJ (2008). Similarity effect and optimal control of multiple-choice decision making. *Neuron* 60: 1153–1168.
Fuster JM (1973). Unit activity in prefrontal cortex during delayed-response performance: neuronal correlates of

transient memory. *Joural of Neurophysiology* 36: 61–78.
Fuster JM (2000). *Memory Systems in the Brain.* Raven Press, New York.
Fuster JM (2008). *The Prefrontal Cortex.* Academic Press, London, 4th edn.
Fuster JM & Jervey JP (1982). Neuronal firing in the inferotemporal cortex of the monkey in a visual memory task. *Journal of Neuroscience* 2: 361–375.
Gabbott PL, Warner TA, Jays PR, & Bacon SJ (2003). Areal and synaptic interconnectivity of prelimbic (area 32), infralimbic (area 25) and insular cortices in the rat. *Brain Research* 993: 59–71.
Gaffan D (1992). Amygdala and the memory of reward. In Aggleton JP, editor, *The Amygdala*, chap. 18, 471–483. Wiley-Liss, New York.
Gaffan D, Saunders RC, Gaffan EA, Harrison S, Shields C, & Owen MJ (1984). Effects of fornix section upon associative memory in monkeys: role of the hippocampus in learned action. *Quarterly Journal of Experimental Psychology* 36B: 173–221.
Gainotti G (2012). Unconscious processing of emotions and the right hemisphere. *Neuropsychologia* 50: 205–218.
Gallagher HL & Frith CD (2003). Functional imaging of 'theory of mind'. *Trends in Cogntive Neuroscience* 7: 77–83.
Gallagher M (2000). The amygdala and associative learning. In Aggleton JP, editor, *The Amygdala: a Functional Analysis*, chap. 6, 213–287. Oxford University Press, Oxford, 2nd edn.
Gallagher M & Holland PC (1992). Understanding the function of the central nucleus: is simple conditioning enough? In Aggleton JP, editor, *The Amygdala: Neurobiological Aspects of Emotion, Memory, and Mental Dysfunction*, 307–321. Wiley-Liss, New York.
Gallagher M & Holland PC (1994). The amygdala complex: multiple roles in associative learning and attention. *Proceedings of the National Academy of Sciences USA* 91: 11771–11776.
Gallistel CR & Beagley G (1971). Specificity of brain-stimulation reward in the rat. *Journal of Comparative and Physiological Psychology* 76: 199–205.
Gallo M, Gamiz F, Perez-Garcia M, Del Moral RG, & Rolls ET (2013). Taste and olfactory status in a gourmand with a right amygdala lesion. *Neurocase* doi: 10.1080/13554794.2013.791862.
Gangestad SW & Simpson JA (2000). The evolution of human mating: trade-offs and strategic pluralism. *Behavioural and Brain Sciences* 23: 573–644.
Gangestad SW & Thornhill R (1999). Individual differences in developmental precision and fluctuating asymmetry: a model and its implications. *Journal of Evolutionary Biology* 12: 402–416.
Garcia J (1989). Food for Tolman: cognition and cathexis in context. In Archer T & Nilsson LG, editors, *Aversion, Avoidance and Anxiety*, 45–85. Erlbaum, Hillsdale, NJ.
Garcia JR, MacKillop J, Aller EL, Merriwether AM, Wilson DS, & Lum JK (2010). Associations between dopamine d4 receptor gene variation with both infidelity and sexual promiscuity. *PLoS ONE* 5: e14162.
Gardiner CW (1985). *Handbook of Stochastic Methods.* Springer, New York.
Gardner E (1988). The space of interactions in neural network models. *Journal of Physics A* 21: 257–270.
Gawin FH (1991). Cocaine addiction: psychology and neurophysiology. *Science* 251: 1580–1586.
Gazzaniga MS (1988). Brain modularity: towards a philosophy of conscious experience. In Marcel AJ & Bisiach E, editors, *Consciousness in Contemporary Science*, chap. 10, 218–238. Oxford University Press, Oxford.
Gazzaniga MS (1995). Consciousness and the cerebral hemispheres. In Gazzaniga MS, editor, *The Cognitive Neurosciences*, chap. 92, 1392–1400. MIT Press, Cambridge, MA.
Gazzaniga MS & LeDoux J (1978). *The Integrated Mind.* Plenum, New York.
Ge T, Feng J, Grabenhorst F, & Rolls ET (2012). Componential Granger causality, and its application to identifying the source and mechanisms of the top-down biased activation that controls attention to affective vs sensory processing. *Neuroimage* 59: 1846–1858.
Gemba H, Sasaki K, & Brooks VB (1986). Error potentials in limbic cortex (anterior cingulate area 24) of monkeys during motor learning. *Neuroscience Letters* 8: 223–227.
Gennaro RJ (2004). *Higher Order Theories of Consciousness.* John Benjamins, Amsterdam.
George MS, Ketter TA, Parekh PI, Herscovitch P, & Post RM (1996). Gender differences in regional cerebral blood flow during transient self-induced sadness or happiness. *Biological Psychiatry* 40: 859–871.
Georges-François P, Rolls ET, & Robertson RG (1999). Spatial view cells in the primate hippocampus: allocentric view not head direction or eye position or place. *Cerebral Cortex* 9: 197–212.
Georgiadis JR & Kringelbach ML (2012). The human sexual response cycle: brain imaging evidence linking sex to other pleasures. *Progress in Neurobiology* 98: 49–81.
Georgiadis JR, Kortekaas R, Kuipers R, Nieuwenburg A, Pruim J, Reinders AA, & Holstege G (2006). Regional cerebral blood flow changes associated with clitorally induced orgasm in healthy women. *European Journal of Neuroscience* 24: 3305–3316.
Gerfen CR & Surmeier DJ (2011). Modulation of striatal projection systems by dopamine. *Annual Reviews of Neuroscience* 34: 441–466.
Gerstner W, Kreiter AK, Markram H, & Herz AV (1997). Neural codes: firing rates and beyond. *Proceedings of the National Academy of Sciences USA* 94: 12740–12741.
Gewirtz JC & Davis M (1998). Application of Pavlovian higher-order conditioning to the analysis of the neural

substrates of fear conditioning. *Neuropharmacology* 37: 453–459.
Ghashghaei HT & Barbas H (2002). Pathways for emotion: interactions of prefrontal and anterior temporal pathways in the amygdala of the rhesus monkey. *Neuroscience* 115: 1261–1279.
Gibbs J, Fauser DJ, Rowe EA, Rolls BJ, Rolls ET, & Maddison SP (1979). Bombesin suppresses feeding in rats. *Nature* 282: 208–210.
Gibbs J, Maddison SP, & Rolls ET (1981). Satiety role of the small intestine examined in sham-feeding rhesus monkeys. *Journal of Comparative and Physiological Psychology* 95: 1003–1015.
Gintis H (2003). The hitchhiker's guide to altruism: genes, culture, and the internalization of norms. *Journal of Theoretical Biology* 220: 407–418.
Gintis H (2007). A framework for the unification of the behavioral sciences. *Behavioral and Brain Sciences* 30: 1–16.
Gintis H (2011). Gene-culture coevolution and the nature of human sociality. *Philosophical Transactions of the Royal Society London B Biological Sciences* 366: 878–888.
Giocomo LM & Hasselmo ME (2007). Neuromodulation by glutamate and acetylcholine can change circuit dynamics by regulating the relative influence of afferent input and excitatory feedback. *Molecular Neurobiology* 36: 184–200.
Giza BK & Scott TR (1983). Blood glucose selectively affects taste-evoked activity in rat nucleus tractus solitarius. *Physiology and Behaviour* 31: 643–650.
Giza BK & Scott TR (1987a). Intravenous insulin infusions in rats decrease gustatory-evoked responses to sugars. *American Journal of Physiology* 252: R994–R1002.
Giza BK & Scott TR (1987b). Blood glucose level affects perceived sweetness intensity in rats. *Physiology and Behaviour* 41: 459–464.
Giza BK, Scott TR, & Vanderweele DA (1992). Administration of satiety factors and gustatory responsiveness in the nucleus tractus solitarius of the rat. *Brain Research Bulletin* 28: 637–639.
Giza BK, Deems RO, Vanderweele DA, & Scott TR (1993). Pancreatic glucagon suppresses gustatory responsiveness to glucose. *American Journal of Physiology* 265: R1231–7.
Glascher J, Adolphs R, Damasio H, Bechara A, Rudrauf D, Calamia M, Paul LK, & Tranel D (2012). Lesion mapping of cognitive control and value-based decision making in the prefrontal cortex. *Proceedings of the National Academy of Sciences U S A* 109: 14681–14686.
Glausier JR & Lewis DA (2013). Dendritic spine pathology in schizophrenia. *Neuroscience* doi: 10.1016/j.neuroscience.2012.04.044.
Gleen JF & Erickson RP (1976). Gastric modulation of gustatory afferent activity. *Physiology and Behaviour* 16: 561–568.
Glickman SE & Schiff BB (1967). A biological theory of reinforcement. *Psychological Review* 74: 81–109.
Glimcher P (2003). The neurobiology of visual-saccadic decision making. *Annual Review of Neuroscience* 26: 133–179.
Glimcher P (2004). *Decisions, Uncertainty, and the Brain.* MIT Press, Cambridge, MA.
Glimcher P (2005). Indeterminacy in brain and behavior. *Annual Review of Psychology* 56: 25–56.
Glimcher P (2011a). *Foundations of Neuroeconomic Analysis.* Oxford University Press, Oxford.
Glimcher PW (2011b). Understanding dopamine and reinforcement learning: the dopamine reward prediction error hypothesis. *Proceedings of the National Academy of Sciences U S A* 108 Suppl 3: 15647–15654.
Glimcher PW, Camerer CF, Fehr E, & Poldrack RA, editors (2009). *Neuroeconomics. Decision Making and the Brain.* Academic Press, London.
Glover GH (1999). Deconvolution of impulse response in event-related BOLD fMRI. *Neuroimage* 9: 416–429.
Gnadt JW & Andersen RA (1988). Memory related motor planning activity in posterior parietal cortex of macaque. *Experimental Brain Research* 70: 216–220.
Goetz AT & Shackelford TK (2009). Sexual conflict in humans: Evolutionary consequences of asymmetric parental investment and paternity uncertainty. *Animal Biology* 59: 449–456.
Goff DC & Coyle JT (2001). The emerging role of glutamate in the pathophysiology and treatment of schizophrenia. *American Journal of Psychiatry* 158: 1367–1377.
Gold J & Shadlen M (2000). Representation of a perceptual decision in developing oculomotor commands. *Nature* 404: 390–394.
Gold JI & Shadlen MN (2001). Neural computations that underlie decisions about sensory stimuli. *Trends in Cognitive Science* 5: 10–16.
Gold JI & Shadlen MN (2002). Banburismus and the brain: decoding the relationship between sensory stimuli, decisions, and reward. *Neuron* 36: 299–308.
Gold JI & Shadlen MN (2007). The neural basis of decision making. *Annual Review of Neuroscience* 30: 535–574.
Goldbach M, Loh M, Deco G, & Garcia-Ojalvo J (2008). Neurodynamical amplification of perceptual signals via system-size resonance. *Physica D* 237: 316–323.
Goldberg DE (1989). *Genetic Algorithms in Search, Optimization and Machine Learning.* Addison-Wesley Publishing Company, Inc.
Goldman PS & Nauta WJH (1977). An intricately patterned prefronto-caudate projection in the rhesus monkey.

Journal of Comparative Neurology 171: 369–386.
Goldman-Rakic P (1994). Working memory dysfunction in schizophrenia. *Journal of Neuropsychology and Clinical Neuroscience* 6: 348–357.
Goldman-Rakic P (1995). Cellular basis of working memory. *Neuron* 14: 477–485.
Goldman-Rakic PS (1996). The prefrontal landscape: implications of functional architecture for understanding human mentation and the central executive. *Philosophical Transactions of the Royal Society B* 351: 1445–1453.
Goldman-Rakic PS (1999). The physiological approach: functional architecture of working memory and disordered cognition in schizophrenia. *Biological Psychiatry* 46: 650–661.
Goleman D (1995). *Emotional Intelligence*. Bantam, New York.
Goodale MA (2004). Perceiving the world and grasping it: dissociations between conscious and unconscious visual processing. In Gazzaniga MS, editor, *The Cognitive Neurosciences III*, 1159–1172. MIT Press, Cambridge, MA.
Goodglass H & Kaplan E (1979). Assessment of cognitive deficit in brain-injured patient. In Gazzaniga MS, editor, *Handbook of Behavioural Neurobiology*, vol. 2, Neuropsychology, 3–22. Plenum, New York.
Gosnell BA & Levine AS (2009). Reward systems and food intake: role of opioids. *International Journal of Obesity (London)* 33 Suppl 2: S54–S58.
Gothard KM, Battaglia FP, Erickson CA, Spitler KM, & Amaral DG (2007). Neural responses to facial expression and face identity in the monkey amygdala. *Journal of Neurophysiology* 97: 1671–1683.
Gottfried JA, O'Doherty J, & Dolan RJ (2003). Encoding predictive reward value in human amygdala and orbitofrontal cortex. *Science* 301: 1104–1107.
Gould SJ (1985). *Ontogeny and Phylogeny*. Harvard University Press, Boston.
Gould SJ & Lewontin RC (1979). The spandrels of San Marco and the Panglossian paradigm; a critique of the adaptationist programme. *Proceedings of the Royal Society of London B* 205: 581–598.
Grabenhorst F & Rolls ET (2008). Selective attention to affective value alters how the brain processes taste stimuli. *European Journal of Neuroscience* 27: 723–729.
Grabenhorst F & Rolls ET (2009). Different representations of relative and absolute subjective value in the human brain. *Neuroimage* 48: 258–268.
Grabenhorst F & Rolls ET (2010). Attentional modulation of affective vs sensory processing: functional connectivity and a top down biased activation theory of selective attention. *Journal of Neurophysiology* 104: 1649–1660.
Grabenhorst F & Rolls ET (2011). Value, pleasure, and choice systems in the ventral prefrontal cortex. *Trends in Cognitive Sciences* 15: 56–67.
Grabenhorst F & Rolls ET (2013). The representation of oral fat texture in the human somatosensory cortex. *Human Brain Mapping* doi: 10.1002/hbm.22346.
Grabenhorst F, Rolls ET, Margot C, da Silva M, & Velazco MI (2007). How pleasant and unpleasant stimuli combine in the brain: odor combinations. *Journal of Neuroscience* 27: 13532–13540.
Grabenhorst F, Rolls ET, & Bilderbeck A (2008a). How cognition modulates affective responses to taste and flavor: top-down influences on the orbitofrontal and pregenual cingulate cortices. *Cerebral Cortex* 18: 1549–1559.
Grabenhorst F, Rolls ET, & Parris BA (2008b). From affective value to decision-making in the prefrontal cortex. *European Journal of Neuroscience* 28: 1930–1939.
Grabenhorst F, D'Souza A, Parris BA, Rolls ET, & Passingham RE (2010a). A common neural scale for the subjective value of different primary rewards. *Neuroimage* 51: 1265–1274.
Grabenhorst F, Rolls ET, Parris BA, & D'Souza A (2010b). How the brain represents the reward value of fat in the mouth. *Cerebral Cortex* 20: 1082–1091.
Grabenhorst F, Hernadi I, & Schultz W (2012). Prediction of economic choice by primate amygdala neurons. *Proceedings of the National Academy of Sciences U S A* 109: 18950–18955.
Grafen A (1990a). Biological signals as handicaps. *Journal of Theoretical Biology* 144: 517–546.
Grafen A (1990b). Sexual selection unhandicapped by the Fisher process. *Journal of Theoretical Biology* 144: 473–516.
Graham HN (1992). Green tea composition, consumption and polyphenol chemistry. *Preventative Medicine* 21: 334–350.
Gray JA (1970). The psychophysiological basis of introversion-extraversion. *Behaviour Research and Therapy* 8: 249–266.
Gray JA (1975). *Elements of a Two-Process Theory of Learning*. Academic Press, London.
Gray JA (1981). Anxiety as a paradigm case of emotion. *British Medical Bulletin* 37: 193–197.
Gray JA (1987). *The Psychology of Fear and Stress*. Cambridge University Press, Cambridge, 2nd edn.
Gray JA, Young AMJ, & Joseph MH (1997). Dopamine's role. *Science* 278: 1548–1549.
Gray MA, Beacher FD, Minati L, Nagai Y, Kemp AH, Harrison NA, & Critchley HD (2012). Emotional appraisal is influenced by cardiac afferent information. *Emotion* 12: 180–191.
Gray TS, Piechowski RA, Yracheta JM, Rittenhouse PA, Betha CL, & Van der Kar LD (1993). Ibotenic acid lesions in the bed nucleus of the stria terminalis attenuate conditioned stress-induced increases in prolactin, ACTH and corticosterone. *Neuroendocrinology* 57: 517–524.
Graybiel AM & Kimura M (1995). Adaptive neural networks in the basal ganglia. In Houk JC, Davis JL, &

Beiser DG, editors, *Models of Information Processing in the Basal Ganglia*, chap. 5, 103–116. MIT Press, Cambridge, MA.

Green D & Swets J (1966). *Signal Detection Theory and Psychophysics*. Wiley, New York.

Green MF (1996). What are the functional consequences of neurocognitive deficits in schizophrenia? *American Journal of Psychiatry* 153: 321–330.

Greenberg BD, Li Q, Lucas FR, Hu S, Sirota LA, Benjamin J, Lesch KP, Hamer D, & Murphy DL (2000). Association between the serotonin transporter promoter polymorphism and personality traits in a primarily female population sample. *American Journal of Medical Genetics* 96: 202–216.

Greenberg D, Smith GP, & Gibbs J (1990). Intraduodenal infusions of fats elicit satiety in sham-feeding rats. *American Journal of Physiology* 259: 110–118.

Griffin DR (1992). *Animal Minds*. University of Chicago Press, Chicago.

Grill HJ & Norgren R (1978). Chronically decerebrate rats demonstrate satiation but not bait shyness. *Science* 201: 267–269.

Gross CG, Bender DB, & Gerstein GL (1979). Activity of inferior temporal neurons in behaving monkeys. *Neuropsychologia* 17: 215–229.

Gross CG, Desimone R, Albright TD, & Schwartz EL (1985). Inferior temporal cortex and pattern recognition. *Experimental Brain Research* Suppl. 11: 179–201.

Grossberg S (1988). Non-linear neural networks: principles, mechanisms, and architectures. *Neural Networks* 1: 17–61.

Grossman SP (1967). *A Textbook of Physiological Psychology*. Wiley, New York.

Grossman SP (1973). *Essentials of Physiological Psychology*. Wiley, New York.

Groves PM (1983). A theory of the functional organization of the neostriatum and the neostriatal control of voluntary movement. *Brain Research Reviews* 5: 109–132.

Groves PM, Garcia-Munoz M, Linder JC, Manley MS, Martone ME, & Young SJ (1995). Elements of the intrinsic organization and information processing in the neostriatum. In Houk JC, Davis JL, & Beiser DG, editors, *Models of Information Processing in the Basal Ganglia*, chap. 4, 51–96. MIT Press, Cambridge, MA.

Grueninger WE, Kimble DP, Grueninger J, & Levine S (1965). GSR and corticosteroid response in monkeys with frontal ablations. *Neuropsychologia* 3: 205–216.

Guest S, Grabenhorst F, Essick G, Chen Y, Young M, McGlone F, de Araujo I, & Rolls ET (2007). Human cortical representation of oral temperature. *Physiology and Behavior* 92: 975–984.

Guo K, Smith C, Powell K, & Nicholls K (2012). Consistent left gaze bias in processing different facial cues. *Psychological Research* 76: 263–269.

Gurney K, Prescott TJ, & Redgrave P (2001a). A computational model of action selection in the basal ganglia I: A new functional anatomy. *Biological Cybernetics* 84: 401–410.

Gurney K, Prescott TJ, & Redgrave P (2001b). A computational model of action selection in the basal ganglia II: Analysis and simulation of behaviour. *Biological Cybernetics* 84: 411–423.

Guyenet SJ & Schwartz MW (2012). Clinical review: Regulation of food intake, energy balance, and body fat mass: implications for the pathogenesis and treatment of obesity. *Journal of Clinical Endocrinology and Metabolism* 97: 745–755.

Haber SN & Knutson B (2009). The reward circuit: linking primate anatomy and human imaging. *Neuropsychopharmacology* 35: 4–26.

Hadland KA, Rushworth MFS, Gaffan D, & Passingham RE (2003). The effect of cingulate lesions on social behaviour and emotion. *Neuropsychologia* 41: 919–931.

Hafner H, Maurer K, Loffler W, an der Heiden W, Hambrecht M, & Schultze-Lutter F (2003). Modeling the early course of schizophrenia. *Schizophrenia Bulletin* 29: 325–340.

Hahn JD & Swanson LW (2010). Distinct patterns of neuronal inputs and outputs of the juxtaparaventricular and suprafornical regions of the lateral hypothalamic area in the male rat. *Brain Research Reviews* 64: 14–103.

Haid D, Widmayer P, Voigt A, Chaudhari N, Boehm U, & Breer H (2013). Gustatory sensory cells express a receptor responsive to protein breakdown products (GPR92). *Histochemistry and Cell Biology* 140: 137–145.

Hailman JP (1967). How an instinct is learned. *Scientific American* 221(6): 98–108.

Hajnal A, Takenouchi K, & Norgren R (1999). Effect of intraduodenal lipid on parabrachial gustatory coding in awake rats. *Journal of Neuroscience* 19: 7182–7190.

Halgren E (1992). Emotional neurophysiology of the amygdala within the context of human cognition. In Aggleton JP, editor, *The Amygdala*, chap. 7, 191–228. Wiley-Liss, New York.

Hamani C, Mayberg H, Snyder B, Giacobbe P, Kennedy S, & Lozano AM (2009). Deep brain stimulation of the subcallosal cingulate gyrus for depression: anatomical location of active contacts in clinical responders and a suggested guideline for targeting. *Journal of Neurosurgery* 111: 1209–1215.

Hamani C, Mayberg H, Stone S, Laxton A, Haber S, & Lozano AM (2011). The subcallosal cingulate gyrus in the context of major depression. *Biological Psychiatry* 69: 301–308.

Hamann S & Canli T (2004). Individual differnces in emotion processing. *Current Opinion in Neurobiology* 14: 233–238.

Hamer DH & Copeland P (1998). *Living with our Genes: Why they matter more than you think*. Doubleday, New

York.
Hamilton JP, Chen MC, & Gotlib IH (2013). Neural systems approaches to understanding major depressive disorder: an intrinsic functional organization perspective. *Neurobiology of Disease* 52: 4–11.
Hamilton WD (1964). The genetical evolution of social behaviour. *Journal of Theoretical Biology* 7: 1–52.
Hamilton WD (1996). *Narrow Roads of Gene Land.* W. H. Freeman, New York.
Hamilton WD & Zuk M (1982). Heritable true fitness and bright birds: a role for parasites. *Science* 218: 384–387.
Hampton AN & O'Doherty JP (2007). Decoding the neural substrates of reward-related decision making with functional MRI. *Proceedings of the National Academy of Sciences USA* 104: 1377–1382.
Hampton RR (2001). Rhesus monkeys know when they can remember. *Proceedings of the National Academy of Sciences of the USA* 98: 5539–5362.
Hanes DP & Schall JD (1996). Neural control of voluntary movement initiation. *Science* 274: 427–430.
Harcourt AH, Harvey PH, Larson SG, & Short RV (1981). Testis weight, body weight and breeding system in primates. *Nature* 293: 55–57.
Harcourt AH, Purvis A, & Liles L (1995). Sperm competition: mating system, not breeding season, affects testes size of primates. *Functional Ecology* 9: 468–476.
Harlow CM (1986). *Learning to Love: The Selected Papers of HF Harlow.* Praeger, New York.
Harlow HF & Stagner R (1933). Psychology of feelings and emotion. *Psychological Review* 40: 84–194.
Harlow JM (1848). Passage of an iron rod though the head. *Boston Medical and Surgical Journal* 39: 389–393.
Harrison NA, Gray MA, Gianaros PJ, & Critchley HD (2010). The embodiment of emotional feelings in the brain. *Journal of Neuroscience* 30: 12878–12884.
Hasselmo ME & Bower JM (1993). Acetylcholine and memory. *Trends in Neurosciences* 16: 218–222.
Hasselmo ME & Sarter M (2011). Modes and models of forebrain cholinergic neuromodulation of cognition. *Neuropsychopharmacology* 36: 52–73.
Hasselmo ME, Rolls ET, & Baylis GC (1989a). The role of expression and identity in the face-selective responses of neurons in the temporal visual cortex of the monkey. *Behavioural Brain Research* 32: 203–218.
Hasselmo ME, Rolls ET, Baylis GC, & Nalwa V (1989b). Object-centered encoding by face-selective neurons in the cortex in the superior temporal sulcus of the monkey. *Experimental Brain Research* 75: 417–429.
Hasselmo ME, Schnell E, & Barkai E (1995). Learning and recall at excitatory recurrent synapses and cholinergic modulation in hippocampal region CA3. *Journal of Neuroscience* 15: 5249–5262.
Hatfield T, Han JS, Conley M, Gallagher M, & Holland P (1996). Neurotoxic lesions of basolateral, but not central, amygdala interfere with Pavlovian second-order conditioning and reinforcer devaluation effects. *Journal of Neuroscience* 16: 5256–5265.
Hauser MD (1996). *The Evolution of Communication.* MIT Press, Cambridge, MA.
Haxby JV, Hoffman EA, & Gobbini MI (2002). Human neural systems for face recognition and social communication. *Biological Psychiatry* 51: 59–67.
Hayden BY, Nair AC, McCoy AN, & Platt ML (2008). Posterior cingulate cortex mediates outcome-contingent allocation of behavior. *Neuron* 60: 19–25.
Hayden BY, Pearson JM, & Platt ML (2011). Neuronal basis of sequential foraging decisions in a patchy environment. *Nature Neuroscience* 14: 933–939.
Haynes JD & Rees G (2005a). Predicting the orientation of invisible stimuli from activity in human primary visual cortex. *Nature Neuroscience* 8: 686–691.
Haynes JD & Rees G (2005b). Predicting the stream of consciousness from activity in human visual cortex. *Current Biology* 15: 1301–1307.
Haynes JD & Rees G (2006). Decoding mental states from brain activity in humans. *Nature Reviews Neuroscience* 7: 523–534.
Haynes JD, Sakai K, Rees G, Gilbert S, Frith C, & Passingham RE (2007). Reading hidden intentions in the human brain. *Current Biology* 17: 323–328.
Hebb DO (1949). *The Organization of Behavior: a Neuropsychological Theory.* Wiley, New York.
Heberlein AS, Padon AA, Gillihan SJ, Farah MJ, & Fellows LK (2008). Ventromedial frontal lobe plays a critical role in facial emotion recognition. *Journal of Cognitive Neuroscience* 20: 721–733.
Hebert MA, Ardid D, Henrie JA, Tamashiro K, Blanchard DC, & Blanchard RJ (1999). Amygdala lesions produce analgesia in a novel, ethologically relevant acute pain test. *Physiology and Behavior* 67: 99–105.
Hedges JH, Gartshteyn Y, Kohn A, Rust NC, Shadlen MN, Newsome WT, & Movshon JA (2011). Dissociation of neuronal and psychophysical responses to local and global motion. *Current Biology* 21: 2023–2028.
Heekeren HR, Marrett S, Bandettini PA, & Ungerleider LG (2004). A general mechanism for perceptual decision-making in the human brain. *Nature* 431: 859–862.
Heekeren HR, Marrett S, & Ungerleider LG (2008). The neural systems that mediate human perceptual decision making. *Nature Reviews Neuroscience* 9: 467–479.
Heimer L, Switzer RD, & Van Hoesen GW (1982). Ventral striatum and ventral pallidum. Components of the motor system? *Trends in Neurosciences* 5: 83–87.
Heims HC, Critchley HD, Dolan R, Mathias CJ, & Cipolotti L (2004). Social and motivational functioning is not critically dependent on feedback of autonomic responses: neuropsychological evidence from patients with

pure autonomic failure. *Neuropsychologia* 42: 1979–1988.
Heistermann M, Ziegler T, van Schaik CP, Launhardt K, Winkler P, & Hodges JK (2001). Loss of oestrus, concealed ovulation and paternity confusion in free-ranging Hanuman langurs. *Proceedings of the Royal Society of London B* 268: 2445–2451.
Heitmann BL, Westerterp KR, Loos RJ, Sorensen TI, O'Dea K, Mc Lean P, Jensen TK, Eisenmann J, Speakman JR, Simpson SJ, Reed DR, & Westerterp-Plantenga MS (2012). Obesity: lessons from evolution and the environment. *Obesity Reviews* 13: 910–922.
Hempel CM, Hartman KH, Wang XJ, Turrigiano GG, & Nelson SB (2000). Multiple forms of short-term plasticity at excitatory synapses in rat medial prefrontal cortex. *Journal of Neurophysiology* 83: 3031–3041.
Hernandez A, Zainos A, & Romo R (2002). Temporal evolution of a decision-making process in medial premotor cortex. *Neuron* 33: 959–972.
Hertz JA, Krogh A, & Palmer RG (1991). *Introduction to the Theory of Neural Computation.* Addison-Wesley, Wokingham, UK.
Herz RS & von Clef J (2001). The influence of verbal labeling on the perception of odors: evidence for olfactory illusions? *Perception* 30: 381–391.
Herzog AG & Van Hoesen GW (1976). Temporal neocortical afferent connections to the amygdala in the rhesus monkey. *Brain Research* 115: 57–69.
Hestrin S, Sah P, & Nicoll R (1990). Mechanisms generating the time course of dual component excitatory synaptic currents recorded in hippocampal slices. *Neuron* 5: 247–253.
Heyes C (2008). Beast machines? Questions of animal consciousness. In Weiskrantz L & Davies M, editors, *Frontiers of Consciousness*, chap. 9, 259–274. Oxford University Press, Oxford.
Hick WE (1952). On the rate of gain of information. *Quarterly Journal of Experimental Psychology* 4: 11–26.
Hikosaka K & Watanabe M (2000). Delay activity of orbital and lateral prefrontal neurons of the monkey varying with different rewards. *Cerebral Cortex* 10: 263–271.
Hines M (2010). Sex-related variation in human behavior and the brain. *Trends in Cognitive Sciences* 14: 448–456.
Hladik CM (1978). Adaptive strategies of primates in relation to leaf-eating. In Montgomery GG, editor, *The Ecology of Arboreal Folivores*, 373–395. Smithsonian Institute Press, Washington, DC.
Hoebel BG (1969). Feeding and self-stimulation. *Annals of the New York Academy of Sciences* 157: 757–778.
Hoebel BG (1997). Neuroscience, and appetitive behavior research: 25 years. *Appetite* 29: 119–133.
Hoebel BG, Rada P, Mark GP, Parada M, Puig de Parada M, Pothos E, & Hernandez L (1996). Hypothalamic control of accumbens dopamine: a system for feeding reinforcement. In Bray G & Ryan D, editors, *Molecular and Genetic Aspects of Obesity*, vol. 5, 263–280. Louisiana State University Press, Baton Rouge, LA.
Hoge EA, Ivkovic A, & Fricchione GL (2012). Generalized anxiety disorder: diagnosis and treatment. *BMJ* 345: e7500.
Hohmann GW (1966). Some effects of spinal cord lesions on experienced emotional feelings. *Psychophysiology* 3: 143–156.
Holland JH (1975). *Adaptation in Natural and Artificial Systems.* The University of Michigan Press, Michigan, USA.
Holland PC & Gallagher M (1999). Amygdala circuitry in attentional and representational processes. *Trends in Cognitive Sciences* 3: 65–73.
Holland PC & Gallagher M (2003). Double disosociation of the effects of lesions of basolateral and central amygdala on conditioned stimulus-potentiated feeding and Pavlovian-instrumental transfer. *European Journal of Neuroscience* 17: 1680–1694.
Holland PC & Gallagher M (2004). Amygdala-frontal interactions and reward expectancy. *Current Opinion in Neurobiology* 14: 148–155.
Holland PC & Straub JJ (1979). Differential effects of two ways of devaluing the unconditioned stimulus after pavlovian appetitive conditioning. *Journal of Experimental Psychology* 5: 65–78.
Holman JG & Mackintosh NJ (1981). The control of appetitive instrumental responding does not depend on classical conditioning to the discriminative stimulus. *Quarterly Journal of Experimental Psychology B* 33: 21–31.
Hölscher C & Rolls ET (2002). Perirhinal cortex neuronal activity is actively related to working memory in the macaque. *Neural Plasticity* 9: 41–51.
Hölscher C, Jacob W, & Mallot HA (2003a). Reward modulates neuronal activity in the hippocampus of the rat. *Behavioural Brain Research* 142: 181–191.
Hölscher C, Rolls ET, & Xiang JZ (2003b). Perirhinal cortex neuronal activity related to long term familiarity memory in the macaque. *European Journal of Neuroscience* 18: 2037–2046.
Hopfield JJ (1982). Neural networks and physical systems with emergent collective computational abilities. *Proceedings of the National Academy of Sciences USA* 79: 2554–2558.
Hopfield JJ & Herz AV (1995). Rapid local synchronization of action potentials: toward computation with coupled integrate-and-fire neurons. *Proceedings of the National Academy of Sciences USA* 92: 6655–6662.
Hornak J, Rolls ET, & Wade D (1996). Face and voice expression identification in patients with emotional and behavioural changes following ventral frontal lobe damage. *Neuropsychologia* 34: 247–261.
Hornak J, Bramham J, Rolls ET, Morris RG, O'Doherty J, Bullock PR, & Polkey CE (2003). Changes in emotion

after circumscribed surgical lesions of the orbitofrontal and cingulate cortices. *Brain* 126: 1691–1712.
Hornak J, O'Doherty J, Bramham J, Rolls ET, Morris RG, Bullock PR, & Polkey CE (2004). Reward-related reversal learning after surgical excisions in orbitofrontal and dorsolateral prefrontal cortex in humans. *Journal of Cognitive Neuroscience* 16: 463–478.
Hornykiewicz O (1973). Dopamine in the basal ganglia: its role and therapeutic implications including the use of L-Dopa. *British Medical Bulletin* 29: 172–178.
Horvath TL (2005). The hardship of obesity: a soft-wired hypothalamus. *Nature Neuroscience* 8: 561–565.
Horvitz JC (2000). Mesolimbocortical and nigrostriatal dopamine responses to salient non-reward events. *Neuroscience* 96: 651–656.
Horwitz B & Tagamets MA (1999). Predicting human functional maps with neural net modeling. *Human Brain Mapping* 8: 137–142.
Horwitz B, Tagamets MA, & McIntosh AR (1999). Neural modeling, functional brain imaging, and cognition. *Trends in Cognitive Sciences* 3: 85–122.
Houk JC, Adams JL, & Barto AC (1995). A model of how the basal ganglia generates and uses neural signals that predict reinforcement. In Houk JC, Davies JL, & Beiser DG, editors, *Models of Information Processing in the Basal Ganglia*, chap. 13, 249–270. MIT Press, Cambridge, MA.
Houthakker HS (1950). Revealed preference and the utility function. *Economica* 17: 159–174.
Hoyle RH, Fejfar MC, & Miller JD (2000). Personality and sexual risk taking: a quantitative review. *Journal of Personality* 68: 1203–1231.
Hrdy SB (1996). The evolution of female orgasms: logic please but no atavism. *Animal Behaviour* 52: 851–852.
Hrdy SB (1999). *Mother Nature: Natural Selection and the Female of the Species*. Chatto and Windus, London.
Hughes J (1975). Isolation of an endogenous compound from the brain with pharmacological properties similar to morphine. *Brain Research* 88: 293–308.
Hughes J, Smith TW, Kosterlitz HW, Fothergill LA, Morgan BA, & Morris HR (1975). Identification of two related pentapeptides from the brain with potent opiate antagonist activity. *Nature* 258: 577–579.
Huk AC & Shadlen MN (2005). Neural activity in macaque parietal cortex reflects temporal integration of visual motion signals during perceptual decision making. *Journal of Neuroscience* 25: 10420–10436.
Hull EM, Meisel RL, & Sachs BD (2002). Male sexual behavior. In Pfaff DW, Arnold AP, Etgen AM, Fahrbach SE, & Rubin RT, editors, *Hormones, Brain and Behavior*, vol. 1, chap. 1, 3–137. Academic Press, San Diego, CA.
Humphrey NK (1980). Nature's psychologists. In Josephson BD & Ramachandran VS, editors, *Consciousness and the Physical World*, 57–80. Pergamon, Oxford.
Humphrey NK (1986). *The Inner Eye*. Faber, London.
Hunt JN (1980). A possible relation between the regulation of gastric emptying and food intake. *American Journal of Physiology* 239: G1–G4.
Hunt JN & Stubbs DF (1975). The volume and energy content of meals as determinants of gastric emptying. *Journal of Physiology* 245: 209–225.
Ikeda K (1909). On a new seasoning. *Journal of the Tokyo Chemistry Society* 30: 820–836.
Imamura K, Mataga N, & Mori K (1992). Coding of odor molecules by mitral/tufted cells in rabbit olfactory bulb. I. Aliphatic compounds. *Journal of Neurophysiology* 68: 1986–2002.
Insabato A, Pannunzi M, Rolls ET, & Deco G (2010). Confidence-related decision-making. *Journal of Neurophysiology* 104: 539–547.
Insausti R, Amaral DG, & Cowan WM (1987). The entorhinal cortex of the monkey. II. Cortical afferents. *Journal of Comparative Neurology* 264: 356–395.
Ishai A, Ungerleider LG, Martin A, & Haxby JV (2000). The representation of objects in the human occipital and temporal cortex. *Journal of Cognitive Neuroscience* 12: 35–51.
Ishizu T & Zeki S (2011). Toward a brain-based theory of beauty. *PLoS ONE* 6: e21852.
Ishizu T & Zeki S (2013). The brain's specialized systems for aesthetic and perceptual judgment. *European Journal of Neuroscience* 37: 1413–14120.
Ito M (1984). *The Cerebellum and Neural Control*. Raven Press, New York.
Ito M (1989). Long-term depression. *Annual Review of Neuroscience* 12: 85–102.
Ito M (1993a). Synaptic plasticity in the cerebellar cortex and its role in motor learning. *Canadian Journal of Neurological Science* Suppl. 3: S70–S74.
Ito M (1993b). Cerebellar mechanisms of long-term depression. In Baudry M, Thompson RF, & Davis JL, editors, *Synaptic Plasticity: Molecular, Cellular and Functional Aspects*, chap. 6, 117–128. MIT Press, Cambridge, MA.
Iversen LL, Iversen SD, Bloom FE, & Roth RH, editors (2009). *Introduction to Neuropharmacology*. Oxford University Press, Oxford.
Iversen SD (1979). Behaviour after neostriatal lesions in animals. In Divac I, editor, *The Neostriatum*, 195–210. Pergamon, Oxford.
Iversen SD (1984). Behavioural effects of manipulation of basal ganglia neurotransmitters. In *Functions of the Basal Ganglia. CIBA Foundation Symposium*, vol. 107, 183–195. Pitman, London.

Iversen SD & Mishkin M (1970). Perseverative interference in monkey following selective lesions of the inferior prefrontal convexity. *Experimental Brain Research* 11: 376–386.

Izard CE (1971). *The Face of Emotion*. Meredity, New York.

Izard CE (1993). Four systems for emotion activation: cognitive and non-cognitive processes. *Psychological Review* 100: 68–90.

Jackendoff R (2002). *Foundations of Language*. Oxford University Press, Oxford.

Jacob S, McClintock MK, Zelano B, & Ober C (2002). Paternally inherited HLA alleles are associated with women's choice of male odour. *Nature Genetics* 30: 175–179.

Jacobsen CF (1936). The functions of the frontal association areas in monkeys. *Comparative Psychology Monographs* 13: 1–60.

Jahanshahi M, Jenkins IH, Brown RG, Marsden CD, Passingham RE, & Brooks DJ (1995). Self-initiated versus externally triggered movements. I: an investigation using measurement of regional cerebral blood flow with PET and movement-related potentials in normal and Parkinson's disease subjects. *Brain* 118: 913–933.

Jahanshahi M, Dinberger G, Fuller R, & Frith CD (2000). The role of the dorsolateral prefrontal cortex in random number generation: a study with positron emission tomography. *Neuroimage* 12: 713–725.

Jahr C & Stevens C (1990). Voltage dependence of NMDA-activated macroscopic conductances predicted by single-channel kinetics. *Journal of Neuroscience* 10: 3178–3182.

James W (1884). What is an emotion? *Mind* 9: 188–205.

Jarvis CD & Mishkin M (1977). Responses of cells in the inferior temporal cortex of monkeys during visual discrimination reversals. *Society for Neuroscience Abstracts* 3: 1794.

Jenni DA & Collier G (1972). Polyandry in the American jacana. *The Auk* 89: 743–765.

Jezek K, Henriksen EJ, Treves A, Moser EI, & Moser MB (2011). Theta-paced flickering between place-cell maps in the hippocampus. *Nature* 278: 246–249.

Johansen JP, Tarpley JW, LeDoux JE, & Blair HT (2010). Neural substrates for expectation-modulated fear learning in the amygdala and periaqueductal gray. *Nature Neuroscience* 13: 979–986.

Johansen-Berg H, Gutman DA, Behrens TE, Matthews PM, Rushworth MF, Katz E, Lozano AM, & Mayberg HS (2008). Anatomical connectivity of the subgenual cingulate region targeted with deep brain stimulation for treatment-resistant depression. *Cerebral Cortex* 18: 1374–1383.

Johns T & Duquette M (1991). Detoxification and mineral supplementation as functions of geophagy. *American Journal of Clinical Nutrition* 53: 448–456.

Johnson-Laird PN (1988). *The Computer and the Mind: An Introduction to Cognitive Science*. Harvard University Press, Cambridge, MA.

Johnston VS & Franklin M (1993). Is beauty in the eyes of the beholder? *Ethology and Sociobiology* 13: 73–85.

Johnston VS, Hagel R, Franklin M, Fink B, & Grammer K (2001). Male facial attractiveness: evidence for hormone-mediated adaptive design. *Evolution and Human Behaviour* 22: 251–267.

Johnstone S & Rolls ET (1990). Delay, discriminatory, and modality specific neurons in striatum and pallidum during short-term memory tasks. *Brain Research* 522: 147–151.

Jones B & Mishkin M (1972). Limbic lesions and the problem of stimulus–reinforcement associations. *Experimental Neurology* 36: 362–377.

Jones EG & Peters A, editors (1984). *Cerebral Cortex, Functional Properties of Cortical Cells*, vol. 2. Plenum, New York.

Jones EG & Powell TPS (1970). An anatomical study of converging sensory pathways within the cerebral cortex of the monkey. *Brain* 93: 793–820.

Jones-Gotman M & Zatorre RJ (1988). Olfactory identification in patients with focal cerebral excision. *Neuropsychologia* 26: 387–400.

Jonsson FU, Olsson H, & Olsson MJ (2005). Odor emotionality affects the confidence in odor naming. *Chemical Senses* 30: 29–35.

Jouandet M & Gazzaniga MS (1979). The frontal lobes. In Gazzaniga MS, editor, *Handbook of Behavioural Neurobiology*, vol. 2, Neuropsychology, 25–59. Plenum, New York.

Julius D & Basbaum AL (2001). Molecular mechansims of nociception. *Nature* 413: 203–210.

Jurgens U (2002). Neural pathways underlying vocal control. *Neuroscience and Biobehavioral Reviews* 26: 235–258.

Kable JW & Glimcher PW (2007). The neural correlates of subjective value during intertemporal choice. *Nature Neuroscience* 10: 1625–1633.

Kable JW & Glimcher PW (2009). The neurobiology of decision: consensus and controversy. *Neuron* 63: 733–745.

Kacelnik A & Brito e Abreu F (1998). Risky choice and Weber's Law. *Journal of Theoretical Biology* 194: 289–298.

Kadohisa M, Rolls ET, & Verhagen JV (2004). Orbitofrontal cortex neuronal representation of temperature and capsaicin in the mouth. *Neuroscience* 127: 207–221.

Kadohisa M, Rolls ET, & Verhagen JV (2005a). The primate amygdala: neuronal representations of the viscosity, fat texture, grittiness and taste of foods. *Neuroscience* 132: 33–48.

Kadohisa M, Rolls ET, & Verhagen JV (2005b). Neuronal representations of stimuli in the mouth: the primate insular taste cortex, orbitofrontal cortex, and amygdala. *Chemical Senses* 30: 401–419.

Kagan J (1966). Reflection-impulsivity: the generality of dynamics of conceptual tempo. *Journal of Abnormal*

Psychology 1: 917–924.
Kagel JH, Battalio RC, & Green L (1995). *Economic Choice Theory: An Experimental Analysis of Animal Behaviour.* Cambridge University Press, Cambridge.
Kahneman D & Tversky A (1979). Prospect theory: An analysis of decision under risk. *Econometrica* 47: 263–292.
Kahneman D & Tversky A (1984). Choices, values, and frames. *American Psychologist* 4: 341–350.
Kahneman D, Knetch JL, & Thaler RH (1990). Experimental tests of the endowment effect and tests of the Coase theorem. *Journal of Political Economy* 98: 1325–1348.
Kahneman D, Wakker PP, & Sarin R (1997). Back to Bentham? - Explorations of experienced utility. *Quarterly Journal of Economics* 112: 375–405.
Kandel ER, Schwartz JH, Jessell TM, Siegelbaum SA, & Hudspeth AJ, editors (2012). *Principles of Neural Science.* McGraw-Hill, New York, 5th edn.
Kanwisher N, McDermott J, & Chun MM (1997). The fusiform face area: a module in human extrastriate cortex specialized for face perception. *Journal of Neuroscience* 17: 4301–4311.
Kapp BS, Whalen PJ, Supple WF, & Pascoe JP (1992). Amygdaloid contributions to conditioned arousal and sensory information processing. In Aggleton JP, editor, *The Amygdala*, chap. 8, 229–245. Wiley-Liss, New York.
Kappeler PM & van Schaik CP (2004). Sexual selection in primates: review and selective preview. In Kappeler PM & van Schaik CP, editors, *Sexual Selection in Primates*, chap. 1, 3–23. Cambridge University Press, Cambridge.
Karadi Z, Oomura Y, Nishino H, Scott TR, Lenard L, & Aou S (1990). Complex attributes of lateral hypothalamic neurons in the regulation of feeding of alert monkeys. *Brain Research Bulletin* 25: 933–939.
Karadi Z, Oomura Y, Nishino H, Scott TR, Lenard L, & Aou S (1992). Responses of lateral hypothalamic glucose-sensitive and glucose-insensitive neurons to chemical stimuli in behaving rhesus monkeys. *Journal of Neurophysiology* 67: 389–400.
Karno M, Golding JM, Sorenson SB, & Burnam MA (1988). The epidemiology of obsessive-compulsive disorder in five US communities. *Archives of General Psychiatry* 45: 1094–1099.
Katz LD (2000). Emotion, representation, and consciousness. *Behavioral and Brain Sciences* 23: 204–205.
Kawamura Y & Kare MR, editors (1992). *Umami: a Basic Taste.* Dekker, New York.
Kelley AE (1999). Neural integrative activities of nucleus accumbens subregions in relation to learning and motivation. *Psychobiology* 27: 198–213.
Kelley AE (2004a). Ventral striatal control of appetitive motivation: role in ingestive behaviour and reward-related learning. *Neuroscience and Biobehavioral Reviews* 27: 765–776.
Kelley AE (2004b). Memory and addiction: shared neural circuitry and molecular mechanisms. *Neuron* 44: 161–179.
Kelley AE & Berridge KC (2002). The neuroscience of natural rewards: relevance to addictive drugs. *Journal of Neuroscience* 22: 3306–3311.
Kelly RM & Strick PL (2004). Macro-architecture of basal ganglia loops with the cerebral cortex: use of rabies virus to reveal multisynaptic circuits. *Progress in Brain Research* 143: 449–459.
Keltikangas-Jarvinen L, Elovainio M, Kivimaki M, Lichtermann D, Ekelund J, & Peltonen L (2003). Association between the type 4 dopamine receptor gene polymorphism and novelty seeking. *Psychosomatic Medicine* 65: 471–476.
Keltner D, Oatley K, & Jenkins JM (2013). *Understanding Emotions.* Wiley-Blackwell, Hoboken, NJ, 3rd edn.
Kemp JM & Powell TPS (1970). The cortico-striate projections in the monkey. *Brain* 93: 525–546.
Kennedy DP & Adolphs R (2011). Reprint of: Impaired fixation to eyes following amygdala damage arises from abnormal bottom-up attention. *Neuropsychologia* 49: 589–595.
Kennerley SW & Wallis JD (2009). Encoding of reward and space during a working memory task in the orbitofrontal cortex and anterior cingulate sulcus. *Journal of Neurophysiology* 102: 3352–3364.
Kennerley SW, Walton ME, Behrens TE, Buckley MJ, & Rushworth MF (2006). Optimal decision making and the anterior cingulate cortex. *Nature Neuroscience* 9: 940–947.
Kennerley SW, Dahmubed AF, Lara AH, & Wallis JD (2009). Neurons in the frontal lobe encode the value of multiple decision variables. *Journal of Cognitive Neuroscience* 21: 1162–1178.
Kennerley SW, Behrens TE, & Wallis JD (2011). Double dissociation of value computations in orbitofrontal and anterior cingulate neurons. *Nature Neuroscience* 14: 1581–1589.
Kennis M, Rademaker AR, & Geuze E (2013). Neural correlates of personality: an integrative review. *Neuroscience and Biobehavioural Reviews* 37: 73–95.
Kenrick DT, DaSadalla EK, Groth G, & Trost MR (1990). Evolution, traits, and the stages of human courtship: qualifying the parental investment model. *Journal of Personality* 58: 97–116.
Kepecs A, Uchida N, Zariwala HA, & Mainen ZF (2008). Neural correlates, computation and behavioural impact of decision confidence. *Nature* 455: 227–231.
Kettlewell HBD (1955). Selection experiments on industrial melanism in the Lepidoptera. *Heredity* 9: 323–335.
Keverne EB (1995). Neurochemical changes accompanying the reproductive process; their significance for maternal care in primates and other mammals. In Pryce CR, Martin RD, & Skuse D, editors, *Motherhood in Human and Nonhuman Primates*, 69–77. Karger, Basel.
Keverne EB, Nevison CM, & Martel FL (1997). Early learning and the social bond. *Annals of the New York Academy*

of Science 807: 329–339.
Khalil H (1996). *Nonlinear Systems*. Prentice Hall, Upper Saddle River, NJ.
Kiani R & Shadlen MN (2009). Representation of confidence associated with a decision by neurons in the parietal cortex. *Science* 324: 759–764.
Kievit J & Kuypers HGJM (1975). Subcortical afferents to the frontal lobe in the rhesus monkey studied by means of retrograde horseradish peroxidase transport. *Brain Research* 85: 261–266.
Killcross S & Coutureau E (2003). Coordination of actions and habits in the medial prefrontal cortex of rats. *Cerebral Cortex* 13: 400–408.
Killcross S, Robbins TW, & Everitt BJ (1997). Different types of fear-conditioned behaviour mediated by separate nuclei within amygdala. *Nature* 388: 377–380.
Kim J & Shadlen M (1999). Neural correlates of a decision in the dorsolateral prefrontal cortex of the macaque. *Nature Neuroscience* 2: 176–185.
King BM (2006). The rise, fall, and resurrection of the ventromedial hypothalamus in the regulation of feeding behavior and body weight. *Physiology and Behavior* 87: 221–244.
Kleinfeld D (1986). Sequential state generation by model neural networks. *Proceedings of the National Academy of Sciences of the USA* 83: 9469–9473.
Kling A & Steklis HD (1976). A neural substrate for affiliative behavior in nonhuman primates. *Brain, Behavior, and Evolution* 13: 216–238.
Kling AS & Brothers LA (1992). The amygdala and social behavior. In Aggleton JP, editor, *The Amygdala*, chap. 13, 353–377. Wiley-Liss, New York.
Kluger AN, Siegfried Z, & Ebstein RP (2002). A meta-analysis of the association between DRD4 polymorphism and novelty seeking. *Molecular Psychiatry* 7: 712–717.
Kluver H & Bucy PC (1939). Preliminary analysis of functions of the temporal lobe in monkeys. *Archives of Neurology and Psychiatry* 42: 979–1000.
Knutson B, Adams CM, Fong GW, & Hommer D (2001). Anticipation of increasing monetary reward selectively recruits nucleus accumbens. *Journal of Neuroscience* 21: 1–5.
Knutson B, Delgado MR, & Phillips EM (2009). Representation of subjective value in the striatum. In Glimcher PW, Camerer CF, Fehr E, & Poldrack RA, editors, *Neuroeconomics. Decision Making and the Brain*, chap. 25, 389–406. Academic Press, London.
Kobayashi S (2012). Organization of neural systems for aversive information processing: pain, error, and punishment. *Frontiers in Neuroscience* 6: 136.
Kobayashi S, Pinto de Carvalho O, & Schultz W (2010). Adaptation of reward sensitivity in orbitofrontal neurons. *Journal of Neuroscience* 30: 534–544.
Koch C (1999). *Biophysics of Computation*. Oxford University Press, Oxford.
Koch C (2004). *The Quest for Consciousness*. Roberts, Englewood, CO.
Kohonen T (1977). *Associative Memory: A System Theoretical Approach*. Springer, New York.
Kohonen T (1989). *Self-Organization and Associative Memory*. Springer-Verlag, Berlin, 3rd edn.
Kokko H, Brooks R, McNamara JM, & Houston AI (2002). The sexual selection continuum. *Proceedings of the Royal Society of London B* 269: 1331–1340.
Kokko H, Brooks R, Jennions MD, & Morley J (2003). The evolution of mate choice and mating biases. *Proceedings of the Royal Society of London B* 270: 653–664.
Kolb B & Whishaw IQ (2008). *Fundamentals of Human Neuropsychology*. Worth, New York, 6th edn.
Konorski J (1967). *Integrative Activity of the Brain: An Interdisciplinary Approach*. University of Chicago Press, Chicago.
Koob GF (1992). Dopamine, addiction and reward. *Seminars in the Neurosciences* 4: 139–148.
Koob GF (1996). Hedonic valence, dopamine and motivation. *Molecular Psychiatry* 1: 186–189.
Koob GF & Le Moal M (1997). Drug abuse: hedonic homeostatic dysregulation. *Science* 278: 52–58.
Kosar E, Grill HJ, & Norgren R (1986). Gustatory cortex in the rat. II. Thalamocortical projections. *Brain Research* 379: 342–352.
Koski L & Paus T (2000). Functional connectivity of anterior cingulate cortex within human frontal lobe: a brain mapping meta-analysis. *Experimental Brain Research* 133: 55–65.
Kowalska DM, Bachevalier J, & Mishkin M (1991). The role of the inferior prefrontal convexity in performance of delayed nonmatching-to-sample. *Neuropsychologia* 29: 583–600.
Kralik JD & Hauser MD (2000). A taste of things to come. *Behavioral and Brain Sciences* 23: 207–208.
Kraut RE & Johnson RE (1979). Social and emotional messages of smiling: an ethological approach. *Journal of Personality and Social Psychology* 37: 1539–1553.
Krebs JR & Davies NB (1991). *Behavioural Ecology*. Blackwell, Oxford, 3rd edn.
Krebs JR & Kacelnik A (1991). Decision making. In Krebs JR & Davies NB, editors, *Behavioural Ecology*, chap. 4, 105–136. Blackwell, Oxford, 3rd edn.
Kreps DM (1990). *A Course in Microeconomic Theory*. Princeton University Press, Princeton, N.J.
Krettek JE & Price JL (1974). A direct input from the amygdala to the thalamus and the cerebral cortex. *Brain Research* 67: 169–174.

Krettek JE & Price JL (1977). The cortical projections of the mediodorsal nucleus and adjacent thalamic nuclei in the rat. *Journal of Comparative Neurology* 171: 157–192.
Kringelbach ML & Rolls ET (2003). Neural correlates of rapid reversal learning in a simple model of human social interaction. *Neuroimage* 20: 1371–1383.
Kringelbach ML & Rolls ET (2004). The functional neuroanatomy of the human orbitofrontal cortex: evidence from neuroimaging and neuropsychology. *Progress in Neurobiology* 72: 341–372.
Kringelbach ML, O'Doherty J, Rolls ET, & Andrews C (2003). Activation of the human orbitofrontal cortex to a liquid food stimulus is correlated with its subjective pleasantness. *Cerebral Cortex* 13: 1064–1071.
Krolak-Salmon P, Henaff MA, Isnard J, Tallon-Baudry C, Guenot M, Vighetto A, Bertrand O, & Mauguiere F (2003). An attention modulated response to disgust in human ventral anterior insula. *Annals of Neurology* 53: 446–453.
Krug R, Plihal W, Fehm HL, & Born J (2000). Selective influence of the menstrual cycle on perception of stimuli with reproductive significance: an event-related potential study. *Psychophysiology* 37: 111–122.
Kruger TH, Haake P, Chereath D, Knapp W, Janssen OE, Exton MS, Schedlowski M, & Hartmann U (2003). Specificity of the neuroendocrine response to orgasm during sexual arousal in men. *Journal of Endocrinology* 177: 57–64.
Kuhar MJ, Pert CB, & Snyder SH (1973). Regional distribution of opiate receptor binding in monkey and human brain. *Nature* 245: 447–450.
Kuhn R (1990). Statistical mechanics of neural networks near saturation. In Garrido L, editor, *Statistical Mechanics of Neural Networks*. Springer-Verlag, Berlin.
Kuhn R, Bos S, & van Hemmen JL (1991). Statistical mechanics for networks of graded response neurons. *Physical Review A* 243: 2084–2087.
Kupferman I (2000). Reward: Wanted - a better definition. *Behavioral and Brain Sciences* 23: 208.
Kyl-Heku LM & Buss DM (1996). Tactics as units of analysis in personality psychology: an illustration using tactics of hierarchy negotiation. *Personality and Individual Differences* 21: 497–517.
LaBar KS, Gitelman DR, Parrish TB, Kim YH, Nobre AC, & Mesulam MM (2001). Hunger selectively modulates corticolimbic activation to food stimuli in humans. *Behavioral Neuroscience* 115: 493–500.
Laibson D (1997). Golden eggs and hyperbolic discounting. *Quarterly Journal of Economics* 112: 443–477.
Laland KN & Brown GR (2002). *Sense and Nonsense. Evolutionary Perspectives on Human Behaviour*. Oxford University Press, Oxford.
Laming D (1968). *Information theory of choice reaction time*. Wiley, Chichester.
Lane RD, Sechrest L, Reidel R, Weldon V, Kaszniak A, & Schwartz GE (1996). Impaired verbal and nonverbal emotion recognition in alexithymia. *Psychosomatic Medicine* 58: 203–210.
Lane RD, Fink GR, Chau PML, & Dolan RJ (1997a). Neural activation during selective attention to subjective emotional responses. *Neuroreport* 8: 3969–3972.
Lane RD, Reiman EM, Ahern GL, Schwartz GE, & Davidson RJ (1997b). Neuroanatomical correlates of happiness, sadness, and disgust. *American Journal of Psychiatry* 154: 926–933.
Lane RD, Reiman EM, Bradley MM, Lang PJ, Ahern GL, Davidson RJ, & Schwartz GE (1997c). Neuroanatomical correlates of pleasant and unpleasant emotion. *Neuropsychologia* 35: 1437–1444.
Lane RD, Reiman E, Axelrod B, Yun LS, Holmes AH, & Schwartz G (1998). Neural correlates of levels of emotional awareness. Evidence of an interaction between emotion and attention in the anterior cingulate cortex. *Journal of Cognitive Neuroscience* 10: 525–535.
Lange C (1885). The emotions. In Dunlap E, editor, *The Emotions*. Williams and Wilkins, Baltimore, 1922nd edn.
Langlois JH, Roggman LA, Casey RJ, & Ritter JM (1987). Infant preferences for attractive faces: Rudiments of a stereotype? *Developmental Psychology* 23: 363–369.
Langlois JH, Roggman LA, & Reiser-Danner LA (1990). Infants' differential social responses to attractive and unattractive faces. *Developmental Psychology* 29: 153–159.
Langlois JH, Ritter JM, Roggman LA, & Vaughn LS (1991). Facial diversity and infant preferences for attractive faces. *Developmental Psychology* 27: 79–84.
Langlois JH, Kalakanis L, Rubenstein AJ, Larson A, Hallam M, & Smoot M (2000). Maxims or myths of beauty? A meta-analytic and theoretical review. *Psychological Bulletin* 126: 390–423.
Lanthorn T, Storm J, & Andersen P (1984). Current-to-frequency transduction in CA1 hippocampal pyramidal cells: slow prepotentials dominate the primary range firing. *Experimental Brain Research* 53: 431–443.
Lau H & Rosenthal D (2011). Empirical support for higher-order theories of conscious awareness. *Trends in Cognitive Sciences* 15: 365–373.
Lau HC, Rogers RD, & Passingham RE (2006). On measuring the perceived onsets of spontaneous actions. *Journal of Neuroscience* 26: 7265–7271.
Lawrence AD, Calder AJ, McGowan SW, & Grasby PM (2002). Selective disruption of the recogntion of facial expressions of anger. *NeuroReport* 13: 881–884.
Laxton AW, Neimat JS, Davis KD, Womelsdorf T, Hutchison WD, Dostrovsky JO, Hamani C, Mayberg HS, & Lozano AM (2013). Neuronal coding of implicit emotion categories in the subcallosal cortex in patients with depression. *Biological Psychiatry* doi: 10.1016/j.biopsych.2013.03.029.

Lazarus RS (1991). *Emotion and Adaptation.* Oxford University Press, New York.

Leak GK & Christopher SB (1982). Freudian psychoanalysis and sociobiology: a synthesis. *American Psychologist* 37: 313–322.

LeDoux JE (1987). Emotion. In Plum F & Mountcastle VB, editors, *Handbook of Physiology: The Nervous System*, vol. 5, Higher cortical functions of the brain, 419–459. American Physiological Society, Bethesda MD.

LeDoux JE (1992). Emotion and the amygdala. In Aggleton JP, editor, *The Amygdala*, chap. 12, 339–351. Wiley-Liss, New York.

LeDoux JE (1994). Emotion, memory and the brain. *Scientific American* 220 (June): 50–57.

LeDoux JE (1995). Emotion: clues from the brain. *Annual Review of Psychology* 46: 209–235.

LeDoux JE (1996). *The Emotional Brain.* Simon and Schuster, New York.

LeDoux JE (2000). The amygdala and emotion: a view through fear. In Aggleton JP, editor, *The Amygdala: a Functional Analysis*, chap. 7, 289–310. Oxford University Press, Oxford.

LeDoux JE (2008). Emotional coloration of consciousness: how feelings come about. In Weiskrantz L & Davies M, editors, *Frontiers of Consciousness*, 69–130. Oxford University Press, Oxford.

LeDoux JE (2011). Rethinking the emotional brain. *Neuron* 73: 653–676.

LeDoux JE, Iwata J, Cicchetti P, & Reis DJ (1988). Different projections of the central amygdaloid nucleus mediate autonomic and behavioral correlates of conditioned fear. *Journal of Neuroscience* 8: 2517–2529.

Lehrman DS (1965). Reproductive behavior in the ring dove. *Scientific American* 211: 48–54.

Leibowitz SF & Hoebel BG (1998). Behavioral neuroscience and obesity. In Bray GA, Bouchard C, & James PT, editors, *The Handbook of Obesity*, 313–358. Dekker, New York.

Leite FP & Ratcliff R (2010). Modeling reaction time and accuracy of multiple-alternative decisions. *Attention, Perception and Psychophysics* 72: 246–273.

LeMagnen J (1956). Hyperphagia produced in the white rat by alteration of the peripheral satiety mechanism. *Comptes Rendues Societé Biologie* 150: 32–50.

Lemus L, Hernandez A, Luna R, Zainos A, Nacher V, & Romo R (2007). Neural correlates of a postponed decision report. *Proceedings of the National Academy of Sciences (USA)* 104: 17174–17179.

Leonard CM, Rolls ET, Wilson FAW, & Baylis GC (1985). Neurons in the amygdala of the monkey with responses selective for faces. *Behavioural Brain Research* 15: 159–176.

Lesschaeve I & Noble AC (2005). Polyphenols: factors influencing their sensory properties and their effects on food and beverage preferences. *American Journal of Clinical Nutrition* 81: 330S–335S.

Levenson RW, Ekman P, & Friesen WV (1990). Voluntary facial action generates emotion-specific autonomic nervous system activity. *Psychophysiology* 27: 363–384.

Levin RJ (2002). The physiology of sexual arousal in the human female: a recreational and procreational synthesis. *Archives of Sexual Behaviour* 31: 405–411.

Levine AS & Billington CJ (2004). Opioids as agents of reward-related feeding: a consideration of the evidence. *Physiology and Behaviour* 82: 57–61.

Levy DJ & Glimcher PW (2012). The root of all value: a neural common currency for choice. *Current Opinion in Neurobiology* 22: 1027–1038.

Levy I, Snell J, Nelson AJ, Rustichini A, & Glimcher PW (2010). Neural representation of subjective value under risk and ambiguity. *J Neurophysiol* 103: 1036–1047.

Levy WB (1985). Associative changes in the synapse: LTP in the hippocampus. In Levy WB, Anderson JA, & Lehmkuhle S, editors, *Synaptic Modification, Neuron Selectivity, and Nervous System Organization*, chap. 1, 5–33. Erlbaum, Hillsdale, NJ.

Levy WB & Desmond NL (1985). The rules of elemental synaptic plasticity. In Levy WB, Anderson JA, & Lehmkuhle S, editors, *Synaptic Modification, Neuron Selectivity, and Nervous System Organization*, chap. 6, 105–121. Erlbaum, Hillsdale, NJ.

Lewis DA, Hashimoto T, & Volk DW (2005). Cortical inhibitory neurons and schizophrenia. *Nature Reviews Neuroscience* 6: 312–324.

Li CS & Cho YK (2006). Efferent projection from the bed nucleus of the stria terminalis suppresses activity of taste-responsive neurons in the hamster parabrachial nuclei. *American Journal of Physiology Regul Integr Comp Physiol* 291: R914–R926.

Li CS, Cho YK, & Smith DV (2002). Taste responses of neurons in the hamster solitary nucleus are modulated by the central nucleus of the amygdala. *Journal of Neurophysiology* 88: 2979–2992.

Li JX, Yoshida T, Monk KJ, & Katz DB (2013). Lateral hypothalamus contains two types of palatability-related taste responses with distinct dynamics. *Journal of Neuroscience* 33: 9462–9473.

Li X, Frye MA, & Shelton RC (2012). Review of pharmacological treatment in mood disorders and future directions for drug development. *Neuropsychopharmacology* 37: 77–101.

Libet B (2002). The timing of mental events: Libet's experimental findings and their implications. *Consciousmess and Cognition* 11: 291–299; discussion 304–333.

Liddle PF (1987). The symptoms of chronic schizophrenia: a re-examination of the positive-negative dichotomy. *British Journal of Psychiatry* 151: 145–151.

Lieberman DA, editor (2000). *Learning: Behavior and Cognition.* Wadsworth, Belmont, CA.

Lieberman JA, Perkins D, Belger A, Chakos M, Jarskog F, Boteva K, & Gilmore J (2001). The early stages of schizophrenia: speculations on pathogenesis, pathophysiology, and therapeutic approaches. *Biological Psychiatry* 50: 884–897.

Liebeskind JC & Paul LA (1977). Psychological and physiological mechanisms of pain. *Annual Review of Psychology* 88: 41–60.

Liebeskind JC, Giesler GJ, & Urca G (1985). Evidence pertaining to an endogenous mechanism of pain inhibition in the central nervous system. In Zotterman Y, editor, *Sensory Functions of the Skin*. Pergamon, Oxford.

Liebman JM & Cooper SJ, editors (1989). *Neuropharmacological Basis of Reward*. Oxford University Press, Oxford.

Lim MM, Wang Z, Olazabal DE, Ren X, Terwilliger EF, & Young LJ (2004). Enhanced partner preference in a promiscuous species by manipulating the expression of a single gene. *Nature* 429: 754–757.

Lin W, Ogura T, & Kinnamon SC (2003). Responses to di-sodium guanosine 5′-monophosphate and monosodium L-glutamate in taste receptor cells of rat fungiform papillae. *Journal of Neurophysiology* 89: 1434–1439.

Lo CC & Wang XJ (2006). Cortico-basal ganglia circuit mechanism for a decision threshold in reaction time tasks. *Nature Neuroscience* 9: 956–963.

Logothetis NK (2008). What we can do and what we cannot do with fMRI. *Nature* 453: 869–878.

Logothetis NK, Pauls J, Augath M, Trinath T, & Oeltermann A (2001). Neurophysiological investigation of the basis of the fMRI signal. *Nature* 412: 150–157.

Loh M, Rolls ET, & Deco G (2007a). A dynamical systems hypothesis of schizophrenia. *PLoS Computational Biology* 3: e228. doi:10.1371/journal.pcbi.0030228.

Loh M, Rolls ET, & Deco G (2007b). Statistical fluctuations in attractor networks related to schizophrenia. *Pharmacopsychiatry* 40: S78–84.

Longtin A (1993). Stochastic resonance in neuron models. *Journal of Statistical Physics* 70: 309–327.

Lovibond PF (1983). Facilitation of instrumental behaviour by Pavlovian appetitive conditioned stimulus. *Journal of Experimental Psychology* 9: 225–247.

Lovlie H, Gillingham MAF, Worley K, Pizzari T, & Richardson DS (2013). Cryptic female choice favours sperm from major histocompatibility complex-dissimilar males. *Proceedings of the Royal Society B* 280: 20131296.

Lozano AM, Giacobbe P, Hamani C, Rizvi SJ, Kennedy SH, Kolivakis TT, Debonnel G, Sadikot AF, Lam RW, Howard AK, Ilcewicz-Klimek M, Honey CR, & Mayberg HS (2012). A multicenter pilot study of subcallosal cingulate area deep brain stimulation for treatment-resistant depression. *J Neurosurg* 116: 315–322.

Luce RD (1986). *Response Times: Their Role in Inferring Elementary Mental Organization*. Oxford University Press, New York.

Lujan JL, Chaturvedi A, Choi KS, Holtzheimer PE, Gross RE, Mayberg HS, & McIntyre CC (2013). Tractography-activation models applied to subcallosal cingulate deep brain stimulation. *Brain Stimulation* doi: 10.1016/j.brs.2013.03.008.

Luk CH & Wallis JD (2009). Dynamic encoding of responses and outcomes by neurons in medial prefrontal cortex. *Journal of Neuroscience* 29: 7526–7539.

Luk CH & Wallis JD (2013). Choice coding in frontal cortex during stimulus-guided or action-guided decision-making. *Journal of Neuroscience* 33: 1864–1871.

Lund JS, Angelucci A, & Bressloff PC (2003). Anatomical substrates for functional columns in macaque monkey primary visual cortex. *Cerebral Cortex* 13: 15–24.

Lundy J R F & Norgren R (2004). Activity in the hypothalamus, amygdala, and cortex generates bilateral and convergent modulation of pontine gustatory neurons. *Journal of Neurophysiology* 91: 1143–1157.

Luo Q, Ge T, Grabenhorst F, Feng J, & Rolls ET (2013). Attention-dependent modulation of cortical taste circuits revealed by Granger causality with signal-dependent noise. *PLoS Computational Biology* doi: 10.1371/journal.pcbi.1003265.

Lycan WG (1997). Consciousness as internal monitoring. In Block N, Flanagan O, & Guzeldere G, editors, *The Nature of Consciousness: Philosophical Debates*, 755–771. MIT Press, Cambridge, MA.

Lyness WH, Friedle NM, & Moore KE (1980). Destruction of dopaminergic nerve terminals in nucleus accumbens: effect of D-amphetamine self-administration. *Pharmacology, Biochemistry, and Behavior* 11: 553–556.

Lynn R (2013). Rushton's *r–K* life history theory of race differences in penis length and circumference examined in 113 populations. *Personality and Individual Differences* 55: 261–266.

Ma WJ, Beck JM, Latham PE, & Pouget A (2006). Bayesian inference with probabilistic population codes. *Nature Neuroscience* 9: 1432–1438.

Ma WJ, Beck JM, & Pouget A (2008). Spiking networks for Bayesian inference and choice. *Current Opinion in Neurobiology* 18: 217–222.

Mackey S & Petrides M (2010). Quantitative demonstration of comparable architectonic areas within the ventromedial and lateral orbital frontal cortex in the human and the macaque monkey brains. *European Journal of Neuroscience* 32: 1940–1950.

Mackintosh NJ (1983). *Conditioning and Associative Learning*. Oxford University Press, Oxford.

Maia TV & McClelland JL (2004). A reexamination of the evidence for the somatic marker hypothesis: what participants really know in the Iowa gambling task. *Proceedings of the National Academy of Sciences* 101: 16075–16080.

Maia TV & McClelland JL (2005). The somatic marker hypothesis: still many questions but no answers. *Trends in Cognitive Sciences* 9: 162–164.

Maier A, Logothetis NK, & Leopold DA (2005). Global competition dictates local suppression in pattern rivalry. *Journal of Vision* 5: 668–677.

Malhotra AK, Pinals DA, Weingartner H, Sirocco K, Missar CD, Pickar D, & Breier A (1996). NMDA receptor function and human cognition: the effects of ketamine in healthy volunteers. *Neuropsychopharmacology* 14: 301–307.

Malkova L, Gaffan D, & Murray EA (1997). Excitotoxic lesions of the amygdala fail to produce impairment in visual learning for auditory secondary reinforcement but interfere with reinforcer devaluation effects in rhesus monkeys. *Journal of Neuroscience* 17: 6011–6120.

Malsburg Cvd (1990). A neural architecture for the representation of scenes. In McGaugh JL, Weinberger NM, & Lynch G, editors, *Brain Organization and Memory: Cells, Systems and Circuits*, chap. 19, 356–372. Oxford University Press, New York.

Mangia S, Giove F, Tkac I, Logothetis NK, Henry PG, Olman CA, Maraviglia B, Di Salle F, & Ugurbil K (2009). Metabolic and hemodynamic events after changes in neuronal activity: current hypotheses, theoretical predictions and in vivo NMR experimental findings. *Journal of Cerebral Blood Flow and Metabolism* 29: 441–463.

Markov NT & Kennedy H (2013). The importance of being hierarchical. *Current Opinion in Neurobiology* 23: 187–194.

Markov NT, Vezoli J, Chameau P, Falchier A, Quilodran R, Huissoud C, Lamy C, Misery P, Giroud P, Ullman S, Barone P, Dehay C, Knoblauch K, & Kennedy H (2013). The anatomy of hierarchy: Feedforward and feedback pathways in macaque visual cortex. *Journal of Compparative Neurology* doi: 10.1002/cne.23458.

Markram H & Siegel M (1992). The inositol 1,4,5-triphosphate pathway mediates cholinergic potentiation of rat hippocampal neuronal responses to NMDA. *Journal of Physiology* 447: 513–533.

Markram H & Tsodyks M (1996). Redistribution of synaptic efficacy between neocortical pyramidal neurons. *Nature* 382: 807–810.

Markram H, Lübke J, Frotscher M, & Sakmann B (1997). Regulation of synaptic efficacy by coincidence of postsynaptic APs and EPSPs. *Science* 275: 213–215.

Markram H, Pikus D, Gupta A, & Tsodyks M (1998). Information processing with frequency-dependent synaptic connections. *Neuropharmacology* 37: 489–500.

Marshall J (1951). Sensory disturbances in cortical wounds with special reference to pain. *Journal of Neurology, Neurosurgery and Psychiatry* 14: 187–204.

Marshall JF, Richardson JS, & Teitelbaum P (1974). Nigrostriatal bundle damage and the lateral hypothalamic syndrome. *Journal of Comparative and Physiological Psychology* 87: 808–830.

Marti D, Deco G, Del Giudice P, & Mattia M (2006). Reward-biased probabilistic decision-making: mean-field predictions and spiking simulations. *Neurocomputing* 39: 1175–1178.

Marti D, Deco G, Mattia M, Gigante G, & Del Giudice P (2008). A fluctuation-driven mechanism for slow decision processes in reverberant networks. *PLoS ONE* 3: e2534. doi:10.1371/journal.pone.0002534.

Martin SJ, Grimwood PD, & Morris RG (2000). Synaptic plasticity and memory: an evaluation of the hypothesis. *Annual Review of Neuroscience* 23: 649–711.

Martinez-Garcia M, Rolls ET, Deco G, & Romo R (2011). Neural and computational mechanisms of postponed decisions. *Proceedings of the National Academy of Sciences* 108: 11626–11631.

Masquelier T, Albantakis L, & Deco G (2011). The timing of vision - how neural processing links to different temporal dynamics. *Frontiers in Psychology* 2: 151.

Matsumoto K, Suzuki W, & Tanaka K (2003). Neuronal correlates of goal-based motor selection in the prefrontal cortex. *Science* 301: 229–232.

Matsumoto M & Hikosaka O (2009). Two types of dopamine neuron distinctly convey positive and negative motivational signals. *Nature* 459: 837–841.

Matsumoto M, Matsumoto K, Abe H, & Tanaka K (2007). Medial prefrontal selectivity signalling prediction errors of action values. *Nature Neuroscience* 10: 647–656.

Matthews G & Gilliland K (1999). The personality theories of H.J.Eysenck and J.A.Gray: a comparative review. *Personality and Individual Differences* 26: 583–626.

Matthews G, Zeidner M, & Roberts RD (2002). *Emotional Intelligence: Science and Myth.* MIT Press, Cambridge, MA.

Mayberg HS (1997). Limbic-cortical dysregulation: a proposed model of depression. *Journal of Neuropsychiatry* 9: 471–481.

Mayberg HS (2003). Positron emission tomography imaging in depression: a neural systems perspective. *Neuroimaging Clinics of North America* 13: 805–815.

Mayberg HS, Brannan SK, Mahurin RK, Jerabek PA, Brickman JS, Tekell JL, Silva JA, McGinnis S, Glass TG, Martin CC, & Fox PT (1997). Cingulate function in depression: a potential predictor of treatment response. *NeuroReport* 8: 1057–1061.

Mayberg HS, Liotti M, Brannan SK, McGinnis S, Mahurin RK, Jerabek PA, Silva JA, Tekell JL, Martin CC, Lancaster

JL, & Fox PT (1999). Reciprocal limbic-cortical function and negative mood: converging PET findings in depression and normal sadness. *American Journal of Psychiatry* 156: 675–682.

Mayberg HS, Lozano AM, Voon V, McNeely HE, Seminowicz D, Hamani C, Schwalb JM, & Kennedy SH (2005). Deep brain stimulation for treatment-resistant depression. *Neuron* 45: 651–660.

Mayer JD, Roberts RD, & Barsade SG (2008). Human abilities: emotional intelligence. *Annual Review of Psychology* 59: 507–536.

Maynard Smith J (1982). *Evolution and the Theory of Games*. Cambridge University Press, Cambridge.

Maynard Smith J (1984). Game theory and the evolution of behaviour. *Behavioral and Brain Sciences* 7: 95–125.

Maynard Smith J & Harper D (2003). *Animal Signals*. Oxford University Press, Oxford.

Mayr E (1961). Cause and effect in biology. *Science* 134: 1501–1506.

Mazur JE (2012). *Learning and Behavior*. Pearson, Boston, MA, 7th edn.

Mazurek ME, Roitman JD, Ditterich J, & Shadlen MN (2003). A role for neural integrators in perceptual decision making. *Cerebral Cortex* 13: 1257–1269.

McCabe C & Rolls ET (2007). Umami: a delicious flavor formed by convergence of taste and olfactory pathways in the human brain. *European Journal of Neuroscience* 25: 1855–1864.

McCabe C, Rolls ET, Bilderbeck A, & McGlone F (2008). Cognitive influences on the affective representation of touch and the sight of touch in the human brain. *Social, Cognitive and Affective Neuroscience* 3: 97–108.

McClelland JL & Rumelhart DE (1986). A distributed model of human learning and memory. In McClelland JL & Rumelhart DE, editors, *Parallel Distributed Processing*, vol. 2, chap. 17, 170–215. MIT Press, Cambridge, MA.

McClure SM, Berns GS, & Montague PR (2003). Temporal prediction errors in a passive learning task activate human striatum. *Neuron* 38: 339–346.

McClure SM, Laibson DI, Loewenstein G, & Cohen JD (2004). Separate neural systems value immediate and delayed monetary rewards. *Science* 306: 503–507.

McCormick D, Connors B, Lighthall J, & Prince D (1985). Comparative electrophysiology of pyramidal and sparsely spiny stellate neurons in the neocortex. *Journal of Neurophysiology* 54: 782–806.

McCoy AN & Platt ML (2005a). Expectations and outcomes: decision-making in the primate brain. *Journal of Comparative Physiology A* 191: 201–211.

McCoy AN & Platt ML (2005b). Risk-sensitive neurons in macaque posterior cingulate cortex. *Nature Neuroscience* 8: 1220–1227.

McDonald AJ (1992). Cell types and intrinsic connections to the amygdala. In Aggleton JP, editor, *The Amygdala*, chap. 2, 67–96. Wiley-Liss, New York.

McFadden D (1974). Conditional logit analysis of qualitative choice behavior 105–142.

McFarland DJ & Sibly RM (1975). The behavioural final common path. *Philosophical Transactions of the Royal Society of London B Biological Science* 270: 265–293.

McGinty D & Szymusiak R (1988). Neuronal unit activity patterns in behaving animals: brainstem and limbic system. *Annual Review of Psychology* 39: 135–168.

McLeod P, Plunkett K, & Rolls ET (1998). *Introduction to Connectionist Modelling of Cognitive Processes*. Oxford University Press, Oxford.

McMillen T & Holmes P (2006). The dynamics of choice among multiple alternatives. *Journal of Mathematical Psychology* 50: 30–57.

Mei N (1993). Gastrointestinal chemoreception and its behavioural role. In Booth DA, editor, *The Neurophysiology of Ingestion*, chap. 4, 47–56. Manchester University Press, Manchester.

Mei N (1994). Role of digestive afferents in food intake regulation. In Legg CR & Booth DA, editors, *Appetite, Neural and Behavioural Bases*, chap. 4, 86–97. Oxford University Press, Oxford.

Melzack R & Wall PD (1996). *The Challenge of Pain*. Penguin, Harmondsworth, UK.

Mende-Siedlecki P, Said CP, & Todorov A (2013). The social evaluation of faces: a meta-analysis of functional neuroimaging studies. *Social Cognitive and Affective Neuroscience* 8: 285–299.

Mendez MF (2009). The neurobiology of moral behavior: review and neuropsychiatric implications. *CNS Spectrums* 14: 608–620.

Menon V & Uddin LQ (2010). Saliency, switching, attention and control: a network model of insula function. *Brain Structure and Function* 214: 655–667.

Menzies L, Chamberlain SR, Laird AR, Thelen SM, Sahakian BJ, & Bullmore ET (2008). Integrating evidence from neuroimaging and neuropsychological studies of obsessive-compulsive disorder: The orbitofronto-striatal model revisited. *Neuroscience and Biobehavioral Reviews* 32: 525–549.

Meredith M (2001). Human vomeronasal organ function: a critical review of best and worst cases. *Chemical Senses* 26: 433–445.

Meston CM & Frohlich PF (2000). The neurobiology of sexual function. *Archives of General Psychiatry* 57: 1012–1030.

Mesulam MM (1990). Human brain cholinergic pathways. *Progress in Brain Research* 84: 231–241.

Mesulam MM & Mufson EJ (1982a). Insula of the Old World monkey. I: Architectonics in the insulo-orbito-temporal component of the paralimbic brain. *Journal of Comparative Neurology* 212: 1–22.

Mesulam MM & Mufson EJ (1982b). Insula of the Old World monkey. III. Efferent cortical output and comments on function. *Journal of Comparative Neurology* 212: 38–52.

Metcalfe J & Mischel W (1999). A hot/cool-system analysis of delay of gratification: dynamics of willpower. *Psychological Review* 106: 3–19.

Meunier M, Bachevalier J, & Mishkin M (1997). Effects of orbital frontal and anterior cingulate lesions on object and spatial memory in rhesus monkeys. *Neuropsychologia* 35: 999–1015.

Middleton FA & Strick PL (1994). Anatomical evidence for cerebellar and basal ganglia involvement in higher cognitive function. *Science* 266: 458–461.

Middleton FA & Strick PL (1996a). The temporal lobe is a target of output from the basal ganglia. *Proceedings of the National Academy of Sciences of the USA* 93: 8683–8687.

Middleton FA & Strick PL (1996b). New concepts about the organization of the basal ganglia. In Obeso JA, editor, *Advances in Neurology: The Basal Ganglia and the Surgical Treatment for Parkinson's Disease*. Raven, New York.

Middleton FA & Strick PL (2000). Basal ganglia output and cognition: evidence from anatomical, behavioral, and clinical studies. *Brain and Cognition* 42: 183–200.

Millenson JR (1967). *Principles of Behavioral Analysis*. MacMillan, New York.

Miller EK (2000a). The prefrontal cortex and cognitive control. *Nature Reviews Neuroscience* 1: 59–65.

Miller EK & Cohen JD (2001). An integrative theory of prefrontal cortex function. *Annual Review of Neuroscience* 24: 167–202.

Miller EK & Desimone R (1994). Parallel neuronal mechanisms for short-term memory. *Science* 263: 520–522.

Miller EK, Li L, & Desimone R (1993). Activity of neurons in anterior inferior temporal cortex during a short-term memory task. *Journal of Neuroscience* 13: 1460–1478.

Miller EK, Erickson C, & Desimone R (1996). Neural mechanisms of visual working memory in prefrontal cortex of the macaque. *Journal of Neuroscience* 16: 5154–5167.

Miller GA (1956). The magic number seven, plus or minus two: some limits on our capacity for the processing of information. *Psychological Review* 63: 81–93.

Miller GF (2000b). *The Mating Mind*. Heinemann, London.

Miller KD (1992). Development of orientation columns via competition between ON– and OFF–center inputs. *NeuroReport* 3: 73–76.

Millhouse OE (1986). The intercalated cells of the amygdala. *Journal of Comparative Neurology* 247: 246–271.

Millhouse OE & DeOlmos J (1983). Neuronal configuration in lateral and basolateral amygdala. *Neuroscience* 10: 1269–1300.

Millikan RG (1984). *Language, Thought, and Other Biological Categories: New Foundation for Realism*. MIT Press, Cambridge, MA.

Milner A (2008). Conscious and unconscious visual processing in the human brain. In Weiskrantz L & Davies M, editors, *Frontiers of Consciousness*, chap. 5, 169–214. Oxford University Press, Oxford.

Milner AD & Goodale MA (1995). *The Visual Brain in Action*. Oxford University Press, Oxford.

Milner B (1963). Effects of different brain lesions on card sorting. *Archives of Neurology* 9: 90–100.

Milner B (1982). Some cognitive effects of frontal-lobe lesions in man. *Philosophical Transactions of the Royal Society B* 298: 211–226.

Milton AL, Lee JL, Butler VJ, Gardner R, & Everitt BJ (2008). Intra-amygdala and systemic antagonism of NMDA receptors prevents the reconsolidation of drug-associated memory and impairs subsequently both novel and previously acquired drug-seeking behaviors. *Journal of Neuroscience* 28: 8230–8237.

Minai AA & Levy WB (1993). Sequence learning in a single trial. *International Neural Network Society World Congress of Neural Networks* 2: 505–508.

Mirenowicz J & Schultz W (1996). Preferential activation of midbrain dopamine neurons by appetitive rather than aversive stimuli. *Nature* 279: 449–451.

Mishkin M & Aggleton J (1981). Multiple functional contributions of the amygdala in the monkey. In Ben-Ari Y, editor, *The Amygdaloid Complex*, 409–420. Elsevier, Amsterdam.

Mishkin M & Manning FJ (1978). Non-spatial memory after selective prefrontal lesions in monkeys. *Brain Research* 143: 313–324.

Miyashita Y & Chang HS (1988). Neuronal correlate of pictorial short-term memory in the primate temporal cortex. *Nature* 331: 68–70.

Miyashita Y, Rolls ET, Cahusac PMB, Niki H, & Feigenbaum JD (1989). Activity of hippocampal neurons in the monkey related to a conditional spatial response task. *Journal of Neurophysiology* 61: 669–678.

Moller AP & Thornhill R (1998). Male parental care, differential parental investment by females and sexual selection. *Animal Behaviour* 55: 1507–1515.

Mombaerts P (2006). Axonal wiring in the mouse olfactory system. *Annual Review of Cell and Developmental Biology* 22: 713–737.

Mongillo G, Barak O, & Tsodyks M (2008). Synaptic theory of working memory. *Science* 319: 1543–1546.

Moniz E (1936). *Tentatives Opératoires dans le Traitment de Certaines Psychoses*. Masson, Paris.

Montague PR & Berns GS (2002). Neural economics and the biological substrates of valuation. *Neuron* 36: 265–284.

Montague PR, King-Casas B, & Cohen JD (2006). Imaging valuation models in human choice. *Annual Review of Neuroscience* 29: 417–448.

Monti-Bloch L, Jennings-White C, Dolberg DS, & Berliner DL (1994). The human vomeronasal system. *Psychoneuroendocrinology* 19: 673–686.

Monti-Bloch L, Jennings-White C, & Berliner DL (1998). The human vomeronasal system: a review. *Annals of the New York Academy of Science* 855: 373–389.

Moore HDM, Martin M, & Birkhead TR (1999). No evidence for killer sperm or other selective interactions between human spermatozoa in ejaculates of different males in vitro. *Procedings of the Royal Society of London B* 266: 2343–2350.

Moore HDM, Dvorakova K, Jenkins N, & Breed W (2002). Exceptional sperm cooperation in the wood mouse. *Nature* 418: 174–177.

Moors A, Ellsworth PC, Scherer, & Frijda NH (2013). Appraisal theories of emotion: state of the art and future development. *Emotion Review* 5: 119–124.

Mora F, Sanguinetti AM, Rolls ET, & Shaw SG (1975). Differential effects on self-stimulation and motor behaviour produced by microintracranial injections of a dopamine-receptor blocking agent. *Neuroscience Letters* 1: 179–184.

Mora F, Rolls ET, & Burton MJ (1976a). Modulation during learning of the responses of neurones in the lateral hypothalamus to the sight of food. *Experimental Neurology* 53: 508–519.

Mora F, Rolls ET, Burton MJ, & Shaw SG (1976b). Effects of dopamine-receptor blockade on self-stimulation in the monkey. *Pharmacology, Biochemistry and Behavior* 4: 211–216.

Mora F, Mogenson GJ, & Rolls ET (1977). Activity of neurones in the region of the substantia nigra during feeding. *Brain Research* 133: 267–276.

Mora F, Avrith DB, Phillips AG, & Rolls ET (1979). Effects of satiety on self-stimulation of the orbitofrontal cortex in the monkey. *Neuroscience Letters* 13: 141–145.

Mora F, Avrith DB, & Rolls ET (1980). An electrophysiological and behavioural study of self-stimulation in the orbitofrontal cortex of the rhesus monkey. *Brain Research Bulletin* 5: 111–115.

Morecraft RJ & Tanji J (2009). Cingulofrontal interactions and the cingulate motor areas. In Vogt B, editor, *Cingulate Neurobiology and Disease*, chap. 5, 113–144. Oxford University Press, Oxford.

Morecraft RJ, Geula C, & Mesulam MM (1992). Cytoarchitecture and neural afferents of orbitofrontal cortex in the brain of the monkey. *Journal of Comparative Neurology* 323: 341–358.

Moreno-Bote R, Rinzel J, & Rubin N (2007). Noise-induced alternations in an attractor network model of perceptual bistability. *Journal of Neurophysiology* 98: 1125–1139.

Mori K & Sakano H (2011). How is the olfactory map formed and interpreted in the mammalian brain? *Annual Reviews of Neuroscience* 34: 467–499.

Mori K, Mataga N, & Imamura K (1992). Differential specificities of single mitral cells in rabbit olfactory bulb for a homologous series of fatty acid odor molecules. *Journal of Neurophysiology* 67: 786–789.

Mori K, Nagao H, & Yoshihara Y (1999). The olfactory bulb: coding and processing of odor molecule information. *Science* 286: 711–715.

Moriguchi Y & Komaki G (2013). Neuroimaging studies of alexithymia: physical, affective, and social perspectives. *Biopsychosocial Medicine* 7: 8.

Morris JA, Jordan CL, & Breedlove MS (2004). Sexual differentiation of the vertebrate nervous system. *Nature Neuroscience* 7: 1034–1039.

Morris JS, Frith CD, Perrett DI, Rowland D, Young AW, Calder AJ, & Dolan RJ (1996). A differential neural response in the human amygdala to fearful and happy facial expressions. *Nature* 383: 812–815.

Morris JS, De Gelder B, Weiskrantz L, & Dolan RJ (2001). Differential extrageniculostriate and amygdala responses to presentation of emotional faces in a cortically blind field. *Brain* 124: 1241–1252.

Morris RGM (1989). Does synaptic plasticity play a role in information storage in the vertebrate brain? In Morris RGM, editor, *Parallel Distributed Processing: Implications for Psychology and Neurobiology*, chap. 11, 248–285. Oxford University Press, Oxford.

Morrot G, Brochet F, & Dubourdieu D (2001). The color of odors. *Brain and Language* 79: 309–320.

Mossman JA, Slate J, Birkhead TR, Moore HD, & Pacey AA (2013). Sperm speed is associated with sex bias of siblings in a human population. *Asian Journal of Andrology* 15: 152–154.

Mueser KT & McGurk SR (2004). Schizophrenia. *Lancet* 363: 2063–2072.

Mufson EJ & Mesulam MM (1982). Insula of the Old World monkey II: Afferent cortical input and comments on the claustrum. *Journal of Comparative Neurology* 212: 23–37.

Muir JL, Everitt BJ, & Robbins TW (1994). AMPA-induced excitotoxic lesions of the basal forebrain: a significant role for the cortical cholinergic system in attentional function. *Journal of Neuroscience* 14: 2313–2326.

Munzberg H & Myers MG (2005). Molecular and anatomical determinants of central leptin resistance. *Nature Neuroscience* 8: 566–570.

Murray EA & Izquierdo A (2007). Orbitofrontal cortex and amygdala contributions to affect and action in primates. *Annals of the New York Academy of Sciences* 1121: 273–296.

Murray EA, Gaffan EA, & Flint RW (1996). Anterior rhinal cortex and amygdala: dissociation of their contributions to memory and food preference in rhesus monkeys. *Behavioral Neuroscience* 110: 30–42.

Murray EA, Wise SP, & Rhodes SEV (2011). What can different brains do with reward? In Gottfried JA, editor, *Neurobiology of Sensation and Reward*, chap. 4. CRC Press, Boca Raton (FL).

Nagai Y, Critchley HD, Featherstone E, Trimble MR, & Dolan RJ (2004). Activity in ventromedial prefrontal cortex covaries with sympathetic skin conductance level: a physiological account of a "default mode" of brain function. *Neuroimage* 22: 243–251.

Nakahara H, Amari S, & Hikosaka O (2002). Self-organisation in the basal ganglia with modulation of reinforcement signals. *Neural Computation* 14: 819–844.

Nakamura K, Kawashima R, Ito K, Sugiura M, Kato T, Nakamura A, Hatano K, Nagumo S, Kubota K, Fukuda H, & Kojima S (1999). Activation of the right inferior frontal cortex during assessment of facial emotion. *Journal of Neurophysiology* 82: 1610–1614.

Nauta WJH (1972). Neural associations of the frontal cortex. *Acta Neurobiologica Experimentalis* 32: 125–140.

Nauta WJH & Domesick VB (1978). Crossroads of limbic and striatal circuitry: hypothalamonigral connections. In Livingston KE & Hornykiewicz O, editors, *Limbic Mechanisms*, 75–93. Plenum, New York.

Nemeroff CB (2003). The role of GABA in the pathophysiology and treatment of anxiety disorders. *Psychopharmacology Bulletin* 37: 133–146.

Nesse RM (2000a). Natural selection, mental modules and intelligence. *Novartis Foundation Symposium: The Nature of Intelligence* 233: 96–115.

Nesse RM (2000b). Is depression an adaptation? *Archives of General Psychiatry* 57: 14–20.

Nesse RM & Lloyd AT (1992). The evolution of psychodynamic mechanisms. In Barkow JH, Cosmides L, & Tooby J, editors, *The Adapted Mind*, 601–624. Oxford University Press, New York.

Newcomer JW, Farber NB, Jevtovic-Todorovic V, Selke G, Melson AK, Hershey T, Craft S, & Olney JW (1999). Ketamine-induced NMDA receptor hypofunction as a model of memory impairment and psychosis. *Neuropsychopharmacology* 20: 106–118.

Newman EL, Gupta K, Climer JR, Monaghan CK, & Hasselmo ME (2012). Cholinergic modulation of cognitive processing: insights drawn from computational models. *Frontiers in Behavioural Neuroscience* 6: 24.

Neyman J & Pearson ES (1933). On the problem of the most efficient tests of statistical hypotheses. *Philosophical Transactions of the Royal Society* 231: 289–337.

Nicholls MER, Ellis BE, Clement JG, & Yoshino M (2004). Detecting hemifacial asymmetries in emotional expression with three-dimensional computerised image analysis. *Proceedings of the Royal Society of London B* 271: 663–668.

Nicolaidis S & Rowland N (1975). Systemic vs oral and gastro-intestinal metering of fluid intake. In Peters G & Fitzsimons JT, editors, *Control Mechanisms of Drinking*, 601–624. Springer, Berlin.

Nicolaidis S & Rowland N (1976). Metering of intravenous versus oral nutrients and regulation of energy balance. *American Journal of Physiology* 231: 661–669.

Nicolaidis S & Rowland N (1977). Intravenous self-feeding: long-term regulation of energy balance in rats. *Science* 195: 589–591.

Nicoll RA & Malenka RC (1995). Contrasting properties of two forms of long-term potentiation in the hippocampus. *Nature* 377: 115–118.

Niki H & Watanabe M (1979). Prefrontal and cingulate unit activity during timing behavior in the monkey. *Brain Research* 171: 213–224.

Nishijo H, Ono T, & Nishino H (1988). Single neuron responses in amygdala of alert monkey during complex sensory stimulation with affective significance. *Journal of Neuroscience* 8: 3570–3583.

Nissen E, Uvnas-Moberg K, Svennson K, Stock S, Widstrom AM, & Winberg J (1996). Different patterns of oxytocin, prolactin but not cortisol release during breastfeeding in women delivered by caesarean section or by the vaginal route. *Early Human Development* 45: 103–118.

Niv Y, Duff MO, & Dayan P (2005). Dopamine, uncertainty, and TD learning. *Behavioral and Brain Functions* 1: 6.

Niwa M & Ditterich J (2008). Perceptual decisions between multiple directions of visual motion. *Journal of Neuroscience* 28: 4435–4445.

Noonan MP, Kolling N, Walton ME, & Rushworth MF (2012). Re-evaluating the role of the orbitofrontal cortex in reward and reinforcement. *European Journal of Neuroscience* 35: 997–1010.

Norgren R (1974). Gustatory afferents to ventral forebrain. *Brain Research* 81: 285–295.

Norgren R (1976). Taste pathways to hypothalamus and amygdala. *Journal of Comparative Neurology* 166: 17–30.

Norgren R (1984). Central neural mechanisms of taste. In Darien-Smith I, editor, *Handbook of Physiology - the Nervous System III, Sensory Processes 1*, 1087–1128. American Physiological Society, Washington, DC.

Norgren R (1990). Gustatory system. In Paxinos G, editor, *The Human Nervous System*, 845–861. Academic Press, San Diego.

Norgren R & Leonard CM (1971). Taste pathways in rat brainstem. *Science* 173: 1136–1139.

Norgren R & Leonard CM (1973). Ascending central gustatory pathways. *Journal of Comparative Neurology* 150: 217–238.

Oatley K & Jenkins JM (1996). *Understanding Emotions*. Blackwell, Oxford.

Oatley K & Johnson-Laird PN (1987). Towards a cognitive theory of emotions. *Cognition and Emotion* 1: 29–50.

Oberg RGE & Divac I (1979). "Cognitive" functions of the striatum. In Divac I & Oberg RGE, editors, *The Neostriatum*, 291–314. Pergamon, New York.

O'Brien CP, Childress AR, Ehrman R, & Robbins SJ (1998). Conditioning factors in drug abuse: can they explain compulsion? *Journal of Psychopharmacology* 12: 15–22.

Ochoa G & Jaffe K (1999). On sex, mate selection and the Red Queen. *Journal of Theoretical Biology* 199: 1–9.

Odent M (1999). *The Scientification of Love*. Free Association Books, London.

O'Doherty J, Rolls ET, Francis S, Bowtell R, McGlone F, Kobal G, Renner B, & Ahne G (2000). Sensory-specific satiety related olfactory activation of the human orbitofrontal cortex. *NeuroReport* 11: 893–897.

O'Doherty J, Kringelbach ML, Rolls ET, Hornak J, & Andrews C (2001a). Abstract reward and punishment representations in the human orbitofrontal cortex. *Nature Neuroscience* 4: 95–102.

O'Doherty J, Rolls ET, Francis S, Bowtell R, & McGlone F (2001b). The representation of pleasant and aversive taste in the human brain. *Journal of Neurophysiology* 85: 1315–1321.

O'Doherty J, Deichmann R, Critchley HD, & Dolan RJ (2002). Neural response during anticipation of a primary taste reward. *Neuron* 33: 815–826.

O'Doherty J, Dayan P, Friston KJ, Critchley HD, & Dolan RJ (2003a). Temporal difference models and reward-related learning in the human brain. *Neuron* 38: 329–337.

O'Doherty J, Winston J, Critchley HD, Perrett DI, Burt DM, & Dolan RJ (2003b). Beauty in a smile: the role of the medial orbitofrontal cortex in facial attractiveness. *Neuropsychologia* 41: 147–155.

O'Doherty J, Dayan P, Schultz J, Deichmann R, Friston K, & Dolan RJ (2004). Dissociable roles of ventral and dorsal striatum in instrumental conditioning. *Science* 304: 452–454.

O'Donoghue T & Rabin M (1999). Doing it now or later. *American Economic Review* 89: 103–124.

O'Kane D & Treves A (1992). Why the simplest notion of neocortex as an autoassociative memory would not work. *Network* 3: 379–384.

Olds J (1977). *Drives and Reinforcements: Behavioral Studies of Hypothalamic Functions*. Raven Press, New York.

Ongur D & Price JL (2000). The organisation of networks within the orbital and medial prefrontal cortex of rats, monkeys and humans. *Cerebral Cortex* 10: 206–219.

Ongur D, Ferry AT, & Price JL (2003). Architectonic subdivision of the human orbital and medial prefrontal cortex. *Journal of Comparative Neurology* 460: 425–449.

Ono T & Nishijo H (1992). Neurophysiological basis of the Kluver–Bucy syndrome: responses of monkey amygdaloid neurons to biologically significant objects. In Aggleton JP, editor, *The Amygdala*, chap. 6, 167–190. Wiley-Liss, New York.

Ono T, Nishino H, Sasaki K, Fukuda M, & Muramoto K (1980). Role of the lateral hypothalamus and amygdala in feeding behavior. *Brain Research Bulletin* 5, Suppl.: 143–149.

Ono T, Tamura R, Nishijo H, Nakamura K, & Tabuchi E (1989). Contribution of amygdala and LH neurons to the visual information processing of food and non-food in the monkey. *Physiology and Behavior* 45: 411–421.

Oomura Y & Yoshimatsu H (1984). Neural network of glucose monitoring system. *Journal of the Autonomic Nervous System* 10: 359–372.

Oomura Y, Nishino H, Karadi Z, Aou S, & Scott TR (1991). Taste and olfactory modulation of feeding related neurons in the behaving monkey. *Physiology and Behavior* 49: 943–950.

O'Rahilly S (2009). Human genetics illuminates the paths to metabolic disease. *Nature* 462: 307–314.

Orban GA (2011). The extraction of 3D shape in the visual system of human and nonhuman primates. *Annual Reviews of Neuroscience* 34: 361–388.

Oring LW (1986). Avian polyandry 3: 309–351.

Padoa-Schioppa C (2009). Range-adapting representation of economic value in the orbitofrontal cortex. *Journal of Neuroscience* 29: 14004–14014.

Padoa-Schioppa C (2011). Neurobiology of economic choice: a good-based model. *Annual Review of Neuroscience* 34: 333–359.

Padoa-Schioppa C & Assad JA (2006). Neurons in the orbitofrontal cortex encode economic value. *Nature* 441: 223–226.

Padoa-Schioppa C & Assad JA (2008). The representation of economic value in the orbitofrontal cortex is invariant for changes of menu. *Nature Neuroscience* 11: 95–102.

Pager J (1974). A selective modulation of the olfactory bulb electrical activity in relation to the learning of palatability in hungry and satiated rats. *Physiology and Behavior* 12: 189–196.

Pager J, Giachetti I, Holley A, & LeMagnen J (1972). A selective control of olfactory bulb electrical activity in relation to food deprivation and satiety in rats. *Physiology and Behavior* 9: 573–580.

Palmer J, Huk AC, & Shadlen MN (2005). The effect of stimulus strength on the speed and accuracy of a perceptual decision. *Journal of Vision* 5: 376–404.

Palomero-Gallagher N & Zilles K (2004). Isocortex. In Paxinos G, editor, *The Rat Nervous System*, 729–757. Elsevier Academic Press, San Diego.

Pandya DN (1996). Comparison of prefrontal architecture and connections. *Philosophical Transactions of the Royal Society B* 351: 1423–1432.

Panksepp J (1998). *Affective Neuroscience: The Foundations of Human and Animal Emotions*. Oxford University

Press, New York.
Panksepp J (2011a). The basic emotional circuits of mammalian brains: Do animals have affective lives? *Neuroscience and Biobehavioral Reviews* 35: 1791–1804.
Panksepp J (2011b). Cross-species affective neuroscience decoding of the primal affective experiences of humans and related animals. *PLoS One* 6: e21236.
Panksepp J, Nelson E, & Bekkedal M (1997). Brain systems for the mediation of social separation-distress and social reward. *Annals of the New York Academy of Sciences* 807: 78–100.
Panzeri S, Rolls ET, Battaglia F, & Lavis R (2001). Speed of feedforward and recurrent processing in multilayer networks of integrate-and-fire neurons. *Network: Computation in Neural Systems* 12: 423–440.
Pare D, Quirk GJ, & LeDoux JE (2004). New vistas on amygdala networks in conditioned fear. *Journal of Neurophysiology* 92: 1–9.
Pareto V (1906). *Manuel d'economie politique*. Augustus M Kelley 1971, New York.
Parker GA, Baker RR, & Smith VGF (1972). The origin and evolution of gamete dimorphism and the male-female phenomenon. *Journal of Theoretical Biology* 36: 529–553.
Parker GA, Ball MA, Stockley P, & Gage MJ (1997). Sperm competition games: a prospective analysis of risk assessment. *Proceedings of the Royal Society of London B* 264: 1793–1802.
Pascal RD (1672). *Pensees*. Penguin 1966, New York.
Passingham R (1975). Delayed matching after selective prefrontal lesions in monkeys (Macaca mulatta). *Brain Research* 92: 89–102.
Passingham REP & Wise SP (2012). *The Neurobiology of the Prefrontal Cortex*. Oxford University Press, Oxford.
Paton JJ, Belova MA, Morrison SE, & Salzman CD (2006). The primate amygdala represents the positive and negative value of visual stimuli during learning. *Nature* 439: 865–870.
Patton JH, Stanford MS, & Barratt ES (1995). Factor structure of the Barratt impulsiveness scale. *Journal of Clinical Psychology* 51: 768–774.
Pearce JM (2008). *Animal Learning and Cognition*. Psychology Press, Hove, Sussex, 3rd edn.
Peitgen HO, Jürgens H, & Saupe D (2004). *Chaos and Fractals: New Frontiers of Science*. Springer, New York.
Penn D & Potts WK (1998). Untrained mice discriminate MHC-determined odors. *Physiology and Behaviour* 64: 235–243.
Pennartz CM, Ameerun RF, Groenewegen HJ, & Lopes da Silva FH (1993). Synaptic plasticity in an in vitro slice preparation of the rat nucleus accumbens. *European Journal of Neuroscience* 5: 107–117.
Penton-Voak IS, Perrett DI, Castles DL, Kobayashi T, Burt DM, Murray LK, & Minamisawa R (1999). Menstrual cycle alters faces preference. *Nature* 399: 741–742.
Percheron G, Yelnik J, & François C (1984a). A Golgi analysis of the primate globus pallidus. III. Spatial organization of the striato-pallidal complex. *Journal of Comparative Neurology* 227: 214–227.
Percheron G, Yelnik J, & François C (1984b). The primate striato-pallido-nigral system: an integrative system for cortical information. In McKenzie JS, Kemm RE, & Wilcox LN, editors, *The Basal Ganglia: Structure and Function*, 87–105. Plenum, New York.
Percheron G, Yelnik J, François C, Fenelon G, & Talbi B (1994). Informational neurology of the basal ganglia related system. *Revue Neurologique (Paris)* 150: 614–626.
Perl ER & Kruger L (1996). Nociception and pain: evolution of concepts and observations. In Kruger L, editor, *Pain and Touch*, chap. 4, 180–211. Academic Press, San Diego.
Perrett DI & Rolls ET (1983). Neural mechanisms underlying the visual analysis of faces. In Ewert JP, Capranica RR, & Ingle DJ, editors, *Advances in Vertebrate Neuroethology*, 543–566. Plenum Press, New York.
Perrett DI, Rolls ET, & Caan W (1982). Visual neurons responsive to faces in the monkey temporal cortex. *Experimental Brain Research* 47: 329–342.
Perrett DI, Smith PAJ, Potter DD, Mistlin AJ, Head AS, Milner D, & Jeeves MA (1985). Visual cells in temporal cortex sensitive to face view and gaze direction. *Proceedings of the Royal Society of London, Series B* 223: 293–317.
Perry G, Rolls ET, & Stringer SM (2006). Spatial vs temporal continuity in view invariant visual object recognition learning. *Vision Research* 46: 3994–4006.
Perry G, Rolls ET, & Stringer SM (2010). Continuous transformation learning of translation invariant representations. *Experimental Brain Research* 204: 255–270.
Pessoa L & Adolphs R (2010). Emotion processing and the amygdala: from a 'low road' to 'many roads' of evaluating biological significance. *Nature Reviews Neuroscience* 11: 773–783.
Pessoa L & Padmala S (2005). Quantitative prediction of perceptual decisions during near-threshold fear detection. *Proceedings of the National Academy of Sciences USA* 102: 5612–5617.
Peters J & Buchel C (2009). Overlapping and distinct neural systems code for subjective value during intertemporal and risky decision making. *Journal of Neuroscience* 29: 15727–15734.
Petri HL & Mishkin M (1994). Behaviorism, cognitivism, and the neuropsychology of memory. *American Scientist* 82: 30–37.
Petrides M (1996). Specialized systems for the processing of mnemonic information within the primate frontal cortex. *Philosophical Transactions of the Royal Society of London B* 351: 1455–1462.

Petrides M (2007). The orbitofrontal cortex: novelty, deviation from expectation, and memory. *Annals of the New York Academy of Sciences* 1121: 33–53.

Petrides M & Pandya DN (1988). Association fiber pathways to the frontal cortex from the superior temporal region in the rhesus monkey. *Journal of Comparative Neurology* 273: 52–66.

Petrides M & Pandya DN (1994). Comparative architectonic analysis of the human and macaque frontal cortex. In Grafman J & Boller F, editors, *Handbook of Neuropsychology*, vol. 9, 17–58. Elsevier, Amsterdam.

Petrides M, Tomaiuolo F, Yeterian EH, & Pandya DN (2012). The prefrontal cortex: comparative architectonic organization in the human and the macaque monkey brains. *Cortex* 48: 46–57.

Petrovich P, Petersson KM, Ghatan PH, Ston-Elander S, & Ingvar M (2000). Pain-related cerebral activation is altered by a distracting cognitive task. *Pain* 85: 19–30.

Pfaff DW (1980). *Estrogens and Brain Function*. Springer, New York.

Pfaff DW (1982). Neurobiological mechanisms of sexual behavior. In Pfaff DW, editor, *The Physiological Mechanisms of Motivation*, 287–317. Springer, New York.

Pfaus JG, Damsma G, Nomikos GG, Wenkstern D, Blaha CD, Phillips AG, & Fibiger HC (1990). Sexual behavior enhances central dopamine transmission in the male rat. *Brain Research* 530: 345–348.

Phelps E, O'Connor KJ, Gatenby JC, Gore JC, Grillon C, & Davis M (2001). Activation of the left amygdala to a cognitive representation of fear. *Nature Neuroscience* 4: 437–441.

Phelps EA (2004). Human emotion and memory: interactions of the amygdala and hippocampal complex. *Current Opinion in Neurobiology* 14: 198–202.

Phelps EA (2006). Emotion and cognition: insights from studies of the human amygdala. *Annual Review of Psychology* 57: 27–53.

Phelps EA & LeDoux JE (2005). Contributions of the amygdala to emotion processing: from animal models to human behavior. *Neuron* 48: 175–187.

Phillips AG & Fibiger HC (1989). Neuroanatomical bases of intracranial self-stimulation: untying the Gordian knot. In Liebman JM & Cooper SJ, editors, *The Neuropharmacological Basis of Reward*, 66–105. Oxford University Press, Oxford.

Phillips AG & Fibiger HC (1990). Role of reward and enhancement of conditioned reward in persistence of responding for cocaine. *Behavioral Pharmacology* 1: 269–282.

Phillips AG, Mora F, & Rolls ET (1981). Intra-cerebral self-administration of amphetamine by rhesus monkeys. *Neuroscience Letters* 24: 81–86.

Phillips AG, Pfaus JG, & Blaha CD (1991). Dopamine and motivated behavior: insights provided by in vivo analysis. In Willner P & Scheel-Kruger J, editors, *The Mesolimbic Dopamine System: From Motivation to Action*, chap. 8, 199–224. Wiley, New York.

Phillips ML (2004). Facial processing deficits and social dysfunction: how are they related? *Brain* 127: 1691–1692.

Phillips ML, Young AW, Scott SK, Calder AJ, Andrew C, Giampetro V, Williams SCR, Bullmore ET, Brammer M, & Gray JA (1998). Neural responses to facial and vocal expressions of fear and disgust. *Proceedings of the Royal Society of London B* 265: 1809–1817.

Phillips ML, Drevets WC, Rauch SL, & Lane R (2003a). Neurobiology of emotion perception II: Implications for major psychiatric disorders. *Biological Psychiatry* 54: 515–528.

Phillips ML, Williams LM, Heining M, Herba CM, Russell T, Andrew C, Bullmore ET, Brammer MJ, Williams SC, Morgan M, Young AW, & Gray JA (2004). Differential neural responses to overt and covert presentations of facial expressions of fear and disgust. *Neuroimage* 21: 1484–1496.

Phillips PEM, Stuber GD, Heian MLAV, Wightman RM, & Carelli RM (2003b). Subsecond dopamine release promotes cocaine seeking. *Nature* 422: 614–618.

Phillips RR, Malamut BL, Bachevalier J, & Mishkin M (1988). Dissociation of the effects of inferior temporal and limbic lesions on object discrimination learning with 24-h intertrial intervals. *Behavioural Brain Research* 27: 99–107.

Picciotto MR, Higley MJ, & Mineur YS (2012). Acetylcholine as a neuromodulator: cholinergic signaling shapes nervous system function and behavior. *Neuron* 76: 116–129.

Pickens CL, Saddoris MP, Setlow B, Gallagher M, Holland PC, & Schoenbaum G (2003). Different roles for orbitofrontal cortex and basolateral amygdala in a reinforcer devaluation task. *Journal of Neuroscience* 23: 11078–11084.

Piguet O (2011). Eating disturbance in behavioural-variant frontotemporal dementia. *Journal of Molecuar Neuroscience* 45: 589–593.

Pinker S (1997). *How the Mind Works*. Norton, New York.

Pinker S & Bloom P (1992). Natural language and natural selection. In Barkow JH, Cosmides L, & Tooby J, editors, *The Adapted Mind*, chap. 12, 451–493. Oxford University Press, New York.

Pinto S, Roseberry AG, Liu HY, Diano S, Shanabrough M, Cai XL, Friedman JM, & Horvath TL (2004). Rapid rewiring of arcuate nucleus feeding circuits by leptin. *Science* 304: 110–115.

Pitkanen A (2000). Connectivitiy of the rat amygdaloid complex. In Aggleton JP, editor, *The Amygdala: a Functional Analysis*, chap. 2, 31–116. Oxford University Press, Oxford.

Pitkanen A, Kelly JL, & Amaral DG (2002). Projections from the lateral, basal, and accessory basal nuclei of the

amygdala to the entorhinal cortex in the macaque monkey. *Hippocampus* 12: 186–205.
Pittenger C, Krystal JH, & Coric V (2006). Glutamate-modulating drugs as novel pharmacotherapeutic agents in the treatment of obsessive-compulsive disorder. *NeuroRx* 3: 69–81.
Pittenger C, Bloch MH, & Williams K (2011). Glutamate abnormalities in obsessive compulsive disorder: Neurobiology, pathophysiology, and treatment. *Pharmacology and Therapeutics* 132: 314–332.
Pizzari T, Cornwallis CK, Lovlie H, Jakobsson S, & Birkhead TR (2003). Sophisticated sperm allocation in male fowl. *Nature* 426: 70–74.
Plassmann H, O'Doherty J, & Rangel A (2007). Orbitofrontal cortex encodes willingness to pay in everyday economic transactions. *Journal of Neuroscience* 27: 9984–9988.
Platek SM & Singh D (2010). Optimal waist-to-hip ratios in women activate neural reward centers in men. *PLoS One* 5: e9042.
Platt M & Padoa-Schioppa C (2009). Neuronal representations of value. In Glimcher PW, Camerer CF, Fehr E, & Poldrack RA, editors, *Neuroeconomics. Decision Making and the Brain*, chap. 29, 441–462. Academic Press, London.
Platt ML & Glimcher PW (1999). Neural correlates of decision variables in parietal cortex. *Nature* 400: 233–238.
Pleskac TJ & Busemeyer JR (2010). Two-stage dynamic signal detection: a theory of choice, decision time, and confidence. *Psychological Review* 117: 864–901.
Potts W (2002). Wisdom through immunogenetics. *Nature Genetics* 30: 130–131.
Potts W, Manning J, & Wakeland EK (1991). Mating patterns in seminatural populations of mice influenced by MHC genotype. *Nature* 352: 619–621.
Prelec D (1998). The probability weighting function. *Econometrica* 66: 497–527.
Preuschhof C, Heekeren HR, Taskin B, Schubert T, & Villringer A (2006). Neural correlates of vibrotactile working memory in the human brain. *Journal of Neuroscience* 26: 13231–13239.
Preuss TM (1995). Do rats have prefrontal cortex? The Rose-Woolsey-Akert program reconsidered. *Journal of Cognitive Neuroscience* 7: 1–24.
Preuss TM & Goldman-Rakic PS (1989). Connections of the ventral granular frontal cortex of macaques with perisylvian premotor and somatosensory areas: anatomical evidence for somatic representation in primate frontal association cortex. *Journal of Comparative Neurology* 282: 293–316.
Price J (2006). Connections of orbital cortex. In Zald DH & Rauch SL, editors, *The Orbitofrontal Cortex*, chap. 3, 39–55. Oxford University Press, Oxford.
Price JL & Drevets WC (2012). Neural circuits underlying the pathophysiology of mood disorders. *Trends in Cognitive Science* 16: 61–71.
Price JL, Carmichael ST, Carnes KM, Clugnet MC, & Kuroda M (1991). Olfactory input to the prefrontal cortex. In Davis JL & Eichenbaum H, editors, *Olfaction: A Model System for Computational Neuroscience*, 101–120. MIT Press, Cambridge, MA.
Priest CA & Pfaff DW (1995). Actions of sex steroids on behaviours beyond reproductive reflexes. In *CIBA Foundation Symposium*, vol. 191, 74–84. Pitman, London.
Pritchard TC, Hamilton RB, Morse JR, & Norgren R (1986). Projections of thalamic gustatory and lingual areas in the monkey. *Journal of Comparative Neurology* 244: 213–228.
Pritchard TC, Hamilton RB, & Norgren R (1989). Neural coding of gustatory information in the thalamus of macaca mulatta. *Journal of Neurophysiology* 61: 1–14.
Pritchard TC, Schwartz GJ, & Scott TR (2007). Taste in the medial orbitofrontal cortex of the macaque. *Annals of the New York Academy of Sciences* 1121: 121–135.
Pu W, Guo S, Liua H, Yub Y, Xuea Z, Rolls ET, Feng J, & Liu Z (2013). Schizophrenia: functional disconnection of the precuneus and posterior cingulate cortex, and volition .
Purcell BA, Heitz RP, Cohen JY, Schall JD, Logan GD, & Palmeri TJ (2010). Neurally constrained modeling of perceptual decision making. *Psychological Reviews* 117: 1113–1143.
Quirk GJ, Armony JL, Repa JC, Li XF, & LeDoux JE (1996). Emotional memory: a search for sites of plasticity. *Cold Spring Harbor Symposia on Quantitative Biology* 61: 247–257.
Quiroga RQ, Kreiman G, Koch C, & Fried I (2008). Sparse but not 'grandmother-cell' coding in the medial temporal lobe. *Trends in Cognitive Sciences* 12: 87–91.
Rachlin H (1989). *Judgement, Decision, and Choice: A Cognitive/Behavioural Synthesis*. Freeman, New York.
Rachlin H (2000). *The Science of Self-Control*. Harvard Univeristy Press, Cambridge, MA.
Rada P, Mark GP, & Hoebel BG (1998). Dopamine in the nucleus accumbens released by hypothalamic stimulation-escape behavior. *Brain Research* 782: 228–234.
Rahman S, Sahakian BJ, Hodges JR, Rogers RD, & Robbins TW (1999). Specific cognitive deficits in mild frontal variant frontotemporal dementia. *Brain* 122: 1469–1493.
Rao SC, Rainer G, & Miller EK (1997). Integration of what and where in the primate prefrontal cortex. *Science* 276: 821–824.
Rascovsky K, Hodges JR, & al (2011). Sensitivity of revised diagnostic criteria for the behavioural variant of frontotemporal dementia. *Brain* 134: 2456–2477.
Ratcliff R (1978). Theory of memory retrieval. *Psychological Review* 85: 59–108.

Ratcliff R & McKoon G (2008). The diffusion decision model: theory and data for two-choice decision tasks. *Neural Computation* 20: 873–922.

Ratcliff R & Rouder JF (1998). Modeling response times for two-choice decisions. *Psychological Science* 9: 347–356.

Ratcliff R & Smith PL (2004). A comparison of sequential sampling models for two-choice reaction time. *Psychological Review* 111: 333–367.

Ratcliff R, Zandt TV, & McKoon G (1999). Connectionist and diffusion models of reaction time. *Psychological Reviews* 106: 261–300.

Ratcliff R, Cherian A, & Segraves M (2003). A comparison of macaque behavior and superior colliculus neuronal activity to predictions from models of two-choice decisions. *Journal of Neurophysiology* 90: 1392–1407.

Rawlins JN, Winocur G, & Gray JA (1983). The hippocampus, collateral behavior, and timing. *Behavioral Neuroscience* 97: 857–872.

Reddi BA & Carpenter RH (2000). The influence of urgency on decision time. *Nature Neuroscience* 3: 827–830.

Reddy WM (2001). *The Navigation of Feeling: A Framework for the History of Emotions*. Cambridge University Press, Cambridge.

Redgrave P, Prescott TJ, & Gurney K (1999). Is the short-latency dopamine response too short to signal reward error? *Trends in Neuroscience* 22: 146–151.

Reisenzein R (1983). The Schachter theory of emotion: two decades later. *Psychological Bulletin* 94: 239–264.

Rempel-Clower NL & Barbas H (1998). Topographic organization of connections between the hypothalamus and prefrontal cortex in the rhesus monkey. *Journal of Comparative Neurology* 398: 393–419.

Renart A, Parga N, & Rolls ET (1999a). Backprojections in the cerebral cortex: implications for memory storage. *Neural Computation* 11: 1349–1388.

Renart A, Parga N, & Rolls ET (1999b). Associative memory properties of multiple cortical modules. *Network* 10: 237–255.

Renart A, Parga N, & Rolls ET (2000). A recurrent model of the interaction between the prefrontal cortex and inferior temporal cortex in delay memory tasks. In Solla S, Leen T, & Mueller KR, editors, *Advances in Neural Information Processing Systems*, vol. 12, 171–177. MIT Press, Cambridge, MA.

Renart A, Moreno R, Rocha J, Parga N, & Rolls ET (2001). A model of the IT–PF network in object working memory which includes balanced persistent activity and tuned inhibition. *Neurocomputing* 38–40: 1525–1531.

Renart A, Brunel N, & Wang XJ (2003). Mean field theory of irregularly spiking neuronal populations and working memory in recurrent cortical networks. In Feng J, editor, *Computational Neuroscience: A Comprehensive Approach*, 431–490. Chapman and Hall, Boca Raton, FL.

Rescorla RA (1990a). The role of information about the response–outcome relation in instrumental discrimination learning. *Journal of Experimental Psychology* 16: 262–270.

Rescorla RA (1990b). Evidence for an association between the discriminative stimulus and the response–outcome association in instrumental learning. *Journal of Experimental Psychology* 16: 326–334.

Rescorla RA & Solomon RL (1967). Two-process learning theory: relationships between Pavlovian conditioning and instrumental learning. *Psychology Reviews* 74: 151–182.

Rescorla RA & Wagner AR (1972). A theory of Pavlovian conditioning: the effectiveness of reinforcement and non-reinforcement. In *Classical Conditioning II: Current Research and Theory*, 64–69. Appleton-Century-Crofts, New York.

Reynolds JN & Wickens JR (2002). Dopamine-dependent plasticity of corticostriatal synapses. *Neural Networks* 15: 507–521.

Riani M & Simonotto E (1994). Stochastic resonance in the perceptual interpretation of ambiguous figures: A neural network model. *Physical Review Letters* 72: 3120–3123.

Ridley M (1993a). *The Red Queen: Sex and the Evolution of Human Nature*. Penguin, London.

Ridley M (1993b). *Evolution*. Blackwell, Oxford.

Ridley M (1996). *The Origins of Virtue*. Viking, London.

Ridley M (2003). *Nature via Nurture*. Harper, London.

Ridley RM, Hester NS, & Ettlinger G (1977). Stimulus- and response-dependent units from the occipital and temporal lobes of the unanaesthetized monkey performing learnt visual tasks. *Experimental Brain Research* 27: 539–552.

Ritter S, Li AJ, Wang Q, & Dinh TT (2011). Minireview: The value of looking backward: the essential role of the hindbrain in counterregulatory responses to glucose deficit. *Endocrinology* 152: 4019–4032.

Robbins TW, Cador M, Taylor JR, & Everitt BJ (1989). Limbic-striatal interactions in reward-related processes. *Neuroscience and Biobehavioral Reviews* 13: 155–162.

Robbins TW, Gillan CM, Smith DG, de Wit S, & Ersche KD (2012). Neurocognitive endophenotypes of impulsivity and compulsivity: towards dimensional psychiatry. *Trends in Cognitive Sciences* 16: 81–91.

Roberts DCS, Koob GF, Klonoff P, & Fibiger HC (1980). Extinction and recovery of cocaine self-administration following 6-hydroxydopamine lesions of the nucleus accumbens. *Pharmacology, Biochemistry and Behavior* 12: 781–787.

Robertson RG, Rolls ET, & Georges-François P (1998). Spatial view cells in the primate hippocampus: Effects of removal of view details. *Journal of Neurophysiology* 79: 1145–1156.

Robins LN, Helzer JE, Weissman MM, Orvaschel H, Gruenberg E, Burke JDJ, & Regier DA (1984). Lifetime prevalence of specific psychiatric disorders in three sites. *Archives of General Psychiatry* 41: 949–958.

Robinson MD, Watkins ER, & Harmon-Jones E (2013). *Handbook of Cognition and Emotion*. Guilford, New York.

Robinson TE & Berridge KC (1993). The neural basis of drug craving: an incentive-sensitization theory of addiction. *Brain Research, Brain Research Reviews* 18: 247–291.

Robinson TE & Berridge KC (2003). Addiction. *Annual Review of Psychology* 54: 25–53.

Rockland KS & Pandya DN (1979). Laminar origins and terminations of cortical connections of the occipital lobe in the rhesus monkey. *Brain Research* 179: 3–20.

Rodin J (1976). The role of perception of internal and external signals in the regulation of feeding in overweight and non-obese individuals. *Dahlem Konferenzen, Life Sciences Research Report* 2: 265–281.

Roesch MR & Olson CR (2005). Neuronal activity in primate orbitofrontal cortex reflects the value of time. *Journal of Neurophysiology* 94: 2457–2471.

Roesch MR, Taylor AR, & Schoenbaum G (2006). Encoding of time-discounted rewards in orbitofrontal cortex is independent of value representation. *Neuron* 51: 509–520.

Rogan MT, Staubli UV, & LeDoux JE (1997). Fear conditioning induces associative long-term potentiation in the amygdala. *Nature* 390: 604–607.

Roitman JD & Shadlen MN (2002). Response of neurons in the lateral intraparietal area during a combined visual discrimination reaction time task. *Journal of Neuroscience* 22: 9475–9489.

Rolls BJ (2012a). Dietary strategies for weight management. *Nestle Nutrition Institute Workshop Series* 73: 37–48.

Rolls BJ & Hetherington M (1989). The role of variety in eating and body weight regulation. In Shepherd R, editor, *Handbook of the Psychophysiology of Human Eating*, chap. 3, 57–84. Wiley, Chichester.

Rolls BJ & Rolls ET (1973a). Effects of lesions in the basolateral amygdala on fluid intake in the rat. *Journal of Comparative and Physiological Psychology* 83: 240–247.

Rolls BJ & Rolls ET (1982a). *Thirst*. Cambridge University Press, Cambridge.

Rolls BJ, Rolls ET, Rowe EA, & Sweeney K (1981a). Sensory specific satiety in man. *Physiology and Behavior* 27: 137–142.

Rolls BJ, Rowe EA, Rolls ET, Kingston B, Megson A, & Gunary R (1981b). Variety in a meal enhances food intake in man. *Physiology and Behavior* 26: 215–221.

Rolls BJ, Rowe EA, & Rolls ET (1982a). How sensory properties of foods affect human feeding behavior. *Physiology and Behavior* 29: 409–417.

Rolls BJ, Rowe EA, & Rolls ET (1982b). How flavour and appearance affect human feeding. *Proceedings of the Nutrition Society* 41: 109–117.

Rolls BJ, Van Duijenvoorde PM, & Rowe EA (1983a). Variety in the diet enhances intake in a meal and contributes to the development of obesity in the rat. *Physiology and Behavior* 31: 21–27.

Rolls BJ, Van Duijenvoorde PM, & Rolls ET (1984a). Pleasantness changes and food intake in a varied four course meal. *Appetite* 5: 337–348.

Rolls ET (1975). *The Brain and Reward*. Pergamon Press, Oxford.

Rolls ET (1976). The neurophysiological basis of brain-stimulation reward. In Wauquier A & Rolls ET, editors, *Brain-Stimulation Reward*, 65–87. North Holland, Amsterdam.

Rolls ET (1979). Effects of electrical stimulation of the brain on behaviour. *Psychology Surveys* 2: 151–169.

Rolls ET (1981a). Processing beyond the inferior temporal visual cortex related to feeding, learning, and striatal function. In Katsuki Y, Norgren R, & Sato M, editors, *Brain Mechanisms of Sensation*, chap. 16, 241–269. Wiley, New York.

Rolls ET (1981b). Central nervous mechanisms related to feeding and appetite. *British Medical Bulletin* 37: 131–134.

Rolls ET (1981c). Responses of amygdaloid neurons in the primate. In Ben-Ari Y, editor, *The Amygdaloid Complex*, 383–393. Elsevier, Amsterdam.

Rolls ET (1982). Neuronal mechanisms underlying the formation and disconnection of associations between visual stimuli and reinforcement in primates. In Woody CD, editor, *Conditioning: Representation of Involved Neural Functions*, 363–373. Plenum, New York.

Rolls ET (1984). Neurons in the cortex of the temporal lobe and in the amygdala of the monkey with responses selective for faces. *Human Neurobiology* 3: 209–222.

Rolls ET (1986a). A theory of emotion, and its application to understanding the neural basis of emotion. In Oomura Y, editor, *Emotions. Neural and Chemical Control*, 325–344. Japan Scientific Societies Press; and Karger, Tokyo; and Basel.

Rolls ET (1986b). Neural systems involved in emotion in primates. In Plutchik R & Kellerman H, editors, *Emotion: Theory, Research, and Experience*, vol. 3: Biological Foundations of Emotion, chap. 5, 125–143. Academic Press, New York.

Rolls ET (1986c). Neuronal activity related to the control of feeding. In Ritter R, Ritter S, & Barnes C, editors, *Feeding Behavior: Neural and Humoral Controls*, chap. 6, 163–190. Academic Press, New York.

Rolls ET (1987). Information representation, processing and storage in the brain: analysis at the single neuron level. In Changeux JP & Konishi M, editors, *The Neural and Molecular Bases of Learning*, 503–540. Wiley,

Chichester.
Rolls ET (1989a). Information processing in the taste system of primates. *Journal of Experimental Biology* 146: 141–164.
Rolls ET (1989b). Functions of neuronal networks in the hippocampus and neocortex in memory. In Byrne JH & Berry WO, editors, *Neural Models of Plasticity: Experimental and Theoretical Approaches*, chap. 13, 240–265. Academic Press, San Diego, CA.
Rolls ET (1989c). The representation and storage of information in neuronal networks in the primate cerebral cortex and hippocampus. In Durbin R, Miall C, & Mitchison G, editors, *The Computing Neuron*, chap. 8, 125–159. Addison-Wesley, Wokingham, England.
Rolls ET (1990a). Functions of neuronal networks in the hippocampus and of backprojections in the cerebral cortex in memory. In McGaugh J, Weinberger N, & Lynch G, editors, *Brain Organization and Memory: Cells, Systems and Circuits*, chap. 9, 184–210. Oxford University Press, New York.
Rolls ET (1990b). A theory of emotion, and its application to understanding the neural basis of emotion. *Cognition and Emotion* 4: 161–190.
Rolls ET (1990c). Theoretical and neurophysiological analysis of the functions of the primate hippocampus in memory. *Cold Spring Harbor Symposia in Quantitative Biology* 55: 995–1006.
Rolls ET (1992a). Neurophysiology and functions of the primate amygdala. In Aggleton JP, editor, *The Amygdala*, chap. 5, 143–165. Wiley-Liss, New York.
Rolls ET (1992b). Neurophysiological mechanisms underlying face processing within and beyond the temporal cortical visual areas. *Philosophical Transactions of the Royal Society* 335: 11–21.
Rolls ET (1992c). The processing of face information in the primate temporal lobe. In Bruce V & Burton M, editors, *Processing Images of Faces*, chap. 3. Ablex, Norwood, NJ. 41–68.
Rolls ET (1993). The neural control of feeding in primates. In Booth D, editor, *Neurophysiology of Ingestion*, chap. 9, 137–169. Pergamon, Oxford.
Rolls ET (1994a). Neurophysiology and cognitive functions of the striatum. *Revue Neurologique (Paris)* 150: 648–660.
Rolls ET (1994b). Brain mechanisms for invariant visual recognition and learning. *Behavioural Processes* 33: 113–138.
Rolls ET (1995a). A theory of emotion and consciousness, and its application to understanding the neural basis of emotion. In Gazzaniga MS, editor, *The Cognitive Neurosciences*, chap. 72, 1091–1106. MIT Press, Cambridge, MA.
Rolls ET (1995b). Central taste anatomy and neurophysiology. In Doty R, editor, *Handbook of Olfaction and Gustation*, chap. 24, 549–573. Dekker, New York.
Rolls ET (1996a). A theory of hippocampal function in memory. *Hippocampus* 6: 601–620.
Rolls ET (1996b). The orbitofrontal cortex. *Philosophical Transactions of the Royal Society B* 351: 1433–1444.
Rolls ET (1997a). Brain mechanisms of vision, memory, and consciousness. In Ito M, Miyashita Y, & Rolls E, editors, *Cognition, Computation, and Consciousness*, chap. 6, 81–120. Oxford University Press, Oxford.
Rolls ET (1997b). Consciousness in neural networks? *Neural Networks* 10: 1227–1240.
Rolls ET (1997c). Taste and olfactory processing in the brain and its relation to the control of eating. *Critical Reviews in Neurobiology* 11: 263–287.
Rolls ET (1999a). *The Brain and Emotion*. Oxford University Press, Oxford.
Rolls ET (1999b). Spatial view cells and the representation of place in the primate hippocampus. *Hippocampus* 9: 467–480.
Rolls ET (1999c). The functions of the orbitofrontal cortex. *Neurocase* 5: 301–312.
Rolls ET (2000a). Précis of The Brain and Emotion. *Behavioral and Brain Sciences* 23: 177–233.
Rolls ET (2000b). The orbitofrontal cortex and reward. *Cerebral Cortex* 10: 284–294.
Rolls ET (2000c). Functions of the primate temporal lobe cortical visual areas in invariant visual object and face recognition. *Neuron* 27: 205–218.
Rolls ET (2000d). Neurophysiology and functions of the primate amygdala, and the neural basis of emotion. In Aggleton JP, editor, *The Amygdala: Second Edition. A Functional Analysis*, chap. 13, 447–478. Oxford University Press, Oxford.
Rolls ET (2000e). Memory systems in the brain. *Annual Review of Psychology* 51: 599–630.
Rolls ET (2000f). Hippocampo-cortical and cortico-cortical backprojections. *Hippocampus* 10: 380–388.
Rolls ET (2001a). The representation of umami taste in the human and macaque cortex. *Sensory Neuron* 3: 227–242.
Rolls ET (2001b). The rules of formation of the olfactory representations found in the orbitofrontal cortex olfactory areas in primates. *Chemical Senses* 26: 595–604.
Rolls ET (2002). A theory of emotion, its functions, and its adaptive value. In Trappl R, Petta P, & Payr S, editors, *Emotions in Humans and Artifacts*, chap. 2, 11–32. MIT Press, Cambridge, Mass.
Rolls ET (2003). Consciousness absent and present: a neurophysiological exploration. *Progress in Brain Research* 144: 95–106.
Rolls ET (2004a). The operation of memory systems in the brain. In Feng J, editor, *Computational Neuroscience: A Comprehensive Approach*, chap. 16, 491–534. CRC Press (UK), London.

Rolls ET (2004b). Invariant object and face recognition. In Chalupa LM & Werner JS, editors, *The Visual Neurosciences*, 1165–1178. MIT Press, Cambridge, Mass.

Rolls ET (2004c). The functions of the orbitofrontal cortex. *Brain and Cognition* 55: 11–29.

Rolls ET (2004d). A higher order syntactic thought (HOST) theory of consciousness. In Gennaro RJ, editor, *Higher Order Theories of Consciousness*, chap. 7, 137–172. John Benjamins, Amsterdam.

Rolls ET (2004e). Convergence of sensory systems in the orbitofrontal cortex in primates and brain design for emotion. *The Anatomical Record Part A* 281: 1212–1225.

Rolls ET (2004f). Taste, olfactory, texture and temperature multimodal representations in the brain, and their relevance to the control of appetite. *Primatologie* 6: 5–32.

Rolls ET (2005a). What are emotions, why do we have emotions, and what is their computational basis in the brain? In Fellous JM & Arbib MA, editors, *Who Needs Emotions? The Brain Meets the Robot*, chap. 5, 117–146. Oxford University Press, New York.

Rolls ET (2005b). *Emotion Explained.* Oxford University Press, Oxford.

Rolls ET (2006a). Consciousness absent and present: a neurophysiological exploration of masking. In Ogmen H & Breitmeyer BG, editors, *The First Half Second*, chap. 6, 89–108. MIT Press, Cambridge, MA.

Rolls ET (2006b). The neurophysiology and functions of the orbitofrontal cortex. In Zald DH & Rauch SL, editors, *The Orbitofrontal Cortex*, chap. 5, 95–124. Oxford University Press, Oxford.

Rolls ET (2006c). Brain mechanisms underlying flavour and appetite. *Philosophical Transactions of the Royal Society B* 361: 1123–1136.

Rolls ET (2007a). The representation of information about faces in the temporal and frontal lobes of primates including humans. *Neuropsychologia* 45: 124–143.

Rolls ET (2007b). The affective neuroscience of consciousness: higher order syntactic thoughts, dual routes to emotion and action, and consciousness. In Zelazo PD, Moscovitch M, & Thompson E, editors, *Cambridge Handbook of Consciousness*, chap. 29, 831–859. Cambridge University Press, New York.

Rolls ET (2007c). Sensory processing in the brain related to the control of food intake. *Proceedings of the Nutrition Society* 66: 96–112.

Rolls ET (2007d). A neuro-biological approach to emotional intelligence. In Matthews G, Zeidner M, & Roberts R, editors, *The Science of Emotional Intelligence*, chap. 3, 72–100. Oxford University Press, Oxford.

Rolls ET (2007e). Understanding the mechanisms of food intake and obesity. *Obesity Reviews* 8: 67–72.

Rolls ET (2007f). Invariant representations of objects in natural scenes in the temporal cortex visual areas. In Funahashi S, editor, *Representation and Brain*, chap. 3, 47–102. Springer, Tokyo.

Rolls ET (2007g). A computational neuroscience approach to consciousness. *Neural Networks* 20: 962–982.

Rolls ET (2008a). The representation of flavor in the brain. In Basbaum A, Keneko A, Shepherd GM, & Westheimer G, editors, *The Senses - A Comprehensive Reference. Vol. 4 Olfaction and Taste. Eds. Firestein, S. and Beauchamp, G. K.*, chap. 4.26, 469–478. Elsevier, Oxford.

Rolls ET (2008b). *Memory, Attention, and Decision-Making. A Unifying Computational Neuroscience Approach.* Oxford University Press, Oxford.

Rolls ET (2008c). Emotion, higher order syntactic thoughts, and consciousness. In Weiskrantz L & Davies M, editors, *Frontiers of Consciousness*, chap. 4, 131–167. Oxford University Press, Oxford.

Rolls ET (2008d). Face representations in different brain areas, and critical band masking. *Journal of Neuropsychology* 2: 325–360.

Rolls ET (2008e). Functions of the orbitofrontal and pregenual cingulate cortex in taste, olfaction, appetite and emotion. *Acta Physiologica Hungarica* 95: 131–164.

Rolls ET (2009a). The neurophysiology and computational mechanisms of object representation. In Dickinson S, Tarr M, Leonardis A, & Schiele B, editors, *Object Categorization: Computer and Human Vision Perspectives*, chap. 14, 257–287. Cambridge University Press, Cambridge.

Rolls ET (2009b). From reward value to decision-making: neuronal and computational principles. In Dreher JC & Tremblay L, editors, *Handbook of Reward and Decision-Making*, chap. 5, 95–130. Academic Press, New York.

Rolls ET (2009c). Functional neuroimaging of umami taste: what makes umami pleasant. *American Journal of Clinical Nutrition* 90: 803S–814S.

Rolls ET (2009d). The anterior and midcingulate cortices and reward. In Vogt B, editor, *Cingulate Neurobiology and Disease*, chap. 8, 191–206. Oxford University Press, Oxford.

Rolls ET (2010a). Noise in the brain, decision-making, determinism, free will, and consciousness. In Perry E, Collerton D, Ashton H, & Lebeau F, editors, *New Horizons in the Neuroscience of Consciousness*, 113–120. John Benjamins, Amsterdam.

Rolls ET (2010b). A computational theory of episodic memory formation in the hippocampus. *Behavioural Brain Research* 215: 180–196.

Rolls ET (2010c). The affective and cognitive processing of touch, oral texture, and temperature in the brain. *Neuroscience and Biobehavioral Reviews* 34: 237–245.

Rolls ET (2010d). Taste, olfactory and food texture processing in the brain and the control of appetite. In LDube, ABechara, ADagher, ADrewnowski, JLeBel, PJames, & RYYada, editors, *Obesity Prevention*, chap. 4,

41–56. Academic Press, London.

Rolls ET (2011a). Consciousness, decision-making, and neural computation. In Cutsuridis V, Hussain A, & Taylor JG, editors, *Perception-Action Cycle: Models, architecture, and hardware*, chap. 9, 287–333. Springer, Berlin.

Rolls ET (2011b). Taste, olfactory, and food texture reward processing in the brain and obesity. *International Journal of Obesity* 35: 550–561.

Rolls ET (2011c). Face neurons. In Calder AJ, Rhodes G, Johnson MH, & Haxby JV, editors, *The Oxford Handbook of Face Perception*, chap. 4, 51–75. Oxford University Press, Oxford.

Rolls ET (2011d). A neurobiological basis for affective feelings and aesthetics. In Schellekens E & Goldie P, editors, *The Aesthetic Mind: Philosophy and Psychology*, chap. 8, 116–165. Oxford University Press, Oxford.

Rolls ET (2011e). The neural representation of oral texture including fat texture. *Journal of Texture Studies* 42: 137–156.

Rolls ET (2011f). Chemosensory learning in the cortex. *Frontiers in Systems Neuroscience* 5: 78 (1–13).

Rolls ET (2012b). Glutamate, obsessive-compulsive disorder, schizophrenia, and the stability of cortical attractor neuronal networks. *Pharmacology, Biochemistry and Behavior* 100: 736–751.

Rolls ET (2012c). Taste, olfactory, and food texture reward processing in the brain and the control of appetite. *Proceedings of the Nutrition Society* 71: 488–501.

Rolls ET (2012d). *Neuroculture: On the Implications of Brain Science*. Oxford University Press, Oxford.

Rolls ET (2012e). Invariant visual object and face recognition: neural and computational bases, and a model, VisNet. *Frontiers in Computational Neuroscience* 6: 1–70.

Rolls ET (2012f). Advantages of dilution in the connectivity of attractor networks in the brain. *Biologically Inspired Cognitive Architectures* 1: 44–54.

Rolls ET (2012g). Willed action, free will, and the stochastic neurodynamics of decision-making. *Frontiers in Integrative Neuroscience* 6: 68.

Rolls ET (2013a). A biased activation theory of the cognitive and attentional modulation of emotion. *Frontiers in Human Neuroscience* 7: 74.

Rolls ET (2013b). On the relation between the mind and the brain: a neuroscience perspective. *Philosophia Scientiae* 17: 31–70.

Rolls ET (2013c). A quantitative theory of the functions of the hippocampal CA3 network in memory. *Frontiers in Cellular Neuroscience* 7: 98.

Rolls ET (2013d). What are emotional states, and why do we have them? *Emotion Review* 5: 241–247.

Rolls ET (2013e). Brain processing of reward for touch, temperature, and oral texture. In Olausson H, Wessberg J, Morrison I, & McGlone F, editors, *Affective Touch and the Neurophysiology of CT Afferents*. Springer, Berlin.

Rolls ET (2014a). Central neural integration of taste, smell and other sensory modalities. In Doty RL, editor, *Handbook of Olfaction and Gustation: Modern Perspectives*, chap. 44. Dekker, New York, 3rd edn.

Rolls ET (2014b). Neurobiological foundations of art and aesthetics. In Nadal M, Huston JP, Agnati L, Mora F, & Cela-Conde CJ, editors, *Art, Aesthetics and the Brain*. Oxford University Press, Oxford.

Rolls ET (2014c). Neuroculture: art, aesthetics, and the brain. *Rendiconti Lincei Scienze Fisiche e Naturali* in press.

Rolls ET (2014d). *Emotion and Decision-Making Explained*. Oxford University Press, Oxford.

Rolls ET (2014e). Limbic systems for emotion and for memory, but no single limbic system. *Cortex* .

Rolls ET & Baylis GC (1986). Size and contrast have only small effects on the responses to faces of neurons in the cortex of the superior temporal sulcus of the monkey. *Experimental Brain Research* 65: 38–48.

Rolls ET & Baylis LL (1994). Gustatory, olfactory and visual convergence within the primate orbitofrontal cortex. *Journal of Neuroscience* 14: 5437–5452.

Rolls ET & de Waal AWL (1985). Long-term sensory-specific satiety: evidence from an Ethiopian refugee camp. *Physiology and Behavior* 34: 1017–1020.

Rolls ET & Deco G (2002). *Computational Neuroscience of Vision*. Oxford University Press, Oxford.

Rolls ET & Deco G (2006). Attention in natural scenes: neurophysiological and computational bases. *Neural Networks* 19: 1383–1394.

Rolls ET & Deco G (2010). *The Noisy Brain: Stochastic Dynamics as a Principle of Brain Function*. Oxford University Press, Oxford.

Rolls ET & Deco G (2011a). A computational neuroscience approach to schizophrenia and its onset. *Neuroscience and Biobehavioral Reviews* 35: 1644–1653.

Rolls ET & Deco G (2011b). Prediction of decisions from noise in the brain before the evidence is provided. *Frontiers in Neuroscience* 5: 33.

Rolls ET & Grabenhorst F (2008). The orbitofrontal cortex and beyond: from affect to decision-making. *Progress in Neurobiology* 86: 216–244.

Rolls ET & Johnstone S (1992). Neurophysiological analysis of striatal function. In Vallar G, Cappa S, & Wallesch C, editors, *Neuropsychological Disorders Associated with Subcortical Lesions*, chap. 3, 61–97. Oxford University Press, Oxford.

Rolls ET & Kesner RP (2006). A theory of hippocampal function, and tests of the theory. *Progress in Neurobiology* 79: 1–48.

Rolls ET & McCabe C (2007). Enhanced affective brain representations of chocolate in cravers vs non-cravers. *European Journal of Neuroscience* 26: 1067–1076.

Rolls ET & Milward T (2000). A model of invariant object recognition in the visual system: learning rules, activation functions, lateral inhibition, and information-based performance measures. *Neural Computation* 12: 2547–2572.

Rolls ET & Rolls BJ (1973b). Altered food preferences after lesions in the basolateral region of the amygdala in the rat. *Journal of Comparative and Physiological Psychology* 83: 248–259.

Rolls ET & Rolls BJ (1977). Activity of neurones in sensory, hypothalamic and motor areas during feeding in the monkey. In Katsuki Y, Sato M, Takagi S, & Oomura Y, editors, *Food Intake and Chemical Senses*, 525–549. University of Tokyo Press, Tokyo.

Rolls ET & Rolls BJ (1982b). Brain mechanisms involved in feeding. In Barker L, editor, *Psychobiology of Human Food Selection*, chap. 3, 33–62. AVI Publishing Company, Westport, Connecticut.

Rolls ET & Rolls JH (1997). Olfactory sensory-specific satiety in humans. *Physiology and Behavior* 61: 461–473.

Rolls ET & Scott TR (2003). Central taste anatomy and neurophysiology. In Doty R, editor, *Handbook of Olfaction and Gustation*, chap. 33, 679–705. Dekker, New York, 2nd edn.

Rolls ET & Stringer SM (2000). On the design of neural networks in the brain by genetic evolution. *Progress in Neurobiology* 61: 557–579.

Rolls ET & Stringer SM (2001a). Invariant object recognition in the visual system with error correction and temporal difference learning. *Network: Computation in Neural Systems* 12: 111–129.

Rolls ET & Stringer SM (2001b). A model of the interaction between mood and memory. *Network: Computation in Neural Systems* 12: 89–109.

Rolls ET & Stringer SM (2005). Spatial view cells in the hippocampus, and their idiothetic update based on place and head direction. *Neural Networks* 18: 1229–1241.

Rolls ET & Stringer SM (2006). Invariant visual object recognition: a model, with lighting invariance. *Journal of Physiology – Paris* 100: 43–62.

Rolls ET & Stringer SM (2007). Invariant global motion recognition in the dorsal visual system: a unifying theory. *Neural Computation* 19: 139–169.

Rolls ET & Tovee MJ (1994). Processing speed in the cerebral cortex and the neurophysiology of visual masking. *Proceedings of the Royal Society, B* 257: 9–15.

Rolls ET & Tovee MJ (1995). Sparseness of the neuronal representation of stimuli in the primate temporal visual cortex. *Journal of Neurophysiology* 73: 713–726.

Rolls ET & Treves A (1990). The relative advantages of sparse versus distributed encoding for associative neuronal networks in the brain. *Network* 1: 407–421.

Rolls ET & Treves A (1998). *Neural Networks and Brain Function.* Oxford University Press, Oxford.

Rolls ET & Treves A (2011). The neuronal encoding of information in the brain. *Progress in Neurobiology* 95: 448–490.

Rolls ET & Webb TJ (2012). Cortical attractor network dynamics with diluted connectivity. *Brain Research* 1434: 212–225.

Rolls ET & Williams GV (1987a). Sensory and movement-related neuronal activity in different regions of the primate striatum. In Schneider JS & Lidsky TI, editors, *Basal Ganglia and Behavior: Sensory Aspects and Motor Functioning*, 37–59. Hans Huber, Bern.

Rolls ET & Williams GV (1987b). Neuronal activity in the ventral striatum of the primate. In Carpenter MB & Jayamaran A, editors, *The Basal Ganglia II – Structure and Function – Current Concepts*, 349–356. Plenum, New York.

Rolls ET & Xiang JZ (2005). Reward–spatial view representations and learning in the primate hippocampus. *Journal of Neuroscience* 25: 6167–6174.

Rolls ET & Xiang JZ (2006). Spatial view cells in the primate hippocampus, and memory recall. *Reviews in the Neurosciences* 17: 175–200.

Rolls ET, Kelly PH, & Shaw SG (1974a). Noradrenaline, dopamine and brain-stimulation reward. *Pharmacology, Biochemistry and Behavior* 2: 735–740.

Rolls ET, Rolls BJ, Kelly PH, Shaw SG, & Dale R (1974b). The relative attenuation of self-stimulation, eating and drinking produced by dopamine-receptor blockade. *Psychopharmacologia (Berlin)* 38: 219–310.

Rolls ET, Burton MJ, & Mora F (1976). Hypothalamic neuronal responses associated with the sight of food. *Brain Research* 111: 53–66.

Rolls ET, Judge SJ, & Sanghera M (1977). Activity of neurones in the inferotemporal cortex of the alert monkey. *Brain Research* 130: 229–238.

Rolls ET, Sanghera MK, & Roper-Hall A (1979a). The latency of activation of neurons in the lateral hypothalamus and substantia innominata during feeding in the monkey. *Brain Research* 164: 121–135.

Rolls ET, Thorpe SJ, Maddison S, Roper-Hall A, Puerto A, & Perrett D (1979b). Activity of neurones in the neostriatum and related structures in the alert animal. In Divac I & Oberg R, editors, *The Neostriatum*, 163–182. Pergamon Press, Oxford.

Rolls ET, Burton MJ, & Mora F (1980). Neurophysiological analysis of brain-stimulation reward in the monkey.

Brain Research 194: 339–357.
Rolls ET, Perrett DI, Caan AW, & Wilson FAW (1982c). Neuronal responses related to visual recognition. *Brain* 105: 611–646.
Rolls ET, Rolls BJ, & Rowe EA (1983b). Sensory-specific and motivation-specific satiety for the sight and taste of food and water in man. *Physiology and Behavior* 30: 185–192.
Rolls ET, Thorpe SJ, & Maddison SP (1983c). Responses of striatal neurons in the behaving monkey. 1. Head of the caudate nucleus. *Behavioural Brain Research* 7: 179–210.
Rolls ET, Thorpe SJ, Boytim M, Szabo I, & Perrett DI (1984b). Responses of striatal neurons in the behaving monkey. 3. Effects of iontophoretically applied dopamine on normal responsiveness. *Neuroscience* 12: 1201–1212.
Rolls ET, Baylis GC, & Leonard CM (1985). Role of low and high spatial frequencies in the face-selective responses of neurons in the cortex in the superior temporal sulcus. *Vision Research* 25: 1021–1035.
Rolls ET, Murzi E, Yaxley S, Thorpe SJ, & Simpson SJ (1986). Sensory-specific satiety: food-specific reduction in responsiveness of ventral forebrain neurons after feeding in the monkey. *Brain Research* 368: 79–86.
Rolls ET, Scott TR, Sienkiewicz ZJ, & Yaxley S (1988). The responsiveness of neurones in the frontal opercular gustatory cortex of the macaque monkey is independent of hunger. *Journal of Physiology* 397: 1–12.
Rolls ET, Miyashita Y, Cahusac PMB, Kesner RP, Niki H, Feigenbaum J, & Bach L (1989a). Hippocampal neurons in the monkey with activity related to the place in which a stimulus is shown. *Journal of Neuroscience* 9: 1835–1845.
Rolls ET, Sienkiewicz ZJ, & Yaxley S (1989b). Hunger modulates the responses to gustatory stimuli of single neurons in the caudolateral orbitofrontal cortex of the macaque monkey. *European Journal of Neuroscience* 1: 53–60.
Rolls ET, Yaxley S, & Sienkiewicz ZJ (1990). Gustatory responses of single neurons in the orbitofrontal cortex of the macaque monkey. *Journal of Neurophysiology* 64: 1055–1066.
Rolls ET, Hornak J, Wade D, & McGrath J (1994a). Emotion-related learning in patients with social and emotional changes associated with frontal lobe damage. *Journal of Neurology, Neurosurgery and Psychiatry* 57: 1518–1524.
Rolls ET, Tovee MJ, Purcell DG, Stewart AL, & Azzopardi P (1994b). The responses of neurons in the temporal cortex of primates, and face identification and detection. *Experimental Brain Research* 101: 474–484.
Rolls ET, Critchley HD, Mason R, & Wakeman EA (1996a). Orbitofrontal cortex neurons: role in olfactory and visual association learning. *Journal of Neurophysiology* 75: 1970–1981.
Rolls ET, Critchley HD, & Treves A (1996b). The representation of olfactory information in the primate orbitofrontal cortex. *Journal of Neurophysiology* 75: 1982–1996.
Rolls ET, Critchley HD, Wakeman EA, & Mason R (1996c). Responses of neurons in the primate taste cortex to the glutamate ion and to inosine 5′-monophosphate. *Physiology and Behavior* 59: 991–1000.
Rolls ET, Robertson RG, & Georges-François P (1997a). Spatial view cells in the primate hippocampus. *European Journal of Neuroscience* 9: 1789–1794.
Rolls ET, Treves A, Foster D, & Perez-Vicente C (1997b). Simulation studies of the CA3 hippocampal subfield modelled as an attractor neural network. *Neural Networks* 10: 1559–1569.
Rolls ET, Treves A, Tovee M, & Panzeri S (1997c). Information in the neuronal representation of individual stimuli in the primate temporal visual cortex. *Journal of Computational Neuroscience* 4: 309–333.
Rolls ET, Treves A, & Tovee MJ (1997d). The representational capacity of the distributed encoding of information provided by populations of neurons in the primate temporal visual cortex. *Experimental Brain Research* 114: 149–162.
Rolls ET, Critchley HD, Browning A, & Hernadi I (1998a). The neurophysiology of taste and olfaction in primates, and umami flavor. *Annals of the New York Academy of Sciences* 855: 426–437.
Rolls ET, Treves A, Robertson RG, Georges-François P, & Panzeri S (1998b). Information about spatial view in an ensemble of primate hippocampal cells. *Journal of Neurophysiology* 79: 1797–1813.
Rolls ET, Critchley HD, Browning AS, Hernadi A, & Lenard L (1999a). Responses to the sensory properties of fat of neurons in the primate orbitofrontal cortex. *Journal of Neuroscience* 19: 1532–1540.
Rolls ET, Tovee MJ, & Panzeri S (1999b). The neurophysiology of backward visual masking: information analysis. *Journal of Cognitive Neuroscience* 11: 335–346.
Rolls ET, Stringer SM, & Trappenberg TP (2002). A unified model of spatial and episodic memory. *Proceedings of The Royal Society B* 269: 1087–1093.
Rolls ET, Aggelopoulos NC, & Zheng F (2003a). The receptive fields of inferior temporal cortex neurons in natural scenes. *Journal of Neuroscience* 23: 339–348.
Rolls ET, Franco L, Aggelopoulos NC, & Reece S (2003b). An information theoretic approach to the contributions of the firing rates and the correlations between the firing of neurons. *Journal of Neurophysiology* 89: 2810–2822.
Rolls ET, Kringelbach ML, & De Araujo IET (2003c). Different representations of pleasant and unpleasant odours in the human brain. *European Journal of Neuroscience* 18: 695–703.
Rolls ET, O'Doherty J, Kringelbach ML, Francis S, Bowtell R, & McGlone F (2003d). Representations of pleasant and painful touch in the human orbitofrontal and cingulate cortices. *Cerebral Cortex* 13: 308–317.

Rolls ET, Verhagen JV, & Kadohisa M (2003e). Representations of the texture of food in the primate orbitofrontal cortex: neurons responding to viscosity, grittiness, and capsaicin. *Journal of Neurophysiology* 90: 3711–3724.

Rolls ET, Aggelopoulos NC, Franco L, & Treves A (2004). Information encoding in the inferior temporal visual cortex: contributions of the firing rates and the correlations between the firing of neurons. *Biological Cybernetics* 90: 19–32.

Rolls ET, Browning AS, Inoue K, & Hernadi S (2005a). Novel visual stimuli activate a population of neurons in the primate orbitofrontal cortex. *Neurobiology of Learning and Memory* 84: 111–123.

Rolls ET, Franco L, & Stringer SM (2005b). The perirhinal cortex and long-term familiarity memory. *Quarterly Journal of Experimental Psychology B* 58: 234–245.

Rolls ET, Xiang JZ, & Franco L (2005c). Object, space and object-space representations in the primate hippocampus. *Journal of Neurophysiology* 94: 833–844.

Rolls ET, Critchley HD, Browning AS, & Inoue K (2006a). Face-selective and auditory neurons in the primate orbitofrontal cortex. *Experimental Brain Research* 170: 74–87.

Rolls ET, Franco L, Aggelopoulos NC, & Jerez JM (2006b). Information in the first spike, the order of spikes, and the number of spikes provided by neurons in the inferior temporal visual cortex. *Vision Research* 46: 4193–4205.

Rolls ET, Grabenhorst F, Margot C, da Silva M, & Velazco MI (2008a). Selective attention to affective value alters how the brain processes olfactory stimuli. *Journal of Cognitive Neuroscience* 20: 1815–1826.

Rolls ET, Grabenhorst F, & Parris B (2008b). Warm pleasant feelings in the brain. *Neuroimage* 41: 1504–1513.

Rolls ET, Loh M, & Deco G (2008c). An attractor hypothesis of obsessive-compulsive disorder. *European Journal of Neuroscience* 28: 782–793.

Rolls ET, Loh M, Deco G, & Winterer G (2008d). Computational models of schizophrenia and dopamine modulation in the prefrontal cortex. *Nature Reviews Neuroscience* 9: 696–709.

Rolls ET, McCabe C, & Redoute J (2008e). Expected value, reward outcome, and temporal difference error representations in a probabilistic decision task. *Cerebral Cortex* 18: 652–663.

Rolls ET, Grabenhorst F, & Franco L (2009). Prediction of subjective affective state from brain activations. *Journal of Neurophysiology* 101: 1294–1308.

Rolls ET, Critchley H, Verhagen JV, & Kadohisa M (2010a). The representation of information about taste and odor in the primate orbitofrontal cortex. *Chemosensory Perception* 3: 16–33.

Rolls ET, Grabenhorst F, & Deco G (2010b). Choice, difficulty, and confidence in the brain. *Neuroimage* 53: 694–706.

Rolls ET, Grabenhorst F, & Deco G (2010c). Decision-making, errors, and confidence in the brain. *Journal of Neurophysiology* 104: 2359–2374.

Rolls ET, Grabenhorst F, & Parris BA (2010d). Neural systems underlying decisions about affective odors. *Journal of Cognitive Neuroscience* 10: 1068–1082.

Rolls ET, Webb TJ, & Deco G (2012). Communication before coherence. *European Journal of Neuroscience* 36: 2689–2709.

Rolls ET, Dempere-Marco L, & Deco G (2013). Holding multiple items in short term memory: a neural mechanism. *PLoS One* 8: e61078.

Romo R & Salinas E (2001). Touch and go: Decision-making mechanisms in somatosensation. *Annual Review of Neuroscience* 24: 107–137.

Romo R & Salinas E (2003). Flutter discrimination: Neural codes, perception, memory and decision making. *Nature Reviews Neuroscience* 4: 203–218.

Romo R, Hernandez A, Zainos A, Lemus L, & Brody C (2002). Neural correlates of decision-making in secondary somatosensory cortex. *Nature Neuroscience* 5: 1217–1225.

Romo R, Hernandez A, Zainos A, & Salinas E (2003). Correlated neuronal discharges that increase coding efficiency during perceptual discrimination. *Neuron* 38: 649–657.

Romo R, Hernandez A, & Zainos A (2004). Neuronal correlates of a perceptual decision in ventral premotor cortex. *Neuron* 41: 165–173.

Rosenberg DR, MacMaster FP, Keshavan MS, Fitzgerald KD, Stewart CM, & Moore GJ (2000). Decrease in caudate glutamatergic concentrations in pediatric obsessive-compulsive disorder patients taking paroxetine. *Journal of the American Academy of Child and Adolescent Psychiatry* 39: 1096–1103.

Rosenberg DR, MacMillan SN, & Moore GJ (2001). Brain anatomy and chemistry may predict treatment response in paediatric obsessive–compulsive disorder. *International Journal of Neuropsychopharmacology* 4: 179–190.

Rosenberg DR, Mirza Y, Russell A, Tang J, Smith JM, Banerjee SP, Bhandari R, Rose M, Ivey J, Boyd C, & Moore GJ (2004). Reduced anterior cingulate glutamatergic concentrations in childhood OCD and major depression versus healthy controls. *Journal of the American Academy of Child and Adolescent Psychiatry* 43: 1146–1153.

Rosenkilde CE (1979). Functional heterogeneity of the prefrontal cortex in the monkey: a review. *Behavioral and Neural Biology* 25: 301–345.

Rosenkilde CE, Bauer RH, & Fuster JM (1981). Single unit activity in ventral prefrontal cortex in behaving monkeys. *Brain Research* 209: 375–394.

Rosenthal D (1990). A theory of consciousness. *ZIF Report 40/1990. Zentrum für Interdisziplinaire Forschung, Bielefeld* 40. Reprinted in Block, N., Flanagan, O. and Guzeldere, G. (eds.) (1997) *The Nature of Consciousness: Philosophical Debates*. MIT Press, Cambridge MA, pp. 729–853.
Rosenthal DM (1986). Two concepts of consciousness. *Philosophical Studies* 49: 329–359.
Rosenthal DM (1993). Thinking that one thinks. In Davies M & Humphreys GW, editors, *Consciousness*, chap. 10, 197–223. Blackwell, Oxford.
Rosenthal DM (2004). Varieties of higher order theory. In Gennaro RJ, editor, *Higher Order Theories of Consciousness*, 17–44. John Benjamins, Amsterdam.
Rosenthal DM (2005). *Consciousness and Mind.* Oxford University Press, Oxford.
Rosenthal DM (2012). Higher-order awareness, misrepresentation, and function. *Philosophical Transactions of the Royal Society B: Biological Sciences* 367: 1424–1438.
Roxin A & Ledberg A (2008). Neurobiological models of two-choice decision making can be reduced to a one-dimensional nonlinear diffusion equation. *PLoS Computational Biology* 4(3): e1000046.
Royet JP, Zald D, Versace R, Costes N, Lavenne F, Koenig O, Gervais R, Routtenberg A, Gardner EI, & Huang YH (2000). Emotional responses to pleasant and unpleasant olfactory, visual, and auditory stimuli: a positron emission tomography study. *Journal of Neuroscience* 20: 7752–7759.
Rozin P & Kalat JW (1971). Specific hungers and poison avoidance as adaptive specializations of learning. *Psychological Review* 78: 459–486.
Rudebeck PH & Murray EA (2011). Dissociable effects of subtotal lesions within the macaque orbital prefrontal cortex on reward-guided behavior. *Journal of Neuroscience* 31: 10569–10578.
Rudebeck PH, Behrens TE, Kennerley SW, Baxter MG, Buckley MJ, Walton ME, & Rushworth MF (2008). Frontal cortex subregions play distinct roles in choices between actions and stimuli. *Journal of Neuroscience* 28: 13775–13785.
Rumelhart DE, Hinton GE, & Williams RJ (1986). Learning internal representations by error propagation. In Rumelhart DE, McClelland JL, & the PDP Research Group, editors, *Parallel Distributed Processing: Explorations in the Microstructure of Cognition*, vol. 1, chap. 8, 318–362. MIT Press, Cambridge, MA.
Rupp HA & Wallen K (2009). Sex-specific content preferences for visual sexual stimuli. *Archives in Sexual Behavior* 38: 417–426.
Rushworth MF, Noonan MP, Boorman ED, Walton ME, & Behrens TE (2011). Frontal cortex and reward-guided learning and decision-making. *Neuron* 70: 1054–1069.
Rushworth MF, Kolling N, Sallet J, & Mars RB (2012). Valuation and decision-making in frontal cortex: one or many serial or parallel systems? *Current Opinion in Neurobiology* 22: 946–955.
Rushworth MFS, Hadland KA, Paus T, & Sipila PK (2002). Role of the human medial frontal cortex in task-switching: a combined fMRI and TMS study. *Journal of Neurophysiology* 87: 2577–2592.
Rushworth MFS, Hadland KA, Gaffan D, & Passingham RE (2003). The effect of cingulate cortex lesions on task switching and working memory. *Journal of Cognitive Neuroscience* 15: 338–353.
Rushworth MFS, Walton ME, Kennerley SW, & Bannerman DM (2004). Action sets and decisions in the medial frontal cortex. *Trends in Cognitive Sciences* 8: 410–417.
Rushworth MFS, Behrens TE, Rudebeck PH, & Walton ME (2007a). Contrasting roles for cingulate and orbitofrontal cortex in decisions and social behaviour. *Trends in Cognitive Sciences* 11: 168–176.
Rushworth MFS, Buckley MJ, Behrens TE, Walton ME, & Bannerman DM (2007b). Functional organization of the medial frontal cortex. *Current Opinion in Neurobiology* 17: 220–227.
Russchen FT, Amaral DG, & Price JL (1985). The afferent connections of the substantia innominata in the monkey, Macaca fascicularis. *Journal of Comparative Neurology* 242: 1–27.
Rusting C & Larsen R (1998). Personality and cognitive processing of affective information. *Personality and Social Psychology Bulletin* 24: 200–213.
Rutishauser U, Tudusciuc O, Neumann D, Mamelak AN, Heller AC, Ross IB, Philpott L, Sutherling WW, & Adolphs R (2011). Single-unit responses selective for whole faces in the human amygdala. *Current Biology* 21: 1654–1660.
Rylander G (1948). Personality analysis before and after frontal lobotomy. *Association for Research into Nervous and Mental Disorders* 27 (The Frontal Lobes): 691–705.
Saint-Cyr JA, Ungerleider LG, & Desimone R (1990). Organization of visual cortical inputs to the striatum and subsequent outputs to the pallido-nigral complex in the monkey. *Journal of Comparative Neurology* 298: 129–156.
Saleem KS, Kondo H, & Price JL (2008). Complementary circuits connecting the orbital and medial prefrontal networks with the temporal, insular, and opercular cortex in the macaque monkey. *Journal of Comparative Neurology* 506: 659–693.
Salin P & Prince D (1996). Spontaneous GABA-A receptor mediated inhibitory currents in adult rat somatosensory cortex. *Journal of Neurophysiology* 75: 1573–1588.
Salzman D, Britten K, & Newsome W (1990). Cortical microstimulation influences perceptual judgements of motion direction. *Nature* 364: 174–177.
Samuelson PA (1938). A note on the pure theory of consumers' behavior. *Economica* 51: 61–71.

Sanfey AG, Rilling JK, Aronson JA, Nystrom LE, & Cohen JD (2003). The neural basis of economic decision-making in the ultimatum game. *Science* 300: 1755–1758.

Sanghera MK, Rolls ET, & Roper-Hall A (1979). Visual responses of neurons in the dorsolateral amygdala of the alert monkey. *Experimental Neurology* 63: 610–626.

Saper CB, Loewy AD, Swanson LW, & Cowan WM (1976). Direct hypothalamo-autonomic connections. *Brain Research* 117: 305–312.

Sara SJ & Bouret S (2012). Orienting and reorienting: the locus coeruleus mediates cognition through arousal. *Neuron* 76: 130–141.

Sato T, Kawamura T, & Iwai E (1980). Responsiveness of inferotemporal single units to visual pattern stimuli in monkeys performing discrimination. *Experimental Brain Research* 38: 313–319.

Savic I (2001). Smelling of odorous sex hormone-like compounds causes sex-differentiated hypothalamic activations in humans. *Neuron* 31: 661–668.

Savic I (2002). Imaging of brain activation by odorants in humans. *Current Opinion in Neurobiology* 12: 455–461.

Savic I, Berglund H, Gulyas B, & Roland P (2001). Smelling of odorous sex hormones-like compounds causes sex-differentiated hypothalamic activations in humans. *Neuron* 31: 661–668.

Schachter S (1971). Importance of cognitive control in obesity. *American Psychologist* 26: 129–144.

Schachter S & Singer J (1962). Cognitive, social and physiological determinants of emotional state. *Psychological Review* 69: 378–399.

Schacter GB, Yang CR, Innis NK, & Mogenson GJ (1989). The role of the hippocampal–nucleus accumbens pathway in radial-arm maze performance. *Brain Research* 494: 339–349.

Schaefer ML, Young DA, & Restrepo D (2001). Olfactory fingerprints for major histocompatibility complex-determined body odors. *Journal of Neuroscience* 21: 2481–2487.

Schaefer ML, Yamazaki K, Osada K, Restrepo D, & Beauchamp GK (2002). Olfactory fingerprints for major histocompatibility complex-determined body odors II: Relationship among odor maps, genetics, odor composition, and behavior. *Journal of Neuroscience* 22: 9513–9521.

Schall J (2001). Neural basis of deciding, choosing and acting. *Nature Review Neuroscience* 2: 33–42.

Scherer K (2009). The dynamic architecture of emotion: Evidence for the component process model. *Cognition and Emotion* 23: 1307–1351.

Scherer KS (1999). Appraisal theory. In Dalgleish T & Power MJ, editors, *Handbook of Cognition and Emotion*, 637–663. Wiley, New York.

Scherer KS (2001). The nature and study of appraisal. A review of the issues. In Scherer KS, Schorr A, & Johnstone T, editors, *Appraisal Processes in Emotion*, 369–391. Oxford University Press, Oxford.

Scherer KS, Schorr A, & Johnstone T, editors (2001). *Appraisal Processes in Emotion*. Oxford University Press, Oxford.

Scheuerecker J, Ufer S, Zipse M, Frodl T, Koutsouleris N, Zetzsche T, Wiesmann M, Albrecht J, Bruckmann H, Schmitt G, Moller HJ, & Meisenzahl EM (2008). Cerebral changes and cognitive dysfunctions in medication-free schizophrenia – An fMRI study. *Journal of Psychiatric Research* 42: 469–476.

Schiller D, Monfils MH, Raio CM, Johnson DC, LeDoux JE, & Phelps EA (2010). Preventing the return of fear in humans using reconsolidation update mechanisms. *Nature* 463: 49–53.

Schirmer A, Zysset S, Kotz SA, & von Cramon YD (2004). Gender differences in the activation of inferior frontal cortex during emotional speech perception. *Neuroimage* 21: 1114–1123.

Schliebs R & Arendt T (2011). The cholinergic system in aging and neuronal degeneration. *Behavioral Brain Research* 221: 555–563.

Schmitt DP (2004). The big five related to risky sexual behaviour across 10 world regions: differential personality associations of sexual promiscuity and relationship infidelity. *European Journal of Personality* 18: 301–319.

Schoenbaum G & Eichenbaum H (1995). Information encoding in the rodent prefrontal cortex. I. Single-neuron activity in orbitofrontal cortex compared with that in pyriform cortex. *Journal of Neurophysiology* 74: 733–750.

Schoenbaum G, Roesch MR, Stalnaker TA, & Takahashi YK (2009). A new perspective on the role of the orbitofrontal cortex in adaptive behaviour. *Nature Reviews Neuroscience* 10: 885–892.

Schultz W (1998). Predictive reward signal of dopamine neurons. *Journal of Neurophysiology* 80: 1–27.

Schultz W (2004). Neural coding of basic reward terms of animal learning theory, game theory, microeconomics and behavioural ecology. *Current Opinion in Neurobiology* 14: 139–147.

Schultz W (2006). Behavioral theories and the neurophysiology of reward. *Annual Review of Psychology* 57: 87–115.

Schultz W (2013). Updating dopamine reward signals. *Current Opinion in Neurobiology* 23: 229–238.

Schultz W, Apicella P, Scarnati E, & Ljungberg T (1992). Neuronal activity in the ventral striatum related to the expectation of reward. *Journal of Neuroscience* 12: 4595–4610.

Schultz W, Apicella P, Romo R, & Scarnati E (1995a). Context-dependent activity in primate striatum reflecting past and future behavioral events. In Houk JC, Davis JL, & Beiser DG, editors, *Models of Information Processing in the Basal Ganglia*, chap. 2, 11–27. MIT Press, Cambridge, MA.

Schultz W, Romo R, Ljunberg T, Mirenowicz J, Hollerman JR, & Dickinson A (1995b). Reward-related signals carried by dopamine neurons. In Houk JC, Davis JL, & Beiser DG, editors, *Models of Information Processing*

in the Basal Ganglia, chap. 12, 233–248. MIT Press, Cambridge, MA.
Schultz W, Dayan P, & Montague PR (1997). A neural substrate of prediction and reward. *Science* 275: 1593–1599.
Schultz W, Tremblay L, & Hollerman JR (2003). Changes in behavior-related neuronal activity in the striatum during learning. *Trends in Neurosciences* 26: 312–328.
Schwaber JS, Kapp BS, Higgins GA, & Rapp PR (1982). Amygdaloid and basal forebrain direct connections with the nucleus of the solitary tract and the dorsal motor nucleus. *Journal of Neuroscience* 2: 1424–1438.
Schwartz MW & Porte D (2005). Diabetes, obesity, and the brain. *Science* 307: 375–379.
Scott SK, Young AW, Calder AJ, Hellawell DJ, Aggleton JP, & Johnson M (1997). Impaired auditory recognition of fear and anger following bilateral amygdala lesions. *Nature* 385: 254–257.
Scott TR (2011). Learning through the taste system. *Frontiers in Systems Neuroscience* 5: 87.
Scott TR & Giza BK (1987). A measure of taste intensity discrimination in the rat through conditioned taste aversions. *Physiology and Behaviour* 41: 315–320.
Scott TR & Giza BK (1992). Gustatory control of ingestion. In Booth DA, editor, *The Neurophysiology of Ingestion*. Manchester University Press, Manchester.
Scott TR & Small DM (2009). The role of the parabrachial nucleus in taste processing and feeding. *Annals of the New York Academy of Sciences* 1170: 372–377.
Scott TR, Yaxley S, Sienkiewicz ZJ, & Rolls ET (1986a). Taste responses in the nucleus tractus solitarius of the behaving monkey. *Journal of Neurophysiology* 55: 182–200.
Scott TR, Yaxley S, Sienkiewicz ZJ, & Rolls ET (1986b). Gustatory responses in the frontal opercular cortex of the alert cynomolgus monkey. *Journal of Neurophysiology* 56: 876–890.
Scott TR, Karadi Z, Oomura Y, Nishino H, Plata-Salaman CR, Lenard L, Giza BK, & Aou S (1993). Gustatory neural coding in the amygdala of the alert monkey. *Journal of Neurophysiology* 69: 1810–1820.
Scott TR, Yan J, & Rolls ET (1995). Brain mechanisms of satiety and taste in macaques. *Neurobiology* 3: 281–292.
Seamans JK & Yang CR (2004). The principal features and mechanisms of dopamine modulation in the prefrontal cortex. *Progress in Neurobiology* 74: 1–58.
Seigel M & Auerbach JM (1996). Neuromodulators of synaptic strength. In Fazeli MS & Collingridge GL, editors, *Cortical Plasticity*, chap. 7, 137–148. Bios, Oxford.
Seleman LD & Goldman-Rakic PS (1985). Longitudinal topography and interdigitation of corticostriatal projections in the rhesus monkey. *Journal of Neuroscience* 5: 776–794.
Seligman ME (1970). On the generality of the laws of learning. *Psychological Review* 77: 406–418.
Seltzer B & Pandya DN (1989). Frontal lobe connections of the superior temporal sulcus in the rhesus monkey. *Journal of Comparative Neurology* 281: 97–113.
Sem-Jacobsen CW (1968). *Depth-Electrographic Stimulation of the Human Brain and Behavior: From Fourteen Years of Studies and Treatment of Parkinson's Disease and Mental Disorders with Implanted Electrodes*. C. C. Thomas, Springfield, IL.
Sem-Jacobsen CW (1976). Electrical stimulation and self-stimulation in man with chronic implanted electrodes. Interpretation and pitfalls of results. In Wauquier A & Rolls ET, editors, *Brain-Stimulation Reward*, 505–520. North-Holland, Amsterdam.
Setlow B, Gallagher M, & Holland PC (2002). The basolateral complex of the amygdala is necessary for acquisition but not expression of CS motivational value in appetitive Pavlovian second-order conditioning. *European Journal of Neuroscience* 15: 1841–1853.
Seymour B, O'Doherty J, Dayan P, Koltzenburg M, Jones AK, Dolan RJ, Friston KJ, & Frackowiak RS (2004). Temporal difference models describe higher-order learning in humans. *Nature* 429: 664–667.
Shackelford TK & Goetz AT (2007). Adaptation to sperm competition in humans. *Current Directions in Psychological Science* 16: 47–50.
Shackelford TK, Le Blanc GL, Weekes-Shackelford VA, Bleske-Rechek AL, Euler HA, & Hoier S (2002). Psychological adaptation to human sperm competition. *Evolution and Human Behaviour* 23: 123–138.
Shadlen MN & Newsome WT (1996). Motion perception: seeing and deciding. *Proceedings of the National Academy of Sciences U S A* 93: 628–633.
Shadlen MN & Newsome WT (2001). Neural basis of a perceptual decision in the parietal cortex (area LIP) of the rhesus monkey. *Journal of Neurophysiology* 86: 1916–1936.
Shallice T (1982). Specific impairments of planning. *Philosophical Transactions of the Royal Society of London B* 298: 199–209.
Shallice T & Burgess P (1996). The domain of supervisory processes and temporal organization of behaviour. *Philosophical Transactions of the Royal Society B*, 351: 1405–1411.
Shallice T & Burgess PW (1991). Deficits in strategy application following frontal lobe damage in man. *Brain* 114: 727–741.
Shang Y, Claridge-Chang A, Sjulson L, Pypaert M, & Miesenböck G (2007). Excitatory local circuits and their implications for olfactory processing in the fly antennal lobe. *Cell* 128: 601–612.
Sheinberg DL & Logothetis NK (2001). Noticing familiar objects in real world scenes: The role of temporal cortical neurons in natural vision. *Journal of Neuroscience* 21: 1340–1350.
Shepherd GM (2004). *The Synaptic Organisation of the Brain*. Oxford University Press, Oxford, 5th edn.

Shepherd GM & Grillner S, editors (2010). *Handbook of Brain Microcircuits*. Oxford University Press, Oxford.

Shergill SS, Brammer MJ, Williams SC, Murray RM, & McGuire PK (2000). Mapping auditory hallucinations in schizophrenia using functional magnetic resonance imaging. *Archives of General Psychiatry* 57: 1033–1038.

Shiino M & Fukai T (1990). Replica-symmetric theory of the nonlinear analogue neural networks. *Journal of Physics A: Mathematical and General* 23: L1009–L1017.

Shima K & Tanji J (1998). Role for cingulate motor area cells in voluntary movement selection based on reward. *Science* 13: 1335–1338.

Shimura T & Shimokochi M (1990). Involvement of the lateral mesencephalic tegmentum in copulatory behavior of male rats: neuron activity in freely moving animals. *Neuroscience Research* 9: 173–183.

Shizgal P & Arvanitogiannis A (2003). Gambling on dopamine. *Science* 299: 1856–1858.

Short RV (1998). Review of R. R. Baker and M. A. Bellis, Human Sperm Competition: Copulation, Masturbation and Infidelity. *European Sociobiological Society Newsletter* 47: 20–23.

Sigala N & Logothetis NK (2002). Visual categorisation shapes feature selectivity in the primate temporal cortex. *Nature* 415: 318–320.

Simmen-Tulberg B & Moller AP (1993). The relationship between concealed ovulation and mating systems in anthropoid primates: a phylogenetic analysis. *American Naturalist* 141: 1–25.

Simmons JM, Ravel S, Shidara M, & Richmond BJ (2007). A comparison of reward-contingent neuronal activity in monkey orbitofrontal cortex and ventral striatum: guiding actions toward rewards. *Annals of the New York Academy of Sciences* 1121: 376–394.

Simmons JM, Minamimoto T, Murray EA, & Richmond BJ (2010). Selective ablations reveal that orbital and lateral prefrontal cortex play different roles in estimating predicted reward value. *Journal of Neuroscience* 30: 15878–15887.

Simmons LW, Firman RC, Rhodes G, & Peters M (2004). Human sperm competition: testis size, sperm production and rate of extra-pair copulations. *Animal Behaviour* 68: 297–302.

Singer P (1981). *The Expanding Circle: Ethics and Sociobiology*. Oxford University Press, Oxford.

Singer T, Seymour B, O'Doherty J, Kaube H, Dolan RJ, & Frith CD (2004). Empathy for pain involves the affective but not sensory components of pain. *Science* 303: 1157–1162.

Singer W (1987). Activity-dependent self-organization of synaptic connections as a substrate for learning. In Changeux JP & Konishi M, editors, *The Neural and Molecular Bases of Learning*, 301–335. Wiley, Chichester.

Singer W (1995). Development and plasticity of cortical processing architectures. *Science* 270: 758–764.

Singer W (1999). Neuronal synchrony: A versatile code for the definition of relations? *Neuron* 24: 49–65.

Singh D (1993). Adaptive significance of female physical attractiveness: role of waist-to-hip ratio. *Journal of Personality and Social Psychology* 65: 293–307.

Singh D (1995). Female health, attractiveness, and desirability for relationships: role of breast asymmetry and waist-to-hip ratio. *Ethology and Sociobiology* 16: 465–481.

Singh D & Bronstad MP (2001). Female body odour is a potential cue to ovulation. *Proceedings of the Royal Society of London B* 268: 797–801.

Singh D & Luis S (1995). Ethnic and gender consensus for the effect of waist-to-hip ratio on judgements of women's attractiveness. *Human Nature* 6: 51–65.

Singh D & Young RK (1995). Body weight, waist-to-hip ratio, breasts and hips: role in judgements of female attractiveness and desirability for relationships. *Ethology and Sociobiology* 16: 483–507.

Singh D, Meyer W, Zambarano RJ, & Hurlbert DF (1998). Frequency and timing of coital orgasm in women desirous of becoming pregnant. *Archives of Sexual Behaviour* 27: 15–29.

Sisk CL & Foster DL (2004). The neural basis of puberty and adolescence. *Nature Neuroscience* 7: 1040–1047.

Small DM (2010). Taste representation in the human insula. *Brain Structre and Function* 214: 551–561.

Small DM & Scott TR (2009). Symposium overview: What happens to the pontine processing? Repercussions of interspecies differences in pontine taste representation for tasting and feeding. *Annals of the New York Academy of Science* 1170: 343–346.

Small DM, Zald DH, Jones-Gotman M, Zatorre RJ, Petrides M, & Evans AC (1999). Human cortical gustatory areas: a review of functional neuroimaing data. *NeuroReport* 8: 3913–3917.

Small DM, Bender G, Veldhuizen MG, Rudenga K, Nachtigal D, & Felsted J (2007). The role of the human orbitofrontal cortex in taste and flavor processing. *Annals of the New York Academy of Sciences* 1121: 136–151.

Smerieri A, Rolls ET, & Feng J (2010). Decision time, slow inhibition, and theta rhythm. *Journal of Neuroscience* 30: 14173–14181.

Smith P & Ratcliff R (2004). Psychology and neurobiology of simple decisions. *Trends in Neurosciences* 23: 161–168.

Smith R, Fadok RA, Purcell M, Liu S, Stonnington C, Spetzler RF, & Baxter LC (2011). Localizing sadness activation within the subgenual cingulate in individuals: a novel functional mri paradigm for detecting individual differences in the neural circuitry underlying depression. *Brain Imaging and Behavior* 5: 229–239.

Smith RL (1984). Human sperm competiton. In Smith RL, editor, *Sperm Competition and the Evolution of Animal Mating Systems*, 601–660. Academic Press, London.

Smith-Swintosky VL, Plata-Salaman CR, & Scott TR (1991). Gustatory neural coding in the monkey cortex: stimulus quality. *Journal of Neurophysiology* 66: 1156–1165.

Sobel N, Prabhakaran V, Hartley CA, Desmond JE, Glover GH, Sullivan EV, & Gabrieli JD (1999). Blind smell: brain activation induced by an undetected air-borne chemical. *Brain* 122: 209–217.

Softky WR & Koch C (1993). The highly irregular firing of cortical cells is inconsistent with temporal integration of random EPSPs. *Journal of Neuroscience* 13: 334–350.

Soltani A & Wang XJ (2006). A biophysically based neural model of matching law behavior: melioration by stochastic synapses. *Journal of Neuroscience* 26: 3731–3744.

Somerville LH, Hare T, & Casey BJ (2011). Frontostriatal maturation predicts cognitive control failure to appetitive cues in adolescents. *Journal of Cognitive Neuroscience* 23: 2123–2134.

Sompolinsky H & Kanter I (1986). Temporal association in asymmetric neural networks. *Physical Review Letters* 57: 2861–2864.

Spiegler BJ & Mishkin M (1981). Evidence for the sequential participation of inferior temporal cortex and amygdala in the acquisition of stimulus–reward associations. *Behavioural Brain Research* 3: 303–317.

Spiridon M, Fischl B, & Kanwisher N (2006). Location and spatial profile of category-specific regions in human extrastriate cortex. *Human Brain Mapping* 27: 77–89.

Spruston N, Jonas P, & Sakmann B (1995). Dendritic glutamate receptor channel in rat hippocampal CA3 and CA1 pyramidal neurons. *Journal of Physiology* 482: 325–352.

Squire LR (1992). Memory and the hippocampus: A synthesis from findings with rats, monkeys and humans. *Psychological Review* 99: 195–231.

Squire LR, Stark CEL, & Clark RE (2004). The medial temporal lobe. *Annual Review of Neuroscience* 27: 279–306.

Starkstein SE & Robinson RG (1991). The role of the frontal lobe in affective disorder following stroke. In Eisenberg HM, editor, *Frontal Lobe Function and Dysfunction*, 288–303. Oxford University Press, New York.

Stefanacci L, Suzuki WA, & Amaral DG (1996). Organization of connections between the amygdaloid complex and the perirhinal and parahippocampal cortices in macaque monkeys. *Journal of Comparative Neurology* 375: 552–582.

Stein NL, Trabasso T, & Liwag M (1994). The Rashomon phenomenon: personal frames and future-oriented appraisals in memory for emotional events. In Haith MM, Benson JB, Roberts RJ, & Pennington BF, editors, *Future Oriented Processes*. University of Chicago Press, Chicago.

Steiner JE, Glaser D, Hawilo ME, & Berridge KC (2001). Comparative expression of hedonic impact: affective reactions to taste by human infants and other primates. *Neuroscience and Biobehavioral Reviews* 25: 53–74.

Stellar E (1954). The physiology of motivation. *Psychological Review* 61: 5–22.

Stemmler DG (1989). The autonomic differentiation of emotions revisited: convergent and discriminant validation. *Psychophysiology* 26: 617–632.

Stent GS (1973). A psychological mechanism for Hebb's postulate of learning. *Proceedings of the National Academy of Sciences USA* 70: 997–1001.

Stephan KE, Weiskopf N, Drysdale PM, Robinson PA, & Friston KJ (2007). Comparing hemodynamic models with DCM. *Neuroimage* 38: 387–401.

Stern CE & Passingham RE (1995). The nucleus accumbens in monkeys (Macaca fascicularis): III. Reversal learning. *Experimental Brain Research* 106: 239–247.

Stern CE & Passingham RE (1996). The nucleus accumbens in monkeys (Macaca fascicularis): II. Emotion and motivation. *Behavioural Brain Research* 75: 179–193.

Stewart SE, Fagerness JA, Platko J, Smoller JW, Scharf JM, Illmann C, Jenike E, Chabane N, Leboyer M, Delorme R, Jenike MA, & Pauls DL (2007). Association of the SLC1A1 glutamate transporter gene and obsessive-compulsive disorder. *American Journal of Medical Genetics B: Neuropsychiatric Genetics* 144: 1027–1033.

Stocks NG (2000). Suprathreshold stochastic resonance in multilevel threshold systems. *Physical Review Letters* 84: 2310–2313.

Stone M (1960). Models for choice-reaction time. *Psychometrika* 25: 251–260.

Stone VE, Baron-Cohen S, Calder A, Keane J, & Young A (2003). Acquired theory of mind impairments in individuals with bilateral amygdala lesions. *Neuropsychologia* 41: 209–220.

Strauss E & Moscowitsch M (1981). Perception of facial expressions. *Brain and Language* 13: 308–332.

Strick PL, Dum RP, & Picard N (1995). Macro-organization of the circuits connecting the basal ganglia with the cortical motor areas. In Houk JC, Davis JL, & Beiser DG, editors, *Models of Information Processing in the Basal Ganglia*, chap. 6, 117–130. MIT Press, Cambridge, MA.

Stringer SM & Rolls ET (2000). Position invariant recognition in the visual system with cluttered environments. *Neural Networks* 13: 305–315.

Stringer SM & Rolls ET (2002). Invariant object recognition in the visual system with novel views of 3D objects. *Neural Computation* 14: 2585–2596.

Stringer SM & Rolls ET (2008). Learning transform invariant object recognition in the visual system with multiple stimuli present during training. *Neural Networks* 21: 888–903.

Stringer SM, Perry G, Rolls ET, & Proske JH (2006). Learning invariant object recognition in the visual system with continuous transformations. *Biological Cybernetics* 94: 128–142.

Stringer SM, Rolls ET, & Tromans JM (2007). Invariant object recognition with trace learning and multiple stimuli present during training. *Network: Computation in Neural Systems* 18: 161–187.

Strongman KT (2003). *The Psychology of Emotion.* Wiley, New York, 5th edn.

Stuss DT (2011). Functions of the frontal lobes: relation to executive functions. *Journal of the International Neuropsychology Society* 17: 759–65.

Sugrue LP, Corrado GS, & Newsome WT (2005). Choosing the greater of two goods: neural currencies for valuation and decision making. *Nature Reviews Neuroscience* 6: 363–375.

Suri RE & Schultz W (1998). Learning of sequential movements by neural network model with dopamine-like reinforcement signal. *Experimental Brain Research* 121: 350–354.

Suri RE & Schultz W (2001). Temporal difference model reproduces anticipatory neural activity. *Neural Computation* 13: 841–862.

Sutherland S (1997). Emotional displays. *Nature* 390: 458.

Sutton RS & Barto AG (1981). Towards a modern theory of adaptive networks: expectation and prediction. *Psychological Review* 88: 135–170.

Sutton RS & Barto AG (1990). Time-derivative models of Pavlovian reinforcement. In Gabriel M & Moore J, editors, *Learning and Computational Neuroscience*, 497–537. MIT Press, Cambridge, MA.

Sutton RS & Barto AG (1998). *Reinforcement Learning.* MIT Press, Cambridge, MA.

Suzuki K, Simpson KA, Minnion JS, Shillito JC, & Bloom SR (2010). The role of gut hormones and the hypothalamus in appetite regulation. *Endocrinology Journal* 57: 359–372.

Suzuki WA & Amaral DG (1994). Perirhinal and parahippocampal cortices of the macaque monkey – cortical afferents. *Journal of Comparative Neurology* 350: 497–533.

Suzuki WA, Miller EK, & Desimone R (1997). Object and place memory in the macaque entorhinal cortex. *Journal of Neurophysiology* 78: 1062–1081.

Swaddle JP & Reierson GW (2002). Testosterone increases perceived dominance but not attractiveness in human males. *Proceedings of the Royal Society of London B* 269: 2285–2289.

Swash M (1989). John Hughlings Jackson: a historical introduction. In Kennard C & Swash M, editors, *Hierarchies in Neurology*, chap. 1, 3–10. Springer, London.

Szabo M, Almeida R, Deco G, & Stetter M (2004). Cooperation and biased competition model can explain attentional filtering in the prefrontal cortex. *European Journal of Neuroscience* 19: 1969–1977.

Szabo M, Deco G, Fusi S, Del Giudice P, Mattia M, & Stetter M (2006). Learning to attend: Modeling the shaping of selectivity in infero-temporal cortex in a categorization task. *Biological Cybernetics* 94: 351–365.

Tabuchi E, Mulder AB, & Wiener SI (2003). Reward value invariant place responses and reward site associated activity in hippocampal neurons of behaving rats. *Hippocampus* 13: 117–132.

Tagamets M & Horwitz B (1998). Integrating electrophysical and anatomical experimental data to create a large-scale model that simulates a delayed match-to-sample human brain study. *Cerebral Cortex* 8: 310–320.

Taira K & Rolls ET (1996). Receiving grooming as a reinforcer for the monkey. *Physiology and Behavior* 59: 1189–1192.

Takagi SF (1991). Olfactory frontal cortex and multiple olfactory processing in primates. In Peters A & Jones EG, editors, *Cerebral Cortex*, vol. 9, 133–152. Plenum Press, New York.

Takeda K & Funahashi S (2002). Prefrontal task-related activity representing visual cue location or saccade direction in spatial working memory tasks. *Journal of Neurophysiology* 87: 567–588.

Talbot W, Darian-Smith I, Kornhuber H, & Mountcastle VB (1968). The sense of fluttervibration: comparison of the human capacity response patterns of mechanoreceptive afferents from the monkey hand. *Journal of Neurophysiology* 31: 301–334.

Tamietto M, Pullens P, de Gelder B, Weiskrantz L, & Goebel R (2012). Subcortical connections to human amygdala and changes following destruction of the visual cortex. *Current Biology* 22: 1449–55.

Tanabe T, Iino M, & Takagi SF (1975a). Discrimination of odors in olfactory bulb, pyriform-amygdaloid areas, and orbitofrontal cortex of the monkey. *Journal of Neurophysiology* 38: 1284–1296.

Tanabe T, Yarita H, Iino M, Ooshima Y, & Takagi SF (1975b). An olfactory projection area in orbitofrontal cortex of the monkey. *Journal of Neurophysiology* 38: 1269–1283.

Tanaka D (1973). Effects of selective prefrontal decortication on escape behavior in the monkey. *Brain Research* 53: 161–173.

Tanaka K, Saito C, Fukada Y, & Moriya M (1990). Integration of form, texture, and color information in the inferotemporal cortex of the macaque. In Iwai E & Mishkin M, editors, *Vision, Memory and the Temporal Lobe*, chap. 10, 101–109. Elsevier, New York.

Tanaka SC, Doya K, Okada G, Ueda K, Okamoto Y, & Yamawaki S (2004). Prediction of immediate and future rewards differentially recruits cortico-basal ganglia loops. *Nature Neuroscience* 7: 887–893.

Tanner J W P & Swets JA (1954). A decision-making theory of visual detection. *Psychological Review* 61: 401–409.

Terenius L & Johansson B (2010). The opioid systems–panacea and nemesis. *Biochemical and Biophysical Research Communications* 396: 140–142.

Tessman I (1995). Human altruism as a courtship display. *Oikos* 74: 157–158.

Thierry AM, Tassin JP, Blanc G, & Glowinski J (1976). Selective activation of mesocortical DA system by stress. *Nature* 263: 242–244.

Thomas DM, Bouchard C, Church T, Slentz C, Kraus WE, Redman LM, Martin CK, Silva AM, Vossen M, Westerterp K, & Heymsfield SB (2012). Why do individuals not lose more weight from an exercise intervention at a defined dose? An energy balance analysis. *Obesity Reviews* 13: 835–847.

Thornhill R (1983). Cryptic female choice and its implications in the scorpionfly *Harpobittacus nigriceps*. *American Naturalist* 122: 765–788.

Thornhill R & Gangestad SW (1996). The evolution of human sexuality. *Trends in Ecology and Evolution* 11: 98–102.

Thornhill R & Gangstad SW (1999). The scent of symmetry: a human sex pheromone that signals fitness? *Evolution and Human Behaviour* 20: 175–201.

Thornhill R & Grammer K (1999). The body and face of woman: one ornament that signals quality? *Evolution and Human Behaviour* 20: 105–120.

Thornhill R, Gangestad SW, & Comer R (1995). Human female orgasm and mate fluctuating asymmetry. *Animal Behaviour* 50: 1601–1615.

Thorpe SJ, Maddison S, & Rolls ET (1979). Single unit activity in the orbitofrontal cortex of the behaving monkey. *Neuroscience Letters* S3: S77.

Thorpe SJ, Rolls ET, & Maddison S (1983). Neuronal activity in the orbitofrontal cortex of the behaving monkey. *Experimental Brain Research* 49: 93–115.

Tiffany ST & Drobes DJ (1990). Imagery and smoking urges: the manipulation of affective content. *Addiction and Behaviour* 15: 531–539.

Tiihonen J, Kuikka J, Kupila J, Partanen K, Vainio P, Airaksinen J, Eronen M, Hallikainen T, Paanila J, Kinnunen I, & Huttunen J (1994). Increase in cerebral blood flow of right prefrontal cortex in man during orgasm. *Neuroscience Letters* 170: 241–243.

Tinbergen N (1951). *The Study of Instinct*. Oxford University Press, Oxford.

Tinbergen N (1963). On aims and methods of ethology. *Zeitschrift fur Tierpsychologie* 20: 410–433.

Tinbergen N, Broekhuysen GJ, Feekes F, Houghton JCW, Kruuk H, & Szule E (1967). Egg shell removal by black-headed gull *Larus ribibundus*. *Behaviour* 19: 74–117.

Tobler PN, Dickinson A, & Schultz W (2003). Coding of predicted reward omission by dopamine neurons in a conditioned inhibition paradigm. *Journal of Neuroscience* 23: 10402–10410.

Tomkins SS (1995). *Exploring Affect: The Selected Writings of Sylvan S. Tomkins*. Cambridge University Press, New York.

Tovee MJ & Rolls ET (1992). Oscillatory activity is not evident in the primate temporal visual cortex with static stimuli. *Neuroreport* 3: 369–372.

Tovee MJ & Rolls ET (1995). Information encoding in short firing rate epochs by single neurons in the primate temporal visual cortex. *Visual Cognition* 2: 35–58.

Tovee MJ, Rolls ET, Treves A, & Bellis RP (1993). Information encoding and the responses of single neurons in the primate temporal visual cortex. *Journal of Neurophysiology* 70: 640–654.

Tovee MJ, Rolls ET, & Azzopardi P (1994). Translation invariance and the responses of neurons in the temporal visual cortical areas of primates. *Journal of Neurophysiology* 72: 1049–1060.

Tovee MJ, Rolls ET, & Ramachandran VS (1996). Rapid visual learning in neurones of the primate temporal visual cortex. *NeuroReport* 7: 2757–2760.

Townsend JT & Ashby FG (1983). *The Stochastic Modeling of Elementary Psychological Processes*. Cambridge University Press, Cambridge.

Tranel D, Bechara A, & Denburg NL (2002). Asymmetric functional roles of right and left ventromedial prefrontal cortices in social conduct, decision-making and emotional processing. *Cortex* 38: 589–612.

Trappenberg TP, Rolls ET, & Stringer SM (2002). Effective size of receptive fields of inferior temporal visual cortex neurons in natural scenes. In Dietterich TG, Becker S, & Gharamani Z, editors, *Advances in Neural Information Processing Systems*, vol. 14, 293–300. MIT Press, Cambridge, MA.

Tremblay L & Schultz W (1998). Modifications of reward expectation-related neuronal activity during learning in primate striatum. *Journal of Neurophysiology* 80: 964–977.

Tremblay L & Schultz W (1999). Relative reward preference in primate orbitofrontal cortex. *Nature* 398: 704–708.

Tremblay L & Schultz W (2000). Modifications of reward expectation-related neuronal activity during learning in primate orbitofrontal cortex. *Journal of Neurophysiology* 83: 1877–1885.

Treves A (1991a). Dilution and sparse encoding in threshold-linear nets. *Journal of Physics A: Mathematical and General* 24: 327–335.

Treves A (1991b). Are spin-glass effects relevant to understanding realistic auto-associative networks? *Journal of Physics A* 24: 2645–2654.

Treves A (1993). Mean-field analysis of neuronal spike dynamics. *Network* 4: 259–284.

Treves A (1995). Quantitative estimate of the information relayed by the Schaffer collaterals. *Journal of Computational Neuroscience* 2: 259–272.

Treves A & Rolls ET (1991). What determines the capacity of autoassociative memories in the brain? *Network* 2: 371–397.

Treves A & Rolls ET (1992). Computational constraints suggest the need for two distinct input systems to the hippocampal CA3 network. *Hippocampus* 2: 189–199.

Treves A & Rolls ET (1994). A computational analysis of the role of the hippocampus in memory. *Hippocampus* 4: 374–391.

Treves A, Rolls ET, & Simmen M (1997). Time for retrieval in recurrent associative memories. *Physica D* 107: 392–400.

Treves A, Panzeri S, Rolls ET, Booth M, & Wakeman EA (1999). Firing rate distributions and efficiency of information transmission of inferior temporal cortex neurons to natural visual stimuli. *Neural Computation* 11: 601–631.

Trivers R (1971). The evolution of reciprocal altruism. *Quarterly Review of Biology* 46: 35–57.

Trivers R (1974). Parent-offspring conflict. *American Zoologist* 14: 249–264.

Trivers RL (1976). Foreword. In *The Selfish Gene by R. Dawkins*. Oxford University Press, Oxford.

Trivers RL (1985). *Social Evolution*. Benjamin, Cummings, CA.

Troisi A & Carosi M (1998). Female orgasm rate increases with male dominance in Japanese macaque. *Animal Behaviour* 56: 1261–1266.

Tsao DY & Livingstone MS (2008). Mechanisms of face perception. *Annual Reviews of Neuroscience* 31: 411–437.

Tsao DY, Freiwald WA, Tootell RB, & Livingstone MS (2006). A cortical region consisting entirely of face-selective cells. *Science* 311: 617–618.

Tuckwell H (1988). *Introduction to Theoretical Neurobiology*. Cambridge University Press, Cambridge.

Tversky A & Kahneman D (1981). The framing of decisions and the psychology of choice. *Science* 211: 453–458.

Tversky A & Kahneman D (1992). Advances in prospect theory – cumulative representation of uncertainty. *Journal of Risk and Uncertainty* 5: 297–323.

Ubhi K & Masliah E (2013). Alzheimer's disease: recent advances and future perspectives. *Journal of Alzheimer's Disease* 33 Suppl 1: S185–S194.

Udry JR & Eckland BK (1984). Benefits of being attractive: differential pay-offs for men and women. *Psychological Reports* 54: 47–56.

Ullsperger M & von Cramon DY (2001). Subprocesses of performance monitoring: a dissociation of error processing and response competition revealed by event-related fMRI and ERPs. *Neuroimage* 14: 1387–1401.

Uma-Pradeep K, Geervani P, & Eggum BO (1993). Common Indian spices: nutrient composition, consumption and contribution to dietary value. *Plant Foods and Human Nutrition* 44: 138–148.

Ungerstedt U (1971). Adipsia and aphagia after 6-hydroxydopamine induced degeneration of the nigrostriatal dopamine system. *Acta Physiologia Scandinavica* 81 (Suppl. 367): 95–122.

Usher M & McClelland J (2001). On the time course of perceptual choice: the leaky competing accumulator model. *Psychological Reviews* 108: 550–592.

Uvnas-Moberg K (1997). Physiological and endocrine effects of social contact. *Annals of the New York Academy of Sciences* 807: 146–163.

Uvnas-Moberg K (1998). Oxytocin may mediate the benefits of positive social interaction and emotions. *Psychneuroendocrinology* 23: 819–835.

Valenstein ES (1974). *Brain Control. A Critical Examination of Brain Stimulation and Psychosurgery*. Wiley, New York.

van den Heuvel OA, Veltman DJ, Groenewegen HJ, Cath DC, van Balkom AJ, van Hartskamp J, Barkhof F, & van Dyck R (2005). Frontal-striatal dysfunction during planning in obsessive-compulsive disorder. *Archives of General Psychiatry* 62: 301–309.

Van der Kooy D, Koda LY, McGinty JF, Gerfen CR, & Bloom FE (1984). The organization of projections from the cortex, amygdala, and hypothalamus to the nucleus of the solitary tract in rat. *Journal of Comparative Neurology* 224: 1–24.

Van Hoesen GW (1981). The differential distribution, diversity and sprouting of cortical projections to the amygdala in the rhesus monkey. In Ben-Ari Y, editor, *The Amygdaloid Complex*, 77–90. Elsevier, Amsterdam.

Van Hoesen GW, Yeterian EH, & Lavizzo-Mourey R (1981). Widespread corticostriate projections from temporal cortex of the rhesus monkey. *Journal of Comparative Neurology* 199: 205–219.

van Veen V, Cohen JD, Botvinick MM, Stenger AV, & Carter CS (2001). Anterior cingulate cortex, conflict monitoring, and levels of processing. *Neuroimage* 14: 1302–1308.

Vandekerckhove J & Tuerlinckx F (2007). Fitting the Ratcliff diffusion model to experimental data. *Psychonomic Bulletin and Review* 14: 1011–1026.

vandenBerghe PL & Frost P (1986). Skin colour preferences, sexual dimorphism and sexual selection: a case for gene culture evolution. *Ethnic and Racial Studies* 9: 87–113.

Veale DM, Sahakian BJ, Owen AM, & Marks IM (1996). Specific cognitive deficits in tests sensitive to frontal lobe dysfunction in obsessive-compulsive disorder. *Psychological Medicine* 26: 1261–1269.

Verhagen JV, Rolls ET, & Kadohisa M (2003). Neurons in the primate orbitofrontal cortex respond to fat texture independently of viscosity. *Journal of Neurophysiology* 90: 1514–1525.

Verhagen JV, Kadohisa M, & Rolls ET (2004). The primate insular taste cortex: neuronal representations of the viscosity, fat texture, grittiness, and the taste of foods in the mouth. *Journal of Neurophysiology* 92: 1685–1699.

Vickers D (1970). Evidence for an accumulator model of psychophysical discrimination. *Ergonomics* 13: 37–58.

Vickers D (1979). *Decision Processes in Visual Perception*. Academic Press, New York.

Vickers D & Packer J (1982). Effects of alternating set for speed or accuracy on response time, accuracy and confidence in a unidimensional discrimination task. *Acta Psychologica* 50: 179–197.

Voellm BA, De Araujo IET, Cowen PJ, Rolls ET, Kringelbach ML, Smith KA, Jezzard P, Heal RJ, & Matthews PM (2004). Methamphetamine activates reward circuitry in drug naive human subjects. *Neuropsychopharmacology* 29: 1715–1722.

Vogt BA, editor (2009). *Cingulate Neurobiology and Disease*. Oxford University Press, Oxford.

Vogt BA & Sikes RW (2000). The medial pain system, cingulate cortex, and parallel processing of nociceptive information. *Progress in Brain Research* 122: 223–235.

Vogt BA, Derbyshire S, & Jones AKP (1996). Pain processing in four regions of human cingulate cortex localized with co-registered PET and MR imaging. *European Journal of Neuroscience* 8: 1461–1473.

Vogt BA, Berger GR, & Derbyshire SWG (2003). Structural and functional dichotomy of human midcingulate cortex. *European Journal of Neuroscience* 18: 3134–3144.

Volk DW & Lewis DA (2013). Prenatal ontogeny as a susceptibility period for cortical GABA neuron disturbances in schizophrenia. *Neuroscience* 248C: 154–164.

Volkow ND, Wang GJ, Tomasi D, & Baler RD (2013). Obesity and addiction: neurobiological overlaps. *Obesity Reviews* 14: 2–18.

von Neumann J & Morgenstern O (1944). *The Theory of Games and Economic Behavior*. Princeton University Press, Princeton.

Waelti P, Dickinson A, & Schultz W (2001). Dopamine responses comply with basic assumptions of formal learning theory. *Nature* 412: 43–48.

Wagner H (1989). The peripheral physiological differentiation of emotions. In Wagner H & Manstead A, editors, *Handbook of Social Psychophysiology*, 77–98. Wiley, Chichester.

Wald A (1947). *Sequential Analysis*. Wiley, New York.

Wallis G & Rolls ET (1997). Invariant face and object recognition in the visual system. *Progress in Neurobiology* 51: 167–194.

Wallis JD & Miller EK (2003). Neuronal activity in primate dorsolateral and orbital prefrontal cortex during performance of a reward preference task. *European Journal of Neuroscience* 18: 2069–2081.

Wallis JD, Anderson KC, & Miller EK (2001). Single neurons in prefrontal cortex encode abstract rules. *Nature* 411: 953–956.

Walton ME, Bannerman DM, & Rushworth MFS (2002). The role of rat medial frontal cortex in effort-based decision making. *Journal of Neuroscience* 22: 10996–11003.

Walton ME, Bannerman DM, Alterescu K, & Rushworth MFS (2003). Functional specialization within medial frontal cortex of the anterior cingulate for evaluating effort-related decisions. *Journal of Neuroscience* 23: 6475–6479.

Walton ME, Devlin JT, & Rushworth MF (2004). Interactions between decision making and performance monitoring within prefrontal cortex. *Nature Neuroscience* 7: 1259–1265.

Wang XJ (1999). Synaptic basis of cortical persistent activity: the importance of NMDA receptors to working memory. *Journal of Neuroscience* 19: 9587–9603.

Wang XJ (2001). Synaptic reverberation underlying mnemonic persistent activity. *Trends in Neurosciences* 24: 455–463.

Wang XJ (2002). Probabilistic decision making by slow reverberation in cortical circuits. *Neuron* 36: 955–968.

Wang XJ (2008). Decision making in recurrent neuronal circuits. *Neuron* 60: 215–234.

Wang XJ (2010). Neurophysiological and computational principles of cortical rhythms in cognition. *Physiological Reviews* 90: 1195–1268.

Wang XJ, Tegner J, Constantinidis C, & Goldman-Rakic PS (2004). Division of labor among distinct subtypes of inhibitory neurons in a cortical microcircuit of working memory. *Proceedings of the National Academy of Sciences USA* 101: 1368–1373.

Wang Y, Markram H, Goodman PH, Berger TK, Ma J, & Goldman-Rakic PS (2006). Heterogeneity in the pyramidal network of the medial prefrontal cortex. *Nature Neuroscience* 9: 534–542.

Watanabe K, Lauwereyns J, & Hikosaka O (2003). Neural correlates of rewarded and unrewarded eye movements in the primate caudate nucleus. *Journal of Neuroscience* 23: 10052–10057.

Watkins LH, Sahakian BJ, Robertson MM, Veale DM, Rogers RD, Pickard KM, Aitken MR, & Robbins TW (2005). Executive function in Tourette's syndrome and obsessive-compulsive disorder. *Psychological Medicine* 35: 571–582.

Watson JB (1929). *Psychology: From the Standpoint of a Behaviorist*. Lippincott, Philadelphia, 3rd edn.

Watson JB (1930). *Behaviorism: Revised Edition*. University of Chicago Press, Chicago.

Webb TJ, Rolls ET, Deco G, & Feng J (2011). Noise in attractor networks in the brain produced by graded firing rate

representations. *PLoS One* 6: e23620.
Wedell N, Gage MJ, & Parker G (2002). Sperm competition, male prudence and sperm limited females. *Proceedings of the Royal Society of London B* 260: 245–249.
Weiner KS & Grill-Spector K (2013). Neural representations of faces and limbs neighbor in human high-level visual cortex: evidence for a new organization principle. *Psychological Research* 77: 74–97.
Weisenfeld K (1993). An introduction to stochastic resonance. *Annals of the New York Academy of Sciences* 706: 13–25.
Weiskrantz L (1956). Behavioral changes associated with ablation of the amygdaloid complex in monkeys. *Journal of Comparative and Physiological Psychology* 49: 381–391.
Weiskrantz L (1968). Emotion. In Weiskrantz L, editor, *Analysis of Behavioural Change*, 50–90. Harper and Row, New York.
Weiskrantz L (1997). *Consciousness Lost and Found.* Oxford University Press, Oxford.
Weiskrantz L (1998). *Blindsight.* Oxford University Press, Oxford, 2nd edn.
Weiskrantz L (2009). Is blindsight just degraded normal vision? *Experimental Brain Research* 192: 413–416.
Weiskrantz L & Saunders RC (1984). Impairments of visual object transforms in monkeys. *Brain* 107: 1033–1072.
Weiss AP & Heckers S (1999). Neuroimaging of hallucinations: a review of the literature. *Psychiatry Research* 92: 61–74.
Weiss F & Koob GF (2001). Drug addiction: functional neurotoxicity of the brain reward systems. *Neurotoxicity Research* 3: 145–156.
Weissman MM, Bland RC, Canino GJ, Greenwald S, Hwu HG, Lee CK, Newman SC, Oakley-Browne MA, Rubio-Stipec M, Wickramaratne PJ, et al. (1994). The cross national epidemiology of obsessive compulsive disorder. The Cross National Collaborative Group. *Journal of Clinical Psychiatry* 55 Suppl: 5–10.
Welford AT, editor (1980). *Reaction Times.* Academic Press, London.
Werner G & Mountcastle V (1965). Neural activity in mechanoreceptive cutaneous afferents: stimulus-response relations, Weber functions, and information transmission. *Journal of Neurophysiology* 28: 359–397.
West RA & Larson CR (1995). Neurons of the anterior mesial cortex related to faciovocal activity in the awake monkey. *Journal of Neurophysiology* 74: 1856–1869.
Whalen PJ & Phelps EA (2009). *The Human Amygdala.* Guilford, New York.
Wheeler EZ & Fellows LK (2008). The human ventromedial frontal lobe is critical for learning from negative feedback. *Brain* 131: 1323–1331.
Whitelaw RB, Markou A, Robbins TW, & Everitt BJ (1996). Excitotoxic lesions of the basolateral amygdala impair the acquisition of cocaine-seeking behaviour under a second-order schedule of reinforcement. *Psychopharmacology* 127: 213–224.
Whiten A & Byrne RW (1997). *Machiavellian Intelligence II: Extensions and Evaluations.* Cambridge University Press, Cambridge.
Wickens J & Kotter R (1995). Cellular models of reinforcement. In Houk JC, Davis JL, & Beiser DG, editors, *Models of Information Processing in the Basal Ganglia*, chap. 10, 187–214. MIT Press, Cambridge, MA.
Wickens JR, Begg AJ, & Arbuthnott GW (1996). Dopamine reverses the depression of rat corticostriatal synapses which normally follows high-frequency stimulation of cortex in vitro. *Neuroscience* 70: 1–5.
Wiech K & Tracey I (2013). Pain, decisions, and actions: a motivational perspective. *Frontiers in Neuroscience* 7: 46.
Wilks DC, Besson H, Lindroos AK, & Ekelund U (2011). Objectively measured physical activity and obesity prevention in children, adolescents and adults: a systematic review of prospective studies. *Obesity Reviews* 12: 119–129.
Williams GV, Rolls ET, Leonard CM, & Stern C (1993). Neuronal responses in the ventral striatum of the behaving macaque. *Behavioural Brain Research* 55: 243–252.
Wilson CJ (1995). The contribution of cortical neurons to the firing pattern of striatal spiny neurons. In Houk JC, Davis JL, & Beiser DG, editors, *Models of Information Processing in the Basal Ganglia*, chap. 3, 29–50. MIT Press, Cambridge, MA.
Wilson DA & Sullivan RM (2011). Cortical processing of odor objects. *Neuron* 72: 506–519.
Wilson EO (1975). *Sociobiology: The New Synthesis.* Harvard University Press, Cambridge, MA.
Wilson FAW & Rolls ET (1990a). Neuronal responses related to the novelty and familiarity of visual stimuli in the substantia innominata, diagonal band of broca and periventricular region of the primate. *Experimental Brain Research* 80: 104–120.
Wilson FAW & Rolls ET (1990b). Neuronal responses related to reinforcement in the primate basal forebrain. *Brain Research* 509: 213–231.
Wilson FAW & Rolls ET (1990c). Learning and memory are reflected in the responses of reinforcement-related neurons in the primate basal forebrain. *Journal of Neuroscience* 10: 1254–1267.
Wilson FAW & Rolls ET (1993). The effects of stimulus novelty and familiarity on neuronal activity in the amygdala of monkeys performing recognition memory tasks. *Experimental Brain Research* 93: 367–382.
Wilson FAW & Rolls ET (2005). The primate amygdala and reinforcement: a dissociation between rule-based and associatively-mediated memory revealed in amygdala neuronal activity. *Neuroscience* 133: 1061–1072.

Wilson FAW, O'Sclaidhe SP, & Goldman-Rakic PS (1993). Dissociation of object and spatial processing domains in primate prefrontal cortex. *Science* 260: 1955–1958.
Wilson RI & Nicoll RA (2002). Endocannabinoid signalling in the brain. *Science* 296: 678–682.
Winkielman P & Berridge KC (2003). What is an unconscious emotion? *Cognition and Emotion* 17: 181–211.
Winkielman P & Berridge KC (2005). Unconscious affective reactions to masked happy versus angry faces influence consumption behavior and judgments of value. *Personality and Social Psychology Bulletin* 31: 111–135.
Winn P, Tarbuck A, & Dunnett SB (1984). Ibotenic acid lesions of the lateral hypothalamus: comparison with electrolytic lesion syndrome. *Neuroscience* 12: 225–240.
Winn P, Clark A, Hastings M, Clark J, Latimer M, Rugg E, & Brownlee B (1990). Excitotoxic lesions of the lateral hypothalamus made by N-methyl-D-aspartate in the rat: behavioural, histological and biochemical analyses. *Experimental Brain Research* 82: 628–636.
Winslow JT & Insel TR (2004). Neuroendrocrine basis of social recognition. *Current Opinion in Neurobiology* 14: 248–253.
Wise SP (2008). Forward frontal fields: phylogeny and fundamental function. *Trends in Neuroscience* 31: 599–608.
Wolkin A, Sanfilipo M, Wolf AP, Angrist B, Brodie JD, & Rotrosen J (1992). Negative symptoms and hypofrontality in chronic schizophrenia. *Archives of General Psychiatry* 49: 959–965.
Wong K & Wang XJ (2006). A recurrent network mechanism of time integration in perceptual decisions. *Journal of Neuroscience* 26: 1314–1328.
Wong KF & Huk AC (2008). Temporal dynamics underlying perceptual decision making: insights from the interplay between an attractor model and parietal neurophysiology. *Frontiers in Neuroscience* 2: 245–254.
Wong KF, Huk AC, Shadlen MN, & Wang XJ (2007). Neural circuit dynamics underlying accumulation of time-varying evidence during perceptual decision making. *Frontiers in Computational Neuroscience* 1: 6.
Woods SC (2012). Metabolic signals and food intake. Forty years of progress. *Appetite* doi: 10.1016/j.appet.2012.08.016.
Wrangham RW (1993). The evolution of sexuality in chimpanzees and bonobos. *Human Nature* 4: 47–49.
Wu CC, Sacchet MD, & Knutson B (2012). Toward an affective neuroscience account of financial risk taking. *Frontiers in Neuroscience* 6: 159.
Wyatt TD (2014). *Pheromones and Animal Behaviour*. Cambridge University Press, Cambridge, 2nd edn.
Wynne-Edwards KE (2001). Hormonal changes in mammalian fathers. *Hormones and Behaviour* 40: 139–145.
Xiang Z, Huguenard J, & Prince D (1998). GABA-A receptor mediated currents in interneurons and pyramidal cells of rat visual cortex. *Journal of Physiology* 506: 715–730.
Yamaguchi S (1967). The synergistic taste effect of monosodium glutamate and disodium 5′-inosinate. *Journal of Food Science* 32: 473–478.
Yamaguchi S & Kimizuka A (1979). Psychometric studies on the taste of monosodium glutamate. In Filer LJ, Garattini S, Kare MR, Reynolds AR, & Wurtman RJ, editors, *Glutamic Acid: Advances in Biochemistry and Physiology*, 35–54. Raven Press, New York.
Yamamoto S, Kim HF, & Hikosaka O (2013). Reward value-contingent changes of visual responses in the primate caudate tail associated with a visuomotor skill. *Journal of Neuroscience* 33: 11227–11238.
Yan J & Scott TR (1996). The effect of satiety on responses of gustatory neurons in the amygdala of alert cynomolgus macaques. *Brain Research* 740: 193–200.
Yang Y, Paspalas CD, Jin LE, Picciotto MR, Arnsten AF, & Wang M (2013). Nicotinic $\alpha 7$ receptors enhance NMDA cognitive circuits in dorsolateral prefrontal cortex. *Proceedings of the National Academy of Sciences U S A* 110: 12078–12083.
Yaxley S, Rolls ET, Sienkiewicz ZJ, & Scott TR (1985). Satiety does not affect gustatory activity in the nucleus of the solitary tract of the alert monkey. *Brain Research* 347: 85–93.
Yaxley S, Rolls ET, & Sienkiewicz ZJ (1988). The responsiveness of neurones in the insular gustatory cortex of the macaque monkey is independent of hunger. *Physiology and Behavior* 42: 223–229.
Yaxley S, Rolls ET, & Sienkiewicz ZJ (1990). Gustatory responses of single neurons in the insula of the macaque monkey. *Journal of Neurophysiology* 63: 689–700.
Yelnik J (2002). Functional anatomy of the basal ganglia. *Movement Disorders* 17 Suppl 3: S15–S21.
Yeterian EH, Pandya DN, Tomaiuolo F, & Petrides M (2012). The cortical connectivity of the prefrontal cortex in the monkey brain. *Cortex* 48: 58–81.
Yokel RA & Wise RA (1975). Increased lever pressing for amphetamine after pimozide in rats: implications for a dopamine theory of reinforcement. *Science* 187: 547–549.
Young AW, Aggleton JP, Hellawell DJ, Johnson M, Broks P, & Hanley JR (1995). Face processing impairments after amygdalotomy. *Brain* 118: 15–24.
Young AW, Hellawell DJ, Van de Wal C, & Johnson M (1996). Facial expression processing after amygdalotomy. *Neuropsychologia* 34: 31–39.
Young KA, Gobrogge KL, Liu Y, & Wang Z (2011). The neurobiology of pair bonding: insights from a socially monogamous rodent. *Frontiers in Neuroendocrinology* 32: 53–69.
Young LJ & Wang Z (2004). The neurobiology of pairbonding. *Nature Neuroscience* 7: 1048–1054.
Zahavi A (1975). Mate selection: a selection for a handicap. *Journal of Theoretical Biology* 53: 205–214.

Zahavi A & Zahavi A (1997). *The Handicap Principle: A Missing Piece of Darwin's Puzzle.* Oxford University Press, Oxford.

Zald DH & Rauch SL, editors (2006). *The Orbitofrontal Cortex.* Oxford University Press, Oxford.

Zatorre RJ & Jones-Gotman M (1991). Human olfactory discrimination after unilateral frontal or temporal lobectomy. *Brain* 114: 71–84.

Zatorre RJ, Jones-Gotman M, Evans AC, & Meyer E (1992). Functional localization of human olfactory cortex. *Nature* 360: 339–340.

Zatorre RJ, Jones-Gotman M, & Rouby C (2000). Neural mechanisms involved in odor pleasantness and intensity judgments. *NeuroReport* 11: 2711–2716.

Zeller AC (1987). Communication by sight and smell. In Smuts BS, Cheney DL, Seyfarth RM, Wrangham RW, & Stuhsaker TT, editors, *Primate Societies*, 433–439. University of Chicago Press, London.

Zhang M, Gosnell BA, & Kelley AE (1998). Intake of high-fat food is selectively enhanced by mu opioid receptor stimulation within the nucleus accumbens. *Journal of Pharmacology and Experimental Therapeutics* 285: 908–914.

Zhao GQ, Zhang Y, Hoon MA, Chandrashekar J, Erlenbach I, Ryba NJ, & Zucker CS (2003). The receptors for mammalian sweet and umami taste. *Cell* 115: 255–266.

Zink CF, Pagnoni G, Martin ME, Dhamala M, & Berns GS (2003). Human striatal responses to salient nonrewarding stimuli. *Journal of Neuroscience* 23: 8092–8097.

Zink CF, Pagnoni G, Martin-Skurski ME, Chappelow JC, & Berns GS (2004). Human striatal responses to monetary reward depend on saliency. *Neuron* 42: 509–517.

Zucker RS & Regehr WG (2002). Short-term synaptic plasticity. *Annual Review of Physiology* 64: 355–405.

Zuckerman M (1994). *Psychobiology of Personality.* Cambridge University Press, New York.

Zuckerman M & Kuhlman DM (2000). Personality and risk-taking: common biosocial factors. *Journal of Personality* 68: 999–1029.

Index

Appendix 4 Colour Plates

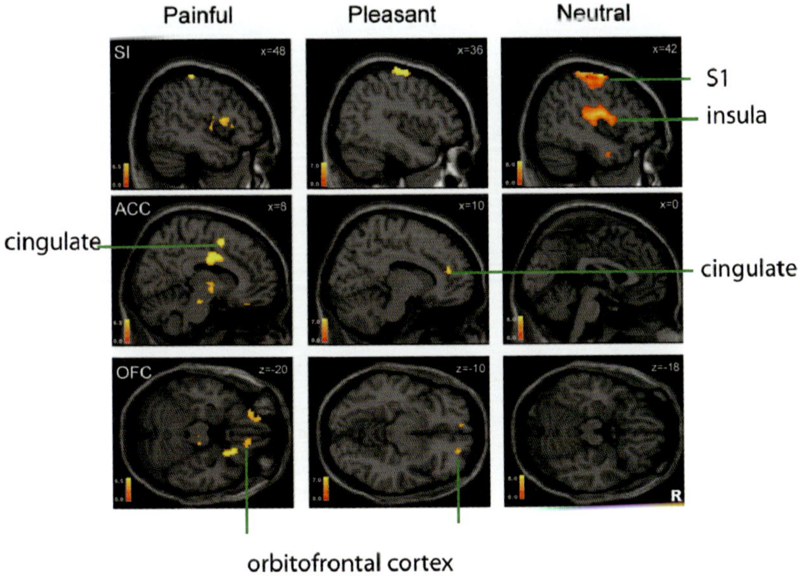

Fig. 4.4 Brain activation to painful, pleasant and neutral touch of the human brain. Top row – somatosensory cortex S1/insula; middle row – cingulate cortex; bottom row – orbitofrontal cortex. The full caption is with the figure in the main text.

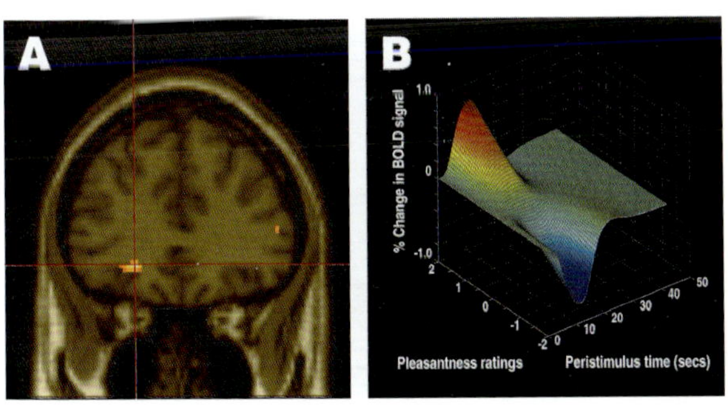

4.23 Areas of the human orbitofrontal cortex with activations correlating with pleasantness ratings for food in the mouth produced by selective devaluation by feeding one food to satiety in a sensory-specific satiety paradigm. The full caption is with the figure in the main text.

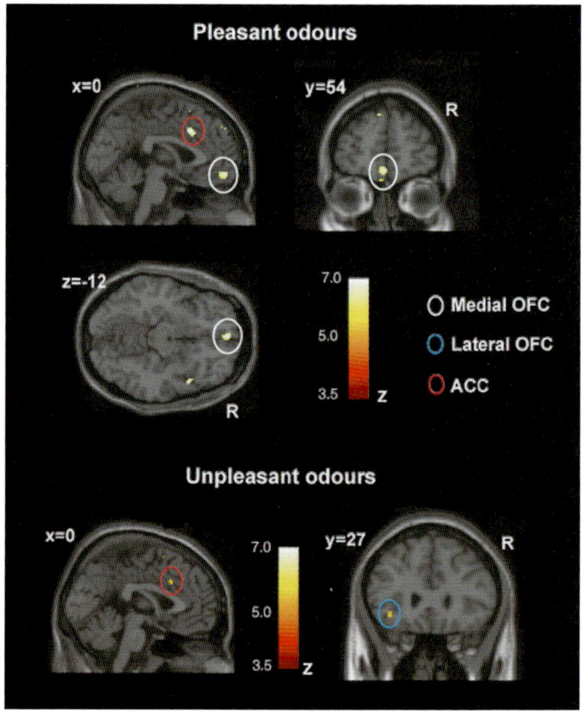

Fig. 4.26 The representation of pleasant and unpleasant odours in the human brain. Above – Group conjunction for 3 pleasant odours. Below – Group conjunction results for 3 unpleasant odours. OFC – orbitofrontal cortex; ACC – anterior cingulate cortex. The full caption is with the figure in the main text.

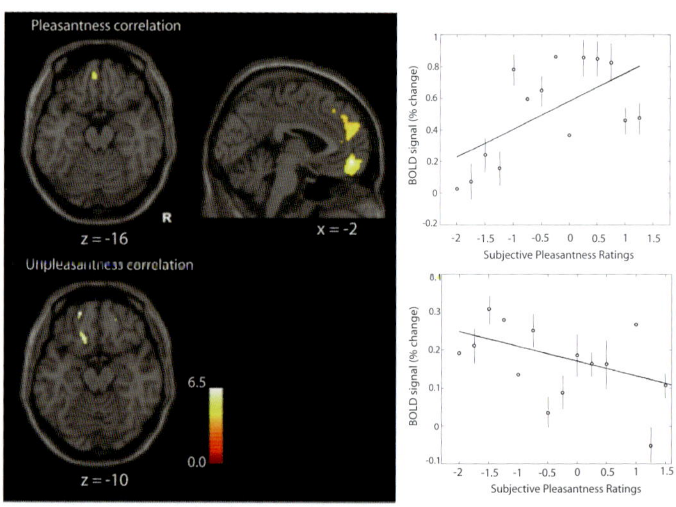

Fig. 4.27 The representation of pleasant and unpleasant odours in the human brain. Correlation of the BOLD signal with the subjective pleasantness ratings in the medial orbitofrontal cortex and anterior cingulate cortex (above), and with the unpleasantness more laterally in the orbitofrontal cortex (below). The full caption is with the figure in the main text.

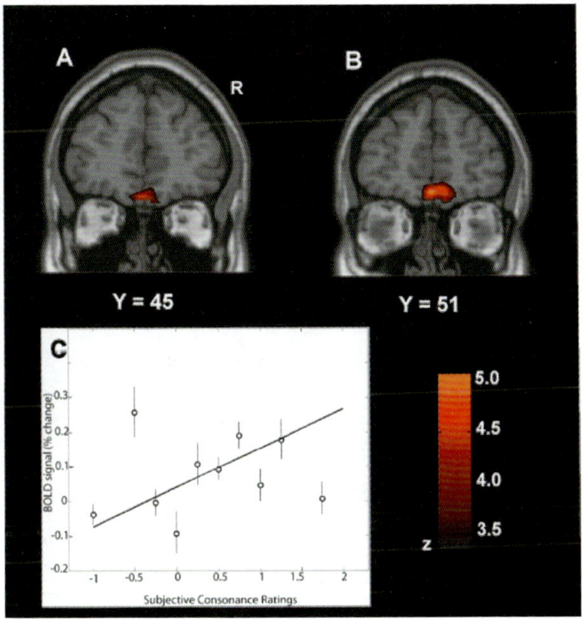

Fig. 4.30 Flavour formation in the human brain, shown by cross-modal olfactory–taste convergence. Activations in the medial orbitofrontal cortex correlated with olfactory–taste consonance are shown in A and C, and with pleasantness in B. The full caption is with the figure in the main text.

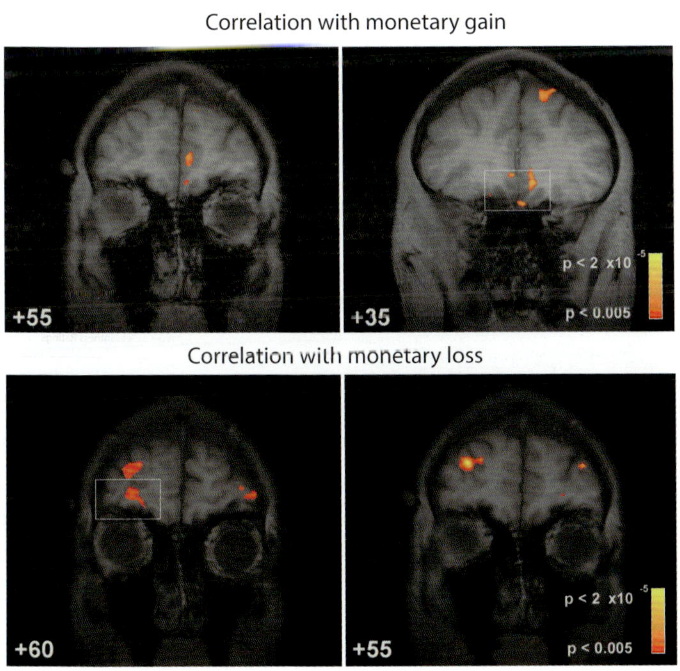

Fig. 4.35 Correlation of brain activations with the amount of money won (upper right, medial orbitofrontal cortex) or lost (lower left, lateral orbitofrontal cortex) in a visual discrimination reversal task with probabilistic monetary reward and loss. The full caption is with the figure in the main text.

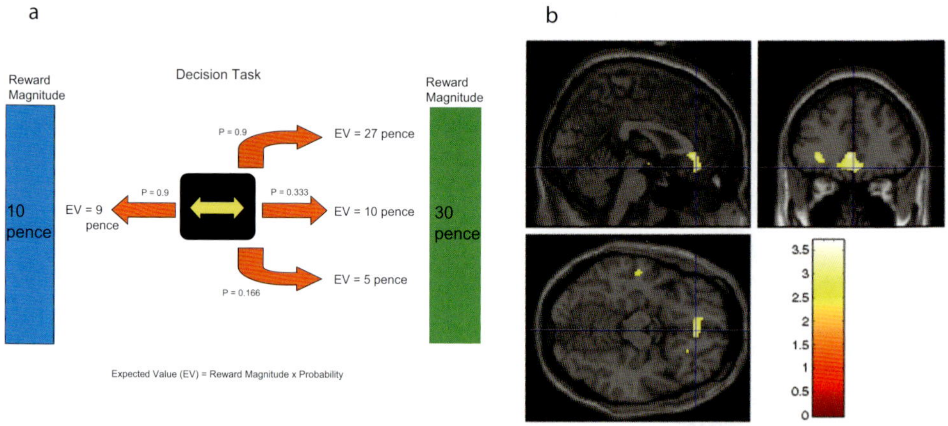

Fig. 4.37 Decision-making under risk in a probabilistic monetary reward task. (a) Expected Value (EV) = probability (P) x Reward outcome Magnitude. (b) Medial orbitofrontal cortex showing in a conjunction analysis where there were correlations both with Expected Value and with Reward outcome Magnitude. The full caption is with the figure in the main text.

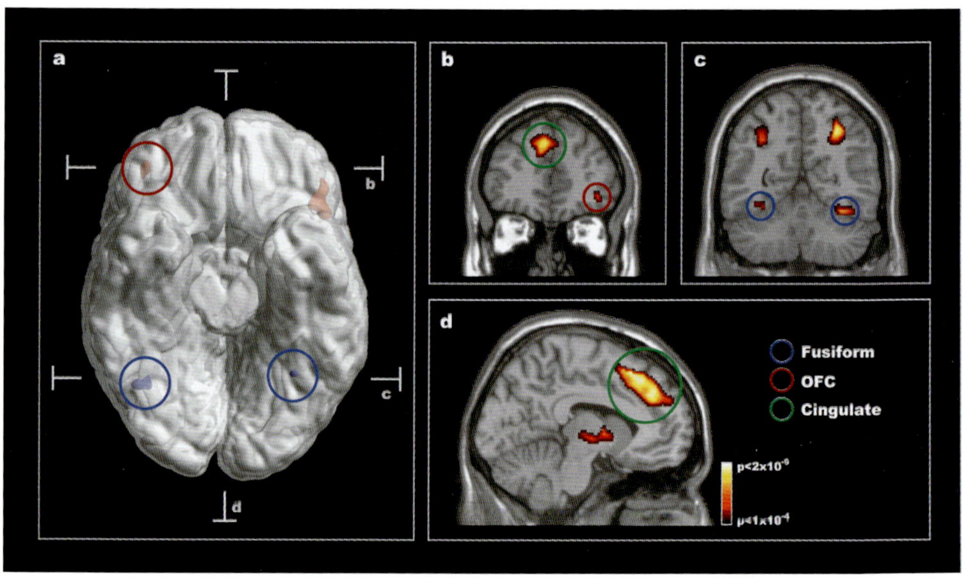

Fig. 4.40 Social reversal: Activations are found in the lateral orbitofrontal cortex (red circle) and cingulate cortex (green) when a face expression changes indicating that choice behaviour should reverse. Activations in the fusiform face area (blue circles) occurred to faces independently of reversal. The full caption is with the figure in the main text.

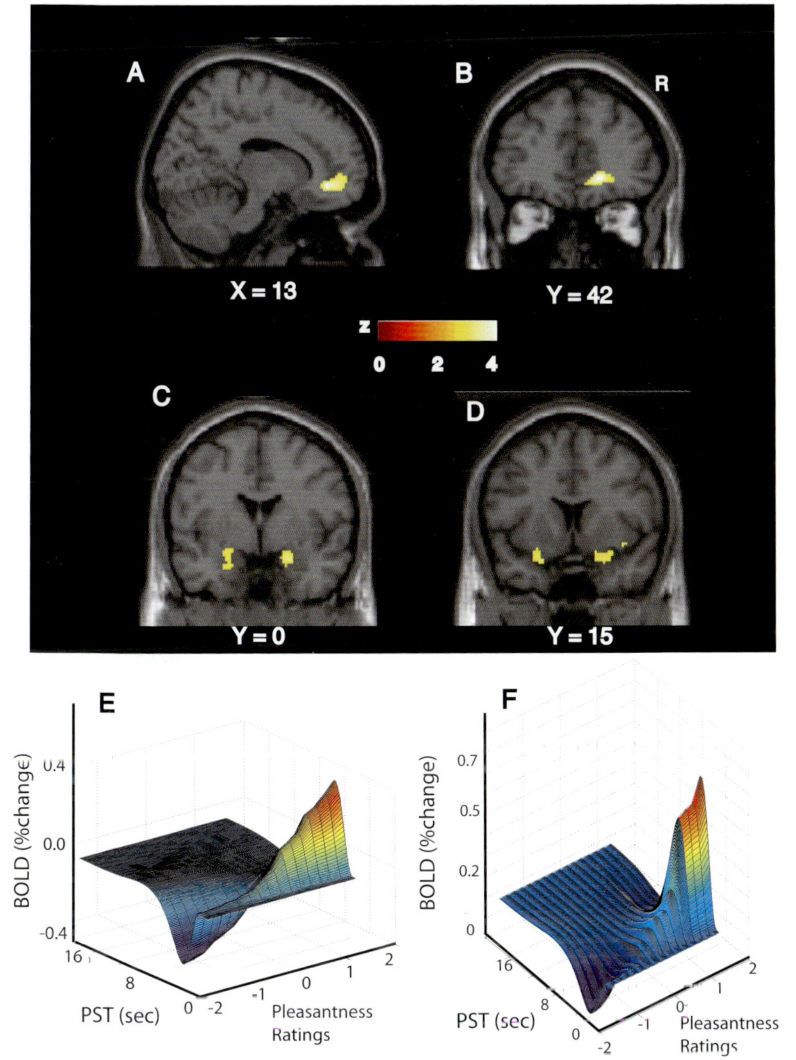

Fig. 4.43 Cognition and emotion. Group (random) effects analysis showing the brain regions where the BOLD signal was correlated with pleasantness ratings given to the test odour. The pleasantness ratings were being modulated by the word labels. (A) Activations in the rostral anterior cingulate cortex, in the region adjoining the medial OFC, shown in a sagittal slice. (B) The same activation shown coronally. (C) Bilateral activations in the amygdala. (D) These activations extended anteriorly to the primary olfactory cortex. The image was thresholded at $p<0.0001$ uncorrected in order to show the extent of the activation. (E) Parametric plots of the data averaged across all subjects showing that the percentage BOLD change (fitted) correlates with the pleasantness ratings in the region shown in A and B. The parametric plots were very similar for the primary olfactory region shown in D. PST – Post-stimulus time (s). (F) Parametric plots for the amygdala region shown in C. (After DeAraujo, Rolls, Velazco, Margot and Cayeux 2005.)

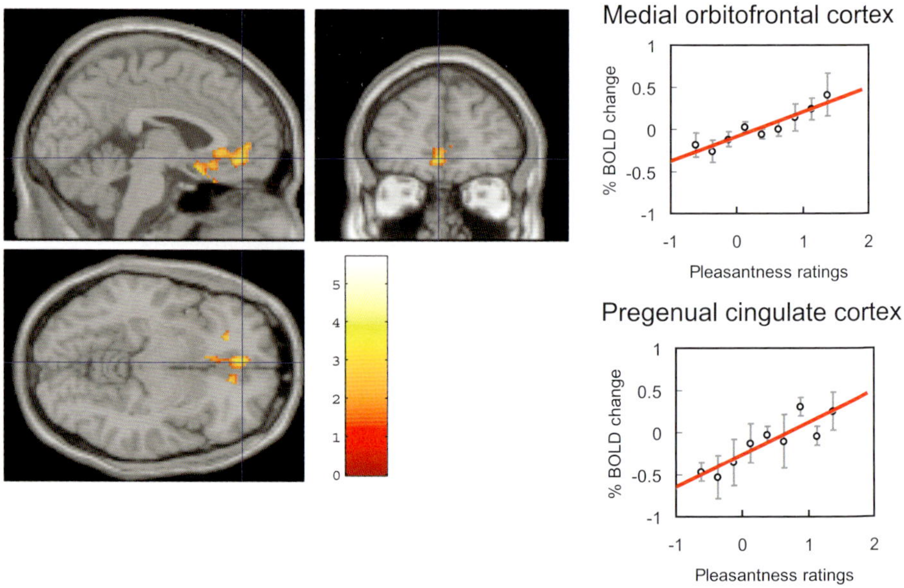

Fig. 4.44 Top-down attention and emotion. Effect of paying attention to the pleasantness of a taste. Left: A significant difference related to the taste period was found in the medial orbitofrontal cortex at [-6 14 -20] z=3.81 p<0.003 (towards the back of the area of activation shown) and in the pregenual cingulate cortex at [-4 46 -8] z=2.90 p<0.04 (at the cursor). Right upper: The correlation between the subjective pleasantness ratings and the activation (% BOLD change) in the orbitofrontal cortex (r=0.94, df=8, p<<0.001). Right lower: The correlation between the pleasantness ratings and the activation (% BOLD change) in the pregenual cingulate cortex r=0.89, df=8, p=0.001). The taste stimulus, monosodium glutamate, was identical on all trials. (After Grabenhorst and Rolls 2008.)

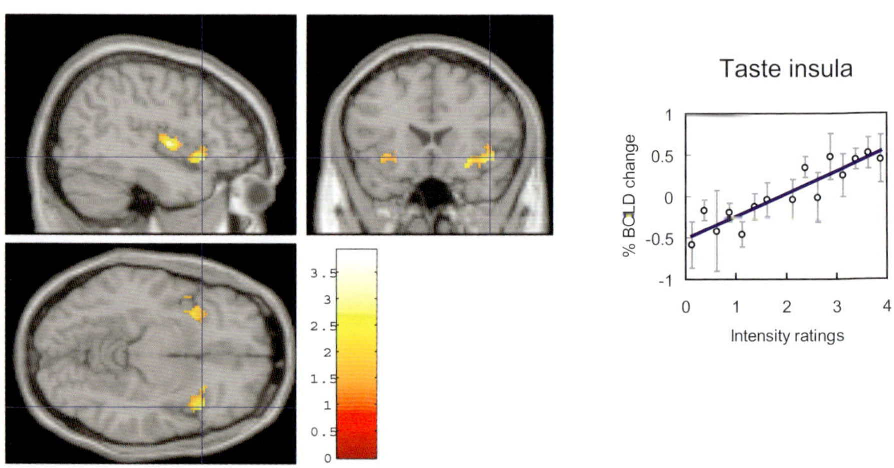

Fig. 4.45 Top-down attention and emotion. Left: Effect of paying attention to the intensity of a taste. Top: A significant difference related to the taste period was found in the taste insula at [42 18 -14] z=2.42 p<0.05 (indicated by the cursor) and in the mid insula at [40 -2 4] z=3.03 p<0.025. Right: The correlation between the intensity ratings and the activation (% BOLD change) in the taste insula (r=0.91, df=14, p<<0.001). The taste stimulus, monosodium glutamate, was identical on all trials. (After Grabenhorst and Rolls 2008.)

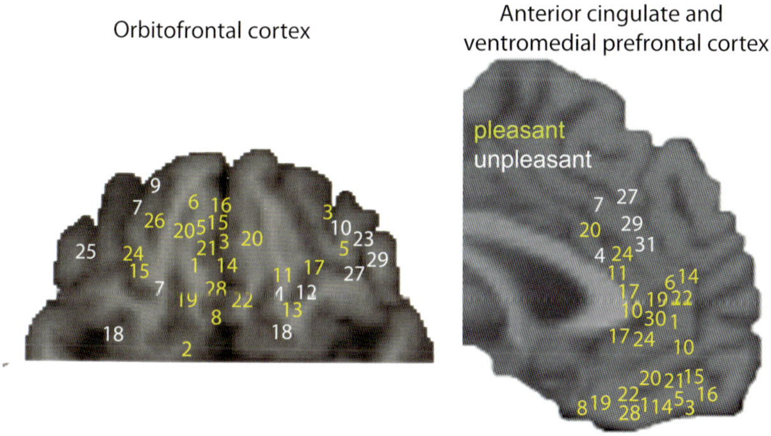

Fig. 4.47 Maps of subjective pleasure in the human orbitofrontal cortex (ventral view) and anterior cingulate and ventromedial prefrontal cortex (sagittal view). Yellow: activations correlated with subjective pleasantness. White: activations correlated with subjective unpleasantness. Taste: 1, 2; odor: 3-10; flavor: 11-16; oral texture: 17, 18; chocolate: 19; water: 20; wine: 21; oral temperature: 22, 23; somatosensory temperature: 24, 25; the sight of touch: 26, 27; facial attractiveness: 28, 29; erotic pictures: 30; laser-induced pain: 31. (See the supplementary material of Grabenhorst and Rolls 2011 for the references to the original studies.) The full caption is with the figure in the main text.

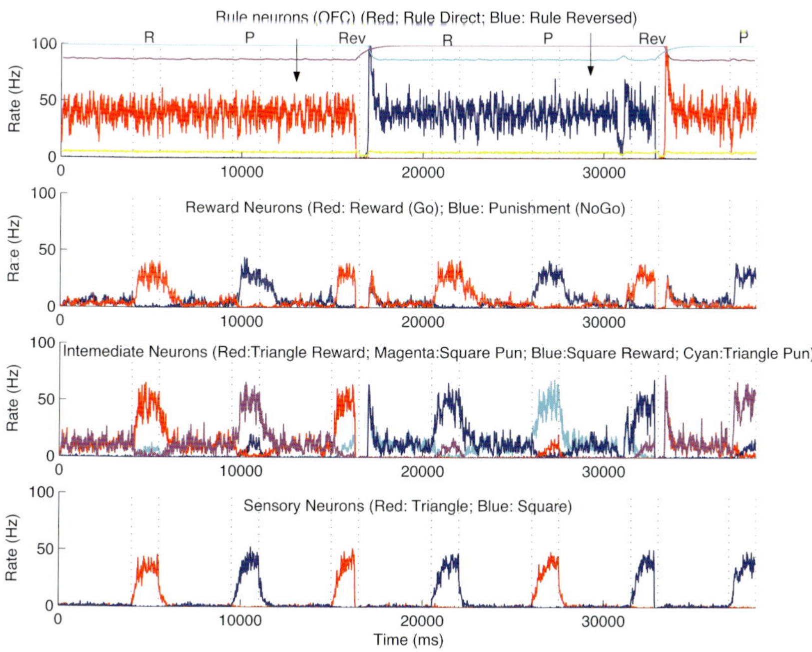

Fig. 4.53 Reward reversal model: Time course of the averaged population activity for all neural pools (sensory, intermediate (stimulus–reward), Reward/Punishment, and Rule) for the network in Fig. 4.52. The full caption is with the figure in the main text.

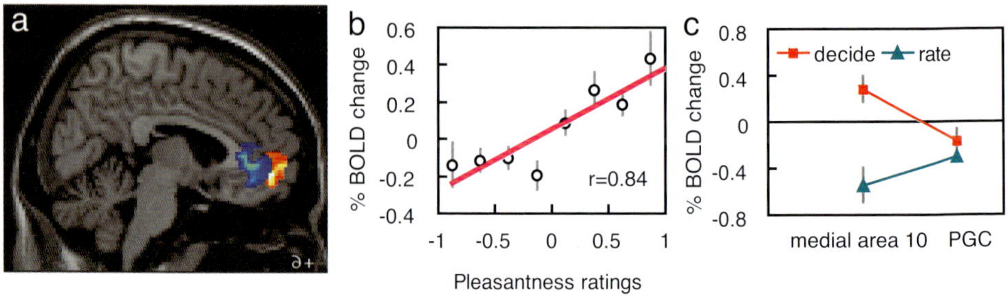

Fig. 4.66 Value-related decision-making and medial prefrontal cortex area 10. (a) A contrast between all trials on which decisions were made and all trials on which ratings were made between thermal stimuli showed a significant effect in the medial prefrontal cortex area 10, as indicated in red ([6 54 -8]). This contrast showed no significant difference in the pregenual cingulate cortex. However, in the pregenual cingulate cortex, as shown in blue, there was a strong and significant correlation with the pleasantness ratings ([4 38 -2]). (b) Shows that the % BOLD signal in the pregenual cingulate cortex was correlated with the pleasantness ratings on the trials on which ratings were made (r=0.84, df=7, p=0.005). (c) Compares the activations (mean ± sem) in medial area 10 with those in the pregenual cingulate cortex (PGC) for decision and rating trials. There was a significant interaction (p=0.015). (After Grabenhorst, Rolls and Parris 2008.)

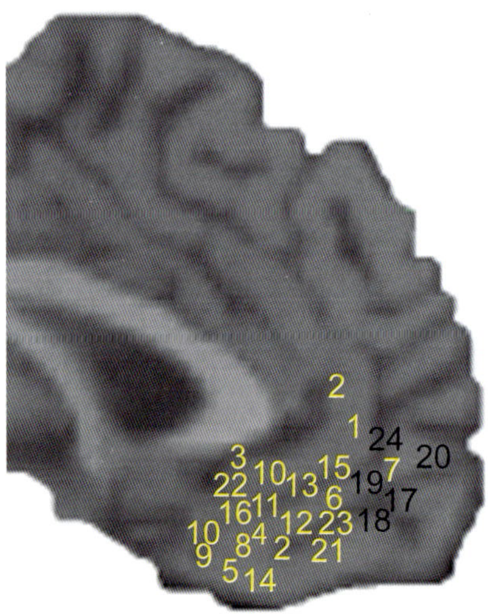

Fig. 4.67 Value-related decision-making and the ventromedial prefrontal cortex. Activations implicated primarily representing value are in yellow; and in value-based decision-making are in black. The full caption is with the figure in the main text.

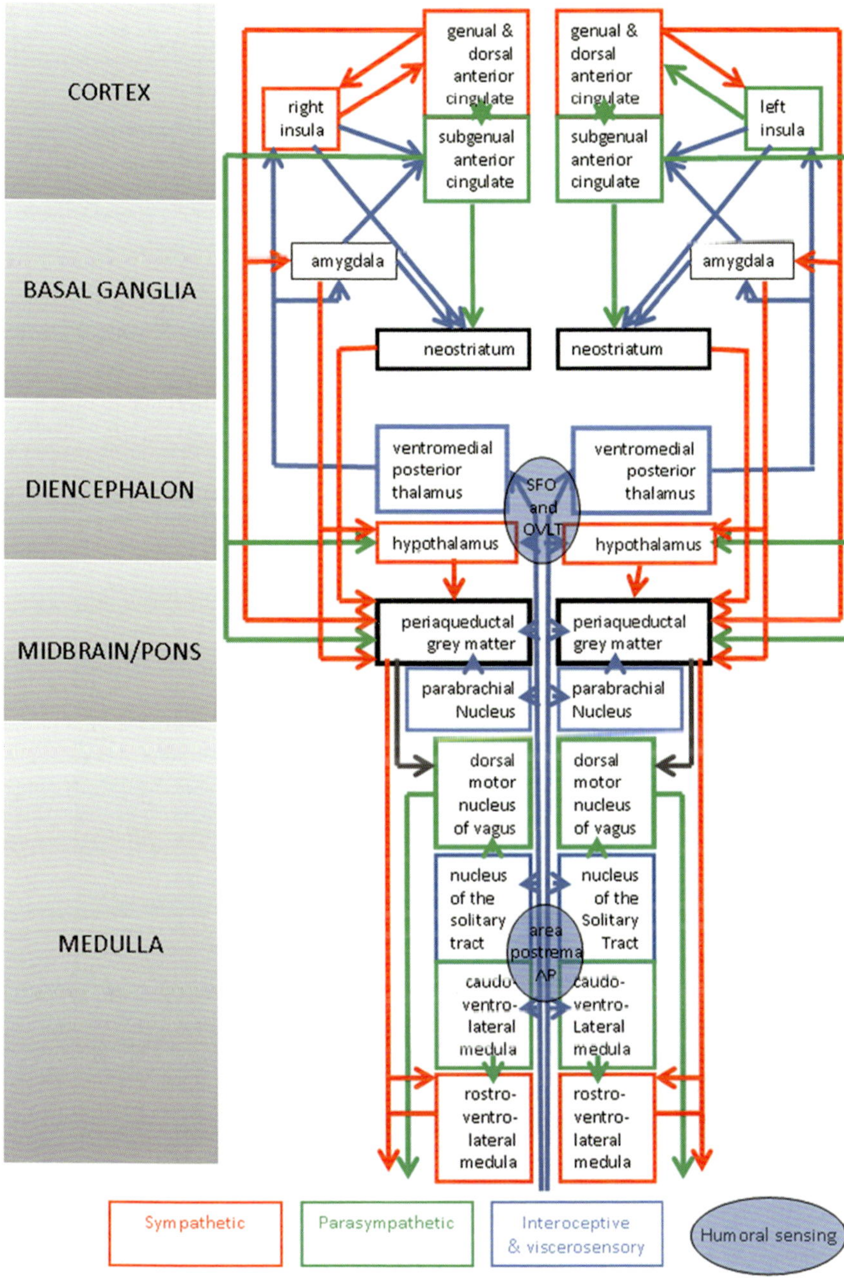

Fig. 4.68 Afferent and efferent neural pathways mediating autonomic system function. Brain regions are linked according to their association with visceral afferent sympathetic and parasympathetic function. SFO: Subfornical organ. OVLT: organum vasculosum of the lamina terminalis. (From Critchley and Harrison 2013.)

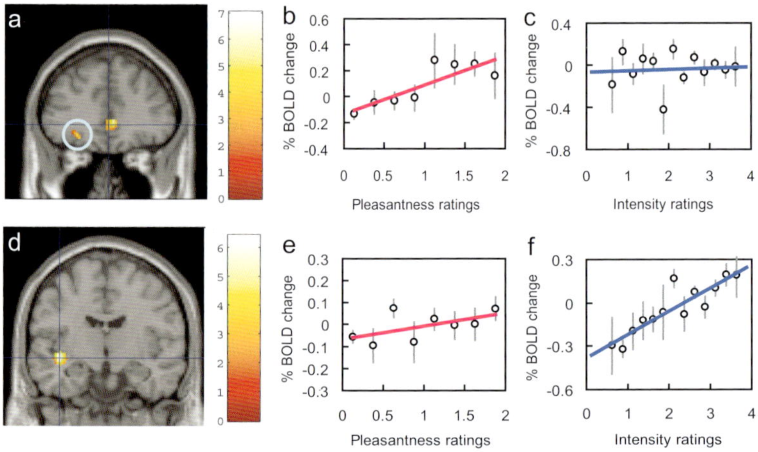

Fig. 4.69 Representation of the pleasantness but not intensity of thermal stimuli applied to the hand in the orbitofrontal cortex (top), and of the intensity but not the pleasantness in the mid ventral (somatosensory) insular cortex (bottom). The full caption is with the figure in the main text.

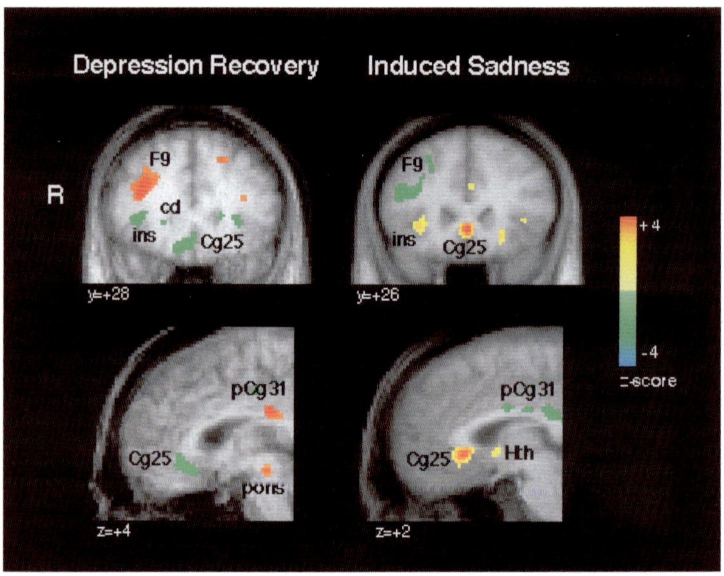

Fig. 4.70 Changes in the subgenual cingulate area (Cg25) associated with the recovery from depression (left), and with the induction of a mood state of sadness (right). Left images: Z-score maps demonstrating changes in regional glucose metabolism (fluorodeoxyglucose PET) in depressed patients following 6 weeks of treatment with the antidepressant fluoxetine. Upper: coronal view; lower, sagittal view). Green indicates that the change is a decrease, and red or yellow an increase (see calibration bar on far right). Right images: changes in regional cerebral blood flow (oxygen-15 water PET) in healthy volunteers 10 min after induction of acute sadness. The recovery from depression and the induction of sadness produce opposite changes in Cg25. Reciprocal changes were seen in a dorsal part of the prefrontal cortex, labelled F9. F, frontal; cd, caudate nucleus; ins, anterior insula; Cg25, subgenual cingulate; Hth, hypothalamus; pCG31, posterior cingulate; R, right. (After Mayberg et al. 1999.)

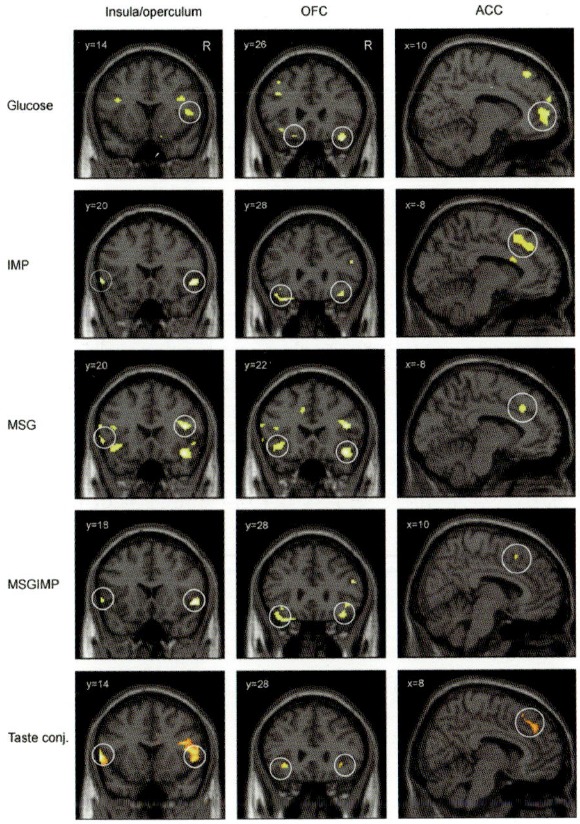

Fig. 5.14 Activation of the human primary taste cortex in the insula/frontal operculum; the orbitofrontal cortex (OFC); and the anterior cingulate cortex (ACC) by taste. The stimuli used included glucose, two umami taste stimuli (monosodium glutamate (MSG) and inosine monophosphate (IMP)), and a mixture of the two umami stimuli. Taste conj. refers to a conjunction analysis over all the taste stimuli. (After De Araujo et al 2003.) The full caption is with the figure in the main text.

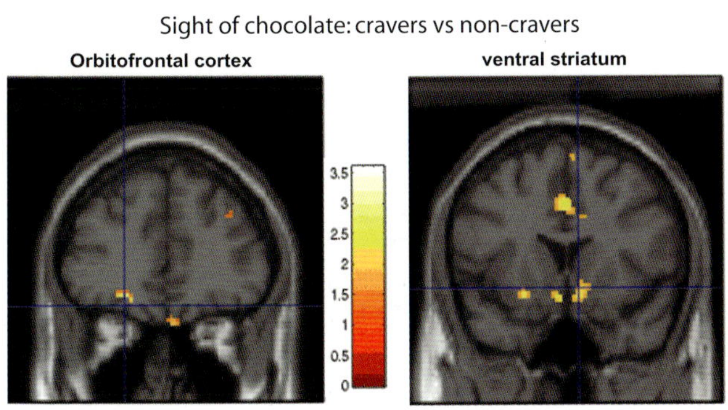

Fig. 5.21 The sight of chocolate produced more activation of mid and medial parts of the orbitofrontal cortex in chocolate cravers than non-cravers (e.g. [-28 42 -10] at the crosshairs), and in the ventral striatum ([-4 16 -12]). (After Rolls and McCabe 2007.) The full caption is with the figure in the main text.

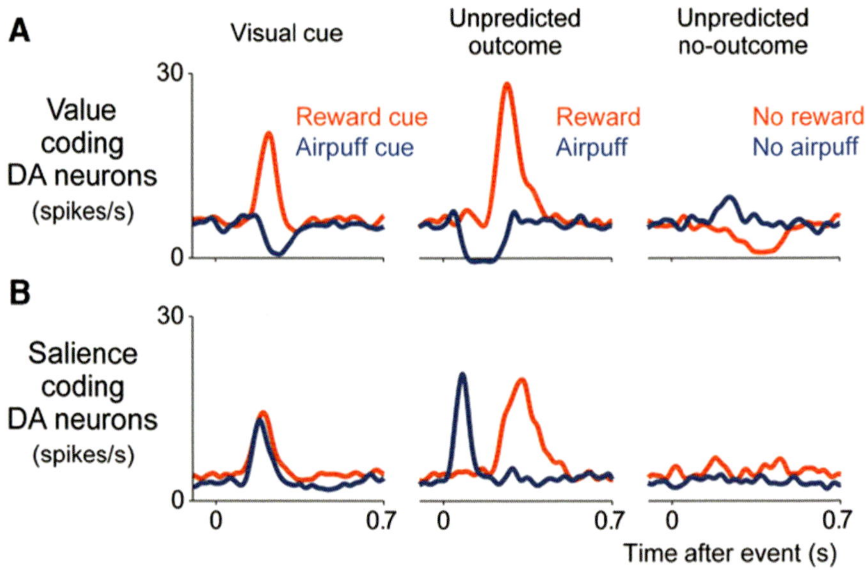

Fig. 6.3 Responses of different types of dopamine neuron. (A) Reward prediction error neurons (see text). (B) Neurons activated by aversive and also by rewarding stimuli, sometime called motivational salience neurons (see text). (After Matsumoto and Hikosaka 2009.) The full caption is with the figure in the main text.

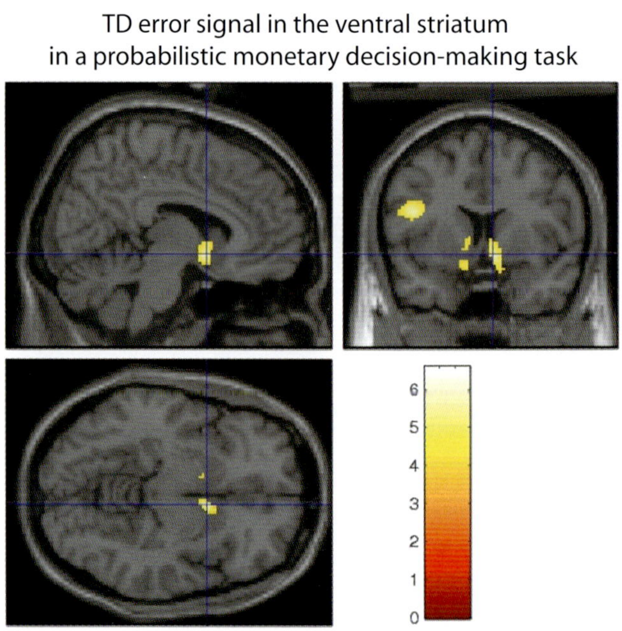

Fig. 6.9 Temporal Difference (TD) error signal in the ventral striatum in a probabilistic monetary decision-making task. The correlation between the TD error and the activation in the nucleus accumbens was significant in a group random effects analysis fully corrected at the cluster level with $p<0.048$ (voxel $z=3.84$) at MNI coordinates [8 8 –8]. The task is illustrated in Fig. 4.37. (From Rolls, McCabe and Redoute 2008.) The full caption is with the figure in the main text.

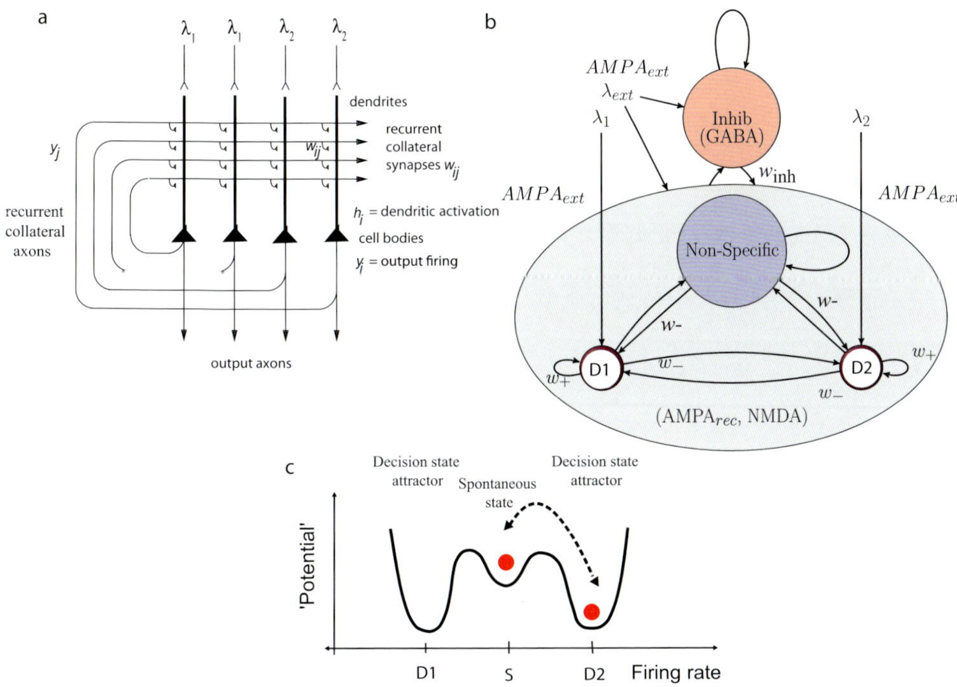

Fig. 8.1 (a) Attractor or autoassociation single network architecture for decision-making. The cell body of each neuron is shown as a triangle (like a cortical pyramidal cell), the dendrite is vertical, and receives recurrent collateral synaptic connections w_{ij} from the other neurons. The evidence for decision 1 is applied via the λ_1 inputs, and for decision 2 via the λ_2 inputs. The synaptic weights w_{ij} have been associatively modified during training in the presence of λ_1 and at a different time of λ_2. When λ_1 and λ_2 are applied, each attractor competes through the inhibitory interneurons (not shown), until one wins the competition, and the network falls into one of the high firing rate attractors that represents the decision. The noise in the network caused by the random spiking times of the neurons (for a given mean rate) means that on some trials, for given inputs, the neurons in the decision 1 (D1) attractor are more likely to win, and on other trials the neurons in the decision 2 (D2) attractor are more likely to win. This makes the decision-making probabilistic, for, as shown in (c), the noise influences when the system will jump out of the spontaneous firing stable (low energy) state S, and whether it jumps into the high firing state for decision 1 (D1) or decision 2 (D2). (b) The architecture of the integrate-and-fire network used to model decision-making (see text). The synaptic weights between the neural populations (decision pools D1 and D2, the nos-specific pool, and the inhibitory pool are 1 except where indicated. In particular, the recurrent weights, indicated by a recurrent arrow, between the neurons within an attractor decision-making pool have strong weights w_+, and between the different pools have the weak strength w_-. (c) A multistable 'effective energy landscape' for decision-making with stable states shown as low 'potential' basins. Even when the inputs are being applied to the network, the spontaneous firing rate state is stable, and noise provokes transitions from the low firing rate spontaneous state S into the high firing rate decision attractor state D1 or D2. If the noise is greater, the escaping time to a decision state, and thus the decision or reaction time, will be shorter (see Rolls and Deco 2010).

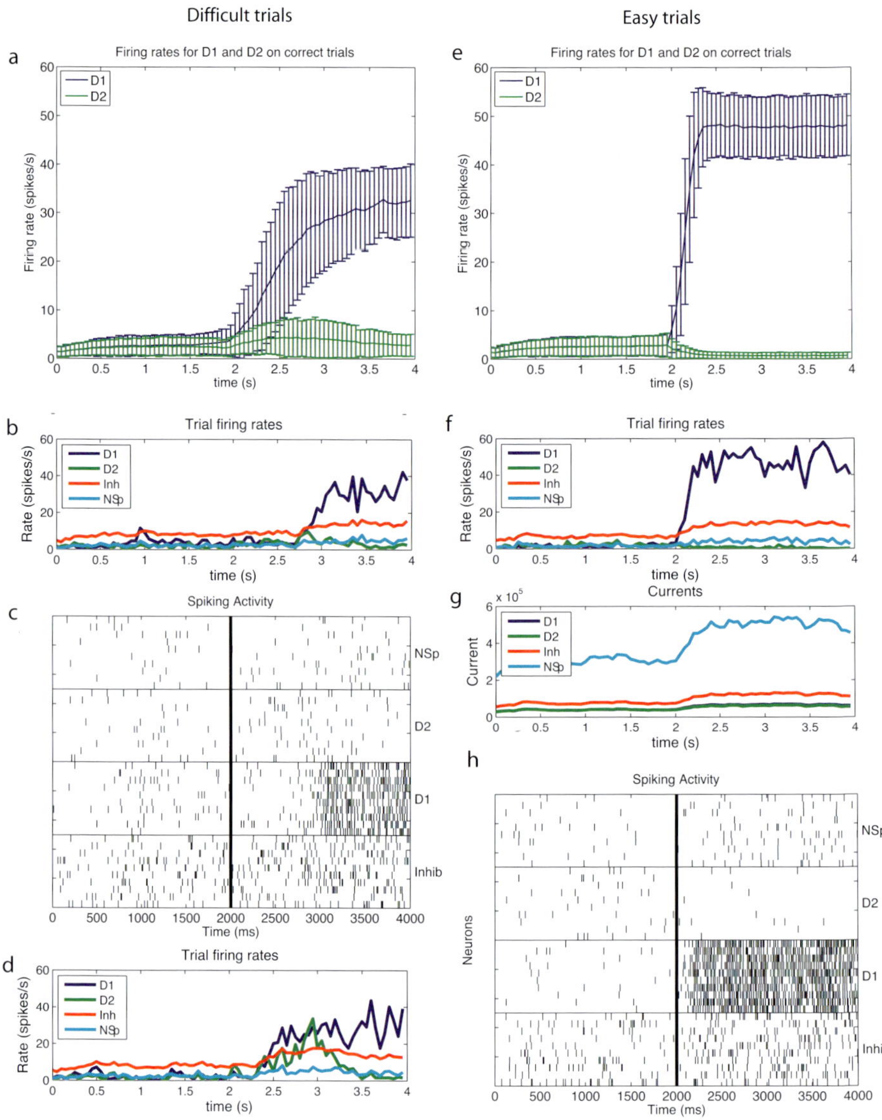

Fig. 8.14 (a) and (e) Firing rates (mean ± sd) for difficult (ΔI=0) and easy (ΔI=160) trials. The period 0–2 s is the spontaneous firing, and the decision cues were turned on at time = 2 s. The mean was calculated over 1000 trials. D1: firing rate of the D1 population of neurons on correct trials on which the D1 population won. D2: firing rate of the D2 population of neurons on the correct trials on which the D1 population won. A correct trial was one in which in which the mean rate of the D1 attractor averaged > 10 spikes/s for the last 1000 ms of the simulation runs. (b) The mean firing rates of the four populations of neurons on a difficult trial. Inh is the inhibitory population that uses GABA as a transmitter. NSp is the non-specific population of neurons (see Fig. 8.13). (c) Rastergrams for the trial shown in b. 10 neurons from each of the four pools of neurons are shown. (d) The firing rates on another difficult trial (ΔI=0) showing prolonged competition between the D1 and D2 attractors until the D1 attractor finally wins after approximately 1100 ms. (f) Firing rate plots for the 4 neuronal populations on a single easy trial (ΔI=160). (g) The synaptic currents in the four neuronal populations on the trial shown in f. (h) Rastergrams for the easy trial shown in f and g. 10 neurons from each of the four pools of neurons are shown. (After Rolls, Grabenhorst and Deco 2010b.)

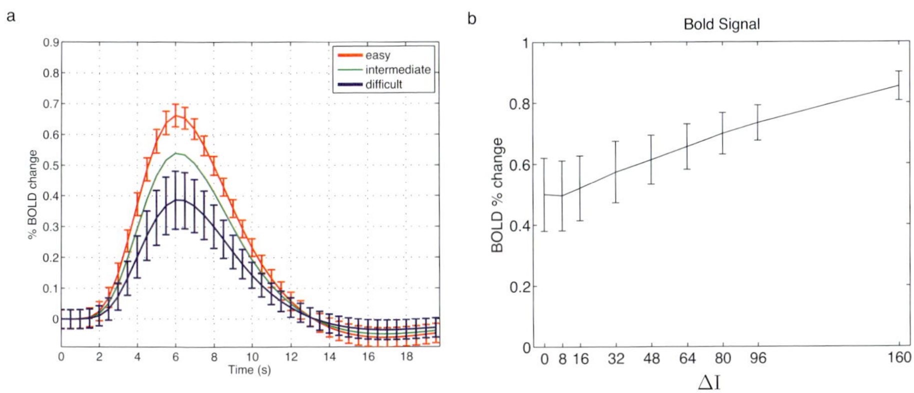

Fig. 8.17 The percentage change in the simulated BOLD signal on easy trials (ΔI=160 spikes/s), on intermediate trials (ΔI=80), and on difficult trials (ΔI=0). The mean $\pm$ sd are shown for the easy and difficult trials. The percentage change in the BOLD signal was calculated from the firing rates of the D1 and D2 populations, and analogous effects were found with calculation from the synaptic currents averaged for example across all 4 populations of neurons. (b) The percentage change in the BOLD signal (peak mean $\pm$ sd) averaged across correct and incorrect trials as a function of ΔI. ΔI=0 corresponds to difficult, and ΔI=160 corresponds to easy. The percent change was measured as the change from the level of activity in a period of 1 s immediately before the decision cues were applied at t=0 s, and was calculated from the firing rates of the neurons in the D1 and D2 populations. The BOLD per cent change scaling is arbitrary, and is set so that the lowest value for the peak of a BOLD response is 0.5%. (After Rolls, Grabenhorst and Deco 2010b.)

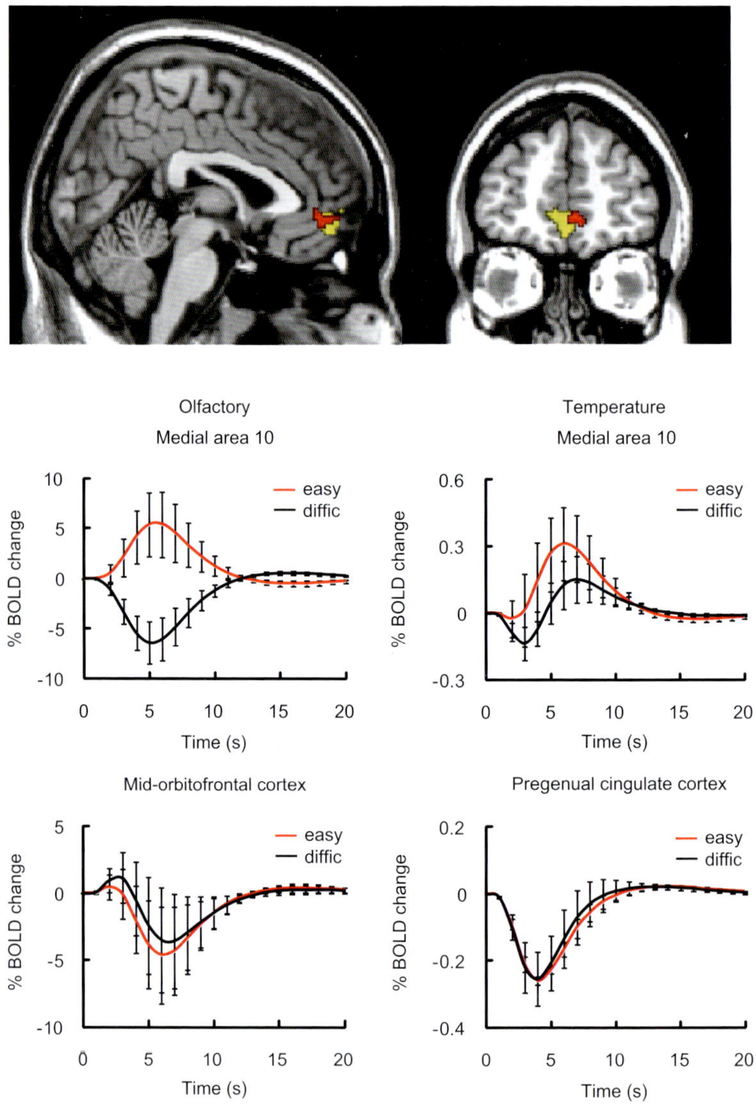

Fig. 8.19 Top: Medial prefrontal cortex area 10 activated on easy vs difficult trials in the olfactory pleasantness decision task (yellow) and the thermal pleasantness decision task (red). Middle: experimental data showing the BOLD signal in medial area 10 on easy and difficult trials of the olfactory affective decision task (left) and the thermal affective decision task (right). This medial area 10 was a region identified by other criteria (see text) as being involved in choice decision-making. Bottom: The BOLD signal for the same easy and difficult trials, but in parts of the pregenual cingulate and mid-orbitofrontal cortex implicated by other criteria (see text) in representing the subjective reward value of the stimuli on a continuous scale, but not in making choice decisions between the stimuli, or about whether to choose the stimulus in future. (After Rolls, Grabenhorst and Deco 2010b.)

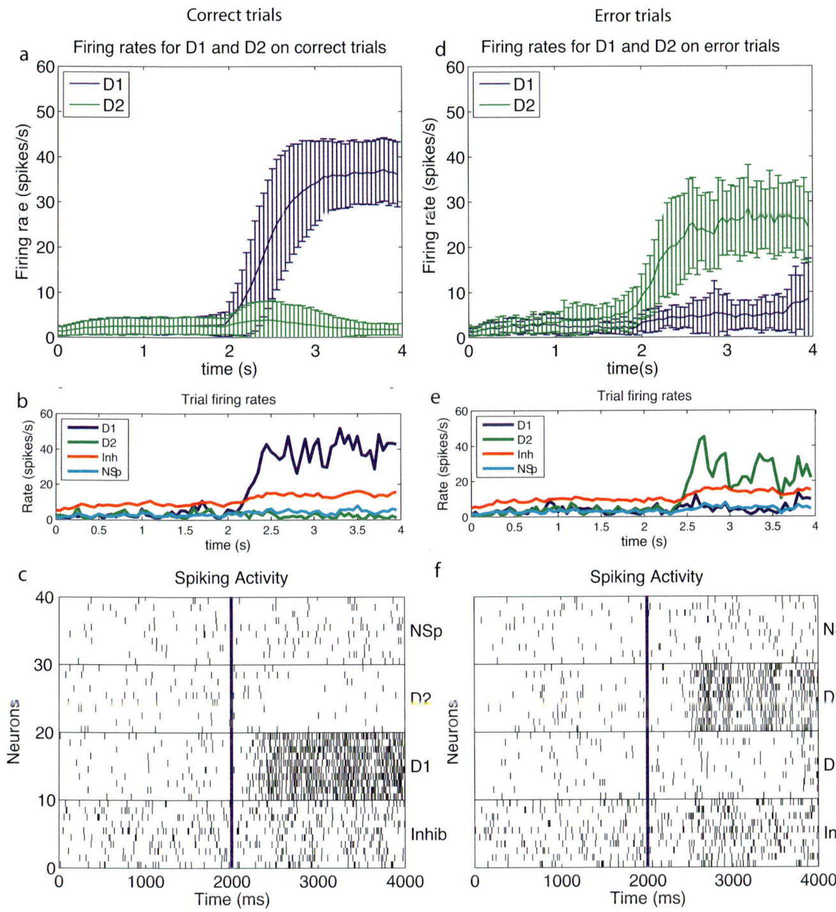

Fig. 8.21 (a and d) Firing rates (mean $\pm$ sd) for correct and error trials for an intermediate level of difficulty (ΔI=32). The period 0–2 s is the spontaneous firing, and the decision cues were turned on at time = 2 s. The means were calculated over 1000 trials. D1: firing rate of the D1 population of neurons, which is the correct population. D2: firing rate of the D2 population of neurons, which is the incorrect population. A correct trial was one in which in which the mean rate of the D1 attractor averaged $>$ 10 spikes/s for the last 1000 ms of the simulation runs. (Given the attractor nature of the network and the parameters used, the network reached one of the attractors on >90% of the 1000 trials, and this criterion clearly separated these trials, as indicated by the mean rates and standard deviations for the last 1 s of the simulation as shown.) (b and e) The firing rates of the four populations of neurons on a single trial for a correct (b) and incorrect (e) decision. Inh is the inhibitory population that uses GABA as a transmitter. NSp is the non-specific population of neurons. (c and f) Rastergrams for the trials shown in (b) and (e). 10 neurons from each of the four pools of neurons are shown. (After Rolls, Grabenhorst and Deco 2010c.)

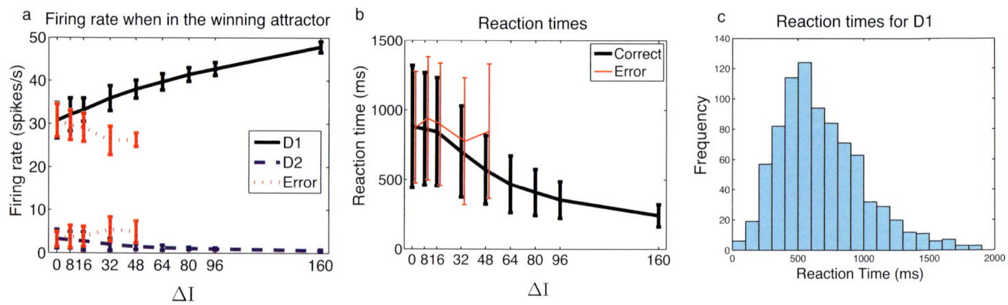

Fig. 8.22 (a) Firing rates (mean $\pm$ sd) on correct and error trials when in the winning attractor as a function of ΔI. ΔI=0 corresponds to difficult, and ΔI=160 corresponds to easy. The firing rates on correct trials for the winning population D1 are shown by solid lines, and for the losing population D2 by dashed lines. All the results are for 1000 simulation trials for each parameter value, and all the results shown are statistically highly significant. The results on error trials are shown by the dotted red lines, and in this case the D2 attractor wins, and the D1 attractor loses the competition. (There were no error trials for values of ΔI=64 Hz or above.) (b) Reaction times (mean $\pm$ sd) for the D1 population to win on correct trials (thick line), and for D2 to win on error trials (thin line), as a function of the difference in inputs ΔI to D1 and D2. The plot for the error trials has been offset by a small amount so that its values can be seen clearly. ΔI=0 corresponds to difficult, and ΔI=160 corresponds to easy. (c) The distribution of reaction times for the model for ΔI=32 illustrating the long tail of slow responses. Reaction times are shown for 837 correct trials, the level of performance was 95.7% correct, and the mean reaction time was 701 ms. (After Rolls, Grabenhorst and Deco 2010c.)

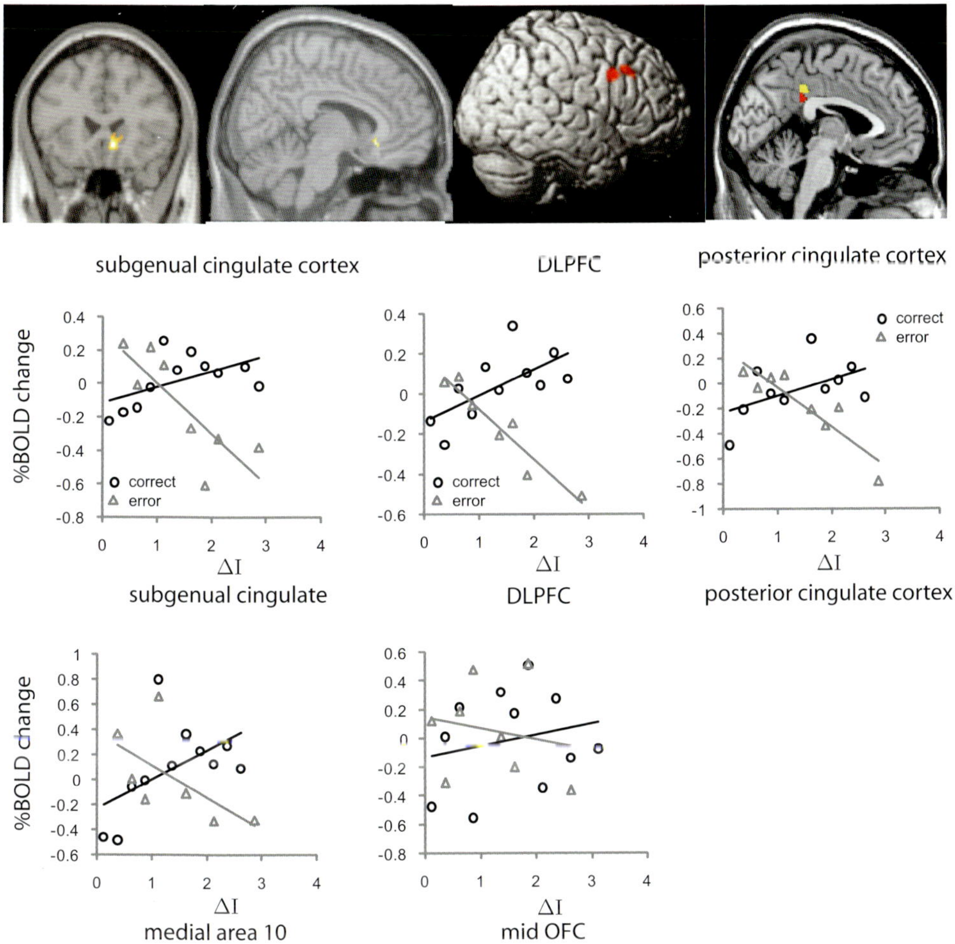

Fig. 8.25 Above. The subgenual cingulate cortex (with coronal and parasaggittal slices), dorsolateral prefrontal cortex (DLPFC) and posterior cingulate cortex regions with the percentage change in the BOLD signal positively correlated with ΔI on correct trials, and negatively correlated on error trials. Below: Separate regression plots for the relation between the BOLD signal and ΔI on correct and on error trials for these regions and for the medial prefrontal cortex area 10, and for a control region, the mid-orbitofrontal cortex (mid OFC) in which effects were not found. The regression plots show for discretized values of ΔI (averaged across subjects) the BOLD signal as a function of ΔI for correct and incorrect trials. For example, for the posterior cingulate cortex the signs of the correlations ($r = 0.51$ on correct trials, and $r = -0.91$ on error trials) are as predicted for a decision-making area of the brain, and are significantly different ($p<0.001$). The medial prefrontal cortex coordinates used for extracting the data were [-4 54 -6] with a 10 mm sphere around this location, the site in the same subjects for the peak of the contrast for easy – difficult trials (Rolls, Grabenhorst and Deco 2010b). The same region [2 50 -12] showed more activity when binary decisions were made compared to when ratings were made in the same subjects (Rolls, Grabenhorst and Deco 2010b). (After Rolls, Grabenhorst and Deco 2010c.)

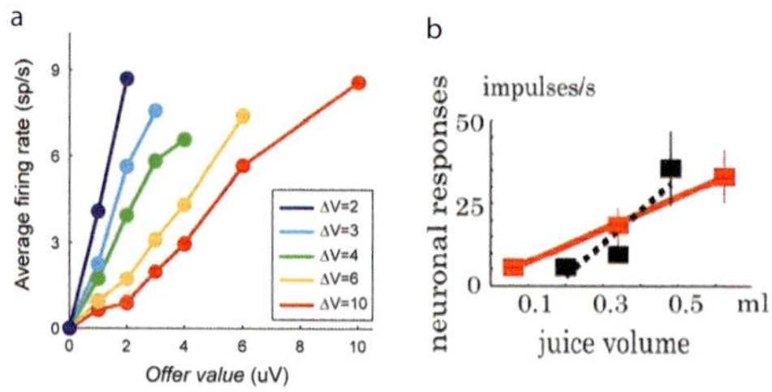

Fig. 9.7 Scaling of value: a representation of relative reward value. (a) Padoa-Schioppa (2009) found that some neurons in the orbitofrontal cortex that encode the offer value of different types of juice adapt their sensitivity to the value range of juice rewards available in a given session, while keeping their neuronal activity range constant. Each line shows the average neuronal response for a given value range. Reproduced with permission. (b) Kobayashi et al. (2010) found that neurons in the orbitofrontal cortex adapt their sensitivity of value coding to the statistical distribution of reward values, in that the reward sensitivity slope adapted to the standard deviation of the probability distribution of juice volumes. These findings indicate that the range of the value scale in the orbitofrontal cortex can be adjusted to reflect the range of rewards that are available at a given time. Reproduced with permission.

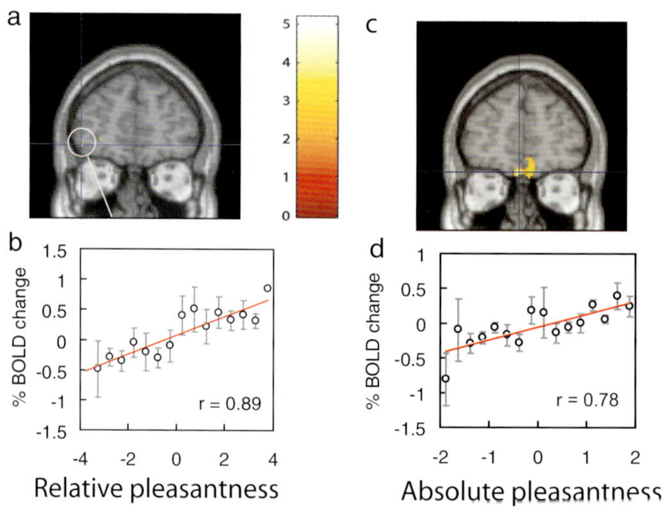

Fig. 9.8 Absolute and relative value representations in the human orbitofrontal cortex. On each trial, the subjects rated the pleasantness (value) of the second odour of a pair of 4 odours used in the experiment. (a-b) Relative pleasantness: positive correlation between the BOLD signal and the difference in pleasantness of the second odor compared to the first odour. (a) A significant correlation was found in the anterior lateral orbitofrontal cortex at [-44 48 -8]. (b) There was a positive correlation between the BOLD signal in this brain region measured at the time of the second odour and the difference in the pleasantness of the second odour compared to the first (i.e. positive values on the abscissa are when the second odour is more pleasant) (r=0.89). (c-d) Absolute pleasantness: positive correlation between the BOLD signal and the absolute value of the pleasantness ratings given to the (second) odour in (c) the medial orbitofrontal cortex [-2 50 -20]. (d) The correlation between the BOLD signal in the medial orbitofrontal cortex and the pleasantness ratings (r=0.78). (After Grabenhorst and Rolls 2009.)

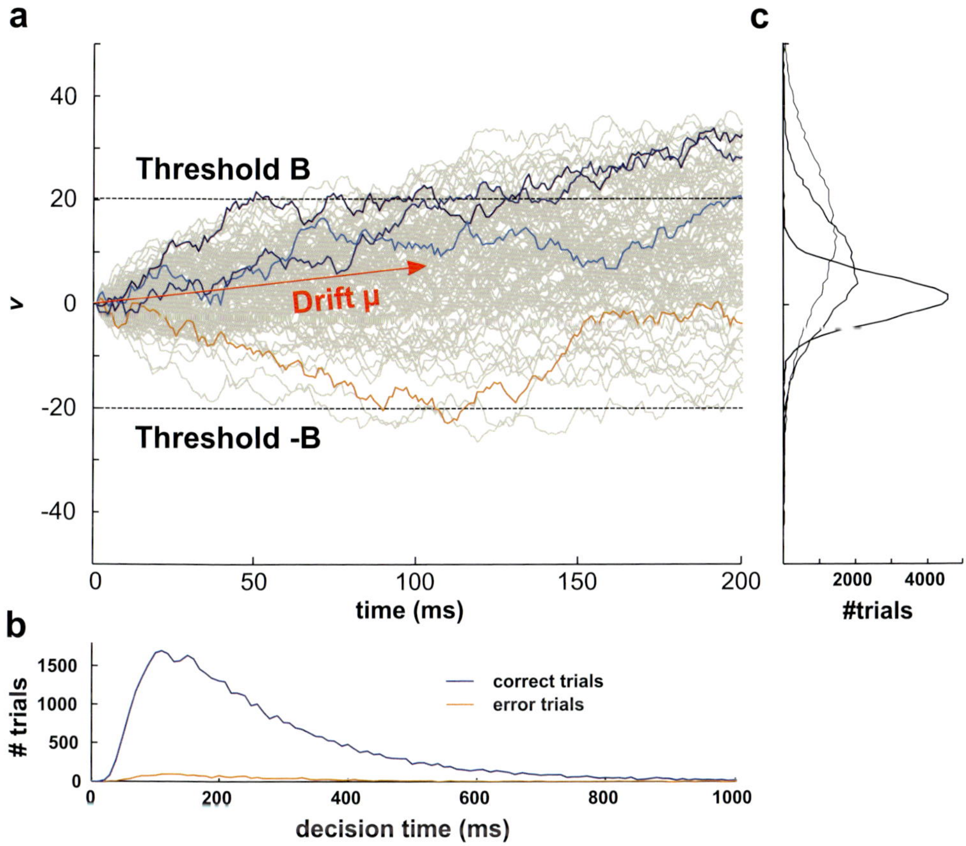

Fig. B.2 Basic drift diffusion model. (a) 100 example traces of the time evolution of $v(t)$. Three correct trials are labelled in blue, one error trial in orange. (b) Left-skewed RT Histograms of correct and error choices from 50,000 trials. (c) The variance of ν increases with time. The distribution of ν for 50,000 trials is given for t = 20 ms, 100 ms and 200 ms (bold to narrow lines). Model parameters: $\mu = 0.07$, $\sigma = 1$, $dt = 1$ ms, $B = 20$. (From Deco, Rolls, Albantakis and Romo 2013.)

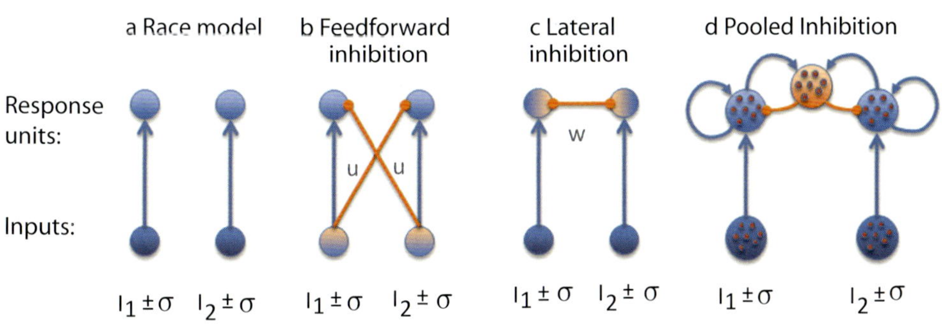

Fig. B.3 Two-alternative forced choice (2AFC) decision models with two integrators. The connections that terminate with arrows denote excitatory connections, and those that terminate with circles denote inhibitory connections. The two inputs to each of the four models are $I_1 \pm \sigma$ and $I_2 \pm \sigma$. (Adapted from Bogacz et al. 2006.)

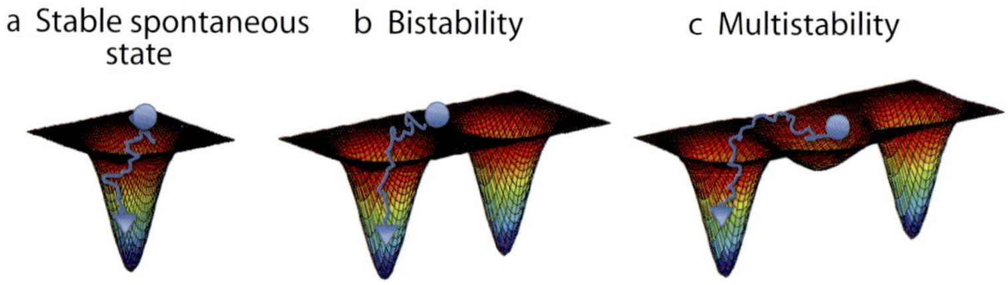

Fig. B.4 Schematic representation of possible attractor configurations in the attractor network of binary decision-making. With multistability, two decision states and the spontaneous state are all stable fixed points, or attractors, shown as valleys in the 'energy landscape'. The full caption is with the figure in the main text.

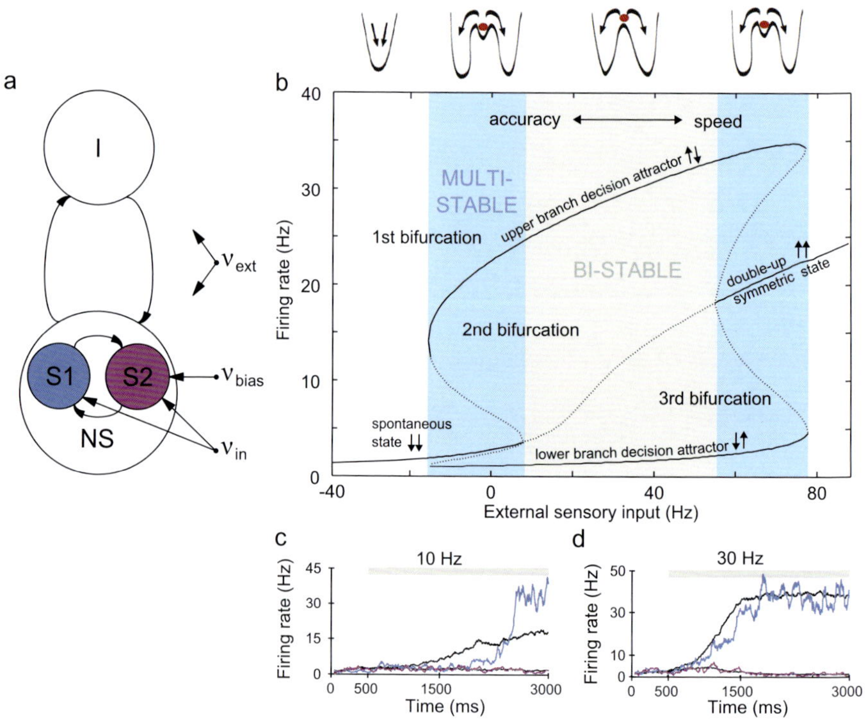

Fig. B.5 Biophysically-realistic attractor network of decision-making. (a) Schematic representation of the network. The excitatory neurons are organized into three pools: the nonselective neurons (NS) and the two selective, decision-making, pools (S1, S2) that receive the inputs encoding each stimulus (with rate ν_{in} in the terminology of this Appendix). An additional bias (ν_{bias}) can be applied to one of the two selective pools. All neurons also receive an input (ν_{ext}) that simulates the spontaneous activity in the surrounding cerebral cortex. (b) Stable (solid lines) and unstable (dotted lines) fixed points depend on the external sensory input. They were calculated with the mean-field approximation of the network (Brunel and Wang, 2001). (c,d) Single trial (colored traces) and mean (black, averaged over 20 trials) temporal evolution of the firing rate of the selective pools for different inputs, denoted by the gray bars ($\nu_{\text{bias}} = 0$). (c) Noise-induced transition from the spontaneous state to the decision state (with low inputs, in the multistable regime). (d) Input-driven transition (in the bistable regime). Simulations were performed with a synaptic strength of $w_+ = 1.68$ within selective populations; all other parameters were taken from Wang (2002). (Adapted with permission from Masquelier et al. 2011.)

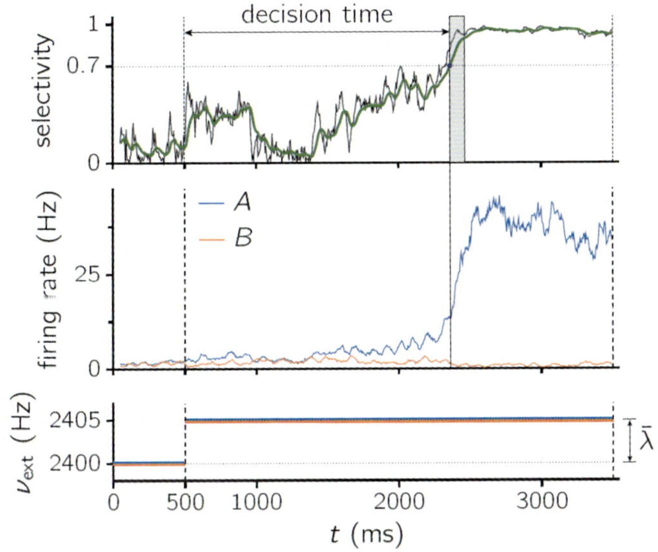

Fig. B.6 Development of the selectivity index (top), the average activity of populations A and B (middle), and the stimulation applied (bottom), for a single decision-making trial with a stable spontaneous state (the 'multistable regime'). The green line in the top panel is the low-pass filtered selectivity. (The selectivity index was $\mid \nu_1 - \nu_2 \mid / (\nu_1 + \nu_2)$.) From 0 to 500 ms no stimulation was applied (λ =0). From 500 ms to the end of the trial, λ was set to a constant value different from zero ($\nu_{\text{ext}} = \nu_0 + \lambda$ for the selective cells). The decision time, DT, was the time between stimulus onset and the time at which the low-pass filtered selectivity index crossed the threshold of 0.7 and stayed above it for at least 100 ms. The shaded area shows the time window within which the signal (green line) was required to be greater than the threshold. N = 2000, w_+ = 1.75, λ = 5 Hz. (After Marti et al. 2008.)

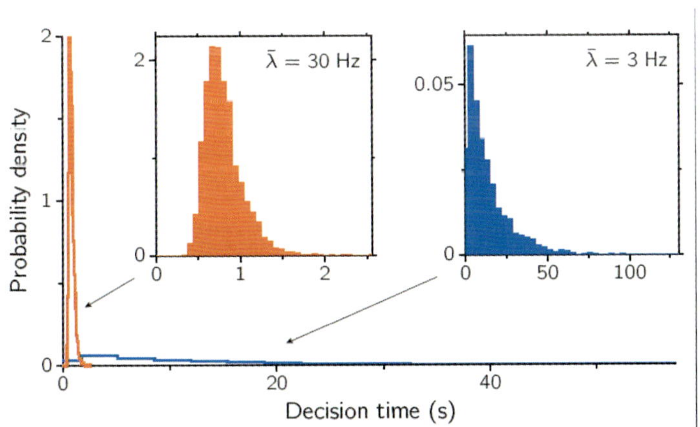

Fig. B.7 Distributions of decision times for a regime with a spontaneous stable state (blue, right, λ = 3 Hz) and without a spontaneous stable state (red, left, λ = 30 Hz), from a sample of 4000 trials each. The two insets show the distributions separately (note the different scales). N = 4500, w_+ = 1.75. (After Marti et al. 2008.)

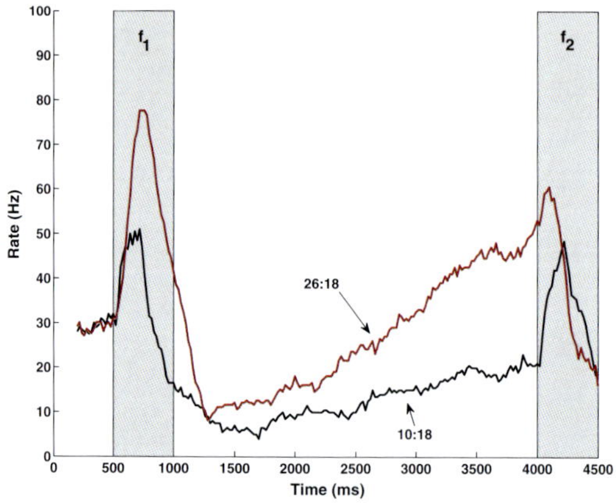

Fig. B.8 Activity of a single neuron of the ‘partially differential’ type recorded in the ventral premotor cortex (VPC) during a vibrotactile decision-making task, after Romo et al. (2004). f_2 was in both cases 18 Hz. When f_1 was 26 Hz (red plot), the firing rate during f_1, and at the end of the delay period, and during the comparison period when f_2 was being applied was higher than when f_1 was 10 Hz (black plot). The full caption is with the figure in the main text.

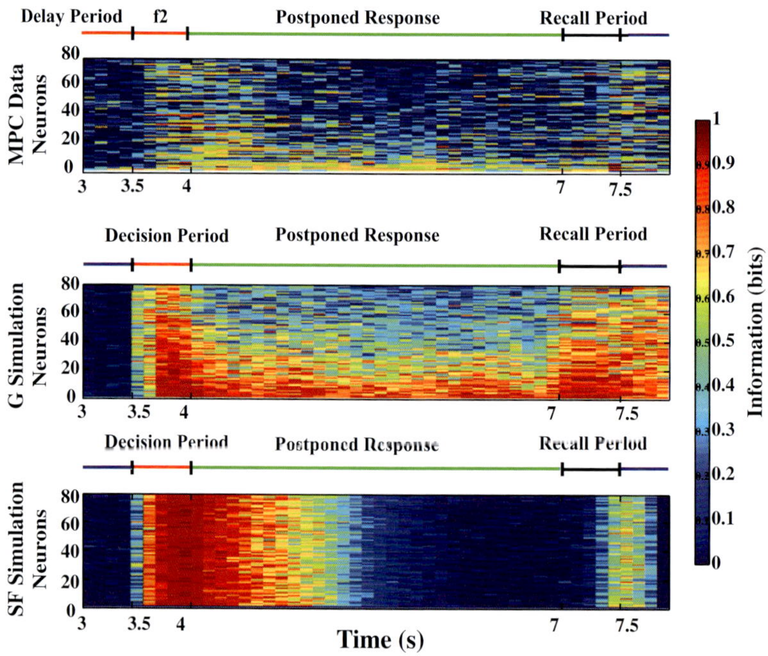

Fig. B.9 Postponed response decision-making. The f_2 stimuli providing the evidence on the basis of which a decision could be made were applied from 3.5–4.0 s, and the postponed response after a delay period from 4.0–7.0 s could be started at 7.0 s. Mutual information analyses between the firing rate and the response are shown, with each row a separate neuron. Top – 80 neurons from the medial premotor cortex. Middle – simulation using graded firing rates. Bottom – Synaptic Facilitation simulation. The full caption is with the figure in the main text.